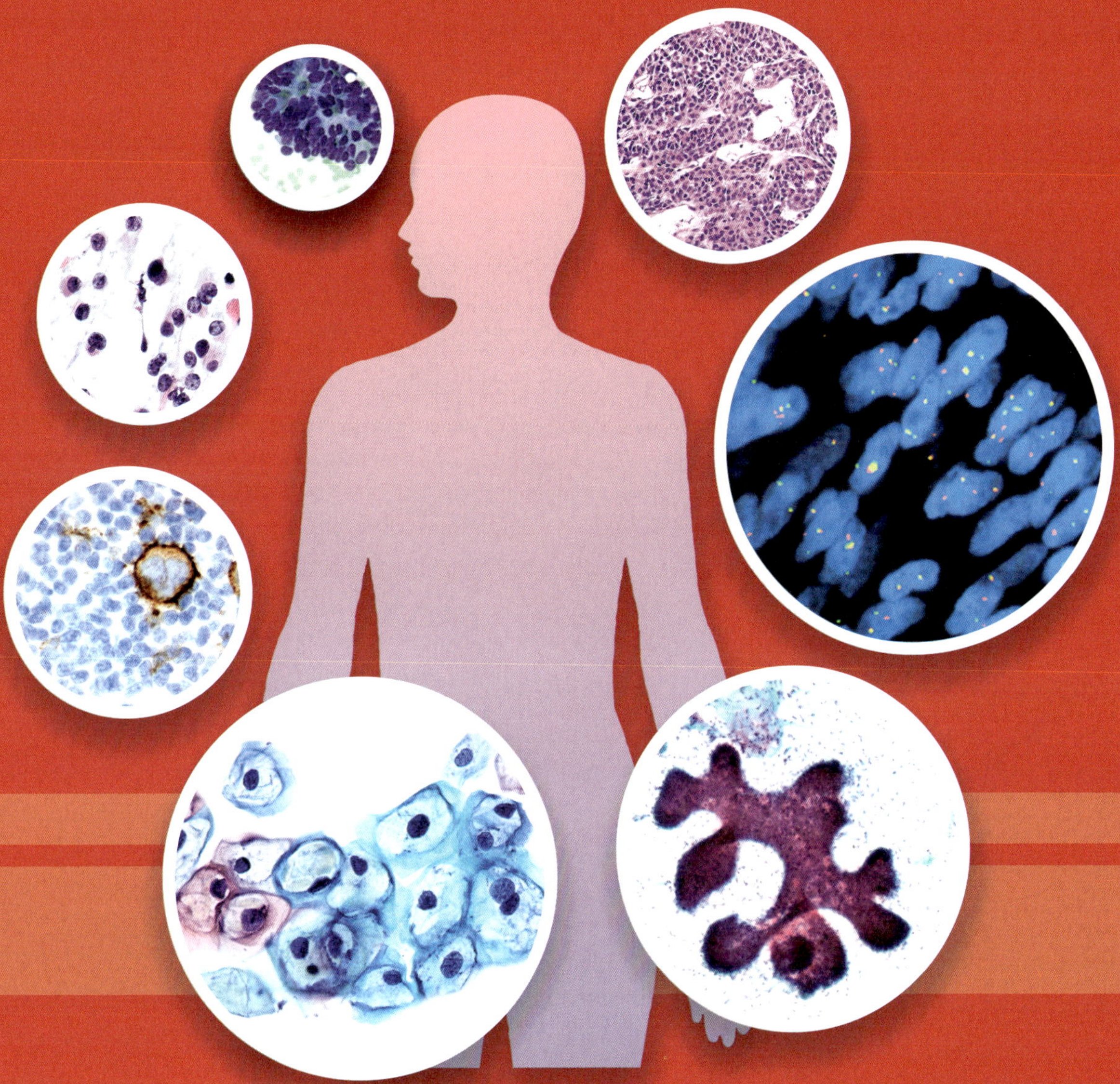

Diagnostic Pathology

Cytopathology

Mody | Thrall | Krishnamurthy

Ge | Gorman | Takei

ELSEVIER

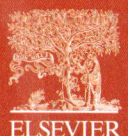

THIRD EDITION

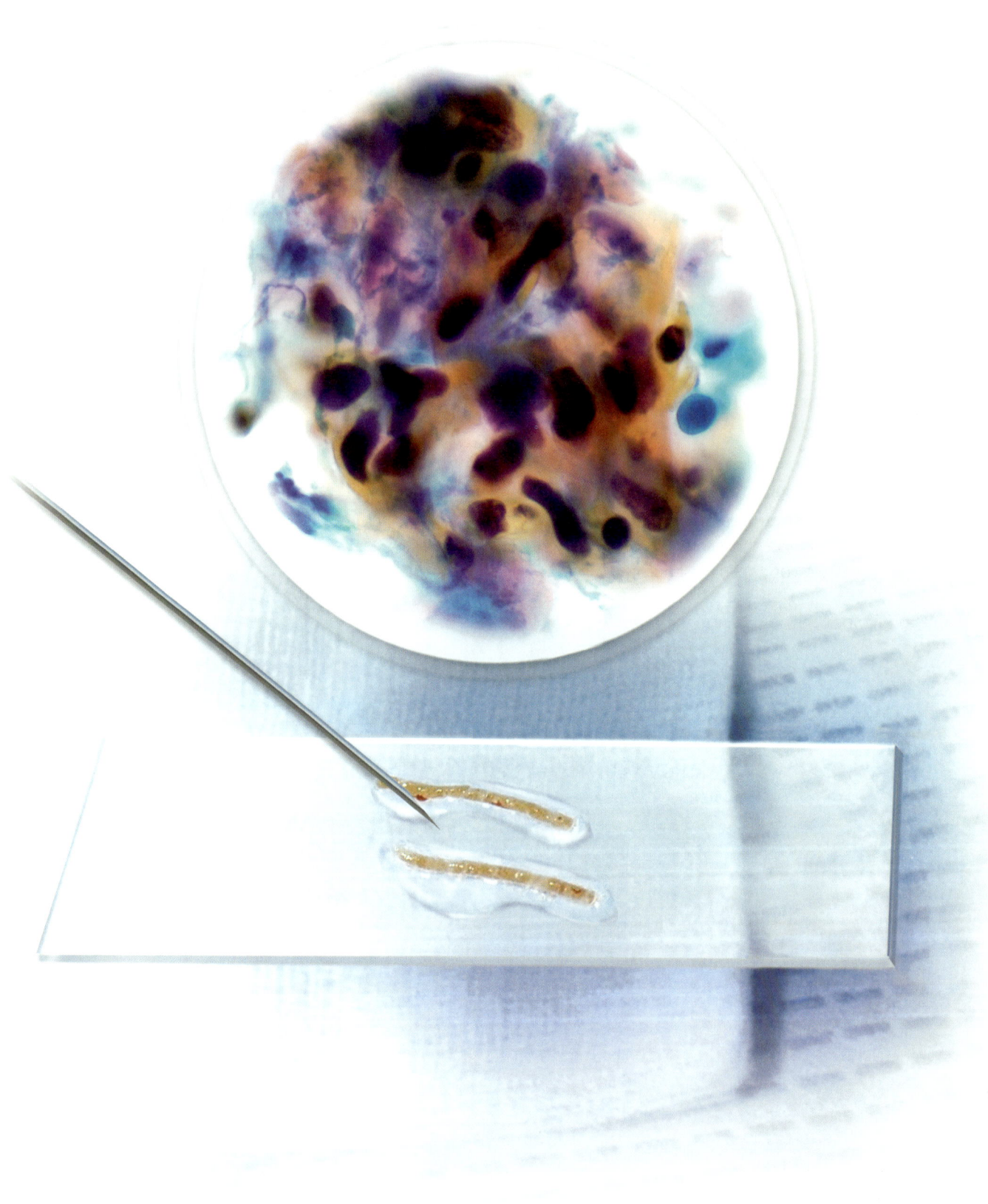

Diagnostic Pathology
Cytopathology

Third Edition

Dina R. Mody, MD
Director of Cytopathology
The Ibrahim Ramzy Chair in Pathology
Department of Pathology and Genomic Medicine
Houston Methodist Hospital
Houston, Texas
Professor of Pathology and Laboratory Medicine
Weill Cornell Medicine
Cornell University
New York, New York

Michael J. Thrall, MD
Cytopathology Fellowship Director
Department of Pathology and Genomic Medicine
Houston Methodist Hospital
Houston, Texas
Professor of Pathology and Laboratory Medicine
Weill Cornell Medicine
Cornell University
New York, New York

Savitri Krishnamurthy, MD
Professor of Pathology
The University of Texas MD Anderson Cancer Center
Houston, Texas

Yimin Ge, MD
Professor of Pathology and
Laboratory Medicine
Department of Pathology
and Genomic Medicine
Houston Methodist Hospital
Houston, Texas
Weill Cornell Medicine
Cornell University
New York, New York

Blythe K. Gorman, MD
Associate Professor
Department of Pathology
and Genomic Medicine
Houston Methodist Hospital
Houston Methodist Institute
for Academic Medicine
Houston, Texas
Weill Cornell Medicine
Cornell University
New York, New York
Assistant Adjunct Professor
Texas A&M University School of Medicine
Bryan, Texas

Hidehiro Takei, MD
Professor
Director of Anatomic Pathology
Department of Pathology
and Translational Pathobiology
Louisiana State University
Health Shreveport
Shreveport, Louisiana

Elsevier
1600 John F. Kennedy Blvd.
Ste 1800
Philadelphia, PA 19103-2899

DIAGNOSTIC PATHOLOGY: CYTOPATHOLOGY, THIRD EDITION

ISBN: 978-0-323-87867-8

Copyright © 2023 by Elsevier. All rights reserved.

No part of this publication may be reproduced or transmitted in any form or by any means, electronic or mechanical, including photocopying, recording, or any information storage and retrieval system, without permission in writing from the publisher. Details on how to seek permission, further information about the Publisher's permissions policies and our arrangements with organizations such as the Copyright Clearance Center and the Copyright Licensing Agency, can be found at our website: www.elsevier.com/permissions.

This book and the individual contributions contained in it are protected under copyright by the Publisher (other than as may be noted herein).

Notices

Practitioners and researchers must always rely on their own experience and knowledge in evaluating and using any information, methods, compounds or experiments described herein. Because of rapid advances in the medical sciences, in particular, independent verification of diagnoses and drug dosages should be made. To the fullest extent of the law, no responsibility is assumed by Elsevier, authors, editors or contributors for any injury and/or damage to persons or property as a matter of products liability, negligence or otherwise, or from any use or operation of any methods, products, instructions, or ideas contained in the material herein.

Previous edition copyrighted 2018.

Library of Congress Control Number: 2022941707

Printed in Canada by Friesens, Altona, Manitoba, Canada

Last digit is the print number: 9 8 7 6 5 4 3 2 1

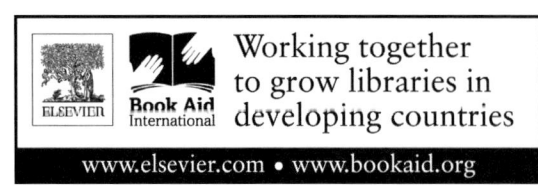

Dedications

This book is dedicated to all the patients and professionals from whom I have learned over a 40-plus-years career in the Texas Medical Center. To the late Drs. Harlan J. Spjut and Malcolm McGavran, who kindled my interest in pathology; Dr. Ramzy, my mentor in cytopathology; and my peer mentors, Diane and Mary. Special thanks to cytologists, colleagues, residents, and fellows at Houston Methodist Hospital, whose queries kept me intellectually curious. Special thanks to my family, who stood by me.

DRM

This book is dedicated to my late mother, Kay, who never failed to offer encouragement and support. I also wish to honor my mentor, Dr. Pambuccian, who inspired so many budding pathologists before his untimely passing. Thank you to Dr. Mody for giving me this opportunity, as well as to my colleagues at Houston Methodist, at MD Anderson, and around the world, who have contributed to this effort.

MJT

This book is dedicated to the patients who provided their tissues that enabled me to study and practice cytopathology and surgical pathology; to my trainees, pathology colleagues, clinicians, and technologists, who have been instrumental in keeping me engaged, stimulated, and passionate about my practice of pathology; and to my loving family, who have supported me in all my endeavors.

SK

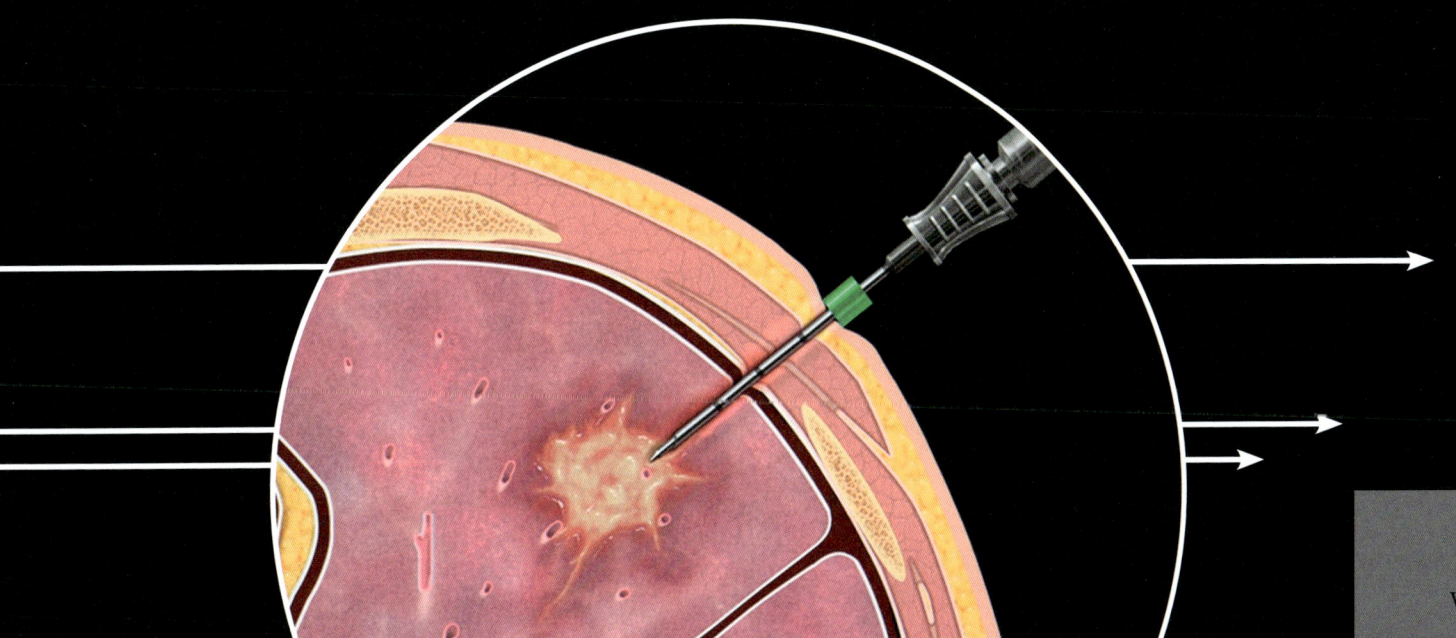

Additional Contributors

Mojgan Amrikachi, MD
Associate Professor
Department of Pathology
and Genomic Medicine
Houston Methodist Hospital
Houston, Texas
Weill Cornell Medicine
Cornell University
New York, New York

Patricia Chévez-Barrios, MD
Chair in Ocular Pathology
Director, Ophthalmic
Pathology Program
Department of Pathology
and Genomic Medicine
Houston Methodist Hospital
Houston, Texas
Professor of Pathology and
Laboratory Medicine and
Ophthalmology
Weill Cornell Medicine
Cornell University
New York, New York

Susan L. Haley, MD
Assistant Professor
Department of Pathology and
Genomic Medicine
Houston Methodist Hospital
Houston, Texas
Weill Cornell Medicine
Cornell University
New York, New York

Elizabeth M. Jacobi, MD
Staff Pathologist
Houston Methodist Hospital
Houston, Texas
Assistant Professor of Pathology and
Laboratory Medicine
Weill Cornell Medicine
Cornell University
New York, New York

Ekene I. Okoye, MD
Associate Professor
Department of Pathology and
Genomic Medicine
Houston Methodist Hospital
Houston, Texas
Weill Cornell Medicine
Cornell University
New York, New York

Suzanne Z. Powell, MD
Chief of Neuropathology
Vice-Chair for Education
Department of Pathology
and Genomic Medicine
Houston Methodist Hospital
Houston, Texas
Professor of Pathology
and Laboratory Medicine
Weill Cornell Medicine
Cornell University
New York, New York
Texas A&M University
School Medicine
Bryan, Texas

Andreana L. Rivera, MD
Pathologist
Department of Pathology
and Genomic Medicine
Houston Methodist Hospital
Houston, Texas

Mary R. Schwartz, MD
Jack L. Titus Chair in Pathology
Deputy Chair and Medical Director
Anatomic Pathology
Houston Methodist Hospital
Clinical Professor of Pathology
Baylor College of Medicine
Houston, Texas

Yuko Sugiyama, MD, PhD, FIAC
Director
Cytology Department
Vice Director
Department of Gynecology
Cancer Institute Hospital (JFCR)
Tokyo, Japan

Paula J. Woodward, MD
David G. Bragg, MD and Marcia R.
Bragg Presidential Endowed Chair
in Oncologic Imaging
Professor of Radiology
and Imaging Sciences
University of Utah School
of Medicine
Salt Lake City, Utah

Other Contributors

Rose Anton, MD
Houston Methodist Hospital
Houston, Texas

George G. Birdsong, MD
Emory University
Atlanta, Georgia

Nancy P. Caraway, MD
The University of Texas
MD Anderson Cancer Center
Houston, Texas

Nikolaos Chantziantoniou, PhD, ART(CSMLS), CFIAC
CellPathology Plus
Ontario, Canada

Donna M. Coffey, MD
Weill Cornell Medicine
New York, New York

Mukul K. Divatia, MD
Houston Methodist Hospital
Houston, Texas

Ming Guo, MD
The University of Texas
MD Anderson Cancer Center
Houston, Texas

Shubhada Kane, MD
Tata Memorial Hospital
Parel, Mumbai, India

Uma Kundu, MD
The University of Texas
MD Anderson Cancer Center
Houston, Texas

Gene Landon, MD
The University of Texas
MD Anderson Cancer Center
Houston, Texas

Norma Quintanilla, MD
Texas Children's Hospital
Houston, Texas

Debora A. Smith, CT(ASCP)
Houston Methodist Hospital
Houston, Texas

Nour Sneige, MD
The University of Texas
MD Anderson Cancer Center
Houston, Texas

John M. Stewart, MD, PhD
The University of Texas
MD Anderson Cancer Center
Houston, Texas

Ashraf Thabet, MD
Massachusetts General Hospital
Boston, Massachusetts

Jun Zhang, MD, MS
Mayo Clinic
Phoenix, Arizona

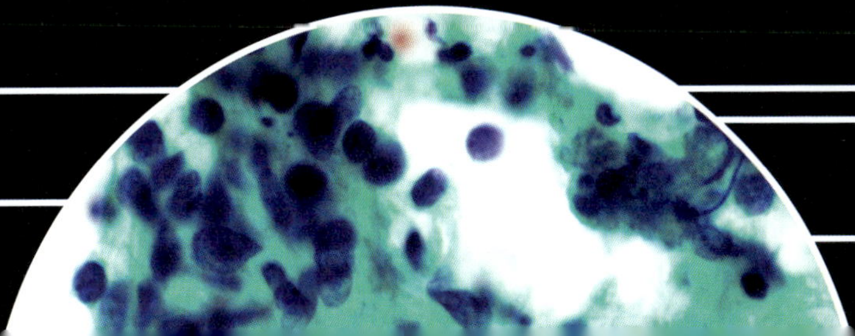

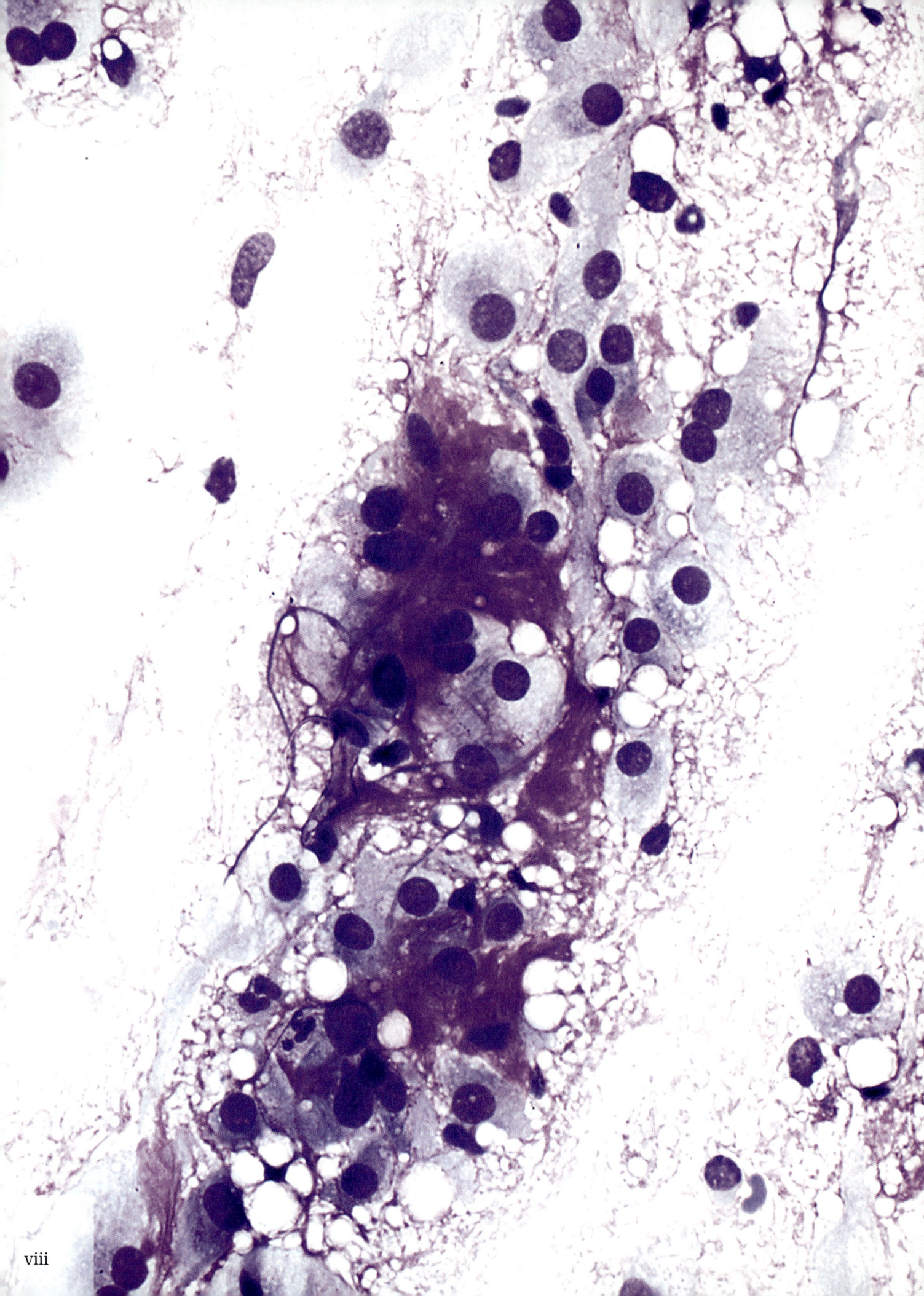

viii

Preface

The practice of pathology has witnessed a paradigm shift in the past 20 years. Successful diagnosis, including ancillary studies and prognostic and predictive biomarkers, is now expected, even with very small tissue samples. Modern imaging technologies enable the procurement of fine-needle aspiration cytology and miniscule core needle biopsies. Ancillary immunophenotyping and molecular testing have significantly advanced in the last decade, and these techniques can be successfully applied using cytology and small biopsy specimens. In many instances, cytopathology and small biopsies are often the only specimens available for testing, and are used to guide clinical management and prognosis. Currently, cytopathology professionals rapidly evaluate these minute specimens in real time onsite or remotely while the patient is undergoing the procedure. This book strives to meet the needs of cytopathology trainees, as well as established professionals, so that they can handle cytopathology and small biopsy specimens with a sound knowledge base of the field, as they perform the ever more difficult task of successfully triaging cytology and small biopsy material.

This comprehensive cytopathology textbook is written in the easy-to-access format popularized by the Amirsys (now Elsevier) surgical pathology, histology, and radiology textbooks. It is written with the busy cytopathology professional, as well as trainees, in mind. The classification schemes and reporting terminologies have been updated based on recent developments. The "key facts" provide quick criteria and facts needed for diagnosis or adequate evaluation at the time of procedure, whereas the main chapter is written in a consistent, thorough, succinct, and synoptic format, which is easy to read, up-to-date, and full of information.

The book covers all aspects of cytology, including gynecologic and nongynecologic exfoliative specimens, fine-needle aspiration, neuropathology squash preparations, ophthalmic cytopathology, quality improvement, instrumentation, immunohistochemistry, and molecular testing as they apply to cytology, cell blocks, and miniscule biopsy specimens.

It is a labor of love from many busy and experienced cytology professionals, and we hope you enjoy reading it.

Dina R. Mody, MD
Director of Cytopathology
The Ibrahim Ramzy Chair in Pathology
Department of Pathology and Genomic Medicine
Houston Methodist Hospital
Houston, Texas
Professor of Pathology and Laboratory Medicine
Weill Cornell Medicine
Cornell University
New York, New York

Michael J. Thrall, MD
Cytopathology Fellowship Director
Department of Pathology and Genomic Medicine
Houston Methodist Hospital
Houston, Texas
Professor of Pathology and Laboratory Medicine
Weill Cornell Medicine
Cornell University
New York, New York

Savitri Krishnamurthy, MD
Professor of Pathology
The University of Texas MD Anderson Cancer Center
Houston, Texas

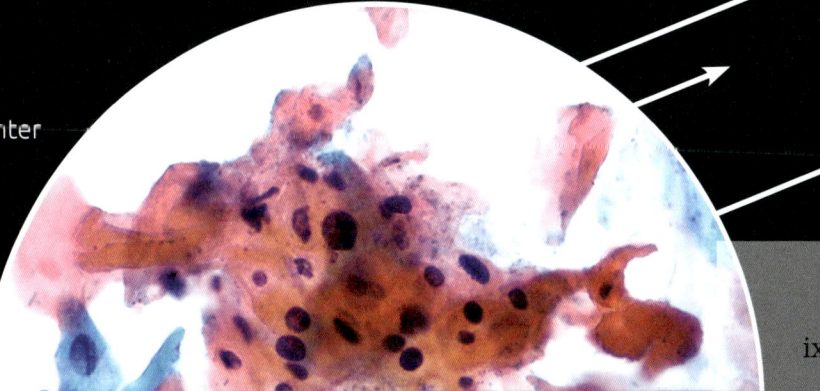

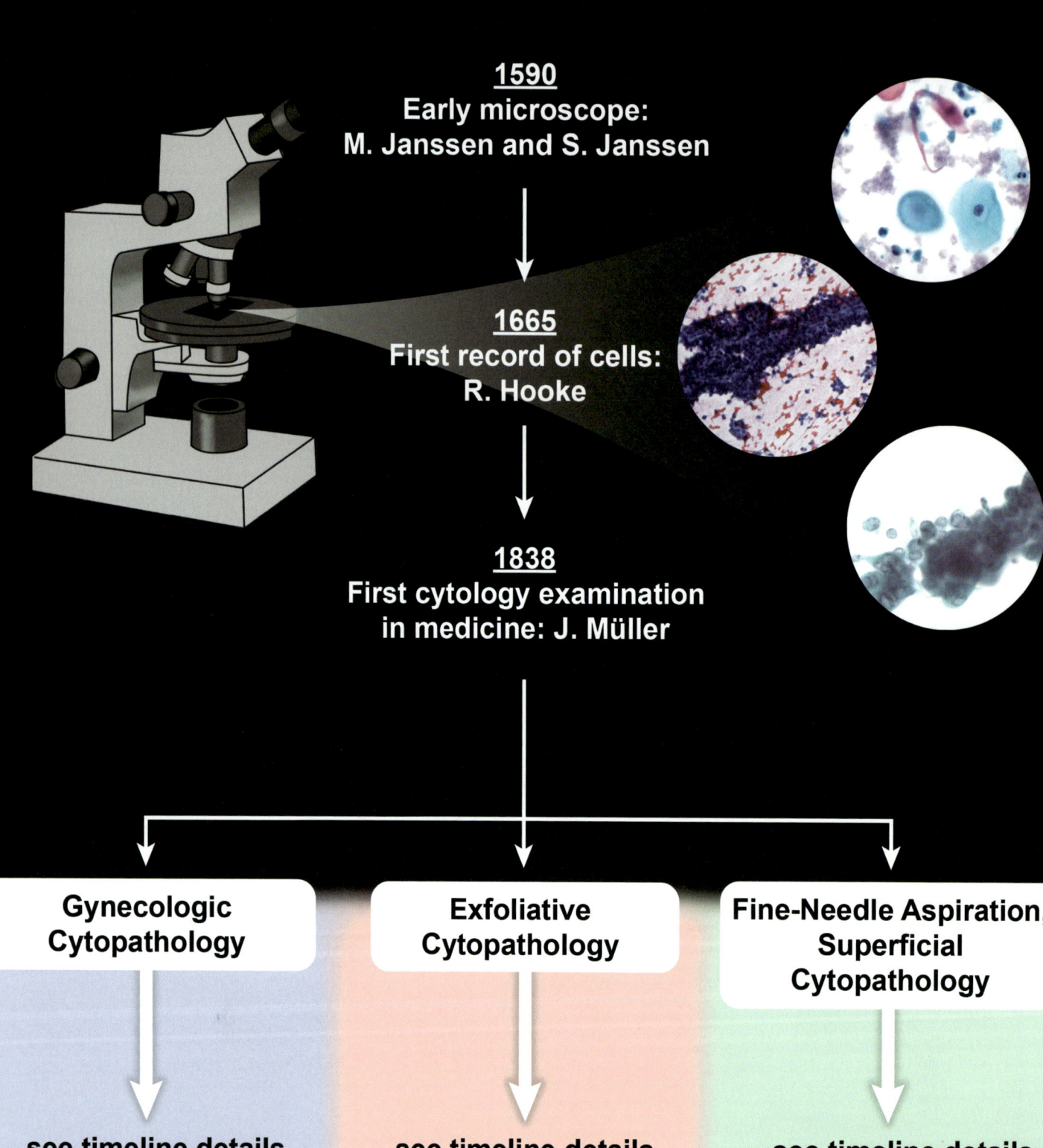

Acknowledgments

LEAD EDITOR
Megg Morin, BA

LEAD ILLUSTRATOR
Laura C. Wissler, MA

TEXT EDITORS
Arthur G. Gelsinger, MA
Rebecca L. Bluth, BA
Nina Themann, BA
Terry W. Ferrell, MS
Kathryn Watkins, BA
Shannon Kelly, MA

ILLUSTRATIONS
Lane R. Bennion, MS
Richard Coombs, MS

IMAGE EDITORS
Jeffrey J. Marmorstone, BS
Lisa A. M. Steadman, BS

ART DIRECTION AND DESIGN
Cindy Lin, BFA

PRODUCTION EDITORS
Emily C. Fassett, BA
John Pecorelli, BS

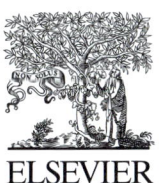

ELSEVIER

Sections

PART I: Gynecologic Cytopathology
SECTION 1: **Overview**
SECTION 2: **Benign and Infectious Conditions**
SECTION 3: **Squamous Cell Abnormalities and Mimics**
SECTION 4: **Glandular Cell Abnormalities and Mimics**
SECTION 5: **Extrauterine Carcinomas and Other Malignancies of Female Genital Tract**
SECTION 6: **Molecular Testing in Gynecologic Cytology**
SECTION 7: **Directly Sampled Endometrial Cytology**
SECTION 8: **Anal Cytology**

PART II: Exfoliative Cytopathology
SECTION 1: **Respiratory Tract, Including Lung FNAs**
SECTION 2: **Gastrointestinal Tract**
SECTION 3: **Cerebrospinal Fluid**
SECTION 4: **Pleural, Peritoneal, Pericardial, and Pelvic Fluid and Washings**
SECTION 5: **Urinary Cytology**

PART III: Fine-Needle Aspiration, Superficial
SECTION 1: **Overview**
SECTION 2: **Thyroid Gland**
SECTION 3: **Parathyroid Gland**
SECTION 4: **Lymph Nodes**
SECTION 5: **Salivary Gland**
SECTION 6: **Breast**
SECTION 7: **Skin and Subcutaneous Cytology**

PART IV: Fine-Needle Aspiration, Deep Organs and Tissues
SECTION 1: **Overview**
SECTION 2: **Mediastinum**
SECTION 3: **Liver**
SECTION 4: **Kidney**
SECTION 5: **Adrenal Gland**
SECTION 6: **Pancreas**
SECTION 7: **Bone**
SECTION 8: **Soft Tissue**
SECTION 9: **Ophthalmic and Neuropathology**

PART V: Management and Ancillary Testing
SECTION 1: **Cytopreparatory and Quality Management**
SECTION 2: **Ancillary Testing**

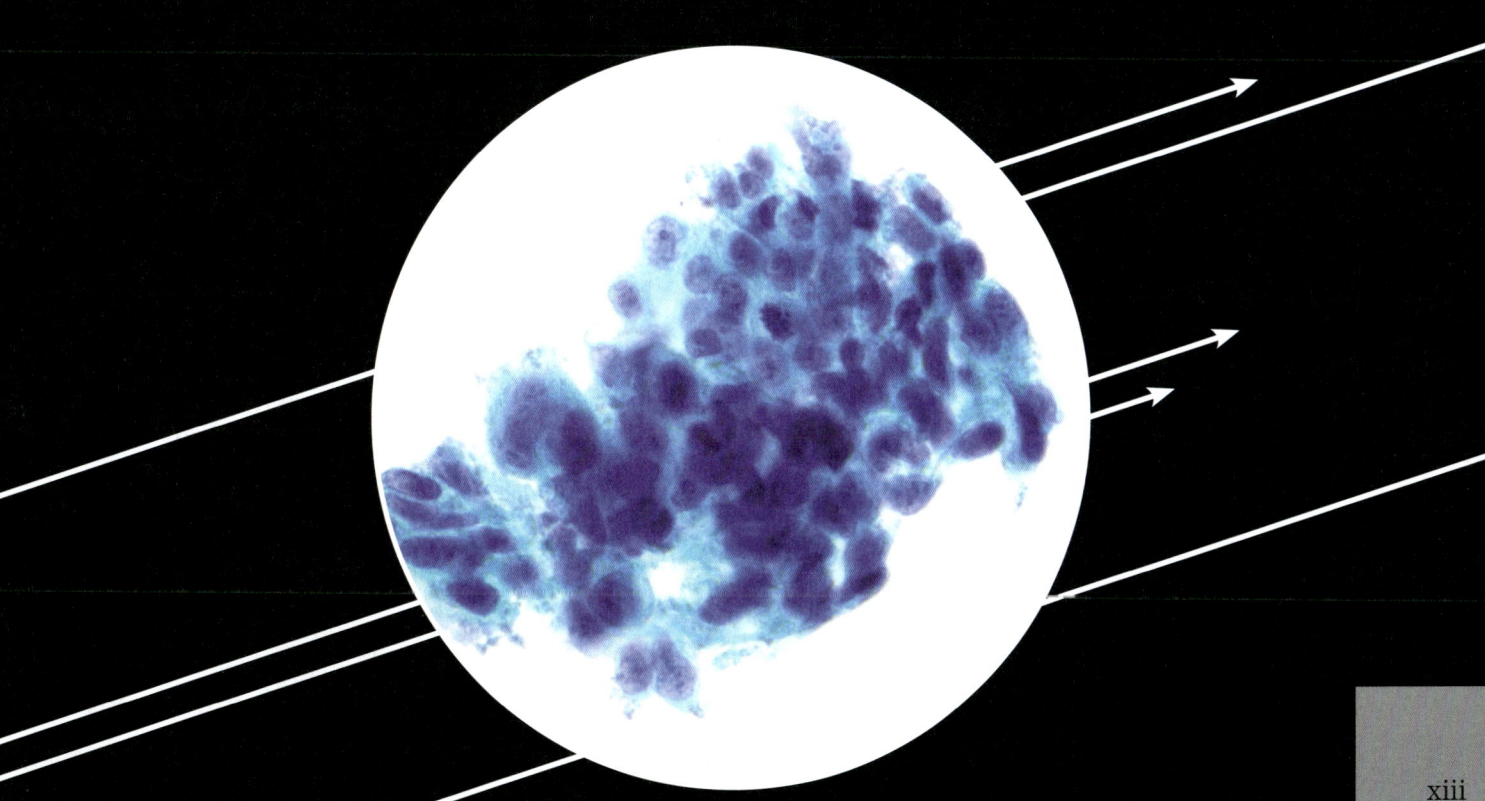

TABLE OF CONTENTS

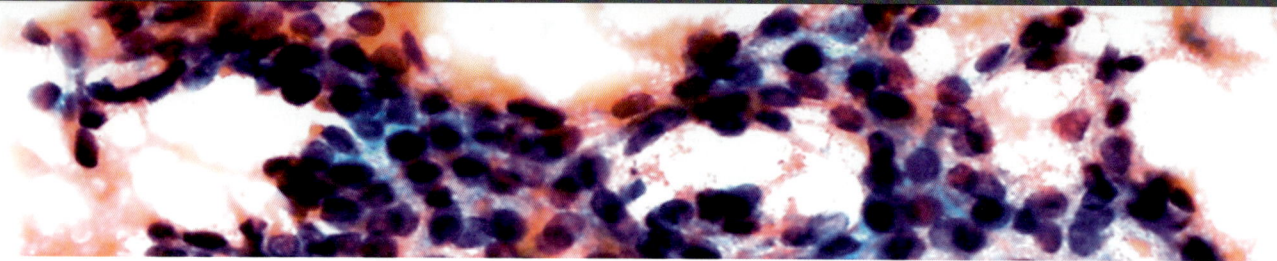

Part I: Gynecologic Cytopathology

SECTION 1: OVERVIEW

- 4 **Pap Test and Cervical Cancer Screening: History and Reporting Terminology**
  Nikolaos Chantziantoniou, PhD, ART(CSMLS), CFIAC and Dina R. Mody, MD
- 8 **Cytopreparation, Instrumentation, and Automated Screening in Gynecologic Cytology**
  Michael J. Thrall, MD and Debora A. Smith, CT(ASCP)
- 10 **Specimen Adequacy in Cervicovaginal Cytology**
  Dina R. Mody, MD and George G. Birdsong, MD

SECTION 2: BENIGN AND INFECTIOUS CONDITIONS

- 14 **Normal Pap Test**
  Nikolaos Chantziantoniou, PhD, ART(CSMLS), CFIAC and Dina R. Mody, MD
- 16 **Infectious and Other Organisms in Pap Tests**
  Nikolaos Chantziantoniou, PhD, ART(CSMLS), CFIAC and Dina R. Mody, MD
- 18 **Nonneoplastic Findings, Mimics, and Artifacts**
  Ekene I. Okoye, MD and Dina R. Mody, MD

SECTION 3: SQUAMOUS CELL ABNORMALITIES AND MIMICS

- 28 **Low-Grade Squamous Intraepithelial Lesion and Mimics**
  Dina R. Mody, MD
- 30 **High-Grade Squamous Intraepithelial Lesion and Mimics**
  Dina R. Mody, MD and Ekene I. Okoye, MD
- 34 **Atypical Squamous Cells of Undetermined Significance**
  Nikolaos Chantziantoniou, PhD, ART(CSMLS), CFIAC and Dina R. Mody, MD
- 36 **Atypical Squamous Cells, Cannot Rule Out High-Grade Squamous Intraepithelial Lesion**
  Dina R. Mody, MD and Nikolaos Chantziantoniou, PhD, ART(CSMLS), CFIAC
- 38 **Squamous Cell Carcinoma of Cervix, Variants and Mimics**
  Dina R. Mody, MD

SECTION 4: GLANDULAR CELL ABNORMALITIES AND MIMICS

- 46 **Endocervical Adenocarcinoma In Situ, Variants and Mimics**
  Dina R. Mody, MD
- 52 **Endocervical Adenocarcinoma, Variants and Mimics**
  Dina R. Mody, MD
- 56 **Adenocarcinoma, Gastric Type**
  Dina R. Mody, MD
- 58 **Endometrial Cancers: Usual Types, Variants, and Mimics**
  Ekene I. Okoye, MD and Dina R. Mody, MD
- 64 **Atypical Glandular Cells: Endocervicals, Endometrials, and Glandulars, NOS**
  Dina R. Mody, MD
- 70 **Endometrial Cells in Pap Test and Glandular Cells Status Post Hysterectomy**
  Dina R. Mody, MD and Ekene I. Okoye, MD

SECTION 5: EXTRAUTERINE CARCINOMAS AND OTHER MALIGNANCIES OF FEMALE GENITAL TRACT

- 74 **Extrauterine Carcinomas and Presentations in Cervicovaginal Cytology**
  Dina R. Mody, MD
- 76 **Neuroendocrine Carcinoma of Cervix**
  Dina R. Mody, MD
- 78 **Other Uncommon Malignancies in Cervicovaginal Cytology**
  Dina R. Mody, MD

SECTION 6: MOLECULAR TESTING IN GYNECOLOGIC CYTOLOGY

- 84 **HPV and Other Molecular Testing in Gynecologic Cytology**
  Michael J. Thrall, MD

SECTION 7: DIRECTLY SAMPLED ENDOMETRIAL CYTOLOGY

- 90 **Directly Sampled Endometrial Cytology**
  Yuko Sugiyama, MD, PhD, FIAC and Dina R. Mody, MD

SECTION 8: ANAL CYTOLOGY

- 96 **Anal Cytology**
  Michael J. Thrall, MD

TABLE OF CONTENTS

Part II: Exfoliative Cytopathology

SECTION 1: RESPIRATORY TRACT, INCLUDING LUNG FNAS

- 100 Specimen Types in Respiratory Cytology and Adequacy Criteria
  Michael J. Thrall, MD
- 102 Benign and Reactive Changes
  Michael J. Thrall, MD
- 106 *Pneumocystis* Pneumonia and Mimics
  Michael J. Thrall, MD
- 108 Fungal Organisms in Respiratory Cytology
  Michael J. Thrall, MD
- 110 Parasitic Organisms in Respiratory Cytology
  Michael J. Thrall, MD
- 112 Viral Infections (Cytomegalovirus, Herpesvirus, and Others)
  Michael J. Thrall, MD
- 114 Mycobacteria and Other Bacterial Infections
  Michael J. Thrall, MD
- 116 Sarcoidosis and Other Immune-Related Conditions
  Michael J. Thrall, MD
- 118 Pulmonary Alveolar Proteinosis and Mimics
  Michael J. Thrall, MD
- 120 Miscellaneous Findings, Including Contaminants
  Michael J. Thrall, MD
- 122 Adenocarcinoma
  Michael J. Thrall, MD
- 126 Squamous Cell Carcinoma
  Michael J. Thrall, MD
- 128 Small Cell Carcinoma
  Michael J. Thrall, MD
- 130 Large Cell Neuroendocrine Carcinoma
  Michael J. Thrall, MD
- 132 Carcinoid and Atypical Carcinoid
  Michael J. Thrall, MD
- 134 Rare Benign and Low Malignant Potential Tumors
  Michael J. Thrall, MD
- 136 Rare Malignant Tumors
  Michael J. Thrall, MD
- 138 NUT Carcinoma
  Michael J. Thrall, MD
- 139 *SMARCA4*-Deficient Undifferentiated Tumor
  Michael J. Thrall, MD
- 140 Pulmonary Lymphoma
  Michael J. Thrall, MD
- 142 Pulmonary Metastasis
  Michael J. Thrall, MD

SECTION 2: GASTROINTESTINAL TRACT

- 146 Specimen Types in Gastrointestinal Cytology and Normal Cellular Components
  Blythe K. Gorman, MD
- 148 Parasitic Infections
  Blythe K. Gorman, MD
- 150 Viral Infections
  Blythe K. Gorman, MD
- 152 Esophagitis and Barrett Esophagus
  Blythe K. Gorman, MD
- 154 Esophageal Adenocarcinoma
  Blythe K. Gorman, MD
- 156 Esophageal Squamous Cell Carcinoma
  Blythe K. Gorman, MD
- 158 Gastritis and Intestinal Metaplasia
  Blythe K. Gorman, MD
- 160 Gastric Adenocarcinoma
  Blythe K. Gorman, MD
- 162 Gastric Lymphoma
  Blythe K. Gorman, MD
- 164 Ampulla/Bile Duct/Pancreatic Duct Reactive Changes
  Blythe K. Gorman, MD
- 166 Ampulla/Bile Duct/Pancreatic Duct Adenocarcinoma
  Blythe K. Gorman, MD
- 168 Colorectal Adenoma/Carcinoma
  Blythe K. Gorman, MD
- 170 Neuroendocrine Tumor/Carcinoma
  Blythe K. Gorman, MD
- 172 Spindle Cell Neoplasms of Gastrointestinal Tract, Including Gastrointestinal Stromal Tumors
  Blythe K. Gorman, MD

SECTION 3: CEREBROSPINAL FLUID

- 176 Normal Cerebrospinal Fluid and Contamination by Normal Elements
  Hidehiro Takei, MD
- 180 Infectious Meningitis
  Hidehiro Takei, MD
- 182 Aseptic and Mollaret Meningitis
  Hidehiro Takei, MD
- 184 Subarachnoid Hemorrhage
  Hidehiro Takei, MD
- 186 Neurodegenerative Diseases
  Hidehiro Takei, MD
- 188 Primary Brain Tumors
  Hidehiro Takei, MD
- 190 Leukemia and Lymphoma
  Hidehiro Takei, MD
- 192 Metastasis in Cerebrospinal Fluid
  Hidehiro Takei, MD

SECTION 4: PLEURAL, PERITONEAL, PERICARDIAL, AND PELVIC FLUID AND WASHINGS

- 196 Normal Cellular Components, Reactive Mesothelial Proliferations, and Reporting Terminology
  Donna M. Coffey, MD and Michael J. Thrall, MD
- 200 Infectious Conditions
  Donna M. Coffey, MD and Michael J. Thrall, MD
- 202 Autoimmune Diseases
  Donna M. Coffey, MD and Michael J. Thrall, MD
- 204 Malignant Effusion, Mesothelioma
  Donna M. Coffey, MD and Michael J. Thrall, MD
- 208 Malignant Effusion, Carcinomas
  Donna M. Coffey, MD and Michael J. Thrall, MD

TABLE OF CONTENTS

212 **Malignant Effusion, Sarcomas**
Donna M. Coffey, MD, Nour Sneige, MD, and Michael J. Thrall, MD

214 **Lymphoid Effusions and Lymphomas**
Donna M. Coffey, MD and Michael J. Thrall, MD

216 **Primary Effusion Lymphoma**
John M. Stewart, MD, PhD and Michael J. Thrall, MD

218 **Endometriosis and Endosalpingiosis**
Donna M. Coffey, MD, Nour Sneige, MD, and Michael J. Thrall, MD

220 **Ovarian Neoplasms**
Donna M. Coffey, MD and Michael J. Thrall, MD

222 **Immunocytochemistry, Histochemistry, and Other Ancillary Techniques**
Donna M. Coffey, MD and Michael J. Thrall, MD

SECTION 5: URINARY CYTOLOGY

228 **Normal Urinary Cytology, Specimen Types, and Reporting Terminology**
Michael J. Thrall, MD and Rose Anton, MD

232 **Ileal Conduit Specimens**
Rose Anton, MD and Michael J. Thrall, MD

234 **Noninfectious Benign Conditions**
Rose Anton, MD and Michael J. Thrall, MD

236 **Infectious Benign Conditions**
Rose Anton, MD and Michael J. Thrall, MD

238 **Reactive Urothelial Changes**
Rose Anton, MD and Michael J. Thrall, MD

240 **Low-Grade Urothelial Lesions**
Rose Anton, MD and Michael J. Thrall, MD

241 **Atypical Urothelial Cells**
Michael J. Thrall, MD

242 **High-Grade Urothelial Dysplasia/Carcinoma/Carcinoma In Situ**
Rose Anton, MD and Michael J. Thrall, MD

244 **Squamous Cell Carcinoma of Urinary Bladder**
Rose Anton, MD, Nour Sneige, MD, and Michael J. Thrall, MD

246 **Adenocarcinoma of Urinary Bladder**
Rose Anton, MD, Nour Sneige, MD, and Michael J. Thrall, MD

248 **Other Malignancies in Urinary Cytology**
Rose Anton, MD, Nour Sneige, MD, and Michael J. Thrall, MD

250 **Renal Pelvic Cytology**
Blythe K. Gorman, MD and Michael J. Thrall, MD

252 **Ancillary Testing, UroVysion, and Others**
Gene Landon, MD, Nancy P. Caraway, MD, and Michael J. Thrall, MD

Part III: Fine-Needle Aspiration, Superficial

SECTION 1: OVERVIEW

256 **Superficial Aspiration Technique**
Rose Anton, MD and Dina R. Mody, MD

SECTION 2: THYROID GLAND

260 **Ultrasound-Guided Thyroid Fine-Needle Aspiration**
Paula J. Woodward, MD

266 **Thyroid Fine-Needle Aspiration Reporting Terminology and Specimen Adequacy**
Dina R. Mody, MD

268 **Adenomatous (Benign Follicular) Nodule**
Mojgan Amrikachi, MD and Dina R. Mody, MD

270 **Chronic Lymphocytic/Hashimoto Thyroiditis**
Mojgan Amrikachi, MD and Dina R. Mody, MD

272 **Granulomatous Thyroiditis**
Mojgan Amrikachi, MD and Dina R. Mody, MD

274 **Graves Disease/Diffuse Toxic Goiter**
Mukul K. Divatia, MD and Dina R. Mody, MD

275 **Pigmented Thyroid Lesions and Crystals**
Mukul K. Divatia, MD and Dina R. Mody, MD

276 **Atypia of Undetermined Significance/Follicular Lesion of Undetermined Significance**
Dina R. Mody, MD

280 **Follicular Neoplasm/Suspicious for a Follicular Neoplasm**
Dina R. Mody, MD

284 **Follicular Neoplasm, Oncocytic (Hürthle Cell) Type**
Mojgan Amrikachi, MD and Dina R. Mody, MD

286 **Papillary Thyroid Carcinoma, Classic Subtype**
Mojgan Amrikachi, MD and Dina R. Mody, MD

290 **Papillary Thyroid Carcinoma Subtypes**
Mojgan Amrikachi, MD and Dina R. Mody, MD

298 **Medullary Thyroid Carcinoma**
Mojgan Amrikachi, MD and Dina R. Mody, MD

302 **Poorly Differentiated Thyroid Carcinoma**
Susan L. Haley, MD and Dina R. Mody, MD

304 **Anaplastic Thyroid Carcinoma**
Susan L. Haley, MD and Dina R. Mody, MD

306 **Thyroid Lymphoma**
Susan L. Haley, MD and Dina R. Mody, MD

308 **Metastatic Carcinoma to Thyroid**
Susan L. Haley, MD and Dina R. Mody, MD

310 **Other Nonneoplastic and Neoplastic Thyroid Lesions Encountered on Thyroid FNA**
Mojgan Amrikachi, MD and Dina R. Mody, MD

SECTION 3: PARATHYROID GLAND

318 **Parathyroid Cyst, Adenoma, and Carcinoma**
Susan L. Haley, MD, Rose Anton, MD, and Dina R. Mody, MD

SECTION 4: LYMPH NODES

OVERVIEW

324 **Lymph Node Aspiration: Indications, Techniques, and Reporting**
Rose Anton, MD and Dina R. Mody, MD

326 **FNA Sample Prep and Triage in Evaluating Suspected Lymphoma**
John M. Stewart, MD, PhD and Savitri Krishnamurthy, MD

TABLE OF CONTENTS

BENIGN, INFECTIOUS, AND REACTIVE HYPERPLASIA

- 328 **Inflammatory and Reactive Lymphoid Hyperplasia**
  Rose Anton, MD and Savitri Krishnamurthy, MD
- 330 **Granulomatous Lymphadenitis, Infectious and Sarcoid**
  Rose Anton, MD and Savitri Krishnamurthy, MD
- 334 **Rosai-Dorfman Disease**
  Rose Anton, MD, John M. Stewart, MD, PhD, and Savitri Krishnamurthy, MD

METASTATIC MALIGNANCIES

- 336 **Metastatic Malignancies (Carcinoma, Melanoma)**
  Rose Anton, MD and Dina R. Mody, MD
- 338 **HPV-Positive Head and Neck Squamous Cell Carcinoma**
  Mary R. Schwartz, MD and Dina R. Mody, MD

NODAL B-CELL LYMPHOMA

- 342 **Small Lymphocytic Lymphoma**
  Nancy P. Caraway, MD, John M. Stewart, MD, PhD, and Savitri Krishnamurthy, MD
- 344 **Lymphoplasmacytic Lymphoma**
  Nancy P. Caraway, MD, John M. Stewart, MD, PhD, and Savitri Krishnamurthy, MD
- 346 **Mantle Cell Lymphoma**
  Nancy P. Caraway, MD, John M. Stewart, MD, PhD, and Savitri Krishnamurthy, MD
- 348 **Nodal Marginal Zone Lymphoma**
  Nancy P. Caraway, MD, John M. Stewart, MD, PhD, and Savitri Krishnamurthy, MD
- 350 **Follicular Lymphoma**
  Nancy P. Caraway, MD, John M. Stewart, MD, PhD, and Savitri Krishnamurthy, MD
- 352 **Burkitt Lymphoma**
  Nancy P. Caraway, MD, John M. Stewart, MD, PhD, and Savitri Krishnamurthy, MD
- 354 **Large B-Cell Lymphoma**
  Nancy P. Caraway, MD, John M. Stewart, MD, PhD, and Savitri Krishnamurthy, MD

EXTRANODAL B-CELL LYMPHOMA

- 356 **Plasmacytoma**
  Nancy P. Caraway, MD, John M. Stewart, MD, PhD, and Savitri Krishnamurthy, MD
- 358 **Mediastinal Large B-Cell Lymphoma**
  Nancy P. Caraway, MD, John M. Stewart, MD, PhD, and Savitri Krishnamurthy, MD
- 360 **Plasmablastic Lymphoma**
  John M. Stewart, MD, PhD, Nancy P. Caraway, MD, and Savitri Krishnamurthy, MD

T-CELL LYMPHOMA

- 362 **Peripheral T-Cell Lymphoma**
  Nancy P. Caraway, MD, John M. Stewart, MD, PhD, and Savitri Krishnamurthy, MD
- 364 **Mycosis Fungoides**
  Nancy P. Caraway, MD, John M. Stewart, MD, PhD, and Savitri Krishnamurthy, MD
- 366 **Angioimmunoblastic Lymphoma**
  Nancy P. Caraway, MD, John M. Stewart, MD, PhD, and Savitri Krishnamurthy, MD
- 368 **ALK(+) Anaplastic Large Cell Lymphoma**
  Nancy P. Caraway, MD, John M. Stewart, MD, PhD, and Savitri Krishnamurthy, MD
- 370 **T-Cell Lymphoblastic Lymphoma**
  Nancy P. Caraway, MD, John M. Stewart, MD, PhD, and Savitri Krishnamurthy, MD

HODGKIN LYMPHOMA

- 372 **Nodular Lymphocyte-Predominant Hodgkin Lymphoma**
  Nancy P. Caraway, MD, John M. Stewart, MD, PhD, and Savitri Krishnamurthy, MD
- 374 **Classic Hodgkin Lymphoma**
  Nancy P. Caraway, MD, John M. Stewart, MD, PhD, and Savitri Krishnamurthy, MD

SECTION 5: SALIVARY GLAND

OVERVIEW

- 378 **Approach to Interpretation of Salivary Gland Aspiration Biopsies and Reporting Terminology (Milan System)**
  Dina R. Mody, MD

BENIGN LESIONS

- 382 **Normal Salivary Gland and Sialadenitis on Aspiration**
  Rose Anton, MD and Dina R. Mody, MD
- 384 **Cysts**
  Rose Anton, MD and Dina R. Mody, MD
- 386 **Pleomorphic Adenoma**
  Rose Anton, MD and Dina R. Mody, MD
- 388 **Warthin Tumor**
  Rose Anton, MD and Dina R. Mody, MD
- 390 **Myoepithelioma**
  Rose Anton, MD and Dina R. Mody, MD
- 391 **Oncocytoma, Salivary Gland**
  Dina R. Mody, MD

MALIGNANT NEOPLASMS

- 392 **Adenoid Cystic Carcinoma**
  Rose Anton, MD and Dina R. Mody, MD
- 394 **Acinic Cell Carcinoma**
  Rose Anton, MD and Dina R. Mody, MD
- 396 **Mucoepidermoid Carcinoma**
  Rose Anton, MD and Dina R. Mody, MD
- 398 **Basaloid Neoplasms, Benign and Malignant**
  Hidehiro Takei, MD and Dina R. Mody, MD
- 400 **Carcinoma Ex Pleomorphic Adenoma**
  Hidehiro Takei, MD
- 402 **Adenocarcinoma, NOS**
  Hidehiro Takei, MD

TABLE OF CONTENTS

- **404** Polymorphous Adenocarcinoma
  Hidehiro Takei, MD and Dina R. Mody, MD
- **406** Salivary Duct Carcinoma
  Hidehiro Takei, MD and Dina R. Mody, MD
- **408** Secretory Carcinoma
  Michael J. Thrall, MD
- **410** Myoepithelial Carcinoma
  Shubhada Kane, MD and Michael J. Thrall, MD
- **411** Cribriform Adenocarcinoma
  Shubhada Kane, MD and Michael J. Thrall, MD
- **412** Metastatic Carcinoma
  Hidehiro Takei, MD
- **414** Primary and Metastatic Nonepithelial Tumors
  Dina R. Mody, MD and Hidehiro Takei, MD

SECTION 6: BREAST

OVERVIEW
- **418** Role of Fine-Needle Aspiration of Breast, Techniques and Triple Test
  Savitri Krishnamurthy, MD

BENIGN BREAST LESIONS
- **420** Inflammatory and Granulomatous Conditions
  Savitri Krishnamurthy, MD
- **422** Fat Necrosis
  Savitri Krishnamurthy, MD
- **424** Nonproliferative and Proliferative Changes in Breast
  Savitri Krishnamurthy, MD
- **428** Radial Scar/Complex Sclerosing Lesion
  Savitri Krishnamurthy, MD
- **430** Gynecomastia
  Savitri Krishnamurthy, MD
- **432** Mucocele-Like Lesion
  Savitri Krishnamurthy, MD

BENIGN NEOPLASMS
- **434** Fibroadenoma
  Savitri Krishnamurthy, MD
- **438** Granular Cell Tumor of Breast
  Savitri Krishnamurthy, MD
- **440** Papillary Neoplasms
  Savitri Krishnamurthy, MD
- **446** Myofibroblastoma, Mammary
  Savitri Krishnamurthy, MD

MALIGNANT NEOPLASMS
- **448** Ductal Carcinoma and Variants of Invasive Mammary Carcinoma
  Savitri Krishnamurthy, MD
- **456** Lobular Carcinoma
  Savitri Krishnamurthy, MD
- **458** Phyllodes Tumor
  Savitri Krishnamurthy, MD
- **460** Angiosarcoma and Other Sarcomas
  Savitri Krishnamurthy, MD
- **464** Lymphomas and Metastatic Tumors
  Savitri Krishnamurthy, MD

NIPPLE DISCHARGE
- **466** Cytology Specimens for Risk Assessment of Breast Cancer
  Savitri Krishnamurthy, MD

SECTION 7: SKIN AND SUBCUTANEOUS CYTOLOGY
- **470** Cutaneous and Adnexal Cytology
  Mary R. Schwartz, MD and Dina R. Mody, MD

Part IV: Fine-Needle Aspiration, Deep Organs and Tissues

SECTION 1: OVERVIEW
- **476** Techniques and Modalities of Deep Aspiration Biopsies
  Paula J. Woodward, MD and Ashraf Thabet, MD

SECTION 2: MEDIASTINUM

OVERVIEW
- **482** Anatomic Compartments and Constituent Tumors
  Ming Guo, MD and Savitri Krishnamurthy, MD

NONNEOPLASTIC LESIONS
- **484** Mediastinal Cysts and Inflammatory Lesions
  Ming Guo, MD and Savitri Krishnamurthy, MD

NEOPLASMS
- **486** Thymoma
  Ming Guo, MD and Savitri Krishnamurthy, MD
- **488** Thymic Carcinoma
  Ming Guo, MD and Savitri Krishnamurthy, MD
- **490** Germ Cell Tumors
  Ming Guo, MD and Savitri Krishnamurthy, MD
- **492** Neurogenic Tumors
  Ming Guo, MD and Savitri Krishnamurthy, MD
- **494** Metastatic Tumors of Mediastinum
  Ming Guo, MD and Savitri Krishnamurthy, MD

SECTION 3: LIVER

OVERVIEW
- **498** Cytology of Normal Liver
  Elizabeth M. Jacobi, MD, Rose Anton, MD, and Michael J. Thrall, MD
- **500** Inflammatory and Infectious Conditions of Liver
  Elizabeth M. Jacobi, MD, Rose Anton, MD, and Michael J. Thrall, MD

BENIGN HEPATIC NEOPLASMS
- **502** Hepatocellular Adenoma
  Elizabeth M. Jacobi, MD, Rose Anton, MD, and Michael J. Thrall, MD

TABLE OF CONTENTS

504 **Focal Nodular Hyperplasia**
Elizabeth M. Jacobi, MD, Rose Anton, MD, and Michael J. Thrall, MD

506 **Hemangioma, Liver**
Elizabeth M. Jacobi, MD, Rose Anton, MD, and Michael J. Thrall, MD

MALIGNANT NEOPLASMS

508 **Hepatocellular Carcinoma**
Elizabeth M. Jacobi, MD, Rose Anton, MD, and Michael J. Thrall, MD

510 **Hepatoblastoma**
Elizabeth M. Jacobi, MD, Rose Anton, MD, and Michael J. Thrall, MD

512 **Liver Metastasis**
Elizabeth M. Jacobi, MD, Rose Anton, MD, and Michael J. Thrall, MD

SECTION 4: KIDNEY

OVERVIEW

516 **Cytology of Normal Kidney**
Yimin Ge, MD

BENIGN LESIONS AND NEOPLASMS

518 **Renal Cysts**
Yimin Ge, MD

520 **Angiomyolipoma**
Yimin Ge, MD

522 **Oncocytoma, Kidney**
Yimin Ge, MD

524 **Metanephric Adenoma**
Yimin Ge, MD and Jun Zhang, MD, MS

526 **Metanephric Stromal Tumor**
Yimin Ge, MD and Norma Quintanilla, MD

527 **Xanthogranulomatous Pyelonephritis/Malakoplakia**
Yimin Ge, MD

MALIGNANT NEOPLASMS

528 **Clear Cell Renal Cell Carcinoma**
Yimin Ge, MD

532 **Papillary Renal Cell Carcinoma**
Yimin Ge, MD

534 **Clear Cell Papillary Renal Cell Carcinoma**
Michael J. Thrall, MD

536 **Chromophobe Renal Cell Carcinoma**
Yimin Ge, MD

538 ***TFE3*- and *TFEB*-Rearranged Renal Cell Carcinomas**
Michael J. Thrall, MD

540 **Collecting Duct Carcinoma**
Yimin Ge, MD and Jun Zhang, MD, MS

541 **Renal Medullary Carcinoma**
Yimin Ge, MD

542 **Mucinous Tubular and Spindle Cell Carcinoma of Kidney**
Yimin Ge, MD

543 **Carcinoid Tumor**
Yimin Ge, MD

544 **Primary Renal Sarcomas in Adults**
Yimin Ge, MD and Jun Zhang, MD, MS

545 **Renal Lymphomas**
Yimin Ge, MD and Jun Zhang, MD, MS

546 **Nephroblastoma (Wilms Tumor)**
Yimin Ge, MD, Jun Zhang, MD, MS, and Norma Quintanilla, MD

548 **Clear Cell Sarcoma of Kidney**
Yimin Ge, MD and Norma Quintanilla, MD

550 **Congenital Mesoblastic Nephroma**
Yimin Ge, MD and Norma Quintanilla, MD

552 **Rhabdoid Tumor of Kidney**
Yimin Ge, MD and Norma Quintanilla, MD

553 **Metastatic Tumors to Kidney**
Yimin Ge, MD

TUMORS OF RENAL PELVIS

554 **Urothelial Carcinoma**
Yimin Ge, MD

SECTION 5: ADRENAL GLAND

OVERVIEW

558 **Cytology of Normal Adrenal Gland**
Yimin Ge, MD

ADRENAL CORTICAL LESIONS

560 **Adrenal Cortical Adenoma**
Yimin Ge, MD

562 **Adrenal Cortical Carcinoma**
Yimin Ge, MD

564 **Metastatic Tumors to Adrenal Gland**
Yimin Ge, MD

ADRENAL MEDULLARY LESIONS

566 **Pheochromocytoma**
Yimin Ge, MD

SECTION 6: PANCREAS

OVERVIEW

570 **Cytology of Normal Pancreas**
Uma Kundu, MD and Dina R. Mody, MD

572 **Pancreaticobiliary Cytology Reporting Terminology, Cyst Evaluation**
Dina R. Mody, MD and Mary R. Schwartz, MD

NONNEOPLASTIC LESIONS

574 **Pancreatitis**
Uma Kundu, MD and Dina R. Mody, MD

576 **Lymphoepithelial Cyst of Pancreas**
Dina R. Mody, MD

577 **Intra- and Peripancreatic Splenules**
Dina R. Mody, MD

NEOPLASMS

578 **Serous Microcystic Adenoma**
Uma Kundu, MD and Savitri Krishnamurthy, MD

TABLE OF CONTENTS

580 **Mucinous Cystic Neoplasm**
Uma Kundu, MD and Savitri Krishnamurthy, MD

582 **Intraductal Papillary Mucinous Neoplasm**
Uma Kundu, MD and Savitri Krishnamurthy, MD

584 **Solid Pseudopapillary Neoplasm**
Gene Landon, MD and Savitri Krishnamurthy, MD

586 **Pancreatic Neuroendocrine Tumor**
Gene Landon, MD and Savitri Krishnamurthy, MD

588 **Pancreatic Ductal Adenocarcinoma**
Gene Landon, MD and Savitri Krishnamurthy, MD

590 **Unusual Variants of Ductal Carcinoma**
Savitri Krishnamurthy, MD

594 **Acinar Cell Carcinoma**
Savitri Krishnamurthy, MD

596 **Lymphoma and Secondary Tumors of Pancreas**
Savitri Krishnamurthy, MD

SECTION 7: BONE

OVERVIEW

600 **Approach to Cytologic/Small Biopsy Diagnosis of Primary Bone Tumors**
Dina R. Mody, MD

NEOPLASMS

602 **Chondromas of Bone and Soft Tissue**
Mukul K. Divatia, MD and Dina R. Mody, MD

604 **Chondroblastoma**
Dina R. Mody, MD

606 **Giant Cell Tumor**
Dina R. Mody, MD

608 **Osteoblastoma**
Dina R. Mody, MD

610 **Adamantinoma**
Dina R. Mody, MD

612 **Langerhans Cell Histiocytosis**
Dina R. Mody, MD

614 **Chordoma**
Dina R. Mody, MD

616 **Osteosarcoma**
Savitri Krishnamurthy, MD

620 **Chondrosarcoma**
Savitri Krishnamurthy, MD

624 **Ewing Sarcoma**
Savitri Krishnamurthy, MD

628 **Bone Lymphoma**
Dina R. Mody, MD

630 **Metastatic Tumors of Bone**
Dina R. Mody, MD

SECTION 8: SOFT TISSUE

OVERVIEW

634 **Approach to Cytologic/Small Biopsy Diagnosis of Primary Soft Tissue Lesions**
Dina R. Mody, MD

ADIPOCYTIC TUMORS

636 **Benign Adipose Tissue Tumors**
Uma Kundu, MD and Savitri Krishnamurthy, MD

638 **Liposarcoma**
Uma Kundu, MD and Savitri Krishnamurthy, MD

FIBROBLASTIC/MYOFIBROBLASTIC LESIONS

642 **Fibrosarcoma**
Uma Kundu, MD and Savitri Krishnamurthy, MD

644 **Myofibroblastoma**
Savitri Krishnamurthy, MD

646 **Low-Grade Myofibroblastic Sarcoma**
Uma Kundu, MD and Savitri Krishnamurthy, MD

FIBROHISTIOCYTIC TUMORS

648 **Giant Cell Tumor of Tendon Sheath**
Uma Kundu, MD and Savitri Krishnamurthy, MD

650 **Undifferentiated Pleomorphic Sarcoma**
Uma Kundu, MD and Savitri Krishnamurthy, MD

TUMORS OF MUSCLE ORIGIN

652 **Smooth Muscle Tumors**
Gene Landon, MD and Savitri Krishnamurthy, MD

654 **Skeletal Muscle Tumors**
Gene Landon, MD and Savitri Krishnamurthy, MD

VASCULAR TUMORS

658 **Hemangioma, Soft Tissue**
Gene Landon, MD and Michael J. Thrall, MD

660 **Epithelioid Hemangioendothelioma**
Gene Landon, MD and Michael J. Thrall, MD

662 **Angiosarcoma**
Gene Landon, MD and Savitri Krishnamurthy, MD

OTHER TUMORS

664 **Other Reactive and Neoplastic Soft Tissue Entities**
Dina R. Mody, MD

666 **Mesenchymal Chondrosarcoma**
Dina R. Mody, MD

667 **Solitary Fibrous Tumor**
Dina R. Mody, MD

668 **Intramuscular Myxoma**
Gene Landon, MD and Savitri Krishnamurthy, MD

670 **Synovial Sarcoma**
Gene Landon, MD and Savitri Krishnamurthy, MD

672 **Epithelioid Sarcoma**
Gene Landon, MD and Savitri Krishnamurthy, MD

674 **Alveolar Soft Part Sarcoma**
Uma Kundu, MD and Savitri Krishnamurthy, MD

676 **Clear Cell Sarcoma of Soft Tissue**
Uma Kundu, MD and Savitri Krishnamurthy, MD

678 **Desmoplastic Small Round Cell Tumor**
Uma Kundu, MD and Savitri Krishnamurthy, MD

TABLE OF CONTENTS

SECTION 9: OPHTHALMIC AND NEUROPATHOLOGY

- 682 **Approach to Ophthalmic Cytology**
  Patricia Chévez-Barrios, MD
- 686 **Ophthalmic Cytopathology, Infectious**
  Patricia Chévez-Barrios, MD
- 690 **Ophthalmic Cytopathology, Neoplastic**
  Patricia Chévez-Barrios, MD
- 696 **Neuropathology Squash Preparations, Infectious**
  Andreana L. Rivera, MD, Suzanne Z. Powell, MD, and Hidehiro Takei, MD
- 700 **Neuropathology Squash Preparations, Glial Neoplasms**
  Suzanne Z. Powell, MD, Andreana L. Rivera, MD, and Hidehiro Takei, MD
- 704 **Neuropathology Squash Preparations, Nonglial Neoplasms**
  Andreana L. Rivera, MD, Suzanne Z. Powell, MD, and Hidehiro Takei, MD

Part V: Management and Ancillary Testing

SECTION 1: CYTOPREPARATORY AND QUALITY MANAGEMENT

- 710 **Cytopreparatory Techniques and Instrumentation in Nongynecologic Cytology**
  Debora A. Smith, CT(ASCP) and Dina R. Mody, MD
- 716 **Quality Improvement and Laboratory Management for Cytopathology**
  Debora A. Smith, CT(ASCP) and Dina R. Mody, MD

SECTION 2: ANCILLARY TESTING

- 724 **Immunocytochemistry**
  Savitri Krishnamurthy, MD
- 728 **Molecular Techniques**
  Savitri Krishnamurthy, MD

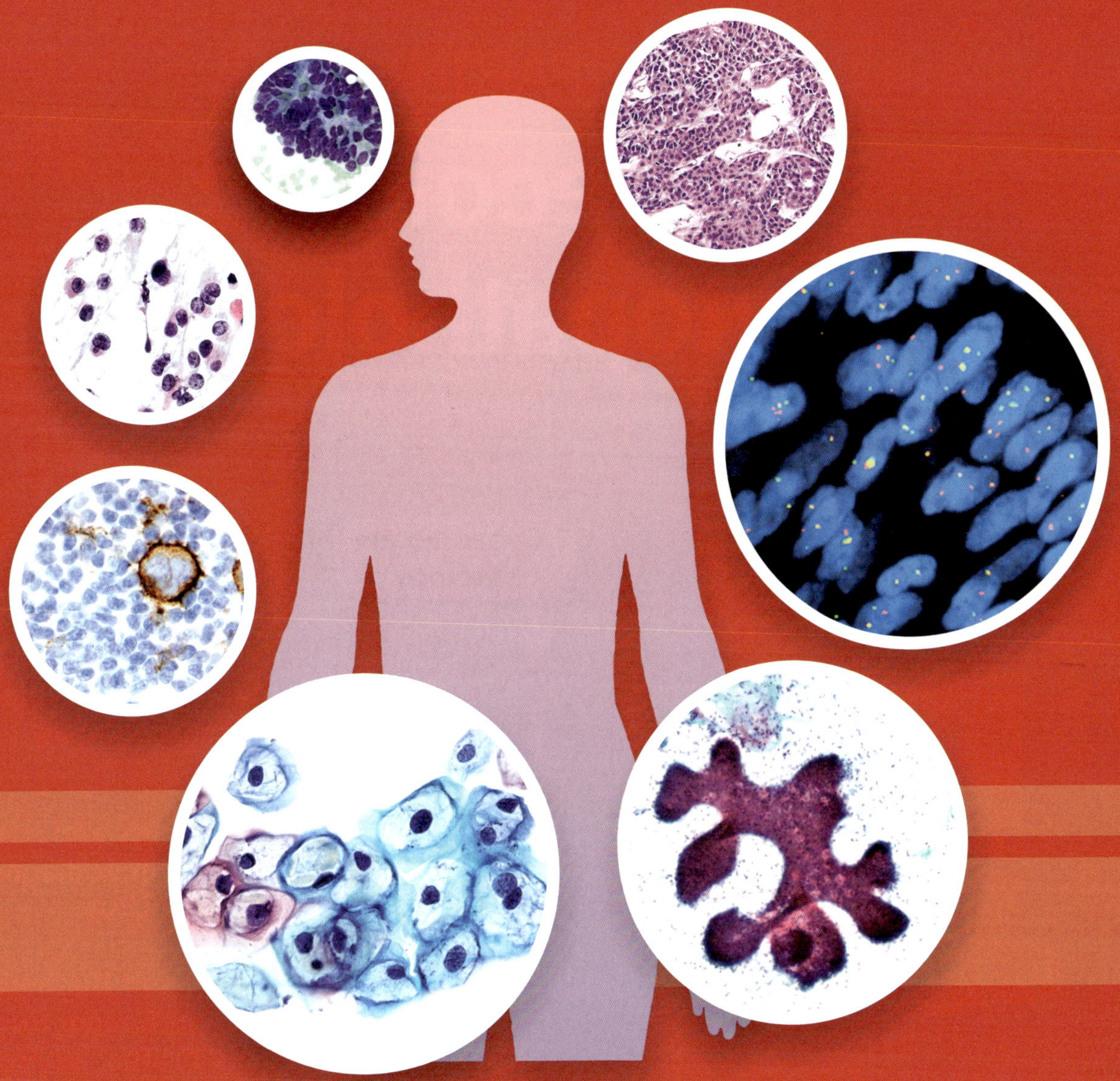

Diagnostic Pathology

Cytopathology

MODY | THRALL | KRISHNAMURTHY
Ge | Gorman | Takei

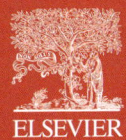

THIRD EDITION

PART I
Gynecologic Cytopathology

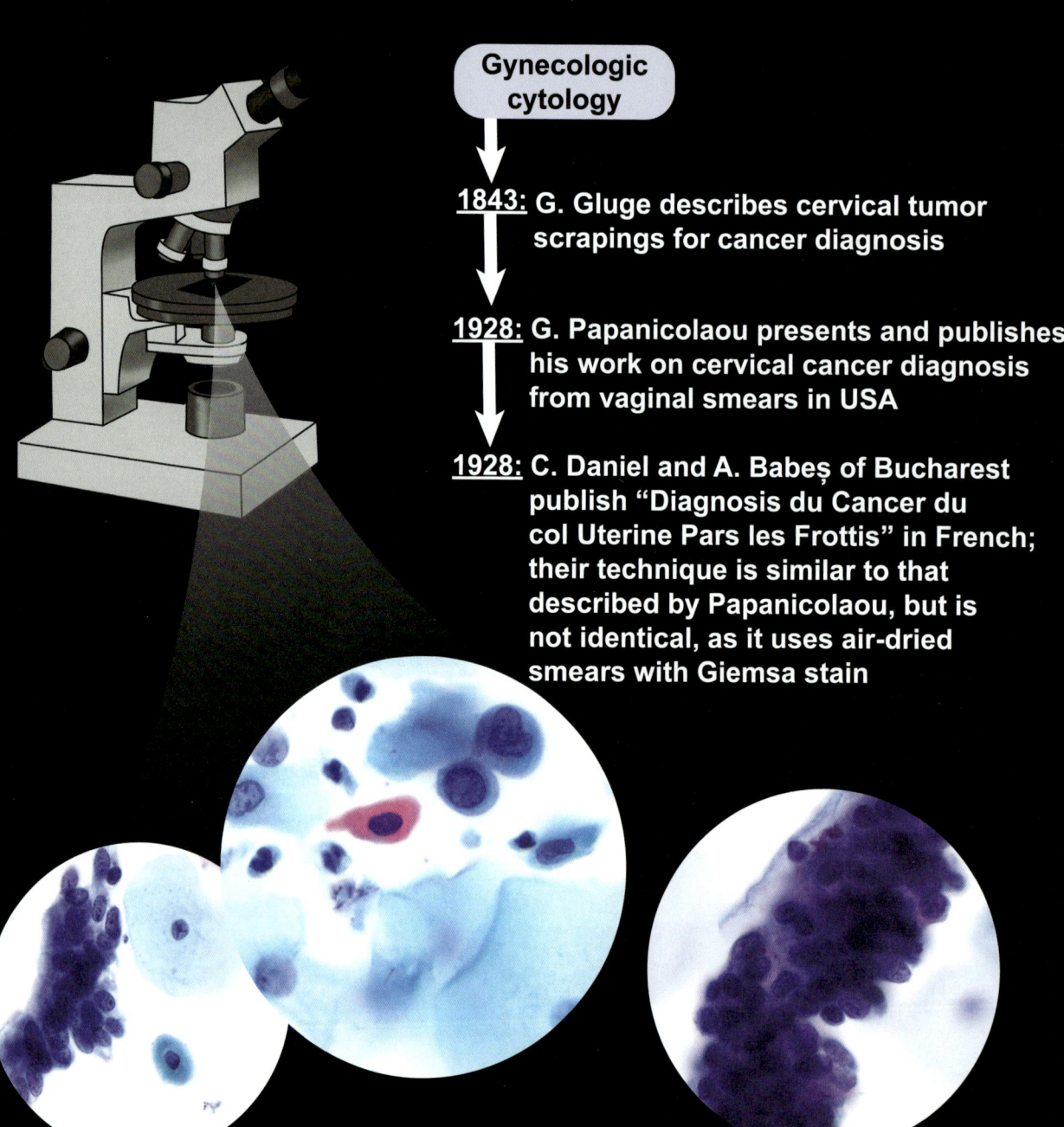

Gynecologic cytology

1843: G. Gluge describes cervical tumor scrapings for cancer diagnosis

1928: G. Papanicolaou presents and publishes his work on cervical cancer diagnosis from vaginal smears in USA

1928: C. Daniel and A. Babeș of Bucharest publish "Diagnosis du Cancer du col Uterine Pars les Frottis" in French; their technique is similar to that described by Papanicolaou, but is not identical, as it uses air-dried smears with Giemsa stain

PART I
SECTION 1
Overview

Pap Test and Cervical Cancer Screening: History and Reporting Terminology	4
Cytopreparation, Instrumentation, and Automated Screening in Gynecologic Cytology	8
Specimen Adequacy in Cervicovaginal Cytology	10

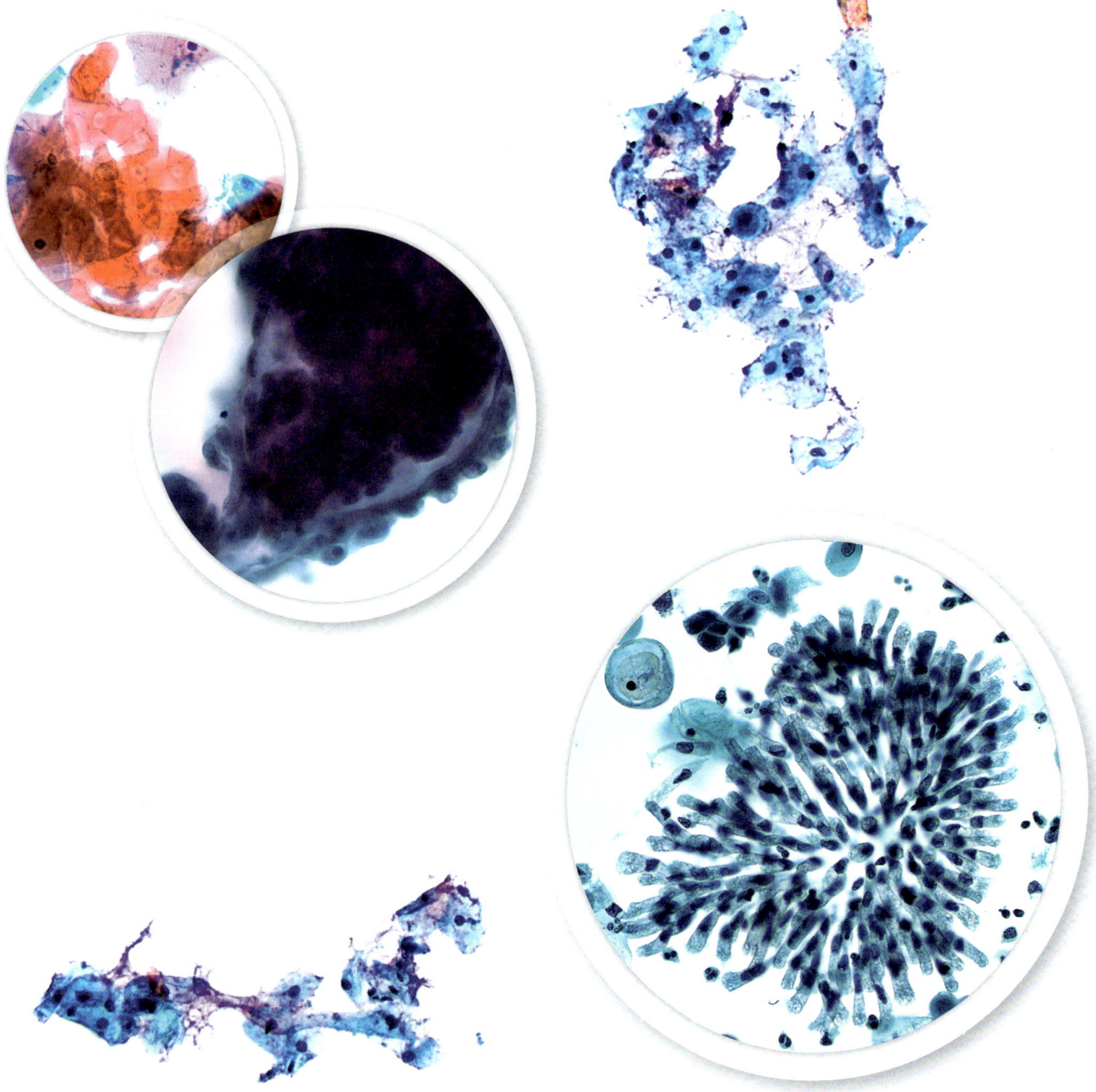

Pap Test and Cervical Cancer Screening: History and Reporting Terminology

TERMINOLOGY

Definitions

- Pap test: Simple, widely accepted, and noninvasive screening procedure designed to detect subclinical squamous epithelial lesions
  - Cervical cells are collected during pelvic examination
  - Ideally, lesions are identified at stage of precursors to cervical cancer
  - Most successful cancer screening test, reducing morbidity and mortality from cervical cancer
- Pap test screening has significantly reduced morbidity and mortality due to invasive cervical cancer
  - Primarily in developed global regions supported by well-managed screening programs
  - One of most successful cervical cancer screening methods ever devised
  - Screening test or diagnostic test in patients with history of cervical pathology
  - Testament to Dr. Papanicolaou's fundamental work establishing diagnostic cytopathology overall

HISTORY

Dr. George Nicholas Papanicolaou

- Credited for his work to develop vaginal smear method, multichromatic Pap stain, and refinement of these tools to facilitate clinical screening practices that detect early cervical cancer
- Born in Kymi, Greece on May 13, 1883
- After receiving MD degree from University of Athens in 1904, pursued graduate work studying sex differentiation and determination of *Daphnia* flies at University of Jena in Germany
- Attained doctorate degree in 1910, then devoted his life to academic and scientific research
- On October 19, 1913, he and his wife, Mary Papanicolaou, emigrated to New York to work and study

Cervical Cancer Screening and Prevention: Milestones and Breakthroughs

1914	Dr. George Papanicolaou emigrates to USA and starts research at Cornell
1928	Papanicolaou publishes findings on detection of cancer cells using vaginal smears in humans
1943	Papanicolaou and Traut monograph
1954	American Cancer Society endorses Pap test
1960	Pap smear widely available in USA
1965	First reports characterize double-stranded HPV virus
1974	zur Hausen publishes link between cervical cancer and HPV
1976	Meisels and Fortin postulate koilocytes are viral cytopathic effect of HPV infection
1983	HPV-16, HPV-18 detection in cervical cancer by Dr. zur Hausen
1988	CLIA '88 cytology mandates and first Bethesda Conference for cytology reporting
1996–2000	ALTS trial (USA) with Hybrid Capture II (Digene)
2006	FDA approves first prophylactic HPV vaccine (Gardasil 4)
2008	Dr. zur Hausen awarded Nobel Prize for Medicine
2014	FDA approval of cobas platform (Roche) for primary HPV screening
2017	Implementation of primary HPV screening in some countries

We are approaching 100 years since the 1st description of abnormal gynecologic cytology by Papanicolaou, the foundation of one of the most successful screening methods in history. The recognition of the role of HPV in cervical cancer by zur Hausen almost 50 years ago started a 2nd wave of innovation that has led to vaccination efforts and an ever-growing utilization of molecular tests. Today we are in the midst of a revolutionary transition to HPV-based screening.

Pap Test and Cervical Cancer Screening: History and Reporting Terminology

FIRST NATIONAL CYTOLOGY CONFERENCE
Boston (1948)
- Conclusions reached by Papanicolaou and Traut were reproduced by other investigators
- Yet vaginal smear method remained unappealing to most pathologists
  - Therefore, in 1945, newly established American Cancer Society initiated campaign to educate profession regarding effectiveness of method
- Papanicolaou felt that instruction should ensue from 1 source
  - Thus, he organized and taught 1st tutorial in exfoliative cytology in New York Cornell Medical Center in September 1947
- In response, American Cancer Society sponsored 1st National Cytology Conference in Boston in 1948
  - Resolved that despite optional biopsy, vaginal smear method was sufficient to detect early uterine cancer before it was obvious and before emergence of cervical cancer symptoms
- Papanicolaou remained concerned over any widespread sampling in absence of greater interpretive knowledge and acceptance amongst practicing pathologists and cytologists

PAP CLASS REPORTING SYSTEM
Introduced in 1948
- Smear technique coupled with Pap staining gained acceptance in realm of diagnostic nongynecologic cytopathology (i.e., urine, sputum, gastric, effusion, and breast)
- Though, emergence of particular false-negative and false-positive cases disturbed Papanicolaou immensely
- It occurred to him that method and its widening application required dedicated language by which to communicate both cytomorphology and ensuing diagnosis
- In 1948, Papanicolaou introduced reporting system based on 5 arbitrary, ill-defined categories by which vaginal smears may be classified
  - 1st reporting system designed for gynecologic cytology, later named Papanicolaou Classification System (a.k.a. Pap Class System)
  - Reporting categories communicated sense of confidence as to whether smears reflected malignancy
    - Suggested single, linear cascade of epithelial cell abnormalities arising from normal to cancerous epithelia
  - 5 classes (I, II, III, IV, and V) conveyed following findings
    - I: Normal
    - II: Inflammatory
    - III: Suspicious of malignancy
    - IV: Strongly suggestive of malignancy
    - V: Definitely malignant

ATLAS OF EXFOLIATIVE CYTOLOGY
Published in 1954
- Despite new reporting strategy, Papanicolaou realized yet another deficiency as reporting classifications lacked cytomorphologic reflection
- Therefore, he and Hashime Murayama embarked upon fundamental work leading up to their magnum opus
  - "The Atlas of Exfoliative Cytology," published in 1954 by Commonwealth Fund, Harvard University Press
    - Remains masterpiece composed of remarkable color plates of cells defining Pap classifications and their relevant cytomorphologic terms, mosaics, and margins
    - Emphasized ongoing refinement of Papanicolaou staining procedure

DYSPLASIA REPORTING SYSTEM
Formalized in 1962
- Diagnostic data that emerged from cervical cancer screening programs suggested that precursor lesions differed from invasive cancer
  - Precursor lesions occur in younger females
  - Not all precursor lesions progress to invasive cancer
  - Untreated lesions do not necessarily advance to cancer
  - Some precursor lesions regress
  - Precursor lesions demonstrate variable cytologic and histologic characteristics, hence grades
- These revelations came soon after Papanicolaou's death
- Dr. James Reagan formalized Dysplasia Reporting System in 1962
- His reporting system was designed upon premise that dysplasia is neoplastic, intraepithelial, cervical lesion (of various grades) of uncertain prognosis, in contrast with carcinoma in situ (CIS), which he regarded obligate precursor lesion to invasive cervical cancer
- In contrast to Pap class system, Reagan's approach suggested distinct categories of intraepithelial lesions
- Although dysplasia nomenclature became accepted by most pathologists, others objected
  - Argued that system could not adequately distinguish carcinoma in situ (CIS) from likely high-grade lesions with surface differentiation
  - Dysplasia nomenclature was associated with poor interobserver reproducibility

CERVICAL INTRAEPITHELIAL NEOPLASIA REPORTING SYSTEM
Proposed in 1967
- It was also becoming evident that regardless of morphologic appearance, any precursor cervical lesion may potentially progress to invasive cancer
  - But frequency of likely progression may differ between low- and high-grade lesions
- Understanding of cervical pathobiology prompted Dr. R. M. Richart to propose alternate approach in 1967
  - Cervical Intraepithelial Neoplasia (CIN) reporting system
    - Nomenclature consisted initially of 3 CIN grades: CIN 1 (slight/mild dysplasia), CIN 2 (moderate dysplasia), and CIN 3 (severe dysplasia and CIS)
  - Essentially, CIN 3 category reflected high-grade lesion with strong likelihood of progression to invasive cancer
    - By combining severe dysplasia with CIS, it simplified oftentimes difficult differentiation between these dysplastic cells

Pap Test and Cervical Cancer Screening: History and Reporting Terminology

THE BETHESDA SYSTEM FOR REPORTING

National Cancer Institute Conference (1988)

- Both dysplasia and CIN reporting systems reflected perception of cervical pathobiologic continuum through to invasive cervical cancer
- All of these reporting systems featured ill-defined cytologic interpretive categories, yet discriminated koilocytotic atypia from true precursor dysplastic lesions
- Nevertheless, cervicovaginal smear method (i.e., conventional Pap test) was effective as screening tool despite its technical and reporting limitations
- Recognition of human papillomavirus (HPV) in cervical carcinogenesis stimulated new insights
- There was also need for uniform reporting language linking cytologic interpretations and practitioner follow-up
- National Cancer Institute convened conference in 1988 resulting in The Bethesda System (TBS) for reporting
  o Featured 2 groups of cervical squamous intraepithelial lesions based on biologic behavior of HPV infection and specific subtypes involved
  o Introduced bipartite concept of cervical precursor neoplasia: Low-grade and high-grade squamous intraepithelial lesions (LSIL and HSIL, respectively)
    – 2 distinct biologic entities rather than initially perceived biologic continuum
  o Also intended to improve interobserver and intraobserver variability by reducing diagnostic categories
    – LSIL reflected mild dysplasia and CIN 1; HSIL + moderate dysplasia, severe dysplasia, and CIS, i.e., CIN 2 and 3
  o Introduced means to communicate atypical, inconclusive findings/diagnostic uncertainty
  o 1st reporting system to address phenomenon of cytomorphologic overlap possible between benign cellular changes and dysplastic cellular changes
  o This problem now reported through specific phrasing
    – Atypical squamous cells of undetermined significance (ASC-US) and atypical squamous cells, cannot exclude HSIL (ASC-H)
    – Atypical glandular cells (AGC)
  o Also advocated definitions and diagnostic criteria of reporting categories and recommended follow-up and patient management

The Bethesda System for Reporting Cervicovaginal Cytology (2001 and 2015 Versions, Which Are Nearly Same)

- Specimen adequacy
  o Satisfactory for evaluation (mention presence or absence of endocervical/transformation zone)
  o Unsatisfactory for evaluation (specify reason)
    – Specimen rejected/not processed (specify reason)
    – Specimen processed and examined but unsatisfactory for evaluation of epithelial cell abnormality (specify reason)
- General categorization (optional)
  o Negative for intraepithelial lesion or malignancy (NILM)
  o Epithelial cell abnormality
  o Other
- Interpretation
- NILM
  o Organisms
    – Trichomonas vaginalis
    – Fungal organisms, morphologically consistent with Candida species
    – Shift in flora suggestive of bacterial vaginosis
    – Bacteria morphologically consistent with Actinomyces species
    – Cellular changes consistent with herpes simplex virus
  o Nonneoplastic findings (optional to report)
    – Reactive cellular changes associated with inflammation (including typical repair)
    – Radiation changes, follicular cervicitis, metaplasias, keratotic changes
    – Intrauterine contraceptive device-related changes
    – Atrophy and atrophic vaginitis
    – Glandular cells status post hysterectomy
  o Endometrial cells in females ≥ 45 years
    – Specify if negative for squamous intraepithelial lesion or malignancy
- Epithelial cell abnormalities
  o Squamous cell
    – Atypical squamous cells
      □ Of undetermined significance (ASC-US)
      □ Cannot rule out high-grade squamous intraepithelial lesion (ASC-H)
    – LSIL encompassing HPV/mild dysplasia/CIN 1
    – HSIL encompassing moderate dysplasia, severe dysplasia, carcinoma in situ; CIN 2 and CIN 3
    – Squamous cell carcinoma
  o Glandular cell
    – AGC, (specify if endocervical, endometrial, or not otherwise specified)
      □ AGC, favor neoplastic (specify if endocervical or NOS)
    – Adenocarcinoma in situ (AIS)
    – Adenocarcinoma
      □ Endocervical, endometrial, extrauterine, or not otherwise specified
  o Other malignant neoplasms (specify)
- Automated review and ancillary testing (include as appropriate)
- Educational notes and suggestions (optional)

HPV MOLECULAR TESTING

Evolving Role of HPV Testing in Screening

- ASC-US/LSIL triage study (ALTS) aimed to determine appropriate follow-up recommendations (Nov 1996-2000)
  o Trial revealed that cervical preinvasive precursor lesions may be classified as
    – (A) HPV infection with regressive potential (i.e., LSIL)
    – (B) dysplastic lesion with progressive potential to cancer due to HPV-induced pathobiology (HSIL)
- Reflex testing for high-risk (HR) HPV for ASC-US triage and HPV subtypes (cotesting in females ≥ 30)
  o Lesion delineation, appropriate patient follow-up, and Pap test rescreening frequency established based on combination of Pap and HPV results (risk stratification)

Pap Test and Cervical Cancer Screening: History and Reporting Terminology

- Molecular testing for HPV subtypes in effort to resolve diagnostic uncertainty and appropriately triage patients
- Trials for use of HPV as primary screen completed with move to primary HPV screening initiated; screening intervals and triage modalities vary
- HPV-vaccinated population entering screening age, possibly necessitating alternate screening strategies
  o Screening strategies, intervals, and triage will be different from nonvaccinated population
  o Colposcopy may not remain gold standard in vaccinated
  o Alternate strategies may be needed
- 2014 Cobas platform approved in USA for primary HPV screening using ThinPrep; SurePath approved subsequently
- 2017 primary HPV screening with reflex cytology introduced in parts of Europe, UK, Australia and others
- 2020 American Cancer society endorses primary HPV screening.
  o Current acceptance is low and most prefer co-testing in females over 30 years

HPV Vaccination

- Prophylactic vaccines (bivalent, quadrivalent, and more recently against 9 HR-HPV types) have been available in past decade
- Clinical results are very promising for preventing infection by types 16, 18, 6, and 11, and more
- Some cross protection against related types also noted
- HPV vaccination recommended for girls and boys between ages 9-12 in USA
- Risk-based screening strategy using history, Pap, and HPV results in USA
- Whether colposcopy will remain gold standard remains to be seen once large lesions from types 16 and 18 are eradicated

EVOLUTION OF PAP TEST

Conventional Smear to Liquid-Based Cytology

- Since its inception, conventional vaginal smear Pap test has undergone technical metamorphosis in parallel with expanding application and reporting language evolution

- Exfoliated cells in cervical secretions, or those physically removed from cervical epithelia by collection devices, may be rinsed, suspended, and wet-fixed in preservative reagents
  o Thereafter, may be processed yielding randomized populations of cells placed onto glass slides through dedicated automated systems
- Liquid-based technology also supports computerized image-based detection and categorization of abnormal cells by minimizing obscuration by blood, mucus, and inflammatory cells
  o Potentially improving observer confidence, diagnostic accuracy, and productivity
  o HPV and other molecular testing from residual in vial became feasible

Primary HR-HPV screening

- 1st FDA approved test in USA in 2014
- Parts of Australia and Europe and UK already moved to primary HPV screening with cytology as triage; USA starting to move to primary HPV screen
- Currently more expensive than cytology but prices anticipated to drop
- Self collection and rapid HPV testing trials in low-resource settings underway and initial results appear to be promising

SELECTED REFERENCES

1. Lu KL et al: Cytomorphologic features of pediatric-type follicular lymphoma on fine needle aspiration biopsy: case series and a review of the literature. J Am Soc Cytopathol. ePub, 2022
2. Fontham ETH et al: Cervical cancer screening for individuals at average risk: 2020 guideline update from the American Cancer Society. CA Cancer J Clin. 70(5):321-46, 2020
3. Nayar R et al: Moving forward-the 2019 ASCCP risk-based management consensus guidelines for abnormal cervical cancer screening tests and cancer precursors and beyond: implications and suggestions for laboratories. J Am Soc Cytopathol. 9(4):291-303, 2020
4. Durdu, M: History of Cytology in Durdu M: Cutaneous Cytology and Tzanck Smear Test. 1st ed. Springer, 2019
5. Cazacu IM et al: A quarter century of EUS-FNA: progress, milestones, and future directions. Endosc Ultrasound. 7(3):141-60, 2018
6. Nayar R et al: The Bethesda System for Reporting Cervical Cytology: Definitions, Criteria, and Explanatory Notes. 3rd ed. Springer, 2015

Comparison of Reporting Terminology for Normal and Abnormal Cytology Categories

Reporting nomenclature	Squamous epithelial cell alterations / interpretations					
Papanicolaou classification system	Pap class I: Normal cells	Pap class II: Inflammatory	Pap class III: Suspicious of malignancy	Pap class IV: Strongly suggestive malignancy		Pap class V: Definitely malignant
Dysplasia reporting system	Normal		Mild dysplasia	Moderate dysplasia	Severe dysplasia	Carcinoma in situ	Squamous cell carcinoma
Cervical intraepithelial neoplasia system	Normal		CIN 1	CIN 2	CIN 3	Squamous cell carcinoma
Bethesda reporting system	Negative for intraepithelial lesion or malignancy (NILM)	NILM Non-neoplastic findings, organisms, reactive cellular changes associated with inflammation typical repair	LSIL Low-grade squamous intraepithelial lesion	HSIL High-grade squamous intraepithelial lesion		Squamous cell carcinoma
	← Atypical squamous cells of undetermined significance (ASC-US, ASC-H) →					

(Left) The cervicovaginal cytology reporting changed over a 60-year period, starting with Dr. Papanicolaou's classes. Pap classes I & II correspond to normal in the dysplasia and CIN reporting and finally NILM under The Bethesda System (TBS). Although the first 3 systems are linear, TBS is nonlinear. It introduced atypical squamous cells, which can include changes from benign to the neoplastic spectrum. (Right) Preneoplastic and neoplastic reporting are shown in various shades of increasing severity.

Cytopreparation, Instrumentation, and Automated Screening in Gynecologic Cytology

PAP TEST SCREENING SAMPLE COLLECTION

Patient Instructions to Optimize Specimen
- Schedule testing to avoid menstruation, optimally 2 weeks after start of last menstrual period
- Avoid vaginal medications, douches, and intercourse prior to appointment

Specimen Collection Recommendations
- Use speculum lubricated only with water
- Excess mucus or discharge should be removed prior to sampling
- Obtain sample before application of acetic acid or Lugol iodine
- Sampling should include ectocervix and endocervix

Broom
- Single device with longer central bristles for endocervical canal and shorter outer bristles for ectocervix
- 3-5 rotations are needed

Spatula and Brush
- One 360° turn of spatula and one 90° turn of brush
- Brush should be inserted with some bristles still visible to avoid endometrial sampling
- Plastic spatulas are preferred to wood spatulas due to less cell entrapment

Cotton Swab
- Not recommended due to cell entrapment and poor sampling

Slide Preparation
- Conventional smears must be prepared immediately and fixed with alcohol by spray or immersion
  - Slide quality is highly dependent on collecting practitioner
- Liquid-based tests require additional processing in laboratory to make slide
  - Automation allows for uniform mass processing of specimens

TEST TYPES

Conventional Pap Smears
- Specimens are manually smeared onto glass slide
- Cells are often clumped, making screening more difficult and concentrating abnormal cells in clusters
- Blood, inflammatory cells, and mucus are frequently abundant and may obscure cells
- Fixation is sometimes delayed, causing artifacts
- Traditional inexpensive method
- Requires additional collection vial for human papillomavirus or other testing

Liquid-Based Pap Tests
- Specimens are collected in vial of liquid for automated laboratory processing
- Fixative and processing remove most blood, inflammatory cells, debris, and mucus
- Cells are dispersed randomly on slide, facilitating screening and computer image analysis
- ThinPrep
  - Squamous cells distributed in thin layer requiring few focus changes
  - 20-mm diameter of circle of cells
  - Some specimens with abundant mucus or debris may have "holes" due to clogging of filter during processing
  - Uses PreservCyt Solution (methanol based)
  - Predominant liquid-based method for nongynecologic specimens
  - Sold by Hologic, Inc.
- SurePath
  - Squamous cells in dense layer requiring much up-and-down focusing
  - 13-mm diameter of circle of cells
  - Uses SurePath Preservative Fluid (21.7% ethanol, 1.2% methanol, and 1.1% isopropanol)
  - Not approved or validated for as many molecular tests as ThinPrep
  - Sold by Becton, Dickinson and Co. (BD)

ThinPrep Flow Chart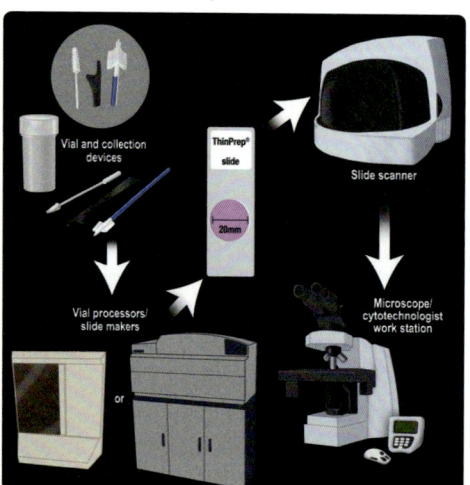

SurePath Flow Chart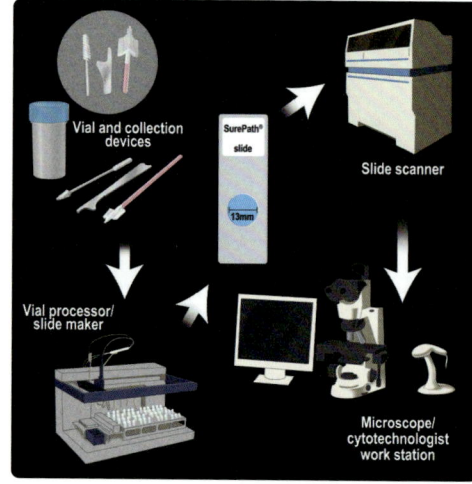

(Left) *A flow chart for ThinPrep specimen processing shows the equipment needed to collect the cervicovaginal specimen, concentrate cells from the vial onto a slide, and perform imager-assisted screening.* **(Right)** *SurePath processing is similar to ThinPrep, but note the smaller area of cells on the slide and the monitor for visual display of imager fields of view. The slide scanner can also accommodate conventional smears.*

Cytopreparation, Instrumentation, and Automated Screening in Gynecologic Cytology

Comparison of Conventional Pap Smears and Liquid-Based Pap Tests

Function	Conventional Pap Smear	ThinPrep	SurePath
Prelaboratory processing	Collection devices smeared onto glass slide and fixed	Collection devices rinsed in methanol-based solution	Collection device heads dropped into ethanol-based solution
Means of breaking up clumps	Smearing action	Vial is agitated by cylinder	Sample is vortexed and passes though small-orifice syringe
Means of cell distribution	Smearing action	Vacuum filtration with automated density monitoring	Centrifugation followed by gravity sedimentation
Automated processing	None	Up to 80 vials at 1 time	Up to 48 vials at 1 time
Size of screening area	Variable, usually most of slide	20-mm circle	13-mm circle
Cells needed for adequacy	8,000-12,000	5,000 (3-4 per 40x field); 2,000 for vaginal and postmenopausal	5,000 (7-9 per 40x field); 2,000 for vaginal and postmenopausal
Automated screening	FocalPoint GS Imaging System	ThinPrep Imaging System	FocalPoint GS Imaging System

ADVANTAGES OF LIQUID-BASED PREPARATIONS

Lower Unsatisfactory Rates
- Simplified sample collection with fewer opportunities for error
- Better processing that removes obscuring elements and distributes squamous cells evenly
- Reprocessing of vial is possible if single slide is unsatisfactory

Facilitates Automated Screening
- Liquid-based technology was originally developed for this purpose

Residual Fluid Available for Ancillary Testing
- Human papillomavirus cotesting or reflex testing
- Gonorrhea, chlamydia, and vaginitis testing
- Cell blocks for morphology or immunocytochemistry

Easier to Screen
- Most cytologists prefer liquid-based Pap tests
- Questionable whether outcomes are improved
  - Small early studies supported increased sensitivity
  - Later metaanalysis failed to show better performance characteristics than those of conventional smears

AUTOMATED SCREENING

Principle
- Pap test slides undergo image analysis that is computerized
- Proprietary algorithms identify most suspicious cells and select associated fields of view

Platforms
- ThinPrep Imaging System
  - 22 fields of view
- BD FocalPoint GS Imaging System
  - 10 fields of view + 1 field for glandular cells
  - Assigns quintile rankings for risk that may aid quality assurance
  - Can be used for SurePath or conventional Pap tests

Cytotechnologist Review
- Fields of view are presented by special robotic microscope
- If no cytologic abnormalities in selected fields of view, no additional screening is needed
  - Each such case counts as 1/2 slide for purpose of calculating workload screening totals (in USA)
  - Reduced screening time per slide increases productivity, especially in low-risk populations
- Abnormalities prompt complete slide rescreening
  - This combined automated and manual screening counts as 1.5 slides for purpose of calculating workload screening totals (in USA)
- U.S. Food and Drug Administration (FDA) sets limit of 100 slides per day for screening based on manufacturer-sponsored studies
  - In these studies, automated screening outperformed manual screening for detection of abnormalities
  - Later trials conducted with lower cytotechnologist productivity expectations show equivalent or lesser performance of automated screening
- American Society of Cytopathology (ASC) has created workload guidelines for automated screening
  - Cytotechnologists should not screen Pap tests for > 7 hours per day
  - Average cytotechnologist screening rate of ≤ 70 slides per day
  - Full manual review rate of 15% of cases or 2x epithelial cell abnormality rate

SELECTED REFERENCES

1. Thrall MJ: Automated screening of Papanicolaou tests: a review of the literature. Diagn Cytopathol. 47(1):20-7, 2019
2. Kitchener HC et al: A study of cellular counting to determine minimum thresholds for adequacy for liquid-based cervical cytology using a survey and counting protocol. Health Technol Assess. 19(22):i-xix, 1-64, 2015
3. Elsheikh TM et al: American Society of Cytopathology workload recommendations for automated Pap test screening: developed by the productivity and quality assurance in the era of automated screening task force. Diagn Cytopathol. 41(2):174-8, 2013
4. Renshaw AA et al: Assessment of manual workload limits in gynecologic cytology: reconciling data from 3 major prospective trials of automated screening devices. Am J Clin Pathol. 139(4):428-33, 2013
5. Whitlock EP et al: Liquid-based cytology and human papillomavirus testing to screen for cervical cancer: a systematic review for the U.S. Preventive Services Task Force. Ann Intern Med. 155(10):687-97, W214-5, 2011
6. Siebers AG et al: Comparison of liquid-based cytology with conventional cytology for detection of cervical cancer precursors: a randomized controlled trial. JAMA. 302(16):1757-64, 2009
7. Arbyn M et al: Liquid compared with conventional cervical cytology: a systematic review and meta-analysis. Obstet Gynecol. 111(1):167-77, 2008

Specimen Adequacy in Cervicovaginal Cytology

ADEQUACY REPORTING CATEGORIES

Satisfactory
- Presence or absence of endocervical/transformation zone component should be mentioned
- Quality indicators, such as partially obscuring inflammation, blood, and foreign material, should be mentioned

Unsatisfactory
- Specimen rejected or not processed
  - Provide reason: Broken slide, no identifiers, empty vial
- Specimen prepared and evaluated but unsatisfactory
  - Provide reason: Scant squamous cellularity; inflammation, blood, or foreign material that obscures > 75% of cells
  - If any epithelial cell abnormalities are noted, then specimen is considered adequate and reported
  - Presence of organisms or endometrial cells can be reported in unsatisfactory specimen

SQUAMOUS CELLULARITY CRITERIA

Conventional Pap Smear
- 8,000-12,000 well-visualized, well-preserved squamous epithelial cells are required
  - This range is an estimate, not precise cell count
    - Endocervical cells and obscured squamous cells should be excluded from this estimate
    - Metaplastic and parabasal cells are considered
- Squamous cellular threshold is lower for postmenopausal and hysterectomized female patients
- Widely available reference images created by Dr. Birdsong can be used for comparison to estimate cellularity

Liquid-Based Preparations (LBP)
- Minimum of 5,000 well-visualized and preserved squamous cells is required for adequate specimen
  - This number is an estimate, and no counting is required
- If specimen is considered to be of borderline cellularity
  - Estimated cellularity can be obtained by counting number of cells per 40x HPF

Low Squamous Cellularity, SurePath

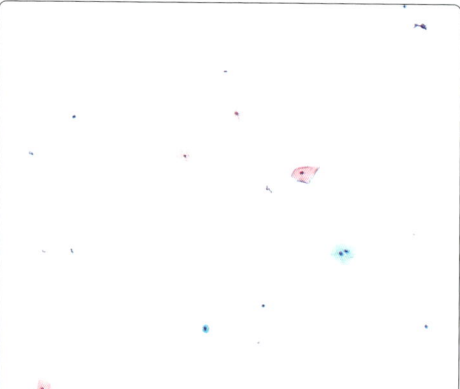

Unsatisfactory, ThinPrep

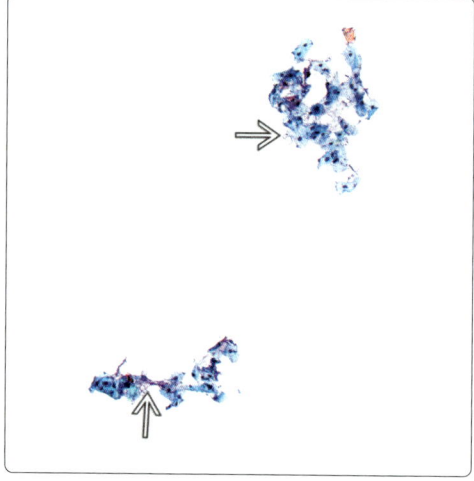

(Left) This representative image from a SurePath Pap test using the 10X objective is an obvious example of unsatisfactory Pap test due to low squamous cellularity. **(Right)** This ThinPrep Pap test seen with the 10X objective is an example of unsatisfactory Pap test due to low squamous cellularity. Lubricant gel ➡ causes clumping of cells and obstructs the pores of the membrane filter resulting in few cells being deposited on the slide. Reprocessing can overcome this problem in some cases.

Squamous Cell Carcinoma on SurePath

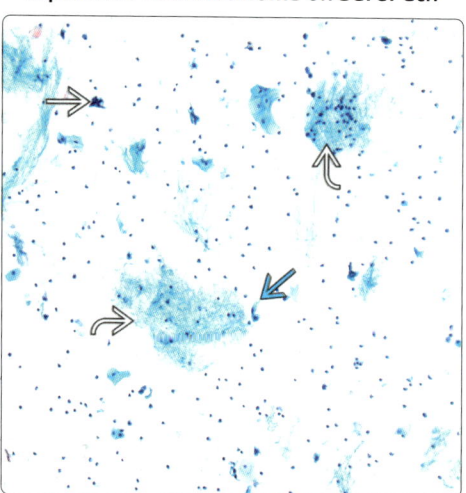

ThinPrep With Atrophy

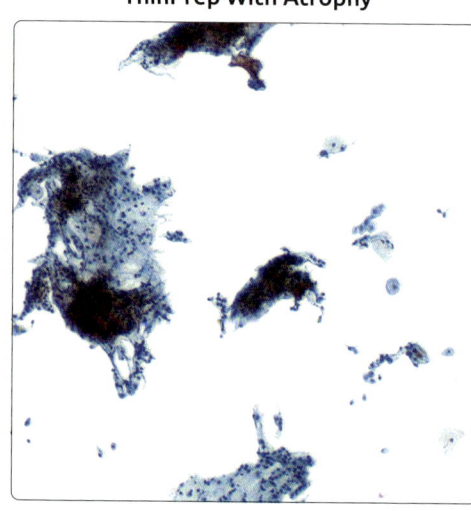

(Left) Cellularity is below the threshold for adequacy in this SurePath Pap. Abundant tumor diathesis ➡ is present; careful examination revealed scattered pleomorphic cells ➡ and tadpole cells ➡ diagnostic for invasive squamous cell carcinoma. **(Right)** ThinPrep Pap shows atrophy. A lower cellularity threshold can be applied to Pap tests from postmenopausal patients, those with total hysterectomy, or female patients treated with radiation or chemotherapy for malignancy. (Courtesy G. Birdsong, MD.)

Specimen Adequacy in Cervicovaginal Cytology

- o Use minimum of 10 fields along diameter to include center of slide
- Average number of cells/40x HPF is estimated
- Holes or acellular areas should be taken into consideration when estimating
- For ThinPrep slides, 3-4 squamous cells/40x HPF in 10 fields across are considered adequate [field number (FN): 20 or 22 eyepiece]
- For SurePath slides, range is 7-9 cells/40x HPF in 10 fields across (FN: 20 or 22 eyepiece)
- Number of cells/unit area is higher for SurePath slides than for ThinPrep slides; this is of no clinical significance
- Specimens with low cellularity can be reprepared after lysing excessive blood or removing obscuring factors
- Adequacy of reprepared slide is judged independently and not cumulatively
- If slide is deemed unsatisfactory, reason should be clearly stated as to whether it was low squamous cellularity or obscuring factors, such as blood, inflammation, or lubricant
- Lower cellularity is acceptable for hysterectomized or postmenopausal specimens with atrophy, posttreatment Paps looking for residual/recurrent malignancy
  - o However, < 2,000 cells is always unsatisfactory
- Female-to-male transgender population tend to have atrophy and low threshold for adequacy may be acceptable
- Even when initial low-power scan shows low cellularity, slide must be examined carefully for rare or scattered dysplastic cells

ENDOCERVICAL/TRANSFORMATION ZONE (EC/TZ) COMPONENT

Cellularity

- Adequate EC/TZ requires 10 well-visualized endocervical or metaplastic cells, either singly or in clusters
- In LBP, endocervical cells are dispersed and hence need careful evaluation
- If high-grade lesion or cancer is present, reporting of EC/TZ is not necessary
- Degenerated cells in mucus or parabasal cells do not count toward EC/TZ component

- It may be difficult to assess EC/TZ in atrophic specimens, and comment can be made to that effect
- Analysis of published data has shown no association between lack of EC/TZ component and missed high-grade squamous intraepithelial lesions
- Human papillomavirus (HPV) testing results are not affected by presence or absence of EC/TZ

Special Pointers in Adequacy Evaluation

- Percentage of obscured squamous cells is evaluated, not percentage of slide covered by obscuring inflammation
- > 75% of obscured squamous cells is unsatisfactory, provided no epithelial cell abnormality
- If 50-75% of cells are obscured, specimen is satisfactory but statement about obscuring factor needs to be made
- Nuclear preservation is key for evaluation, hence cytolysis or cytoplasmic factors can be mentioned as quality indicators in satisfactory specimen

MANAGEMENT

American Society for Colposcopy and Cervical Pathology (ASCCP) Guidelines

- Repeat Pap in 2-4 months is warranted for unsatisfactory
  - o Colposcopy recommended if 2 consecutive unsatisfactory cytologies
- Women ≥ 30 years with high-risk-HPV(+) or HPV-16 or 18 (+) can be referred to colposcopy
- For absent/insufficient EC/TZ with negative Pap, HPV testing is preferred for women ≥ 30 years
- Women 21-29 years with negative cytology and no EC/TZ, continue routine screening
- HPV test (-) on unsatisfactory specimen is not reliable
  - o If HPV test is (+), females require additional follow-up

SELECTED REFERENCES

1. Plummer RM et al: Cervical Papanicolaou tests in the female-to-male transgender population: should the adequacy criteria be revised in this population? An Institutional Experience. J Am Soc Cytopathol. 10(3):255-60, 2021

Unsatisfactory ThinPrep

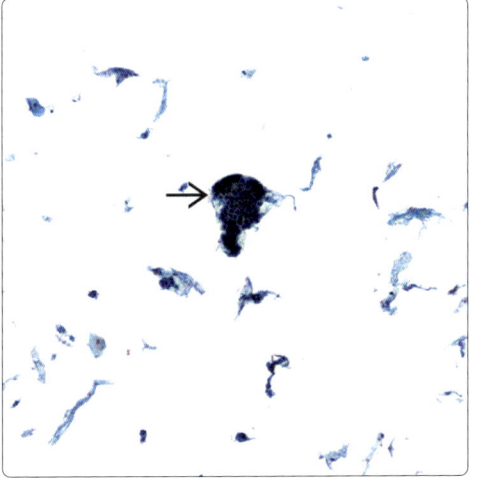

ThinPrep Pap With Borderline Squamous Cellularity

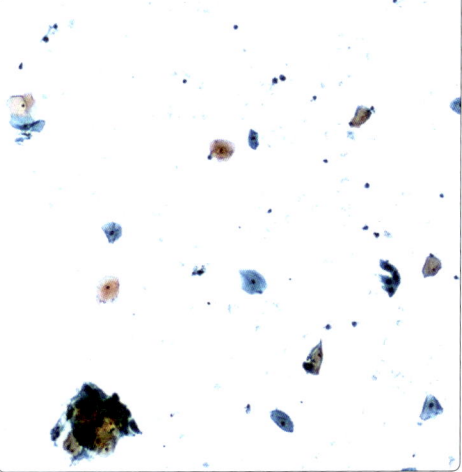

(Left) This example of an unsatisfactory ThinPrep Pap shows a sheet of endocervical cells ⇥ but a lack of squamous cellularity. *(Courtesy G. Birdsong, MD.)* *(Right)* This ThinPrep Pap shows borderline squamous cellularity at 4 squamous cells/40x high-power field, 10 fields across. This corresponds to just over 5,000 squamous cells. On SurePath, 2x the number of cells per field are required for adequacy. *(Courtesy G. Birdsong, MD.)*

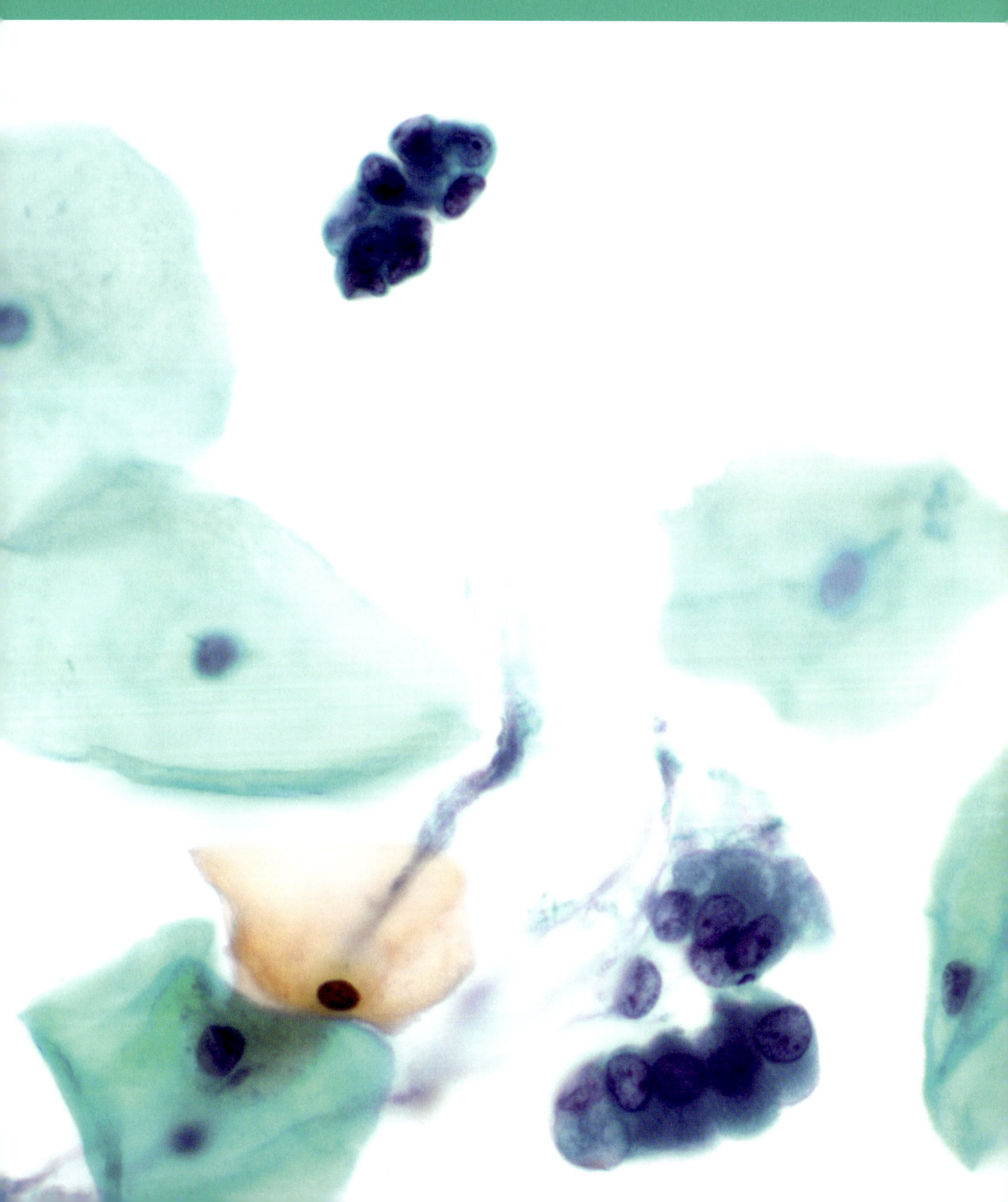

PART I
SECTION 2
Benign and Infectious Conditions

Normal Pap Test	14
Infectious and Other Organisms in Pap Tests	16
Nonneoplastic Findings, Mimics, and Artifacts	18

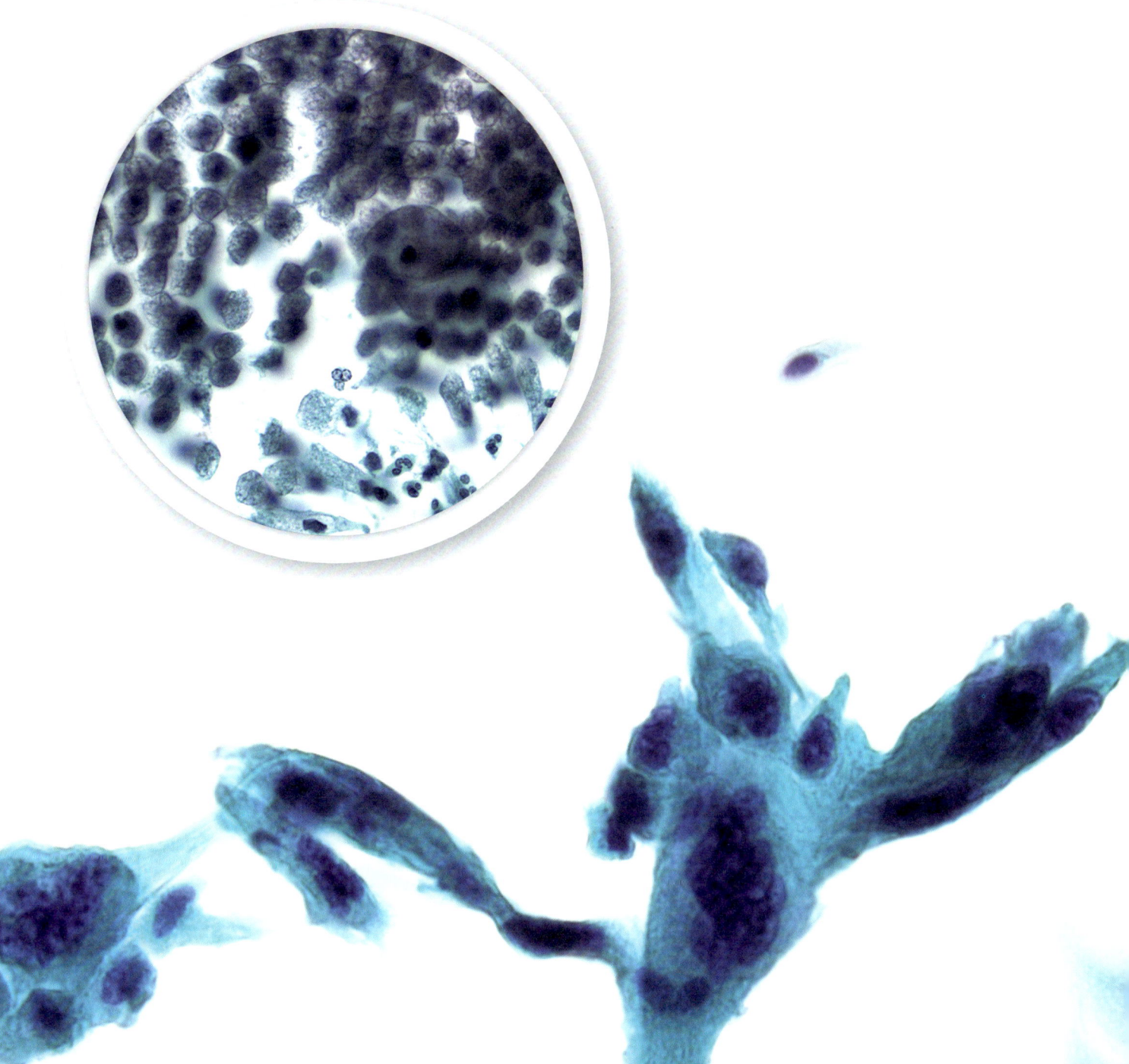

Normal Pap Test

TERMINOLOGY

Abbreviations
- Papanicolaou (Pap) test

BACKGROUND

Cell Types
- Type and maturity of epithelial cells identified in Pap tests depend upon sampling devices used and female's
  - Age
  - Hormonal and menstrual status
  - Extent of ectopy (ectropion)
  - Extent of transformation zone
  - Location of squamocolumnar junctions
  - Epithelial integrity or trauma
- Most cervical squamous carcinomas arise from cervical transformation zone (squamocolumnar junctions)
  - Sampling is confirmed by either endocervical cells or squamous metaplastic cells

PHYSIOLOGY/HISTOLOGY

Cervix
- Lined by 3 epithelial types
  - Mature (native) nonkeratinizing, stratified squamous epithelium
  - Simple columnar mucus-producing epithelium (lining most of endocervical canal)
  - New (de novo) squamous metaplastic epithelium (forming squamocolumnar junctions between glandular columnar cells and native squamous cells within transformation zone areas of cervix)

CYTOPATHOLOGY

Squamous Cells
- Basal squamous cells
  - Small, round squamous cells
  - Infrequently seen; typically in background of inflammation

Normal Epithelial Cell Sizes and Morphology

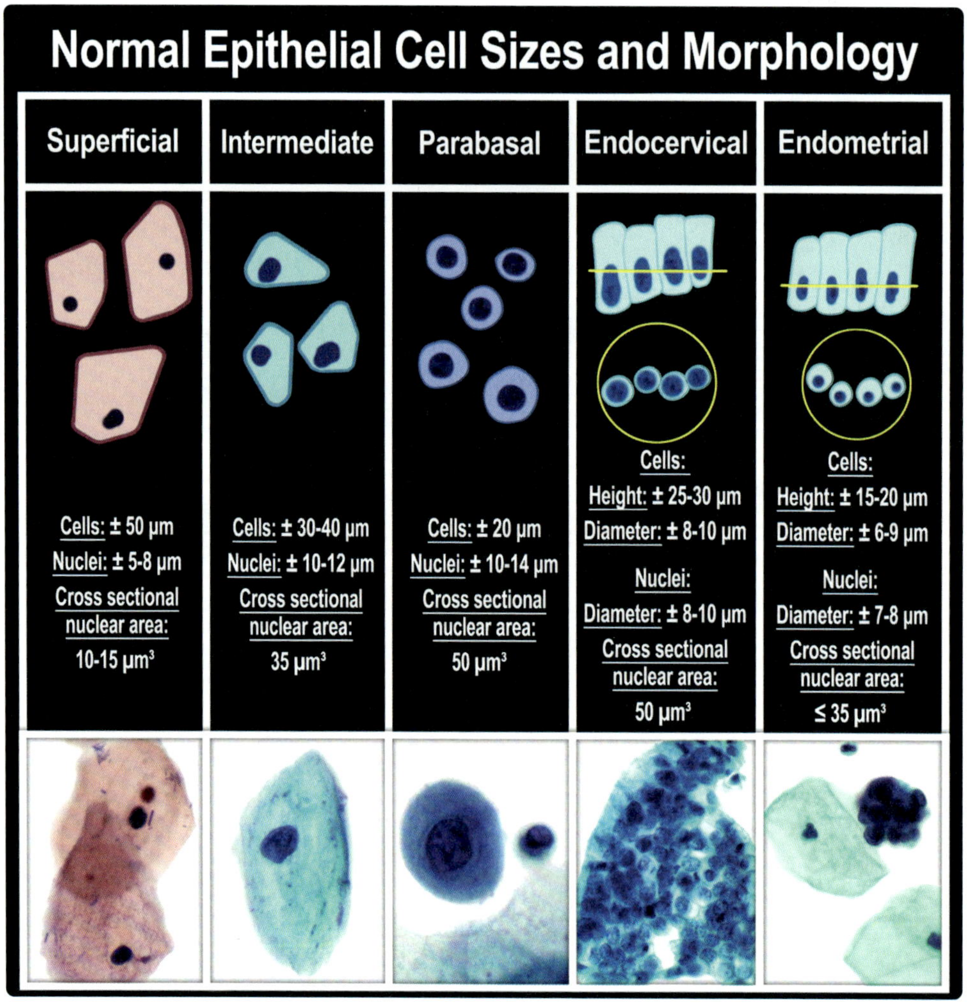

	Superficial	Intermediate	Parabasal	Endocervical	Endometrial
Cells	± 50 µm	± 30-40 µm	± 20 µm	Height: ± 25-30 µm; Diameter: ± 8-10 µm	Height: ± 15-20 µm; Diameter: ± 6-9 µm
Nuclei	± 5-8 µm	± 10-12 µm	± 10-14 µm	Diameter: ± 8-10 µm	Diameter: ± 7-8 µm
Cross sectional nuclear area	10-15 µm³	35 µm³	50 µm³	50 µm³	≤ 35 µm³

Graphic and images depict the various normal cellular components seen on a Pap smear/test. The cell sizes (and dimensions) and how they relate to each other are shown in the drawings. Actual pictures of superficial, intermediate, parabasal, endocervical, and endometrial cells are shown below the drawings. The pictures are not of the same magnification.

Normal Pap Test

- Parabasal squamous cells
  - Round to oval cells
  - Distinct cell borders when seen singly, indistinct cell borders when seen in sheets particularly in atrophic female patients (syncytial morphology)
  - With advanced epithelial atrophy, dryness, and inflammation, parabasal cells may show dense basophilic or orangeophilic cytoplasm with pyknotic nuclei in background of cellular debris, proteinaceous material, and inflammatory cells (atrophic vaginitis)
- Intermediate squamous cells
  - Large, flat, polygonal cells
  - Seen singly or in sheets of variable sizes
  - Under influence of hormones and accumulating glycogen, cytoplasm may appear bulbous with folded edges (navicular cells)
  - In luteal menstrual phase, *Lactobacilli* (normal flora) convert glycogen into lactic acid, lowering vaginal fluid pH and fragmenting intermediate-cell cytoplasm, leading to naked nuclei in background of cytoplasmic debris with bacterial rods (bacterial cytolysis)
- Superficial squamous cells
  - Large, flat, polygonal cells (slightly larger than intermediate cells)
- Hyperkeratotic squamous cells
  - Similar morphology to superficial squamous cells
  - Nuclei absent, forming "ghost" nuclear zones
- Parakeratotic squamous cells
  - Similar size to parabasal cells
  - Pyknotic nuclei

Endocervical Cells

- Endocervical reserve cells
  - Subcolumnar, undifferentiated, bipotential cells
  - Small, fragile cells, frequently spindle-shaped
  - Usually associated with endocervical cells
    - Rarely noted in absence of reserve cell hyperplasia
- Endocervical columnar cells
  - Mucus-producing columnar cells, sharp cell borders
  - Palisading or honeycomb morphology depending on angle of view
  - With secretory activity cytoplasm is abundant due to mucin accumulation compressing nucleus to basal end
  - Occasional cells ciliated with luminal surface terminal bars and pink-red cilia

Squamous Metaplastic Cells

- Immature squamous metaplastic cells
  - Arising from undifferentiated, subcolumnar, reserve cell hyperplasia
  - Cells may be seen isolated (with well-defined cell borders) or in cohesive groups or sheets (with ill-defined cell borders)
  - May have spider-like morphology as desmosomes get detached during sampling
- Mature squamous metaplastic cells
  - Arising from immature squamous metaplasia
  - Cells may be seen isolated or in loosely cohesive groups or sheets (with well-defined cell borders)
  - Frequently noted intracellular junctions
- Florid squamous metaplastic cells (tissue repair)
  - Hyperplasia of mature squamous metaplastic cells with mitotic activity
  - Significance: Attempt to rapidly repair epithelial trauma secondary to surgery, cervicitis, infection, foreign bodies (e.g., IUD), or endocervical polyps

Endometrial Cells

- Endometrial, glandular epithelial cells
  - Exfoliated endometrial cells travel through endocervical canal and emerge at cervical os; frequently seen with marked degeneration
  - May be accompanied by histiocytes (stromal cells) of endometrial origin at end of menstruation (exodus)

SELECTED REFERENCES

1. Williams MPA et al: Cytomorphologic findings of cervical Pap smears from female-to-male transgender patients on testosterone therapy. Cancer Cytopathol. 128(7):491-8, 2020

Normal Cell Types in Pap Tests

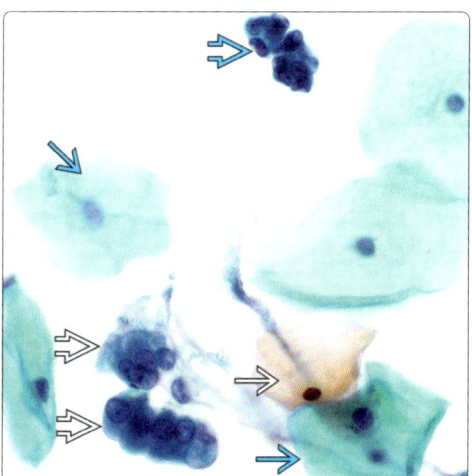

Endocervical Cells, Various Views

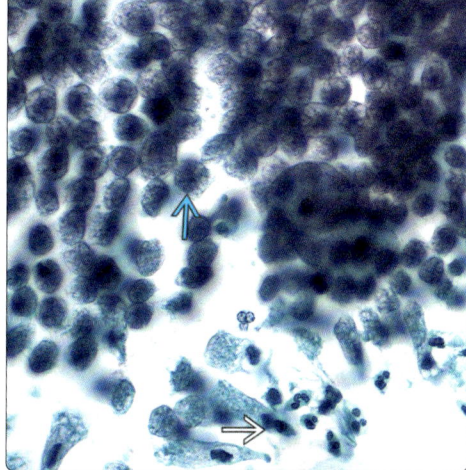

(Left) Superficial ➡, intermediate ➡, endocervical ➡, and endometrial ➡ cells are all seen in this picture for cell size, nuclear size, and nuclear:cytoplasmic ratio comparison. (Right) Endocervical cells viewed sideways show a low nuclear:cytoplasmic ratio with basally placed nuclei ➡. The same cells, when viewed on end, will have a honeycombed appearance to the sheet with mucus caps ➡.

Infectious and Other Organisms in Pap Tests

CLINICAL IMPLICATIONS

Reporting

- Infectious microorganisms in Pap test cytopreparations are reported as nonneoplastic findings
  - Subclassification of "negative for intraepithelial lesion or malignancy" in the Bethesda System for reporting

CYTOPATHOLOGY

Protozoa

- *Trichomonas vaginalis*
  - Primitive, eukaryotic, parasitic protozoan
    - Sexually transmitted disease; may occur in asymptomatic male patients
  - 1/2 of patients may be symptomatic (burning, itching, malodorous vaginal discharge)
  - Organism is pear-shaped (15-30 μm long), frequently staining blue-gray
  - Ill-defined, eccentrically located nucleus
  - Red-staining cytoplasmic granules
    - Infrequently seen flagella
  - Frequently associated with indistinct, small, perinuclear halos in squamous epithelial cells
- Amoeba
  - *Entamoeba histolytica* (from GI tract) and *Entamoeba gingivalis* (from teeth and gums)
  - 15-30 μm in dimension with single nucleus and small central karyosome

Fungi

- Morphologically consistent with *Candida* spp. (candidiasis, moniliasis)
  - Bimorphic fungal organism
  - Patients may be symptomatic (burning, itching, thick, cheesy discharge)
  - Eosinophilic fungal organisms [presenting as single round to oval yeast forms or as elongated yeasts (pseudohyphae)]
  - Yeast forms may be budding and appear connected (bamboo cane appearance)

Trichomonas Vaginalis

Herpes Viral Cytopathic Effect

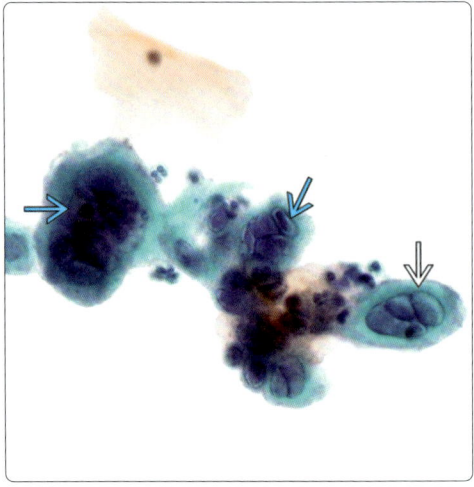

(Left) Liquid-based Pap shows pear-shaped Trichomonas organisms containing a single nucleus ➡, cytoplasmic granules ➡, and a flagellum ➡ that is not easily visualized. (Right) ThinPrep Pap test shows herpes viral cytopathic effect characterized by multinucleation, nuclear molding ➡, and chromatinic clearing. Some cells have distinct eosinophilic intranuclear (Cowdry) inclusions ➡ surrounded by clearing between the inclusion and nuclear membrane.

Cytomegalovirus on Pap Test

Actinomyces

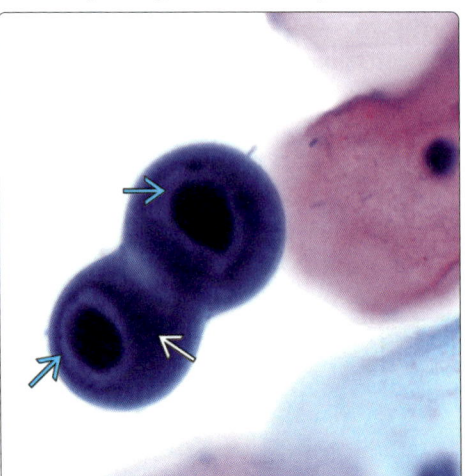
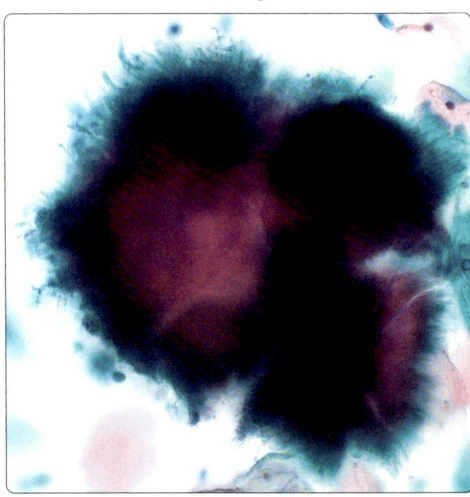

(Left) Surepath Pap shows a very rare example of CMV. The uninucleate cells are enlarged with nuclear and cytoplasmic viral cytopathic effect. The nucleus has a central inclusion surrounded by a halo ➡ The cytoplasm has finely granular cytoplasmic viral effect ➡. (Right) SurePath Pap test shows filamentous bacteria morphologically consistent with the Actinomyces species.

Infectious and Other Organisms in Pap Tests

- Pseudohyphae may appear tangled, evidently piercing squamous epithelial cells (shish-kebab appearance)
- *Torulopsis glabrata* shows small budding yeasts surrounded by clear halo but no pseudohyphae
- Cellular changes in squamous cells include small tight perinuclear halos, hyperkeratosis, and moth-eaten appearance of cytoplasm

Bacteria

- *Lactobacillus* (Döderlein bacilli; normal flora)
  - Rod-shaped bacteria
  - Bacterial enzymes dissolve squamous intermediate cell membranes, releasing glycogen
  - Bacteria convert glycogen to lactic acid, lowering pH; low pH supports *Lactobacilli* growth
  - Enzymatic dissolution of cytoplasm leads to bacterial cytolysis
- Coccobacilli (shift in vaginal flora is suggestive of bacterial vaginosis)
  - Reduction in *Lactobacilli* populations with predominance of coccobacilli (short rods)
  - Associated with bacterial vaginosis (thin, milky, malodorous vaginal discharge)
  - May be due to *Gardnerella vaginalis* or other short coccobacilli, curved bacilli, or mixed bacteria
  - Frequently associated with clue cells (squamous epithelial cells with coccobacilli on them, resulting in dark purple staining and cloudy, filmy appearance)
  - Clue cells are not specific (clinical correlation and microbiologic investigation are required)
- *Leptothrix* (nonpathogenic thread-like bacteria)
  - Much longer than *Lactobacilli*
  - May be associated with trichomonads
  - Not clinically significant (may appear in colonies)
- Filamentous: Bacteria morphologically consistent with *Actinomyces* spp.
  - Gram-positive anaerobic bacteria (normal inhabitants of oral cavity and bowel)
  - Infrequently seen in cervicovaginal samples (but typically related to duration of IUD use in ~ 70% of cases)
  - May rarely cause ascending pelvic actinomycosis
  - Tangled colonies (clumps) of long filamentous bacteria (dark purple-staining, thin, peripheral filaments with Pap stain)

Viruses

- Herpes simplex virus (HSV)
  - Usually HSV type 2 (a.k.a. herpes genitalis; neurodermotropic herpesviruses)
  - Sexually transmitted
  - Causes multiple vesiculopustular or small ulcerative lesions on external genitalia
  - 90% of patients with HSV cervicitis are asymptomatic
  - Cytologically characterized by multinucleation, nuclear molding, and margination of chromatin
- CMV
  - Rare, transient, usually asymptomatic infection in immunocompromised patients
  - Mononuclear cells with nuclear and cytomegaly
  - Basophilic, large intranuclear inclusions surrounded by nuclear clearing with chromatin margination
  - Small granular cytoplasmic particles
- Molluscum Contagiosum
  - Typically affects skin and adnexal structures and is inadvertently picked up by brush at time of Pap
  - Large intracytoplasmic "molluscum body" is characteristic and causes displacement of nucleus

Chlamydia trachomatis

- Obligatory intracellular organisms
- Common sexually transmitted pathogen
  - May cause cervicitis, endometritis
- Nonspecific cytomegaly (interpretations previously included cytoplasmic vacuolization and inflammatory exudates with transformed lymphocytes)
- Microbiologic investigation and specific ancillary staining are required for definitive detection

SELECTED REFERENCES

1. Nayar R et al: The Bethesda System for Reporting Cervical Cytology: Definitions, Criteria, and Explanatory Notes. 3rd ed. Springer, 2015

Candida and Bacterial Vaginosis

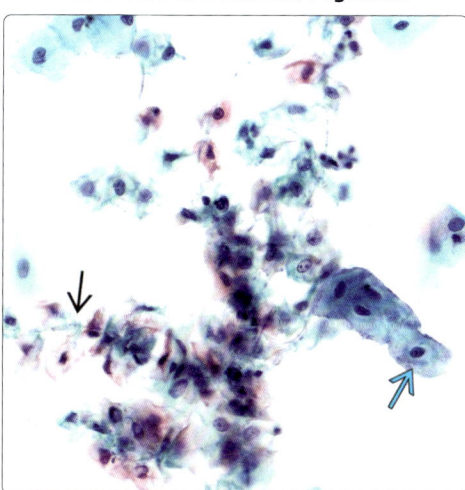

Molluscum Contagiosum

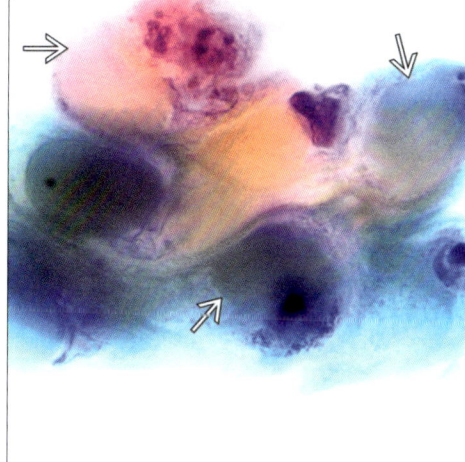

(Left) Liquid-based Pap shows organisms consistent with *Candida* species with spearing of squamous cells ➔ (best appreciated on low magnification). Also note the cells covered by a film of bacteria ➔ consistent with bacterial vaginosis. *(Right)* Liquid-based Pap test shows large intracytoplasmic inclusions ➔. These were inadvertently brushed up from the skin at the time of performing the Pap test.

Nonneoplastic Findings, Mimics, and Artifacts

BENIGN, NONNEOPLASTIC FINDINGS AND MIMICS

Definitions
- Specific alterations in epithelial cell cytomorphology that are benign in nature and associated with inflammation, radiation, and IUD or other nonspecific etiologies

Benign Nonneoplastic Findings
- **Squamous cell inflammatory changes**
    - **Cytoplasmic changes**: Vacuolization (micro- &/or macrovacuolization, indenting nuclei)
    - Leukophagocytosis (engulfed inflammatory cells)
    - Cytolysis (gradual destruction and dissolution of cytoplasm)
    - Perinuclear halo/clearing (perinuclear cytoplasm gets thinner and stains lighter)
    - Alteration in staining reaction (cytoplasmic eosinophilia due to ischemia or degeneration)
    - Condensation (cytoplasm may appear more dense)
    - "Blue blobs" (condensed amorphous cyanophilic bodies) frequently seen in marked atrophy
    - Cytomegaly (with retention of physiologically normal N:C ratios, nuclear symmetry, and nuclear contours)
    - **Nuclear changes**: Enlargement (due to fluid absorption leading to anisonucleosis)
    - Karyomegaly (1.5-2.5x area of reference intermediate-cell nuclei with euchromasia and without nuclear contour irregularities)
    - Chromatinic clearing (leading to open nuclei with visible chromocenters) and hypochromasia
    - Multinucleation, minimal nuclear envelope wrinkling (with more chromatin clumping)
    - Disintegration of nuclear material: Pyknosis (opaqueness), karyorrhexis (nuclear fragmentation)
- **Endocervical cell inflammatory changes**
    - **Cytoplasmic changes**: Cytoplasmic fraying (peripheral disintegration leading to ill-defined cell borders)
    - Total cytoplasmic disintegration (leading to naked nuclei in background of faint mucin)
    - Leukophagocytosis within vacuoles

Moth-Eaten Squamous Cell Cytoplasm

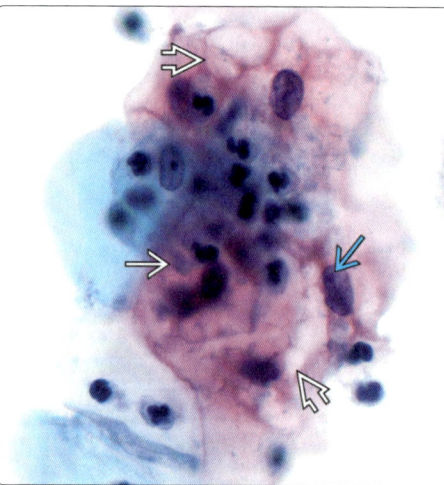

Endocervical Cells With Tubal Metaplasia

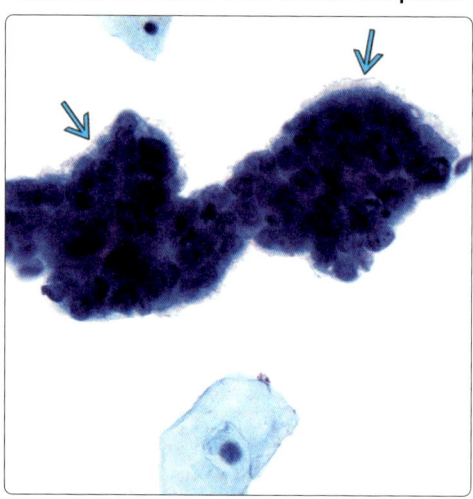

(Left) SurePath Pap test shows squamous cells with a moth-eaten appearance ➡ to the cytoplasm due to inflammation and trichomonads ➡. There is mild nucleomegaly but with hypochromasia. Occasional small nucleoli or chromocenters may be seen ➡. **(Right)** ThinPrep Pap test shows a large group of darkly stained endocervical cells with nuclear crowding and some disorganization. However, note the presence of cilia ➡ on the apical surface, indicating tubal metaplasia.

Repair

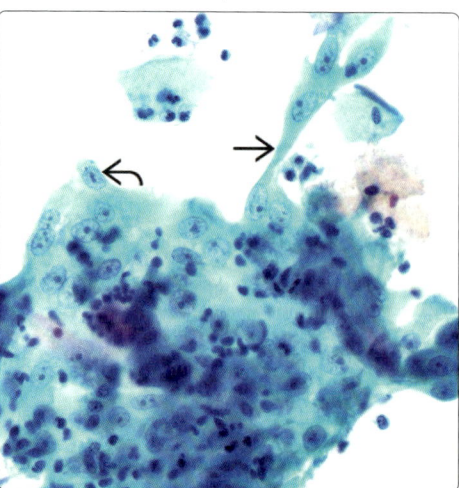

Radiation

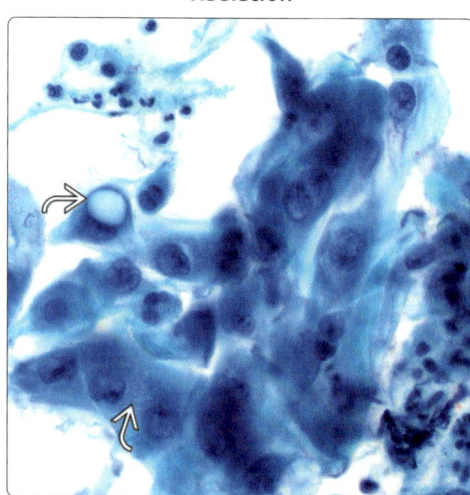

(Left) ThinPrep Pap test shows a flat sheet of cells with classic repair. The cells are drawn out ➡, and there is open nuclear chromatin with hypochromasia and prominent nucleoli ➡. The cells can have inflammatory cells within the cytoplasm as well as overlying them. **(Right)** ThinPrep Pap test shows reactive changes due to radiation in endocervical cells. There is nucleomegaly with corresponding increase in cytoplasm, resulting in normal N:C ratios. Degenerative cytoplasmic vacuoles are another common feature ➡.

Nonneoplastic Findings, Mimics, and Artifacts

- o Ciliocytophthoria (detachment of cilia with terminal bars)
- o Cytomegaly (generalized cellular swelling with retention of physiologically normal N:C ratios and nuclear symmetry)
- o **Nuclear changes**: Karyomegaly (1-2.5x area of reference intermediate-cell nuclei)
- o Marked anisonucleosis (retention of round to oval nuclear shapes)
- o Multinucleation (commonly seen in cervicitis)
- o Minimal nuclear architectural disorganization
- o Chromocenters are more prominent
- o Nucleoli are frequently seen
- o Mitotic figures are frequently seen with regenerative &/or reparative processes
- **Repair**
  - o Changes previously described may be seen in repair
  - o Metaplastic cells may show stretched out processes (spider cells)
  - o Repair tends to occur in flat monolayered sheets with distinct outlines, streaming of cells, and nuclear polarity
  - o In liquid-based (LB) Pap tests, groups tend to round up with less streaming
  - o Prominent nucleoli
- **Radiation changes**
  - o Cytomegaly and karyomegaly with normal N:C ratios
  - o Degenerative changes in nuclei and cytoplasm with smudging and vacuolization
  - o Variation in nuclear size and shape with bi- and multinucleation
  - o Single or multiple nucleoli with coexisting repair
  - o Polychromatic staining of cytoplasm
- **Atrophy and atrophic vaginitis**
  - o Atrophy shows monolayers of parabasal-type cells with increased N:C ratios
  - o Focal nuclear enlargement (up to 3-5x intermediate-cell nucleus) may occur
  - o Cells are normochromatic with evenly distributed chromatin and naked nuclei due to autolysis
  - o Granular inflammatory and basophilic background can result in pseudodiathesis
  - o "Blue blobs" of degenerated parabasal cells &/or inspissated mucus may be seen
  - o Multinucleated giant cells, histiocytes, and parakeratotic cells may be present
- **Parakeratosis**
  - o Miniature, densely orangeophilic, superficial squamous cells seen singly, in sheets, or in whorls
  - o Nuclei are small, dense, and pyknotic in round, oval, or spindle-shaped cells
  - o If nuclear atypia is present, then these are interpreted as atypical parakeratosis and thus fall under atypical squamous cells of undetermined significance (ASC-US)
- **Hyperkeratosis**
  - o Anucleated ghosts of mature squamous cells constitute hyperkeratosis

Tubal Metaplasia/Tuboendometrioid Metaplasia

- Replacement of normal endocervical epithelium by fallopian tube or proliferative endometrium type of epithelium
- Mean age of patients: 39 years
- More often seen post LEEP or conization in younger women
- Epithelium characterized by cuboidal to pseudostratified ciliated cells with terminal bars, intercalated cells, and secretory cells that may show apical vacuoles and snouts
- Focal/patchy p16(+); ProEx C and increased MIB-1 (-) or focally (+); ER/PR/PAX2 and vimentin (+)
- Cytology
  - o Rare groups on Pap test
    - Generally low cellularity
  - o Small sheets and strips with disoriented nuclei with terminal bars and cilia on every cell
  - o Rare strips with nuclear crowding, overlapping, and pseudostratification
  - o Nuclei are round to oval with mild hyperchromasia or washed-out chromatin, unlike those of adenocarcinoma in situ, which are oval to cigar-shaped with coarsely dispersed chromatin
  - o Absent or rare mitosis and absent apoptosis
  - o When viewed en face, nuclei are generally crowded but without nuclear overlap, mitosis, or apoptosis seen in adenocarcinoma in situ
  - o Usually if cilia is not seen en face, isolated ciliated cell with similar nucleus is seen in immediate vicinity
  - o Differential is adenocarcinoma in situ, which is strongly, diffusely p16(+) and MIB-1(+) in > 50% of cells
  - o Tubal metaplasia shows focal or patchy p16(+), and few cells stain with MIB-1

Transitional Cell Metaplasia

- Replacement of normal squamous epithelium of cervix (and rarely vagina) with epithelium resembling transitional/urothelial epithelium
- Occurs in background of atrophy in postmenopausal women
- Epithelium resembles hyperplastic urothelium, is > 10 layers thick, and has disordered streaming appearance
- Lack of "picket fence" vertical orientation of basal layer
- Superficial cells may resemble umbrella cells
- Nuclei are elongated (coffee bean-shaped) and have longitudinal nuclear grooves
- Nuclear size, spacing, and chromatin are uniform without mitosis or apoptosis
- p63(+), p16(-) or patchy, and CK20(-)
- Cytology
  - o Oval, elongated nuclei that can have streaming arrangement
  - o Longitudinal nuclear groove is characteristic
  - o Chromatin is slightly hyperchromatic but evenly distributed without additional nuclear contour irregularities
  - o May be misinterpreted as high-grade squamous intraepithelial lesion (HSIL) or atypical squamous cells, cannot rule out HSIL (ASC-H)
  - o High-risk human papillomavirus (HPV) is negative

Microglandular Hyperplasia

- Benign reactive process of endocervical epithelium secondary to hormonal/progesterone exposure from pregnancy, birth control pills, hormone replacement therapy, or Depo-Provera
- Mostly affects young women; rarely seen post menopause

Nonneoplastic Findings, Mimics, and Artifacts

- Histologically characterized by back-to-back proliferation of endocervical glands with subnuclear &/or supranuclear vacuoles
- Cells are cuboidal to low columnar with rare hobnailing
- Gland lumina contain inflammatory cells or necrosis
- No mitosis or apoptosis; p16(-) or focally (+); HPV(-)
- Cytology
  - Most microglandular hyperplasias resemble repair with inflammation
  - Small parakeratotic cells from center of gland lumina may be seen
  - Rarely resembles atypical repair
  - Polyploidy may result in rare, larger, convoluted nuclei with smudged chromatin pattern
  - LB Pap may show tight clusters/acini with bland nuclei or repair-like changes
  - If nuclear atypia present, may be misinterpreted as atypical endocervical or glandular cells
  - Small parakeratotic cells may be overcalled as keratinizing dysplasia

Follicular Cervicitis

- Benign reactive condition of cervix and vagina characterized by lymphoid follicles under surface epithelium
- Flat cervical mucosa with no characteristic findings
  - Rarely, small bumps on colposcopy
- Cytology
  - Lymphoid aggregates or pools of lymphocytes of varying sizes and shapes
  - Tingible body macrophages are easier to see on conventional Pap smear
  - Can be difficult to see on LB Pap, but small and varying size of cells helps differentiate from HSIL
  - May be mistaken for endometrial cells but have smaller size and different chromatin
  - Differential diagnosis is lymphoma, which is extremely rare in cervicovaginal cytology and has monotonous lymphoid population

Deciduosis

- Decidual transformation of endocervical and endometrial stroma under influence of progesterone from pregnancy
- Typically occurs in 2nd and 3rd trimesters with physiologic regression following delivery
- Histologically characterized by enlarged stromal cells with abundant amphophilic, sometimes vacuolated, cytoplasm
- Overlying squamous epithelium is inflamed and reactive
- Cytology
  - Large polygonal cells, singly or in clusters on conventional smears
  - Abundant eosinophilic or basophilic cytoplasm on conventional smears
  - Large vesicular nuclei with nucleoli but hyperchromatic and smudged if degenerated
  - Cells are better preserved on LB Pap and present singly or in clusters
  - Nuclei can be 3-5x size of intermediate-cell nucleus
  - Nuclear contours can be round and regular or irregular
  - Chromatin can be hyperchromatic or smudged
  - N:C ratios can be low or high, and perinuclear halos may be seen
  - Some large nuclei with nucleoli as well as signet-ring changes may be seen
  - Cytoplasm is abundant and granular and may show vacuolization
  - Isolated cells or groups of cells may be misinterpreted as ASC-US, low-grade squamous intraepithelial lesion (LSIL), ASC-H, or atypical glandular cells
  - Halos surrounding nuclei are usually small and not optically clear like in LSIL
  - Cells are high-risk HPV(-), p16(-), and with low MIB-1 (rare cells)
  - Differential on Pap: Squamous intraepithelial lesion or atypical glandular cells

IUD-Related Changes

- IUDs can cause chronic irritation and inflammation of endocervical canal and endometrium
- Cytology
  - *Actinomyces* colonies and reparative changes can be seen
  - 3D cell balls of high endocervical cells due to irritation and shedding
  - Endocervical cells with large cytoplasmic vacuoles ("bubble gum" vacuoles)
  - Glandular endocervical cells with prominent nucleoli
  - Isolated cells (probably endometrial) resembling HSIL cells with very high N:C ratio but with dark and degenerated chromatin
  - Differential diagnosis: HSIL, atypical glandular cells

Endocervical Glandular Hyperplasia, Diffuse and Lobular

- Benign condition of endocervix with no appreciable mass
- Diffuse laminar endocervical gland hyperplasia (DEGH) involves inner 1/3 of cervical wall with sharply demarcated border
  - Proliferation of benign round to branching endocervical glands with inflammation in deepest part
- Lobular endocervical gland hyperplasia (LEGH) typically involves inner 1/2 of cervical wall
  - Large gland surrounded by small to medium-sized glands
  - LEGH with atypia has papillary projections, budding, or exfoliations
  - May be precursor to gastric-type adenocarcinoma
- Cytology
  - Tall columnar mucinous epithelium with mild nuclear enlargement with nucleoli
  - Cytoplasm may be granular and eosinophilic and may show yellow tinge (gastric foveolar mucin)
  - Can be abundant in sheets to strips but without significant cellular overlap or atypia or mitosis
  - LEGH with atypia will show nuclear enlargement with hyperchromasia with distinct nucleoli
  - Loss of nuclear polarity with apoptosis and mitosis may be seen
  - Main differential is well-differentiated gastric-type adenocarcinoma (a.k.a. minimal deviation adenocarcinoma or adenoma malignum)
    - Both are HPV(-) and HIK1083(+)

Nonneoplastic Findings, Mimics, and Artifacts

Arias-Stella Reaction
- Cytoplasmic and nuclear changes of glandular epithelium associated with pregnancy due to increased gonadotrophin secretion
- Also reported in women with infertility and exogenous hormonal therapy
- More common in endometrium but can involve endocervical glands
- Cytology
  o Enlarged cells with normal N:C ratios
  o Abundant vacuolated or eosinophilic cytoplasm
  o Nuclei are enlarged with irregular nuclear contours
  o Chromatin can range from densely hyperchromatic to vesicular and open with nucleoli
  o Intranuclear cytoplasmic inclusions can often be seen
  o Differential diagnosis: Adenocarcinoma

Rectovaginal Fistula
- Can occur due to rectal carcinoma extending into vagina, Crohn disease, diverticulitis, or surgical mishap
- Cytology
  o Fistulas due to malignancy will have malignant cells and fecal material
  o Benign fistulas will show colonic mucosa with goblet cells on cytology along with feces
  o Goblet cells are also seen in endocervical adenocarcinoma but are cytologically malignant

Pemphigus
- Blistering autoimmune disorder involving skin and squamous mucosal surfaces
- Cytology
  o Cytologic findings are those of repair but with very prominent rectangular nucleoli
  o Reparative changes show very dramatic cytoplasmic processes and spider cells
    – Do not simulate dysplasia or malignancy
  o Clinical correlation is required for diagnosis

Multinucleated Giant Cells/Histiocytes
- Commonly seen in postmenopausal women, post radiation, and post hysterectomy
- Syncytiotrophoblasts in pregnant women may be harbingers of pregnancy loss if many and associated with bleeding
  o Larger cells with many more nuclei than histiocytes

Histiocytes
- Loose clusters of small stromal histiocytes with oval or bean-shaped nuclei with grooves and fine vacuolated cytoplasm
- Nonspecific finding, seen with exodus and other conditions
- May be mistaken for HSIL

Contaminant Fungal Organisms
- *Alternaria*
  o Plant fungus and contaminant on Pap
  o Rarely causes infection in immunocompromised patients
  o Cytology
    – Snowshoe-shaped brown fungus with horizontal and vertical septations
    – 7-10 µm x 24-34 µm in dimensions
- *Geotrichum*
  o Widespread fungus found in food, dairy, soil, water
  o No clinical significance, hence not reported
  o Cytology
    – Hyphae with true septa, 4-6 µm in width
    – Lacks spores or yeast forms

Glycogenation
- Normal component of cells, *Lactobacilli* metabolism of glycogen helps maintain acid pH of vagina
- Can be abundant in pregnancy or due to medroxyprogesterone
- Cytology
  o Navicular cells due to glycogenation may be mistaken for koilocytes, which have optically clear clearing of cytoplasm unlike yellow coloration seen in glycogenation
  o Unlike koilocytes, navicular cells do not show nuclear enlargement and hyperchromasia

ARTIFACTS

Cornflaking
- Common artifact that occurs when mounting medium starts to evaporate prior to coverslipping
- Cytology
  o Brown artifact overlying cells due to air bubbles trapped between cells and coverslip
  o Slightly above plane of focus of cells

Cockleburs
- Artifacts of no clinical significance
- Very rare and seen in pregnancy
- Cytology
  o Yellow crystalline material in spoke-like configuration surrounded by inflammatory cells and histiocytes
  o Contain glycoproteins and calcium

Pollen
- May be mistaken for keratinizing dysplasia or HSIL
- Variations in size, shape, and presence of cell wall are clue to correct interpretation

Fibers and Threads
- From clothing, pads, and tampons
  o May be picked up on Pap
- Easily recognizable as foreign but (rarely) may be mistaken for *Candida* or other fungal organisms

Starch Granules
- Refractile, hexagonal, or pentagonal; best seen with dropped condenser

Lubricant Jelly
- Various types are available, some of which are insoluble and clog pores of membrane filters (ThinPrep) and result in unsatisfactory Pap tests

SELECTED REFERENCES

1. Smith SM et al: Cervical pemphigus vulgaris presenting as postmenopausal bleeding. Int J Gynecol Pathol. 40(5):477-81, 2021
2. Torous VF et al: Interpretation pitfalls and malignant mimics in cervical cytology. J Am Soc Cytopathol. 10(2):115-27, 2021

Nonneoplastic Findings, Mimics, and Artifacts

Pseudodiathesis of Atrophic Vaginitis

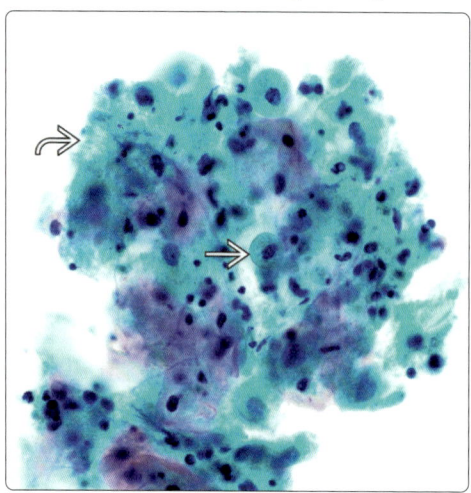

"Blue Blobs" of Atrophy

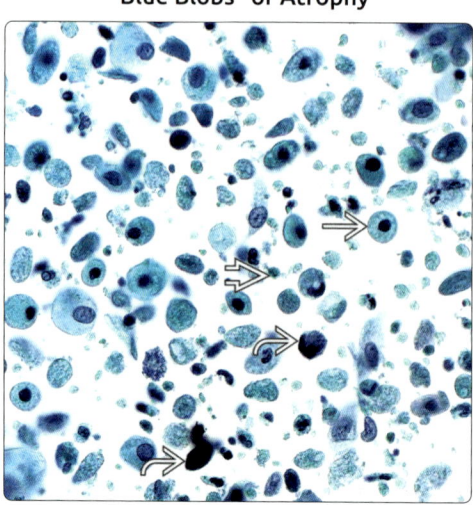

(Left) ThinPrep Pap test shows atrophic vaginitis (AV) with pseudodiathesis ⇨. Unlike conventional smears, the background precipitate seen in AV is cleared in liquid-based preparations, resulting in puddles of pseudodiathesis in which the atrophic parabasal cells ⇨ and debris are found. **(Right)** SurePath Pap test shows "blue blobs" ⇨, which are epithelial cell alterations in AV. Parabasal cells ⇨ with debris ⇨ are seen.

IUD Cells

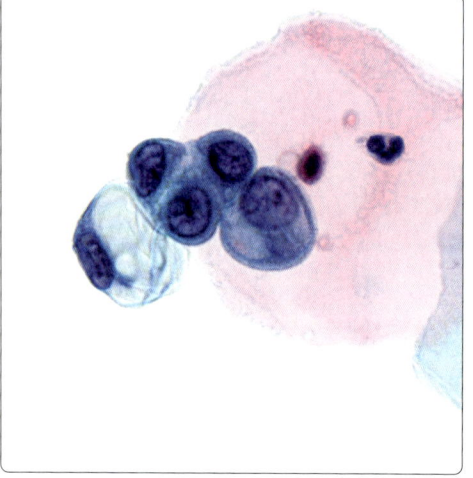

Decidual Cells

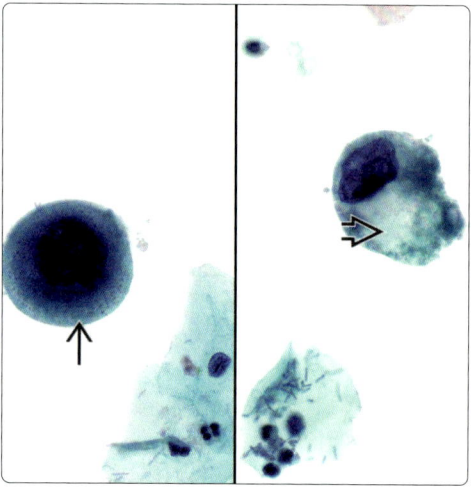

(Left) Cluster of endocervical cells with large cytoplasmic vacuoles is shown; typical appearance of IUD cells. **(Right)** ThinPrep Pap test shows 2 decidual cells with cytoplasm that varies from scant ⇨ to abundant and vacuolated ⇨. The nuclei appear degenerated or smudged without chromatinic details.

Strip of Distorted Endocervical Cells Post LEEP

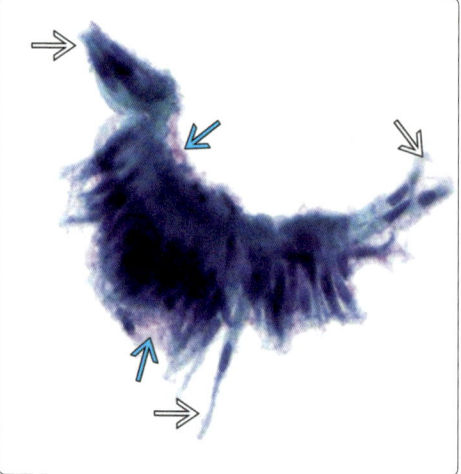

Tubal Metaplasia

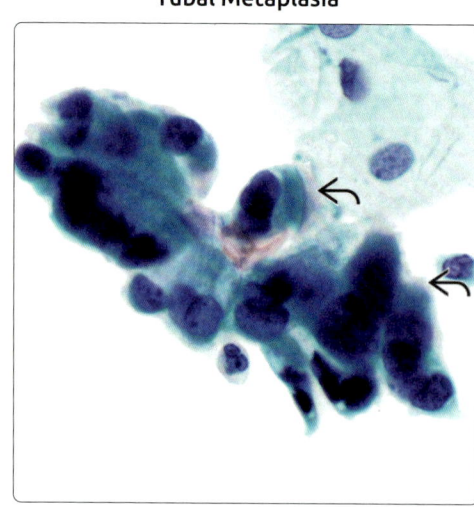

(Left) ThinPrep Pap test performed for endocervical evaluation post LEEP shows endocervical cells with distortion due to cautery. Although worrisome at 1st glance, the cells have low N:C ratios, are stretched/pulled out ⇨, and are lined up like a picket fence. Note the partially autolyzed fresh blood ⇨ from the procedure, which may be mistaken for diathesis. **(Right)** ThinPrep Pap test shows a strip of cells with terminal bars and cilia ⇨ on every cell from a case of tubal metaplasia.

Nonneoplastic Findings, Mimics, and Artifacts

Microglandular Hyperplasia, Polyploidy

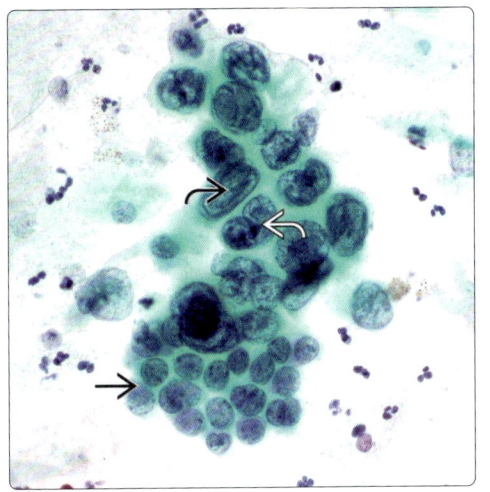

Microglandular Hyperplasia Histology

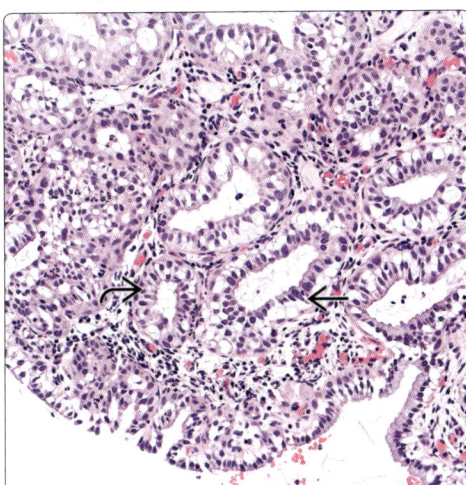

(Left) Pap stain shows normal ⇨ and large endocervical cells with nuclear grooves ⇨, irregularity, and multilobation ⇨ from a case of microglandular hyperplasia (MGH). (Right) H&E stain of polypoid MGH shows back-to-back benign endocervical glands ⇨ with subnuclear vacuoles ⇨ and inflammation.

Transitional Metaplasia

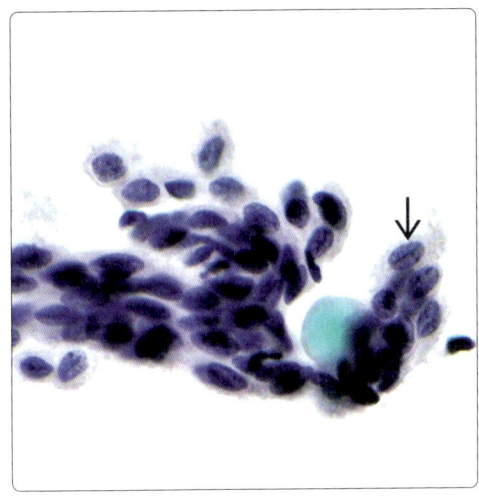

Transitional Metaplasia Histology

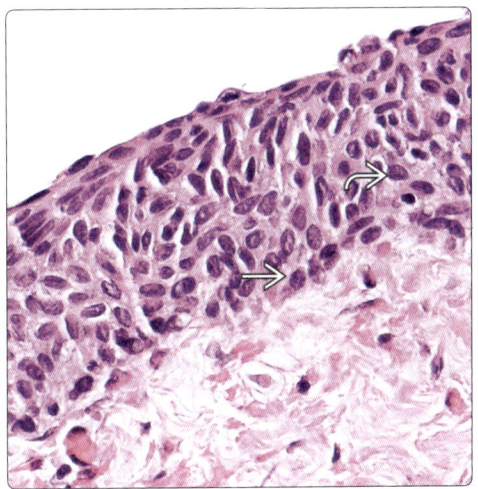

(Left) Transitional cell metaplasia may be mistaken for dysplasia on cytology specimens. Fine, even chromatin and the presence of longitudinal nuclear grooves ⇨ are diagnostic features. (Courtesy B. Howitt, MD.) (Right) H&E-stained section of transitional cell metaplasia in a postmenopausal woman shows that the basal layer ⇨ lacks the "picket fence" arrangement of nuclei, which are instead seen in a disorganized pattern. Longitudinal nuclear grooves are seen in most nuclei ⇨.

Follicular Cervicitis in Liquid-Based Pap

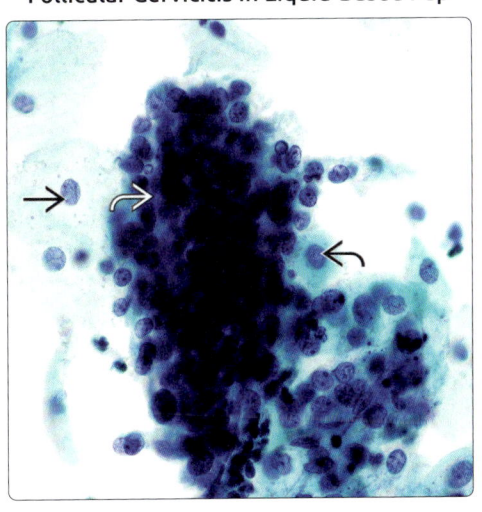

Follicular Cervicitis Histology

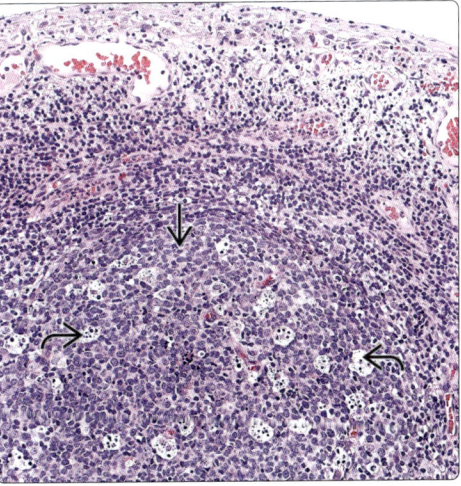

(Left) ThinPrep Pap test shows an aggregate of lymphocytes ⇨ associated with follicular cervicitis. The small size of the cells can be compared with adjacent intermediate-cell ⇨ and parabasal cell ⇨ nuclei. There is variation in nuclear size, and tingible body macrophages are difficult to see on liquid-based preparations. (Right) H&E-stained section of follicular cervicitis shows a large, reactive germinal center ⇨ with tingible body macrophages ⇨, which are easier to see on conventional smears.

Nonneoplastic Findings, Mimics, and Artifacts

Lobular Endocervical Gland Hyperplasia

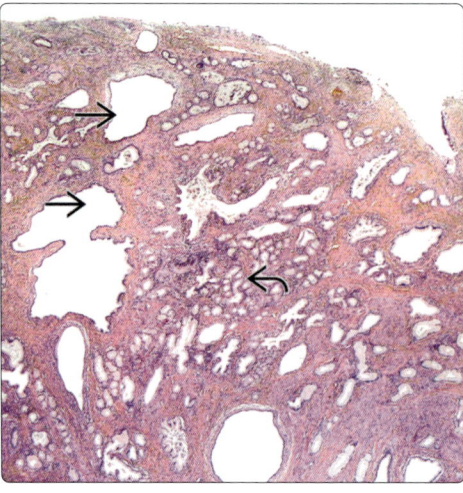

Yellow Gastric-Type Mucin in Lobular Endocervical Gland Hyperplasia

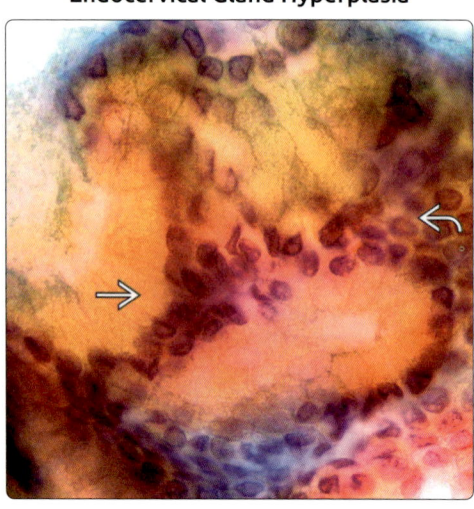

(Left) H&E stain of cervix shows lobular endocervical gland hyperplasia (LEGH) characterized by proliferation of small endocervical glands ⇨ centered around larger glands ⇨. *(Right)* Conventional Pap test of LEGH shows endocervical glands with abundant gastric-type mucin with a slightly yellow tinge ⇨. The nuclei are bland but crowded ⇨ in this histologically confirmed LEGH, originally interpreted as atypical endocervical cells. (Courtesy Y. Sugiyama, MD.)

ThinPrep of Lobular Endocervical Gland Hyperplasia

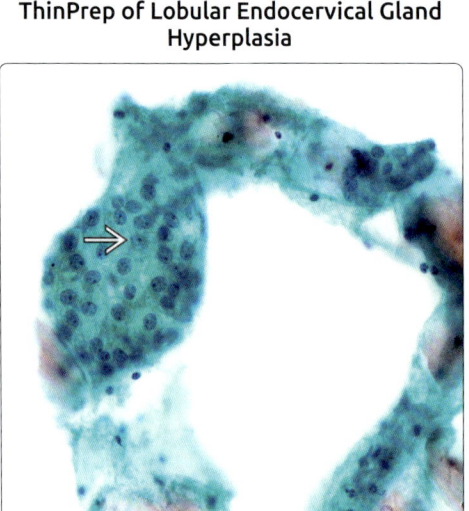

Histiocytes, May Be Mistaken for High-Grade Squamous Intraepithelial Lesion

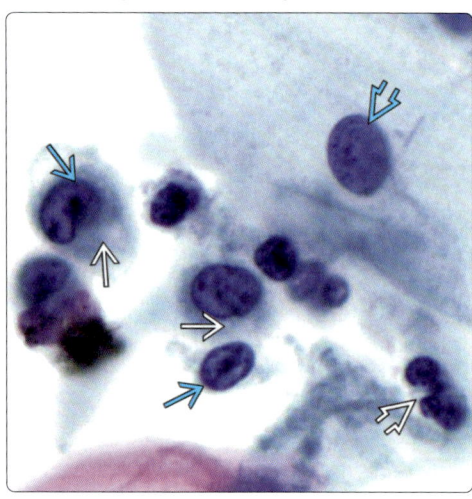

(Left) ThinPrep Pap test shows a 3D cell ball of bland, mucin-producing cells with low N:C ratios, vesicular chromatin, and small regular nucleoli ⇨. (Courtesy Y. Sugiyama, MD.) *(Right)* ThinPrep Pap test shows a collection of histiocytes ⇨ with nuclear folds and flimsy vacuolated cytoplasm ⇨. These are small cells when compared to the size of a nearby intermediate-cell nucleus ⇨ or polymorphonuclear leukocyte ⇨.

Diathermy Artifact

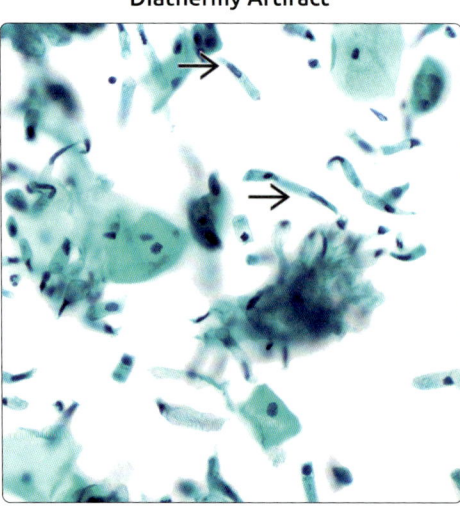

Arias-Stella Cells

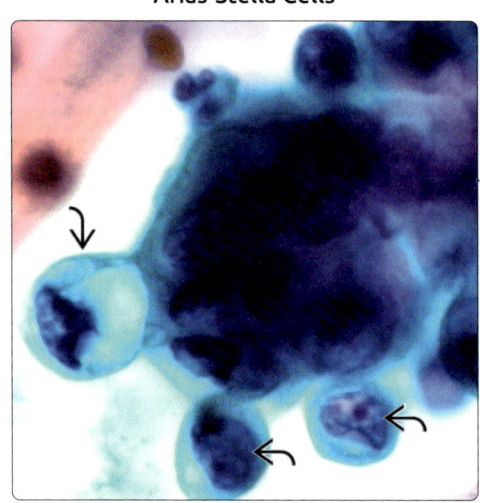

(Left) ThinPrep Pap test shows pencil-thin endocervical cells ⇨, which are artifacts seen due to application of Lugol iodine on the cervix or from diathermy effect post LEEP. *(Right)* ThinPrep Pap test shows very atypical glandular cells ⇨ from a pregnant patient. These cells disappeared 6 months post partum and were felt to represent Arias-Stella reaction. All subsequent Pap tests were normal.

Nonneoplastic Findings, Mimics, and Artifacts

Alternaria
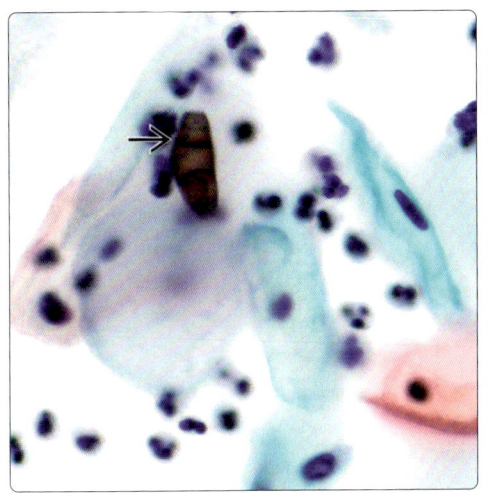

Cocklebur
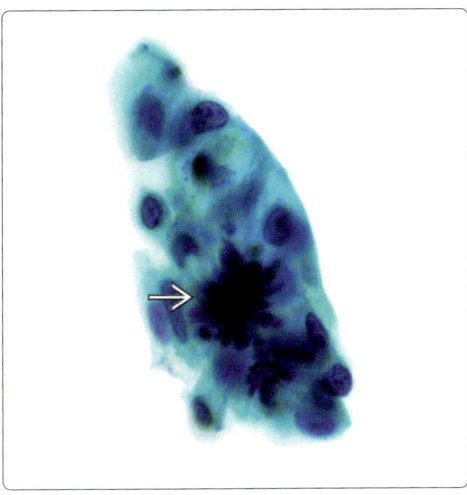

(Left) SurePath Pap test shows a multiseptate brown organism ➡, the characteristic morphology of Alternaria. (Right) ThinPrep Pap test from a pregnant patient shows a cocklebur ➡ characterized by a "spoke-wheeled" crystalline array.

Pollen
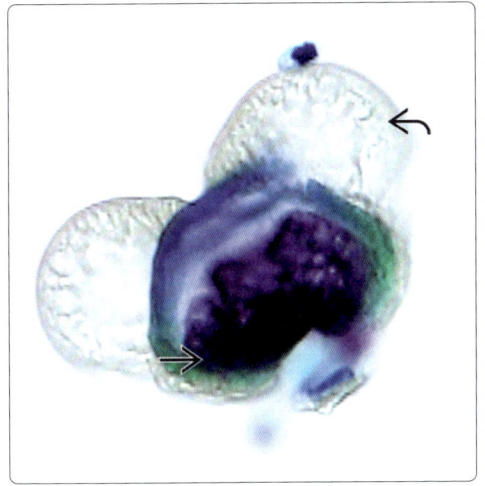

Giant Cell in Postmenopausal Pap Test
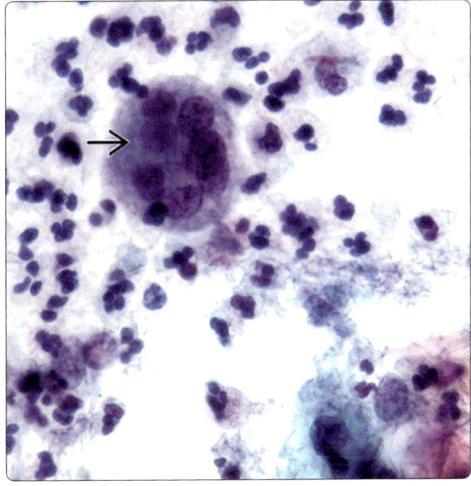

(Left) ThinPrep Pap test shows pollen ➡, which could be mistaken for high-grade squamous intraepithelial lesion (HSIL) or atypical squamous cells, cannot rule out HSIL. The additional structures ➡ in the background indicate the true nature of this object. (Right) ThinPrep Pap test from a postmenopausal woman shows a multinucleated histiocytic giant cell ➡ in an inflammatory background.

Cornflaking
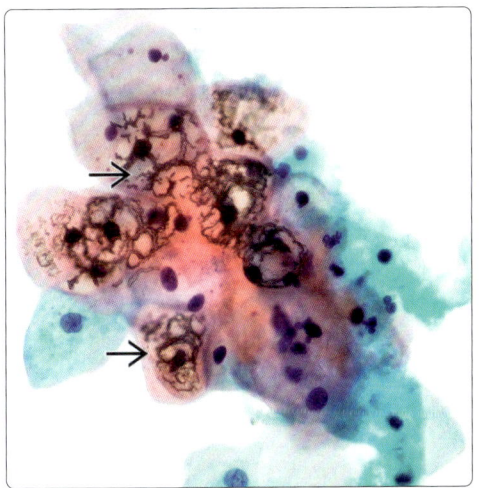

Lubricant Gel
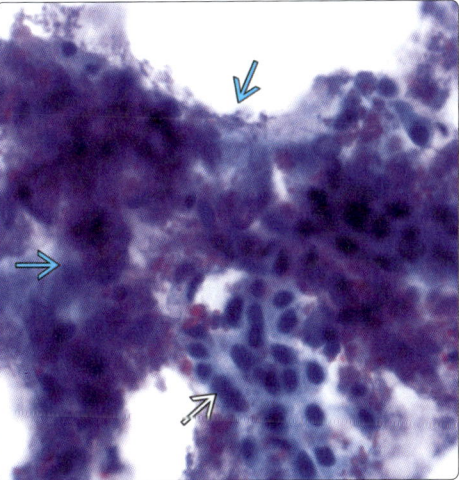

(Left) ThinPrep Pap test shows cornflaking ➡ artifact. This change results from lack of mounting material over the cells in question and has no significance. If excessive, recoverslipping the slide may be helpful to reduce the artifact and improve cell visualization. (Right) ThinPrep Pap test with obscuring purple/pink lubricant gel ➡ is shown. Certain insoluble gels cannot be used with membrane filters as they clog the filter pores and result in obscuring of cellular details. Note the atrophic cells caught up in the gel ➡.

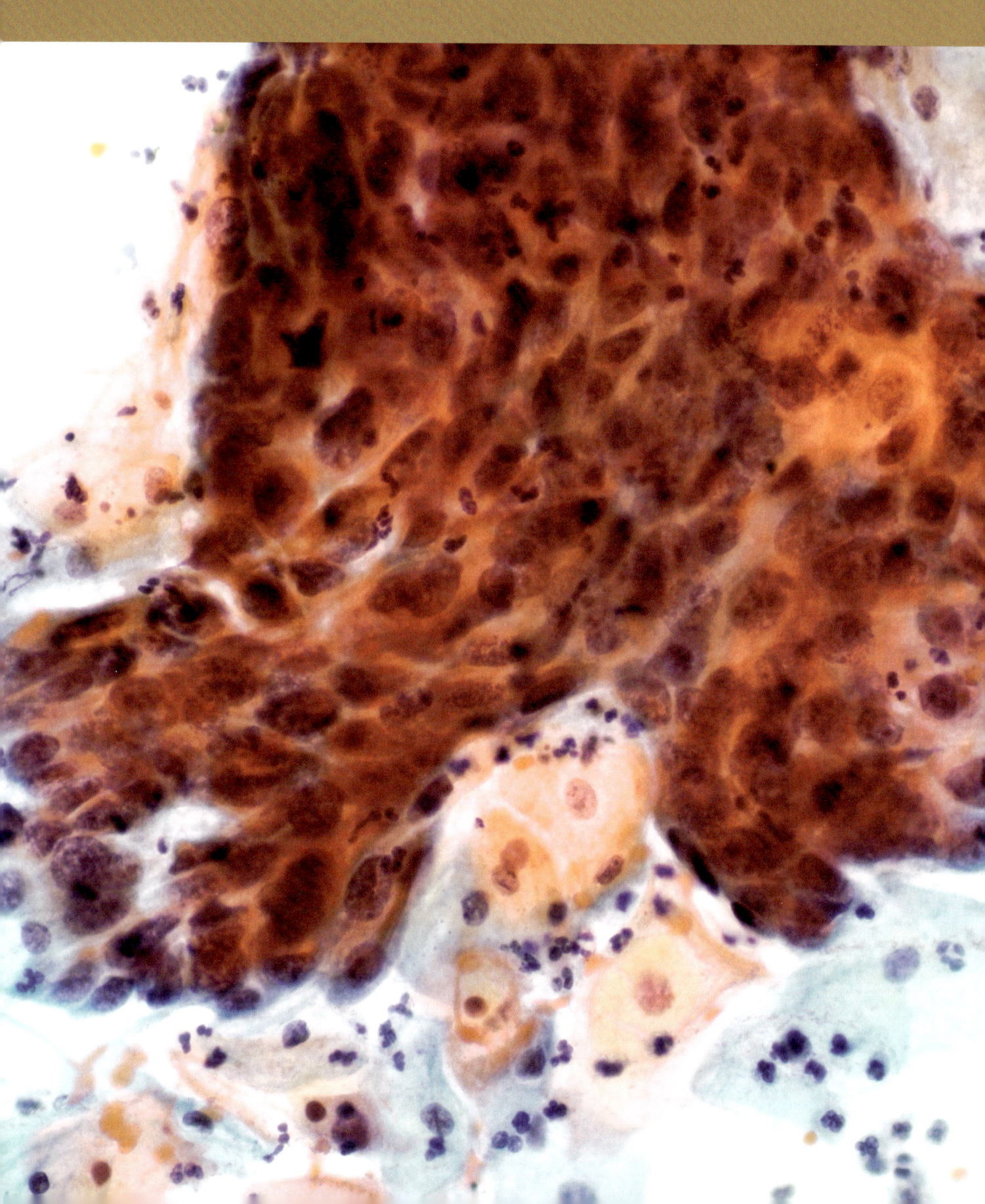

PART I
SECTION 3
Squamous Cell Abnormalities and Mimics

Low-Grade Squamous Intraepithelial Lesion and Mimics	28
High-Grade Squamous Intraepithelial Lesion and Mimics	30
Atypical Squamous Cells of Undetermined Significance	34
Atypical Squamous Cells, Cannot Rule Out High-Grade Squamous Intraepithelial Lesion	36
Squamous Cell Carcinoma of Cervix, Variants and Mimics	38

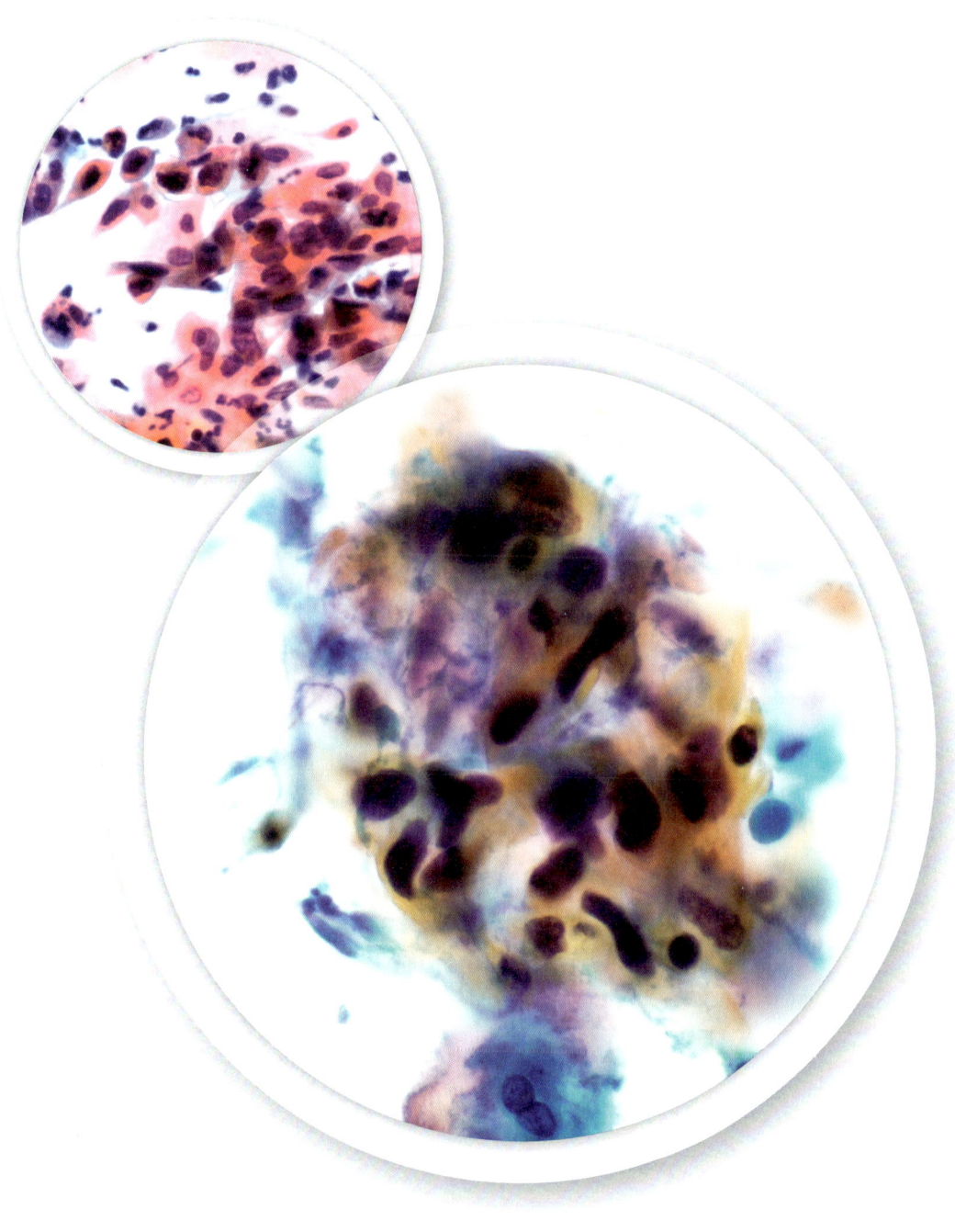

Low-Grade Squamous Intraepithelial Lesion and Mimics

KEY FACTS

TERMINOLOGY
- Squamous cell changes associated with HPV infection
- Includes koilocytosis, mild dysplasia/cervical intraepithelial neoplasia grade 1 (CIN 1)
- Terminology for cytology and histology unified after lower anogenital squamous terminology conference in 2012

ETIOLOGY/PATHOGENESIS
- Most low-grade squamous intraepithelial lesions (LSILs) are due to high-risk HPV (HR-HPV) types (85% per ASC-US Low-Grade Triage Study); others due to low-risk types 6 and 11
- HPV-16 dominates in HR-HPV(+) group

CLINICAL ISSUES
- Asymptomatic; presents as abnormal Pap smear/test
- Often regresses spontaneously over period of 1-2 years
- Persistence is indicator for coexistent high-grade squamous intraepithelial lesion (HSIL), which is biologically independent event

CYTOPATHOLOGY
- Mature cell types (i.e., superficial or intermediate)
- Nuclear enlargement > 3x size (area) of intermediate cell nucleus with mild increase in nucleus:cytoplasm ratio
- Variable hyperchromasia, size, shape, and number (binucleated and multinucleated)
- Coarsely granular and uniformly distributed or densely opaque and smudged
- Nuclear contours are smooth or slightly irregular
- Sharply delineated perinuclear clearing with peripheral rim of densely stained cytoplasm (koilocyte) is characteristic but not requirement for diagnosis
- Cytoplasm may be densely keratinized (orangeophilic)
- Perinuclear halos in absence of nuclear abnormalities do not qualify for a diagnosis of LSIL
- Interpretive traps include navicular cells, radiation changes, early herpes viral changes, tight halos of reactive changes

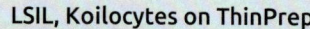

LSIL, Koilocytes on ThinPrep
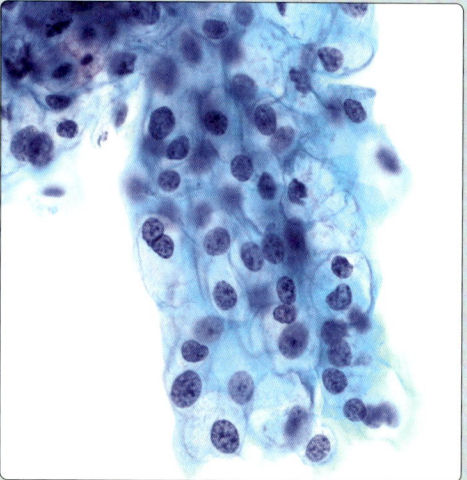

LSIL
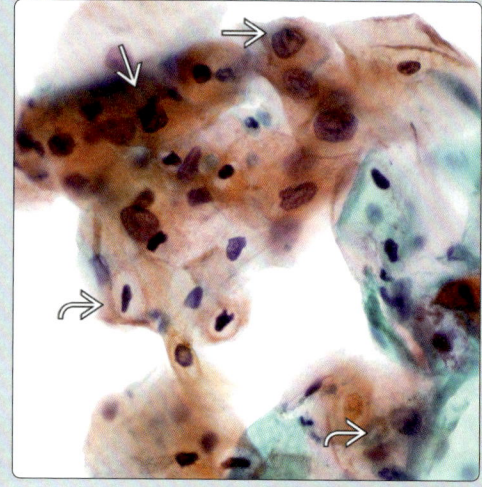

(Left) This ThinPrep Pap test demonstrates a group of uni- and binuclear koilocytes with an optically clear halo and nuclear enlargement, hyperchromasia, and contour irregularities. The nuclei are not centrally located within the halos. (Right) Low-grade squamous intraepithelial lesion (LSIL) on ThinPrep shows cells ➡ without the koilocytic cytoplasmic clearing but with nuclear features, including enlargement, hyperchromasia, and contour irregularities. Koilocytes ➡ are seen in the lower part of the image.

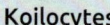

Koilocytes
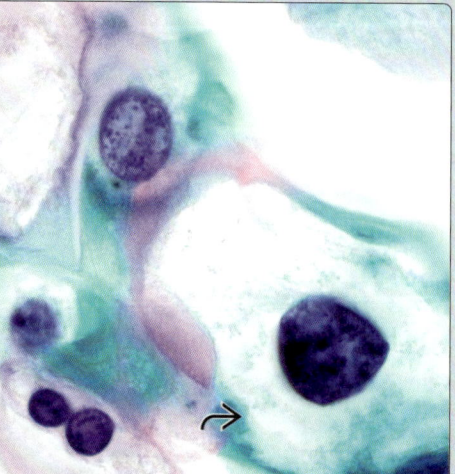

Tight Halos, Not LSIL
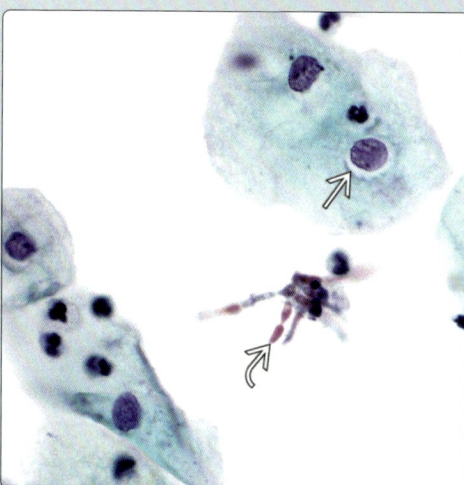

(Left) Koilocytes on SurePath Pap show uni- and binucleation, hyperchromasia, and distinct optically clear cytoplasmic clearing (halos) and peripheral condensation ➡. (Right) Tight halos ➡ from reactive changes secondary to Candida ➡ overgrowth. These reactive halos are small, not optically clear, and the nucleus tends to be centrally located within the halo. Unlike koilocytes, there is no peripheral cytoplasmic condensation.

Low-Grade Squamous Intraepithelial Lesion and Mimics

TERMINOLOGY

Abbreviations
- Low-grade squamous intraepithelial lesion (LSIL)

CLINICAL ISSUES

Presentation, Treatment, and Prognosis
- Often regresses spontaneously over period of 1-2 years

CYTOPATHOLOGY

Cellularity, Pattern, and Background
- Variable cellularity with cells in clumps, small groups, or single in clean or inflammatory background
  - Cases with LSIL and rare cells suggestive of HSIL can be reported as LSIL and ASC-H or just ASC-H or LSIL; cannot rule out HSIL (LSIL-H); Bethesda 2014 does not sanction new category of LSIL-H due to potential confusion

Cells
- Mature cell types (i.e., superficial or intermediate cells)

Nuclear Details
- Nuclear enlargement > 3x size (area) of intermediate cell nucleus with mild increase in nucleus:cytoplasm ratio
- Variable hyperchromasia, size, shape, and number (binucleated and multinucleated)
- Coarsely granular and uniformly distributed or densely opaque and smudged
- Smooth or slightly irregular nuclear contours
- Nucleoli usually absent or inconspicuous

Cytoplasmic Details
- Sharply delineated perinuclear clearing with peripheral rim of densely stained cytoplasm (koilocyte) is characteristic but not requirement for diagnosis
- Cytoplasm may be densely keratinized (orangeophilic)
- Perinuclear halos in absence of nuclear abnormalities do not qualify for diagnosis of LSIL

Cytology-Histology Correlation
- LSIL on biopsy (a.k.a. mild dysplasia or CIN 1)
- Terminology for cytology and histology unified after lower anogenital squamous terminology conference in 2012
- Some overlap with CIN 2 possible
  - Utilize p16 to further clarify issue on histology
  - Lack of block staining = LSIL/CIN 1

ANCILLARY TESTS

PCR
- HR-HPV testing may be useful for triage in certain age groups and clinical scenarios (per ASCCP guidelines)

DIFFERENTIAL DIAGNOSIS

Navicular Cells
- Yellow-tinged, large halo due to glycogen

Hyperkeratosis
- Nuclear changes of LSIL are not seen

Tight Halos Due to Inflammation/Infections
- Slight nuclear enlargement (< 3x) and smooth contours

Herpes Viral Infection
- Early infection may lack characteristic viral cytopathic effect

Radiation Effect
- Nuclear enlargement, chromatinic smudging, altered shapes

Vegetable matter
- Patients with vaginal mesh may very rarely show vegetable-like matter similar to ileal conduit urine specimens in patients using coloplast osteotomy device

SELECTED REFERENCES
1. Staats PN et al: Performance of specific morphologic features in distinguishing low-grade squamous intraepithelial lesions from high-grade squamous intraepithelial lesions in borderline cases: a CAP cytopathology committee multiobserver study. J Am Soc Cytopathol. 11(2):102-13, 2022

Foreign Material Mimicking Koilocytes

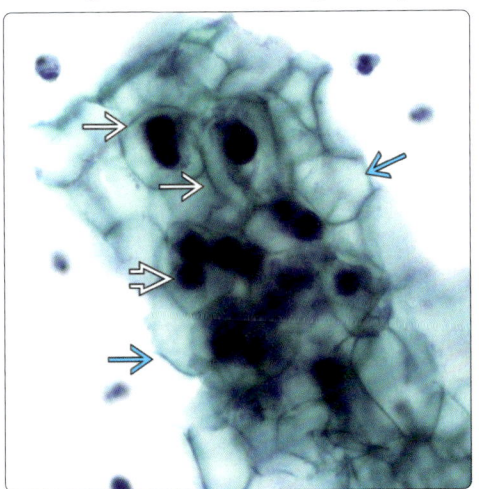

LSIL Mimic, Navicular Cells

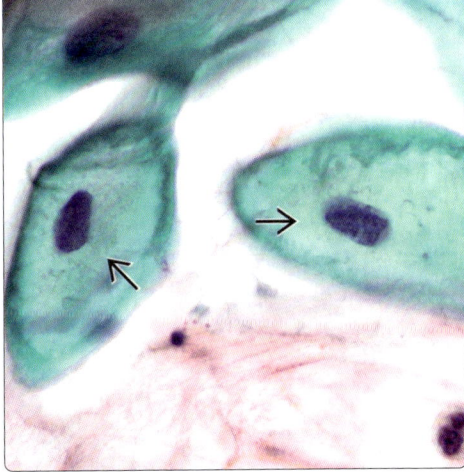

(Left) This ThinPrep Pap test shows koilocyte-like cells ➡ mimicking LSIL in this vaginal specimen. This is foreign material/vegetable-like matter from the mesh used to fix the prolapse at time of hysterectomy. Note the distinct rigid cell walls ➡ and dark nuclei ➡ of the foreign material. *(Right)* Pap smear shows navicular cells with yellow-tinged coloration ➡ to the cytoplasmic clearing. Nuclear changes of LSIL are absent in this mimic.

High-Grade Squamous Intraepithelial Lesion and Mimics

KEY FACTS

CYTOPATHOLOGY
- Usually cellular, multiple patterns on cytology, which include dispersed cell pattern, hyperchromatic crowded groups (HCGs), hypochromatic cell types, stripped nuclei, repair-like patterns, and keratinizing types
- Along mucous streaks or clumps or syncytial aggregates or HCGs if in glands on conventional Paps
- Dispersed cells, singly or in small groups on liquid-based preparations (LBPs); rarely HCGs
- Affects immature/small cells
  - Cell sizes range from small basal to metaplastic-type cells to larger cells that are closer to intermediate cells but with higher N:C ratio
- Hyperchromatic nuclei with nuclear contour irregularities due to indentations and grooves, cerebriform in LBPs
- Nuclear:cytoplasmic ratios can vary from very high in smaller, basal-type cells to lower in metaplastic-type cells but still higher than in low-grade SIL
- Varies from densely keratinized in keratinizing dysplasia (less common) to more delicate and metaplastic with fine vacuoles

ANCILLARY TESTS
- Positive for high-risk HPV types (type 16 predominates in most parts of world, followed by 18)
  - Other high-risk and intermediate-risk HPVs are also causative agents
  - Although these are HPV-driven lesions, 9-19% have tested negative for HPV in real-world experience
  - Low viral copy numbers, interfering substances, test failure, and low cellularity may be reasons for HPV-negative testing

TOP DIFFERENTIAL DIAGNOSES
- Adenocarcinoma in situ and atypical glandular cells, follicular cervicitis, IUD cells, and atrophy and bare nuclei of atrophy

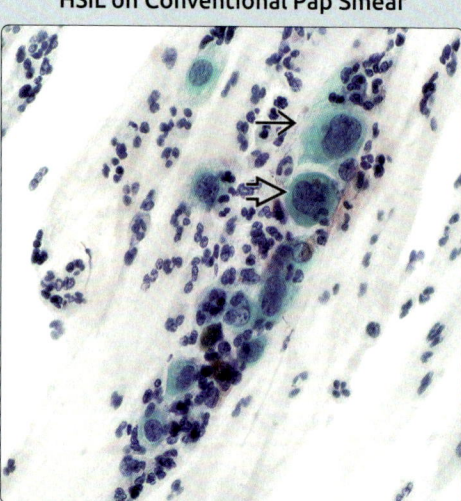

HSIL on Conventional Pap Smear

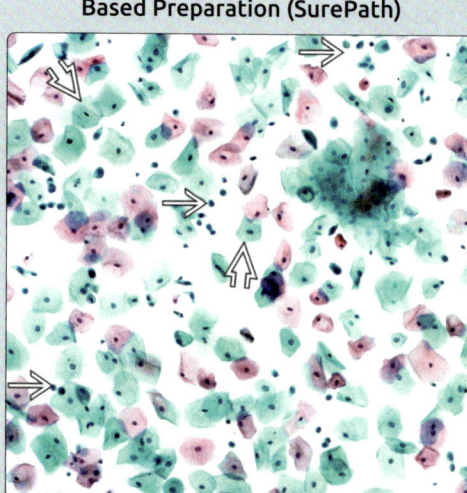

Dispersed Cell Pattern of HSIL on Liquid-Based Preparation (SurePath)

(Left) Conventional Pap shows streaks of mucus with entrapped cells of cervical intraepithelial neoplasia 2 (CIN2) ➔, cervical intraepithelial neoplasia 3 (CIN3) ➔, and inflammatory cells. This characteristic pattern is lost in liquid-based preparations due to cell suspension, mucolysis, and vortexing. (Right) SurePath shows dispersal of small cells of high-grade squamous intraepithelial lesion (HSIL) ➔ between mature superficial and intermediate cells ➔ due to cell suspension, mucolysis, and vortexing.

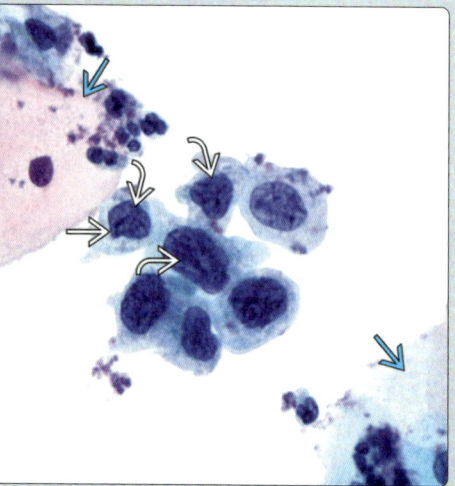

HSIL

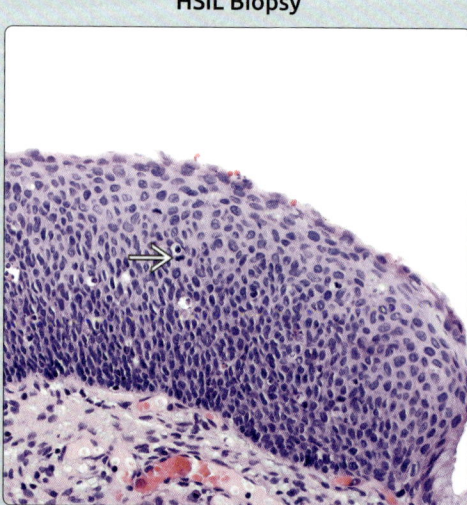

HSIL Biopsy

(Left) ThinPrep Pap test shows a cluster of 7 immature cell types with high N:C ratios, irregular nuclear contours ➔, cerebriform nuclei ➔, and marked hyperchromasia. Contrast with the background mature cells ➔. (Right) H&E of transformation zone with HSIL/CIN3 demonstrates full-thickness replacement by small, immature dysplastic cells with mitosis ➔ and apoptosis.

High-Grade Squamous Intraepithelial Lesion and Mimics

TERMINOLOGY

Abbreviations
- High-grade squamous intraepithelial lesion (HSIL)

Synonyms
- Cervical intraepithelial neoplasia grades 2 and 3 (CIN2 and CIN3); also includes squamous carcinoma in situ

Definitions
- HPV-driven neoplastic conversion of cervical or vaginal squamous epithelium with higher chance of progression to invasive squamous cell carcinoma if left untreated

CYTOPATHOLOGY

Cellularity
- Usually cellular; low cellularity cases with rare/few cells are best classified as atypical squamous cells; cannot rule out HSIL (ASC-H)

Pattern
- On conventional Pap, HSIL cells seen along mucous streaks or as clumps, syncytial aggregates, or hyperchromatic crowded groups (HCGs) if extending into endocervical glands
- Dispersed cells, singly or in small groups, on liquid-based preparations (LBPs)
  - HCGs or rarely hypochromatic on ThinPrep Pap
- Individual single cells are dispersed in empty spaces between superficial and intermediate cells
- Rarely, stripped-bare nuclei of HSIL or repair-like configuration

Background
- Mucous on conventionals, clean on LBPs

Cells
- Affects immature/small cells
  - Cell sizes range from small basal to metaplastic-type cells to larger cells that are closer to intermediate cells but with higher nuclear:cytoplasmic ratios

Nuclear Details
- Hyperchromatic nuclei with nuclear contour irregularities due to indentations and grooves
- Cerebriform nuclei in LBPs
- Nuclear:cytoplasmic ratios can vary from very high in smaller, basal-type cells to lower in metaplastic-type cells but still higher than in low-grade squamous intraepithelial lesion
- Chromatin ranges from fine to coarsely granular
- Nucleoli are usually absent but can be seen in cases where gland extension is present
- Chromatin is much darker in keratinizing dysplasia
- Rare hypochromic HSIL in ThinPrep LBPs with usual Pap stain (not seen with darker Imager Pap stain)

Cytoplasmic Details
- Varies from densely keratinized in keratinizing dysplasia (rare in North America) to more delicate and metaplastic with fine vacuoles
- Can be dense and "hard"/opaque cyanophilic but not orangeophilic in some cases

Adequacy Criteria
- Always adequate if abnormal cells are present
- If only rare cells are present or if qualitatively/quantitatively short of diagnosis of HSIL, interpret as ASC-H

Cell Block Findings
- Can be helpful in certain scenarios to distinguish from glandular or mimic lesions
- Immunohistochemistry for p16 can be helpful in some scenarios

Cytology-Histology Correlation
- Dysplastic cells with nuclear crowding involving > lower 1/3 (CIN2) or > 2/3 (CIN3) surface squamous epithelial thickness
- All HSILs are referred to colposcopy and biopsy
  - Refer to ASCCP management guidelines

ANCILLARY TESTS

PCR
- Positive for high-risk HPV types (type 16, which is predominant, followed by type 18)
- 9-19% may test negative for high-risk HPV types in real-world experience
- Reasons for false-negatives include low viral copy numbers below analytic sensitivity of test, interfering substances, too few cells in specimen, test failure, etc.

DIFFERENTIAL DIAGNOSIS

Adenocarcinoma In Situ and Atypical Glandular Cells
- HSIL lacks polarization, has peripheral flattening of nuclei

Follicular Cervicitis
- Small lymphocytes with some variation

IUD Cells
- Only very rare single cells with history of IUD
- Probably endometrial stromal in origin

Atrophy and Bare Nuclei of Atrophy
- Should not interpret bare nuclei; atrophy lacks nuclear contour abnormalities and hyperchromasia

Other Etiologies for HCGs and Single Cells
- Endometrial cells, decidual cells, repair

Causes for False-Negative Diagnosis/Missed Cases
- Extremely low cellularity, obscuring factors, inadequate sampling, not in field of view for imager screening

SELECTED REFERENCES

1. Staats PN et al: Performance of specific morphologic features in distinguishing low-grade squamous intraepithelial lesions from high-grade squamous intraepithelial lesions in borderline cases: a College of American Pathologists cytopathology committee multiobserver study. J Am Soc Cytopathol. 11(2):102-13, 2022
2. Goyal A et al: Underrecognized patterns of high-grade squamous intraepithelial lesion on ThinPrep preparations. Am J Clin Pathol. 156(2):300-12, 2021
3. Jones R et al: Endocervical glandular involvement is associated with an increased detection rate of high-grade squamous intraepithelial lesions on the Papanicolaou test. J Am Soc Cytopathol. 9(3):137-45, 2020

High-Grade Squamous Intraepithelial Lesion and Mimics

Keratinizing HSIL

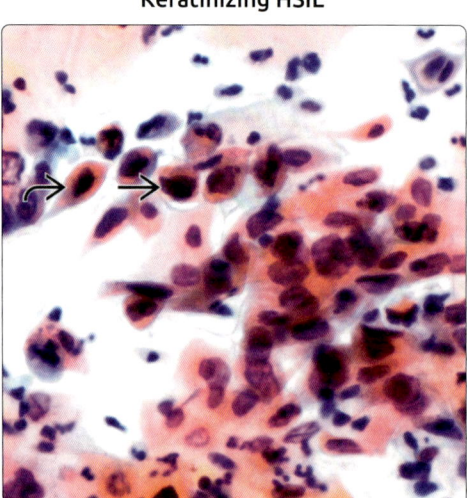

HSIL/CIN2

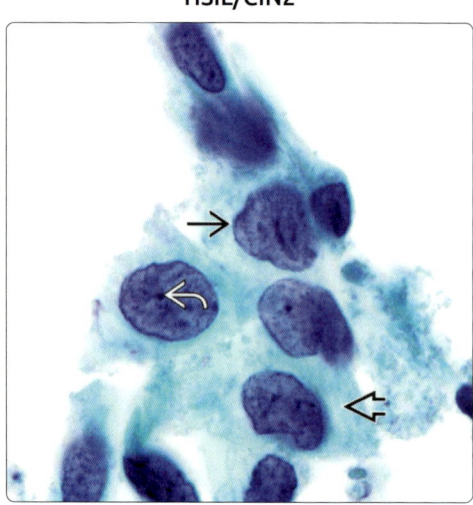

(Left) *Conventional Pap shows keratinizing HSIL. Orangeophilic cells ⇒ with high N:C ratios and dense, dark nuclei with irregular contours ⇒ are shown.* (Right) *ThinPrep Pap test shows HSIL, mostly CIN2, with large nuclei with irregular contours ⇒ and grooves. The chromatin is dispersed with chromocenters ⇒. The cytoplasm ⇒ is more than that seen with CIN3 and is fragile.*

Repair-Like HSIL

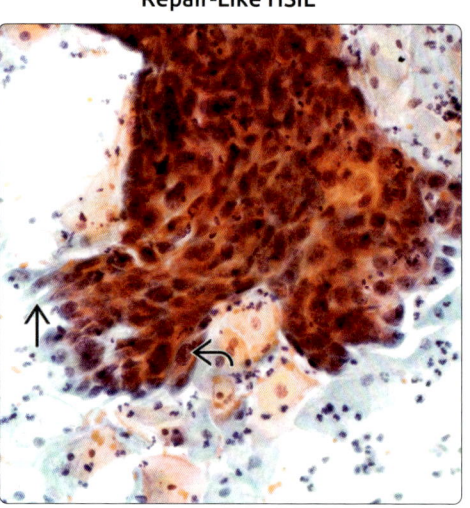

Stripped Nuclear Pattern of HSIL

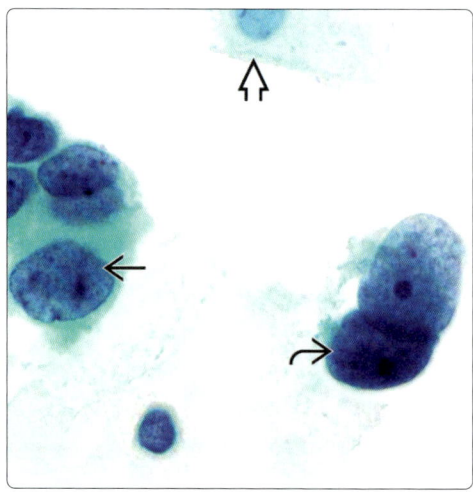

(Left) *Conventional Pap shows a syncytial arrangement of cells where it is difficult to see cell boundaries in the center. However, at the periphery, cell cytoplasm is drawn out ⇒ and resembles repair. The presence of nucleoli ⇒ can also contribute to a misdiagnosis of repair.* (Right) *ThinPrep Pap shows bare nuclei of HSIL ⇒. The diagnosis should be based on intact cells ⇒ with features of HSIL. Note a nearby intermediate cell for size comparison ⇒.*

HSIL, Hyperchromatic Crowded Group Pattern

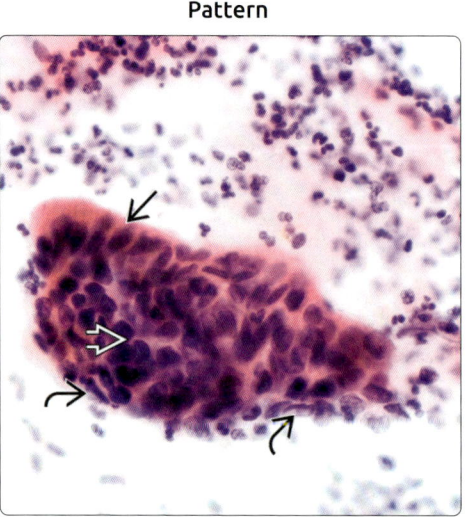

p16/Ki-67 Dual Stain Block-Positive Pattern

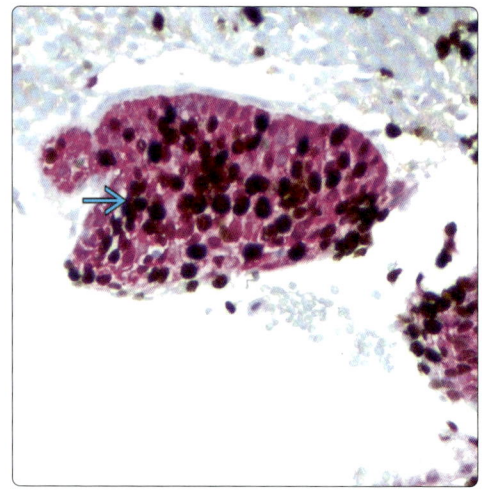

(Left) *Conventional Pap shows a syncytial arrangement of cells ⇒ and overlying benign endocervical cells ⇒ from a case of HSIL with gland extension. Note that the flattening of cells ⇒ along the periphery favors HSIL over adenocarcinoma in situ, where the nuclei are polarized perpendicular to the circumference.* (Right) *Dual p16 (red) and Ki-67 (brown nuclear) ⇒ stain shows full-thickness positivity for both p16 and Ki-67, confirming HSIL/CIN3. The differential was HSIL vs. immature squamous metaplasia.*

High-Grade Squamous Intraepithelial Lesion and Mimics

AIS and HSIL in Same Field of View

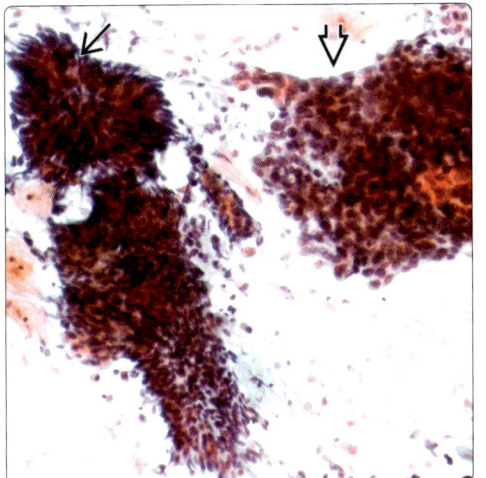

Adenocarcinoma In Situ vs. HSIL

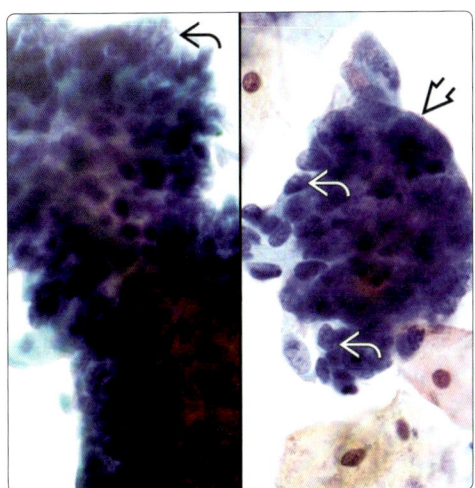

(Left) Conventional Pap shows HSIL ⇨ and adenocarcinoma in situ (AIS) ⇨. Contrast the polarization of the nuclei perpendicular to the circumference in AIS with flattening and parallel to the circumference in HSIL. **(Right)** ThinPrep Pap shows the difference between AIS ⇨ and HSIL with gland extension. The circumference of most HSIL is smooth ⇨ with rare nuclei showing disordered polarization ⇨. Cells of HSIL are round and larger than cells of AIS.

HSIL vs. Follicular Cervicitis

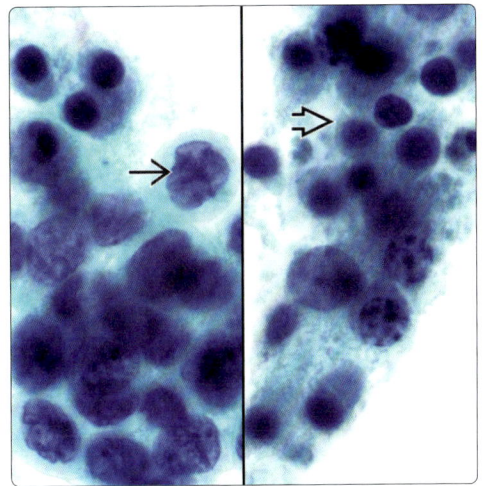

Small Cell HSIL

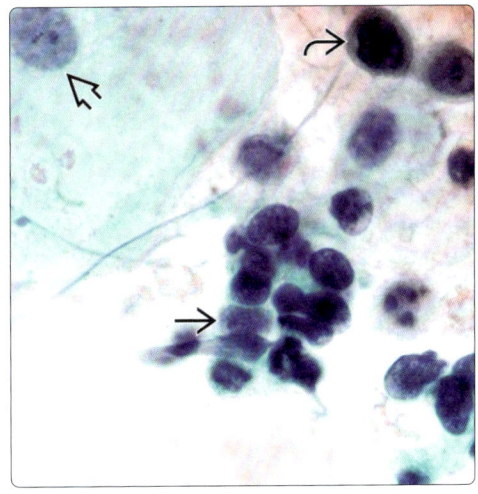

(Left) Composite image contrasts HSIL ⇨ with larger cell size and nuclear contour irregularities with follicular cervicitis ⇨. The nuclei are smaller and varying in size but without the irregular contours and grooves seen in HSIL on this ThinPrep Pap. **(Right)** Conventional Pap shows small cell HSIL ⇨. The small cells with features of HSIL can be compared with conventional nonkeratinizing HSIL ⇨ and an intermediate cell nucleus ⇨. The differential is small cell carcinoma.

HSIL With Atrophy

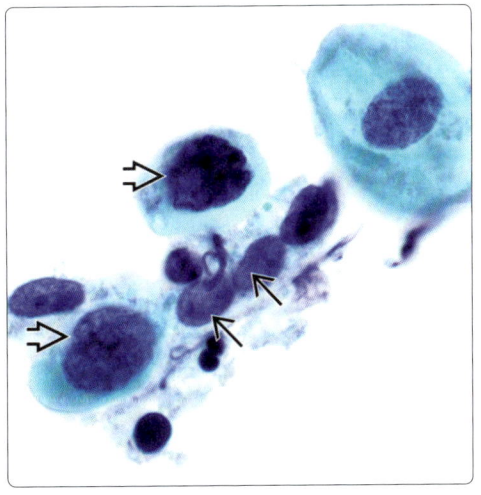

Hypochromatic HSIL, ThinPrep Specific

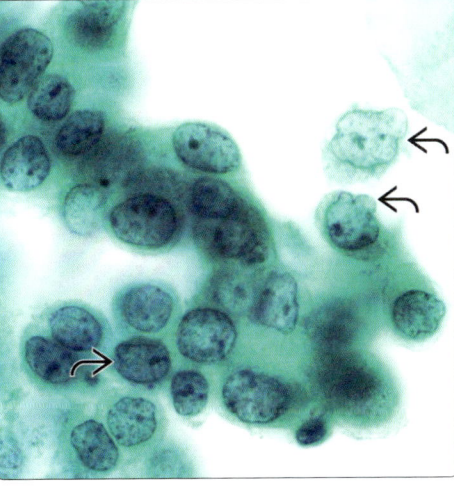

(Left) ThinPrep Pap shows bare nuclei of atrophy ⇨ in contrast with HSIL cells ⇨ in a case with atrophy. Contrast the hyperchromasia and nuclear size and shape in HSIL. **(Right)** ThinPrep Pap with usual (not imager) Pap stain shows hypochromatic HSIL. The nuclei are hypochromic but do show high N:C ratios and contour irregularities ⇨. These are unique to ThinPreps and may be related to the fixative medium. This can be misinterpreted as metaplasia.

Atypical Squamous Cells of Undetermined Significance

KEY FACTS

TERMINOLOGY
- Cytomorphologic changes suggestive of low-grade squamous intraepithelial lesion (LSIL) that are qualitatively or quantitatively short for definitive diagnosis of LSIL

CLINICAL ISSUES
- Atypical squamous cells of undetermined significance (ASC-US) interpretations serve to prompt additional investigations to resolve diagnostic uncertainty
- High-risk human papillomavirus (HR-HPV) testing is preferred modality for triage, except in young patients < 25 years who can be followed irrespective of HPV status
- HPV positivity varies by age; females < 30 years have mean HPV positivity rate of 47.7% and > 30 years have 32.0% positive rate

CYTOPATHOLOGY
- Nuclei have 2.5-3.0x area of normal intermediate squamous cell nuclei (35 µm²) or 2x size of squamous metaplastic cell nucleus (50 µm²)
- Slightly increased nuclear:cytoplasmic ratio
- Mild to minimal nuclear hyperchromasia and variation in contour
- Mild irregularities in nuclear shape
- Large metaplastic or small intermediate cells can be classified as ASC-US if they do not fulfill criteria for cervical intraepithelial neoplasia grade 1 or 2
- Atypical parakeratotic cells are also included if not definitively diagnostic for keratinizing dysplasia
- Basically, these are cases that qualitatively or quantitatively fall short of diagnosis of LSIL
- Atypical repair and atypia in atrophy may also be classified in this category if squamous in origin
- HPV positivity rates and ASC:SIL ratios are important quality indicators for peer comparison of labs and individuals
- Diagnostic pitfalls
  - Atrophy with mild atypia
  - *Candida* and inflammatory changes may mimic ASC-US
  - Robust squamous tissue repair

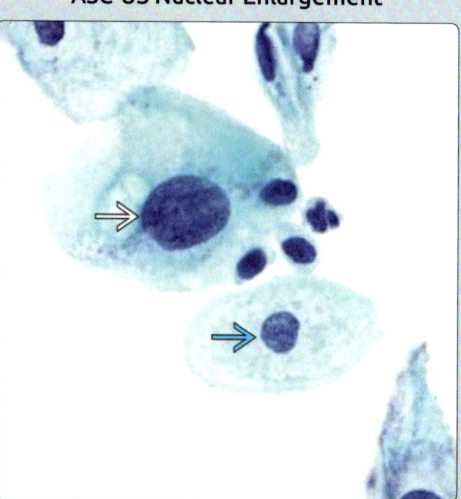

ASC-US Nuclear Enlargement

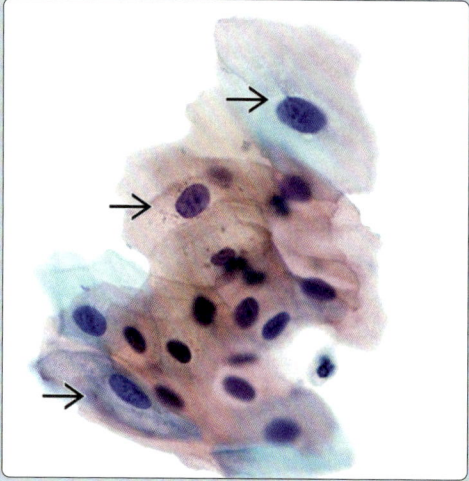

ASC-US in Superficial and Intermediate Cells

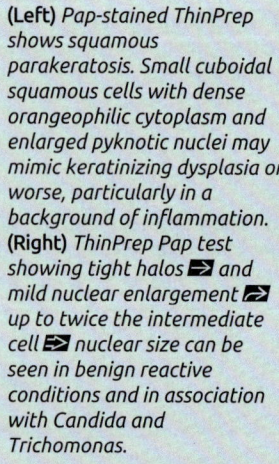

(Left) ThinPrep Pap test shows an intermediate cell with a nucleus ➡ > 2.5 X the size of an adjacent normal nucleus ➡ but also shows degenerative cytoplasmic vacuoles, making it not diagnostic of LSIL. HPV was negative. (Right) ThinPrep Pap test shows superficial and intermediate cells, some with nuclear enlargement and changes that would qualify for a diagnosis of atypical squamous cells of atypical squamous cells of undetermined significance (ASC-US) ➡. HPV was positive, and biopsy showed LSIL.

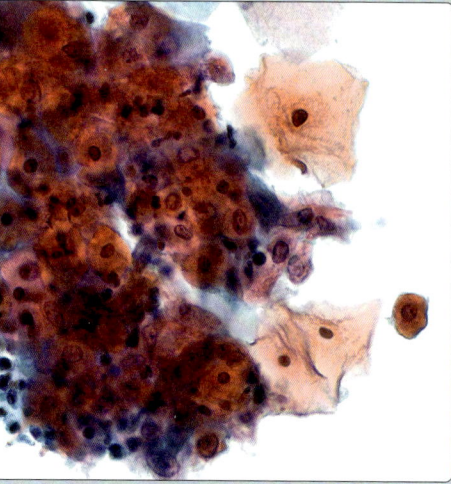

Parakeratotic ASC-US

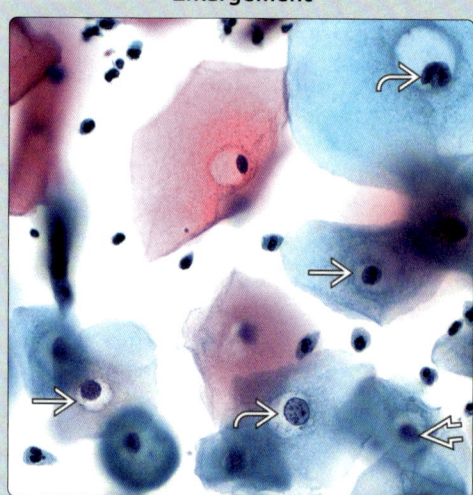

Not ASC-US: Tight Halos and Mild Nuclear Enlargement

(Left) Pap-stained ThinPrep shows squamous parakeratosis. Small cuboidal squamous cells with dense orangeophilic cytoplasm and enlarged pyknotic nuclei may mimic keratinizing dysplasia or worse, particularly in a background of inflammation. (Right) ThinPrep Pap test showing tight halos ➡ and mild nuclear enlargement ➡ up to twice the intermediate cell ➡ nuclear size can be seen in benign reactive conditions and in association with *Candida* and *Trichomonas*.

Atypical Squamous Cells of Undetermined Significance

TERMINOLOGY

Abbreviations
- Atypical squamous cells of undetermined significance (ASC-US) (Bethesda System for reporting)

Definitions
- Cytomorphologic changes suggestive of low-grade squamous intraepithelial lesion (LSIL) that are qualitatively or quantitatively short for definitive diagnosis of LSIL

CLINICAL ISSUES

Management Options, Reporting Rates, and Outcomes
- Recommended investigations may include
  - Repeat Pap test after defined time
  - High-risk human papillomavirus (HR-HPV) testing and triage
    - HR-HPV testing is preferred strategy for triaging ASC-US cases in females > 25 years
    - Based on data from ASC-US Low-Grade Triage Study (ALTS), HPV(+) ASC-US cases on follow-up have same rate of high-grade dysplasia as LSIL cases
    - HR-HPV triage is preferred and more efficient way to triage females and yields same number of cervical intraepithelial neoplasia (CIN) grade 2 and higher cases on follow-up but with 1/2 number of patients being referred for colposcopy
  - Colposcopy and biopsy
  - Management guidelines vary by age groups as well as in different parts of world
- Reporting rates, cytology histology correlation, follow-up
  - HPV positivity varies by age; females < 30 years have mean HPV positivity rate of 47.7% and > 30 years have 32.0% positive rate
  - Benchmarking data are available from College of American Pathologists for ASC-US reporting rates, ASC-US:SIL ratios, and HR-HPV positivity rates
  - Most ASC-US cases turn out to be benign or low grade on colposcopy and biopsy
  - ASC-US median reporting rates for liquid-based and conventional cytology are 5.1% and 2.6%, respectively
  - Based on data from ALTS trial, 25% of females with ASC-US Paps had SIL on follow-up (LSIL: 14%, HSIL: 11%)

CYTOPATHOLOGY

Cells
- Mature (superficial and intermediate) squamous cell types

Nucleus
- 2.5-3.0x area of normal intermediate cell nucleus (35 µm²) or 2x size of squamous metaplastic cell nucleus (50 µm²)
- Slightly increased nuclear:cytoplasmic ratio with mild to minimal hyperchromasia and nuclear contour irregularity
- Mildly irregular chromatin distribution

Other Features
- Atypical parakeratosis characterized by nuclear enlargement and irregularities and dense orangeophilic cytoplasm are also included if not definitively diagnostic for dysplasia
  - Atypical repair and atypia in atrophy may also be classified in this category if squamous in origin
- Conventional and liquid-based Paps have similar appearance except that air drying in smears makes cells appear flatter or may result in normal cells being overcalled
- Large metaplastic or small intermediate cells can also be classified as ASC-US if they do not fulfill criteria for CIN grade 1 or 2
- Inter- and intraobserver variation is highest in this category

DIFFERENTIAL DIAGNOSIS

Diagnostic Pitfalls
- Atrophy, robust squamous repair, inflammatory changes, *Candida* effect

SELECTED REFERENCES
1. Nayar R et al: Moving forward-the 2019 ASCCP risk-based management consensus guidelines for abnormal cervical cancer screening tests and cancer precursors and beyond: implications and suggestions for laboratories. J Am Soc Cytopathol. 9(4):291-303, 2020

ASC-US in Atrophic Pap

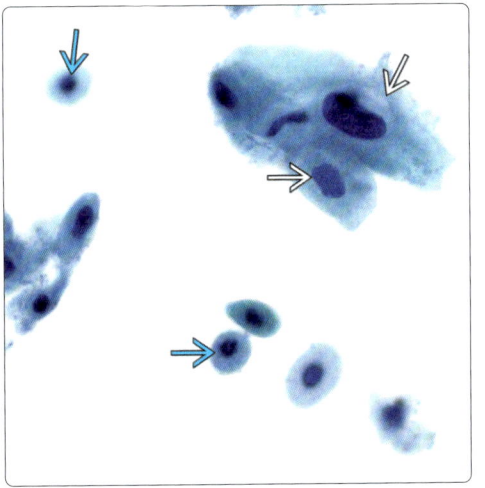

ASC-US vs. Atypical Repair

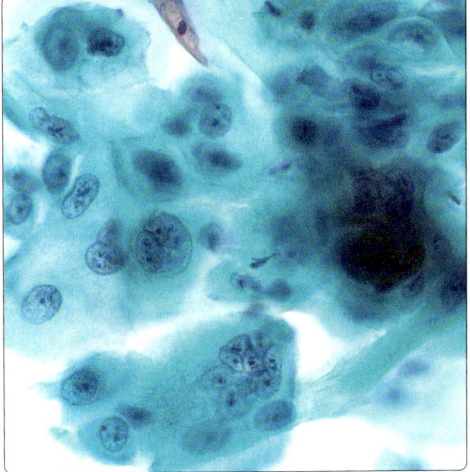

(Left) *Atrophic ThinPrep Pap test with few cells interpreted as ASC-US ➡ is shown. Note the small background parabasal cells in this atrophic Pap test ➡. High-risk HPV was positive, and follow-up biopsy was low-grade squamous intraepithelial lesion.* **(Right)** *SurePath Pap test shows robust squamous metaplasia with "atypical" tissue repair. Karyomegaly, marked anisonucleosis, syncytial architecture, nucleoli, and nuclear molding may mimic LSIL or squamous carcinoma.*

Atypical Squamous Cells, Cannot Rule Out High-Grade Squamous Intraepithelial Lesion

KEY FACTS

CLINICAL ISSUES

- Interpretation of atypical squamous cells (ASC), cannot exclude high-grade squamous intraepithelial lesion (HSIL) (ASC-H), prompts colposcopy and biopsy to rule out possible cervicovaginal HSIL pathology
  - 47% of ASC-H on follow-up will show CIN2(+)
  - Median reporting rate in CAP survey is 0.2% for conventional smears and 0.3% for liquid based
  - Reporting ranges (5-95th percentile) in CAP surveys is 0.0-0.9% for conventionals and SurePath and 0-1% for ThinPreps

CYTOPATHOLOGY

- Patterns similar to HSIL but qualitatively and quantitatively falls short of diagnosis of HSIL
- Dispersed cells, small aggregates with < 10 cells
- Atypical parakeratotic cells in background of atrophy
- Hyperchromatic crowded groups of cells or crowded sheet pattern with difficult-to-visualize individual cells
- Small cells with high nuclear:cytoplasmic (N:C) ratios, atypical immature metaplastic cells
- Karyomegaly in small metaplastic-type cells is ~ 1.5-2.5x area of reference intermediate cell nuclei
- Nuclear contour irregularities and increased N:C ratios that fall short of diagnosis of HSIL

TOP DIFFERENTIAL DIAGNOSES

- Often over- or underdiagnosed in atrophy/atrophic vaginitis
  - Hyperchromasia, contour irregularities in ASC-H as compared with parabasal cells
  - Lack of nuclear overlap in syncytial fragments within plane of focus
- Endometrial cells and histiocytes
  - Small cell size, chromatin help to differentiate
- IDU cells and decidual cells
  - Degenerative changes are key to recognition
- Isolated endocervical cells and artifacts

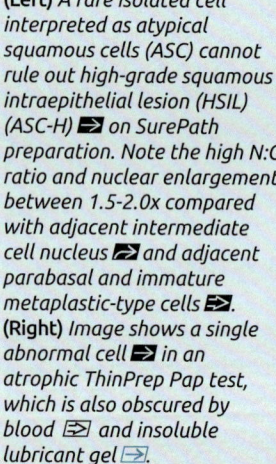

(Left) A rare isolated cell interpreted as atypical squamous cells (ASC) cannot rule out high-grade squamous intraepithelial lesion (HSIL) (ASC-H) ➡ on SurePath preparation. Note the high N:C ratio and nuclear enlargement between 1.5-2.0x compared with adjacent intermediate cell nucleus ➡ and adjacent parabasal and immature metaplastic-type cells ➡. (Right) Image shows a single abnormal cell ➡ in an atrophic ThinPrep Pap test, which is also obscured by blood ➡ and insoluble lubricant gel ➡.

Rare Isolated Cell of ASC-H

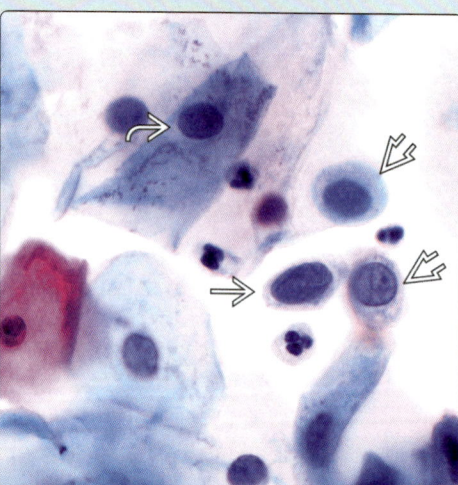

ASC-H in Atrophic Pap With Blood and Gel

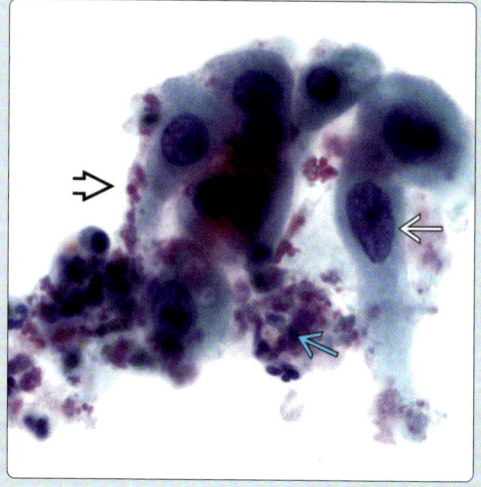

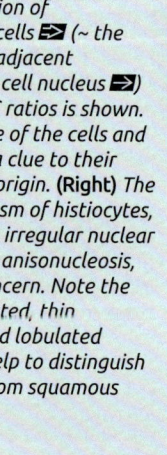

(Left) Collection of endometrial cells ➡ (~ the same size as adjacent intermediate cell nucleus ➡) with high N:C ratios is shown. The small size of the cells and clustering is a clue to their endometrial origin. (Right) The scant cytoplasm of histiocytes, in addition to irregular nuclear contours and anisonucleosis, may raise concern. Note the microvacuolated, thin cytoplasm and lobulated nuclei that help to distinguish histiocytes from squamous cells.

Endometrial Cells Mimicking ASC-H

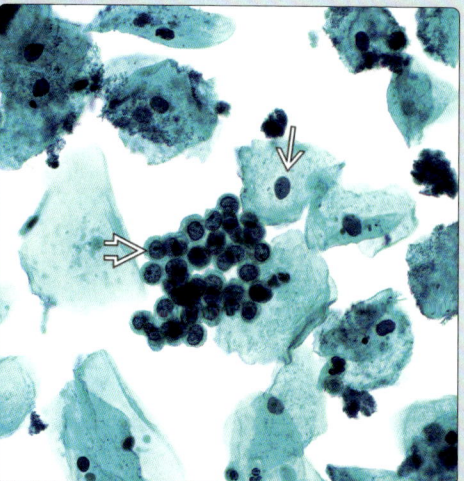

Histiocytes Mimicking ASC-H

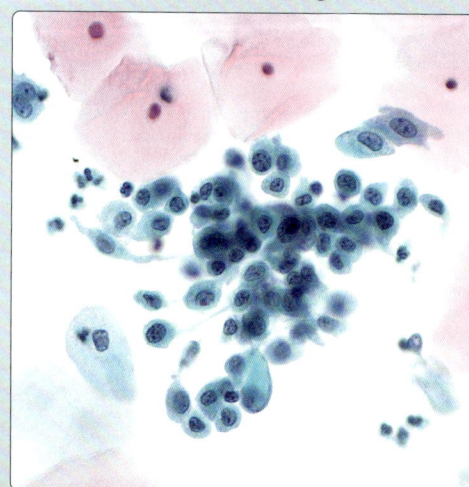

Atypical Squamous Cells, Cannot Rule Out High-Grade Squamous Intraepithelial Lesion

TERMINOLOGY

Abbreviations
- Atypical squamous cells (ASC), cannot exclude high-grade squamous intraepithelial lesion (HSIL) (ASC-H) (Bethesda System for reporting)

CLINICAL ISSUES

Prognosis
- ASC-H is high-risk category and management is colposcopy to rule out high-grade disease
- **Recommended management**
  - Referral to colposcopy and cervical biopsy for patients ≥ 21 years old
  - Further management depends on colposcopy and biopsy findings or lack thereof
    - Please refer to American Society for Colposcopy and Cervical Pathology (ASCCP) management guidelines
- **ASC-H reporting rates and high-risk HPV positivity**
  - Benchmarking data is available from College of American Pathologists (CAP)
  - ASC-H reporting rate is typically ~ 1/10 of atypical squamous cells of undetermined significance (ASC-US) rate and has range of 0.0-1.5% (5th-95th percentile), with median rate of 0.2%
  - 33-84% of ASC-H cases are high-risk HPV(+), with higher positivity rates in younger patients

CYTOPATHOLOGY

Cellularity
- ASC-H reporting is justified when < 10 severely dysplastic squamous epithelial cells are identified

Pattern
- Patterns similar to HSIL [i.e., dispersed single cells, syncytial/crowded sheets, keratinizing atypia, and small cells with increased nuclear:cytoplasmic (N:C) ratios]
- Hyperchromatic crowded groups of cells or crowded sheet pattern with difficult to visualize individual cells
- Cells trapped in mucous streams in conventional smears
- Atypical parakeratotic cells in background of atrophic vaginitis

Cells
- Small cells with high N:C ratios, atypical immature metaplastic cells with nuclear area 1.5-2.5x area of reference intermediate cell nucleus
  - Hyperchromasia, chromatin clumping, minor nuclear contour irregularities
  - Small cell pattern in liquid based shows nuclear size 2-3x that of leukocyte nuclei
  - Cells generally round, cuboidal, or oval but can be elongated and irregular in keratinizing types
- Pleomorphic orangeophilic parakeratotic cells suggestive of keratinizing dysplasia

Cytology-Histology Correlation
- Range of follow-up HSIL rates on biopsy/excision procedures: 12-70%
- Average HSIL on tissue follow-up: ~ 40%

DIFFERENTIAL DIAGNOSIS

Most Common Diagnostic Pitfalls
- Air drying in conventional Pap test smears (naked nuclei, parabasal &/or squamous metaplastic cells, histiocytes)
- Squamous metaplastic cells with benign inflammatory changes
- Atypical (immature) metaplastic cells
- Endometrial cells and histiocytes
- IUD cells and atypia in atrophy/atrophic vaginitis

SELECTED REFERENCES

1. Gonzalez AA et al: The significance of ASC-H and LSIL dual interpretation with risk stratification: one institution experience. J Am Soc Cytopathol. 10(6):565-70, 2021
2. Jenkins TM et al: Role of ancillary techniques in cervical biopsy and endocervical curettage specimens as follow-up to Papanicolaou test results indicating a diagnosis of atypical squamous cells, cannot exclude high-grade squamous intraepithelial lesion, or high-grade squamous intraepithelial lesion. Acta Cytol. 64(1-2):155-65, 2020

ASC-H Pitfall: Decidual Cell
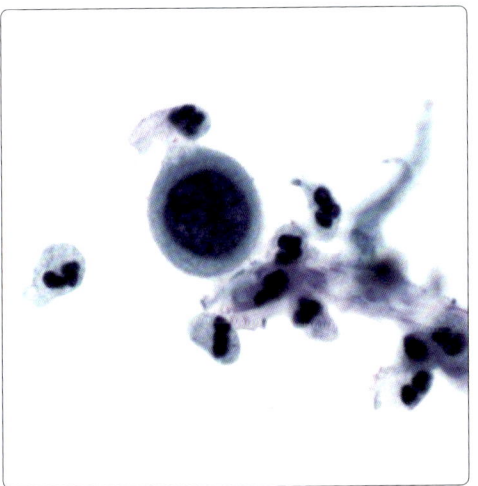

ASC-H Pitfall: Air Drying in Smears
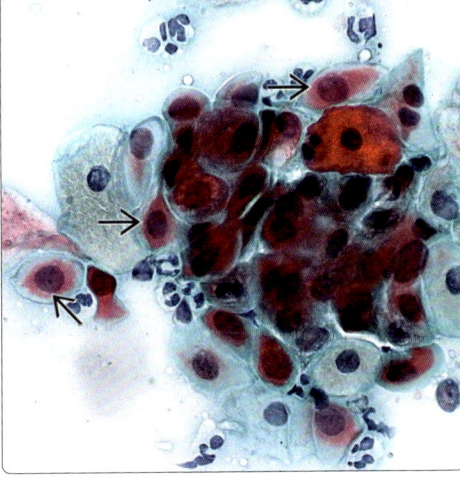

(Left) An isolated single cell with high N:C ratio and dark, smudged chromatin was interpreted as ASC-H. Follow-up was benign, and HPV test was negative. In retrospect, it was felt to be an isolated and degenerated decidual cell, as patient was pregnant at the time. (Right) A conventional Pap smear demonstrates a pitfall related to air-dried squamous metaplastic cells ➡. The pseudoeosinophilic cytoplasm, nuclear pyknosis, and nuclear swelling resulting in the appearance of increased N:C ratios all raise suspicion for HSIL.

Squamous Cell Carcinoma of Cervix, Variants and Mimics

KEY FACTS

CLINICAL ISSUES
- Majority occur from ages 40-55
- Asymptomatic with abnormal Pap smear
- Often epithelial surface abnormalities on colposcopy
- Surgical options are determined by stage
  - Screening has resulted in detection of more superficially invasive carcinoma cases

CYTOPATHOLOGY
- Usually cellular specimen with background diathesis
- Dispersed cells as well as clumps and syncytia
- Type of diathesis varies by preparation type (conventional vs. liquid based) and type of carcinoma (keratinizing vs. nonkeratinizing)
- Hyperchromatic, irregularly shaped squamous cells in keratinizing type
- Pleomorphic and bizarre cells of various sizes and shapes present in background of keratinizing dysplasia
- Nonkeratinizing squamous cell carcinoma (NKSqCas) show large to medium-sized cells, generally uniform with only rare abrupt keratinized cells
- Nucleoli and vesicular chromatin in NKSqCa

ANCILLARY TESTS
- p16 diffusely, strongly positive in majority of high-risk human papillomavirus (HPV) (+) cases
- Although SqCa of cervix is HPV-driven disease, 5-30% will test negative for HPV in real-world scenarios
  - Reasons for negative tests include analytic sensitivity of testing platform, low DNA copy numbers, interfering substances, low epithelial cells, and other reasons resulting in test failure

TOP DIFFERENTIAL DIAGNOSES
- High-grade squamous intraepithelial lesion
- Small cell neuroendocrine carcinoma
- Adenocarcinoma

Bizarre Keratinized Malignant Cell

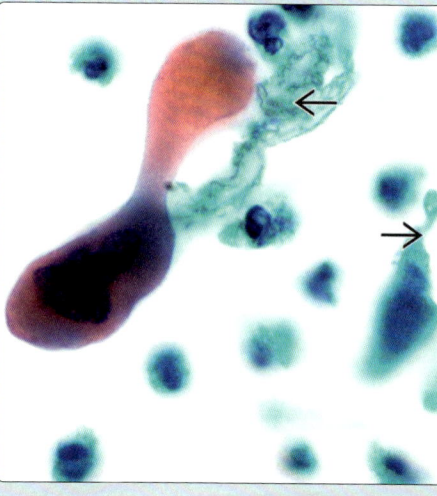

Nonkeratinizing Squamous Cell Carcinoma on Conventional Smear

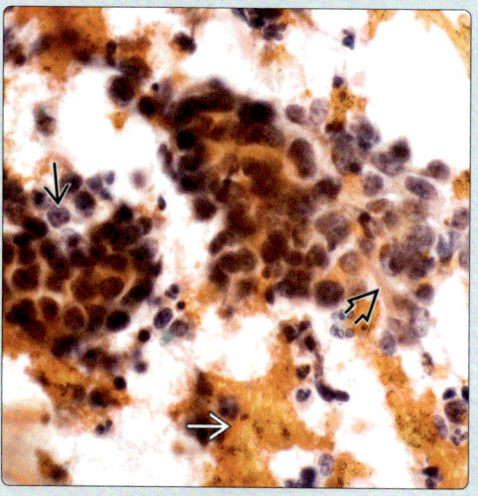

(Left) This bizarre malignant keratinized cell has a long club-shaped tail. Nuclear chromatin is dark with irregular clearing and nuclear contours. Note diathesis ➡, which can be subtle. (Right) Nonkeratinizing SqCa (NKSqCa) in a bloody diathesis ➡ consisting of lysed blood and fibrin is shown. Note nucleoli ➡ and vesicular chromatin of the cells, which are round and irregular with occasional cells showing pulled, a columnar-like cytoplasm ➡.

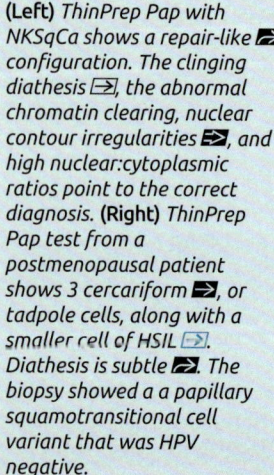

Repair-Like Squamous Cell Carcinoma

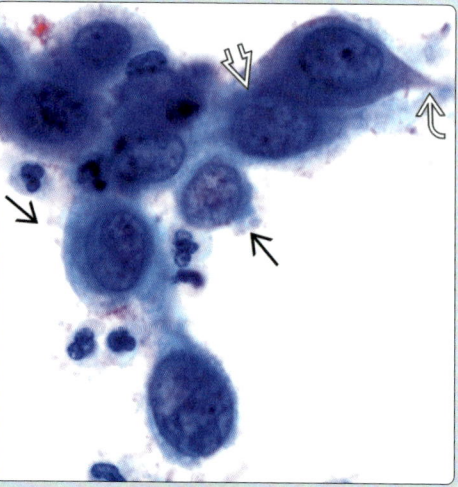

Cerclariform Cells in Papillary Squamotransitional Cell Variant

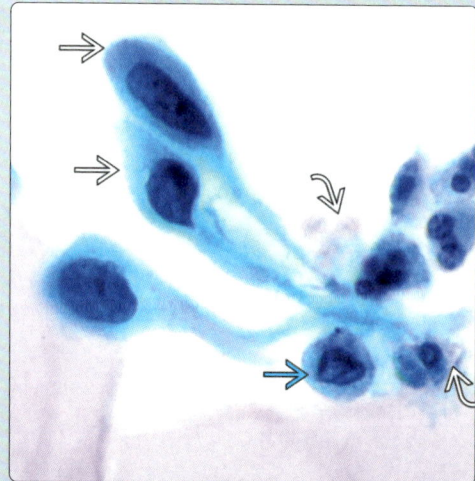

(Left) ThinPrep Pap with NKSqCa shows a repair-like ➡ configuration. The clinging diathesis ➡, the abnormal chromatin clearing, nuclear contour irregularities ➡, and high nuclear:cytoplasmic ratios point to the correct diagnosis. (Right) ThinPrep Pap test from a postmenopausal patient shows 3 cercariform ➡, or tadpole cells, along with a smaller cell of HSIL ➡. Diathesis is subtle ➡. The biopsy showed a a papillary squamotransitional cell variant that was HPV negative.

Squamous Cell Carcinoma of Cervix, Variants and Mimics

TERMINOLOGY

Abbreviations
- Squamous cell carcinoma (SqCa)

Definitions
- Malignant neoplasm originating in or near cervical transformation zone and showing evidence of squamous differentiation

ETIOLOGY/PATHOGENESIS

Human Papillomavirus
- Most commonly high-risk human papillomavirus (HPV) genotypes (HPV-16, HPV-18)
  - Viral proteins E6 and E7 produced after integration of high-risk HPV DNA into host genome
  - Inactivates cell cycle progression leading to cellular immortalization
- Common incident infection in general population
  - Most infections are eliminated by host immune system
  - Increased risk of carcinoma associated with persistent infection

Additional Factors
- Host factors
  - Immunosuppression, HIV positivity, post transplant
- Environmental factors, including smoking
  - Increased risk of HPV acquisition associated with
    - High parity, increased number of lifetime sexual partners, partners with many previous sexual partners

CLINICAL ISSUES

Epidemiology
- Incidence
  - Estimated to be 3.97 per 100,000 person-years (2006-2007)
    - Results in ~ 11,500 new cases per year and 3,500 fatalities per year in USA
    - ↓ 60-70% over preceding 50 years due to improved screening with Pap smear
- Age
  - Majority of cases occur at ages 40-55

Presentation
- Asymptomatic with abnormal Pap smear
- Vaginal bleeding, occasionally pain and vaginal discharge
- On colposcopic examination
  - Atypical, nonbranching vessels (i.e., neovascularization)
  - Ulceration or raised irregular surface
  - Yellow-colored epithelium, firmness on palpation

Natural History
- > 50% of incident and fatal cases were in female patients who had no cytologic screening or inadequate cytologic screening
- Precursor lesions
  - After detection, many regress or persist unchanged
  - Low-grade squamous intraepithelial lesion/cervical intraepithelial neoplasia (CIN) 1
    - Associated with low risk of progression to carcinoma
    - Believed to reflect ongoing HPV infection
  - High-grade squamous intraepithelial lesion (HSIL)/CIN 2, indeterminate risk of progression to carcinoma
  - HSIL/CIN 3, ~ 12% risk of progression to invasive carcinoma

CYTOPATHOLOGY

Cellularity
- Usually cellular specimen with background diathesis in most cases

Pattern
- Dispersed cells as well as clumps and syncytial fragments
- Dispersed population especially in keratinizing SqCa (KSqCa)
- Hyperchromatic crowded groups are more likely in nonkeratinizing SqCa (NKSqCa)

Background
- Diathesis is present in most cases
- Type of diathesis varies by preparation type (conventional vs. liquid based) and type of carcinoma (keratinizing vs. nonkeratinizing)
- Tumor diathesis is less pronounced in KSqCa

Cells
- KSqCa
  - Hyperchromatic, irregularly shaped squamous cells
  - Pleomorphic and bizarre cells of various sizes and shapes present in background of keratinizing dysplasia
  - Keratin pearls, fiber cells, and dyskeratotic cells
  - Foreign-body giant cell response to keratin
  - Occasional mitoses, rarely intercellular bridges
  - Coexistent dysplastic changes (usually keratinizing dysplasia)
- NKSqCa
  - Large- to medium-sized cells, generally uniform with only rare abrupt keratinized cell
  - Groups and syncytia with indistinct cell borders and brisk mitotic activity

Nuclear Details
- KSqCa: Markedly hyperchromatic nuclei with rare nucleoli
  - Some nuclei are ink black, and it may be difficult to view chromatinic characteristics
  - Dark granular irregular chromatin
- NKSqCa: Large nuclei, > 3x intermediate cell nucleus
  - Round nuclei with irregular nuclear borders
  - Naked nuclei and high nuclear:cytoplasmic ratios
  - Coarse, irregularly distributed chromatin with areas of clearing
  - Large/prominent nucleoli, some may be irregular

Cytoplasmic Details
- KSqCa
  - Varying degrees of orangeophilic cytoplasm with bizarre shapes
  - Tadpole shapes with Herxheimer spirals and keratohyaline granules in cytoplasm
- NKSqCa
  - Cells are round or irregular but all more or less equally abnormal in given case
  - Scant cyanophilic cytoplasm without keratinization

Squamous Cell Carcinoma of Cervix, Variants and Mimics

- Rare abruptly keratinized single cells may be seen
- May see focal columnar differentiation, including intracytoplasmic mucin droplets
- Small cell SqCa
  - Small cells with high nuclear:cytoplasmic ratios, no keratinization, mitotically active
  - Most small cell carcinomas are considered neuroendocrine (NE) carcinomas due to presence of NE markers

Adequacy Criteria
- Always adequate if abnormal cells are seen in spite of cellularity
- Malignant cells can hide in diathesis and blood
- Liquid-based samples can be lysed and reprocessed to better demonstrate cells

Cell Block Findings
- May be helpful in liquid-based preparation to sort NE carcinomas with use of immunohistochemistry (IHC) markers

Cytology-Histology Correlation
- Pap may be positive and biopsy negative if lesion is located high in canal
- Most cases of noncorrelation relate to tissue sampling variance
- Real-time correlation at time of biopsy sign-out will avoid delay in diagnosis

MICROSCOPIC

Morphologic Variants
- Spindle cell SqCa
- Lymphoepithelial-like carcinoma
  - Associated with better prognosis compared with conventional SqCa
- Verrucous carcinoma
  - Very minimal cytologic atypia
  - Associated with better prognosis compared with conventional SqCa
  - Less likely high-risk HPV(+)
- Papillary squamous and papillary squamotransitional carcinoma
  - Multilayered epithelium with variable degree of squamous &/or transitional cell differentiation covering true papillae with fibrovascular cores; cercariform/tadpole cells may be seen
- Basaloid squamous carcinoma
  - Small nests of basaloid cells with peripherally palisaded nuclei

ANCILLARY TESTS

Immunohistochemistry
- p63(+), p40(+)
- P16 diffusely, strongly positive in majority of high-risk HPV(+) cases

PCR
- High-risk HPV should be positive; however, real-world testing data shows 5-35% false-negative rates for variety of reasons, including analytic sensitivity of testing platform, low copy numbers, interfering substances, low epithelial cells, and other reasons resulting in test failure

DIFFERENTIAL DIAGNOSIS

DDx of Squamous Cell Carcinoma
- HSIL with inflammation
  - When involving endocervical glands, may mimic invasion
  - May be marked during pregnancy or inflammation for other reasons
  - Lacks nucleoli, broken-down blood, diathesis, and fewer mitoses
- Adenocarcinoma
  - IHC on cell block from residual material will be p40(-) in adenocarcinomas
- Small cell NE carcinoma
  - Mimic of small cell nonkeratinizing carcinoma and basaloid SqCa
  - Mitotically active small cells with nuclear molding is often present
  - p63(-); chromogranin and synaptophysin are often positive
- Epithelioid trophoblastic tumor
  - Features sheets and nests of round to slightly spindle-shaped trophoblasts
  - Within nests, trophoblasts are arranged around necrotic or hyaline-like material
  - Apparent nuclear pleomorphism and nucleoli
  - Inhibin(+), p63(+), HPL(-)
- Atrophy with atypia
  - Usually background of atrophic vaginitis should make one wary
  - Rarely degenerated dyskeratotic squamous cells
- Menstrual pattern endometrium, especially on liquid-based preparations
  - Initial appearance can be alarming, including diathesis
  - Look for geometry to glands, tubular shapes
  - Stromal cells are clue to endometrial etiology
  - Correlate with last menstrual period, if known
  - Cell block from liquid-based preparations can resolve issue
  - p16, ProEx C, and CD10 IHC helps in difficult cases
- Atypical repair
  - Flat sheets, large regular nuclei, no increase in nuclear:cytoplasmic ratio
  - No atypical mitosis or diathesis
- Pemphigus vulgaris and Behçet disease
  - These rare entities can occasionally shed dyskeratotic and abnormal cells
  - Being aware of patient's history helps to avoid pitfalls

SELECTED REFERENCES

1. Lee Y et al: Liquid-based cytology features of papillary squamotransitional cell carcinoma of the uterine cervix. J Pathol Transl Med. 53(5):341-4, 2019

Squamous Cell Carcinoma of Cervix, Variants and Mimics

Keratinizing Squamous Cell Carcinoma on SurePath

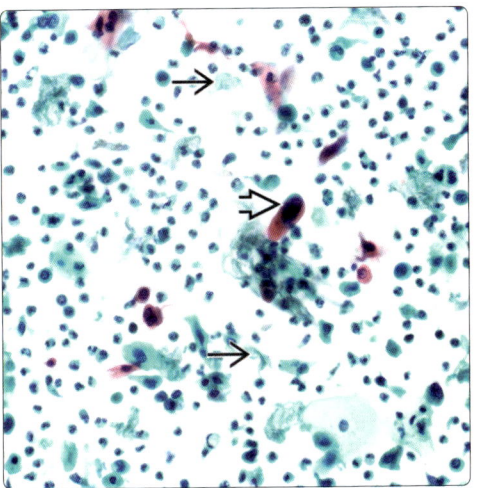

Squamous Cell Carcinoma Difficult to Distinguish From Keratinizing HSIL

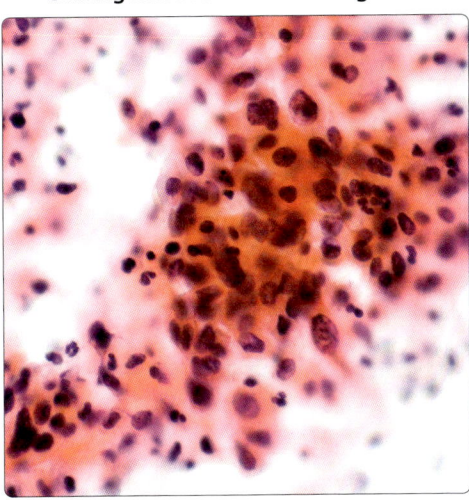

(Left) Keratinizing squamous cell carcinoma (KSqCa) on SurePath Pap test shows a cellular specimen with diathesis ⇨ and inflammation in which large keratinized malignant cells ⇨ are easily seen. (Right) Pap-stained conventional smear shows KSqCa, which, in the absence of diathesis or bizarre tadpole cells, may be difficult to distinguish from a keratinizing high-grade squamous intraepithelial lesion (HSIL).

Bizarre Cells in Squamous Cell Carcinoma

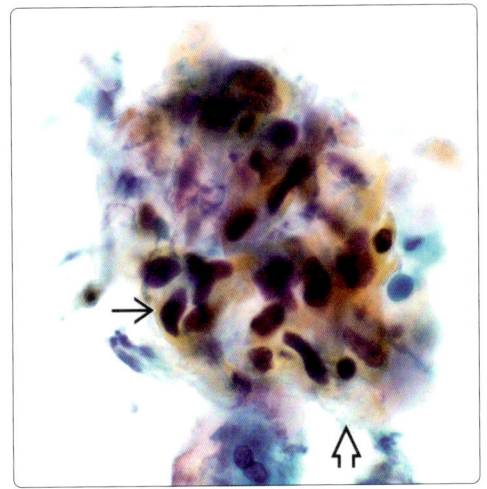

Spindled Malignant Cells

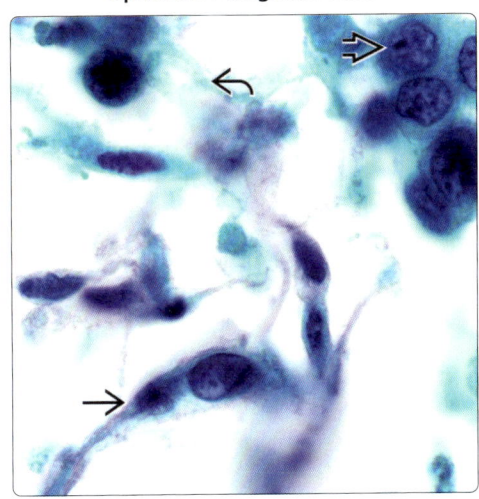

(Left) ThinPrep Pap test shows spindle and bizarre cells ⇨ of a KSqCa. Note the subtle clinging diathesis ⇨ along the periphery with an otherwise clean background. (Right) ThinPrep Pap test shows spindled malignant cells ⇨ and rounded cells ⇨ with nucleoli, irregular nuclear contours, and cyanophilic cytoplasm. Note that keratinized cells do not always stain orange. A subtle diathesis ⇨ is seen.

Fiber Cells of Squamous Cell Carcinoma

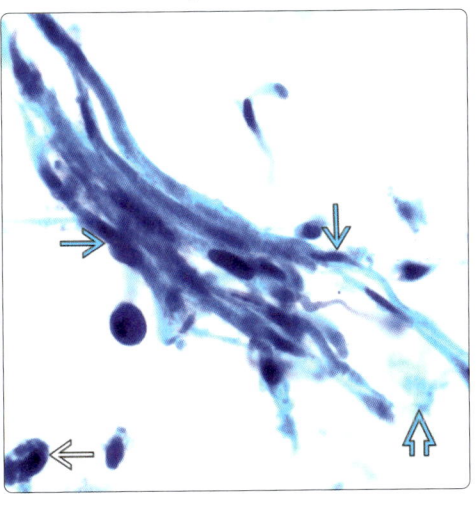

Eosinophilic and Cyanophilic Bizarre Cells

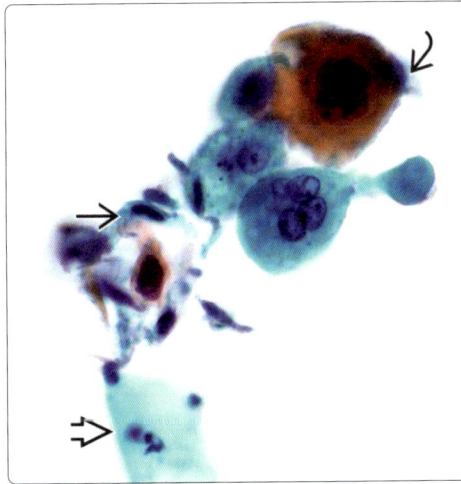

(Left) ThinPrep Pap test shows long skinny cells/fiber cells ⇨ of squamous cell carcinoma. The Pap is atrophic with only parabasal cells ⇨ in the background. The diathesis ⇨ is subtle. (Right) SurePath Pap test shows eosinophilic and cyanophilic bizarre cells along with spindle cells ⇨ with a rare normal squamous cell ⇨ for size comparison. Diathesis is absent or very subtle and of the clinging type ⇨.

Squamous Cell Carcinoma of Cervix, Variants and Mimics

Syncytial Squamous Cell Carcinoma on Conventional Smear

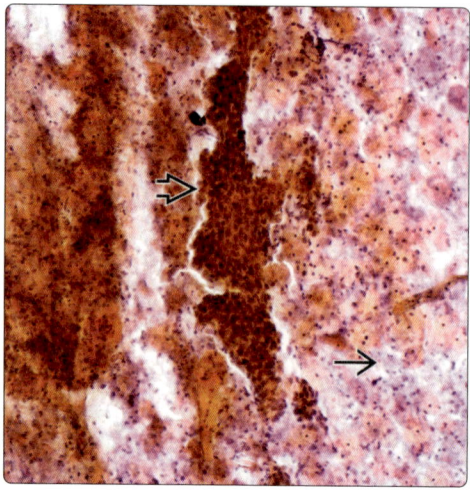

Various Cell Types in Squamous Cell Carcinoma

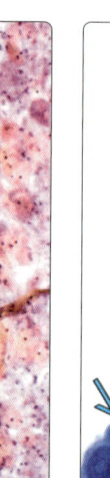

(Left) Conventional Pap shows a large syncytium ➡ of crowded cells such that cell boundaries cannot be separated. Smaller groups are also present in a diffuse precipitate of background diathesis ➡. (Right) SurePath Pap test shows the various cell types in squamous cell carcinoma in a postmenopausal patient. There are eosinophilic keratinizing malignant cells ➡ with low nuclear:cytoplasmic ratios and smaller cells which resemble HSIL ➡. Diathesis is subtle and clinging type ➡.

HSIL-Like Squamous Cell Carcinoma With Diathesis

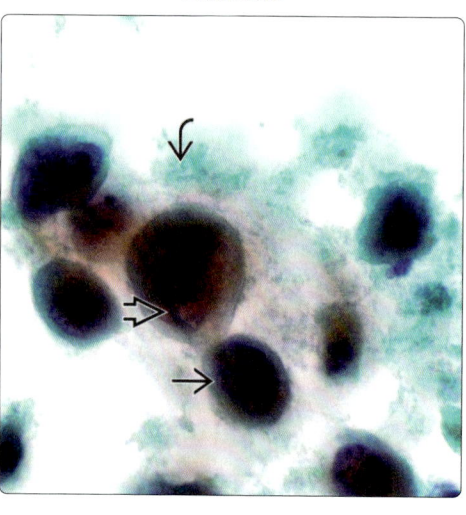

Nonkeratinizing Squamous Cell Carcinoma Histology

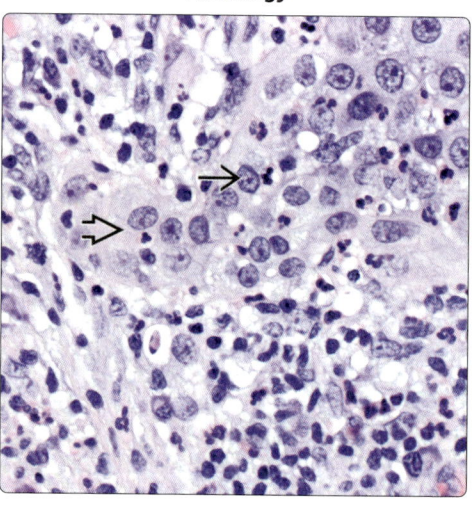

(Left) ThinPrep Pap test shows rounded cells of varying sizes in a precipitate of diathesis ➡. The nuclear contours are irregular with chromatinic clearing and nucleoli in some cells ➡, whereas other cells resemble HSIL ➡. The pleomorphism, nucleoli, and diathesis are clues to the invasive nature of the tumor. (Right) H&E-stained section of nests shows NKSqCa with nucleoli ➡ and paradoxical maturation where the cells acquire increased cytoplasm ➡, unlike HSIL cells.

Nonkeratinizing Squamous Carcinoma With Abrupt Keratinization

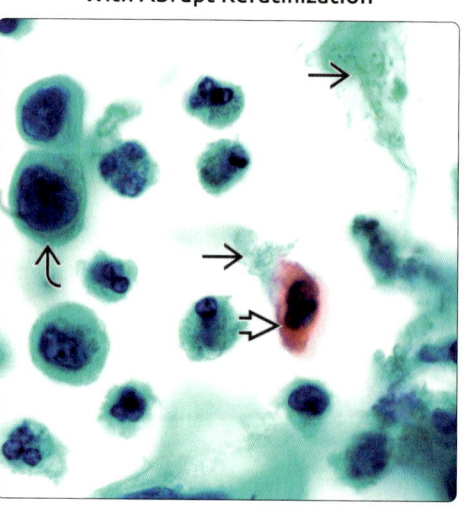

Histology of Nonkeratinizing Squamous Carcinoma With Abrupt Keratinization

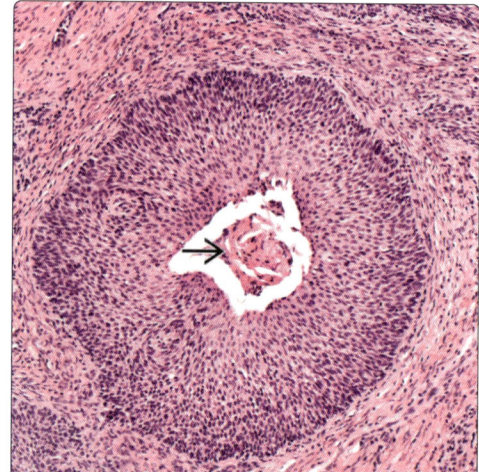

(Left) NKSqCa is shown on SurePath Pap test. Many cells resemble HSIL but with more pleomorphism and irregular chromatinic clearing ➡. The background is wispy, and clinging diathesis is seen ➡. An abruptly keratinized cell ➡ is occasionally encountered. These originate from the center of necrotic nests of tumor. Background inflammatory cells can be used for size comparison. (Right) H&E shows a nest of NKSqCa with abrupt keratinization and necrosis ➡.

Squamous Cell Carcinoma of Cervix, Variants and Mimics

Bloody ThinPrep With Entrapped Cells

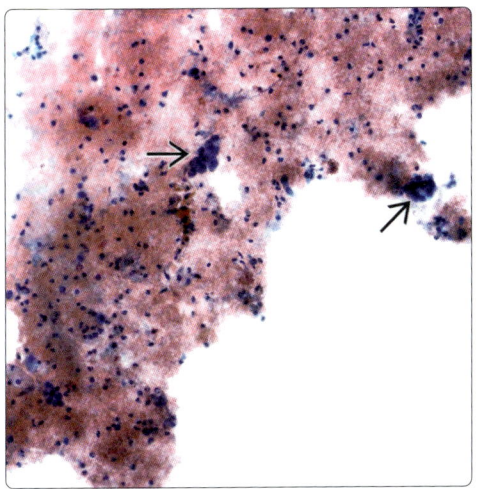

Reprocessed ThinPrep Showing Carcinoma

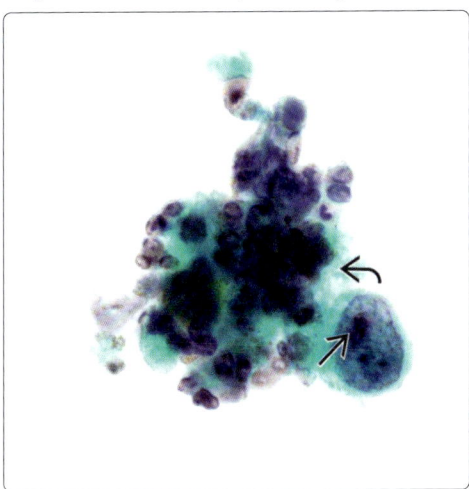

(Left) ThinPrep Pap test shows a bloody circumferential ring with a few entrapped malignant cells ➡. In the absence of abnormal cells, these cases may be misdiagnosed as unsatisfactory. (Right) Reprocessed and lysed ThinPrep Pap test shows a large malignant cell with irregular nuclear outline and large nucleolus ➡ at the edge of diathesis consisting of fibrin and trapped inflammatory cells ➡. Bloody unsatisfactory tests may hide cancers. Lyse and reprep the case.

Postradiation Atypical Repair

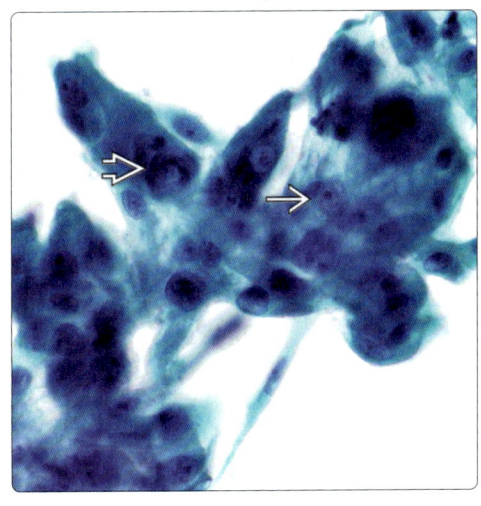

Atrophic Vaginitis on Conventional Smear

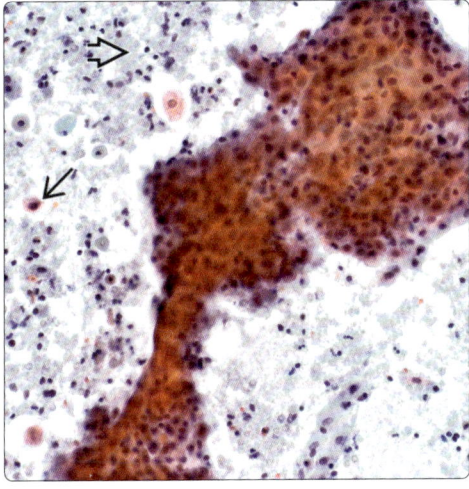

(Left) ThinPrep Pap test shows postradiation atypia characterized by mostly flat sheets of large spindle and polygonal cells with abnormal shapes and sizes, prominent nucleoli ➡, and abnormally smudged chromatin ➡. There is still plenty of cytoplasm with a normal nuclear:cytoplasmic ratio and a clean background. (Right) Conventional Pap smear shows atrophic vaginitis. The background of pseudodiathesis ➡ with dyskeratotic cells ➡ can result in overdiagnosis.

Endometrial Cells With Diathesis

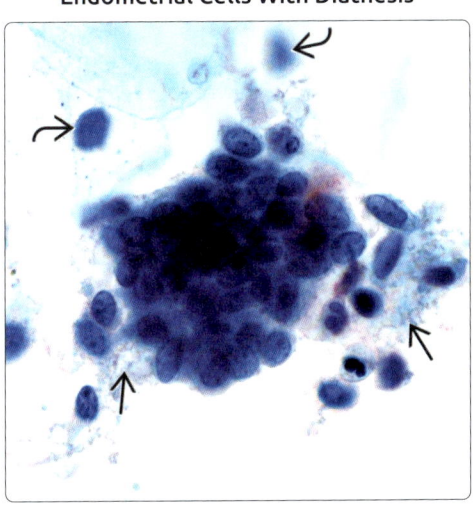

Keratinizing Squamous Cell Carcinoma Without Diathesis

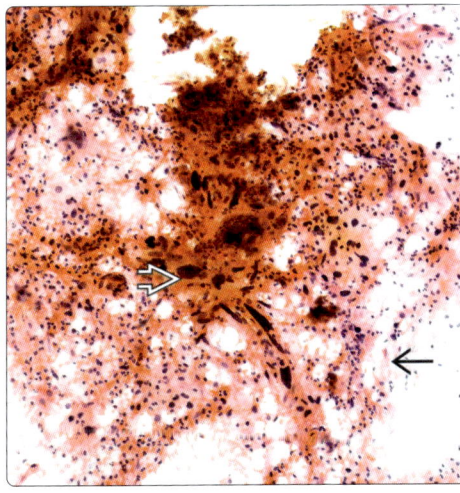

(Left) Endometrial cells with diathesis-like ➡ appearance due to partially lysed blood may be mistaken for SqCa. The small size of the cells compared with the nuclei ➡ of intermediate cells in the background is helpful. Cell blocks from residual material in a liquid-based vial can help. (Right) Conventional Pap smear shows KSqCa with a background of mostly intact red blood cells ➡. The bizarre malignant cells ➡ are easy to recognize even at low magnification, but diathesis may be lacking in KSqCas.

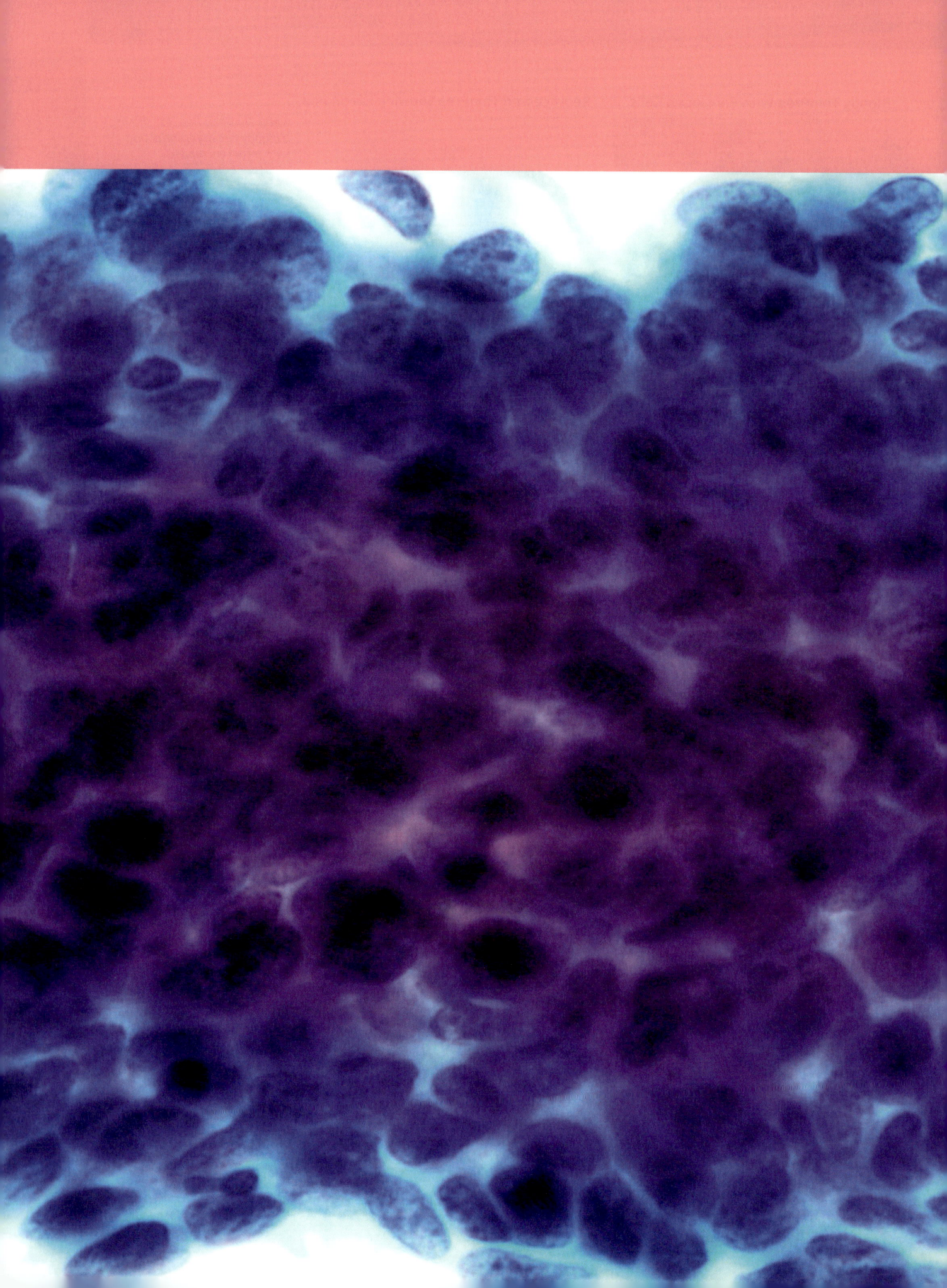

PART I
SECTION 4
Glandular Cell Abnormalities and Mimics

Endocervical Adenocarcinoma In Situ, Variants and Mimics	46
Endocervical Adenocarcinoma, Variants and Mimics	52
Adenocarcinoma, Gastric Type	56
Endometrial Cancers: Usual Types, Variants, and Mimics	58
Atypical Glandular Cells: Endocervicals, Endometrials, and Glandulars, NOS	64
Endometrial Cells in Pap Test and Glandular Cells Status Post Hysterectomy	70

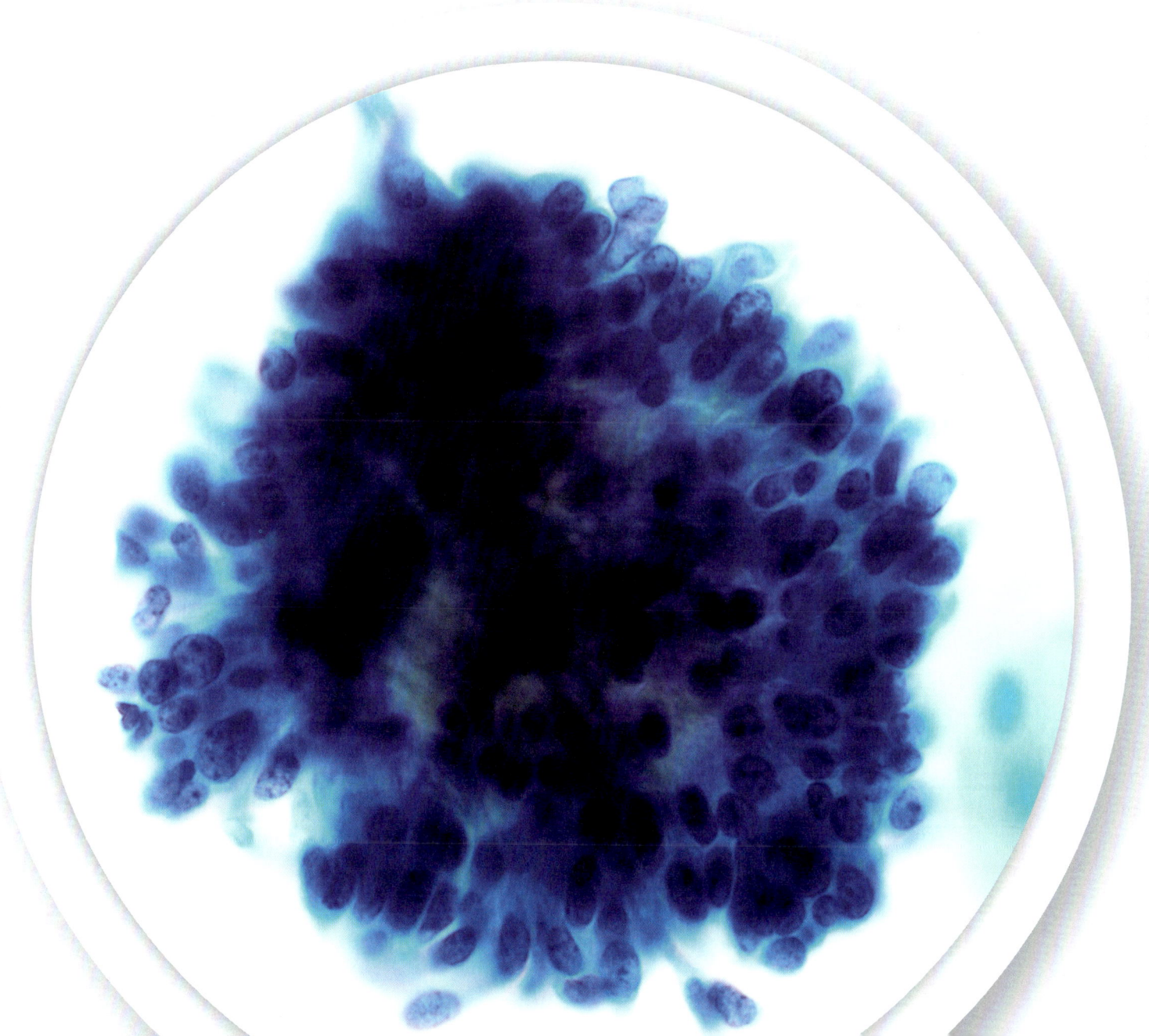

Endocervical Adenocarcinoma In Situ, Variants and Mimics

KEY FACTS

CLINICAL ISSUES
- Mean age: 38 years; WHO classifies as human papillomavirus (HPV)-dependent (~ 90% of cases) and HPV-independent types (gastric)
- Often coexistent squamous intraepithelial lesion in 50-70% of HPV-dependent cases
- Atypical glandular cells or adenocarcinoma in situ (AIS) on Pap test

CYTOPATHOLOGY
- Findings on Pap smear/test
  - Hyperchromatic nuclei in crowded groups (overlapping nuclei) and strips
  - Peripheral feathering of neoplastic cells may be seen, better on conventional than liquid-based Pap tests
  - May form rosette-like structures
  - Sheet, strips, and torn gland forms with polarization of nuclei perpendicular to circumferential axis
- Oval or elongated hyperchromatic nuclei with increased N:C ratios and nuclear overlap/crowding
- Nuclei bulge out from center of cytoplasm, imparting snake egg appearance
- Cytoplasmic characteristics vary based on AIS type
- Most types are mixed
- Endometrioid variant has small cells and lacks cytoplasmic mucin

ANCILLARY TESTS
- High-risk HPV(+) on Pap test, especially HPV-18, HPV-16, 45
- p16 block (+), ProEx C, and Ki-67 (+)

TOP DIFFERENTIAL DIAGNOSES
- High-grade squamous intraepithelial lesion
- Invasive endocervical adenocarcinoma
- Reactive/repair/radiation changes in endocervix
- Tubal metaplasia, polyps, artefacts
- Endometrium/endometriosis, directly sampled

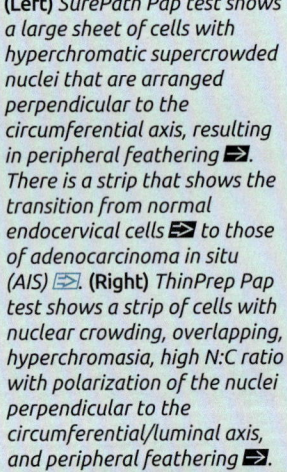

(Left) SurePath Pap test shows a large sheet of cells with hyperchromatic supercrowded nuclei that are arranged perpendicular to the circumferential axis, resulting in peripheral feathering ➡. There is a strip that shows the transition from normal endocervical cells ➡ to those of adenocarcinoma in situ (AIS) ➡. (Right) ThinPrep Pap test shows a strip of cells with nuclear crowding, overlapping, hyperchromasia, high N:C ratio with polarization of the nuclei perpendicular to the circumferential/luminal axis, and peripheral feathering ➡.

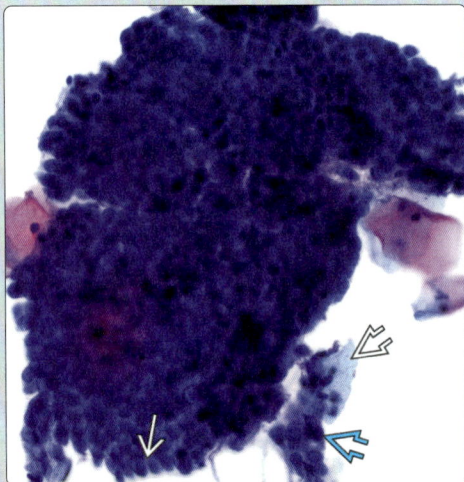

Large Sheet With Nuclear Supercrowding

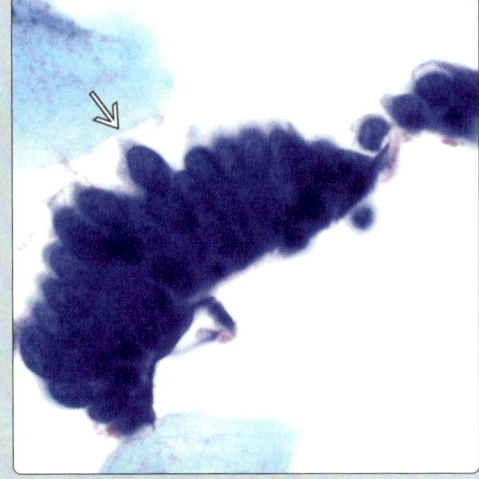

Strip of AIS, HPV-Associated

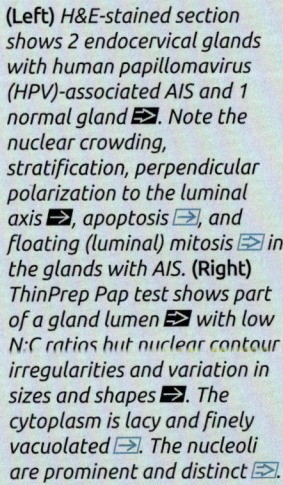

(Left) H&E-stained section shows 2 endocervical glands with human papillomavirus (HPV)-associated AIS and 1 normal gland ➡. Note the nuclear crowding, stratification, perpendicular polarization to the luminal axis ➡, apoptosis ➡, and floating (luminal) mitosis ➡ in the glands with AIS. (Right) ThinPrep Pap test shows part of a gland lumen ➡ with low N:C ratios but nuclear contour irregularities and variation in sizes and shapes ➡. The cytoplasm is lacy and finely vacuolated ➡. The nucleoli are prominent and distinct ➡.

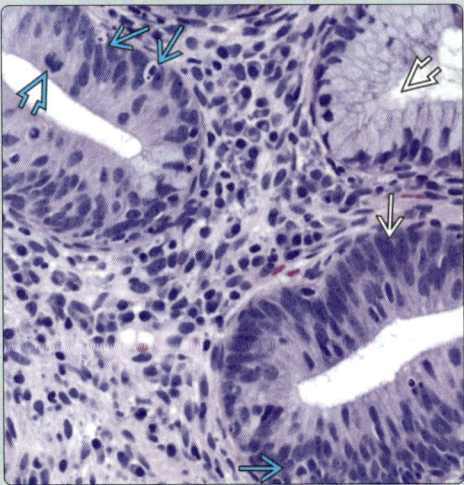

HPV-Associated AIS of Cervix

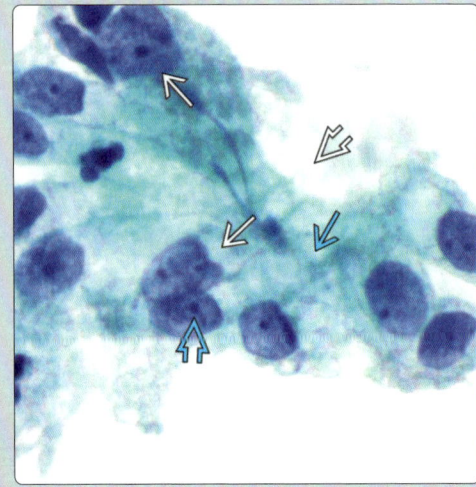

Gland From Gastric-Type AIS

Endocervical Adenocarcinoma In Situ, Variants and Mimics

TERMINOLOGY

Abbreviations
- Adenocarcinoma in situ (AIS)

Definitions
- Neoplastic endocervical glandular precursor of invasive adenocarcinoma
  - WHO classifies AIS into human papillomavirus (HPV)-associated (~ 90%) and HPV-independent gastric type

ETIOLOGY/PATHOGENESIS

Infectious Agents
- High-risk (HPV) infection (80-90%; HPV-18, 16, and 45 most common)

CLINICAL ISSUES

Presentation
- Asymptomatic; rarely, vaginal bleeding
- Atypical glandular/endocervical cells or AIS on Pap smear/test

Treatment
- Excision (cold knife cone), hysterectomy

CYTOPATHOLOGY

Cellularity
- Usually cellular specimens but can be variable
- Hyperchromatic crowded groups and strips
- Clean (liquid-based) or intact RBCs (conventional smears)

Cells
- Sheets, strips, and torn gland forms with polarization of nuclei perpendicular to circumferential or luminal axis
- Peripheral feathering of neoplastic cells due to polarization and wisps of cytoplasm
- May form rosette-like structures, which may be difficult to appreciate on liquid-based preparations
- On liquid-based specimens, sheets will be smaller, and peripheral feathering is muted and appears as peripheral knuckles
- SurePath preparations have more strips and single cells
- Fish tail or bird tail appearance of strips on SurePath
- Endometrioid type of AIS may be difficult due to smaller cells, no cytoplasmic mucin, and subtle strips
- HPV-independent, gastric type of AIS lacks many of features seen in HPV-related AIS and may be missed

Nuclear Details
- Oval, elongated, and hyperchromatic with increased nuclear:cytoplasmic (N:C) ratios and evenly dispersed chromatin
  - All cells are more or less similar with little or no pleomorphism
    - Mitosis and apoptosis may be difficult to appreciate on cytologic samples
- Gastric type of AIS has open vesicular chromatin with nucleoli; mitosis and apoptosis may be subtle/absent

Cytoplasmic Details
- Can vary depending on stain and variant of AIS
  - Eosinophilic or cyanophilic, ± goblet cells
    - Endometrioid types lack mucin, have scant cytoplasm, and may be mistaken for endometrial cells
    - Gastric type has abundant vacuolated gastric-type mucinous cytoplasm (yellow tinge on conventional Paps)

ANCILLARY TESTS

Immunohistochemistry
- p16 (diffuse) (+) in HPV-associated type (~ 90% of cases)
- Ki-67 proliferative index typically high (> 75%)
- Gastric type (not HPV associated) is MUC6 and HIK1083 (+) but HPV(-)

HPV Detection
- PCR or in situ hybridization for HPV-associated types

DIFFERENTIAL DIAGNOSIS

Invasive Endocervical Adenocarcinoma
- Diathesis in background, which varies depending on preparation type
- More rounded vesicular nuclei with nucleoli
- Nuclear pleomorphism and polarization (may be lost)

Reactive Endocervical Glands
- Flat sheets, school of fish appearance
- N:C ratio is preserved
- Usually dispersed chromatin with prominent nucleoli
- Radiation may result in bizarre sizes and shapes with vacuoles but preservation of N:C ratio
- p16 (-) to focally (+)

Tubal Metaplasia
- Very few/rare groups or strips
- Lacks other patterns of AIS
- Chromatin is powdery or watery
- Terminal bars and cilia are key for diagnosis
- No mitosis and apoptosis
- p16 focal/patchy positivity unlike AIS, which stains every cell

Endometriosis or Directly Sampled Lower Uterine Segment
- Geometrically shaped/tubular glands ± plump spindle stromal cells
- Directly sampled endometrium will show strips that lack classic feathering
- Epithelial cells are small and may ball up
- If unlysed, background blood may resemble diathesis and is trap
- Cell block from liquid-based specimens can help in avoiding overcall as adenocarcinoma or AIS
- p16 on cell block is negative or shows rare/patchy positivity

Posttrachelectomy Sampling
- Lower uterine segment is attached to vaginal vault in this fertility-sparing procedure for early cervical cancer
- 1/3 of follow-up Paps will show endometrium

Arias-Stella Reaction
- History of pregnancy or hormonal therapy

Endocervical Adenocarcinoma In Situ, Variants and Mimics

Comparison Between Conventional Pap Smear and Liquid-Based Technologies

Cytologic Criteria	Conventional Smear	ThinPrep	SurePath
Cellularity	Cellular	Variable	Variable
Sheets	Large	Smaller	Small, dispersed
Strips	Present, few	Present, few	Present, many
Feathering	Present, low-power recognition	Present but can be subtle	Present but can be subtle
Rosettes	Present	Present but 3D	Present but subtle
Mitosis/apoptosis	May or may not be present	Difficult to visualize	Difficult to visualize
3D groups	Usually flat	Mostly rounded/3D	Present
Single AIS cells	Unusual	Present, few	Present, many
Nuclear shape	Oval/cigar-shaped	Oval/rounded	Oval
Nucleoli	Absent	Chromocenters/rare	Chromocenters/rare
Background	Clean or intact RBCs	Clean	Clean

Adenocarcinoma In Situ and Mimics

Cytologic Criteria	AIS	HSIL	Repair	Tubal Metaplasia	Directly Sampled Endometrium
Cellularity	Cellular	Usually cellular	Rare fragments	Rare event	Few groups
Hyperchromatic crowded groups	Many	Can be many	Not present	Rare event	Present
Sheets	Many with feathering	Syncytia	Flat sheets	Absent/rare/small	Present, 3D
Nuclear crowding/overlap	Present	Present	Absent	Present but mild	Present
Nuclear polarization perpendicular	Present	Absent	Absent	Present	Can be present
Hyperchromasia	Present	Present	Absent	Mild	Mild
Nuclear shape	Oval/elongated	Round	Round	Oval/cigar-shaped	Oval/cigar-shaped
Peripheral feathering	Present	Absent/focal	Absent	Rare	Absent
Strips	Present	Absent	Absent	Present	Present
Rosettes	Present	Absent	Absent	Absent	May be present
Terminal bars/cilia	Absent	Absent	Absent	Present/diagnostic	May be present
Spindled stroma	Absent	Absent	Absent	Absent	Present
Mitosis/apoptosis	May or may not be present	May be seen	Rare	Absent	May be present
p16	Block-positive pattern	Block-positive pattern	Negative	Patchy positive	Patchy/focal/rare cells positive

AIS = adenocarcinoma in situ; HSIL = high-grade squamous intraepithelial lesion.

- Abundant eosinophilic to vacuolated cytoplasm with preserved N:C ratio
- No mitoses or apoptotic bodies

Endometrial Polyps
- Directly sampled endometrial or lower uterine polyps can have endometrial glandular or stromal fragments

High-Grade Squamous Intraepithelial Lesion
- 50-70% of HPV-associated AIS have coexisting squamous intraepithelial lesion
- Lack of peripheral feathering; instead, peripheral flattening or rounding of hyperchromatic crowded groups (HCGs) of cells
- Cells round instead of columnar and usually larger than cells of AIS
- Cells parallel to circumferential axis of HCG

SELECTED REFERENCES
1. Lashmanova N et al: Endocervical adenocarcinoma in situ-from Papanicolaou test to hysterectomy: a series of 74 cases. J Am Soc Cytopathol. 11(1):13-20, 2022
2. Lin M et al: False-negative Papanicolaou tests in women with biopsy-proven invasive endocervical adenocarcinoma/adenocarcinoma in situ: a retrospective analysis with assessment of interobserver agreement. J Am Soc Cytopathol. 11(1):3-12, 2022
3. Bruehl FK et al: Cytology and curetting diagnosis of endocervical adenocarcinoma. J Am Soc Cytopathol. 9(6):556-62, 2020
4. Niu S et al: Challenges in the Pap diagnosis of endocervical adenocarcinoma in situ. J Am Soc Cytopathol. 8(3):141-8, 2019
5. Nayar R et al: The Bethesda System for Reporting Cervical Cytology: Definitions, Criteria, and Explanatory Notes. 3rd ed. Springer-Verlag, 2015

Endocervical Adenocarcinoma In Situ, Variants and Mimics

AIS Configuration (Large Sheets With Feathering) on Conventional Pap

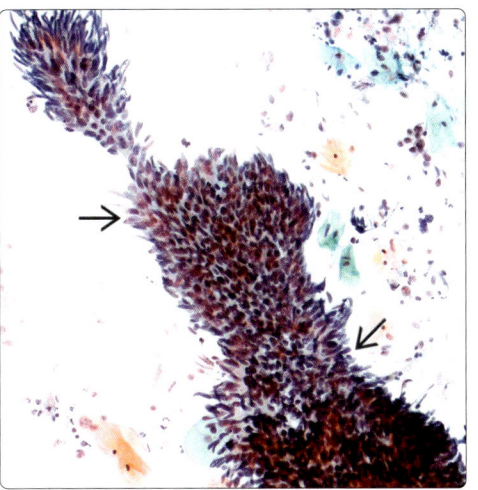

Strips and Torn Glands of AIS on Conventional Pap

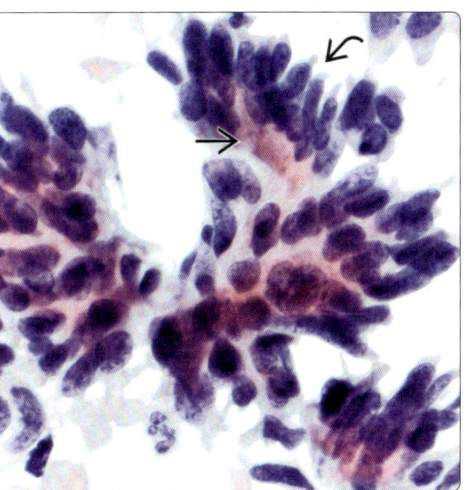

(Left) Large sheets of endocervical cells with nuclear overcrowding, polarization, and peripheral feathering ⇒ are seen on this conventional Pap smear. The background is clean, and no single intact AIS cells are seen. **(Right)** Pap-stained conventional smear shows strips and torn gland forms lined by columnar epithelium. Note the polarization of the nuclei perpendicular to the luminal axis ⇒ and peripheral feathering ⇒.

Strips of AIS Nuclear Details

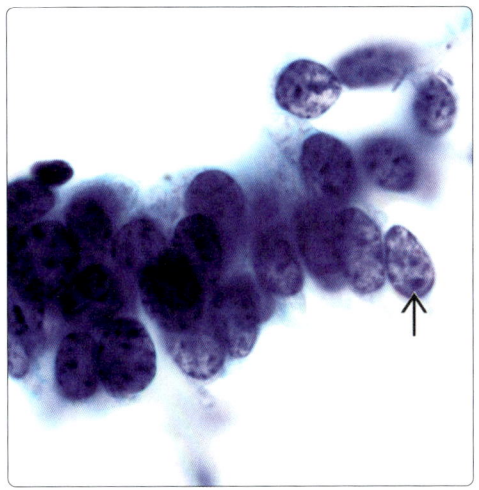

Fish Tail Configuration of AIS Strip on SurePath Pap Test

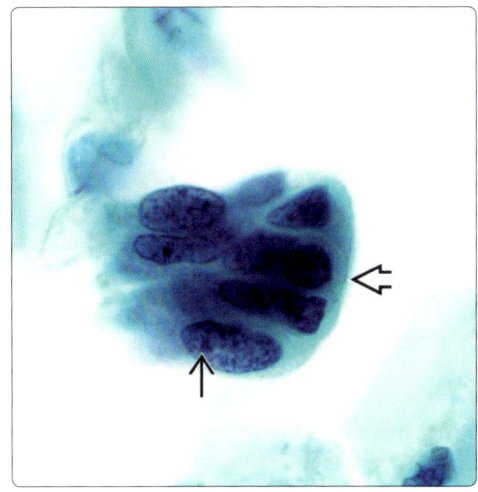

(Left) ThinPrep Pap test shows a strip of AIS. N:C ratio is increased, and nuclear crowding, polarization, and feathering are seen. Nuclei are hyperchromatic and may show chromocenters ⇒ in liquid-based preparations. **(Right)** Fish tail appearance of a short strip of hyperchromatic, crowded, and overlapping cells of AIS splayed out on luminal side ⇒. This is a characteristic appearance on SurePath Paps when seen and is diagnostic. Note the high N:C ratio and small cell size compared to background squamous cells. A rare chromocenter is seen ⇒.

Rosette of AIS With Nuclear Details on Liquid-Based Pap

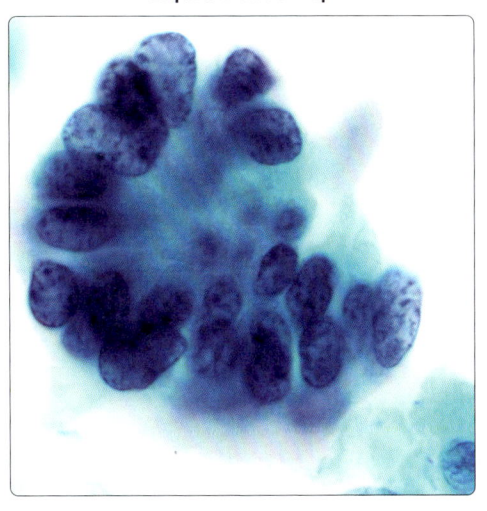

Rosette of AIS on Conventional Pap

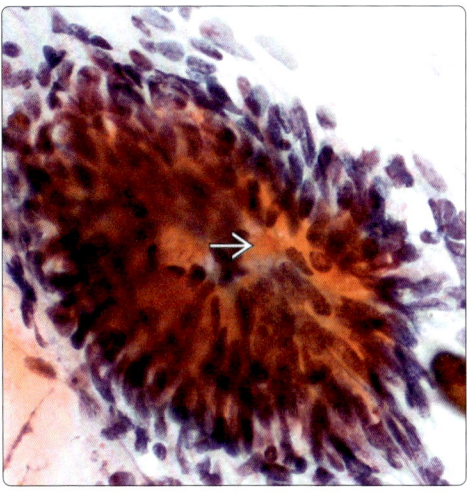

(Left) ThinPrep Pap test shows a rosette of oval nuclei with hyperchromasia, overlapping, high N:C ratios, and dispersed chromatin. Nuclear polarization is perpendicular to the circumferential axis. **(Right)** Conventional Pap shows endocervical AIS with a complete rosette. The oval elongated nuclei with hyperchromasia and overlapping radiate from the center to the periphery, recapitulating an entire gland as seen on histology. Note the fine endocervical-type mucin ⇒.

Endocervical Adenocarcinoma In Situ, Variants and Mimics

Hyperchromatic Crowded Groups of AIS on Liquid-Based Pap

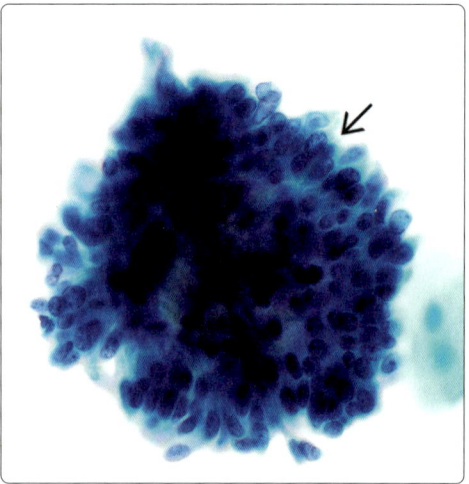

p16 Block Staining Pattern of AIS

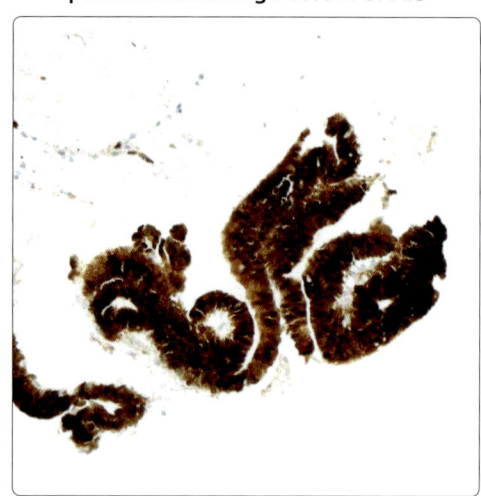

(Left) Large sheet of hyperchromatic crowded endocervical cells with peripheral palisading/feathering ➡ is seen on this SurePath Pap test. Due to the rounding of cells in liquid-based preparations, the center of the sheet is difficult to visualize. (Right) Strips of AIS on cell block of residual Pap test fluid with strong block-positive stain for p16 are shown. Cell blocks can be a useful adjunct in select cases.

Strip of Tubal Metaplasia

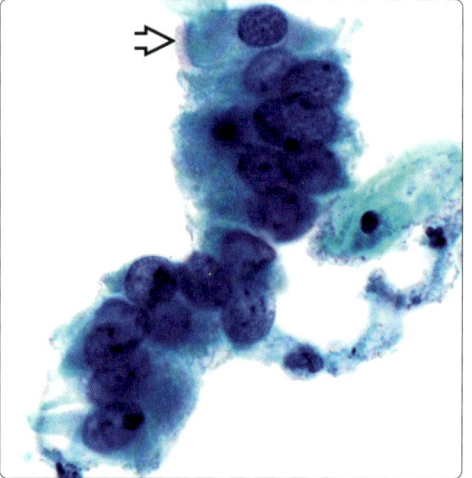

Strip of Tubal Metaplasia With Patchy p16

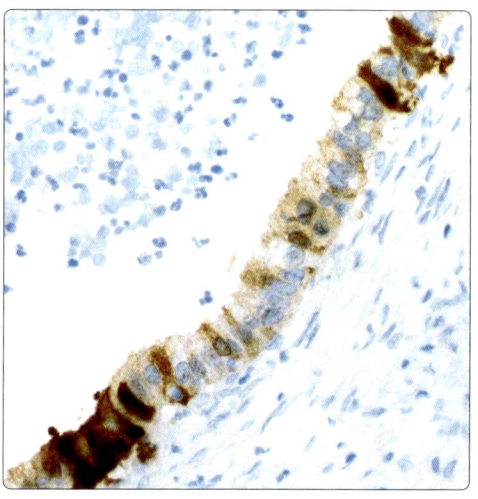

(Left) ThinPrep Pap test shows a rare strip of cells with tubal metaplasia. The terminal bar and cilia are visible only on the very top cell ➡. The nuclei are round, and the N:C ratio is not high. (Right) Contrast the patchy p16 staining pattern of tubal metaplasia with the block staining pattern seen in AIS. Positive p16 in individual glandular cells or small groups must be interpreted with caution.

Hyperchromatic Crowded Group of Cells of Tubal Metaplasia

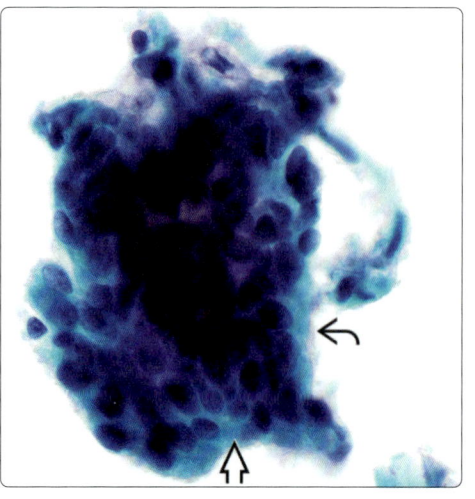

HSIL Presenting as Hyperchromatic Crowded Group on Liquid-Based Pap

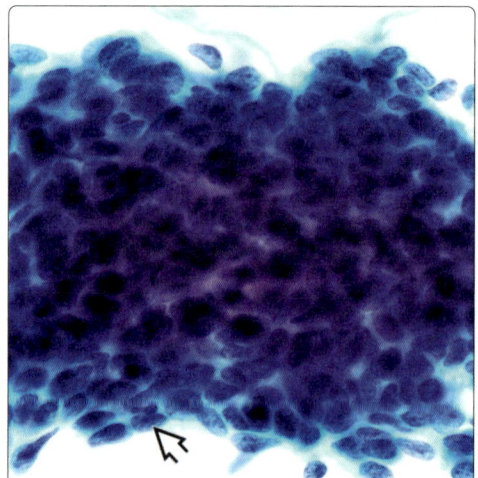

(Left) ThinPrep Pap test shows a crowded sheet. The edge focally shows terminal bars and cilia ➡. The lower edge ➡ shows that the N:C ratio is not increased. These were the only concerning cells in the Pap test with benign follow-up and high-risk HPV(-). (Right) SurePath Pap test shows hyperchromatic syncytium of high-grade squamous intraepithelial lesion (HSIL) cells. There is no nuclear polarization perpendicular to the circumferential axis. The cells flatten out along the periphery ➡. Contrast this with the image of AIS.

Endocervical Adenocarcinoma In Situ, Variants and Mimics

Cervical Endometriosis Mimicking AIS or Adenocarcinoma of Cervix

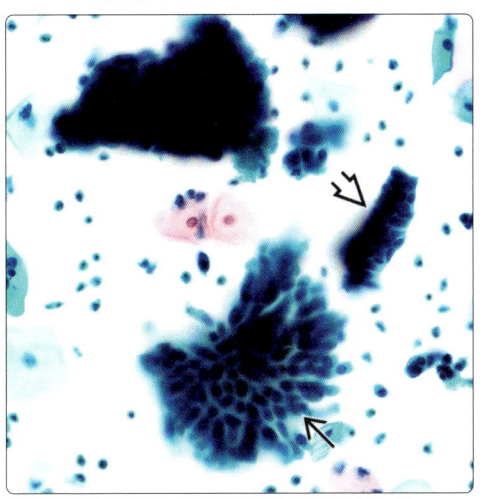

Tubular Endometrial Gland on Pap

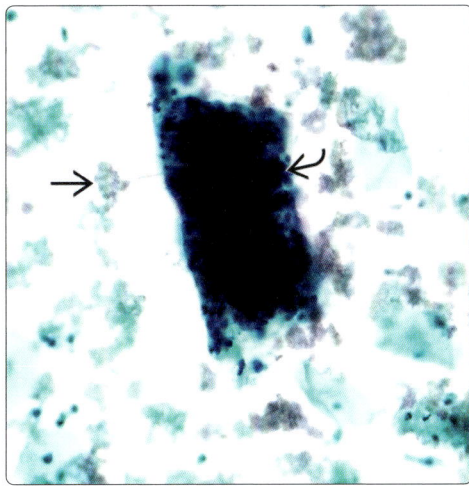

(Left) SurePath Pap test of endometriosis of cervix shows strips ⇨ and sheets of small endometrial cells in an inflammatory background. Some feathering is also noted ⇨. *(Right)* SurePath Pap test of tubular endometrial gland ⇨ shows a bloody background ⇨ that may be worrisome for diathesis. The last menstrual period can be very helpful in such cases. Cell block with p16 staining can help clarify the issue, especially post conization for high-grade dysplasia or AIS.

Endometrial Stromal Fragment on Liquid-Based Pap

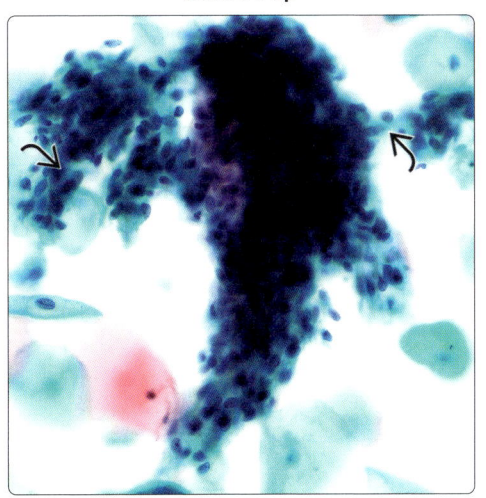

Flat Sheets of Radiation/Repair

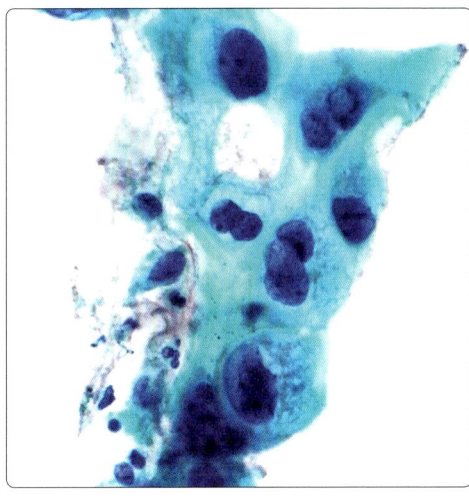

(Left) Endometrial stroma separated from glands on a SurePath Pap test is from a case of cervical endometriosis. The cells are plump and bipolar. Blood vessels ⇨ coursing through stroma is a helpful cytologic feature. Otherwise, cell block on a liquid-based specimen with p16 immunostaining, if necessary, can resolve the issue. *(Right)* ThinPrep Pap test shows a flat sheet of endocervical and metaplastic cells with changes of radiation and repair. N:C ratio is maintained despite abnormal nuclear features.

Arias Stella on Pap

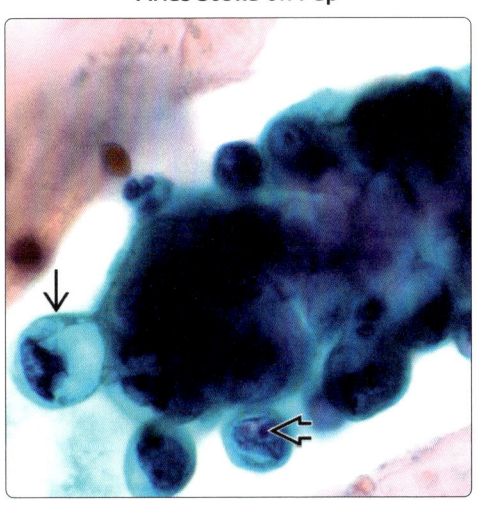

Normal Endocervical Cells With Feathering

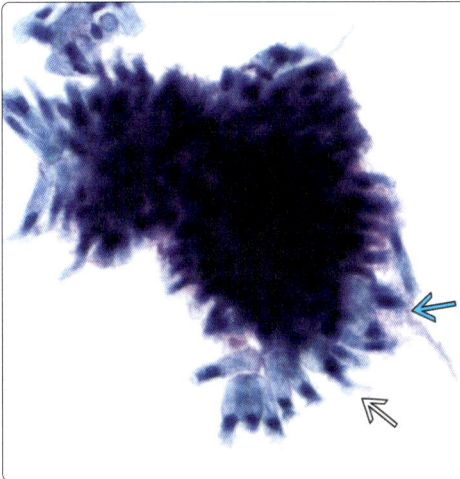

(Left) A pregnant 20-year-old had an Arias-Stella reaction. Large bubbly ⇨ vacuolated cells with nucleoli and abnormal nuclear shapes ⇨ are seen. It was the only group on ThinPrep Pap to disappear on Pap tests after pregnancy. *(Right)* ThinPrep Pap test post LEEP shows a large sheet of normal endocervical cells with low N:C ratios, lack of hyperchromasia, but with feathering at the periphery ⇨. All cells appear stretched and hence distorted from the diathermy. Fresh, partly lysed blood is seen clinging to the periphery of the cluster ⇨.

Endocervical Adenocarcinoma, Variants and Mimics

KEY FACTS

ETIOLOGY/PATHOGENESIS
- High-risk human papillomavirus (HPV) infection (~ 90%)
- Rising relative to squamous cell carcinomas of cervix, 20-30% of cervical cancers

CYTOPATHOLOGY
- Usually cellular irrespective of preparation type (conventional Pap smear vs. liquid based)
- Strips, rosettes, 3D groups, large sheets ± abnormal configurations, single intact malignant cells, cell balls
- Well-differentiated carcinomas and early invasive tumors will resemble adenocarcinoma (ACA) in situ (AIS)
- Columnar configuration of cells arranged in sheets, rosettes, and strips but with some loss of polarity and pleomorphism within group, strip, or rosette
- Chromatin becomes vesicular, and nucleoli appear as tumor becomes invasive
- Nuclear membrane irregularity and pleomorphism increase with increasing grade as does mitotic activity
- Large and irregular or multiple nucleoli with increasing grade and invasiveness
- Cytoplasm is finely vacuolated and diathesis in background
- Diathesis varies by preparation type
- May coexist with squamous intraepithelial lesion or squamous cancer, rarely small cell carcinoma
- Cells from tumors originating high in canal ball up and may be difficult to distinguish from endometrial cancers

ANCILLARY TESTS
- Helpful in differentiating primary
  - Endocervical: HPV, ProEx C, and CEA (+), p16 in block pattern; vimentin, ER, and PR (-)
  - Endometrial: ProEx C and CEA (-), p16 may be patchy; vimentin, ER, and PR (+)

TOP DIFFERENTIAL DIAGNOSES
- AIS ± early invasion, squamous carcinoma, morphologic variants of cervical ACA, endometrial ACA, repair/atypical repair, Arias-Stella reaction, microglandular hyperplasia

Diathesis and Low Power of Endocervical Adenocarcinoma on ThinPrep
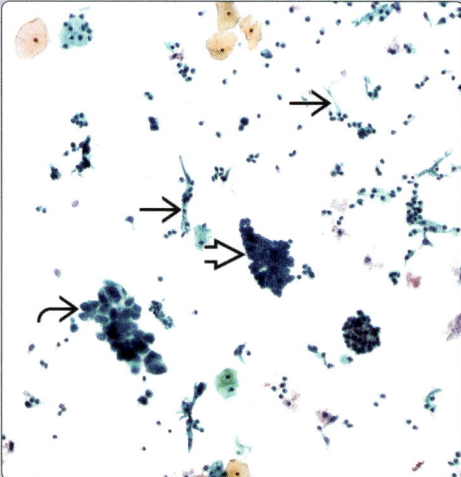

Architectural and Nuclear Features of Endocervical Adenocarcinoma on ThinPrep
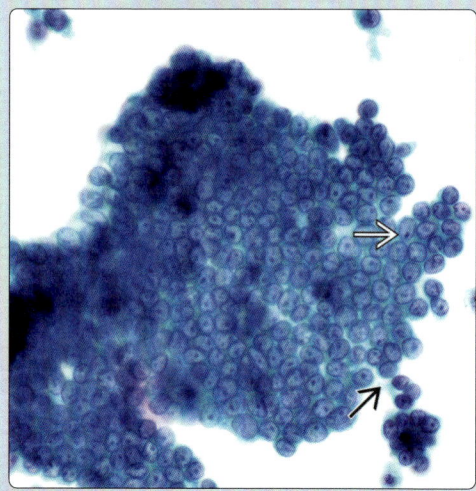

(Left) ThinPrep Pap test, low magnification, shows a wispy diathesis ➡. The sheets and rosettes show nuclear crowding with subtle peripheral feathering ➡ as well as 1 group with more cytoplasm and open chromatin ➡. (Right) This image shows a large sheet with nuclear supercrowding, distinct nuclear membranes, prominent nucleoli ➡, and vesicular chromatin. The diathesis is subtle and of the clinging type ➡ in this ThinPrep Pap of a well-differentiated endocervical adenocarcinoma (ACA).

Endocervical Adenocarcinoma, Retained In Situ Features
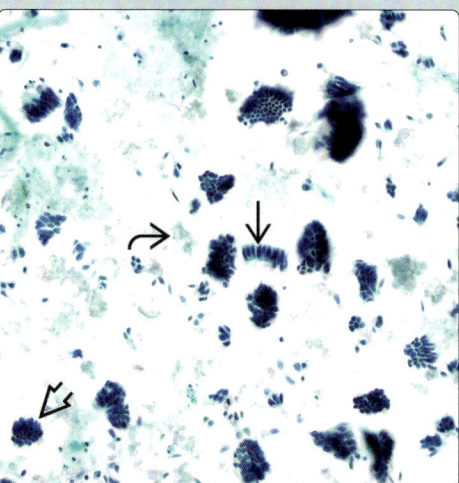

Fish Tail on SurePath
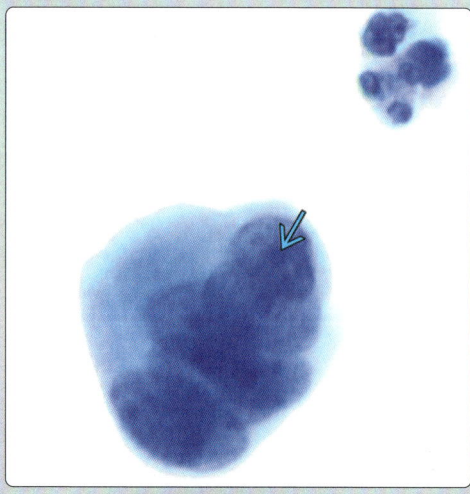

(Left) SurePath Pap test shows a well-differentiated endocervical ACA. Note the features of ACA in situ (AIS) with strips ➡, sheets, and rosettes with nuclear crowding and feathering ➡. The background of "cotton candy" diathesis ➡ indicates invasive ACA. (Right) A fish tail- or bird tail-shaped strip of adenocarcinoma of cervix is shown. The nuclei show pleomorphism and have an open chromatin and prominent nucleoli ➡. Diathesis is lacking in this early invasive ACA.

Endocervical Adenocarcinoma, Variants and Mimics

TERMINOLOGY

Synonyms
- Cervical adenocarcinoma (ACA), HPV-associated (WHO classification), include usual type, villoglandular, signet-ring, stratified mucin producing
- Cervical ACA, HPV-independent, include gastric, clear cell, and mesonephric types

ETIOLOGY/PATHOGENESIS

Infectious Agents
- High-risk human papillomavirus (HPV) infection (~ 90%)
  - HPV-18 > HPV-16 > HPV-45

CLINICAL ISSUES

Epidemiology
- Incidence
  - On rise relative to squamous cell carcinomas (SqCa) of cervix, 20-30% of cervical cancers
- Age
  - Typically late 30s to early 40s

Presentation
- Cervical mass or abnormality visualized on exam (85%)
- Abnormal vaginal bleeding (50-75%)
- Asymptomatic; atypical glandular cells identified on Pap test

Natural History
- Precursor lesion: ACA in situ (AIS)

CYTOPATHOLOGY

Cellularity
- Usually cellular irrespective of preparation type (conventional Pap smear vs. liquid based)
- Small lesions or those high in canal may have low cellularity

Pattern
- Strips, rosettes, 3D groups, large sheets ± abnormal configurations, single intact malignant cells, cell balls
- Pattern depends on whether cells are directly stripped by sampling, shed from higher in canal, or combination of both

Background
- Conventional smear will show bloody or granular diathesis
- ThinPrep can show obscuring or wrinkled tissue paper-like diathesis
  - Another diathesis type is clinging diathesis where fine wisps of degraded blood and fibrin adhere to edge of cells or sheets
- SurePath shows either fluffy "cotton candy" precipitate or subtle precipitate that can be easily missed

Cells
- Well-differentiated carcinomas and early invasive tumors resemble AIS
- Columnar configuration of cells arranged in sheets, rosettes, and strips but with some loss of polarity and pleomorphism within group, strip, or rosette
- Poorly differentiated tumors may be difficult to distinguish from SqCa
- Increase in grade results in increased pleomorphism and loss of features that help distinguish endocervical primary
- Cells from tumors originating high in canal ball up and may be difficult to distinguish from endometrial cancers
- Abnormal squamous cells from coexisting squamous intraepithelial lesion or carcinoma may be seen

Nuclear Details
- Chromatin becomes vesicular, and nucleoli appear as tumor becomes invasive
- Well-differentiated ACAs will have vesicular chromatin with round, large nucleoli, and distinct chromatinic rims
- Nuclear membrane irregularity and pleomorphism increase with increasing grade, as does mitotic activity
- Large and irregular or multiple nucleoli with increasing grade and invasiveness

Cytoplasmic Details
- Amount of cytoplasm and presence or absence of mucin and type of mucin (goblet cells or dispersed) depend on tumor type (usual vs. intestinal vs. endometrioid)

Cell Block Findings
- Helpful in difficult cases or if adenosquamous or neuroendocrine component is suspected
- Immunohistochemistry can help in distinction: p40 for squamous, CD56 for small cell, and ER/PR and vimentin for endometrial primary

ANCILLARY TESTS

Immunohistochemistry
- Helpful in differentiating endocervical vs. endometrial primary
  - Endocervical: p16 strong diffuse (+), ProEx C(+), carcinoembryonic antigen (CEA)(+), vimentin (-), ER(-), PR(-)
  - Endometrial: p16(-) or patchy (+), ProEx C(-), vimentin (+), CEA(-), ER(+), PR(+)

In Situ Hybridization
- HPV is helpful for distinguishing endocervical (+) from endometrial (-) primary

DIFFERENTIAL DIAGNOSIS

Endometrial Adenocarcinoma
- Few, smaller cells shed as tight clusters on cytology

Arias-Stella Reaction
- Rare cells, hormonally related (pregnancy, oral contraceptives, hormone replacement therapy)

Microglandular Hyperplasia
- Younger females
- Bland chromatin, repair-like configuration on cytology
- Small parakeratotic cells, lacks mitosis

SELECTED REFERENCES

1. Pulkkinen J et al: The role of Pap smear in the diagnostics of endocervical adenocarcinoma. APMIS. 129(4):195-203, 2021
2. Stolnicu S et al: Tumor typing of endocervical adenocarcinoma: contemporary review and recommendations from the International Society of Gynecological Pathologists. Int J Gynecol Pathol. 40(Suppl 1):S75-S91, 2021

Endocervical Adenocarcinoma, Variants and Mimics

(Left) *Conventional Pap smear shows a diffuse, even precipitate of diathesis ⇨ in which sheets and strips with feathered edges ⇨ are seen even on this low magnification.* **(Right)** *Conventional Pap shows strips with disordered polarization ⇨ of nuclei and nuclear overlap. A 3D acinar structure with peripheral polarization of nuclei and central mucin is also seen ⇨.*

Endocervical Adenocarcinoma on Conventional Pap

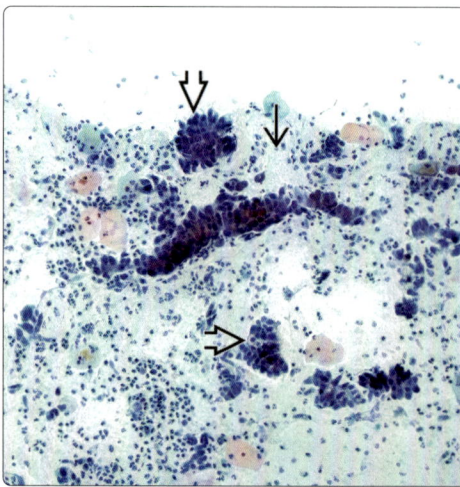

Endocervical Adenocarcinoma Disordered Strips on Conventional Pap

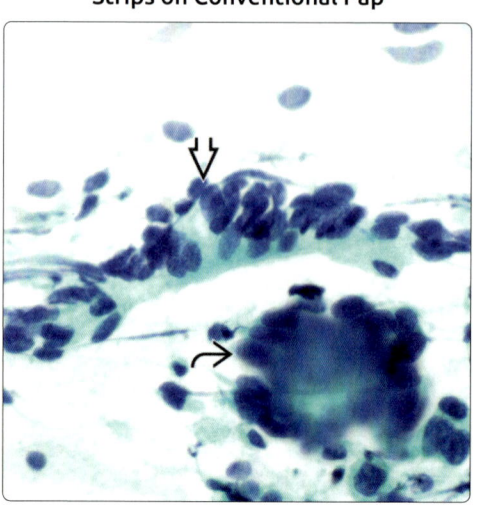

(Left) *ThinPrep Pap test of adenocarcinoma of cervix in a bloody diathesis. Outlines of partially lysed red cells are seen ⇨. The malignant cells are columnar with large nuclei with irregular nuclear outlines, open chromatin, and large nucleoli ⇨.* **(Right)** *Rosettes, short strips ⇨, and single malignant cells ⇨ are shown via conventional Pap. The nuclei have an open chromatin with nucleoli ⇨. The cells have more cytoplasm and nuclear pleomorphism compared with AIS. The fine background precipitate should also be a clue to invasion.*

Adenocarcinoma With Bloody Diathesis

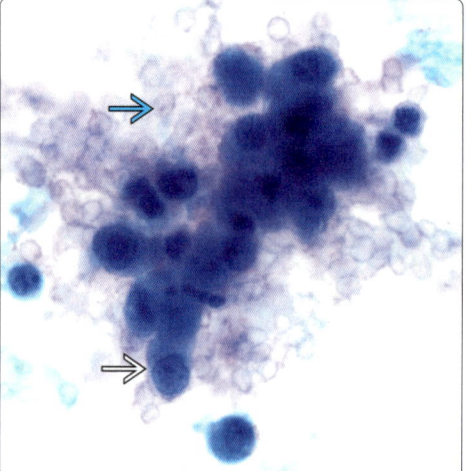

Rosettes of Endocervical Adenocarcinoma

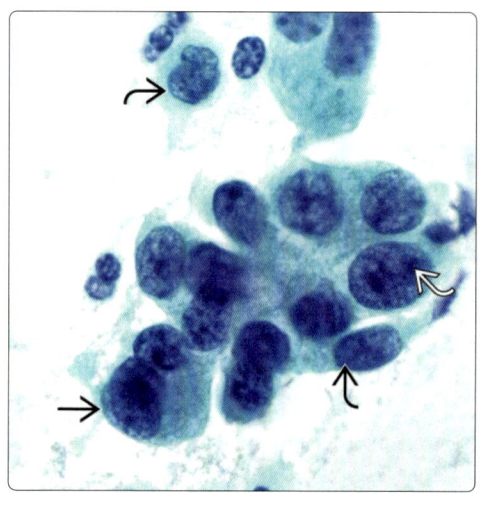

(Left) *Pap smear shows nuclear disorientation in a strip ⇨ with nucleoli and mitotically active ⇨ single malignant cells.* **(Right)** *Low-magnification H&E stain shows superficially invasive papillary villoglandular ACA of the cervix. Note long, slender villi with nuclear crowding and polarization reminiscent of colonic villous tumors.*

Nuclear Disorientation in Endocervical Adenocarcinoma

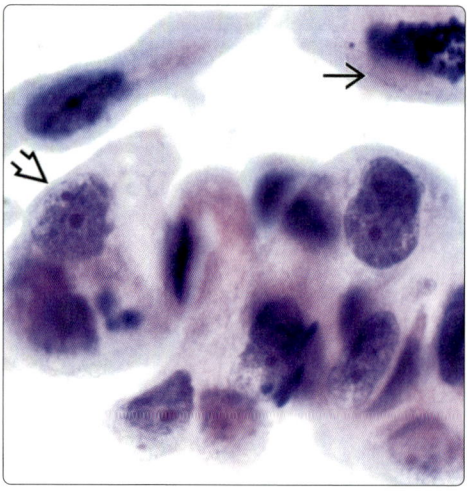

Papillary Villoglandular Adenocarcinoma of Cervix

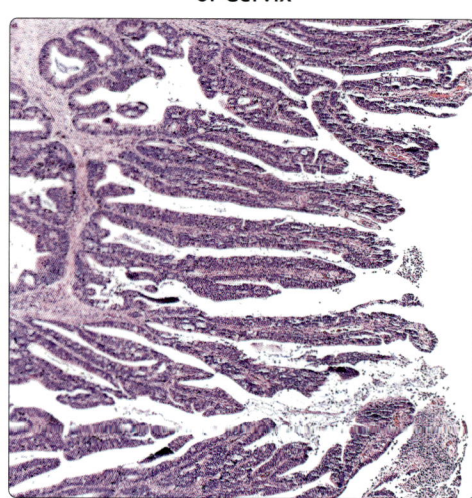

Endocervical Adenocarcinoma, Variants and Mimics

Nuclear Features of Endocervical Adenocarcinoma

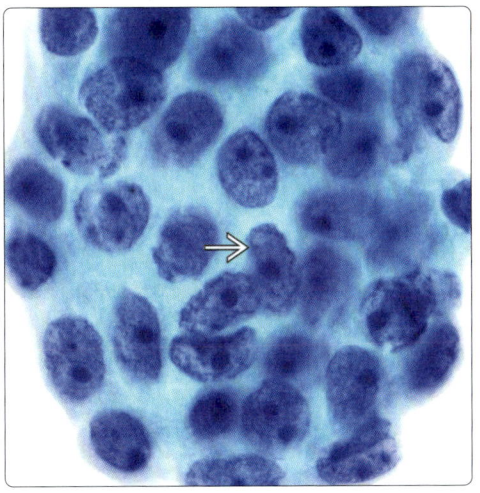

Strip With Open Chromatin and Nucleoli

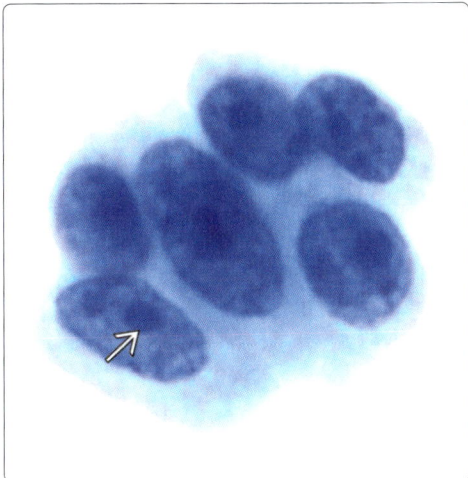

(Left) Pap stain shows a cell ball of endocervical ACA. This is shed from higher in the canal (unlike the directly scraped strips and sheets). The vesicular chromatin, nuclear contour irregularities ➡, and large nucleoli point to invasion in this well-differentiated ACA. **(Right)** SurePath Pap shows a disorganized strip of malignant cells with a vesicular chromatin and huge nucleoli ➡. Contrast this with the strips of AIS on SurePath in the previous chapter.

Repair-Like Features of Endocervical Adenocarcinoma

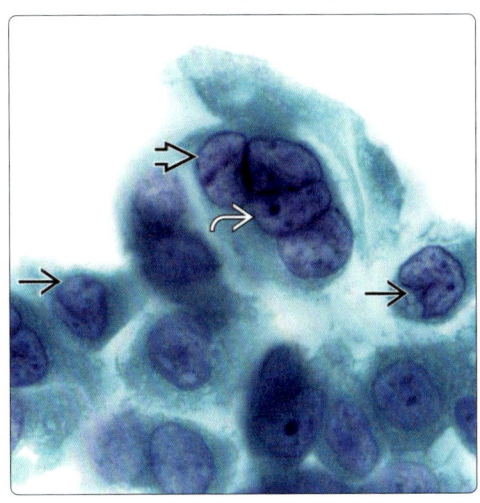

True Repair

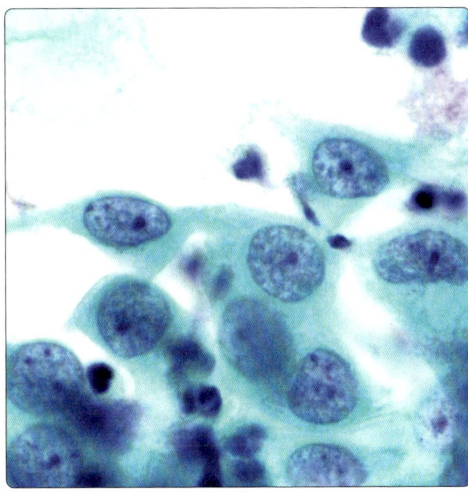

(Left) This image shows invasive endocervical ACA with repair-like configuration on ThinPrep Pap. Unlike repair, there are nuclear contour irregularities ➡ and irregular arrangement of nuclei with some overlapping ➡ vs. others spaced far apart. The chromatinic rims are dark ➡ and distinct with variable nucleoli. **(Right)** ThinPrep Pap test shows flat sheets of repair with evenly spaced cells, regular nuclear contours, hypochromasia with fine chromatin, and uniform nucleoli.

Cervical Endometriosis on Liquid-Based Pap

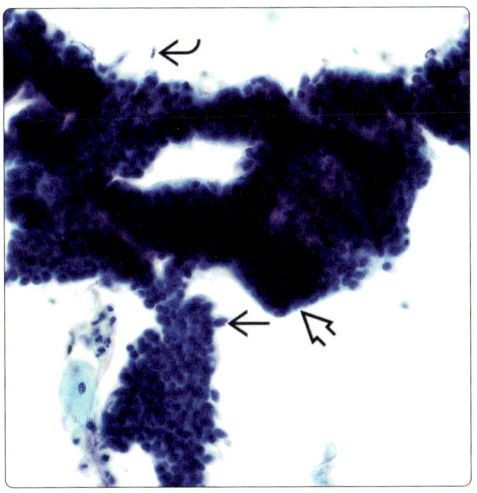

Endometrial Polyp Presenting as Hyperchromatic Crowded Group of Cells

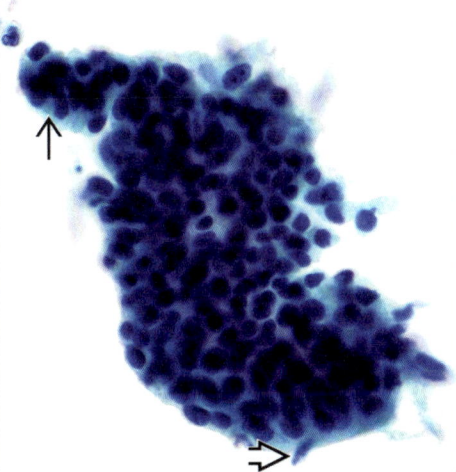

(Left) Directly sampled cervical endometriosis on Pap can be misleading. Bizarre architecture with gland openings but sharp borders ➡ with some focal feathering ➡ is seen. Spindled stromal cells ➡ attached to the large sheets can be a helpful clue if present. A cell block may also be useful. **(Right)** Endometrial cells in sheets and strips ➡ from directly sampled endometrial polyp on Pap can be mistaken for AIS or invasive ACA. Stromal cells ➡ and clinical history aid diagnosis.

Adenocarcinoma, Gastric Type

KEY FACTS

TERMINOLOGY

- Gastric-type adenocarcinoma (GAS): Adenocarcinoma of uterine cervix showing gastric (pyloric) differentiation
  - Shows spectrum from extremely well differentiated [previously called minimal deviation adenocarcinoma (MDA) or adenoma malignum (AM)] to poorly differentiated
  - Hallmark is abundant clear or pale eosinophilic cytoplasm with distinct cell borders

CLINICAL ISSUES

- Vaginal bleeding or mucoid/watery discharge
- May be associated with Peutz-Jeghers syndrome
- MDA/AM considered low end of GAS spectrum
- Poorer prognosis compared with usual HPV-positive endocervical adenocarcinomas
- Will be missed on primary HPV screening
- Incidence in USA is < 5% of all cervical adenocarcinomas, 10-15% worldwide, and up to 25% in Japan

CYTOPATHOLOGY

- Hypercellular with endocervical columnar-type cells with abundant mucin-rich cytoplasm resembling gastric cells
- Large, complex sheets with abnormal configurations
- Few single cytologically malignant cells
- Yellow-tinged mucin may be seen

ANCILLARY TESTS

- CEA and gastric-type mucin (HIK1083/MUC6) positive
- Somatic mutation of *STK11* gene on chromosome 19p (serine threonine kinase gene) if Peutz-Jeghers syndrome
- Not HPV-related, but may be p16 patchy positive (30%)

TOP DIFFERENTIAL DIAGNOSES

- Lobular endocervical gland hyperplasia (LEGH)
- Atypical LEGH and gastric-type adenocarcinoma in situ are considered precursor lesions
- HPV-related endocervical adenocarcinoma

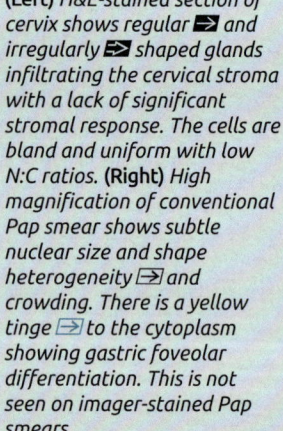

(Left) H&E-stained section of cervix shows regular ➡ and irregularly ➡ shaped glands infiltrating the cervical stroma with a lack of significant stromal response. The cells are bland and uniform with low N:C ratios. (Right) High magnification of conventional Pap smear shows subtle nuclear size and shape heterogeneity ➡ and crowding. There is a yellow tinge ➡ to the cytoplasm showing gastric foveolar differentiation. This is not seen on imager-stained Pap smears.

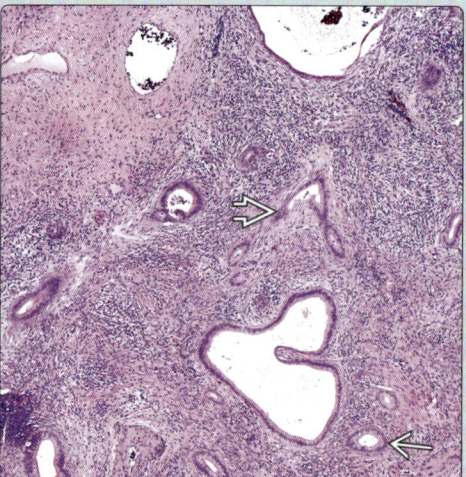

GAS, Well Differentiated

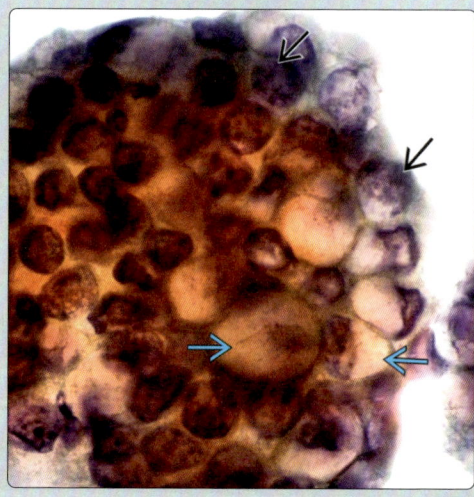

GAS, Well Differentiated

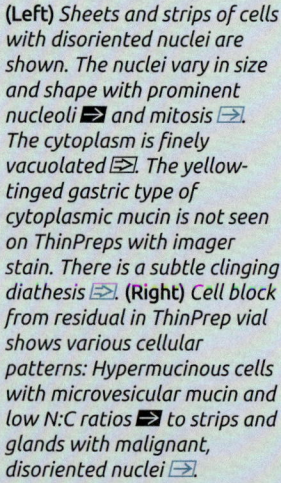

(Left) Sheets and strips of cells with disoriented nuclei are shown. The nuclei vary in size and shape with prominent nucleoli ➡ and mitosis ➡. The cytoplasm is finely vacuolated ➡. The yellow-tinged gastric type of cytoplasmic mucin is not seen on ThinPreps with imager stain. There is a subtle clinging diathesis ➡. (Right) Cell block from residual in ThinPrep vial shows various cellular patterns: Hypermucinous cells with microvesicular mucin and low N:C ratios ➡ to strips and glands with malignant, disoriented nuclei ➡.

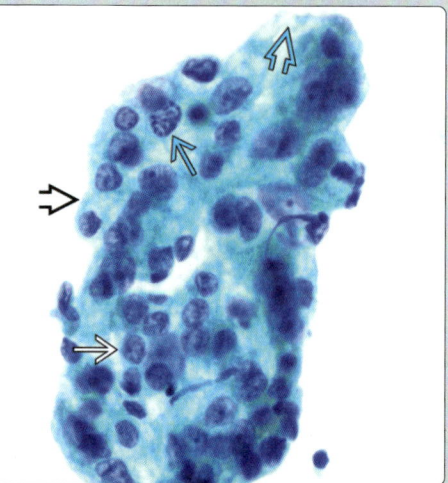

GAS on ThinPrep Imager Stain

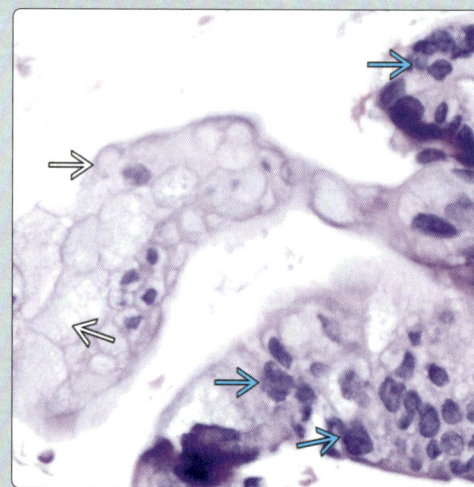

GAS Strips on Cell Block

Adenocarcinoma, Gastric Type

TERMINOLOGY

Abbreviations
- Gastric-type adenocarcinoma (GAS)

Definitions
- Adenocarcinoma of uterine cervix showing gastric (pyloric) differentiation
- Extremely well differentiated [previously called minimal deviation adenocarcinoma (MDA) or adenoma malignum] to poorly differentiated

ETIOLOGY/PATHOGENESIS

Genetic Abnormalities
- May have germline mutations of *STK11* gene (either Peutz-Jeghers syndrome or sporadic)
- Unrelated to HPV; rarely p53 abnormalities, Her2 and *MDM2* gene amplification in some cases

CLINICAL ISSUES

Epidemiology
- Incidence
  - < 5% of all cervical adenocarcinomas in USA, 10-15% worldwide, and up to 25% in Japan; mean age: 50-55 years

Prognosis
- GAS are aggressive tumors: Present at higher stage than HPV-related cervical adenocarcinomas

CYTOPATHOLOGY

Cellularity
- Cellular specimens with abundant mucin

Pattern
- Large sheets, strips of cells and smaller single cells
- Some sheets with abnormal configurations and lumina

Background
- Mucinous &/or bloody diathesis
- Rarer endometrioid variant shows bloody diathesis

Cells
- Mucinous type shows columnar mucin-containing cells resembling gastric foveolar cells
- Cytoplasmic mucin may appear yellow (helpful feature on conventional and nonimager Pap stain); endometrioid variant cells are smaller and lack mucin
- Degree of atypia varies with level of differentiation from almost normal endocervical/gastric foveolar cell appearance to severe atypia in higher grades

Nuclear Details
- Small, bland, basally located with small nucleoli in low grade; more atypical to clearly malignant in high grade
- Mitosis varies depending upon degree of differentiation

Cytoplasmic Details
- Abundant mucin-rich cytoplasm in mucinous type, rarely cilia
- Yellow tinge to mucin in gastric phenotype on usual Pap stain; not seen on imager stains

ANCILLARY TESTS

Immunohistochemistry
- Positive for HIK1083 &/or MUC6

DIFFERENTIAL DIAGNOSIS

Lobular Endocervical Gland Hyperplasia
- Well demarcated, no cytologic atypia, and rare mitoses
- Atypical form and gastric-type adenocarcinoma in situ (AIS) may represent precursor of MDA (both composed of pyloric-type epithelium)

Endocervical Adenocarcinoma, Usual Type
- Obvious cytologic atypia and brisk mitotic activity
- High-risk HPV and p16 positive

SELECTED REFERENCES
1. Schwock J et al: Cytomorphologic features of gastric-type endocervical adenocarcinoma in liquid-based preparations. Acta Cytol. 65(1):56-66, 2021

Drunken Honeycomb

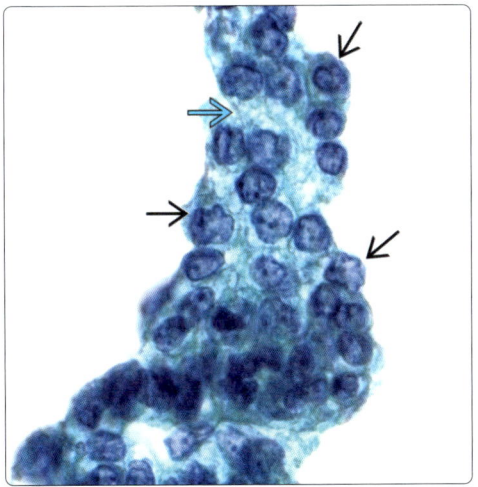

Nuclear and Cytoplasmic Details

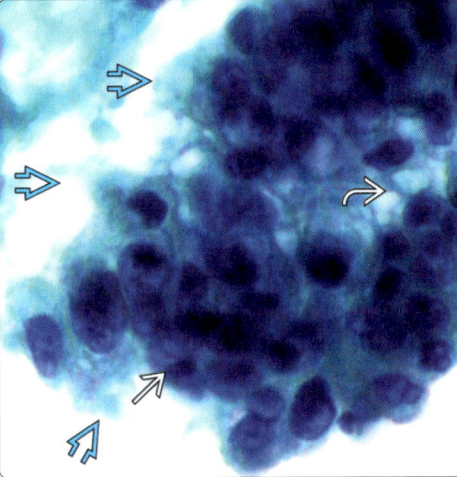

(Left) ThinPrep Pap shows a drunken honeycomb pattern of cells with finely vacuolated cytoplasm ➡, low N:C ratios, and irregular nuclear contours ➡. These cells are more obviously malignant compared with minimal deviation adenocarcinoma (MDA). The tumor was p16 and HPV negative. *(Right)* ThinPrep Pap shows strips and sheets with nuclear crowding, overlapping ➡, and variable N:C ratios. The cytoplasm is hypermucinous in some cells with microvesicles ➡. A clinging diathesis is also seen ➡.

Endometrial Cancers: Usual Types, Variants, and Mimics

KEY FACTS

CLINICAL ISSUES
- Low-grade cancers affect peri- and postmenopausal women and younger women with morbid obesity or polycystic ovarian syndrome
- High-grade cancers seen in postmenopausal women with atrophic endometrium, mean age 60 or older

CYTOPATHOLOGY
- Low-grade endometrial cancers usually have low cellularity
  o Mildly atypical cells in small groups, ~ 2-3x size of normal endometrial cells
  o Nuclei 2-3x size of normal endometrials, with open chromatin and small nucleoli
  o Background shows high estrogen effect, and diathesis may be absent, especially in liquid-based Paps
- High-grade cancers are generally more cellular, as cells are more abundant and dyshesive
  o Cells are more atypical or malignant and larger
  o Large papillary clusters, single malignant cells, and nonviable cells may be seen
  o Large nuclei with prominent nucleoli
  o Background is atrophic, and watery or bloody diathesis is usually present

ANCILLARY TESTS
- Endometrial endometrioid cancers are generally estrogen and progesterone receptor positive, vimentin positive, p53 (strong diffuse positive or completely negative) if serous
- p16 can be patchy or diffuse depending on type (serous cancers show strong and diffuse p16 staining)
- Human papillomavirus (HPV) is negative

TOP DIFFERENTIAL DIAGNOSES
- Endocervical or extrauterine primary malignancy
- Arias-Stella reaction, polyps, atrophy/bare nuclei, IUD cells, atypical repair
- Menstrual endometrium
- Small cell carcinoma

Low-Grade Endometrial Adenocarcinoma

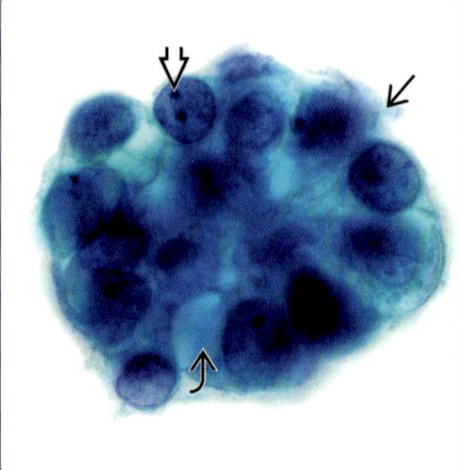

Histology of Low-Grade Endometrial Carcinoma

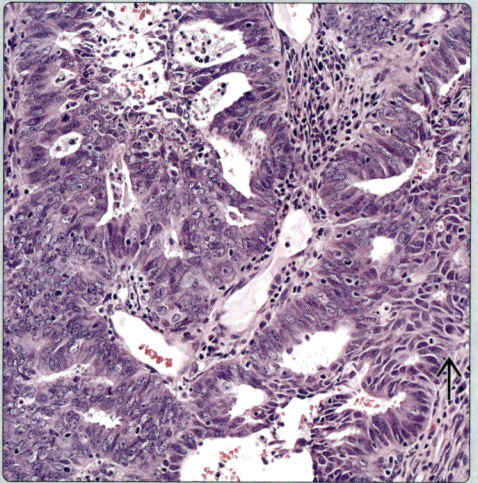

(Left) Pap of FIGO II low-grade endometrial adenocarcinoma (EMACA) shows a rounded cluster of endometrial cells with a subtle clinging diathesis ⇨, nonmucinous cytoplasmic vacuoles ⇨, nuclei with small nucleoli ⇨, and no mitosis. Rare groups of atypical endometrial cells were seen on ThinPrep Pap. (Right) H&E of FIGO II EMACA shows glands arranged back-to-back with cribriforming and smooth luminal contour. Nuclei are tall and columnar; nucleoli are visible. Solid areas ⇨ comprise > 5% of tumor.

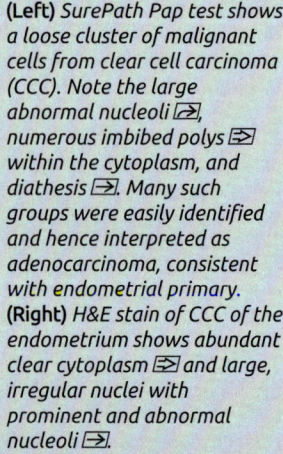

Clear Cell Carcinoma Cytology

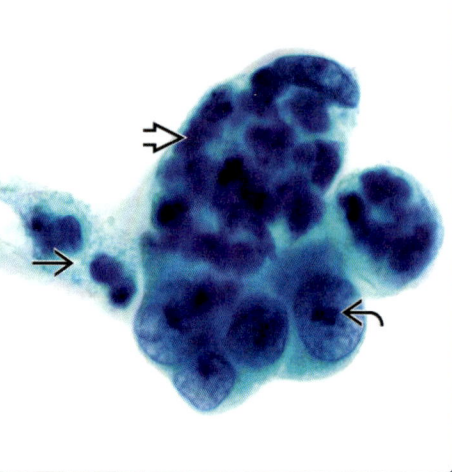

Clear Cell Carcinoma of Endometrium

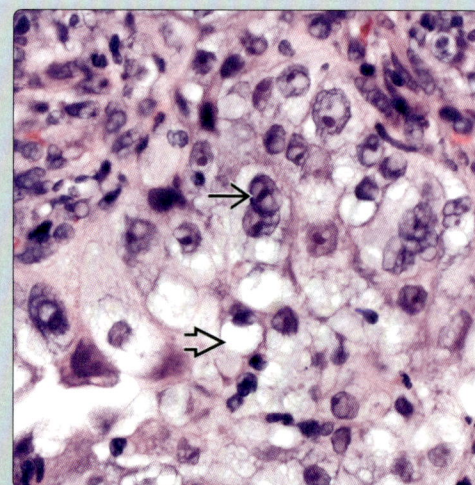

(Left) SurePath Pap test shows a loose cluster of malignant cells from clear cell carcinoma (CCC). Note the large abnormal nucleoli ⇨, numerous imbibed polys ⇨ within the cytoplasm, and diathesis ⇨. Many such groups were easily identified and hence interpreted as adenocarcinoma, consistent with endometrial primary. (Right) H&E stain of CCC of the endometrium shows abundant clear cytoplasm ⇨ and large, irregular nuclei with prominent and abnormal nucleoli ⇨.

Endometrial Cancers: Usual Types, Variants, and Mimics

TERMINOLOGY

Abbreviations
- Endometrioid adenocarcinoma (EMACA)
- Clear cell carcinoma (CCC)
- High-grade serous carcinoma (HGSCA)
- Malignant mixed müllerian tumor (MMMT)
- Undifferentiated carcinoma (UCA)

ETIOLOGY/PATHOGENESIS

2 Types of Endometrial Cancers
- Type I (usually low-grade cancers)
  - Comprise EMACA and other low-grade carcinomas (e.g., mucinous)
  - Arise on basis of unopposed estrogen stimulation (unopposed exogenous or endogenous estrogen, anovulation, polycystic ovaries, obesity)
- Type II (high-grade cancers)
  - Comprise serous carcinoma, CCC, MMMT, UCA
- Recent studies, however, have shown significant heterogeneity within and overlap between type I and II cancers
- Additionally, recent molecular studies have stratified endometrial cancers into 4 genomic types

CLINICAL ISSUES

Presentation
- Type I (low-grade cancers)
  - Peri- and postmenopausal women or younger women with morbid obesity or polycystic ovarian syndrome
  - May be asymptomatic and present with normal or atypical endometrial cells on Pap test
- Type II (high-grade cancers)
  - Postmenopausal women, mean age ≥ 60 years
  - May present with disseminated disease, especially HGSCA, CCC, and MMMT, and obvious malignant cells with diathesis on cytology
  - Background of atrophic endometrium
- Both types present with postmenopausal bleeding &/or serosanguineous vaginal discharge

Prognosis
- Low-grade: Generally good prognosis unless late stage
- High-grade: Generally poorer prognosis, as they often present at later stage and are more aggressive

CYTOPATHOLOGY

Cellularity
- Type I: Usually low cellularity
- Type II: Generally more cellular, as cells are more abundant and dyshesive
- However, if endocervical canal extension is present, cells are directly sampled and hence cellular
  - Thus, distinction from endocervical primary may be difficult

Pattern
- Since cells are shed from above, they tend to clump together and degenerate
  - Hence, present as small groups of cohesive cells with degenerative changes

Background
- Low-grade cancers
  - High estrogenic background
  - Diathesis may be subtle and watery on conventional smears and washed away on liquid-based (clean background)
- High-grade cancers
  - Background of atrophy or atrophic vaginitis
  - Diathesis is bloody or clinging type
  - More obvious even on liquid based
- If tumor involves cervical canal, it can be directly sampled and resemble endocervical primary

Cells
- Low-grade cancer
  - Mildly atypical, in small groups, ~ 2-3x size of normal endometrial cells
  - May shed cells that resemble normal endometrial cells with histiocytes, which are better seen on conventional smears
- High-grade cancer
  - More atypical or obviously malignant and larger
  - Large papillary clusters, single malignant cells, and nonviable cells may be seen on conventional and liquid-based preparations

Nuclear Details
- Low-grade EMACA
  - Nuclei 2-3x that of normal endometrials
  - Open chromatin with small nucleoli
- High-grade cancers
  - Large nuclei with prominent nucleoli
  - Usually recognized as highly atypical/suspicious or malignant

Cytoplasmic Details
- Low-grade cancers
  - Less cytoplasm and often degenerative vacuoles seen; rarely, mucin in low-grade endometrioid of mucinous type
- High-grade cancers
  - High N:C ratios but degenerative vacuoles and obvious malignant features
- Intracytoplasmic inflammatory cells (polys) are characteristic but not specific, as they can also be seen in benign conditions

Adequacy Criteria
- Always adequate if atypical or malignant cells present irrespective of cellularity
- Bloody specimens can overwhelm liquid-based system (especially membrane filters)
  - Result in bloody rim of partially lysed blood and fibrin around circumference with no cells in center
  - If no atypical or malignant cells are seen along rim, best to dilute or lyse sample with glacial acetic acid and repeat prep

Endometrial Cancers: Usual Types, Variants, and Mimics

Cytologic Distinction Between Endocervical and Endometrial Primaries

Features	Endocervical Carcinoma	Endometrial Carcinoma
Cellularity	Hypercellular	Low cellularity
Pattern	Strips, rosettes, large abnormal sheets, peripheral feathering, single malignant cells	Small clusters, rarely papillae or single cells
Diathesis	Visible, type varies by preparation	Watery, absent or subtle
Cell shapes	Oval, columnar, pleomorphic	Round, irregular, smaller
Nuclei	Oval, elongated, pleomorphic	Round, irregular in higher grade
Cytoplasm	Mucin (+)	Degenerative vacuoles, mucin (-)
Squamous intraepithelial lesion or SqCa	Usually present	Absent
High-risk HPV	Positive	Negative

SqCa = squamous cell carcinoma; HPV = human papillomavirus.

Cell Block Findings
- Can be helpful in liquid-based samples to sort endometrial vs. endocervical cancers
  - Especially in younger perimenopausal patients
- Endometrial cancer
  - Generally ER(+), PR(+), and vimentin (+)
- Endocervical primary
  - HPV(+), mCEA(+), and p16(+) (block pattern)

Cytology-Histology Correlation
- Low-grade endometrial cancers
  - Usual cytologic diagnosis is atypical endometrial or glandular cells
  - Rarely, normal-appearing endometrial cells, usually in women > 45
- High-grade cancers
  - Usually called malignant, atypical endometrials, or atypical glandulars favor neoplastic on cytology

ANCILLARY TESTS

Immunohistochemistry
- Endometrial endometrioid cancers are generally ER/PR(+), vimentin (+), p53(+) if serous type
  - Serous cancers show aberrant p53 expression [diffusely positive in at least 75% of cells salpingo-oophorectomy **or** completely absent (null phenotype)], typically ER(-) and PR(-) or weakly (+)
  - CCC usually ER(-) and PR(-), rarely may show aberrant p53 expression
- p16 can be patchy or diffuse depending on type (serous cancers show strong and diffuse p16 staining)
- However, endometrial cancers are not HPV driven
  - Hence, HPV by in situ hybridization or PCR is negative
  - These can be performed on cell blocks from liquid-based specimens in difficult cases

DIFFERENTIAL DIAGNOSIS

Endocervical Primary
- More cellular; strips, rosettes, feathering
- Use immunohistochemistry (IHC) to distinguish in difficult cases or in younger women with lower uterine segment primary

Extrauterine Primary
- Few cells and absent diathesis (unless direct extension) or metastasis; history is usually available
- Morphology different from usual endometrial types

Arias-Stella Reaction
- Rare cells seen in pregnancy or on high-dose Provera

Polyps
- Can rarely be problematic if directly sampled or infarcted and shed very atypical cells with broken-down blood and fibrin

Endometrial Hyperplasia
- Low cellularity of normal or mildly atypical endometrial cells

Menstrual Endometrium
- Problematic in perimenopausal women when last menstrual period is unknown
- Cell blocks on liquid-based specimens and IHC can help
- Stromal cells (if recognized) are clue

Directly Sampled Endometrium/Endometriosis
- Can resemble endocervical or endometrial primary
- Tubular glands and stroma are giveaway
- IHC on cell blocks is helpful in difficult cases

IUD Cells
- Rare cells with "bubblegum" cytoplasm, history of IUD

Atypical Repair
- Flat sheets with distinct cell borders and round regular nuclei and nucleoli

Atrophy/Bare Nuclei
- Pseudodiathesis of atrophic vaginitis is trap
- Bland nuclei with no nucleoli or degenerate vacuoles

Small Cell Carcinoma
- Hypercellularity, diathesis, nuclear molding, small or absent nucleoli, neuroendocrine chromatin, HPV(+)

SELECTED REFERENCES
1. Soslow RA et al: Endometrial carcinoma diagnosis: use of FIGO grading and genomic subcategories in clinical practice: recommendations of the International Society of Gynecological Pathologists. Int J Gynecol Pathol. 38 Suppl 1:S64-74, 2019

Endometrial Cancers: Usual Types, Variants, and Mimics

Low-Grade Endometrial Carcinoma With High Estrogenic Background

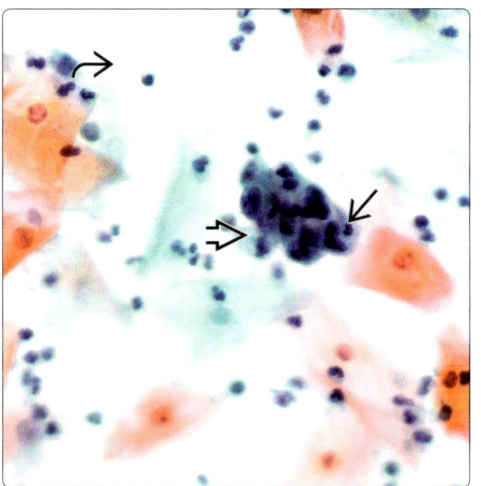

Histology of Low-Grade Endometrial Carcinoma

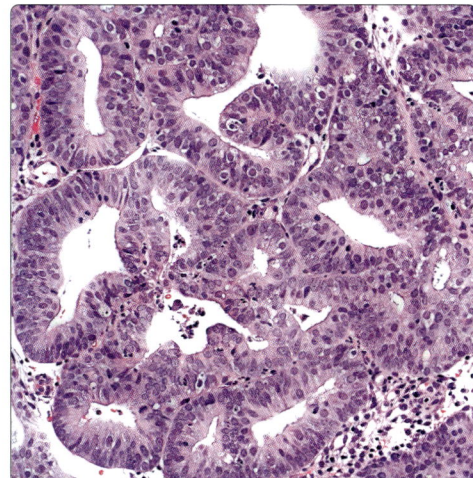

(Left) A conventional Pap smear shows rare cohesive cell groups of small cells in a high-estrogen background of superficial and intermediate cells. Note the polys ➡ in the cytoplasm of cells with degenerate vacuoles ➡. Very subtle diathesis ➡ is difficult to see and may be absent. (Right) H&E stain shows a FIGO I endometrioid EMACA, which is composed of back-to-back glands with tall columnar nuclei. There is minimal nuclear size and shape variation.

Atypical Endometrial Cells Engorged With Polymorphonuclear Leukocytes

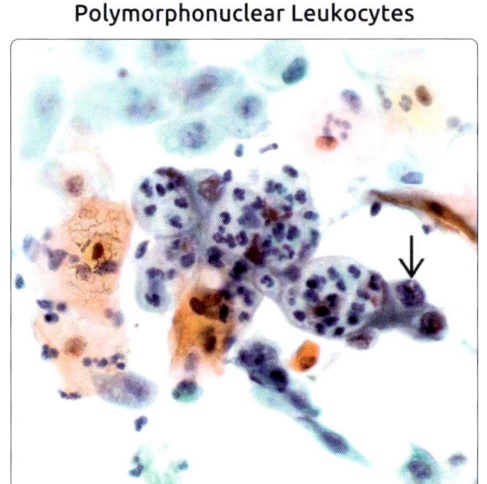

Rare Atypical Endometrial Cells

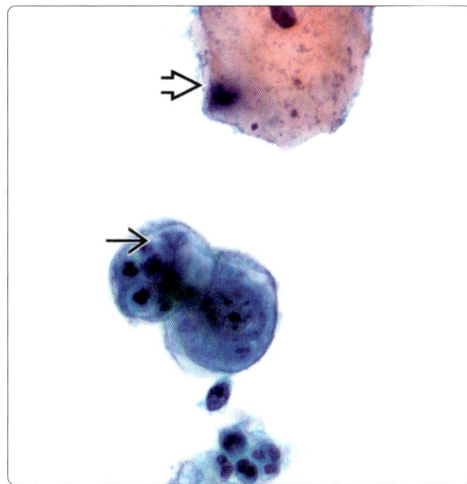

(Left) This conventional Pap smear of low-grade EMACA shows a few groups of small atypical endometrial cells with engulfed polys. Some nuclear contour irregularities ➡ are in a nonatrophic background. (Right) A conventional Pap smear of a postmenopausal woman with a high-estrogen background shows 2 small atypical endometrial cells with degenerative vacuoles ➡, imbibed polys, and a superficial cell ➡ in the background. Biopsy identified a FIGO I EMACA.

Endometrial Cluster With Cytoplasmic Polys

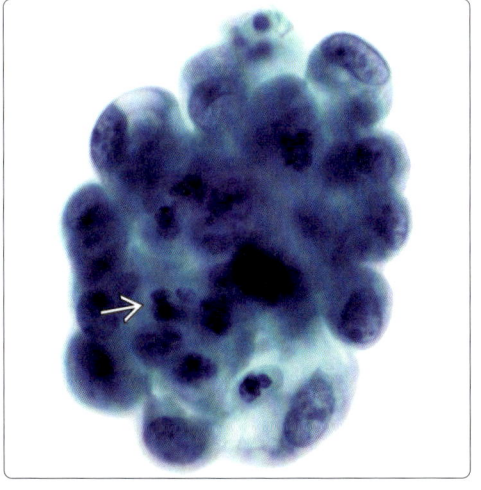

High-Grade Endometrioid Carcinoma With Diathesis

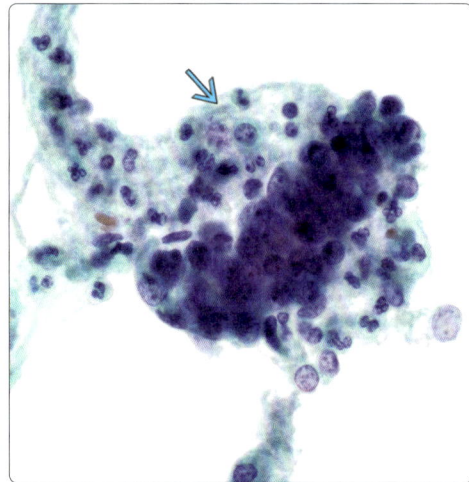

(Left) A large group of endometrial carcinoma cells on ThinPrep Pap shows inflammatory cells in the cytoplasm ➡. The background is clean, as the watery diathesis is easily cleared on liquid-based preparations. (Right) This conventional Pap smear shows a large, tight cluster of endometrial carcinoma cells in an atrophic background and diathesis ➡.

Endometrial Cancers: Usual Types, Variants, and Mimics

Clear Cell Carcinoma on Conventional Smear

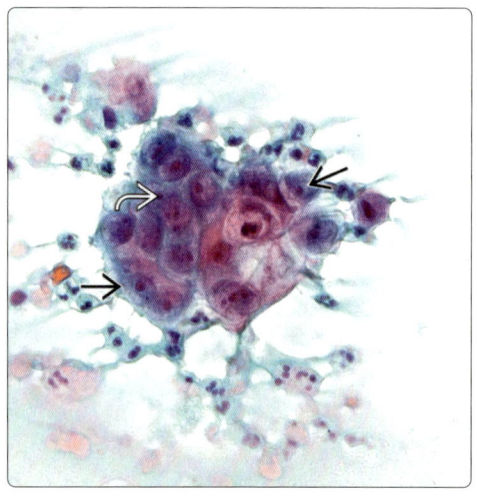

Clear Cell Carcinoma Histology

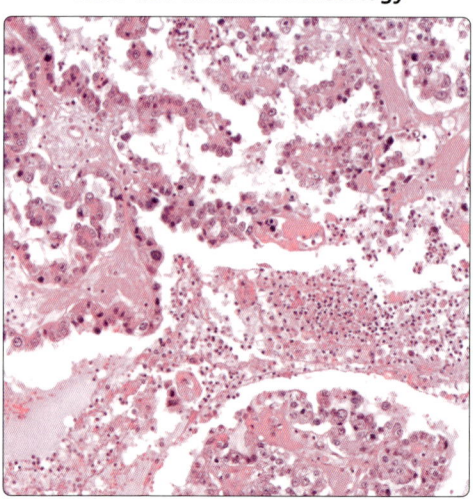

(Left) This is a conventional smear of a CCC. There is a cluster of atypical cells with large nucleoli ➡ and some imbibed neutrophils ➡. Many groups such as this were present. Subsequent biopsy showed a CCC. (Right) Endometrial biopsy of a CCC shows a papillary pattern. It is the nuclear features that make the diagnosis.

Cytology of Malignant Mixed Müllerian Tumor on Conventional Smear

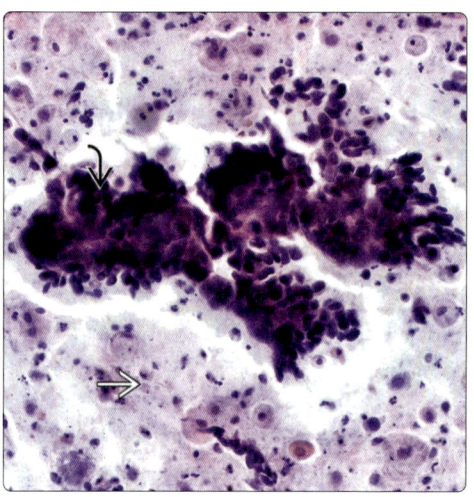

Malignant Mixed Müllerian Tumor

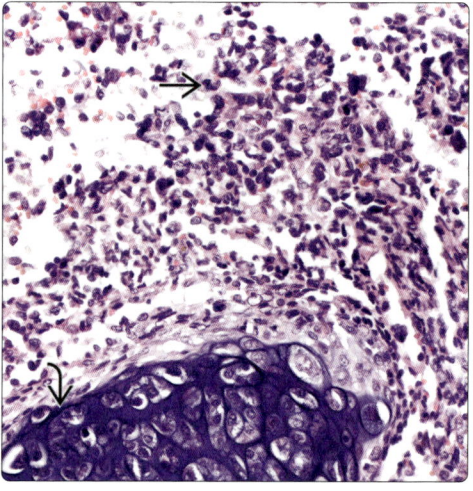

(Left) A conventional Pap smear from a 75-year-old woman who presented with postmenopausal bleeding shows a large and somewhat papillary group ➡ of malignant cells in a background of atrophic vaginitis ➡. Only the high-grade serous component was seen. The sarcomatous and heterologous elements were not present. (Right) H&E stain of malignant mixed müllerian tumor (carcinosarcoma) shows heterologous elements (e.g., cartilage ➡) and extensive necrosis in the background with high-grade cells ➡.

Direct Extension of EMACA to Cervix

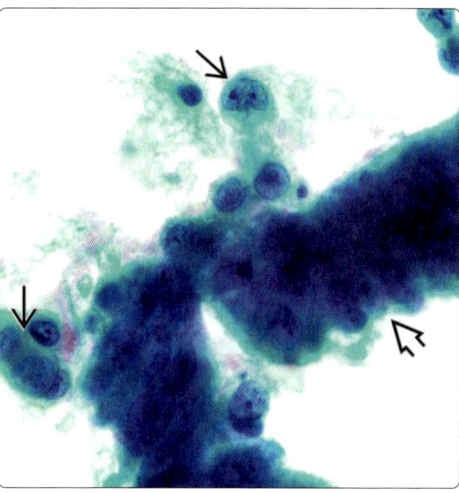

Histology of High-Grade Endometrioid Carcinoma

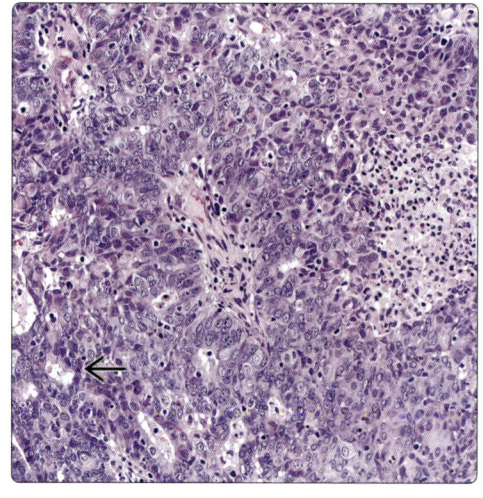

(Left) FIGO III EMACA with extension into the endocervix is seen. Pap test features (e.g., polarized strips ➡ and single malignant cells with diathesis ➡) overlap with those of endocervical cancer. (Right) H&E stain of FIGO III EMACA with a solid component (> 50%) shows that glandular structures ➡ are still visualized. Nuclei are columnar to round with nuclear size variation and visible nucleoli. The cytologic features of the cells in the solid component are similar to the glandular component.

Endometrial Cancers: Usual Types, Variants, and Mimics

High-Grade Endometrial Carcinoma

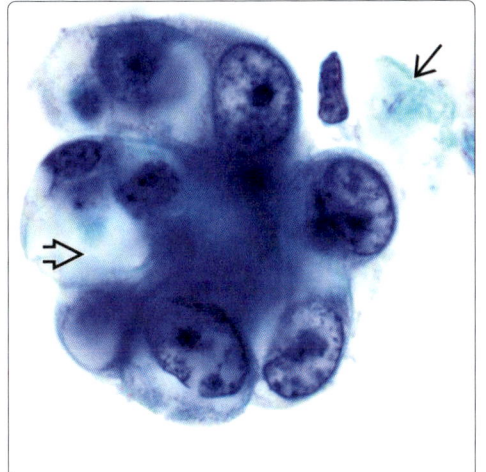

Histology of Serous Carcinoma

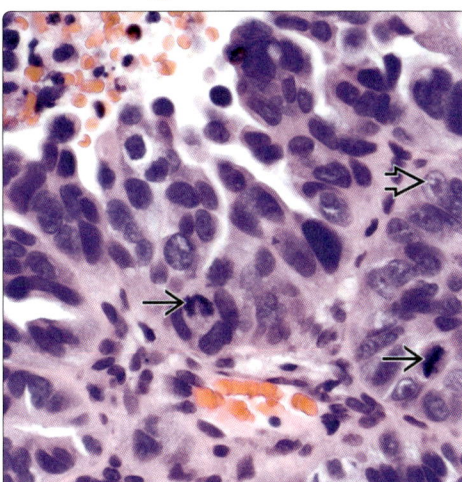

(Left) 3D cell ball on ThinPrep Pap test shows serous carcinoma of endometrium. Note subtle clinging diathesis ⇨, vesicular chromatin, large nucleoli, degenerate vacuoles ⇨, and some nuclear contour irregularities. (Right) Serous carcinoma of the endometrium can be seen on H&E stain. Note the high nuclear grade, pleomorphism, prominent nucleoli ⇨, and increased mitotic activity ⇨.

Endometrial Carcinoma on ThinPrep

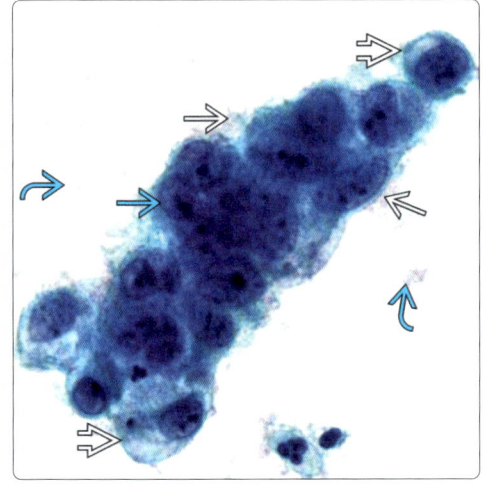

Endometrial Cancer, SurePath

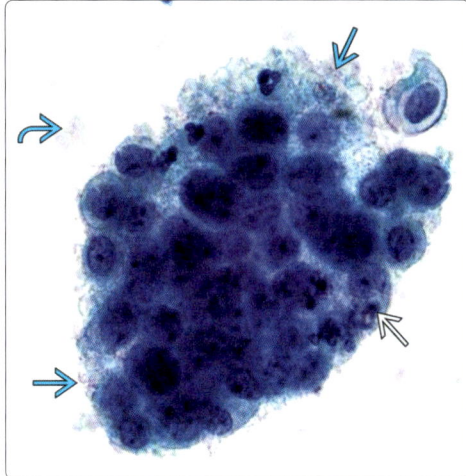

(Left) This ThinPrep image shows a cohesive group of endometrial carcinoma cells with readily visible nucleoli ⇨ and vacuolated delicate cytoplasm ⇨. Note the associated clinging diathesis ⇨. A few flimsy fibrin strands with blood are also seen ⇨ but can be subtle. (Right) This SurePath Pap test shows a cluster of highly atypical endometrial cells with ingested polymorphonuclear leukocytes ⇨. Note the clinging diathesis ⇨ and the background fluffy "cotton candy" diathesis ⇨, which can be very subtle.

High-Grade Endometrial Cancer, ThinPrep

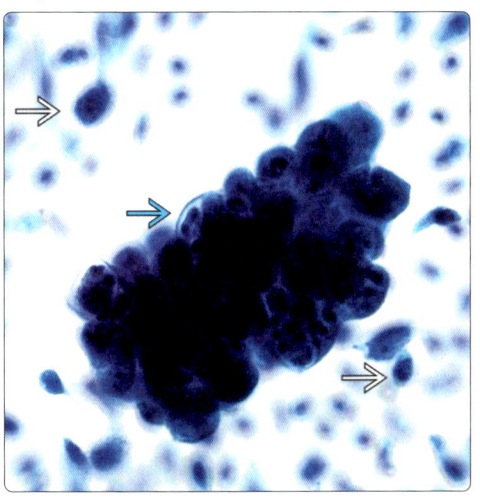

High Grade Endometrial Carcinoma

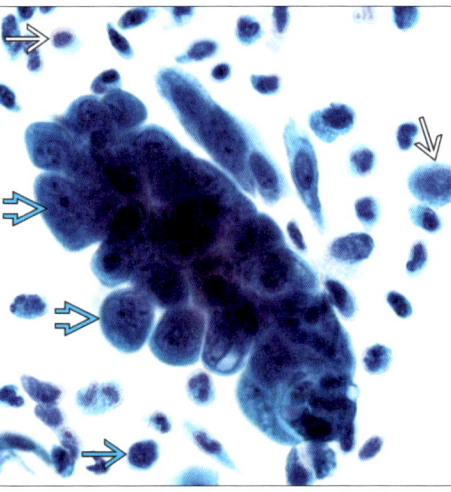

(Left) This papillary hyperchromatic cluster of strikingly malignant cells, some with imbibed polymorphonuclear leukocytes ⇨, sits in a background of single intact malignant cells ⇨. Diathesis may be difficult to appreciate but such findings can still be easily interpreted as malignant. (Right) ThinPrep shows a high-grade endometrial carcinoma cluster in an atrophic background ⇨ that also contains single intact malignant cells ⇨. Diathesis is subtle, but cells are clearly malignant ⇨ with high N:C ratios.

Atypical Glandular Cells: Endocervicals, Endometrials, and Glandulars, NOS

KEY FACTS

CYTOPATHOLOGY

- **Atypical endocervical cells (AEC)**
  - Columnar endocervical-type cells in sheets and strips with some nuclear crowding and overlapping
  - Nuclei 3-5x size of normal endocervical cell nuclei
  - Minimal variation in nuclear size and shape with mild hyperchromasia
  - Rare mitosis, nucleoli/chromocenters may be seen
  - Cytoplasm abundant, but ↑ nuclear:cytoplasmic (N:C) ratios and distinct cell borders may be seen
  - On liquid-based Paps, cells round up; hence, center of group may be difficult to visualize
- **AEC, favor neoplastic (AECN)**
  - Columnar endocervical-type cells presenting as large sheets, strips, and rosettes
  - Nuclear crowding, overlapping, and ↑ N:C ratios
  - Ill-defined or nonexistent cell borders due to overcrowding
  - Nuclear stratification with palisading and peripheral palisading along sheets, strips, and rosettes
  - Hyperchromasia with even chromatin; chromocenters may be better seen on liquid-based Paps
- **Atypical endometrial cells (AEMC)**
  - Small rounded endometrial-type cells presenting in small groups of 5-10 cells (more cohesive on liquid-based Paps)
  - Mildly enlarged nuclei with small nucleoli (more prominent on liquid-based Paps)
  - Slight hyperchromasia, ill-defined cell borders, cytoplasmic vacuoles

REPORTING

- Median reporting rate for atypical glandular category per CAP is 0.1-0.2% for conventional and liquid based
- 25% are HPV(+); of those, 50% will have significant cervical pathology (squamous intraepithelial lesion most frequent)
- This is high-risk reporting category; hence, follow-up with cytology alone is not option

Normal Endocervical Cells

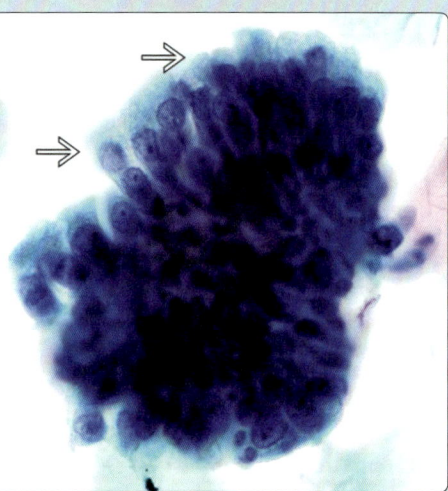

Atypical Endocervical Cells, Favor Neoplastic

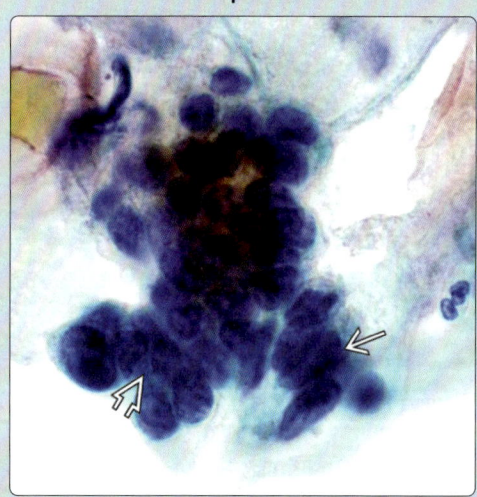

(Left) SurePath Pap test with a thick cluster of normal endocervical cells is shown. The peripheral cells ➡ show low nuclear:cytoplasmic (N:C) ratios, lack of overlapping, and hyperchromasia. Contrast this with the next image. *(Right)* ThinPrep Pap test from a 31-year-old with a rare cluster ➡ and strip ➡ of cells with nuclear hyperchromasia, crowding, overlapping, and high N:C ratios from a case with adenocarcinoma (ACA) in situ found on follow-up is shown.

Normal Endocervical and Shed Endometrial Cells

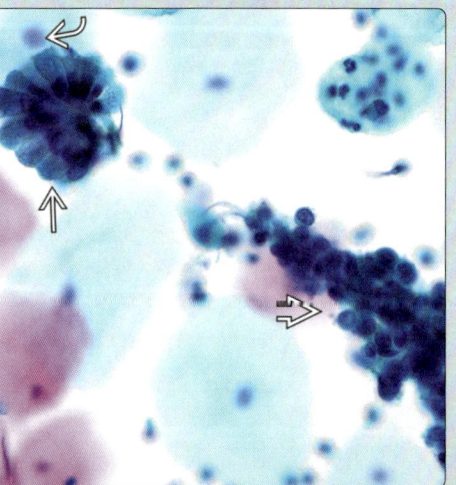

Atypical Endometrial Cells

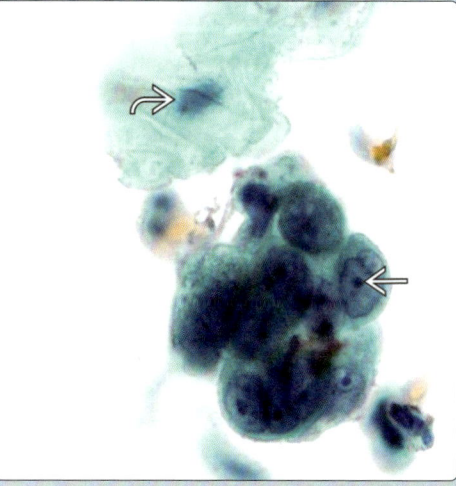

(Left) SurePath Pap test shows normal endocervical cells ➡ with low N:C ratios and distinct cell boundaries. The shed endometrial cells ➡ are small and in clusters. Compare endometrial cell size to a normal intermediate squamous cell nucleus ➡ in the background. *(Right)* ThinPrep Pap test shows a cluster of atypical endometrial cells (AECs) with nuclear contour irregularities and nucleoli ➡. The cells are much larger than the background intermediate squamous cell nucleus ➡.

Atypical Glandular Cells: Endocervicals, Endometrials, and Glandulars, NOS

TERMINOLOGY

Abbreviations
- Atypical glandular cells (AGC), not otherwise specified
- AGC, favor neoplastic (AGCN)

Definitions
- **Atypical endocervical cells (AEC)**
  - Endocervical-type cells with nuclear atypia that exceeds reactive/reparative changes but lack unequivocal features of endocervical adenocarcinoma in situ or adenocarcinoma
  - Can be further qualified as favor neoplastic (AECN) if index of suspicion is high
- **AECN**
  - Endocervical-type cells, morphologic features of which either qualitatively or quantitatively fall short of diagnosis of adenocarcinoma in situ or invasive adenocarcinoma
- **Atypical endometrial cells (AEMC)**
  - Small endometrial-type cells that are abnormal but do not meet criteria for endometrial adenocarcinoma
  - Not further qualified as cytologically may represent wide spectrum of conditions, and it is not possible to predict malignancy based on these features
- **AGC**
  - Generic AGC is used when one cannot tell if cells are endocervical or endometrial in origin
  - Depending upon index of suspicion, those that qualitatively or quantitatively fall short of malignancy can be further qualified as AGCN

CYTOPATHOLOGY

Cellularity
- Usually low in all preparation types

Pattern
- Small, tightly cohesive group of cells or hyperchromatic crowded groups (HCGs)

Background
- Usually clean, rarely bloody or diathesis-like but with only very rare atypical cells

Cells
- **AEC**
  - Columnar endocervical-type cells in sheets and strips with some nuclear crowding and overlapping
  - Nuclei 3-5x size of normal endocervical cell nuclei
  - Minimal variation in nuclear size and shape with mild hyperchromasia
  - Rare mitosis &/or nucleoli/chromocenters may be seen
  - Abundant cytoplasm, but ↑ nuclear:cytoplasmic (N:C) ratios and distinct cell borders may be seen
  - On liquid-based Paps, cells round up; hence, center of group may be difficult to visualize
  - Apply criteria to cells along periphery that are well visualized
- **AECN**
  - Columnar endocervical-type cells presenting as large sheets, strips, and rosettes
  - Nuclear crowding, overlapping, and ↑ N:C ratios
  - Ill-defined or nonexistent cell borders due to overcrowding
  - Nuclear stratification with palisading and peripheral palisading along sheets, strips, and rosettes
  - Hyperchromasia with even chromatin
  - Chromocenters may be better seen on liquid-based Paps
  - Mitosis, especially floating mitosis on luminal side of strip or rosette
  - Architectural features better visualized on conventional Paps, as cells are 3D on liquid-based Paps
- **AEMC**
  - Small, rounded, endometrial-type cells presenting in small groups of 5-10 cells (more cohesive on liquid-based Paps)
  - Mildly enlarged nuclei with small nucleoli (more prominent on liquid-based Paps)
  - Slight hyperchromasia
  - Ill-defined cell borders, scant cytoplasm ± degenerative vacuoles
  - Vacuoles may contain engulfed inflammatory cells
- **AGC**
  - Cellular features beyond those expected with reactive/reparative changes, but exact nature of cells cannot be discerned (i.e., endocervical or endometrial)
  - If index of suspicion for neoplastic process is high, then AGCN can be used

Cell Block Findings
- Cell blocks from liquid-based specimens may be helpful in some cases

Cytology-Histology Correlation
- Reporting rates for AGC are between 0.1-0.9% of all Paps per College of American Pathologists published data
- Incidence of finding clinically significant lesions after diagnosis of any type of AGC abnormality is much higher than that following diagnosis of atypical squamous cells
  - Hence, tissue sampling is a must depending upon guidelines
- In young patients, most frequent significant finding after diagnosis of AGC, AGCN, AEC, or AECN is actually squamous intraepithelial lesion (SIL)
  - If HPV is positive
    - More likely to have cervical lesion like SIL or cervical carcinoma
  - If HPV is negative
    - More likely benign or endometrial pathology, especially in postmenopausal patients
- In older patients with diagnosis of AEMC, preneoplastic/neoplastic finding is usually endometrial hyperplasia or carcinoma
  - Endometrial polyps and disordered proliferative are among more frequent benign histologic correlates
- The older the postmenopausal patient with AEMC or AGC, the greater the likelihood of malignancy

ANCILLARY TESTS

Recommendations
- High-risk HPV testing can be useful in some scenarios as 2nd-line management [~ 25% HPV(+)]

Atypical Glandular Cells:
Endocervicals, Endometrials, and Glandulars, NOS

Reporting Rates for AGCs, College of American Pathologists Benchmarking Data

Pap Test Type	5th Percentile	25th Percentile	Median	75th Percentile	95th Percentile
Conventional (%)	0.0	0.0	0.1	0.2	0.8
ThinPrep (%)	0.0	0.1	0.2	0.3	1.0
SurePath (%)	0.0	0.1	0.2	0.3	0.8
AGC = atypical glandular cells.					

College of American Pathologists Cytopathology checklist 2021.

Relative Distribution of Malignancies in Paps Reported as AGCs*

Study/Year	Total Ca Cases	SqCa Cervix (%)	ACA/AdSQ Ca (%)	Others (%)	EM Ca (%)	Ovary/Tube Ca (%)
Schnatz P, 2006	203.0	5.4	23.6	6.9	57.6	6.4
Zhao C, 2009	44.0	2.3	12.4	n/a	77.2	9.1

*Includes all types of AGCs ± squamous abnormality reported; AGCs = atypical glandular cells; Ca = carcinoma; SqCa = squamous cell carcinoma; ACA = adenocarcinoma; AdSQ = adenosquamous carcinoma; EM = endometrial.

From: Schnatz P et al: Obstet Gynecol. 107(3):701-8, 2006 and Zhao C et al: Gynecol Oncol. 114(3):383-9, 2009.

- ○ HPV positivity varies with age; younger populations tend to have higher positivity rate
- Management of any AGC diagnosis on Pap always includes examination with tissue sampling
  - ○ Follow-up with cytology alone is not acceptable option

DIFFERENTIAL DIAGNOSIS

Tubal Metaplasia
- Terminal bars and cilia are key to diagnosis

Microglandular Hyperplasia
- Usually looks like repair, but nuclear overlap and polyploid cells may be problematic

High-Grade Squamous Intraepithelial Lesion
- Smooth outer contours to HCGs with cellular flattening and lack of polarization

Follicular Cervicitis
- Loose collections of lymphocytes, which are smaller cells and, hence, may be mistaken for AEMC

Endometrial Polyps
- Can shed AEMC or can be mistaken for AGC if directly sampled

Atypical Repair
- Flat sheets and some overlap of nuclei but repair-like configuration

Arias-Stella Reaction
- Patients are pregnant
- Cells resemble endometrials more than endocervicals

IUD Cells
- Bubbly cytoplasm with history of IUD

Menstrual Endometrium or Directly Sampled Endometrium/Endometriosis
- Usually mistaken for atypical endometrials
- Can resemble AEC if directly sampled

Bare Nuclei of Deep Atrophy
- Bland nuclear chromatin
- No cytoplasm
- Mistaken for AEMC

Lobular Endocervical Glandular Hyperplasia
- Abundant cytoplasm with yellowish tinge and large complex sheets; hence, called AEC

Abundant But Bland Hypermucinous Epithelium on Pap
- Rare phenomenon but can be indicator of serious underlying malignancy or benign conditions
- Benign conditions include lesions from endogenous or exogenous estrogens (microglandular hyperplasia/polyps, Arias-Stella reaction of pregnancy)
- Malignant conditions include metastatic low-grade mucinous carcinomas, well-differentiated gastric-type endocervical adenocarcinomas (adenoma malignum/minimal deviation adenocarcinomas), and mucinous endometrial carcinomas extending into cervix/lower uterine segment

SELECTED REFERENCES

1. ASCCP: Risk-based management consensus guidelines for abnormal cervical cancer screening tests and cancer precursors. Reviewed March 11, 2022. Accessed March 11, 2022. www.ASCCP.org/management-guidelines
2. Mantri S et al: Assessment of cytological features of glandular lesions of the cervix on conventional smear preparations-a comprehensive study from a tertiary care hospital. Diagn Cytopathol. 49(3):388-94, 2021
3. Torous VF et al: Interpretation pitfalls and malignant mimics in cervical cytology. J Am Soc Cytopathol. 10(2):115-27, 2021
4. Yucel Polat A et al: Atypical glandular cells in Papanicolaou test: which is more important in the detection of malignancy, architectural or nuclear features? Cytopathology. 32(3):344-52, 2021
5. Zuo T et al: High-risk human papillomavirus testing, genotyping, and histopathologic follow-up in women with abnormal glandular cells on Papanicolaou tests. Am J Clin Pathol. 156(4):569-76, 2021
6. Liu S et al: The reporting rates of atypical glandular cells and their HPV testing and histologic follow-up results: a comparison between ThinPrep and SurePath preparations from a single academic institution. J Am Soc Cytopathol. 8(3):128-32, 2019

Atypical Glandular Cells: Endocervicals, Endometrials, and Glandulars, NOS

Hypermucinous Glandular Epithelium

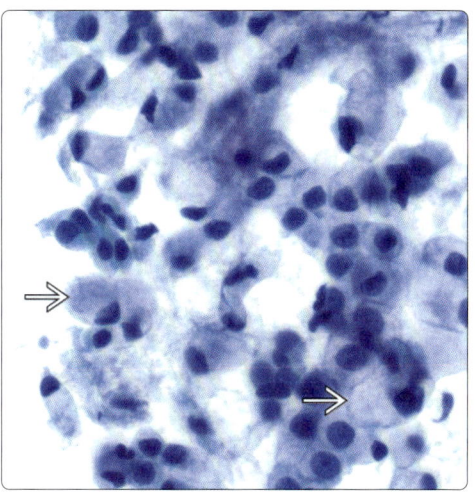

Atypical Glandular Cells, Favor Neoplastic

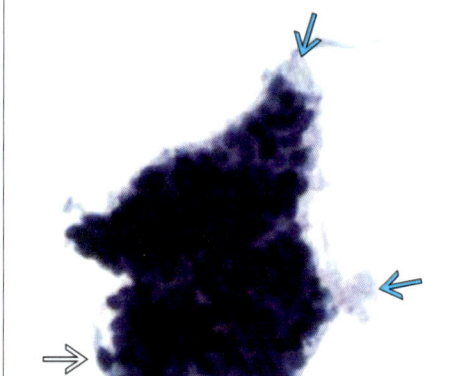

(Left) *Abundant hypermucinous but relatively bland glandular/endocervical cells are shown. Cytoplasm is engorged with mucin ➡. In the absence of history or unequivocal features of malignancy, these can be classified as AEC and warrant further work-up.* (Right) *A bloody and paucicellular ThinPrep Pap test in a 45-year-old shows a single large tight sheet of glandular cells with peripheral feathering ➡ and clinging diathesis ➡. Such cases should not be called unsatisfactory/nondiagnostic in the presence of any atypia.*

Atypical Endocervical Cells, Not Otherwise Specified

Atypical Endocervical Cells, Favor Neoplastic

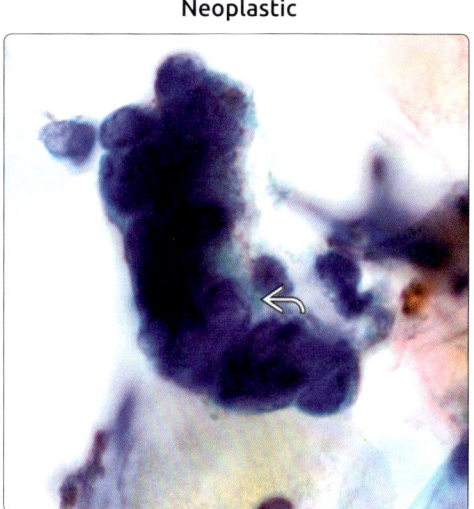

(Left) *ThinPrep Pap with a crowded sheet of endocervical-type cells shows nuclear overlap and increased N:C ratios ➡. Terminal bars and cilia ➡ were not easily visible on this tubal metaplasia, which was interpreted as AEC.* (Right) *ThinPrep Pap with a strip of AEC, favor neoplastic (AECN) shows high N:C ratios, marked nuclear crowding, and polarization perpendicular to the luminal axis ➡. Although these were suspicious for ACA in situ, they were quantitatively insufficient for a definitive diagnosis.*

Atypical Glandular Cells, Favor Neoplastic

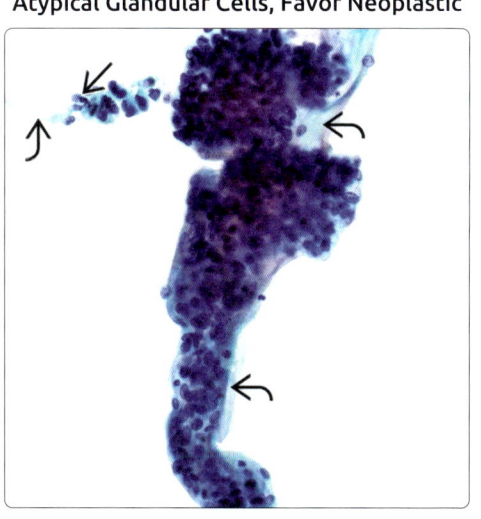

Atypical Endometrial Cells

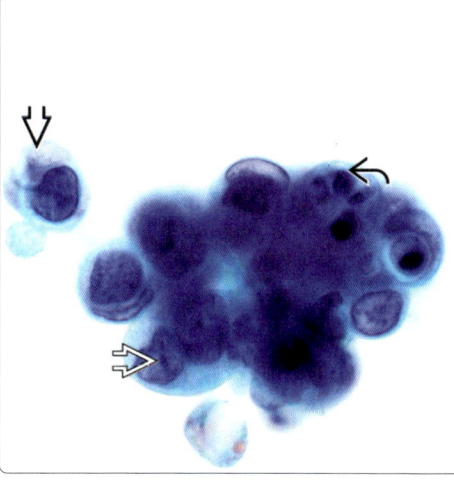

(Left) *ThinPrep Pap shows only a crowded strip of small cells with clinging-type diathesis ➡. 3D clusters and rare small cells ➡ are also noted in an otherwise bloody and hypocellular smear interpreted as AGCN. Biopsy showed endocervical adenocarcinoma (ACA).* (Right) *ThinPrep Pap test shows a tight cluster of small round cells with cytoplasmic vacuoles ➡. Nucleoli ➡, imbibed leukocytes, and lymphocytes ➡ are seen in atypical endometrial cells. Endometrial biopsy showed endometrioid ACA, FIGO grade II.*

Atypical Glandular Cells:
Endocervicals, Endometrials, and Glandulars, NOS

Atypical Endometrial Cells

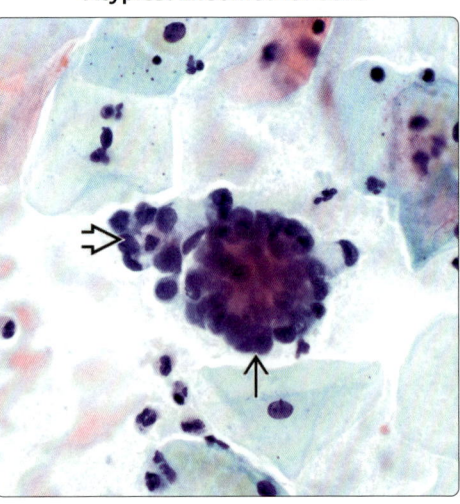

Atypical Endometrial Cells

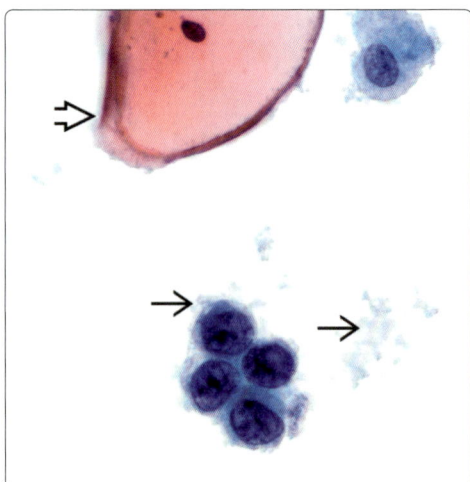

(Left) *Conventional Pap smear shows a large tight cluster ⇒ and a smaller loose group ⇒ of atypical endometrial cells in a high estrogenic background in a postmenopausal patient. Biopsy showed complex hyperplasia with atypia.* (Right) *ThinPrep Pap shows a cluster of 4 small atypical endometrial cells with a subtle diathesis ⇒. A superficial cell ⇒ in the background provides a size comparison. Biopsy revealed a low-grade endometrioid ACA.*

High-Grade Squamous Intraepithelial Lesion

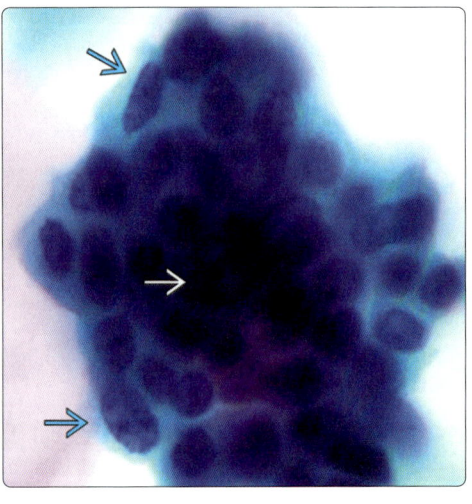

Atypical Endocervical Cells, Favor Neoplastic

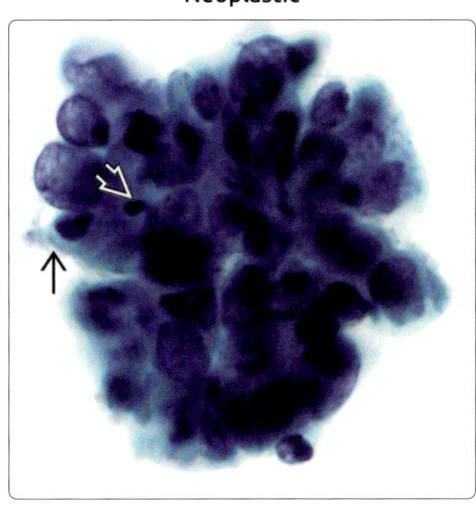

(Left) *SurePath Pap shows a hyperchromatic crowded group of HSIL, most likely with gland extension. The polarization is disordered in the center ⇒, and the cells along the periphery appear to run parallel to the circumference of the group ⇒.* (Right) *ThinPrep Pap with a large cluster of AECN shows variation in nuclear size and shape with evenly distributed hyperchromasia and possible apoptosis ⇒. The terminal bars and cilia ⇒ are difficult to see. Endocervical and endometrial samplings were benign with tubal metaplasia.*

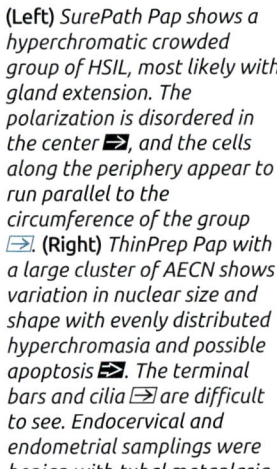

Atypical Endocervical Cells, Favor Neoplastic

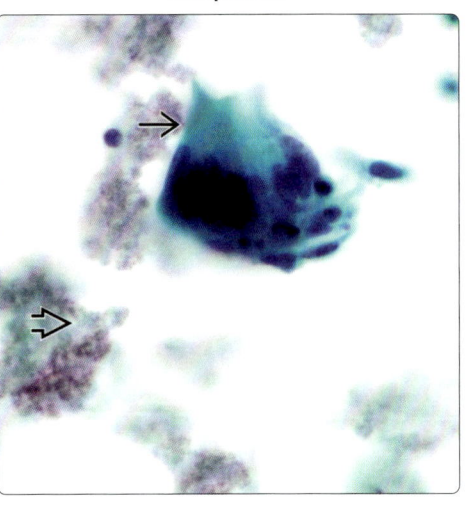

Follicular Cervicitis

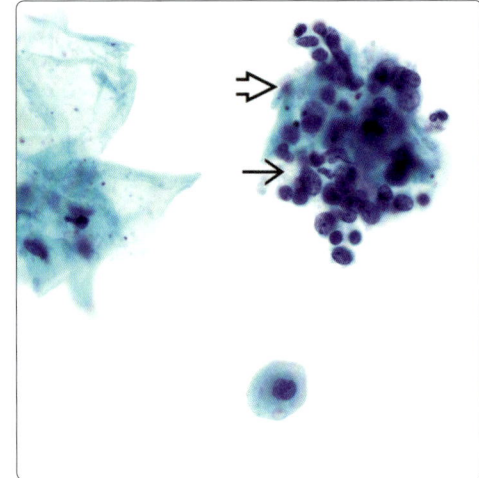

(Left) *SurePath Pap with a strip of AECN shows a bird tail-like configuration ⇒. The N:C ratio is slightly increased with mild hyperchromasia and a bloody background ⇒ in this case of cervical endometriosis.* (Right) *ThinPrep Pap shows loose aggregate of lymphocytes ⇒ of various sizes. Compare the small size of cells with adjacent epithelial cells. Tingible body macrophages ⇒ may be difficult to see on liquid-based Paps of follicular cervicitis and could thereby be misinterpreted as atypical endometrial cells.*

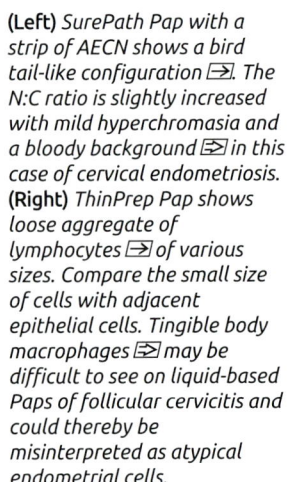

Atypical Glandular Cells: Endocervicals, Endometrials, and Glandulars, NOS

Papillary Villous Endocervicitis

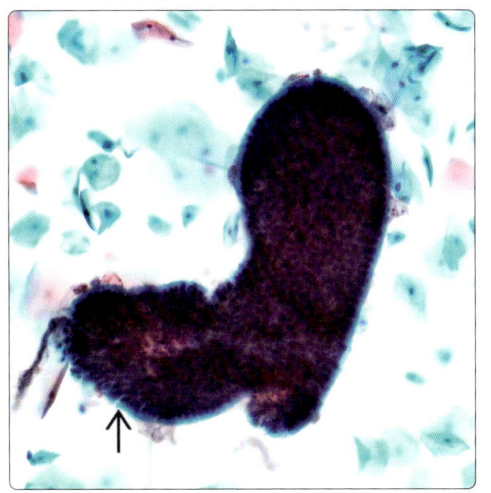

Radiation/Repair

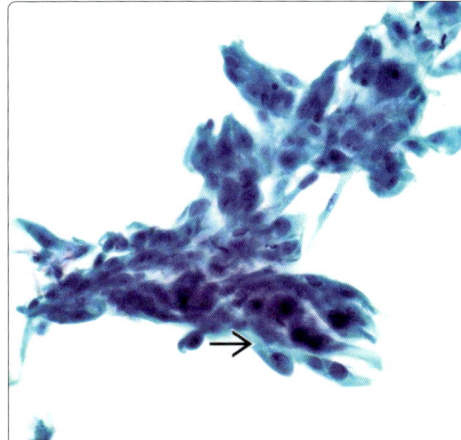

(Left) SurePath Pap shows papillary villous endocervicitis, which was inadvertently interpreted as AEC. Although the center of this cowboy boot-shaped cluster is difficult to visualize, the cells along the periphery are benign with low N:C ratios and proper orientation of normal ➡ but inflamed endocervical cells. *(Right)* Flat sheets of postradiation reparative changes are seen with stretched out cytoplasm ➡ but low N:C ratios on this ThinPrep Pap.

Atypical Lobular Endocervical Glandular Hyperplasia

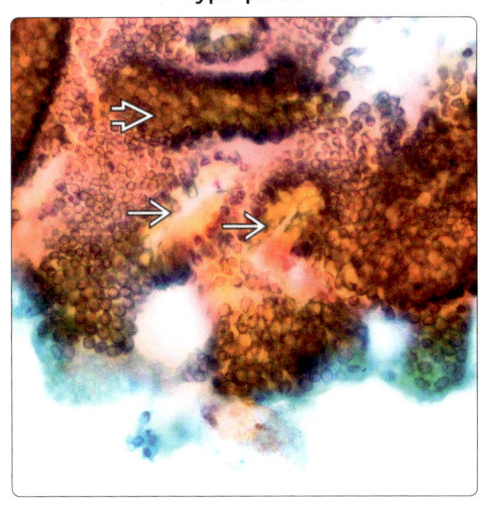

Distorted Endocervical Cells

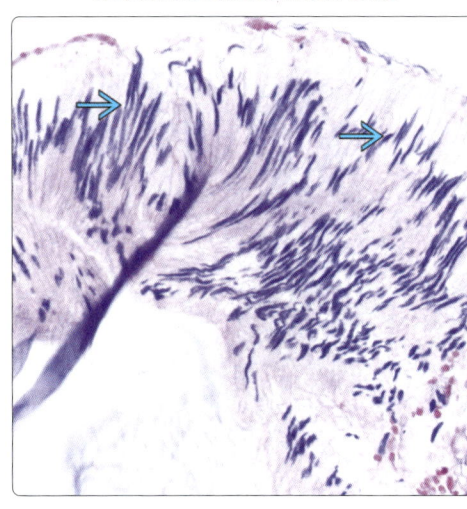

(Left) Pap shows large 3D architecturally complex sheets of crowded but bland mucin-producing endocervical-type cells with intrasheet lumina ➡ and tubular gland forms ➡. This is atypical lobular endocervical glandular hyperplasia, which is considered to be a precursor of minimal deviation ACA. (Courtesy Y. Sugiyama, MD.) *(Right)* H&E-stained section shows a strip of distorted endocervical cells at the loop electrosurgical excision procedure (LEEP) margin with pencil-shaped nuclei ➡.

Atypical Glandular Cells From Polyp

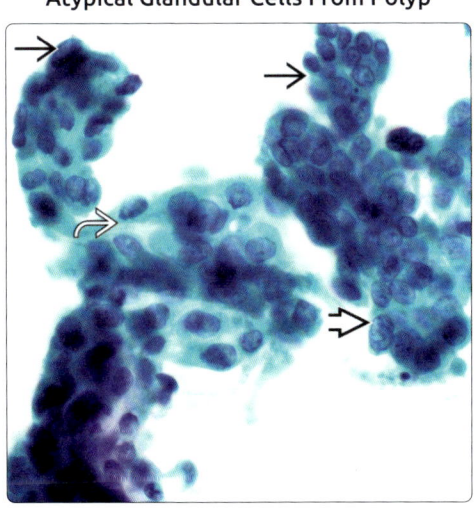

Atrophy With Artifact

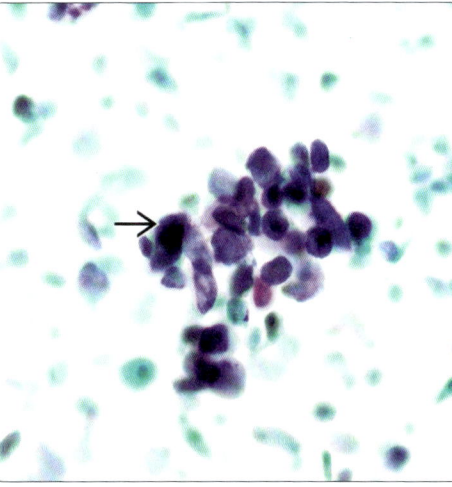

(Left) AGC are seen on ThinPrep Pap from a lower uterine segment polyp, which was inadvertently sampled. There is some glandular crowding ➡ with rosette formation ➡. Some areas resemble repair ➡. *(Right)* Bare nuclei of deep atrophy in this SurePath Pap test can easily be misinterpreted as atypical endometrial cells. The lack of cytoplasm and the bland but overstained nuclei ➡ can contribute to an overcall of atypical endometrial cells.

Endometrial Cells in Pap Test and Glandular Cells Status Post Hysterectomy

KEY FACTS

CYTOPATHOLOGY

- Endometrial cells have different presentations
- **Exfoliated endometrial cells** usually consist of rare groups
  - Endometrial glandular epithelial cells are small, ~ same size as intermediate cell nucleus, with rare nucleoli and vacuolated cytoplasm
  - Reported in women 45 ≥ years per 2014 Bethesda System (nonmenstrual, nonstromal, nonabraded)
- **Directly sampled endometrium or endometriosis** shows large hyperchromatic groups of cells consisting of glandular and stromal cells
  - Cellularity can vary from rare groups to abundant biphasic groups depending upon how vigorously endometrial cells are sampled
- Cervical endometriosis or shortened canal due to previous LEEP or trachelectomy can yield numerous endometrials
  - 1/3 of posttrachelectomy Paps yield directly sampled endometrial cells
- Directly sampled endometrial glandular cells in sheets are small, crowded, but not overlapping in focal plane
  - Glandular cells can show some feathering and strips with nuclear overlap
  - Stromal cells that are spindled may not be attached to glandular cells in liquid-based preparations
  - Mitosis may be seen in proliferative phase
  - Well-demarcated tubular glands and shapes
  - Plump spindled stromal cells with traversing vessels; better visible on conventional smears
- **Menstrual endometrial cells** are abundant if patient bleeding/menstrual
  - Menstrual pattern can be alarming on liquid-based Paps
    - Cell blocks prepared from liquid-based specimens with p16 or ProExC IHC staining can be helpful
- **Glandular cells status post hysterectomy**: Small flat sheets/rare groups of directly sampled bland cells ± mucin
- Glandular cells status post hysterectomy usually have scant cellularity

Endometrial Cells in Pap Test

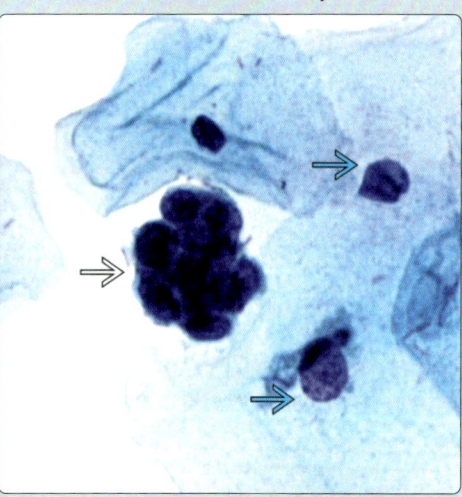

Normal Exfoliated Endometrial Cells

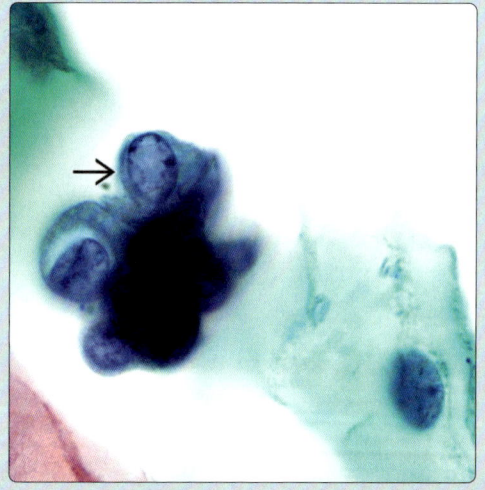

(Left) ThinPrep Pap test shows a tight cluster of endometrial cells ➡. Background intermediate squamous cells are present for nuclear size comparison ➡. *(Right)* SurePath Pap test shows a small cluster of endometrial cells ➡. Cells have a high nuclear:cytoplasmic (N:C) ratio due to scant cytoplasm but with no increase in nuclear size.

Endometrial Cells, Exodus Pattern

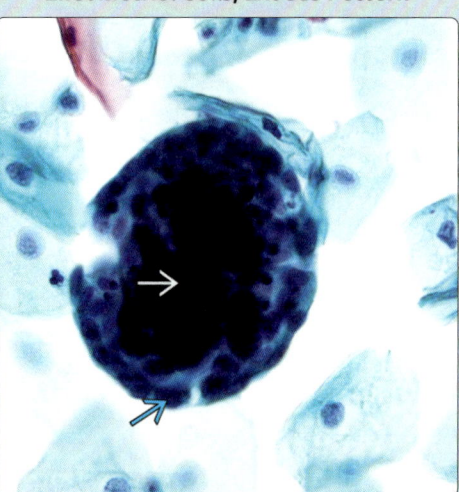

Benign Glandular Cells Post Hysterectomy

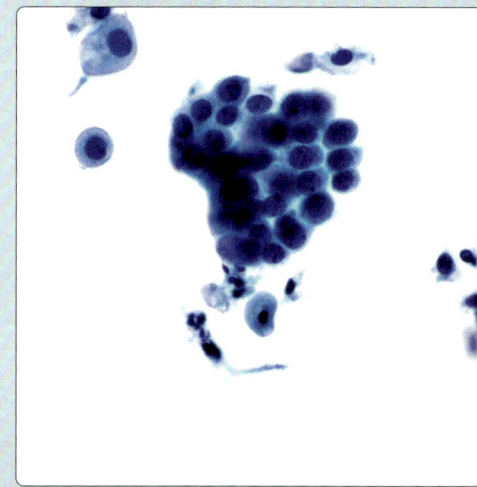

(Left) ThinPrep Pap test shows a cluster of endometrial cells with an exodus pattern typically seen at the end of menstrual flow. There is a 2-layered appearance with central dark and compact endometrial stroma ➡ and outer endometrial glandular cells ➡. *(Right)* SurePath Pap test shows benign glandular cells status post hysterectomy for endometrial cancer. No malignant features are seen.

Endometrial Cells in Pap Test and Glandular Cells Status Post Hysterectomy

TERMINOLOGY

Definitions

- Benign cells found out of phase (endometrial cells) or in situations where they do not belong (post hysterectomy)

CYTOPATHOLOGY

Cellularity

- Exfoliated endometrial cells usually consist of rare groups
  - Only exfoliated endometrial glandular cells in women 45+ years need reporting per 2014 Bethesda System
- Endometrial cells are abundant if patient bleeding/menstrual [no need to report if last menstrual period (LMP) known]
- If directly sampled or abraded, cellularity can vary from rare groups to abundant biphasic groups depending upon how vigorously endometrial cells are sampled
- Cervical endometriosis or shortened canal due to previous LEEP or trachelectomy can yield numerous endometrial cells
- Glandular cells status post hysterectomy usually have scant cellularity

Pattern

- Endometrial cells
  - Few small, tight groups of small cells (5-20 cells) when exfoliated
  - Flat biphasic sheets (can be numerous) if abraded
- Glandular cells status post hysterectomy
  - Rare flat sheet of benign cells without diathesis or necrosis

Background

- Can be clean or bloody (if patient is bleeding or menstrual)
- Usually clean for glandular cells status post hysterectomy (excludes supracervical hysterectomies)

Cells

- Endometrial cells have different presentations
  - Exfoliated cells are small, ~ same size as intermediate cell nucleus, with rare nucleoli and vacuolated cytoplasm
  - Directly sampled endometrium or endometriosis show large hyperchromatic groups of cells consisting of glandular and stromal cells
    - Glandular cells are small and appear crowded but not overlapping in focal plane
    - Stromal cells are spindled and may be attached to glandular groups in conventional preparations but separated in liquid-based preparations
  - Mitosis may be seen if proliferative
  - Well-demarcated tubular glands and shapes
  - Plump, spindle stromal cells with traversing vessels
  - Menstrual pattern can be alarming on liquid-based Paps
    - Abundance of cells with somewhat geometric shapes, stromal breakdown, and blood; therefore, correlation with LMP is key to correct diagnosis
    - In difficult cases, cell block with p16 staining can be helpful
- Glandular cells status post hysterectomy: Small flat sheets or rare groups of directly sampled bland cells ± mucin

Cytology-Histology Correlation

- 2014 Bethesda Reporting System requires reporting of exfoliated, normal endometrial glandular cells in women > 45 years either under "normal" or "other" if standalone finding
  - Post-Bethesda 2001 data and metaanalysis do not support need for follow-up of asymptomatic patients < 45 years due to low yield of significant pathology (hyperplasias or carcinomas)

DIFFERENTIAL DIAGNOSIS

Adenocarcinoma In Situ and Adenocarcinoma

- Sheets, feathering, and rosettes; HPV(+) and p16 block (+)

HSIL, ASC-H, and Squamous Cell Carcinoma

- Nuclear morphology, HPV(+), and p16(+)

SELECTED REFERENCES

1. Hernandez A et al: Reporting of benign endometrial cells in Papanicolaou tests. Am J Clin Pathol. 154(3):381-6, 2020

Directly Sampled Endometrial Cells

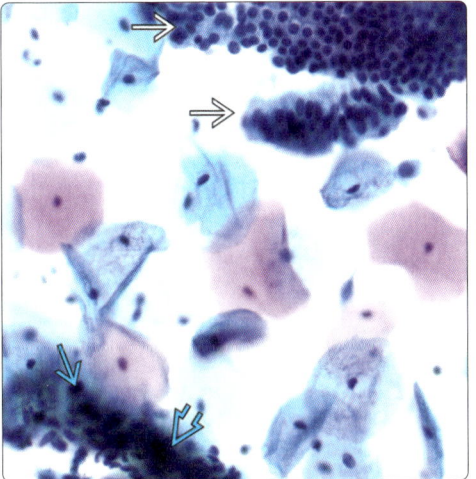

Directly Sampled Cervical Endometriosis

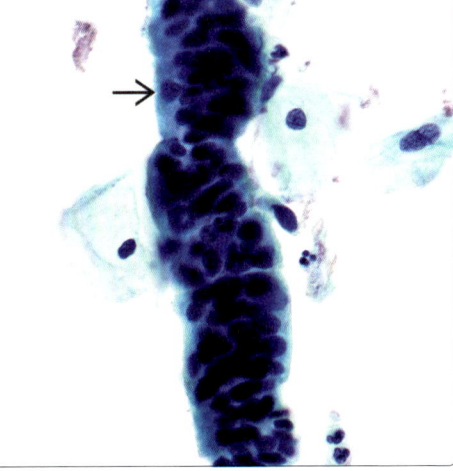

(Left) SurePath Pap test shows dissociated endometrial glandular epithelium ➡ from the endometrial stroma ➡, which has spindle cells with a transgressing vessel ➡. (Right) SurePath Pap test shows a strip of directly sampled cervical endometriosis. There is nuclear overlapping with high N:C ratios and a lack of nuclear polarization. A mitotic figure ➡ is also seen. This is the perfect mimic for adenocarcinoma in situ.

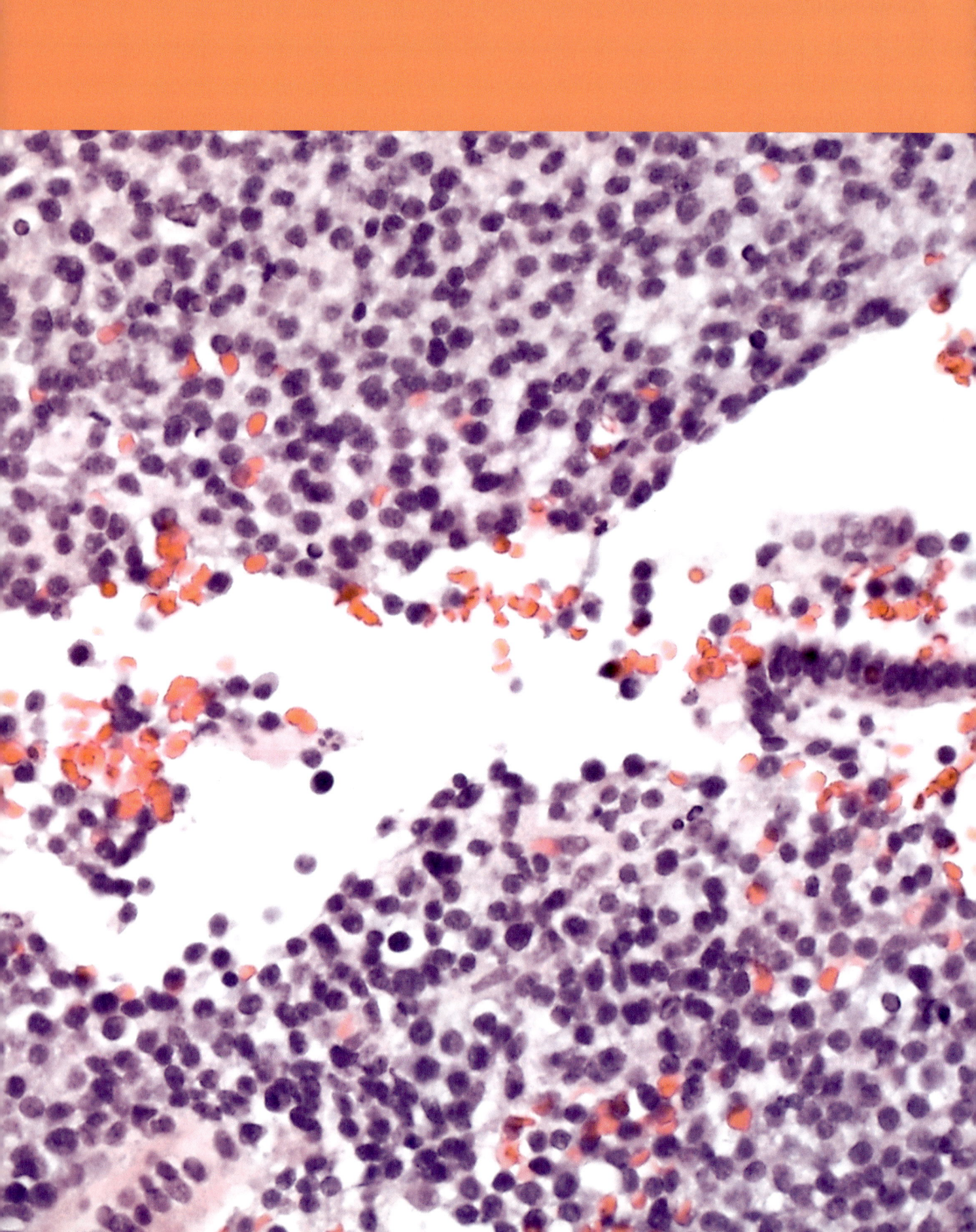

PART I
SECTION 5
Extrauterine Carcinomas and Other Malignancies of Female Genital Tract

Extrauterine Carcinomas and Presentations in Cervicovaginal Cytology	74
Neuroendocrine Carcinoma of Cervix	76
Other Uncommon Malignancies in Cervicovaginal Cytology	78

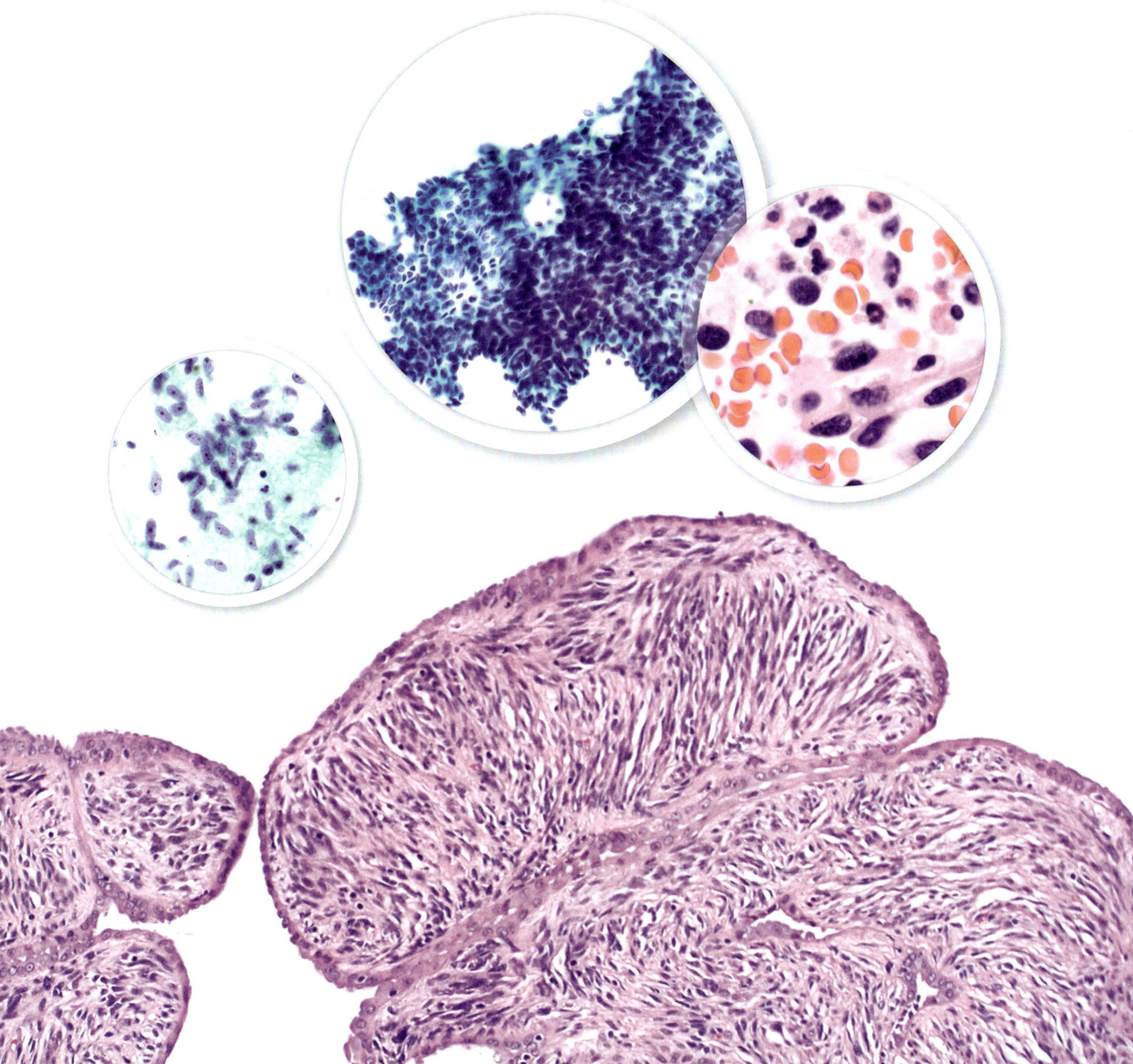

Extrauterine Carcinomas and Presentations in Cervicovaginal Cytology

KEY FACTS

TERMINOLOGY
- Vaginal/cervical metastases may be synchronous or metachronous with primary tumor
- Secondary involvement of vagina must be excluded before diagnosis of vaginal primary

CYTOPATHOLOGY
- Low cellularity if extrauterine carcinoma spreads/floats through fallopian tube and endometrium without metastasis
- Highly cellular if metastasis to vagina or direct extension from rectum or bladder
- Cytologic features depend on primary tumor, extent of spread, ascites, and patency of fallopian tubes
- Clean background if spread via fallopian tube without metastasis; patients may also have ascites
- Diathesis if direct extension or actual metastasis to vagina, endometrium, or cervix due to stromal response
- Morphologically, cells do not belong in environment

ANCILLARY TESTS
- Immunostains can be helpful in confirming diagnosis for tumors originating outside female genital tract
  - e.g., TTF-1 for metastatic lung adenocarcinoma, DOG1 and CD117 for metastatic gastrointestinal stromal tumor, CK20 and CDX2 for metastatic colorectal adenocarcinoma
- Immunostains are often of no use when suspected primary is in female genital tract
  - Primary vaginal adenocarcinoma has same immunophenotype as primary endometrial adenocarcinoma
  - Primary vaginal squamous cell carcinoma has same immunophenotype as primary vulvar or cervical squamous cell carcinoma

TOP DIFFERENTIAL DIAGNOSES
- Adenocarcinoma is most common tumor type to secondarily involve vagina

Ovarian Serous Carcinoma With Psammoma Bodies

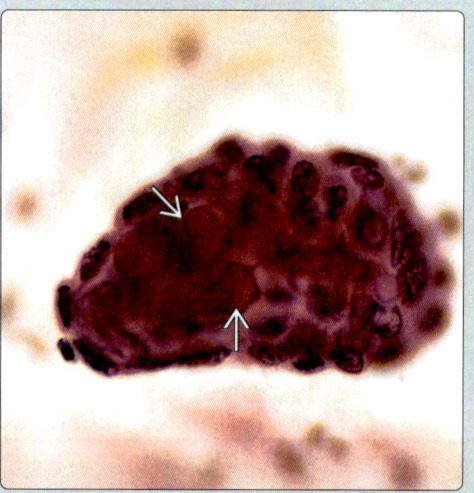

Rectal Carcinoma: Direct Extension

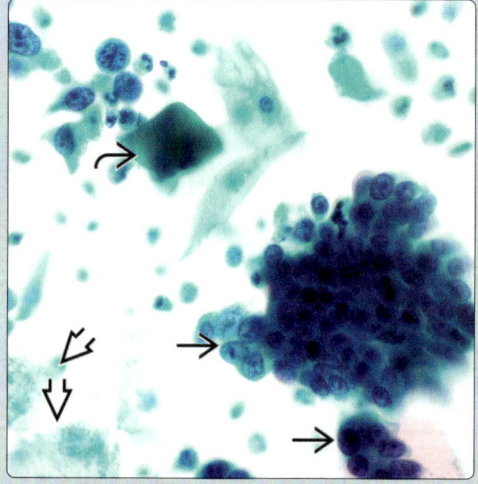

(Left) Conventional Pap stain shows a 3D papillary cluster of ovarian serous papillary carcinoma with psammoma bodies ➡ and a clean background. *(Right)* SurePath Pap stain shows rectal carcinoma and fecal material from a rectovaginal fistula (directly sampled). Note the cancer cells ➡ with rosettes, tumor diathesis ➡, and skeletal muscle fibers ➡.

Fallopian Tube Primary

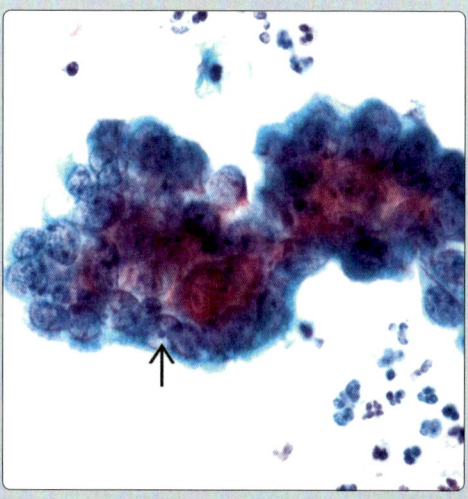

Urothelial Carcinoma

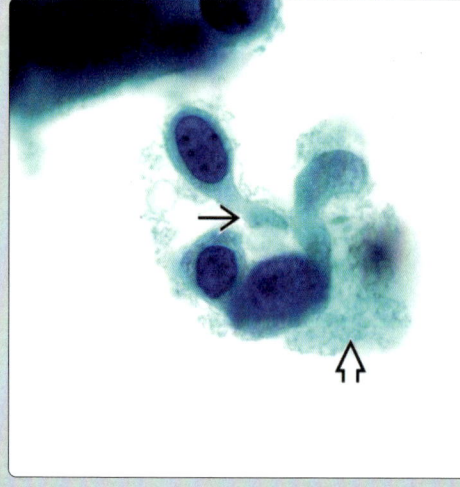

(Left) Conventional Pap stain shows a 3D papillary cluster in a clean background that has traveled from a fallopian tube primary high-grade serous carcinoma. Cells have high nuclear:cytoplasmic ratios, nucleoli ➡, and scant cytoplasm. (Courtesy A. Farnsworth, MBBS, FRCPA.) *(Right)* SurePath Pap stain shows cercariform cells with tail-like extensions ➡ and diathesis ➡ from a metastatic urothelial carcinoma to the vagina.

Extrauterine Carcinomas and Presentations in Cervicovaginal Cytology

TERMINOLOGY

Abbreviations
- Extrauterine carcinoma (ExUCa)

Definitions
- Involvement of vagina (&/or, very rarely, cervix) by secondary malignant neoplasm via metastasis, direct extension, or passing through fallopian tube, endometrial cavity, and cervix without actual metastasis

CLINICAL ISSUES

Presentation
- Incidental finding
  - Vaginal bleeding, symptoms related to mass/metastasis
- Carcinomas more frequent than sarcomas and other metastatic tumors
- Metastatic tumors constitute 90% of all adenocarcinomas in vagina
- In most cases, primary is known

CYTOPATHOLOGY

Cellularity
- Low cellularity if ExUCa floats through fallopian tube without metastasis
- If metastasis to vagina (rarely cervix) or direct extension from rectum or bladder, then very cellular due to direct sampling

Pattern
- Depends upon location and type of primary tumor

Background
- Clean if spread through fallopian tube and endometrium without metastases
  - Patients may have ascites as well
- Diathesis if direct extension or actual metastasis to vagina or (rarely) cervix or endometrium
- Diathesis if direct extension from adjacent organ or fistula

Cells
- Varies by primary site

Cell Block Findings
- Cell blocks from liquid-based specimen can be helpful for immunohistochemical work-up of unknown primary

MICROSCOPIC

Histologic Features
- Resembles primary tumor with respect to architectural and cytologic features

SELECTED REFERENCES

1. Sassi I et al: Uterine cervix metastasis from primary colon adenocarcinoma: a case report and review of the literature. J Med Case Rep. 15(1):486, 2021
2. Wilbur C et al: The Bethesda System for Reporting Cervical Cytology: Definitions, Criteria, and Explanatory Notes. 3rd ed. Springer-Verlag, 2015

Presentation of Extrauterine Malignancies in Cervicovaginal Cytology

Primary Site	Mechanism of Presentation	Cytology	Background	Notes
Ovary	Passing through fallopian tube/endometrium; rarely, metastasis to vagina	Papillae ± psammoma bodies and large nucleoli	Usually clean unless metastasis to cervix or vagina	Rare primary presentation on Pap test
Fallopian tube	Passing through endometrium and cervix	Papillae and high nuclear grade, ± psammoma bodies	Usually clean or watery	Rare primary presentation on Pap test
Bladder	Direct extension or metastasis	Transitional or cercariform cells ± squamous or glandular differentiation	Usually tumor diathesis	p16 and high-risk HPV (-) helps in differentiation from cervical primary
Colon/rectum	Direct extension through rectovaginal septum or fistula or metastasis	Tall columnar cells ± mucin and cigar-shaped nuclei with palisading	Tumor diathesis; fecal material if rectovaginal fistula	CK20 and CDX2 (+); PAX8(-) helpful in diagnosis
Breast	Ascites; rarely, metastasis	Signet-rings, intracytoplasmic targetoid mucin, single files	Usually clean	PAX8(-); ER/PR and GATA3 (+)
Stomach	Ascites, passing through tube; rarely, metastasis	Signet-rings, single files	Usually clean	Usually known history; differential diagnosis is breast carcinoma
Kidney	Metastasis; history usually known	Abundant fragile cytoplasm, large nuclei with nucleoli	Diathesis if metastasis to cervix &/or vagina	PAX8, RCC, and CD10 (+)
Melanoma	Usually metastasis, known history; rarely, primary	Cells can look epithelial, spindle, pleomorphic, amelanotic	Diathesis or clean	S100/HMB-45 (+)
Lymphomas	Involvement by metastasis; rarely, ascites	Dispersed lymphoid population	Diathesis or clean if ascites	Usually known history
Sarcomas	Usually metastasis	Varies by primary type	Tumor diathesis	Primary type usually known

Neuroendocrine Carcinoma of Cervix

KEY FACTS

CLINICAL ISSUES
- Aggressive behavior; often female patients in 30s or 40s

CYTOPATHOLOGY
- Usually hypercellular Pap with tumor cells dominating and brisk mitosis (> 10 mitoses/10 HPF)
- Small, round, oval, or spindle cells with scant cytoplasm and increased nuclear:cytoplasmic ratio
- Nuclei with finely dispersed chromatin or hyperchromasia and inconspicuous nucleoli (salt and pepper chromatin) and numerous apoptoses
- Nuclear molding and crush artifact in conventional Pap
- Liquid-based Pap shows mostly dispersed cell population or small, caterpillar-like linear groups
- Hyperchromatic crowded groups may be seen
- Nuclear contours and chromatinic characteristics different from high-grade squamous intraepithelial lesion or nonkeratinizing squamous cell carcinoma, with which it may coexist
- May be often associated with adenocarcinoma or adenocarcinoma in situ due to human papillomavirus (HPV) type 18 predominance in both
- Large cell neuroendocrine carcinoma has larger cells with more cytoplasm and may show nucleoli

ANCILLARY TESTS
- Neuroendocrine markers (synaptophysin, chromogranin, CD56) variably (+)
- Up to 60% of small cell neuroendocrine carcinoma (SCNEC) can be (-) for chromogranin and synaptophysin
- TTF-1(+) in up to 40% (mostly SCNEC)

TOP DIFFERENTIAL DIAGNOSES
- Metastatic small cell carcinoma
  - History of disseminated disease; HPV(-)
- Basaloid/small cell squamous cell carcinoma
- Large cell neuroendocrine carcinoma
- Bare nuclei of atrophy, follicular cervicitis, menstrual endometrium, endometrial carcinoma

Small Cell Neuroendocrine Carcinoma on Conventional Pap

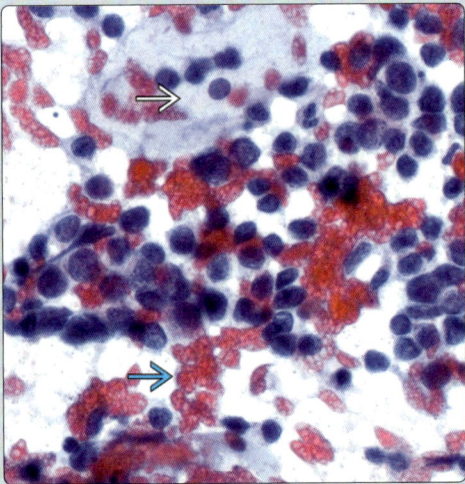

Small Cell Neuroendocrine Carcinoma, Nuclear Molding

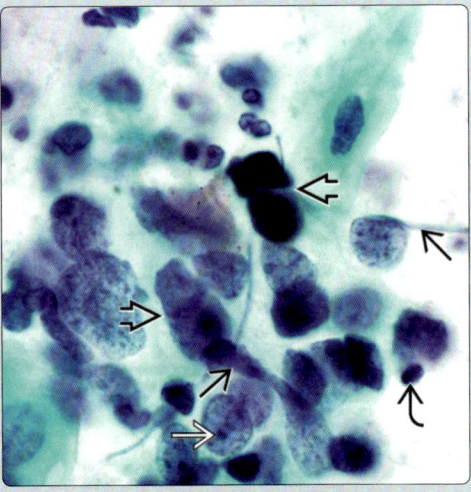

(Left) Pap stain shows overwhelming predominance of the small, round, malignant cells with only a rare normal squamous cell ➡. The bloody diathesis is easily visualized ➡ on conventional Pap. *(Right)* Conventional Pap smear demonstrates nuclear streaking ➡, molding ➡, apoptosis ➡, and small nucleoli ➡ that may be seen in the midst of the characteristic evenly dispersed chromatin.

Small Cell Neuroendocrine Carcinoma on ThinPrep

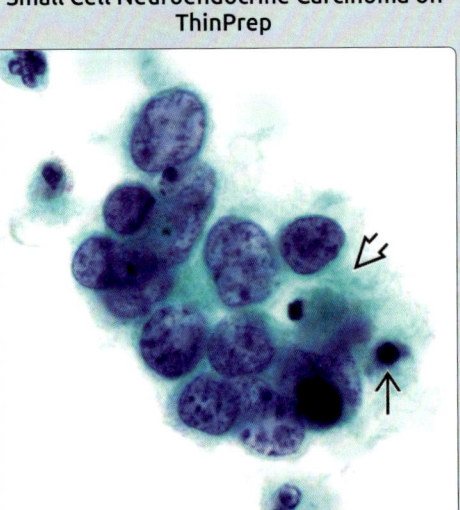

Small Cell Neuroendocrine Carcinoma and Adenocarcinoma

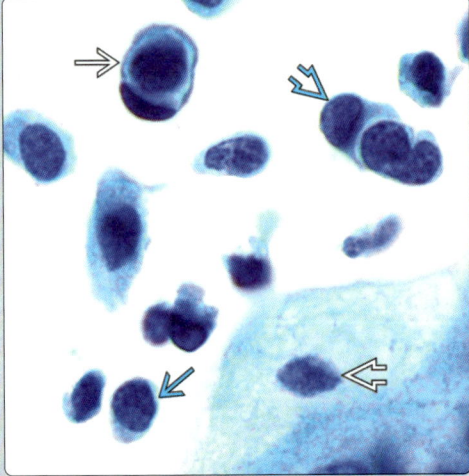

(Left) SCNEC shows hyperchromasia with characteristic chromatin, minimal to no nuclear molding, scant cytoplasm, and apoptosis ➡. A clinging diathesis ➡ is also noted. Some variation in nuclear size is seen absent the significant contour irregularity of HSIL or squamous carcinoma. *(Right)* SurePath Pap shows single ➡ and linear clusters ➡ of cells. Cell-within-cell pattern ➡ of coexistent adenocarcinoma is also seen. An intermediate-cell nucleus ➡ is seen for comparison.

Neuroendocrine Carcinoma of Cervix

TERMINOLOGY

Abbreviations
- Small cell neuroendocrine carcinoma (SCNEC)
- Large cell neuroendocrine carcinoma (LCNEC)

ETIOLOGY/PATHOGENESIS

Infectious Agents
- High-risk human papillomavirus (HPV), type 18 (SCNEC), 16 (LCNEC), or 45 most common

CLINICAL ISSUES

Prognosis
- Poor outcome for all stages with high recurrence rate even when initial good response to neoadjuvant chemotherapy for SCNEC and LCNEC

CYTOPATHOLOGY

Pattern
- Hypercellular, dispersed cells with nuclear molding (less on liquid based) and few hyperchromatic crowded groups

Background
- Bloody diathesis on conventional preparations
  - Can be subtle or clinging type on liquid-based specimens

Cells
- SCNEC 2.0-2.5x size of small lymphocytes, larger in LCNEC
- Scant cytoplasm in SCNEC

Nuclear Details
- Hyperchromatic but dispersed chromatin ± chromocenters
  - Nucleoli are rare (unless LCNEC)
  - Nuclear molding best on conventional preparations; on liquid-based, dispersed or caterpillar-like linear groups

Cell Block Findings
- Cell block from liquid-based specimens is helpful for immunohistochemical confirmation

ANCILLARY TESTS

Immunohistochemistry
- Low molecular weight cytokeratin (punctate staining), EMA, CEA, p16, and p53 variably (+)
- Neuroendocrine markers (synaptophysin, chromogranin, CD56) often (+), TTF-1(+) in up to 40%

DIFFERENTIAL DIAGNOSIS

Metastatic Small Cell Carcinoma (vs. SCNEC)
- Often history of widespread metastases at diagnosis

Squamous Cell Carcinoma With Small &/or Basaloid Cells (vs. SCNEC)
- p40(+), neuroendocrine markers (-)

Adenocarcinoma With Neuroendocrine Features (vs. LCNEC)
- Neuroendocrine markers (-) in glands

Lymphoma/Leukemia (vs. SCNEC and LCNEC)
- Prior history; noncohesive cells; lymphoma markers (+)

Benign Mimics
- Follicular cervicitis, deep atrophy, menstrual endometrium

SELECTED REFERENCES

1. Cimic A et al: Molecular profiling reveals limited targetable biomarkers in neuroendocrine carcinoma of the cervix. Appl Immunohistochem Mol Morphol. 29(4):299-304, 2021
2. Gupta P et al: Cytomorphological features of cervical small cell neuroendocrine carcinoma in SurePath liquid-based cervical samples. Cytopathology. 32(6):813-8, 2021

Cervical Neuroendocrine Tumors and Their Mimics

Tumor/Entity	Cellularity	Cytologic Atypia	Mitosis	Necrosis	Other
Carcinoid (NET G1)	Low	None to mild	Very rare	None	Extremely rare entity
Atypical carcinoid (NET G2)	Low to moderate	Mild to moderate	5-10/HPF on tissue	Minimal/focal	Extremely rare entity
SCNEC	Hypercellular on Pap	Moderate to severe	Brisk, > 10/10 HPF	Extensive	~ 2% of cervical cancers
Large cell neuroendocrine carcinoma	Cellular	Severe	Brisk, > 10/10 HPF	Extensive/geographic on tissue	Rare, mixed with SCNEC, squamous, or adenocarcinoma
Squamous carcinoma (small cell, nonkeratinizing)	Cellular	Moderate to severe	Variable	Tumor diathesis in 50%	Nuclear and chromatinic irregularities compared to SCNEC
Follicular cervicitis	Low	None, cell size can vary	Usually low	None, tingible body macrophages	Small nuclei with size variation in puddles; no molding
Bare nuclei of atrophy	Usually low	None	None	Pseudodiathesis if atrophic vaginitis	Postmenopausal
Endometrial cancer	Low	Low to moderate	None to rare unless high grade	None unless high grade	Postmenopausal or polycystic ovarian syndrome

SCNEC = small cell neuroendocrine carcinoma; NET = neuroendocrine tumor; G1 = grade 1; G2 = grade 2.

Other Uncommon Malignancies in Cervicovaginal Cytology

TERMINOLOGY

Definitions
- Rare malignant neoplasms that are very uncommonly encountered on Pap smears/tests

MELANOMA

General Features
- Primary vaginal melanoma is extremely rare
  - Mostly postmenopausal patients
  - 40% in lower vagina
- Bleeding, discharge, palpable mass
- Vaginal melanomas are not always pigmented and are not associated with pale skin as seen in cutaneous melanomas
- Primary cervical melanoma is even rarer and may be mistaken for sarcoma or carcinoma
- Blue nevi are more common but are stromal, hence not sampled on cytology

Cytology
- Cytology of melanoma on Pap depends on type of melanoma
  - Epithelioid, spindle, pleomorphic, amelanotic
- Tumor diathesis, blood in background
- May show cells resembling high-grade squamous intraepithelial lesion (HSIL) or carcinoma
- History of previous lesions in cervicovaginal tract is helpful as there is field effect for these lesions
- Only 55% of mucosal melanomas contain pigment
- Survival depends upon depth of tumor and extent of spread; generally poor prognosis
- No association with HPV

LYMPHOMA

General Features
- 1% of extranodal lymphomas originate in female genital tract; usually secondary involvement
- Primary lymphomas are mostly non-Hodgkin type, with diffuse large B-cell lymphoma being most common, followed by Burkitt lymphoma and follicular lymphoma
- Diffuse large B-cell lymphoma, Burkitt lymphoma, and follicular lymphoma also predominate in secondary lymphomas to female genital tract
- Primary cervical lymphoma is 3x more likely than endometrial; most are subepithelial and hence not easily detected on exfoliative cytology
- Marker studies are needed for confirmation; cell block may be helpful, but Pap test material is not suitable for flow cytometry due to fixatives in vials

Cytology
- Most present with bleeding and dispersed population of monotonous but atypical lymphocytes
- Obscuring blood and inflammation are problematic
- Differential diagnostic considerations include follicular/chronic cervicitis, small cell carcinoma, and endometrial stromal sarcoma

ADENOSQUAMOUS CARCINOMA

General Features
- Less common than adenocarcinomas
- Worse prognosis
- HPV-18 predominates

Cytology
- Adenocarcinoma resembles usual endocervical type, whereas squamous component can be nonkeratinizing or keratinizing
- Differential is collision tumors and adenoacanthomas
- Glassy cell carcinoma is even rarer variant of poorly differentiated adenosquamous carcinoma
  - Cytologically very malignant, but exact diagnosis is made on tissue sample
  - Large nucleoli, which may be mistaken for Herpes virus or Hodgkin lymphoma
  - Lymphoplasmacytic infiltrate along with eosinophils in background

Melanoma of Cervix Gross Appearance

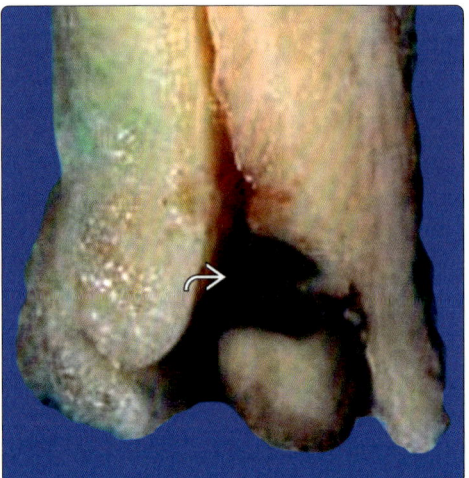

Melanoma Cytology on SurePath

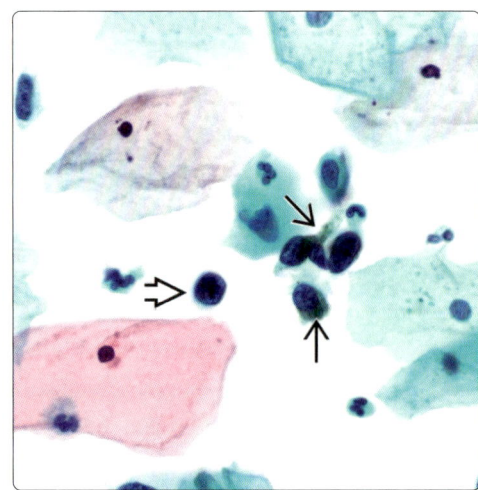

(Left) Gross photograph shows a polypoid, partially pigmented ➔, malignant melanoma of the cervix. (Right) SurePath Pap test shows small, hyperchromatic, round and spindle cells with high nuclear:cytoplasmic ratios. The cytoplasmic melanin pigment ➔ in this case is diagnostic. Amelanotic cells ➔ can be mistaken for a high-grade squamous intraepithelial lesion (HSIL).

Other Uncommon Malignancies in Cervicovaginal Cytology

○ Younger individuals, HPV-18 and 16 predominate

ADENOID CYSTIC CARCINOMA

General Features
- Extremely rare; resembles salivary gland counterpart but poorly differentiated with mitosis and necrosis
- Affects mostly older, postmenopausal women
  ○ Age range: 30-90
- High-risk HPV positive (type 16 predominates)

Cytology
- Presents as hyperchromatic crowded groups and acini with hyaline globules
- Morphologically similar to salivary gland adenoid cystic carcinoma
- Differential includes small cell carcinoma, poorly differentiated squamous cell carcinoma, adenocarcinoma, and endometrial carcinoma

ADENOSARCOMA

General Features
- Rare; can involve cervix or endometrium
- Usually presents as polyp that is inadvertently sampled
- Bland/benign surface glandular epithelium that may show repair-like changes if traumatized
- Underlying stroma is spindled and sarcomatous
- Sarcomatous component may be bland and low grade or higher grade and rarely rhabdoid

Cytology
- Only diagnosable if sampled, in which case it is cytologically recognized as a low- or high-grade nonepithelial spindle cell neoplasm
- Histology and morphology are key to diagnosis

SARCOMAS

General Features
- Very rarely seen on cervicovaginal cytology unless involving cervix or vagina, or, if endometrial, then protruding from cervical os and inadvertently sampled
  ○ Can be carcinosarcomas mixed with epithelial components or pure sarcomas
  ○ Leiomyosarcomas, fibrosarcomas, stromal sarcomas, and rhabdomyosarcomas may occur at this site
  ○ Most present with abnormal spindle cells or bizarre pleomorphic cells
  ○ Difficult to diagnose exact type of sarcoma; immunohistochemical work-up needed on cell block or biopsy

Cytology
- Cellular and hemorrhagic with diathesis when directly sampled
- Pleomorphic population of spindle cells with variable degree of mitotic activity and necrosis
- Low-grade stromal sarcomas may resemble endometrial stroma or even HSIL

ADENOID BASAL CARCINOMA

General Features
- Very rare indolent tumor; affects older postmenopausal women, often non-White women
- Usually diagnosed retrospectively on surgical specimens

Cytology
- Bland basaloid cells with peripheral palisading, rare mitosis, and no necrosis
- Usually associated with HSIL and hence detected on Pap; HPV-16 positive
- Usually not recognized on cytology
  ○ Many may not even involve surface and hence not sampled on cytology

EWING SARCOMA/PRIMITIVE NEUROECTODERMAL TUMOR AND OTHER SMALL ROUND BLUE CELL TUMORS

General Features
- Extremely rare; wide age range but is most common post menopause

Cytology
- Primitive neuroectodermal tumor produces cellular specimens consisting of small round blue cells
- Dark and light cell types with mitosis and apoptosis
- Vesicular chromatin and occasional nucleoli
- Work-up is that of small round blue cell tumors like those under musculoskeletal system
- Differential includes rhabdomyosarcomas and other small round blue cell tumors, including hematopoietic neoplasms

EPITHELIOID TROPHOBLASTIC TUMOR

General Features
- Extremely rare; occurs during reproductive years and is more common in women with history of pregnancy; serum HCG may be elevated

Cytology
- High-risk HPV is negative
- Large cells that cytologically and histologically resemble squamous cell carcinoma

SELECTED REFERENCES

1. Capsa C et al: Primary non-Hodgkin uterine lymphoma of the cervix: a literature review. Medicina (Kaunas). 58(1), 2022
2. Ng JKM et al: Smear detected cervicovaginal melanoma following negative screening-a cautionary tale of rapidly developing malignancy of the lower female genital tract. Cytopathology. 32(6):819-22, 2021
3. Vaziri Fard E et al: Primary synovial sarcoma of the uterine cervix: first case report. Int J Gynecol Pathol. 40(2):196-203, 2021
4. Albert A et al: Primary sarcoma of the cervix: an analysis of patient and tumor characteristics, treatment patterns, and outcomes. J Gynecol Oncol. 31(3):e25, 2020
5. Shi H et al: A clinicopathological and molecular analysis of cervical carcinomas with basaloid features. Histopathology. 76(2):283-95, 2020
6. Zhang Y et al: Ewing's sarcoma of the cervix: a case report and review of literature. Histol Histopathol. 35(5):475-80, 2020
7. Yin C et al: Primary cervical malignant melanoma: 2 cases and a literature review. Int J Gynecol Pathol. 38(2):196-203, 2019

Other Uncommon Malignancies in Cervicovaginal Cytology

Amelanotic Melanoma Cell

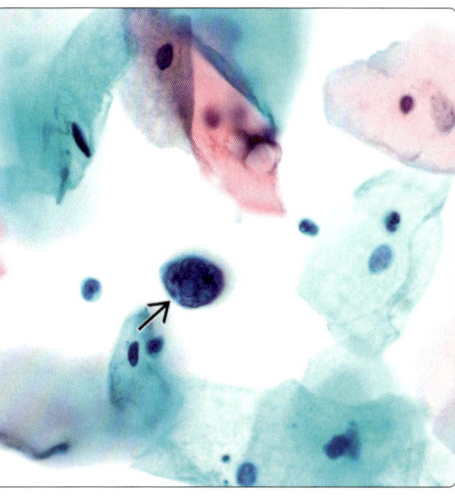

Melanoma Biopsy From Pigmented Area

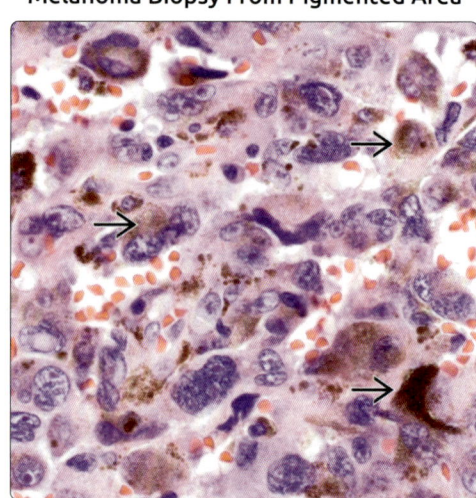

(Left) SurePath Pap test shows a single cell with a high nuclear:cytoplasmic ratio and nuclear contour cerebrations ➔, resembling a cell of HSIL. Other pigmented cells on the same slide pointed to the correct diagnosis of melanoma. **(Right)** Biopsy from the pigmented portion of a melanoma shows easily recognizable, pigmented malignant cells ➔. These bizarre cells were rare or absent on Pap test as they were present high in the canal and not sampled.

Lymphoma in Cervix

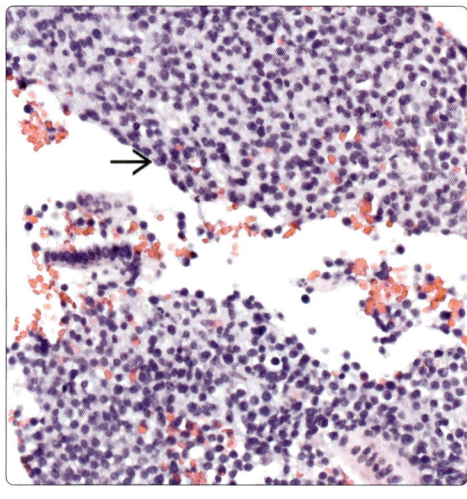

Large B-Cell Lymphoma of Uterus

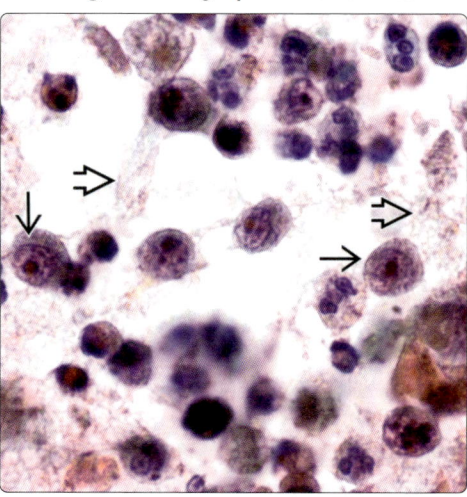

(Left) H&E of non-Hodgkin lymphoma ➔ shows secondary involvement of the cervix and endometrium. Most of the tumor was submucosal and hence not sampled on Pap test. **(Right)** Conventional Pap shows a dispersed population of cells with high nuclear:cytoplasmic ratios, some with prominent nucleoli ➔, in a bloody, diathesis-like background ➔. This was a secondary diffuse large B-cell lymphoma involving the cervix and endometrium.

Adenoid Cystic Carcinoma Sheet of Cells

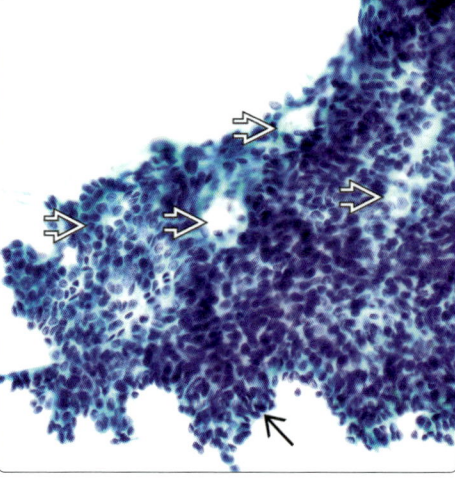

Adenoid Cystic Carcinoma of Cervix

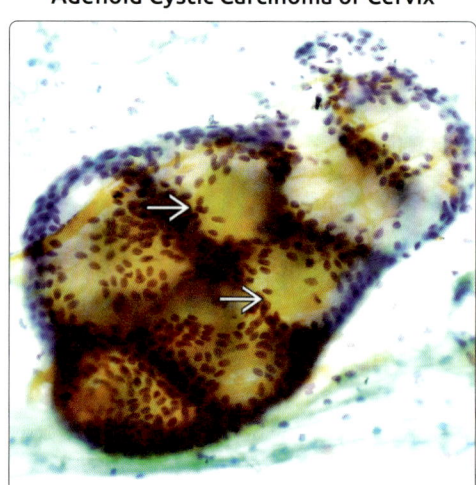

(Left) Pap-stained smear shows adenoid cystic carcinoma with abnormally large sheets of small, basaloid cells with very scant cytoplasm. Note the intrasheet, punched-out circular areas ➔. A hint of peripheral palisading is seen focally ➔. **(Right)** When seen on Pap stain, characteristic Swiss cheese-like, punched-out circular ➔, acellular areas of mucopolysaccharide material surrounded by small blue cells are pathognomic for adenoid cystic carcinoma in the cervix.

Other Uncommon Malignancies in Cervicovaginal Cytology

Adenosarcoma Gross Appearance

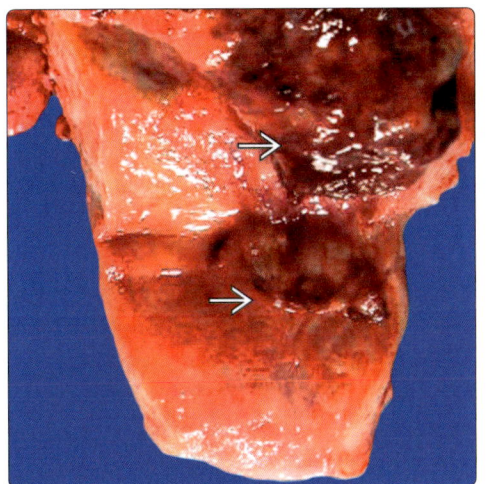

Adenosarcoma Excision

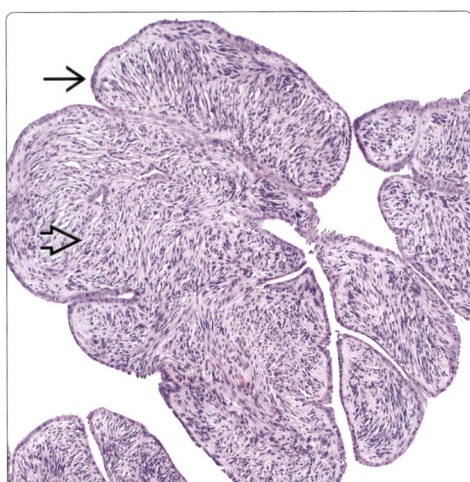

(Left) *Gross photograph shows an adenosarcoma. These tumors can be polypoid and reside in the endometrium or endocervical canal ⇨ or protrude through the os and be inadvertently sampled.* (Right) *H&E shows an adenosarcoma. These tumors have a distinctive, leaf-like architectural pattern. Note the bland surface columnar epithelium ⇨ and underlying pleomorphic spindle cells ⇨ with scattered mitotic figures. The spindle cells are condensed around the benign epithelium.*

Adenosarcoma Epithelial and Stromal Cells

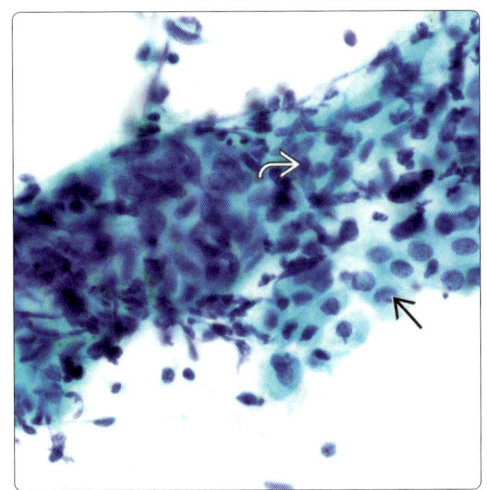

Adenosarcoma Separation of Stroma

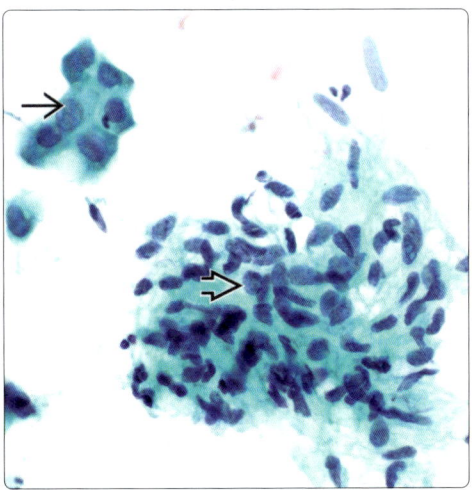

(Left) *Adenosarcoma on Pap stain shows bland surface epithelial cells ⇨ with atypical to malignant underlying spindle neoplastic cells ⇨.* (Right) *Adenosarcoma on Pap stain shows that the bland surface epithelial cells ⇨ are separated from the underlying neoplastic spindle stromal cells ⇨ during the process of smearing or preparation in a liquid-based medium.*

Uterine Leiomyosarcoma

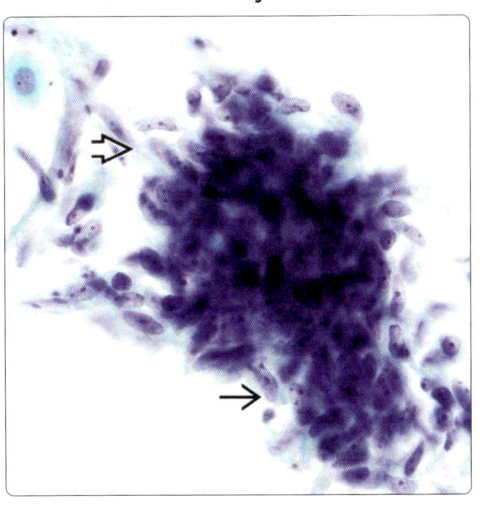

Uterine Sarcoma

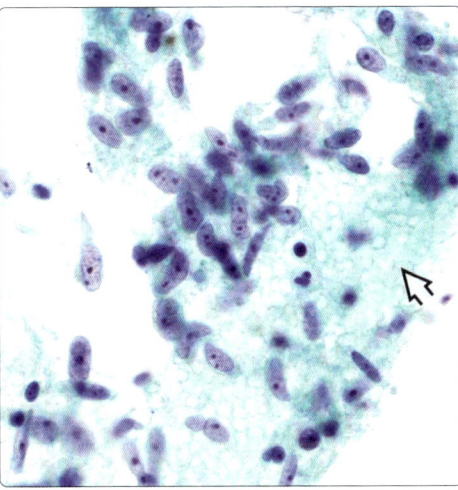

(Left) *Conventional Pap smear from a postmenopausal woman shows a uterine leiomyosarcoma, which was directly sampled. The cells are spindled with high nuclear:cytoplasmic ratios and open chromatin with nucleoli. Some of the nuclei in the plane of focus show rounded or blunt ends ⇨ and tapering cytoplasm ⇨.* (Right) *Pap smear shows sarcoma with dispersed neoplastic spindle cells, mild nuclear contour irregularities, and small nucleoli. Bloody background indicates bleeding &/or diathesis ⇨.*

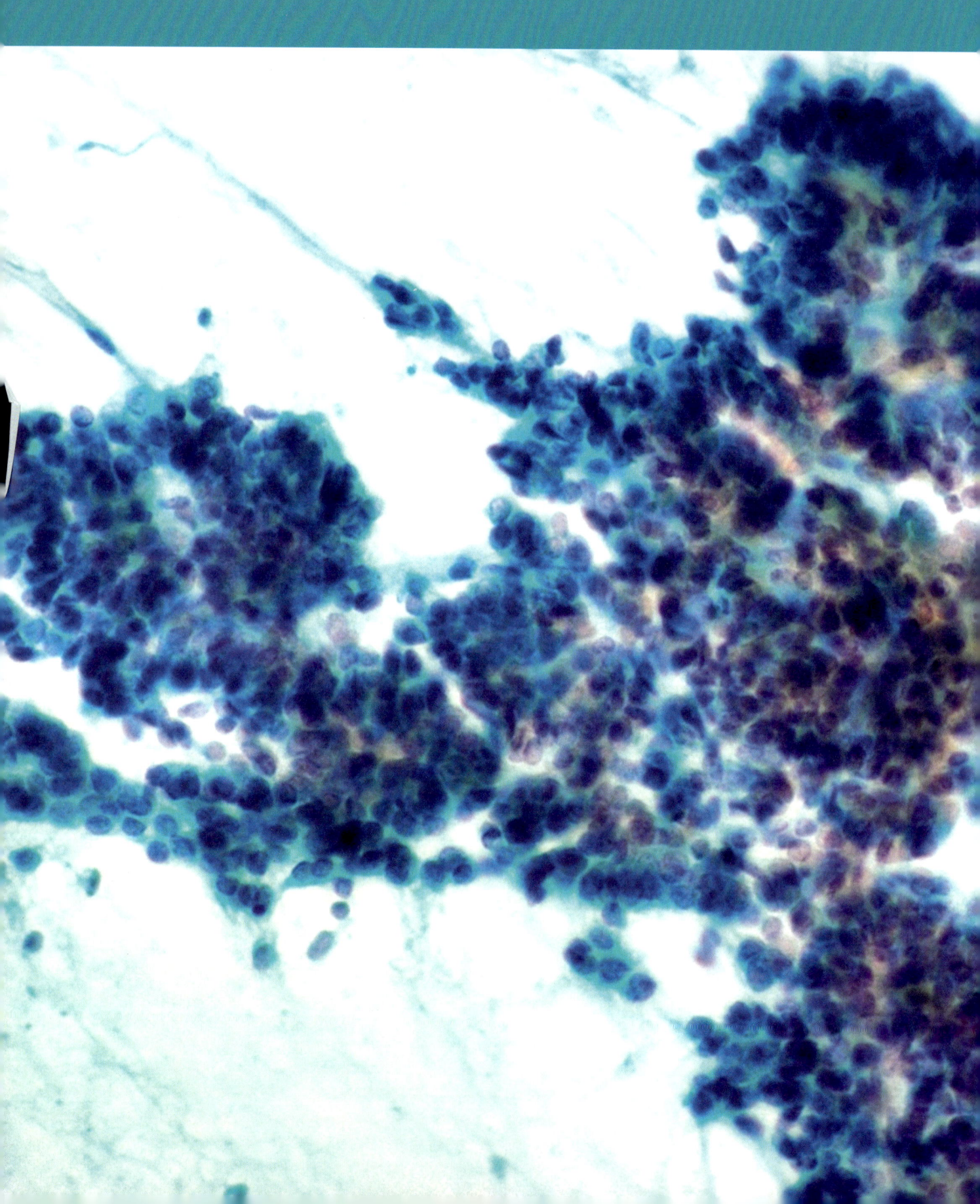

PART I
SECTION 6
Molecular Testing in Gynecologic Cytology

HPV and Other Molecular Testing in Gynecologic Cytology   84

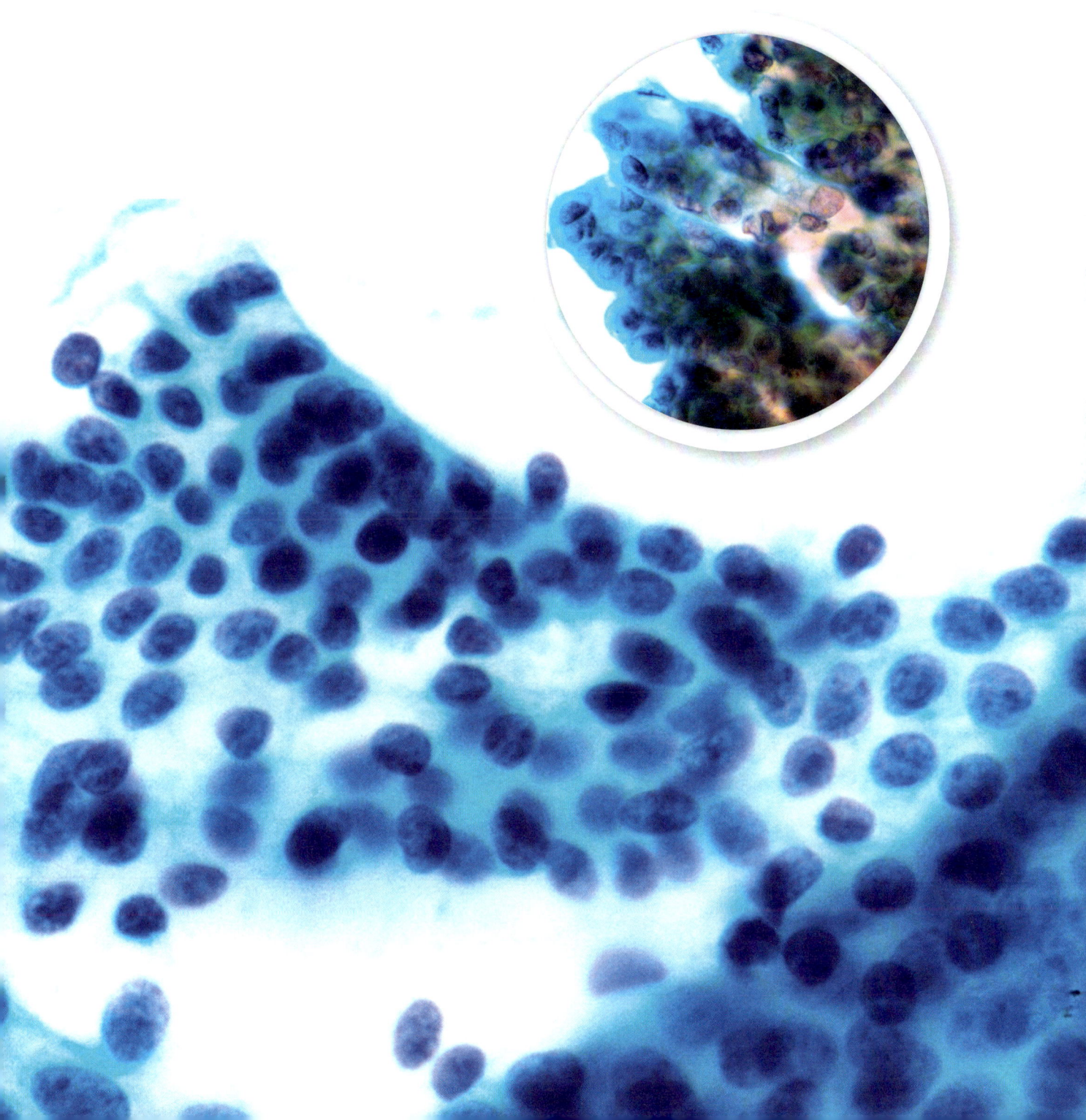

HPV and Other Molecular Testing in Gynecologic Cytology

HUMAN PAPILLOMAVIRUS

Biology and Epidemiology

- Nonenveloped, double-stranded DNA viruses of ~ 7,900 base pairs
- Most common sexually transmitted disease worldwide
- Fundamental cause of cervical cancer in essentially all cases
  - Also important in other anogenital sites and in head and neck squamous cell carcinoma
- Spread by direct contact, usually sexually transmitted in anogenital sites
- > 100 known types differentiated by *L1* gene that encodes viral capsid
- *E6* and *E7* are other key genes that inhibit apoptosis to facilitate viral survival by blocking Rb, p53, and p21, leading to carcinogenesis
- Low-grade squamous intraepithelial lesion (LSIL) is human papillomavirus (HPV) viral cytopathic effect and corresponds to production of viral particles
- High-risk HPV types can be incorporated into host genome and may result in high-grade squamous intraepithelial lesion or carcinoma

Testing

- Residual fluid from liquid-based Pap tests can be used for molecular testing to detect HPV
  - Noncytologic collection kits can also be used, including self-collection kits
    - Self-collection kits may be key to expanding cervical cancer screening to countries without well-established cytologic screening program
  - FDA approval is important for acceptance of molecular testing in USA, though in other countries less regulation is in place
- **Target amplification methods**
  - PCR (Cobas and Onclarity)
    - Segments of DNA are repeatedly copied and recopied by polymerase enzymes to produce large numbers of target genetic sequence

Effect of HPV Proteins on Cell Cycle

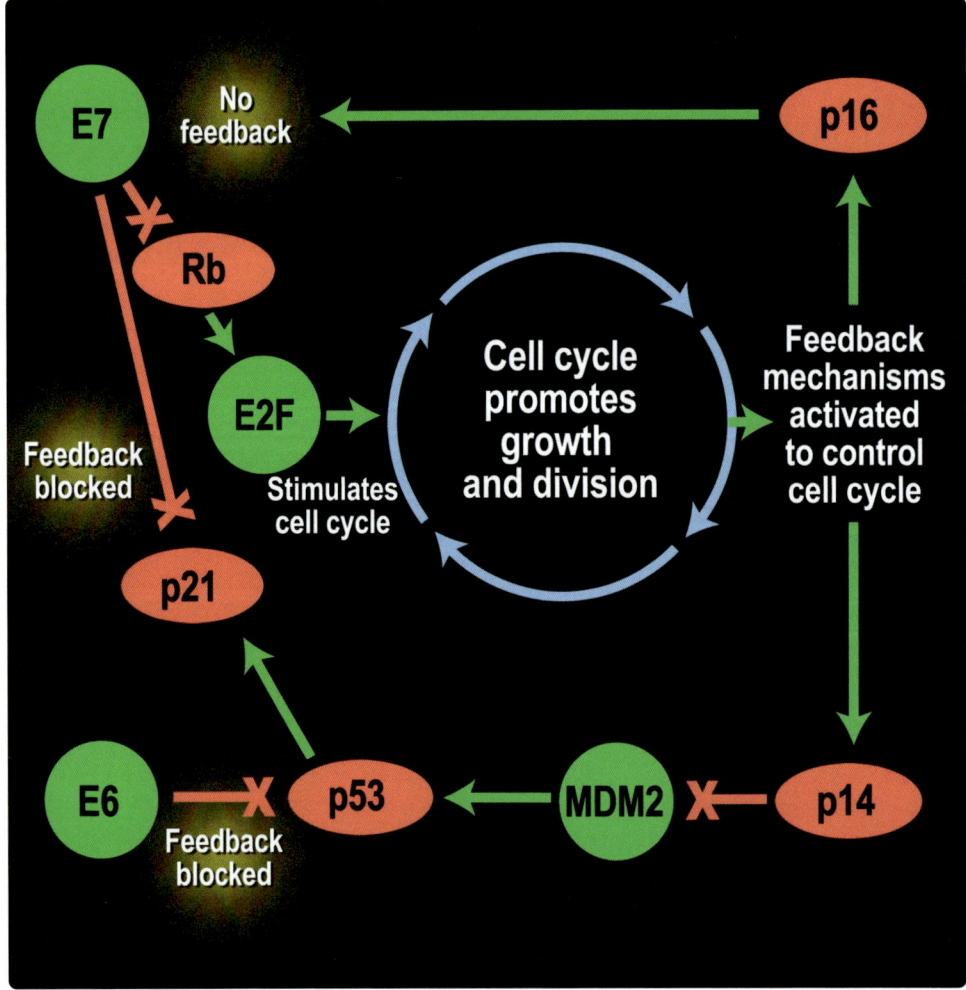

Key mechanisms that drive uncontrolled cell growth and division in HPV-infected cells are highlighted in this simplified graphic. HPV E7 stimulates the cell cycle by binding to Rb and releasing E2F. This in turn activates feedback mechanisms that would ordinarily keep the cell cycle under control. However, HPV E6 halts activity of p53, effectively blocking feedback via the p14 pathway. The p14 pathway is further blocked by E7 inhibition of p21, a cell cycle inhibitor activated by p53. E7 also prohibits p16-mediated feedback by preventing p16 interaction with Rb. This leads to p16 accumulation in the cells.

HPV and Other Molecular Testing in Gynecologic Cytology

- RNA can be detected by PCR if reverse transcription is used first to convert RNA into DNA
- Fluorescent molecules can be used to monitor production of copies for quantitation
- **Transcription-mediated amplification (TMA) (Aptima)**
  - Target RNA is captured by complementary oligomers attached to magnetic particle
  - Reverse transcription of magnet-captured RNA creates DNA that is copied and recopied
  - DNA copies bind to chemiluminescent probes and are detected by luminometer
- These methods offer high sensitivity
- Produce many copies of target that can contaminate laboratory and lead to false-positive results
- Newer, highly automated versions require less technical skill and reduce contamination problems
  - False-positives still occur due to carry-over between vials
- False-negative results are less rare than commonly assumed, due to causes including
  - Interfering substances (blood, lubricants, antifungal creams, etc.)
  - Scant infected cells
  - Low copy numbers of HPV in cells; this phenomenon is observed in significant fraction of invasive squamous cell carcinomas
- **Signal amplification methods**
  - **Hybrid capture technique (Hybrid Capture II)**
    - Target DNA attaches to HPV type-specific RNA probes
    - Antibodies against DNA-RNA hybrids, attached to microplate wells, capture targets and allow for removal of extraneous DNA
    - Probes directed against DNA-RNA hybrids with attached alkaline phosphatase enzymes then indicate presence of target by reacting with chemiluminescent substrates
  - Signal amplification does not result in increased target nucleic acids, eliminating contamination problem
  - Hybrid Capture II has been replaced by newer technologies, but is still important as benchmark
- **HPV typing**
  - High-risk types for carcinogenesis: 16, 18, 31, 33, 35, 39, 45, 51, 52, 56, 58, 59, 68, 73, and 82
    - Some tests examine *L1* gene to maximize sensitivity
    - Some tests target *E6/E7* genes because they are more directly related to risk of malignant progression; therefore, higher specificity
    - Types 16 and 18 are especially common and virulent; triage tests for just these 2 types allow for more aggressive follow-up
    - HPV in situ hybridization staining directed at high-risk types is also available
  - Low-risk types that do not progress to cancer: 6, 11, 40, 42, 43, 44, 54, 61, 70, 72, 81, and CP6108
    - Testing for these types is discouraged but available
  - Other types have intermediate or unknown risk
    - These types are not detected by most tests but pose small risk of cancer progression
- **DNA methylation**
  - FAM19A4/miR124-2 methylation analysis is promising triage method for use in conjunction with HPV screening
  - Negative methylation result could serve as rule out test for cervical carcinoma
- **Immunocytochemistry**
  - Markers, including p16, Ki-67, L1, and MMP-2/topoisomerase II α, have been tested as adjuncts to traditional Pap staining
  - These may increase specificity of Pap tests for high-grade disease but are costly and less sensitive than HPV testing

Indications

- Triage for colposcopy after interpretation of atypical squamous cells of undetermined significance (ASC-US)
  - ASC-US with high-risk HPV positivity has follow-up biopsy rates of high-grade dysplasia similar to LSIL
  - High-risk HPV-negative results are frequently reactive
  - HPV-positive rates in ASC-US can be used as quality assurance and feedback measure in cytology laboratories
- High-risk HPV cotesting with cytology in women ≥ 30 years of age
  - Negative HPV test results combined with negative cytology indicate very low risk of high-grade dysplasia
  - Allows for extended (3-5 year) screening intervals for double-negative women
- Less common uses sanctioned by 2013 guidelines from American Society for Colposcopy and Cervical Cytology (ASCCP)
  - As cotest with cytology after negative or low-grade follow-up colposcopy and biopsy following abnormal cytology, HPV-16 or 18 positivity, or persistent high-risk HPV positivity
  - As cotest with cytology after excision for high-grade dysplasia or adenocarcinoma in situ
    - Test of cure
- Contraindicated in young women
  - Not recommended for female patients < 21 years of age and acceptable but not preferred for women 21-24 years of age (per 2013 ASCCP guidelines)
  - Rationale for guidelines: HPV infection rates are high in young women, but high-grade dysplasia is infrequent
- Primary high-risk HPV screening without cytology or with cytology triage
  - Molecular testing is more readily automated and centralized than cytology
  - Many industrialized countries are adopting HPV-based screening strategies
    - HPV vaccination reduces prevalence of cervical cancer precursor lesions, making cytology screening less effective
    - Molecular testing, with its increased sensitivity, can overcome this problem
    - Reduced prevalence of high-risk HPV in population also means fewer false-positives for molecular testing
    - Referrals to colposcopy may still increase with this strategy, however, limiting its application
  - Cobas and Onclarity have been FDA approved for primary screening with cytology triage
    - This strategy has yet to achieve widespread acceptance in USA
  - HPV-based methods may allow screening to be extended into countries without established cytology workforce

HPV and Other Molecular Testing in Gynecologic Cytology

– These methods remain too expensive for most developing countries

Follow-Up

- HPV is not treated; only dysplastic sequelae are
  ○ Therefore, knowledge of HPV status is useful only to assess risk of dysplasia
- Treatment algorithms are moving toward new paradigm of risk-based management
  ○ 2019 ASCCP management guidelines take into account past screening results as well as current results
  ○ Follow-up decisions are based on immediate and 5-year risk of CIN3+
    – CIN3+ includes cervical intraepithelial neoplasia (CIN) grade 3, adenocarcinoma in situ, and invasive carcinoma
    – CIN3 was chosen as cutoff due to greater specificity for risk of invasive carcinoma than CIN grade 2 or high-grade squamous intraepithelial lesion (HSIL) as whole
  ○ Determination of follow-up is responsibility of treating physician, requiring use of app or ASCCP website
    – Prior screening results unknown to cytology lab may impact follow-up
    – Algorithms are too complicated to memorize, unlike previous versions
    – ASCCP intends to update app/website as new data and new technologies become available, altering algorithm incrementally without waiting to officially announce changes every few years
  ○ 4% risk of immediate CIN3+ is most significant risk level cutoff point
    – Women with ≥ 4% risk go to colposcopy (or possibly expedited treatment if risk > 25%)
    – 4% cutoff approximates risk of single HPV-positive ASC-US screening result
  ○ If immediate risk < 4%, follow-up screening is determined by 5-year risk of CIN 3+
    – Return to screening may be in 1, 3, or 5 years depending on risk level
    – Rescreening at 1 year is now recommended instead of colposcopy for many women with single positive screening result
    – 5-year intervals are recommended for women with negative HPV or cotesting and no prior positive results (< 0.15% 5-year risk)

CHLAMYDIA AND GONORRHEA

Biology and Epidemiology

- *Chlamydia trachomatis*
  ○ Obligate intracellular gram-negative cocci
  ○ Most common bacterial sexually transmitted disease
  ○ Usually asymptomatic, especially in women
  ○ May progress to pelvic inflammatory disease, resulting in infertility or ectopic pregnancy
  ○ May cause pregnancy complications
  ○ May be transmitted to infants during childbirth, resulting in conjunctivitis or pneumonia
- *Neisseria gonorrhoeae*
  ○ Gram-negative diplococci
  ○ Often found with chlamydia but less common
  ○ Usually symptomatic urethritis in males, but often asymptomatic in women
  ○ May progress to pelvic inflammatory disease, resulting in infertility or ectopic pregnancy
  ○ Disseminated disease rarely occurs

Testing

- Specific cervicovaginal swabs are preferred for female molecular testing
- Residual fluid from Pap testing is acceptable
  ○ Facilitates screening because only 1 specimen needs to be collected
- Urine and urethral, rectal, and oropharyngeal swabs can also be tested
- Many molecular testing platforms allow for testing of chlamydia and gonorrhea
  ○ PCR, TMA, and signal amplification methods are available, and many have FDA approval
    – Many of these are designed to run in parallel to HPV testing on same platform
    – Platforms include Aptima, Cobas, and Onclarity

Indications

- In USA, chlamydia screening is recommended for pregnant women, sexually active women ≤ 25 years of age, and women with new or multiple sex partners
- Cost effectiveness of widespread screening is not yet proven, and many countries only do opportunistic testing
- Chlamydia and gonorrhea are often tested and treated together

INFECTIOUS VAGINITIS/CERVICITIS

Biology and Epidemiology

- Bacterial vaginosis
  ○ *Gardnerella vaginalis* (anaerobic gram-variable small coccobacilli responsible for clue cells)
  ○ Other organisms include *Atopobium, Mobiluncus, Prevotella, Ureaplasma, Mycoplasma*, and other anaerobes of gut origin
- *Candida*
  ○ Yeasts that also form pseudohyphae
  ○ Immunosuppression, diabetes, and antibiotic use predispose to infection
- *Trichomonas vaginalis*
  ○ Sexually transmitted unicellular protozoan
- Despite very different organisms, clinical symptoms and implications of these 3 vaginitis causes are similar
  ○ Cause itching, pain, discharge, and malodor
- Herpes simplex virus
  ○ Sexually transmitted with recurrent, blistering sores and asymptomatic viral shedding

Testing

- Molecular methods, including PCR and nucleic acid hybridization, may be used to detect these organisms
- Some laboratories offer self-developed PCR-based vaginitis panels for residual Pap test fluid, but these are not FDA-approved in USA
  ○ Sensitivity and specificity are not well defined, but sensitivity is usually higher than that of cytology

HPV and Other Molecular Testing in Gynecologic Cytology

Comparison of Widely Used HPV Testing Platforms

Name	Method	Types Targeted	Subtyping	Limitations
Hybrid Capture II (Qiagen)	Signal amplification (full genome)	16, 18, 31, 33, 35, 39, 45, 51, 52, 56, 58, 59, 68	No (separate test for 16, 18, and 45)	Needs large volume, no internal positive control, cross-reactivity (types 53, 66, 70, and others)
Aptima (Hologic)	TMA (*E6/E7* RNA)	16, 18, 31, 33, 35, 39, 45, 51, 52, 56, 58, 59, 66, 68	No (separate test for 16, 18, and 45)	ThinPrep specific, cross reactivity (types 62, 70, and others)
Cobas (Roche)	PCR (*L1* DNA)	16, 18, 31, 33, 35, 39, 45, 51, 52, 56, 58, 59, 66, 68	16 and 18	Internal control not epithelium-specific, cross reactivity (types 61, 70, and others)
Onclarity HPV (BD)	PCR (*E6/E7* DNA)	16, 18, 31, 33, 35, 39, 45, 51, 52, 56, 58, 59, 66, 68	16, 18, 31, 45, 51, 52, and others in groups	SurePath specific, internal control not epithelium-specific

HPV = human papillomavirus; TMA = transcription-mediated amplification; NASBA = nucleic acid sequence-based amplification.

Cross-reactivity with low-risk types based on Preisler S et al: BMC Cancer. 16: 510, 2016.

High-Risk HPV-Positive Rates by Cytology Interpretation

Clinical Trial/Survey	Assay	NILM	ASC-US
2012 CAP survey (50th percentile of USA clinical laboratories)	Various; Hybrid Capture II (42.4%), Cervista (37.2%), Cobas (14.9%)	6.5% (≥ 30 years)	38.3%
ALTS trial (USA)	Hybrid Capture II	32.7%	50.6%
ATHENA trial (USA)	Cobas	9.8% (≥ 25 years)	31.8%
CLEAR trial (USA)	Aptima	5.0% (≥ 30 years)	41.8%
CCCaST trial (Canada)	Hybrid Capture II	5.2%	31.0%
ARTISTIC trial (England)	Hybrid Capture II	10.4%	31.1%
POBASCAM trial (Netherlands)	Study-specific PCR	3.6%	27.4%
Swedescreen trial (Sweden)	Study-specific PCR	5.4%	63.6%

ASCCP Management Guidelines Based on Immediate and 5-Year Risk of CIN3+

Risk of CIN3+	Recommended Follow-up
Immediate risk: 60-100%	Expedited treatment preferred
Immediate risk: 25-59%	Expedited treatment or colposcopy acceptable
Immediate risk: 4-24%	Colposcopy recommended
Immediate risk: < 4%; 5-year risk 0.55% or greater	Return in 1 year for screening
5-year risk: 0.15-0.54%	Return in 3 years for screening
5-year risk: < 0.15%	Return in 5 years for screening

American Society for Colposcopy and Cervical Cytology = ASCCP; CIN3+ = cervical intraepithelial neoplasia grade 3, adenocarcinoma in situ, and invasive carcinoma.

Modified from Perkins RB et al: J Low Genit Tract Dis. 24(2):102-31, 2020.

- o Asymptomatic women may have *Gardnerella* or other vaginitis-associated organisms, precluding screening
- o Negative molecular test combined with positive cytology may cause consternation
  - Many cases are attributable to misinterpretation of cytology
  - False-negative molecular results also occur
- TMA method (Aptima) has been FDA approved to detect *Trichomonas* in residual ThinPrep fluid
- FDA-approved methods using test-specific vaginal swabs are also available

SELECTED REFERENCES

1. Nayar R et al: Moving forward-the 2019 ASCCP risk-based management consensus guidelines for abnormal cervical cancer screening tests and cancer precursors and beyond: implications and suggestions for laboratories. J Am Soc Cytopathol. 9(4):291-303, 2020
2. Perkins RB et al: 2019 ASCCP risk-based management consensus guidelines for abnormal cervical cancer screening tests and cancer precursors. J Low Genit Tract Dis. 24(2):102-31, 2020
3. Salazar KL et al: A review of the FDA-approved molecular testing platforms for human papillomavirus. J Am Soc Cytopathol. 8(5):284-92, 2019
4. Workowski KA et al: Sexually transmitted diseases treatment guidelines, 2015. MMWR Recomm Rep. 64(RR-03):1-137, 2015
5. Davey DD et al: 2013 statement on human papillomavirus DNA test utilization. Am J Clin Pathol. 141(4):459-61, 2014

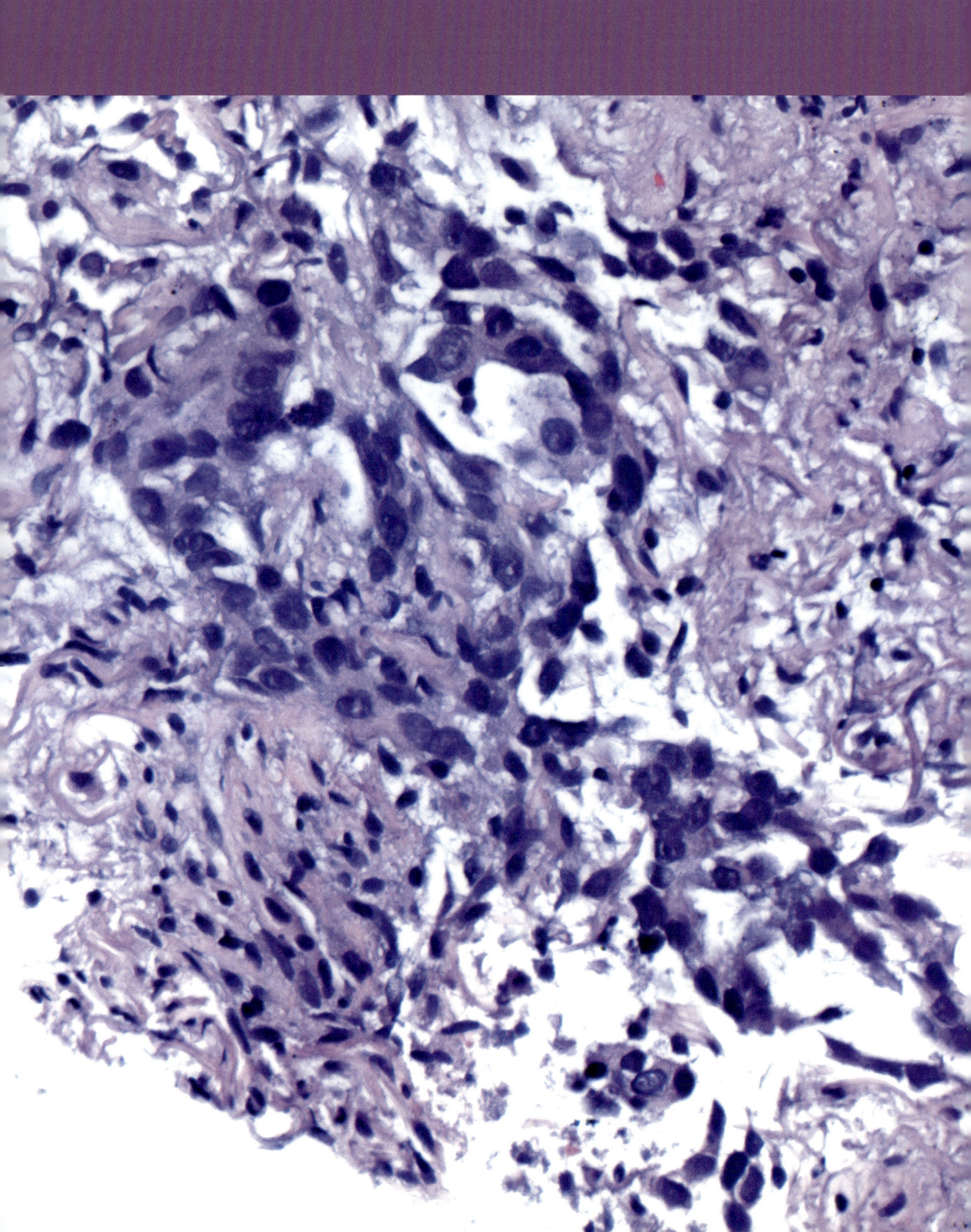

PART I
SECTION 7
Directly Sampled Endometrial Cytology

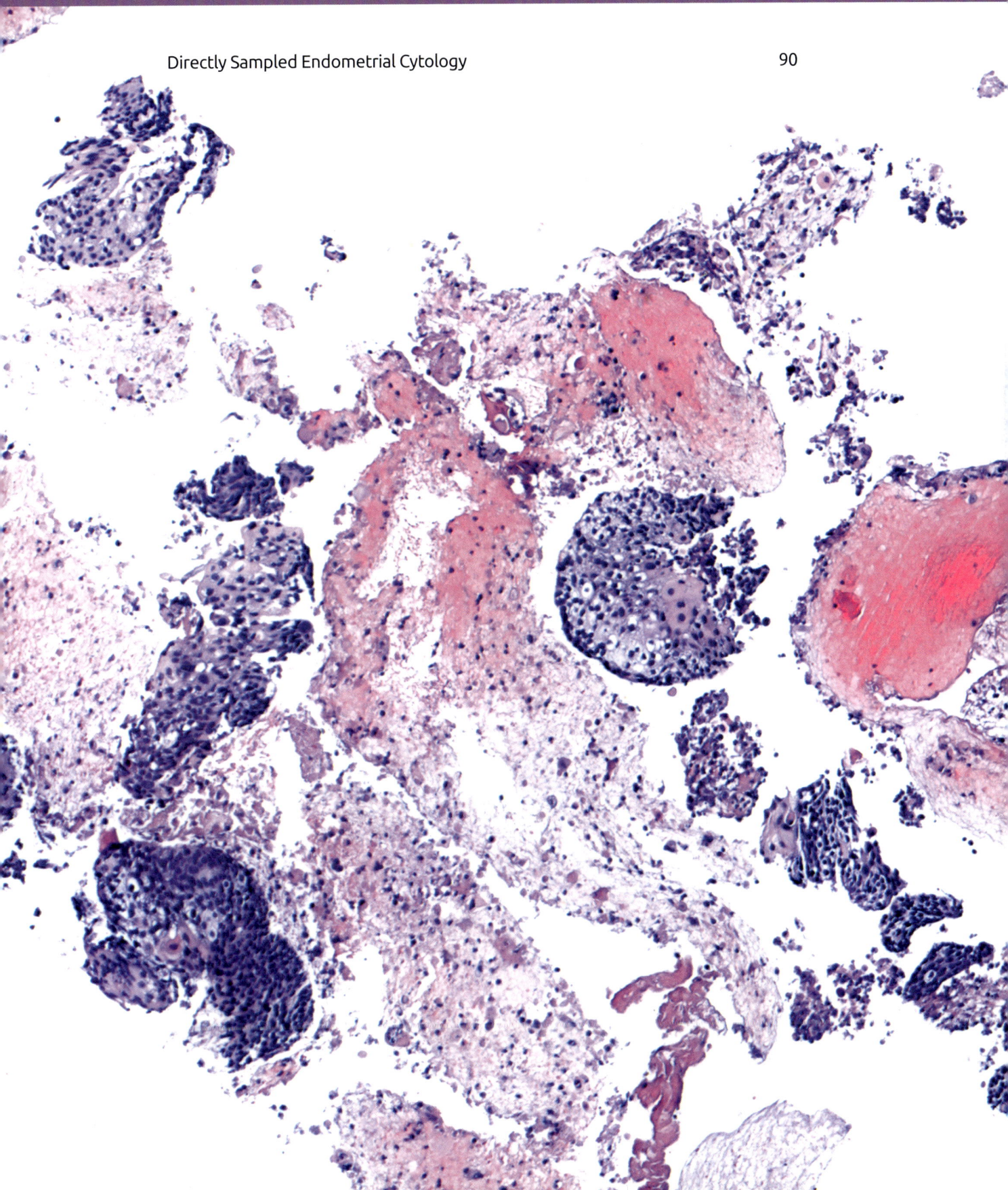

Directly Sampled Endometrial Cytology

TERMINOLOGY

Definitions
- Endometrial cytologic examination with direct endometrial sampling using special endometrial sampler to avoid cervical contamination
- Currently, direct endometrial cytology is most common method of screening for endometrial cancer in Japan

The Yokohama System (TYS) for Reporting Endometrial Cytology
- **Specimen type**
  - Conventional or liquid-based method
- **Specimen adequacy**
  - Satisfactory
  - Unsatisfactory (rejected vs. fully evaluated but unsatisfactory), give reason
- **Result**
  - Unsatisfactory for evaluation: TYS 0
  - Negative for malignant tumors and precursors: TYS 1
    - Proliferative, secretory, menstrual, atrophic endometrium, reactive changes due to IUD, polyps, tamoxifen, stromal breakdown if recognized
  - Atypical endometrial cells of undetermined significance (ATEC-US): TYS 2
  - Endometrial hyperplasia without atypia: TYS 3
  - Atypical endometrial cells, cannot exclude endometrial atypical hyperplasia (EAH)/endometrial intraepithelial neoplasia (EIN) or malignant condition (ATEC-AE): TYS 4
  - EAH/EIN: TYS 5
  - Malignant neoplasm: TYS 6

MICROSCOPIC

Diagnostic Criteria
- Based on cytoarchitecture and conventional cytologic criteria (cellular atypia, arrangement, and background)
- Cell cluster with maximum diameter of ≥ 0.2 mm is defined as cell clump

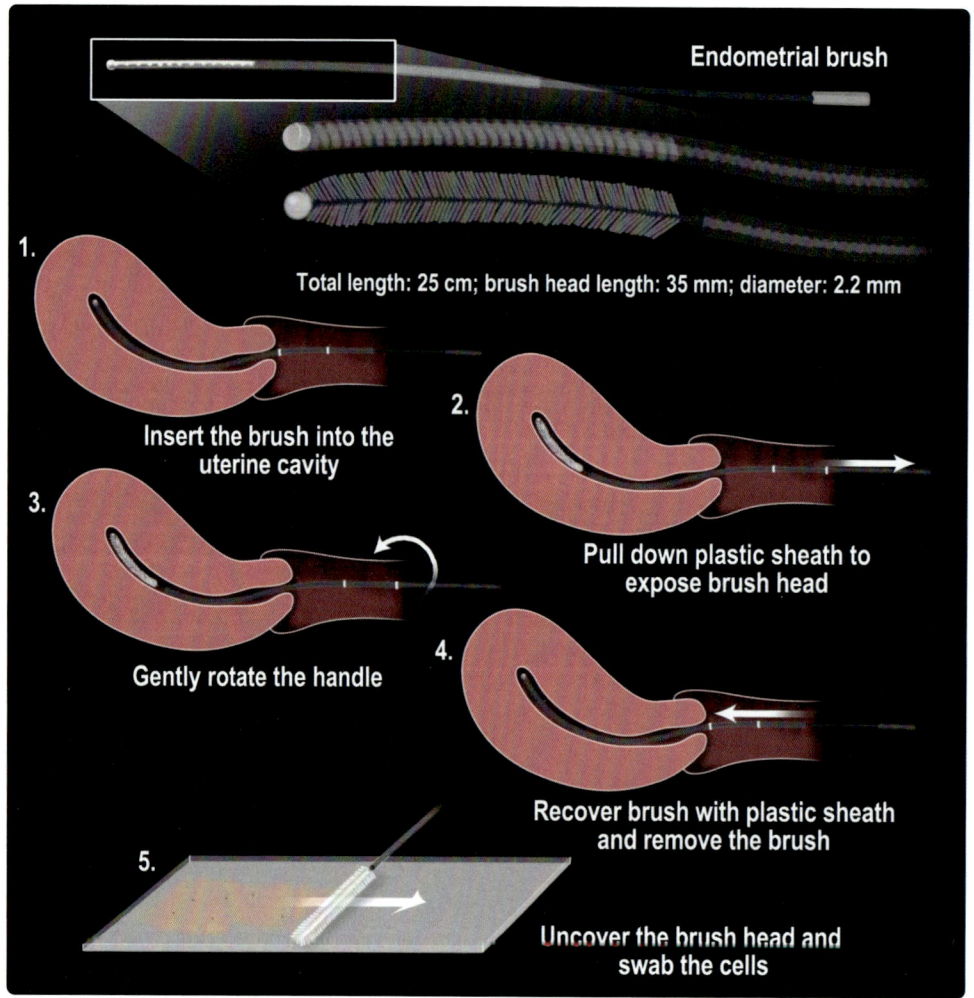

Direct Endometrial Brushing Cytology

Graphic represents direct endometrial brushing cytology procedure and smearing for conventional smears. Material can also be collected in liquid-based medium for liquid-based cytology.

Directly Sampled Endometrial Cytology

Relative Risk and Management of TYS Categories Based on Japanese Studies

Category	Risk of Malignancy (%)	Risk of Atypical Endometrial Hyperplasia (%)	Management
Unsatisfactory for evaluation: TYS 0	No data so far	No data so far	Repeat cytology in 3 months if concern
Negative: TYS 1	0.47	0.20	Clinical follow-up as needed
ATEC-US: TYS 2	No data so far	No data so far	Repeat cytology in 3 months as needed
Endometrial hyperplasia without atypia : TYS 3	18-20	18-20	More follow-up, scope, biopsy
Atypical endometrial cells, cannot exclude AEN/EIN : TYS 4	60	5.7	More aggressive follow-up, scope, biopsy
AEN/EIN: TYS 5	61.5	30.8	More aggressive follow-up, scope, biopsy
Malignant neoplasms: TYS 6	94.5	0.3	More aggressive follow-up, scope, biopsy

TYS = The Yokohama System; ATEC-US = atypical endometrial cells of undetermined significance; AEN = atypical endometrial hyperplasia; EIN = endometrioid intraepithelial neoplasia.

Proliferative Endometrium

- Cell clumps with tube &/or sheet pattern
  - Narrow and straight tubular glands
  - When tubules are open or surface epithelium is sampled, they present as epithelial cells in flat sheets ± mitosis
  - Cells are ovoid to columnar with pseudostratification and dense cytoplasm
  - Abundant stromal cells may adhere to tubular glands but are spindle-shaped and bipolar and have bland nuclei
  - Transversing vessels may be seen in stroma
  - Mitotic activity may be seen in glands or stroma
  - Liquid-based preparations
    - Glands and stromal fragments are usually separated
    - Single stromal cells adherent to glandular cells are usually absent or rare
    - Chromatin is also more open, and chromocenters/nucleoli are easily visible

Secretory Endometrium

- Cell clumps with tube &/or sheet pattern
  - Tubular glands with varying diameter of tubes at ends
    - Maximum diameter is 2x minimum diameter of tubule
  - Honeycomb sheets of endometrial cells with well-defined cell borders and abundant cleared cytoplasm in midsecretory phase
  - Stromal cells adherent to tubular glands and sheets except in liquid-based preparations

Atrophic Endometrium

- Cell clumps with tube &/or sheet pattern
  - Small, narrow, straight, or dilated tubules
  - Sheets with small atrophic cells
  - Scant stromal cells; overall scant cellularity

Endometrial Hyperplasia

- Cell clumps with dilated or branched pattern
- Stromal cells adherent to clumps but may be difficult to see in liquid-based preparations

Endometrial Hyperplasia With Atypia

- Cell clumps with dilated or branched pattern, irregular protrusions
- Margins of cell clumps with irregular outlines, rare isolated cells
- Irregular arrangement of cells within cell clumps
- ≥ 50% abnormal:normal cell clump ratio (minimum 10 clumps needed for evaluation)
- Difficult to correlate with histology and difficult to reproduce

Low-Grade Endometrioid Adenocarcinoma

- Cell clumps with irregular protrusions &/or papillotubular pattern
- No stromal cells adherent to margins of clumps
- Cellular atypia and irregular arrangement within clumps
- Isolated malignant cells with necrotic background, which may be subtle in liquid-based preparations

High-Grade Serous Carcinoma

- Papillary cell clusters with large, atypical, and mitotically active tumor cells with large nucleoli
- Background tumor diathesis (subtle in liquid based)
- Psammoma bodies may or may not be seen

High-Grade Endometrioid Adenocarcinoma

- Irregular cell clusters, background tumor diathesis
- Prominent cytologic atypia and mitosis

Endometrial Stromal Sarcoma

- Bipolar spindled cells without glandular elements
- Transgressing vessels through large tissue fragments

SELECTED REFERENCES

1. Hirai Y et al: The Yokohama System for Reporting Endometrial Cytology. Springer, 2022

Directly Sampled Endometrial Cytology

TYS 1 Proliferative Endometrium
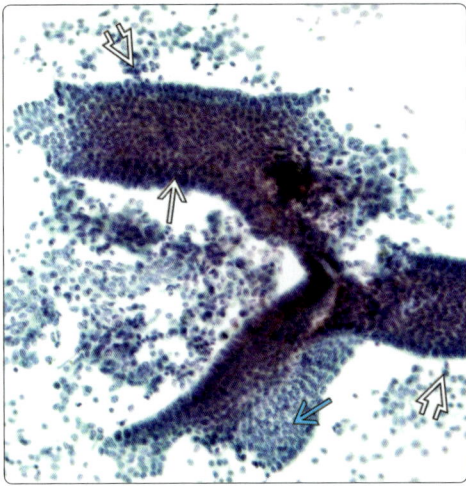

TYS 1 Secretory Endometrium
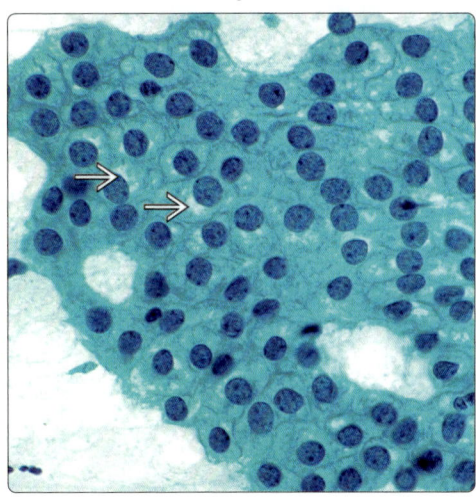

(Left) Directly sampled proliferative endometrium shows tubular ➡ and sheet patterns ➡. Stromal cells are attached along the edge of the tubules and sheets ➡. **(Right)** Pap stain of secretory endometrium shows a honeycomb arrangement of cells. The nuclei are round and regular with tiny nucleoli and subnuclear secretory vacuoles ➡. No mitosis is seen.

TYS 1 Atrophic Endometrium
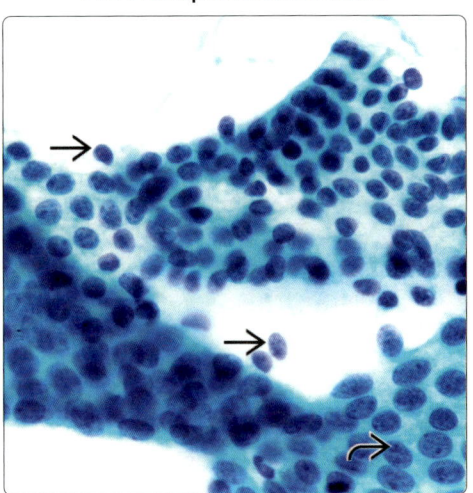

TYS 2 Atypical Endometrial Cells of Undetermined Significance
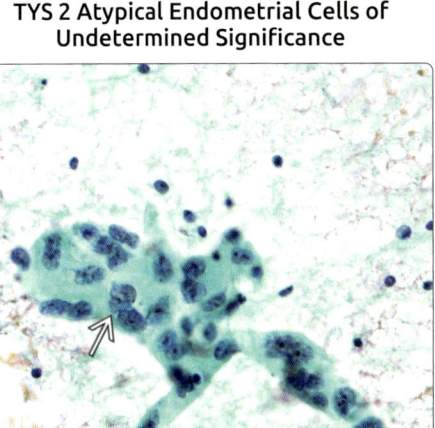

(Left) Pap-stained smear of directly sampled atrophic endometrium shows sheets of cells without secretions and small regular nuclei in a honeycomb pattern. Rare stromal cells ➡ are seen along the edge of the sheet. There is no mitosis or nuclear overlap or atypia. The nucleoli are minute ➡. **(Right)** Pap-stained smear of directly sampled endometrium shows a sheet of atypical endometrial cells ➡ and normal proliferative endometrium ➡. The nuclei of the atypical cells are larger compared to the normal.

TYS 2 Atypical Endometrial Cells of Undetermined Significance
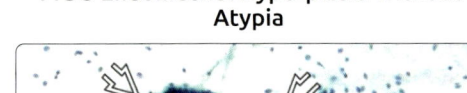
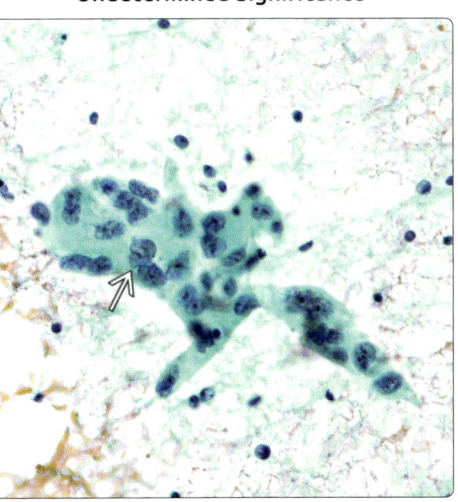

TYS 3 Endometrial Hyperplasia Without Atypia

(Left) Atypical endometrial cells of undetermined significance on higher magnification show larger, irregular, disordered cells ➡. Follow-up was an endometrial polyp. **(Right)** Pap-stained smear shows atypical endometrial cells forming a complex 3D structure with slight architectural abnormality of the cell clumps ➡ and associated stromal cells ➡. Normal atrophic squamous cells ➡ are also present for comparison.

Directly Sampled Endometrial Cytology

TYS 4 Atypical Endometrial Cells, Cannot Exclude EAH/EIN

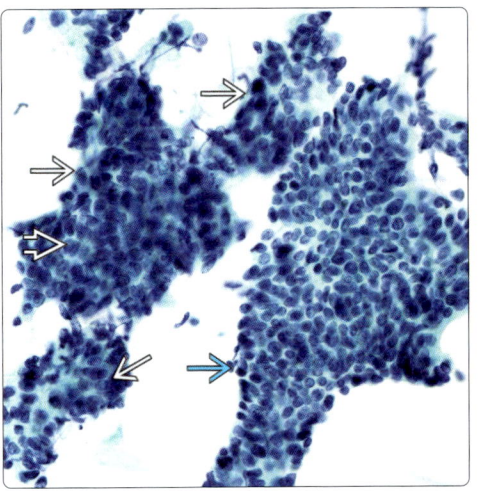

TYS 5 Atypical Endometrial Hyperplasia

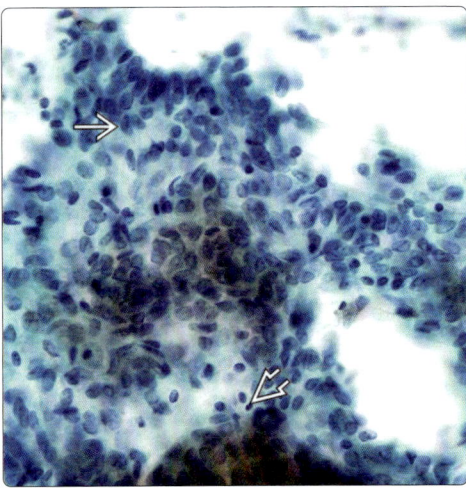

(Left) *Directly sampled endometrium shows 3D cell clumps with atypical architecture of the atypical endometrial cells ➔ and tubular and sheet pattern of atrophic cells ➔. The nuclei ➔ in the atypical cluster are larger than those of the normal cluster.* (Right) *Directly sampled endometrial cytology shows irregular, 3D arrangement of a cell clump with cellular atypia ➔ and neutrophils ➔. Unlike carcinoma (TYS 6), single malignant cells and diathesis are absent.*

Biopsy With Atypical Endometrial Hyperplasia

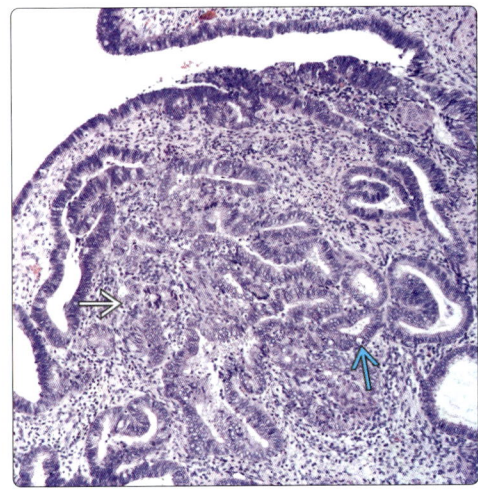

TYS 6 Endometrioid Carcinoma

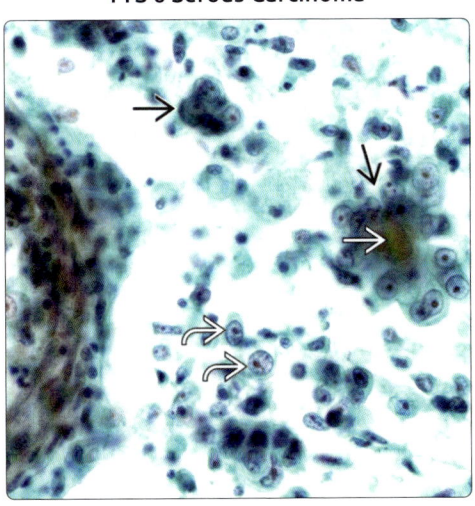

(Left) *H&E-stained endometrial biopsy shows atypical endometrial hyperplasia ➔ with back-to-back irregular gland forms with nuclear atypia and apoptosis ➔.* (Right) *Pap-stained directly sampled high-grade endometrioid adenocarcinoma is shown with single malignant cells ➔, diathesis ➔, and irregular clusters of malignant cells ➔.*

TYS 6 Serous Carcinoma

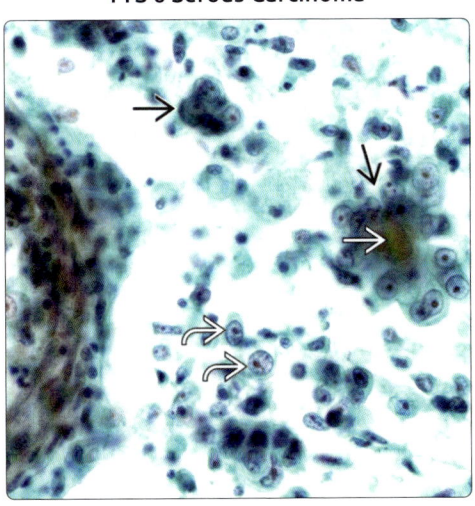

TYS 6 Clear Cell Adenocarcinoma

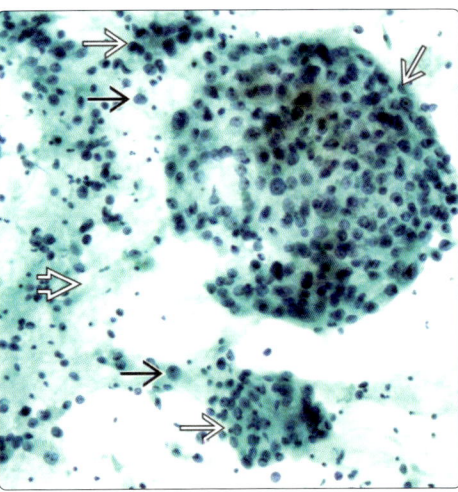

(Left) *Pap-stained direct endometrial sampling of a high-grade serous carcinoma with papillary cell clusters ➔ is shown. There is prominent cytologic atypia with large malignant nuclei and nucleoli ➔. A psammoma body ➔ is also seen.* (Right) *Pap-stained directly sampled endometrium shows cell clumps/balls ➔ as well as single malignant cells ➔ in a background of diathesis ➔.*

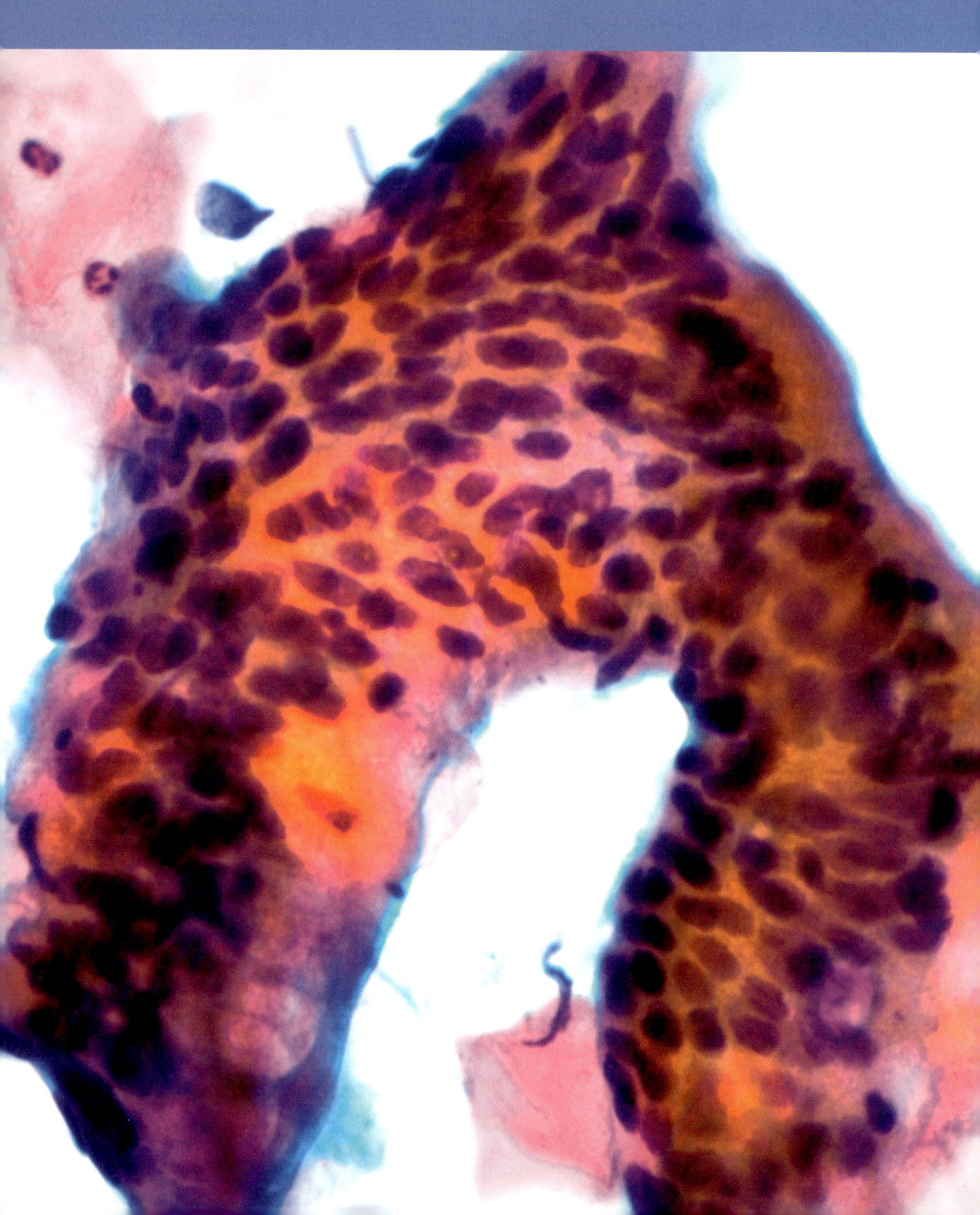

PART I
SECTION 8
Anal Cytology

Anal Cytology

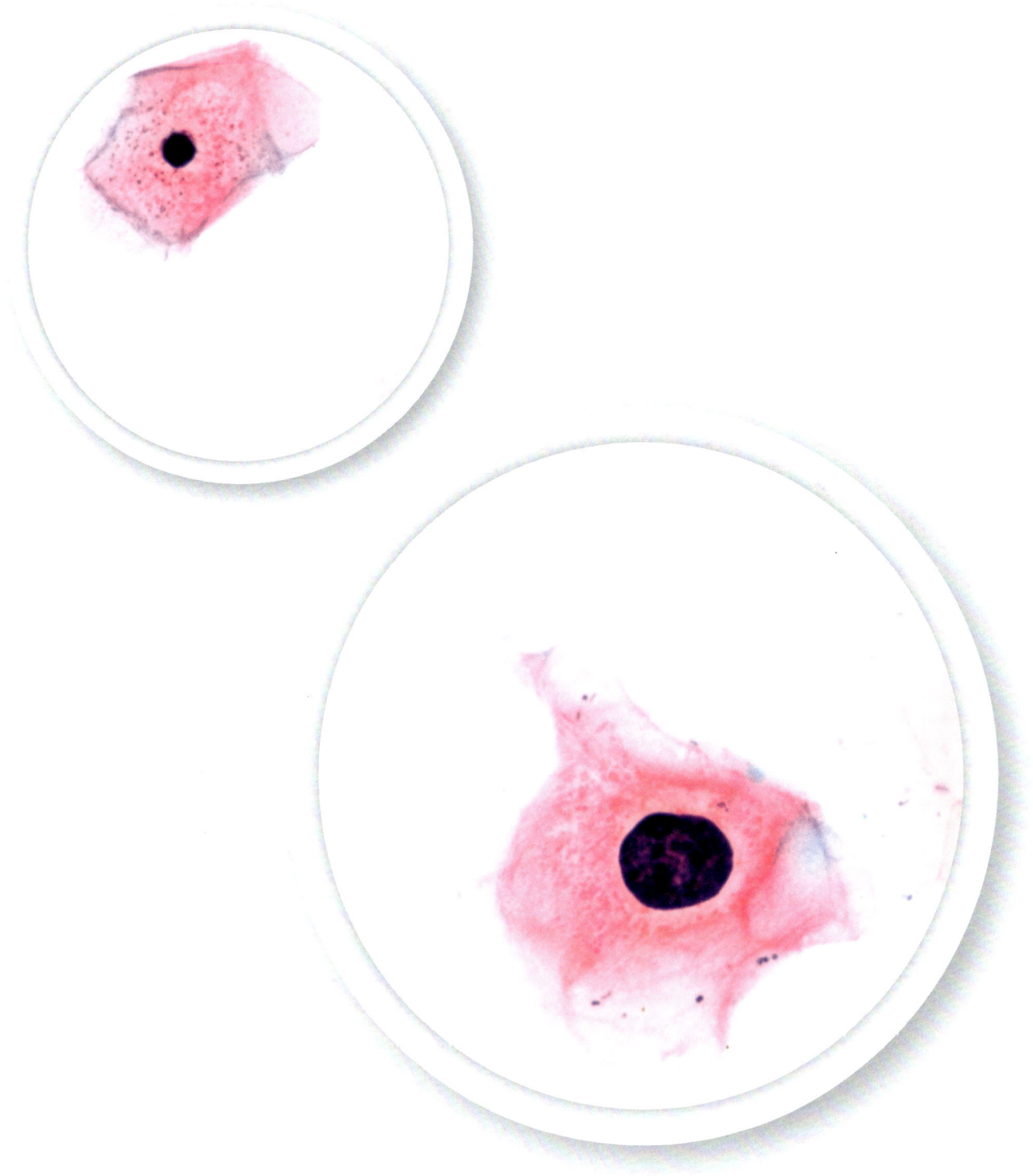

Anal Cytology

KEY FACTS

CLASSIFICATION
- Bethesda Reporting System is used; essentially identical to gynecologic cytology
- LAST guidelines for histology also apply to anal squamous lesions

CLINICAL ISSUES
- Anal squamous intraepithelial lesions are more prevalent in AIDS patients, men who have sex with men, transplant recipients, and women with cervicovaginal or vulvar dysplasia
  - Immune suppression increases risk of progression
- No clear screening guidelines, but only those at high risk get tested
- Follow-up anoscopy is similar in principle to colposcopy
- Treatment of lesions is more difficult than in cervix because excision has more potential to result in clinically significant scarring

CYTOPATHOLOGY
- Relative to cervicovaginal specimens, typically more keratinizing/mature cells are present, including anucleate superficial cells
  - Greater maturation makes interpretation more difficult in many cases
- Low-grade and high-grade squamous intraepithelial lesions have nuclear enlargement, irregularity, and hyperchromasia similar to cervicovaginal specimens
- 2,000-3,000 squamous cells needed for adequacy
- Rectal columnar mucosa or squamous metaplastic mucosa indicates anorectal transformation zone sampling
- Bacteria and fecal debris are frequently present
  - In some instances, debris may compromise adequacy
- *Candida* and herpesvirus, similar to gynecologic cytology, may be present
- Rectal organisms, including amebae or *Enterobius*, may also be seen

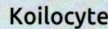

Koilocyte

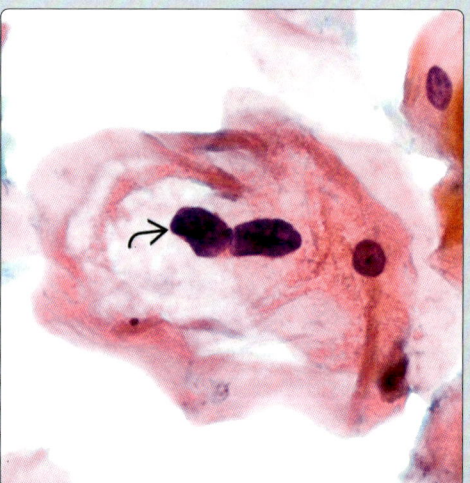

Low-Grade Parakeratotic Lesion

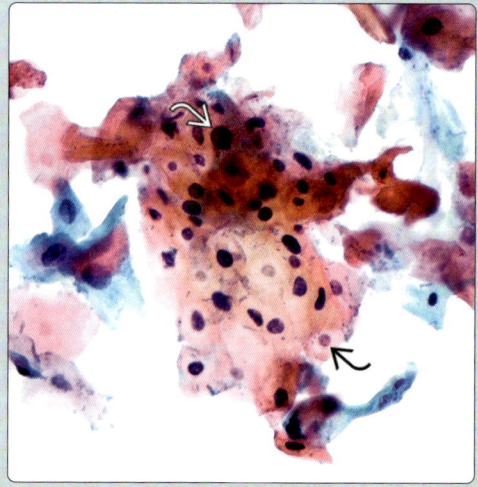

(Left) *Koilocytosis with a perinuclear halo, binucleation, nuclear enlargement, irregularity, and darkening ➡ is diagnostic of a low-grade squamous intraepithelial lesion in anal Pap tests, similar to cervicovaginal specimens.* (Right) *Squamous atypia ➡ is seen alongside nuclear karyorrhexis ➡ in a specimen from a parakeratotic condylomatous lesion.*

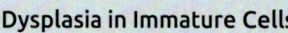

Dysplasia in Immature Cells

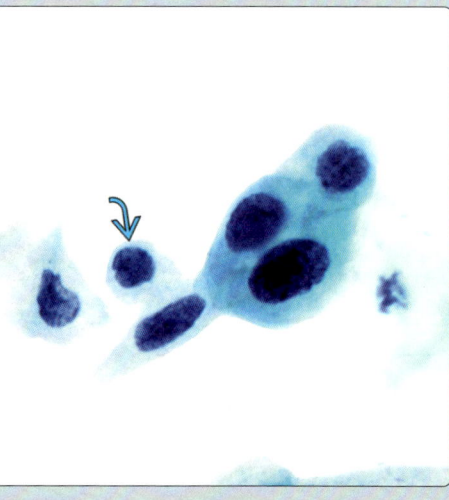

High-Grade Squamous Intraepithelial Lesion

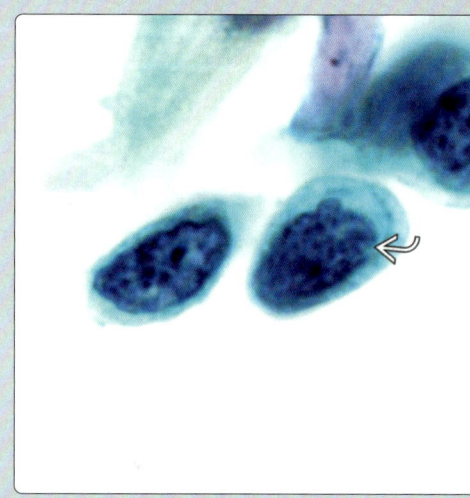

(Left) *Dysplastic changes can also be seen in immature/metaplastic cells, such as those seen here, raising concern for a high-grade squamous intraepithelial lesion in cells with less cytoplasm ➡.* (Right) *Classic features of a high-grade squamous intraepithelial lesion, including high nuclear:cytoplasmic ratio, chromatin clumping, and marked nuclear contour irregularities ➡, are seen in these dysplastic cells.*

Anal Cytology

TERMINOLOGY

Definitions
- Screening cytology for anal squamous cell carcinoma and precursors
- Bethesda reporting terminology mirrors cervicovaginal specimens
  - LAST tissue reporting terminology mirrors Bethesda cytology reporting terminology

ETIOLOGY/PATHOGENESIS

Infectious Agents
- Human papillomavirus, usually type 16, sexually transmitted

CLINICAL ISSUES

Presentation
- Anal dysplasia is more prevalent in AIDS patients, men who have sex with men, transplant recipients, and women with cervicovaginal or vulvar dysplasia
- No clear screening guidelines exist, but some centers do screen high-risk groups
  - Percentage of positive cases is therefore higher than in typical gynecologic screening
- Positive cytology is followed by anoscopy (similar to colposcopy) and biopsy

Laboratory Tests
- Sampling is performed with moistened swab, from distal rectum outward with lateral pressure on anal canal mucosa
  - Dacron or flocked nylon swabs preferred to cotton

Treatment
- Topical agents or ablation for nonsurgical treatment
- Excision limited by stenosis complications and recurrence

CYTOPATHOLOGY

Background
- Bacteria and fecal debris are frequently present, can compromise adequacy
- *Candida*, herpesvirus, amebae, or *Enterobius* organisms may be seen

Cells
- Relative to cervicovaginal specimens, typically more keratinizing/mature cells are present
- Anucleate squamous cells common

Nuclear Details
- Low-grade and high-grade squamous intraepithelial lesions have nuclear enlargement, irregularity, and hyperchromasia similar to cervicovaginal specimens

Cytoplasmic Details
- Low-grade lesions have halos less commonly

Adequacy Criteria
- 2,000-3,000 squamous cells for liquid-based tests
  - 1-2 cells per 40x field for ThinPrep and 3-6 cells per 40x field for SurePath
- Rectal columnar mucosa or squamous metaplastic mucosa indicates anorectal transformation zone sampling

DIFFERENTIAL DIAGNOSIS

Reactive Changes
- Similar to cervicovaginal cytology, there is overlap between reactive and viral changes

DIAGNOSTIC CHECKLIST

Pathologic Interpretation Pearls
- Anal cytology resembles its cervicovaginal counterpart
  - More maturation/keratinization often makes dysplastic changes more subtle

SELECTED REFERENCES

1. Swanson AA et al: Evaluation of high-risk human papillomavirus testing and anal cytology to detect high-grade anal intraepithelial neoplasia. J Am Soc Cytopathol. 10(4):406-13, 2021
2. Morency EG et al: Anal cytology: institutional statistics, correlation with histology, and development of multidisciplinary screening program with review of the current literature. Arch Pathol Lab Med. 143(1):23-9, 2019

Columnar Rectal Mucosa

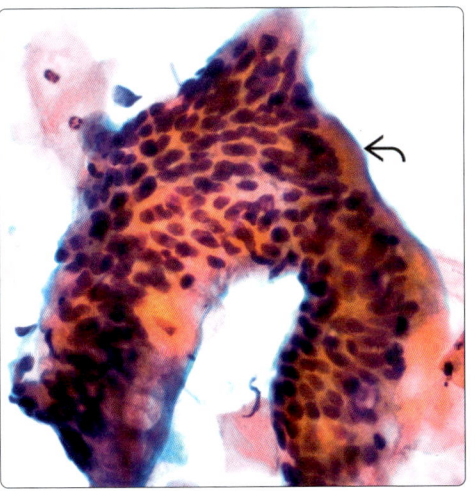

Anucleate Squamous Cells

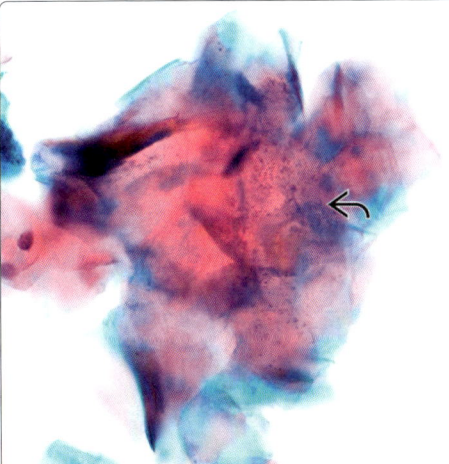

(Left) Rectal mucosa in anal Pap tests has a honeycomb arrangement of nuclei in columnar cells with abundant apical cytoplasm ➔. (Right) Anucleate squamous cells are common in anal Pap tests, reflecting the greater degree of keratinization of the squamous mucosa at this site relative to cervicovaginal specimens. Abundant bacteria ➔ are also commonly seen.

PART II
Exfoliative Cytopathology

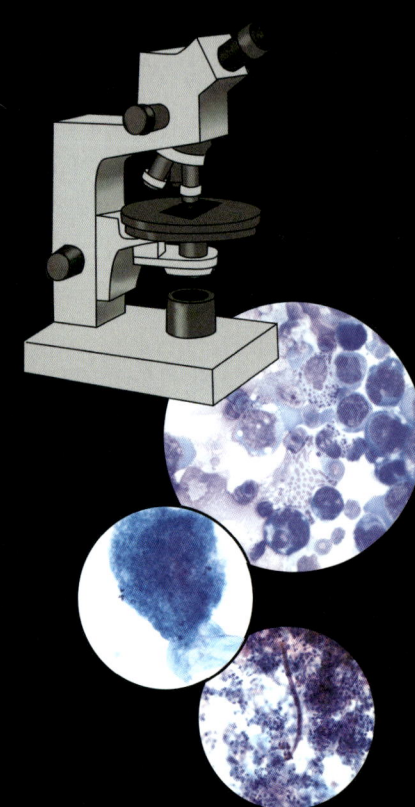

Exfoliative cytology →

1845: H. Lebert
Cytology atlas on effusion, secretions, urine cytology

1845: W. Walsche
Illustrates cancer cells in sputum

1859: W. Lambl
Malignancy diagnosis in urine cytology

1892: F. Ferguson
Urine cytology routine for cancer diagnosis

1896: L. Bahrenburg
Ascites cytology for malignancy

1904: H. Dufour
Malignancy diagnosis in CSF cytology

1909: G. Marini
Gastric cytology

1920: R. Dragallo
Monograph of clinical cytology

1947: A. Tzanck
Dermatologic cytology

1936-1948 Cell block

1950: R. Graham
The Cytologic Diagnosis of Cancer

1963: G. Saccomano
Concentrating respiratory specimens for cancer diagnosis

1980s onward: Histochemistry and immunocytochemistry on cytology

1990s: Automated cytology preparation and staining

2000s: Dawn of molecular testing era in cytology

PART II
SECTION 1
Respiratory Tract, Including Lung FNAs

Specimen Types in Respiratory Cytology and Adequacy Criteria	100
Benign and Reactive Changes	102
Pneumocystis Pneumonia and Mimics	106
Fungal Organisms in Respiratory Cytology	108
Parasitic Organisms in Respiratory Cytology	110
Viral Infections (Cytomegalovirus, Herpesvirus, and Others)	112
Mycobacteria and Other Bacterial Infections	114
Sarcoidosis and Other Immune-Related Conditions	116
Pulmonary Alveolar Proteinosis and Mimics	118
Miscellaneous Findings, Including Contaminants	120
Adenocarcinoma	122
Squamous Cell Carcinoma	126
Small Cell Carcinoma	128
Large Cell Neuroendocrine Carcinoma	130
Carcinoid and Atypical Carcinoid	132
Rare Benign and Low Malignant Potential Tumors	134
Rare Malignant Tumors	136
NUT Carcinoma	138
SMARCA4-Deficient Undifferentiated Tumor	139
Pulmonary Lymphoma	140
Pulmonary Metastasis	142

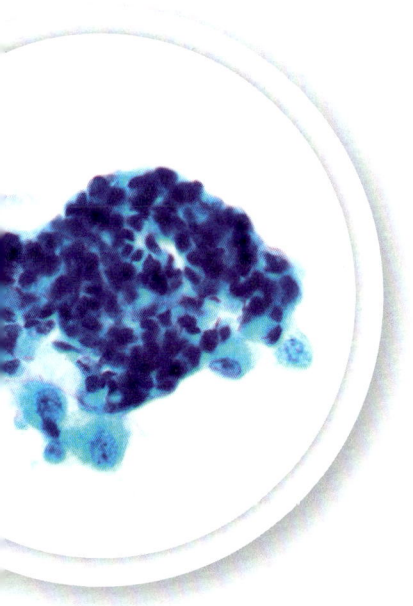
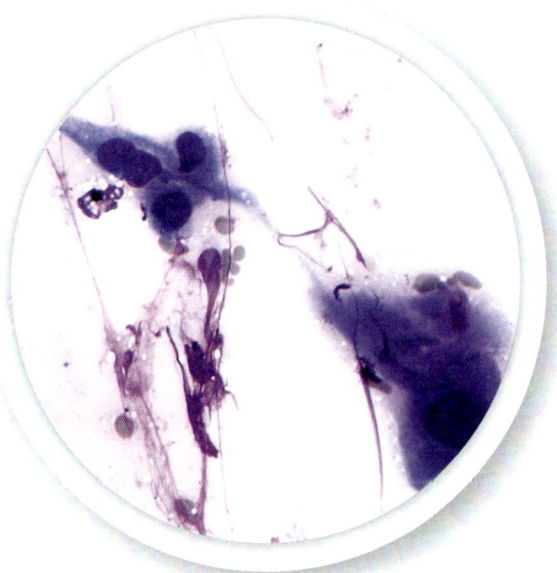
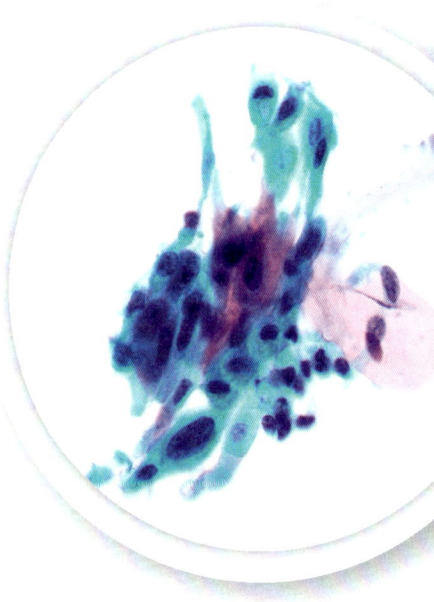

Specimen Types in Respiratory Cytology and Adequacy Criteria

TERMINOLOGY

Definitions

- Sputum
  - Coughed-up lung fluids expectorated by patient either from spontaneous bronchial mucus or from mucus induced by inhaled vapors
- Bronchoalveolar lavage (BAL)
  - Lavage fluid (100-300 mL) collected from alveolated lung parenchyma via bronchoscope wedged into subsegmental bronchus
- Bronchial brushing
  - Bronchial mucosa directly brushed during bronchoscopy
- Bronchial washing
  - Lavage fluid (3-5 mL) collected from area of bronchus
- Endobronchial FNA and core biopsy
  - Sampling from mass lesion using small-bore needle
  - Performed through bronchoscope
    - FNA or core biopsies may be performed using endobronchial ultrasound (EBUS) guidance
    - FNA performed without radiologic guidance known as Wang needle procedure
- Percutaneous FNA and core biopsy
  - Performed under CT or ultrasound guidance using trocar
  - Touch preparations allow for cytologic analysis of cells exfoliated from core biopsy
- Navigation bronchoscopy
  - Uses machine-assisted guidance to sample mass lesion in lung localized by corresponding radiologic scan
  - May be performed for lesions too peripheral to be accessed by transbronchial techniques

EPIDEMIOLOGY

Cancer Screening

- Sputum cytology in conjunction with chest x-ray failed as screening test for lung carcinoma

Tuberculosis Screening

- Sputum and bronchoscopic specimens are often collected in resource-limited world to rule out organisms, especially mycobacteria

CLINICAL IMPLICATIONS

Imaging Findings

- Central lesions, including lymph nodes, are accessible by bronchoscopy
- More peripheral lesions may be detected by BAL but usually require percutaneous CT-guided biopsy or navigation bronchoscopy

MACROSCOPIC

Specimen Handling

- Sputum and bronchoscopic specimens may be alcohol fixed
  - Fresh sputum can be analyzed by pick-and-smear method
- Liquid-based cytology works well for sputum and bronchoscopic specimens
- Collection of transbronchial or percutaneous FNA material in RPMI facilitates flow cytometry if needed to rule out lymphoma
- Touch preparations may be analyzed immediately using Romanowsky stain or rapid Pap stain
  - Additional touch preps for later analysis may counterproductively exfoliate specimen
  - Training in touching technique helps to avoid excessive exfoliation and crush artifact
- Core biopsies may be processed as cell block, especially if too small to be picked up by forceps

MICROSCOPIC

General Features

- Sputum contains cells from lung, including pulmonary macrophages and respiratory mucosa, as well as oral contaminants

Adenocarcinoma in Core Biopsy

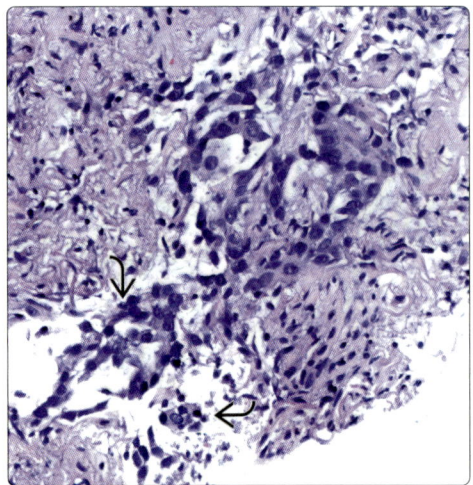

Cell Block of Squamous Carcinoma Biopsy

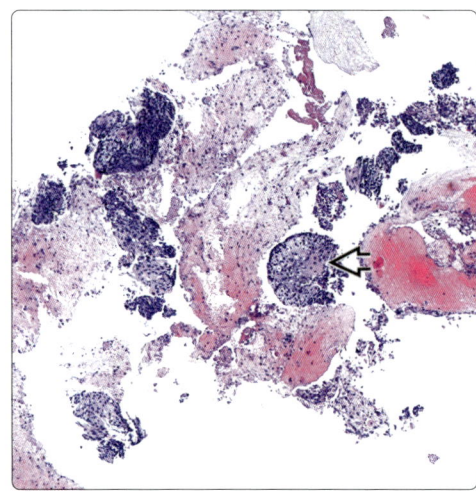

(Left) This H&E-stained core biopsy shows adenocarcinoma with dyscohesion of the malignant cells ➡, a typical finding. Touch preparations for adequacy assessment should be performed carefully by trained personnel to avoid excessive shedding and preserve cells in the biopsy for crucial ancillary studies. *(Right)* This H&E cell block shows squamous cell carcinoma with areas of keratinization ➡. Processing core biopsies with a cell block technique is often the best way to maximize yield in cases with many small fragments.

Specimen Types in Respiratory Cytology and Adequacy Criteria

- o Poor specimens, which are frequent, contain predominantly or only oral contaminants
- BAL should consist predominantly of alveolar macrophages (normally > 80% of cells)
  - o Increased numbers of lymphocytes, neutrophils, or eosinophils may have diagnostic implications even if cells are normal
- Bronchial brushings should contain predominantly bronchial mucosa
- Bronchial washings typically yield mixture of bronchial mucosa and alveolar macrophages
- FNA and core biopsy touch preparations should contain cells that explain target lesion
  - o If peribronchial lymph nodes are targeted, lymphocytes and macrophages may predominate
  - o Transbronchial biopsies may also sample other mediastinal structures

Normal Findings
- Alveolar macrophages
  - o Abundant foamy cytoplasm
    - May contain anthracotic pigment, hemosiderin, or other engulfed material, including lipids
  - o Pale, round or bean-shaped nuclei with nucleoli
  - o Type I pneumocytes are typically not appreciated because they look so similar to macrophages
- Bronchial mucosa
  - o Columnar cells with abundant foamy apical cytoplasm as well as conspicuous terminal bars and cilia
  - o Occasional goblet cells with prominent apical mucin vacuole are interspersed
    - Goblet cell hyperplasia is common benign finding
  - o Nuclei are round with pale chromatin and nucleoli
    - Nuclei should be distributed in basal or pseudostratified configuration
- Oral contaminant
  - o Squamous cells
  - o Organisms, *Actinomyces* and *Candida*, or other bacterial rods and cocci are frequently found in mouth or pharynx
  - o Food particles, including plant matter and skeletal muscle, are also often contaminants

REPORTING CRITERIA

Minimum Requirements
- If there is known mass lesion in area of sampling, cells that explain mass should be present to achieve adequacy
- Sputum requires presence of alveolar macrophages or abnormal cells for adequacy
  - o Ciliated respiratory mucosa may derive from upper respiratory tract
- Bronchoscopic specimens are usually adequate unless they are acellular or have marked obscuration or artifact
  - o BAL specimens with < 50% macrophages may have suboptimal sampling of distal lung parenchyma
- FNA requires lesional cells or cells representative of targeted structure (such as lymph node) to be adequate
  - o Mere diagnosis of malignancy may not be sufficient; adequacy may require sufficient cells for ancillary immunocytochemical &/or molecular work-ups
- Touch preparations of core needle biopsies have adequacy criteria similar to FNA
  - o Combined FNA and core biopsy from same procedure may increase overall adequacy, especially taking into account ancillary studies

PREDICTIVE CANCER TESTING SUMMARY

General Issues
- Sputum is simplest test for lung carcinoma but has poor performance characteristics
  - o Single sputum specimen has low sensitivity for carcinoma (< 30%)
- Bronchoscopy works well for endobronchial lesions or central masses with airway obstruction
  - o Transbronchial biopsy in addition to cytology increases diagnostic yield
  - o EBUS FNA can also be used for mediastinal lymph nodes or other mediastinal structures
    - Now standard of care for evaluation of mediastinal nodes for metastatic carcinoma or sarcoidosis
    - Can also be used in conjunction with flow cytometry to rule out lymphoma
    - Thymoma and other mediastinal tumors can be sampled by this method
  - o Small core needle biopsies for EBUS procedures are now available
    - Not as widely used or accepted as similar needles for gastrointestinal endoscopic ultrasound procedures
    - Role of on-site evaluation for samples from these needles has not been determined
    - May increase yield for ancillary studies; 3-5 biopsy passes recommended
- CT-guided percutaneous biopsy is usually needed for peripheral nodules
  - o Often technically challenging due to tumor size or position relative to vital structures
  - o High rate of associated pneumothorax
  - o FNA and core biopsy have similar diagnostic yield
- Navigation bronchoscopy offers alternate approach to peripheral lesions
  - o May reach areas not accessible to percutaneous biopsy
  - o Less likely to result in pneumothorax than percutaneous biopsy
  - o Needles, forceps, brushes, and lavage may be deployed
  - o This technique is relatively new and has high incidence of nondiagnostic specimens with current technology
- Cytology diagnosis avoids thoracic surgery for wedge resection biopsy

SELECTED REFERENCES

1. Gildea TR et al: The impact of biopsy tool choice and rapid on-site evaluation on diagnostic accuracy for malignant lesions in the prospective: multicenter NAVIGATE study. J Bronchology Interv Pulmonol. 28(3):174-83, 2021
2. Kalinke L et al: The promises and challenges of early non-small cell lung cancer detection: patient perceptions, low-dose CT screening, bronchoscopy and biomarkers. Mol Oncol. 15(10):2544-64, 2021
3. Roy Chowdhuri S et al: Collection and handling of thoracic small biopsy and cytology specimens for ancillary studies: guideline from the College of American Pathologists in collaboration with the American College of Chest Physicians, Association for Molecular Pathology, American Society of Cytopathology, American Thoracic Society, Pulmonary Pathology Society, Papanicolaou Society of Cytopathology, Society of Interventional Radiology, and Society of Thoracic Radiology. Arch Pathol Lab Med. 144(8):933-58, 2020

Benign and Reactive Changes

KEY FACTS

CLINICAL ISSUES
- Reactive cytologic changes often appear in setting of pneumonia and inflammation
- Radiation and chemotherapy changes should be kept in mind in patient with history of malignancy
- Localized changes create diagnostic dilemmas because radiologic patterns for injury and malignancy often overlap

CYTOPATHOLOGY
- Reactive cells may be numerous and predominant or may only be small subpopulation
  - Presence of range of changes from near normal to more atypical may help to support reactive interpretation
- Reactive changes often appear in setting of altered background with inflammation or debris
- Nuclear enlargement, increased pleomorphism, multinucleation, and prominent nucleoli are typical of reactive processes
  - Architectural distortion is also common
- Reactive cells typically have pale nuclei with less chromatin clumping than malignant cells
  - DNA content is not increased, unlike malignancies
- Cilia and terminal bars are indicators of benign changes
- Basal cell hyperplasia is characterized by very small cohesive cells
  - These are usually few
- Creola bodies are rounded aggregates of bronchial cells
  - Can be recognized as benign by analysis of relatively well-visualized cells at edge, which may have cilia
- Radiation and chemotherapy effects frequently result in cytoplasmic enlargement in proportion to nuclear enlargement

TOP DIFFERENTIAL DIAGNOSES
- Adenocarcinoma
- Squamous cell carcinoma
- Small cell carcinoma

Typical Reactive Changes
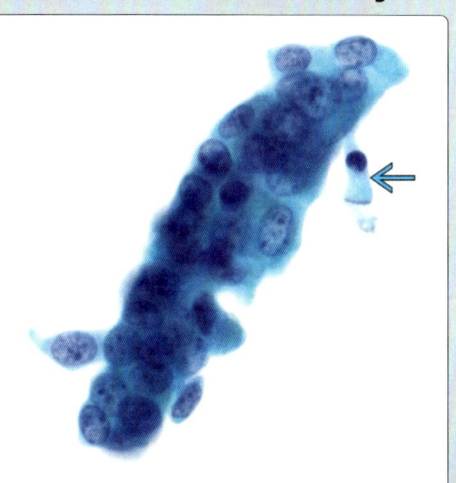

Reactive Changes in Squamous Metaplasia
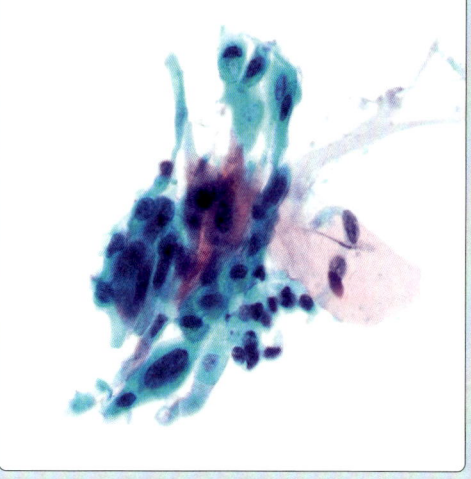

(Left) *Reactive changes seen on this Pap stain are due to organizing pneumonia and include reassuring pale chromatin and prominent nucleoli with striking architectural disorder and nuclear pleomorphism.* (Right) *This Pap-stained cluster illustrates marked atypia in the setting of squamous metaplasia with some cells raising concern for non-small cell carcinoma.*

Radiation-Induced Reactive Changes
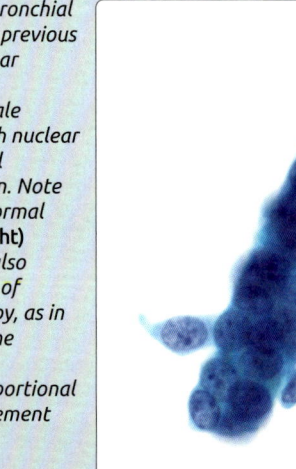

Chemotherapy-Associated Changes
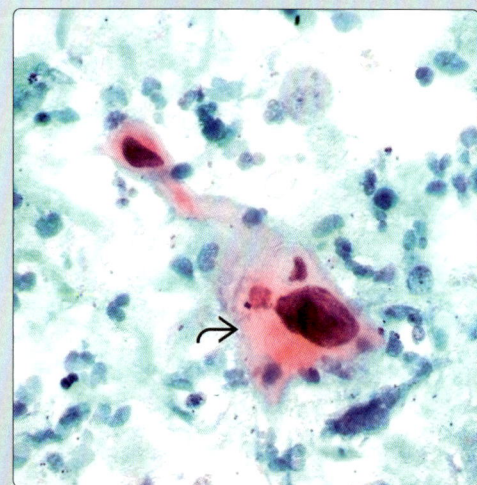

(Left) *This cluster of bronchial cells in a patient with previous radiation shows nuclear enlargement and pleomorphism with pale chromatin and smooth nuclear contours that are well visualized on Pap stain. Note the contrast with a normal bronchial cell ⇨.* (Right) *Reactive atypia may also appear in the context of previous chemotherapy, as in this Pap stain. Note the reassuring abundant cytoplasm that is proportional to the nuclear enlargement ⇨.*

Benign and Reactive Changes

ETIOLOGY/PATHOGENESIS

Reactive Changes
- May be seen in context of any form of lung injury: Chronic or acute, diffuse or localized

CLINICAL ISSUES

Presentation
- Reactive cytologic changes often appear in setting of pneumonia sampled primarily to look for organisms
- Radiation and chemotherapy changes should be kept in mind in specimens from patients with history of malignancy

IMAGING

General Features
- Localized changes create diagnostic dilemmas because of overlapping radiologic patterns for injury and malignancy

CYTOPATHOLOGY

Background
- Normal lung has clean background
- Reactive changes often appear in setting of altered background
  o Increased acute inflammation is frequently feature in samples with reactive change
  o Necrotic debris associated with lung injury may also be seen in setting of reactive changes

Cells
- Normal benign cells
  o Alveolar macrophages
    – Individual round cells with pale, irregular nuclei and abundant, foamy cytoplasm
  o Bronchial cells
    – Cohesive clusters of columnar cells with small nuclei and abundant, apical cytoplasm
    – Terminal bars and cilia are frequent and prominent
    – Occasional goblet cells contain mucin
  o Pneumocytes
    – Type I pneumocytes are not readily recognized, appear same as macrophages
    – Type II pneumocytes are rare in absence of injury
- Reactive cells
  o Goblet cell hyperplasia
    – Increased numbers of mucus-secreting cells associated with chronic bronchial irritation
  o Basal cell (or reserve cell) hyperplasia
    – Very small cells with high nuclear:cytoplasmic ratio and dark, irregular nuclei
  o Squamous metaplasia
    – Scale-like cells with abundant hard or keratinizing cytoplasm and small, round nuclei
  o Reactive glandular cells
    – May be response to inflammatory injury or exposures, such as chemotherapy and radiation
    – Architectural distortion with loss of orderly sheet-like arrangement, nuclear enlargement, increased pleomorphism, multinucleation, and prominent nucleoli are typical changes
    – Nuclear pallor helps to distinguish from malignancy
    – Radiation and chemotherapy effects frequently result in cytoplasmic enlargement in proportion to nuclear enlargement
    – Cilia and terminal bars support benign changes
  o Creola bodies
    – Round, dense clusters of reactive bronchial cells representing detached papillary hyperplasia
    – Cells at edge of cluster should have benign appearance with cilia sometimes apparent
  o Reactive squamous cells
    – Reactive changes in squamous metaplasia include nuclear enlargement and pleomorphism
    – Reactive nuclei retain even chromatin or look glassy

Cytology-Histology Correlation
- Correlation with histology is of tremendous value when trying to differentiate reactive and malignant changes

MICROSCOPIC

Histologic Features
- Some changes in reactive processes, including fibroblast proliferation and hyaline membranes, are more readily seen
- Low-power architecture in histology is usually very helpful to differentiate injury responses from malignancy

DIFFERENTIAL DIAGNOSIS

Adenocarcinoma
- Features of reactive bronchial cells or type II pneumocytes extensively overlap with adenocarcinoma

Squamous Cell Carcinoma
- Reactive squamous cells may mimic carcinoma

Small Cell Carcinoma
- Basal cell hyperplasia may be mistaken for small cell carcinoma, especially if very small cell size is not noted

DIAGNOSTIC CHECKLIST

Pathologic Interpretation Pearls
- Reactive changes extensively overlap with features of malignancy
  o Great care must be taken to avoid false-positives
- Presence of inflammatory background supports reactive change but does not exclude malignancy
- Reactive cells typically have pale nuclei with less chromatin clumping than malignant cells
- Beware of malignancy diagnosis if cilia or terminal bars are present in association with concerning cells
- Basal cell hyperplasia can be distinguished from small cell carcinoma by very small cell size and tight clustering
- Creola bodies can be recognized by analysis of relatively well-visualized cells at edge, which may have cilia

SELECTED REFERENCES

1. Carlier FM et al: Epithelial barrier dysfunction in chronic respiratory diseases. Front Physiol. 12:691227, 2021
2. Saqi A et al: Granulomatous inflammation and organizing pneumonia: role of computed tomography-guided lung fine needle aspirations, touch preparations and core biopsies in the evaluation of common non-neoplastic diagnoses. Cytojournal. 11:2, 2014

Benign and Reactive Changes

(Left) Alveolar macrophages from a Pap-stained bronchoalveolar lavage show the nuclear irregularities typical of this cell type. **(Right)** This cluster of benign bronchial cells from a Pap stain shows basally oriented, uniform small nuclei and a striking terminal bar topped by cilia ⇒.

Alveolar Macrophages
Bronchial Cells

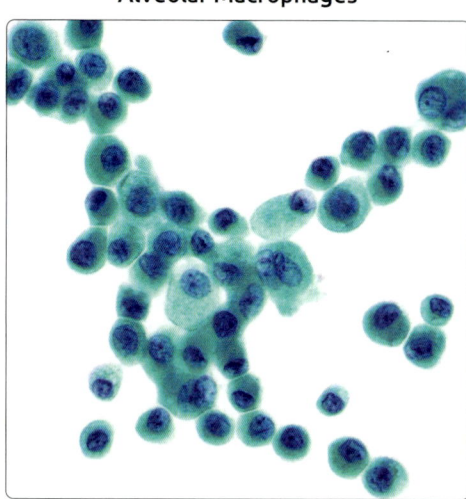

(Left) Benign bronchial cells are numerous in many lung cytology specimens, both exfoliative and aspirated. The keys to identification of the benign nature of these cells during adequacy assessments include recognition of the preserved basal orientation of the nuclei ⇒ and the numerous cilia ⇒ that are metachromatic in Diff-Quik stains. **(Right)** Mucous cell hyperplasia, seen here in a Pap stain, results in an increased number of goblet-type bronchial cells with metachromatic intracytoplasmic mucin ⇒.

Diff-Quik Appearance of Bronchial Cells
Mucous Cell Hyperplasia

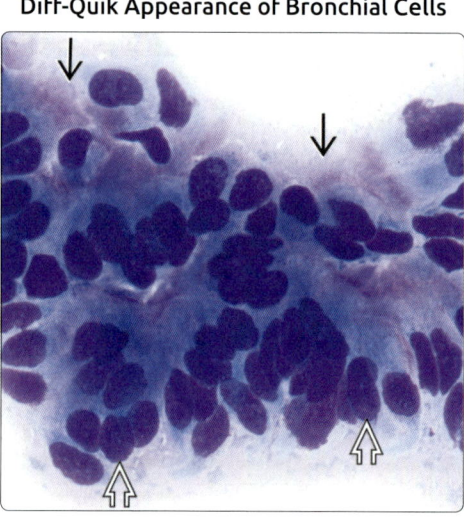

(Left) This aggregate of bronchial cells seen in a lavage ThinPrep shows reassuring features at the periphery, including pale, uniform nuclei, a rim of apical cytoplasm, and cilia ⇒. Numerous similar groups were seen in the specimen, a common occurrence in patients with Creola bodies. **(Right)** Basal cell hyperplasia, as seen in this Pap stain, is characterized by a proliferation of very small cells with dark, irregular nuclei and scant cytoplasm, which may raise concern for small cell carcinoma in the unwary.

Creola Body With Cilia
Basal Cell Hyperplasia

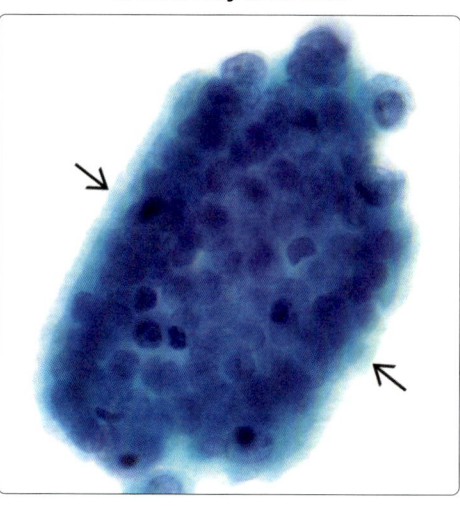
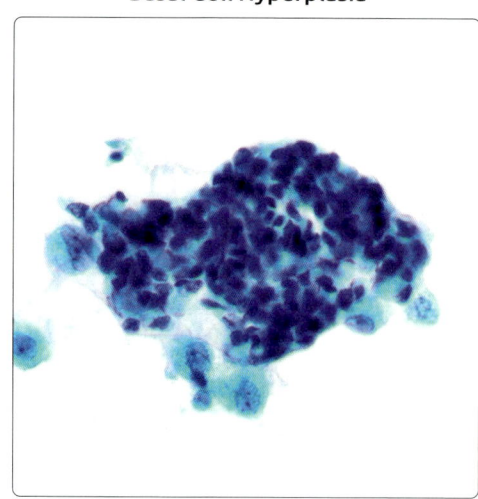

Benign and Reactive Changes

Range of Atypia From Mild to Marked

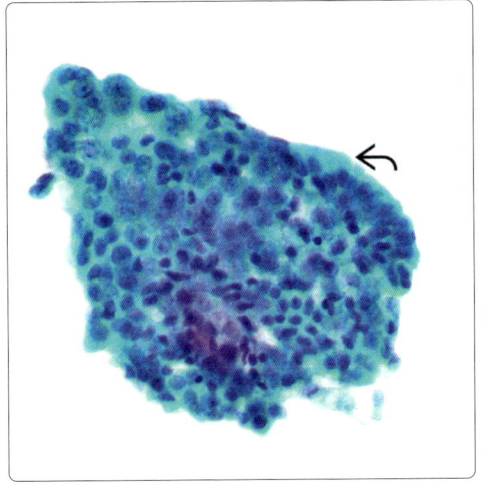

Terminal Bars

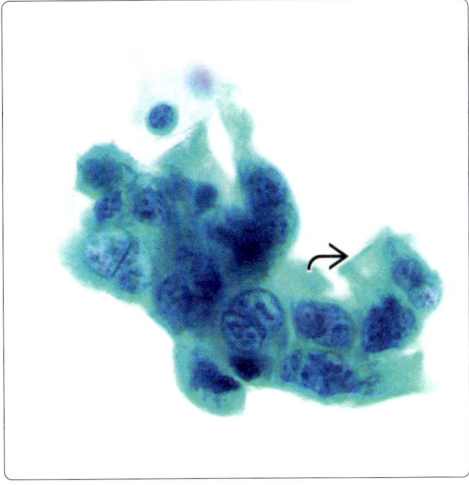

(Left) In some instances, reactive nuclear enlargement and pleomorphism can be easily dismissed because of attached cells that preserve a more normal appearance, such as the well-oriented columnar cells on the edge of this Pap-stained group ⊡. **(Right)** The presence of terminal bars ⊡ &/or cilia are strongly reassuring even in the presence of marked nuclear atypia. This Pap stain demonstrates a prominent terminal bar that should aid the cytologist in making a benign diagnosis.

Associated Acute Inflammation

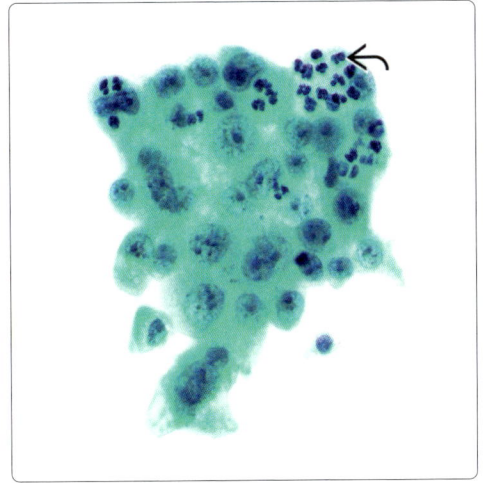

Reactive Changes Enhanced By Diff-Quik

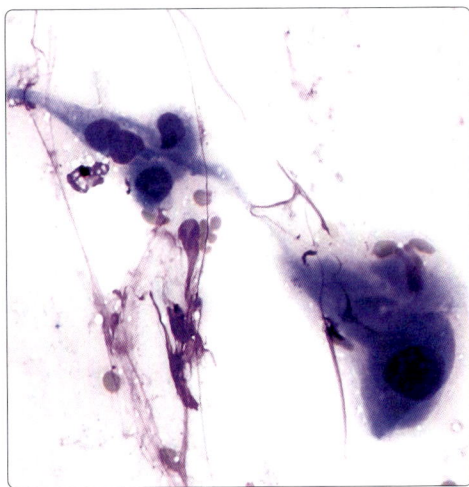

(Left) Reactive changes, such as those seen in this Pap stain, are often found in association with acute inflammation. Intracytoplasmic neutrophils ⊡ do not rule out malignancy but support an interpretation of reactive change. **(Right)** Diff-Quik preparations tend to accentuate the nuclear enlargement and pleomorphism characteristic of reactive changes without allowing for visualization of the chromatin and nucleoli, which makes them quite difficult to interpret in this setting.

Organizing Pneumonia Cytology

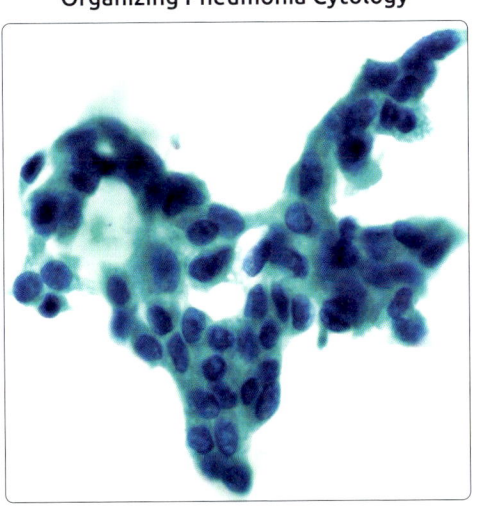

Organizing Pneumonia Histology

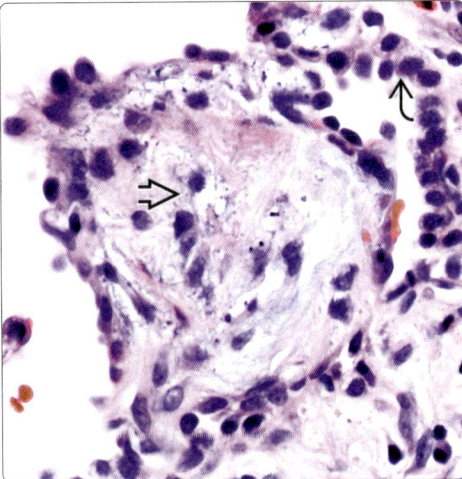

(Left) In some instances, such as this Pap-stained example of reactive atypia associated with organizing pneumonia, the changes may be very difficult to distinguish from well-differentiated adenocarcinoma. **(Right)** In the corresponding resection stained with H&E, similar nuclear atypia can be seen in reactive type II pneumocytes ⊡ lining the residual alveolar wall adjacent to a small plug of granulation tissue ⊡.

Pneumocystis Pneumonia and Mimics

KEY FACTS

CLINICAL ISSUES
- Associated with immune dysfunction, especially HIV/AIDS
- Favorable prognosis when appropriately treated
- Screening for *Pneumocystis* occurs in setting of lung transplantation and in patients with pneumonia not responding to usual therapy
- Among HIV-infected patients, those with CD4 counts < 200 cells/μL are 5x more likely to develop *Pneumocystis* pneumonia (PCP)
- PCR-based molecular testing for PCP has been developed, but since many people are asymptomatic carriers, this methodology is limited by false-positives

CYTOPATHOLOGY
- Alveolar casts of fluffy debris
- On Pap or H&E stains, organisms appear as numerous refractile clear discs (4-7 μm) embedded in clumped amorphous material
- GMS stain highlights cyst organisms with collapsed ovoid morphology and prominent central dot
- Organisms show characteristic "coffee cup" or "crushed ping pong ball" morphology
- Diff-Quik/Romanowsky stains demonstrate central dot but not organism outline
- Increased inflammation and possibly giant cells may be seen in background

TOP DIFFERENTIAL DIAGNOSES
- Other fungal infections
  - Yeasts, including *Histoplasma* and *Cryptococcus*, are closest mimics
  - Mimicking fungi may be intracellular or lack alveolar casts and will show budding yeast forms
- Alveolar proteinosis
  - Lacks organisms and casts stain with PAS

Alveolar Casts

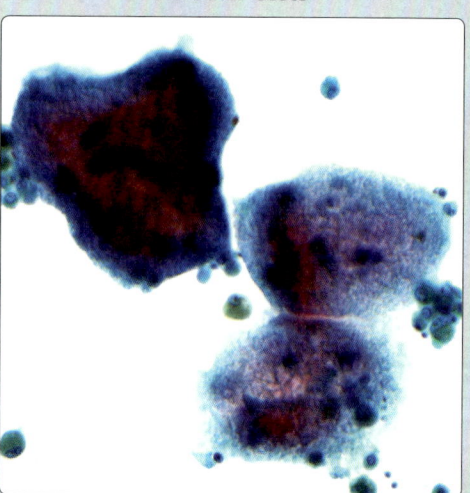

Refractile Organisms

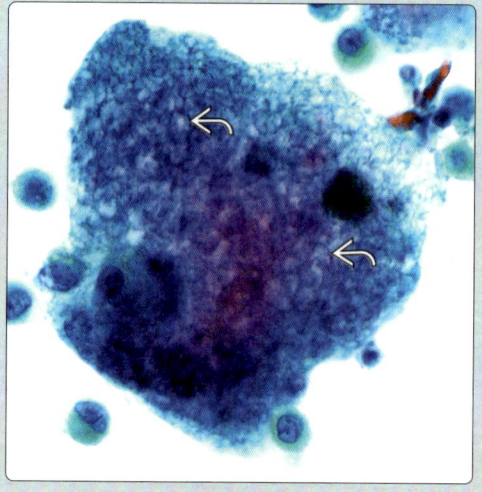

(Left) *Pneumocystis organisms are found within casts that retain the shape of the alveolus during lavage, as seen in this Pap-stained ThinPrep.* (Right) *Refractile organisms can be seen within the Pap-stained casts ➡ at high power, as seen in this example from a ThinPrep specimen. This finding helps to distinguish Pneumocystis casts from mimics, such as alveolar proteinosis.*

Cytospin Appearance

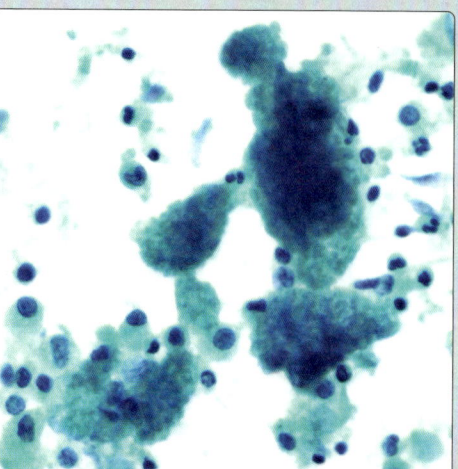

Numerous Casts in Severely Ill Patient

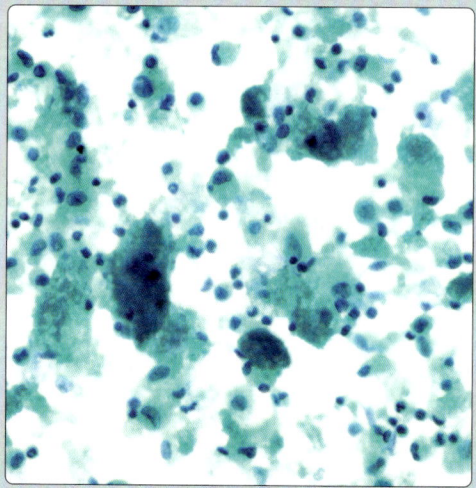

(Left) *On Pap-stained cytospin, the alveolar casts appear blue-green. Note the variability of the size and shape of the casts.* (Right) *In severely ill patients, the casts and cast fragments are numerous and easily seen at low power, such as in this Pap-stained example, in association with macrophages and inflammatory cells.*

Pneumocystis Pneumonia and Mimics

TERMINOLOGY

Abbreviations
- *Pneumocystis* pneumonia (PCP)

CLINICAL ISSUES

Presentation
- Associated with immune dysfunction, especially HIV/AIDS
- Screening for *Pneumocystis* occurs in setting of lung transplantation and in patients with pneumonia not responding to usual therapy

Laboratory Tests
- Among HIV-infected patients, those with CD4 counts < 200 cells/μL are 5x more likely to develop PCP
- PCR-based molecular testing for PCP has been developed, but since many people are asymptomatic carriers, this methodology is limited by false-positives

Natural History
- Infection is acquired by inhalation with primary infection occurring early in life and remaining latent
- Favorable prognosis when appropriately treated

IMAGING

Radiographic Findings
- Ground-glass perihilar or diffuse bilateral airspace consolidation

CYTOPATHOLOGY

Pattern
- Alveolar casts of fluffy debris

Background
- Increased inflammation and possibly giant cells

Cells
- On conventional stains, organisms appear as numerous refractile clear discs (4-7 μm) embedded in clumped amorphous material
- GMS stain highlights cyst organisms with collapsed ovoid morphology and prominent central dot
- Organisms show characteristic "coffee cup" or "crushed ping pong ball" morphology
- Diff-Quik/Romanowsky stains demonstrate central dot but not organism outline

Cytology-Histology Correlation
- Cytology is more sensitive for detection of organisms

DIFFERENTIAL DIAGNOSIS

Other Fungal Infections
- *Histoplasma capsulatum* may show similar morphology to *Pneumocystis*, including central dark dots
- *Cryptococcus neoformans* may also resemble *Pneumocystis* with collapsed ovoid forms
- Mimicking fungi may be intracellular or lack alveolar casts and will show budding yeast forms

Alveolar Proteinosis
- Though clinically very different, both *Pneumocystis* and alveolar proteinosis show alveolar casts in lavage specimens
- Alveolar proteinosis lacks organisms, casts stain with PAS

DIAGNOSTIC CHECKLIST

Pathologic Interpretation Pearls
- Alveolar casts are distinctive, and refractile organisms can be seen on high power with conventional stains
- GMS stains facilitate diagnosis and are helpful for identifying rare organisms in low-level infections
  - Organisms have characteristic central dot and "coffee cup" or "crushed ping pong ball" morphology when viewed from side angle

SELECTED REFERENCES

1. Bateman M et al: Diagnosing Pneumocystis jirovecii pneumonia: a review of current methods and novel approaches. Med Mycol. 58(8):1015-28, 2020
2. Kato H et al: Diagnosis and treatment of Pneumocystis jirovecii pneumonia in HIV-infected or non-HIV-infected patients-difficulties in diagnosis and adverse effects of trimethoprim-sulfamethoxazole. J Infect Chemother. 25(11):920-4, 2019

Pneumocystis Morphology
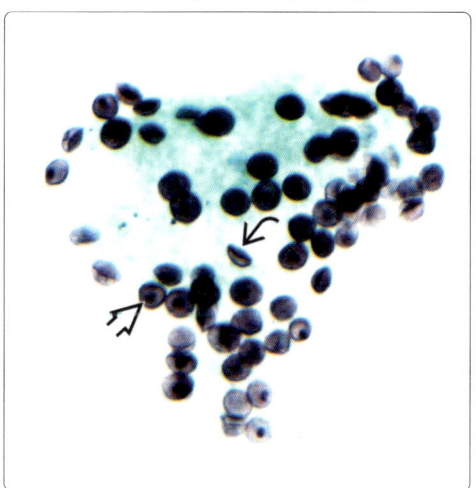

Diff-Quik Staining of Alveolar Cast
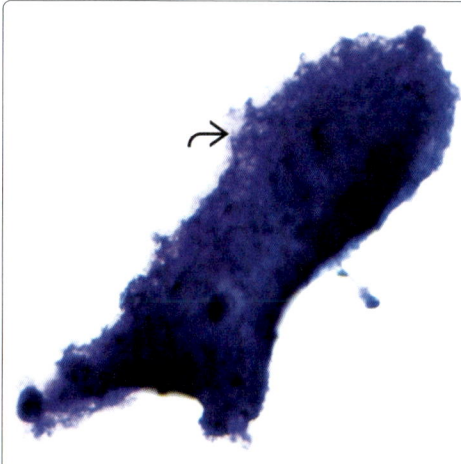

(Left) *Characteristic morphologic features of the Pneumocystis cysts on GMS stain include the central dot ➡ and the collapsed "coffee cup" or "crushed ping pong ball" cross-sectional contour ➡.* **(Right)** *An alveolar cast of Pneumocystis with a "fluffy" periphery ➡ is easily seen by Diff-Quik stain.*

Fungal Organisms in Respiratory Cytology

KEY FACTS

ETIOLOGY/PATHOGENESIS
- AIDS, transplantation, or chemotherapy predispose to severe infections

CYTOPATHOLOGY
- *Aspergillus* have septate straight-edged hyphae (3-6 μm) with acute angle branching
  - Many less common fungi not of *Aspergillus* genus may have identical morphology
- *Zygomyces/Mucor* have ribbon-like, wavy-edged, nonseptate hyphae (4-15 μm) with right angle branching
- *Candida* species, usually contaminants in lung specimens, have yeast or pseudohyphal forms
- Major infectious yeasts include *Cryptococcus*, *Histoplasma*, and *Blastomyces*
  - These can often be differentiated by size, shape, budding pattern, and encapsulation
- Less common yeasts include *Coccidioides*, *Paracoccidioides*, *Talaromyces*, *Emmonsia*, *Emergomyces*, and *Sporothrix*

ANCILLARY TESTS
- GMS and PAS improve sensitivity and morphologic characterization
- Mucicarmine highlights capsule of *Cryptococcus*
- Microbiology laboratories can much more accurately classify organisms than morphology alone, especially among hyphal organisms
  - This may significantly impact upon treatment
  - Caution is indicated in identifying fungal genus in cytology specimens
- Antigen tests for dimorphic fungi often indicate diagnosis prior to cytologic identification

TOP DIFFERENTIAL DIAGNOSES
- Parasitic organisms may resemble yeasts
- Vegetable matter, fibers, and foreign body particles can be confused with fungal forms
- *Pneumocystis* is now recognized as fungus but is generally considered separately

Engulfed *Cryptococcus*

Mucicarmine Stain for *Cryptococcus*

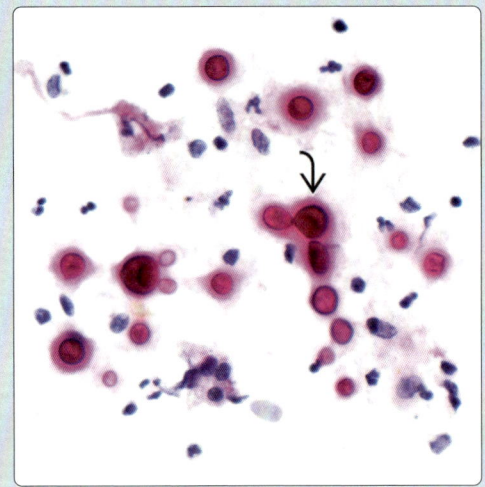

(Left) Cryptococcus yeasts may be seen extracellularly or engulfed within histiocytes, as demonstrated in this Diff-Quik-stained example ➡. (Right) Mucicarmine stain of the same case highlights the thick capsule of Cryptococcus, aiding in differentiation from other fungi ➡. Note the variability of the size and shape of the yeasts, another feature that aids in recognizing Cryptococcus.

Histoplasma in Macrophages

GMS Stain of *Histoplasma*

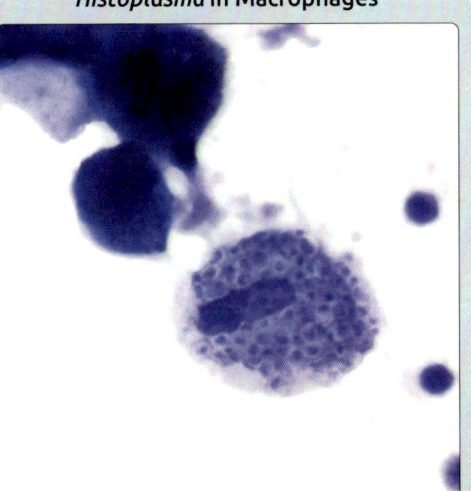
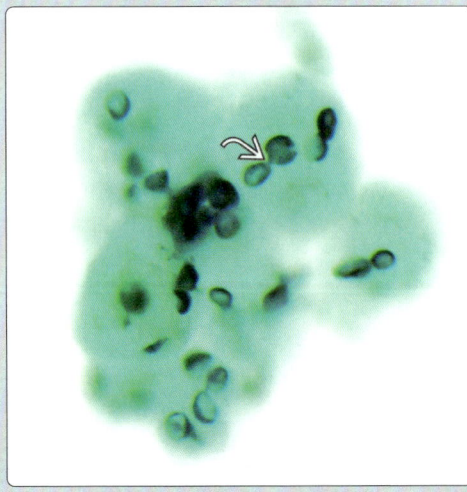

(Left) This Diff-Quik-stained cytospin from a BAL of an HIV patient with pneumonia shows 2 large macrophages with their cytoplasm distended by numerous Histoplasma organisms. Note the capsule-like halos around the organisms. (Right) Fungal organisms within macrophages are highlighted by GMS stain, showing narrow-based budding ➡ that differentiates Histoplasma from Blastomyces. Budding also eliminates Pneumocystis, which is extracellular but has morphologically similar organisms.

Fungal Organisms in Respiratory Cytology

TERMINOLOGY

Definitions
- Infection or colonization of lung by fungal organisms

ETIOLOGY/PATHOGENESIS

Immunosuppression
- AIDS, transplantation, or chemotherapy predispose to severe infections

CLINICAL ISSUES

Presentation
- Ranges from incidental finding to life-threatening pneumonia
- *Aspergillus* may present as allergic bronchopulmonary aspergillosis, chronic pulmonary aspergillosis (including fungus balls in cavitary lesions), or as invasive aspergillosis

CYTOPATHOLOGY

Aspergillus Species and Mimics
- Septate straight-edged hyphae (3-6 μm) with acute angle branching
- Rarely, fruiting bodies in cavity-filling aspergillomas
- Many fungi may have same appearance as *Aspergillus*

Zygomyces/Mucor Species
- Ribbon-like, wavy-edged, nonseptate hyphae (4-15 μm) with right angle branching
- Often empty appearance due to spillage of organelles

Candida Species
- Yeasts and pseudohyphae often seen in association with oral squamous cells and bacteria

Dimorphic Fungi
- *Cryptococcus* is more variable in size than other yeasts
- *Blastomyces* can be distinguished by broad-based budding and thick walls
- *Histoplasma* and *Emergomyces* both small with narrow-based budding
- Large spherules in *Coccidioides* (with endospores), *Paracoccidioides* (with budding), and *Emmonsia*
- *Talaromyces* (*Penicillium*) shows central septation
- *Sporothrix* has elongated "cigar bodies"

ANCILLARY TESTS

Histochemistry
- GMS or PAS highlights fungal forms
- Mucicarmine highlights capsule of *Cryptococcus*

Microbiology Laboratory
- Antigen tests, culture, and PCR provide greater sensitivity and specificity than cytology

DIFFERENTIAL DIAGNOSIS

Other Organisms
- *Toxoplasma* and *Pneumocystis*

Extraneous Debris
- Vegetable matter, fibers, and foreign body particles

DIAGNOSTIC CHECKLIST

Pathologic Interpretation Pearls
- Hyphal organisms can be divided into *Aspergillus*-like and *Mucor*-like categories, but morphology alone is not very reliable for differentiating
- Yeast forms can often be specifically identified on basis of morphology

SELECTED REFERENCES

1. Poplin V et al: Diagnosis of pulmonary infections due to endemic fungi. Diagnostics (Basel). 11(5):856, 2021
2. Van Dyke MCC et al: Fantastic yeasts and where to find them: the hidden diversity of dimorphic fungal pathogens. Curr Opin Microbiol. 52:55-63, 2019

Aspergillus-Like Hyphae

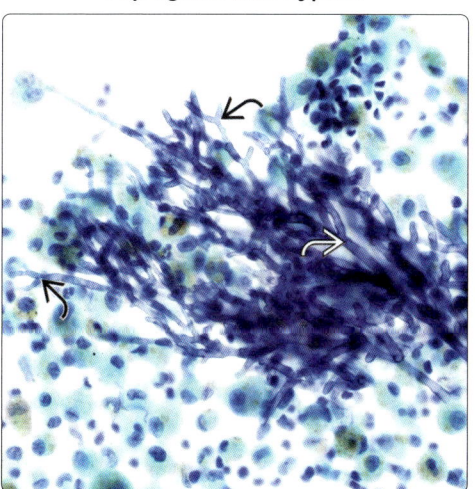

Zygomyces/Mucor-Type Hyphae

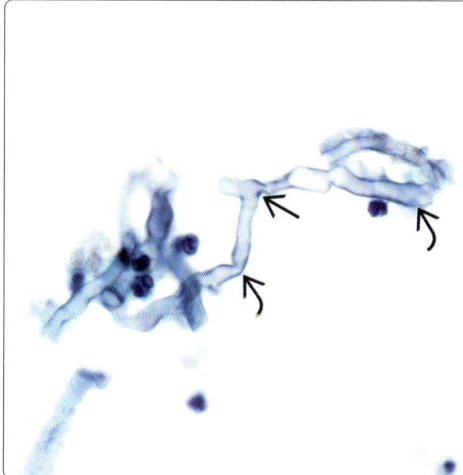

(Left) Pap-stained bronchial specimen contains hyphal organisms of the Aspergillus type with uniform hyphal thickness, septations ➡, and acute angle branching ➡. **(Right)** Pap-stained hyphal organism is of the Zygomyces/Mucor type with variable hyphal thickness ➡, no septations, and right angle branching ➡.

Parasitic Organisms in Respiratory Cytology

KEY FACTS

ETIOLOGY/PATHOGENESIS
- Protozoa (*Toxoplasma*, *Cryptosporidium*, microsporidia, *Entamoeba*), nematodes (*Strongyloides*, *Dirofilaria*, microfilaria), cestodes (*Echinococcus*), and trematodes (*Paragonimus*, *Schistosoma*)

CLINICAL ISSUES
- Parasites numerous enough to be identified in cytology specimens are usually associated with immunosuppression
- *Strongyloides* may be seen in massive numbers in patients with hyperinfection, often associated with steroid treatment
- Disseminated toxoplasmosis is typically associated with AIDS or stem cell/organ transplantation

CYTOPATHOLOGY
- *Strongyloides* filariform larvae (0.2 mm in length) have short, pointed tails and no sheath
- FNA of hydatid cyst may include characteristic protoscolices and hooklets, but biopsy is rarely performed due to risk of rupture
- Characteristic *Paragonimus* or *Schistosoma* eggs may appear in sputum or FNA of granulomatous lesions
- *Toxoplasma* may be identified as free-living, crescent-shaped tachyzoites (5 μm) &/or bradyzoites (2 μm) within pseudocysts (10-50 μm)

ANCILLARY TESTS
- GMS, PAS, Giemsa, or trichrome may help to identify protozoans

TOP DIFFERENTIAL DIAGNOSES
- Vegetable matter, fibers, and other exogenous elements may simulate parasitic forms
- Fungal yeasts may resemble protozoans
- Dirofilarial infarcts and granulomas caused by other protozoans may raise concern for malignancy by radiology

Strongyloides Morphology
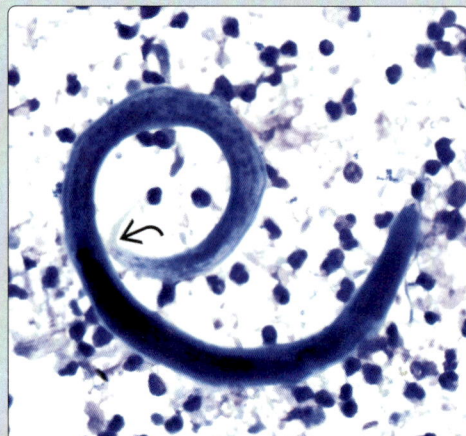

Unstained *Strongyloides* in Pap Stain
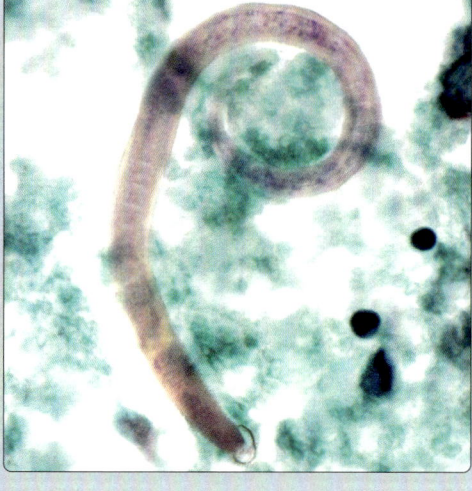

(Left) *Strongyloides* filariform larva, as seen in this Diff-Quik stain, have a characteristic short, pointed tail ➛ and lack a sheath, allowing differentiation from similar small worms. (Right) Pap-stained filariform larva of *Strongyloides* shows limited stain uptake, allowing good visualization of internal structures.

Toxoplasma Bradyzoites
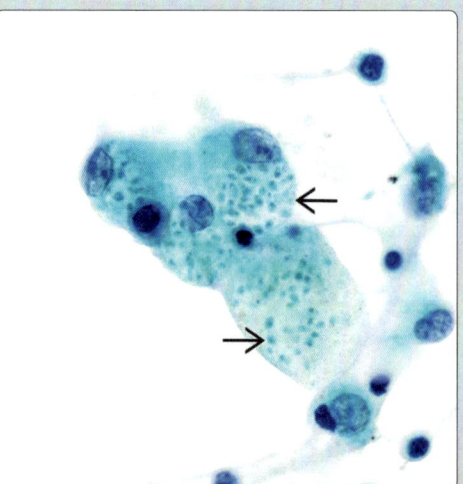

Toxoplasma Highlighted by GMS Stain
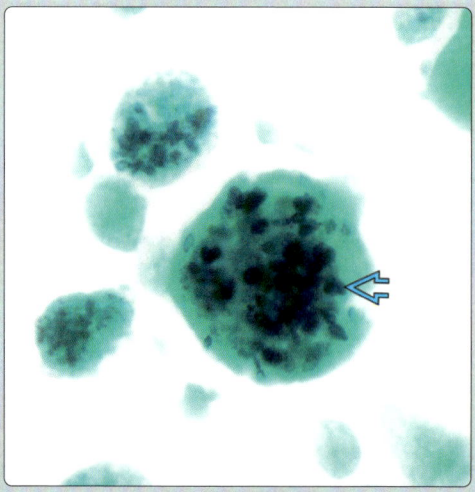

(Left) Bradyzoites of *Toxoplasma* may be seen in Pap-stained preparations, such as this ThinPrep ➛, especially if they are numerous. (Right) GMS may stain *Toxoplasma* organisms positive, as in this example, making differentiation from fungal yeasts, such as *Histoplasma*, difficult ➛.

Parasitic Organisms in Respiratory Cytology

TERMINOLOGY

Definitions
- Infection of lung by parasitic organisms

CLINICAL ISSUES

Presentation
- Parasites numerous enough to be identified in cytology specimens are usually associated with pneumonia in immunocompromised individuals
  - Numerous *Strongyloides* worms are seen in patients with hyperinfection, often due to steroid treatment
  - Disseminated toxoplasmosis is typically associated with AIDS or stem cell/organ transplantation
- Some parasites cause localized inflammatory or granulomatous reaction
  - *Dirofilaria* causes infarcts that look like tumors by radiology
  - *Paragonimus*, *Schistosoma*, or *Echinococcus* may also cause mass lesions

CYTOPATHOLOGY

Strongyloides stercoralis (Threadworm)
- Filariform larvae (0.2 mm in length) have short, pointed tails and no sheath

Dirofilaria immitis (Dog Heartworm)
- Organisms rarely seen in cytology, but FNA biopsies of lesions yield necrotic debris that may mimic malignancy

Echinococcus Species (Hydatid Disease)
- FNA of hydatid cyst may include characteristic protoscolices and hooklets, but biopsy is rarely performed due to risk of rupture

Paragonimus and *Schistosoma* Species
- Characteristic eggs may appear in sputum or FNA of granulomatous lesions

Toxoplasma gondii
- Free-living, crescent-shaped tachyzoites (5 μm) &/or bradyzoites (2 μm) within pseudocysts (10-50 μm)

Entamoeba histolytica
- Trophozoites (10-50 μm) resemble large histiocytes but with small, round nuclei containing karyosomes

ANCILLARY TESTS

Special Stains
- GMS, PAS, Giemsa, or trichrome may help identify protozoans

Laboratory Tests
- PCR, serology, and examination of stool for parasites and eggs

DIFFERENTIAL DIAGNOSIS

Debris
- Vegetable matter, fibers, and other exogenous elements may simulate parasitic forms

Fungi
- Yeasts resemble protozoans, including *Toxoplasma*

Histiocytes
- *Entamoeba* has histiocytoid appearance

Malignancy
- Parasites, such as *Dirofilaria*, *Paragonimus*, *Schistosoma*, and *Echinococcus*, may cause radiologically worrisome mass lesion

SELECTED REFERENCES
1. Krolewiecki A et al: Strongyloidiasis: a neglected tropical disease. Infect Dis Clin North Am. 33(1):135-51, 2019
2. Yoshida A et al: Paragonimus and paragonimiasis in Asia: an update. Acta Trop. 199:105074, 2019
3. Biswas A et al: Human pulmonary dirofilariasis presenting as a solitary pulmonary nodule: a case report and a brief review of literature. Respir Med Case Rep. 10:40-2, 2013

Paragonimus Eggs

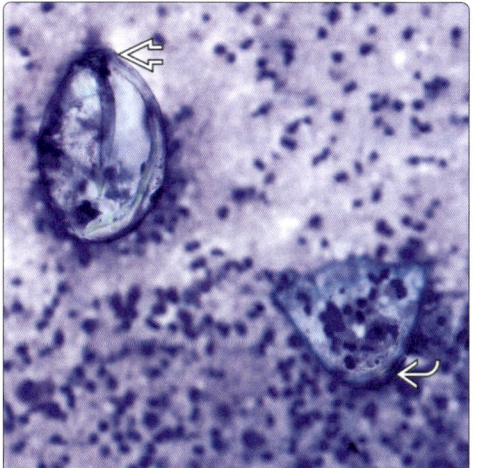

Paragonimus in Histology

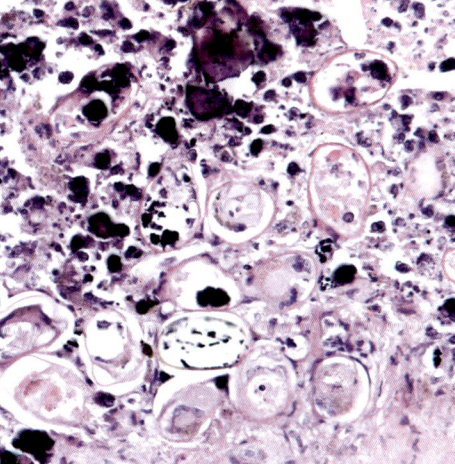

(Left) *Two eggs of the fluke Paragonimus westermani can be seen here in an inflammatory background. Note the thick, yellow-brown shell ➡ with a shouldered operculum ➡.* **(Right)** *A granulomatous response to Paragonimus eggs, shown here in a section stained with H&E, may also present as a mass. (Courtesy C. Moran, MD.)*

Viral Infections (Cytomegalovirus, Herpesvirus, and Others)

KEY FACTS

ETIOLOGY/PATHOGENESIS

- Reproduce within cells, causing injury to pulmonary tissues
- Frequently associated with immunosuppression that allows virus to flourish
- Many common lung viruses, including influenza, parainfluenza, rhinovirus, and coronavirus, do not have distinctive cytologic findings

CLINICAL ISSUES

- Presents as bronchitis or pneumonia
- Acyclovir, ganciclovir, and related medications may be useful
- To degree possible, reversal of drug-related immunosuppression may also lead to improvement

CYTOPATHOLOGY

- Common lung viruses with identifiable cytopathic effect include cytomegalovirus (CMV) and herpesvirus
  - CMV produces nuclear enlargement with prominent intranuclear inclusion and marginated chromatin
  - Herpesvirus shows triad of multinucleation, margination, and molding
- Other viruses that may involve lung and be identified by cytology include adenovirus, respiratory syncytial virus, and measles
  - Consider other viruses when nuclear enlargement and homogenization are seen without typical CMV or herpes features

ANCILLARY TESTS

- CMV, herpesvirus, and adenovirus have specific immunohistochemical stains
- PCR and serology are alternate methods of detection that may be faster and more sensitive

TOP DIFFERENTIAL DIAGNOSES

- Nuclear changes due to inflammation or cytotoxic therapy may mimic viral cytopathic effect

Cytomegalovirus "Owl's Eye" Inclusion
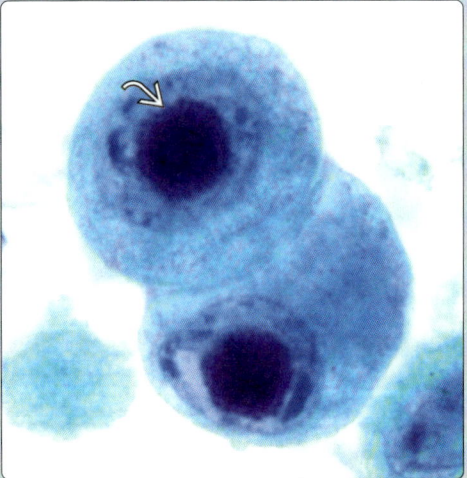

Cytomegalovirus Red Nuclear Inclusion
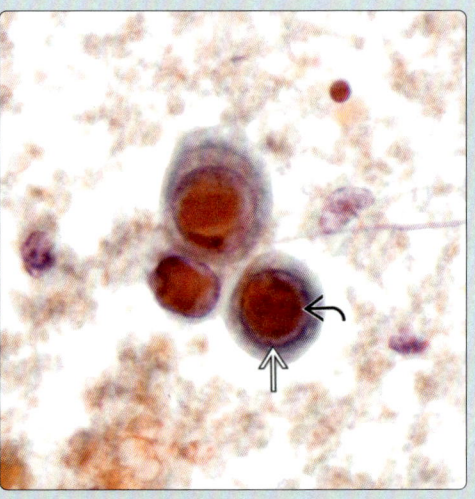

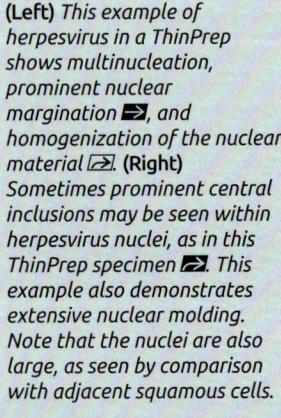

(Left) This example of cytomegalovirus (CMV) from a bronchoalveolar lavage ThinPrep demonstrates the classic "owl's eye" inclusion ➔ within an enlarged nucleus. *(Right)* CMV infection produces classic Cowdry type A nuclear inclusions within a markedly enlarged nucleus ➔. This Pap-stained example has a prominent red inclusion. Peripheral chromatin clumping is also apparent ➔.

Herpesvirus Nuclear Features
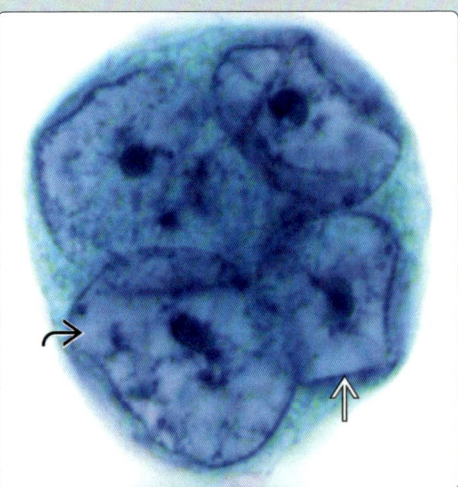

Herpesvirus Nuclear Inclusions
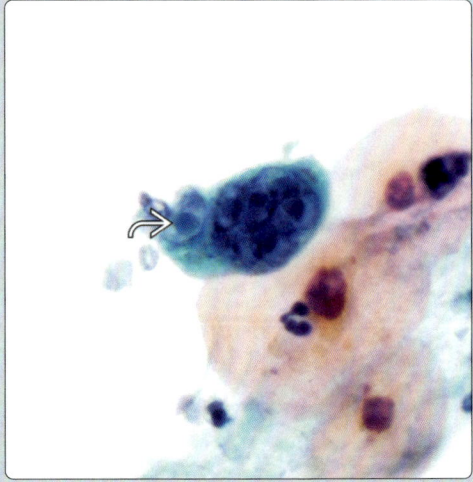

(Left) This example of herpesvirus in a ThinPrep shows multinucleation, prominent nuclear margination ➔, and homogenization of the nuclear material ➔. *(Right)* Sometimes prominent central inclusions may be seen within herpesvirus nuclei, as in this ThinPrep specimen ➔. This example also demonstrates extensive nuclear molding. Note that the nuclei are also large, as seen by comparison with adjacent squamous cells.

Viral Infections (Cytomegalovirus, Herpesvirus, and Others)

ETIOLOGY/PATHOGENESIS

Viral Pathogens
- Frequently associated with immunosuppression that allows virus to flourish
- Cytomegalovirus (CMV) and herpes simplex virus, and related DNA viruses of herpesvirus family, are most commonly identified viruses in lung cytology specimens
- Other viruses that may involve lung, and be identified by cytology include adenovirus, respiratory syncytial virus, and measles virus
- Many common lung viruses, including influenza, parainfluenza, rhinovirus, and coronavirus (including COVID-19), do not have distinctive cytologic findings

CLINICAL ISSUES

Presentation
- Bronchitis or pneumonia

Treatment
- Acyclovir, ganciclovir, and related antiviral medications
- Reversal of immunosuppression to some degree possible

Prognosis
- Outcomes depend on extent of infection and severity of comorbid conditions

CYTOPATHOLOGY

Background
- Increased inflammation and necrotic debris may be noticeable

Cells
- Viral cytopathic effect may be seen in bronchial cells, pneumocytes, or giant cells

Nuclear Details
- CMV produces nuclear enlargement with prominent intranuclear inclusion and marginated chromatin (Cowdry type A body); can also have fine, granular cytoplasmic inclusions
- Herpesvirus (simplex and zoster) has homogenized nuclei that may also contain central inclusion and shows triad of multinucleation, margination, and molding
- Adenovirus produces nuclear enlargement and may have either multiple small inclusions in early stages, or single large inclusion with nuclear margination when fully developed
- Measles virus produces red inclusions in nucleus and cytoplasm

Cytoplasmic Details
- Measles virus and respiratory syncytial virus are associated with cytoplasmic inclusions in giant cells

ANCILLARY TESTS

Immunohistochemistry
- CMV, herpesvirus, and adenovirus have specific immunohistochemical stains

Laboratory Testing
- Cultures, PCR, and serology

DIFFERENTIAL DIAGNOSIS

Reactive Changes
- Nuclear changes due to inflammation or cytotoxic therapy may mimic viral cytopathic effect

DIAGNOSTIC CHECKLIST

Pathologic Interpretation Pearls
- Viral cytopathic effects may have overlapping morphology, especially if only few cells are seen
- Viruses in lung are similar in appearance to same viruses seen in other parts of body

SELECTED REFERENCES
1. Moniz P et al: SARS-CoV-2 and cytomegalovirus co-infections-a case series of critically ill patients. J Clin Med. 10(13):2792, 2021
2. Schildermans J et al: Cytomegalovirus: a troll in the ICU? Overview of the literature and perspectives for the future. Front Med (Lausanne). 7:188, 2020

Adenovirus With Subtle Inclusions

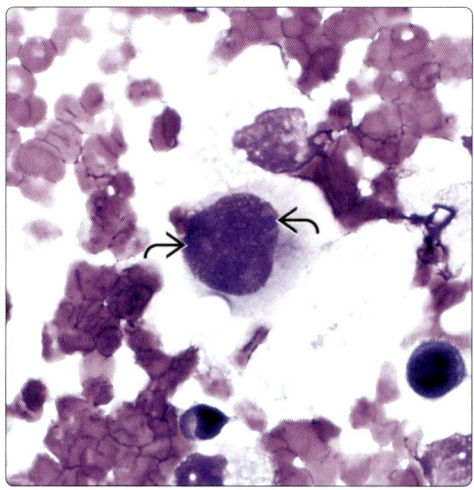

Cytomegalovirus With Blue Inclusion

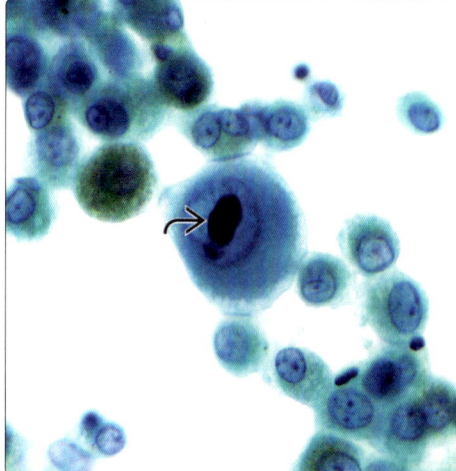

(Left) Some viral changes may be subtle, such as these small intranuclear inclusions ➡ seen on Diff-Quik in a case of adenovirus later confirmed by viral culture. **(Right)** In some instances, such as in this ThinPrep containing CMV, the inclusion ➡ may not stain red, but nuclear enlargement and homogenization aid recognition.

Mycobacteria and Other Bacterial Infections

KEY FACTS

CLINICAL ISSUES
- *Mycobacterium tuberculosis* presents as granulomas
- Nontuberculous mycobacteria (NTM) are most often members of *Mycobacterium avium* complex (MAC) and present as cavitary or nodular/bronchiectatic disease, usually in setting of immune deficiency
- Uncommon bacteria, including *Nocardia* and *Rhodococcus*, may also present in manner similar to NTM, especially in immunocompromised patients
- Other, more common bacteria typically present with pneumonia

CYTOPATHOLOGY
- Necrotic debris is present in many bacterial infections
- Granulomatous inflammation is characterized by epithelioid histiocytes and giant cells
- Acute inflammation manifests as numerous neutrophils
- Reactive bronchial cells &/or type II pneumocytes are frequently present
- Histiocytes have round, bean-shaped, or twisted nuclei with dispersed chromatin
- Histiocytic aggregates form syncytium without clear cytoplasmic borders

ANCILLARY TESTS
- Acid-fast stains enhance detection of mycobacterial organisms but low sensitivity compared with molecular methods or culture

TOP DIFFERENTIAL DIAGNOSES
- Other infections
- Other noninfectious granulomas
  - Sarcoidosis, rheumatoid nodules, and foreign body reactions may look similar to tuberculosis
- Malignancy
  - Reactive cells, epithelioid histiocytes, and necrotic debris may raise concern for malignancy
- Oral contaminant

Necrotizing Granuloma

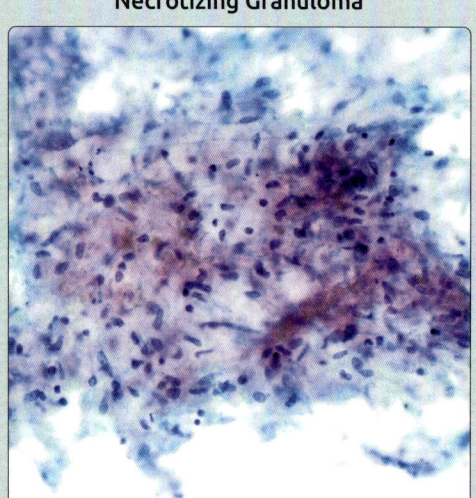

Giant Cells

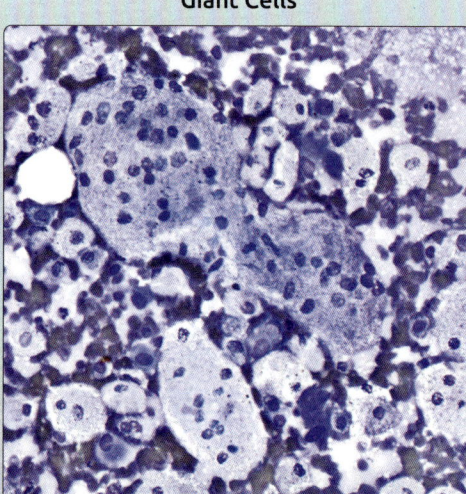

(Left) Pap stain of a necrotizing granuloma shows epithelioid histiocytes with elongated nuclei and fibrillary syncytial cytoplasm that can be seen with clinging necrotic debris. (Right) Giant cells are readily recognizable elements of a specimen from a tuberculous granuloma, such as those seen on this Diff-Quik stain, but they are not specific.

Positive Acid-Fast Stain

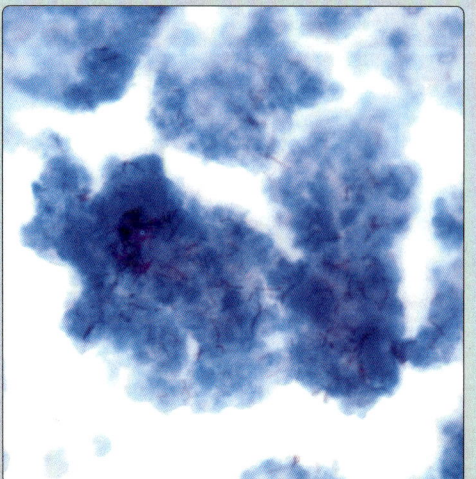

Acid-Fast Bacilli

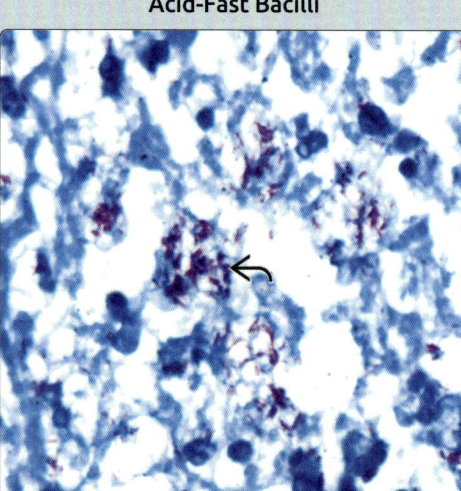

(Left) Kinyoun acid-fast stain of a bronchoalveolar lavage cytospin from a patient with cavitary pneumonia shows numerous rod-like organisms that are staining red. Mycobacterium tuberculosis was confirmed by a PCR test from the same sample. (Right) Numerous small red rods ⮕ diagnostic of mycobacterial infection are seen in this Fite acid-fast stain of a pulmonary granuloma.

Mycobacteria and Other Bacterial Infections

CLINICAL ISSUES

Presentation
- *Mycobacterium tuberculosis* presents as granulomas
  - May be localized or disseminated (miliary)
  - Mediastinal node involvement is often present, and there may be broader systemic involvement, especially in immunocompromised patients
- Nontuberculous mycobacteria (NTM) are most often members of *Mycobacterium avium* complex (MAC)
  - May present as cavitary or nodular/bronchiectatic disease, usually in setting of immune deficiency
  - Some NTM organisms may cause hypersensitivity reaction rather than infection
- Uncommon bacteria, including *Nocardia* and *Rhodococcus*, may also present in manner similar to NTM, especially in immunocompromised patients
- Other, more common bacteria typically present with pneumonia

CYTOPATHOLOGY

Cells
- Granulomatous inflammation is characterized by epithelioid histiocytes and giant cells
- Acute inflammation manifests as numerous neutrophils
- Reactive bronchial cells &/or type II pneumocytes are frequently present

Nuclear Details
- Histiocytes have round, bean-shaped, or twisted nuclei with dispersed chromatin

Cytoplasmic Details
- Histiocytic aggregates form syncytium without clear cytoplasmic borders

ANCILLARY TESTS

Acid-Fast Stains
- Routinely performed to enhance detection of mycobacterial organisms but low sensitivity

Other Microscopy Techniques
- Fluorescent or light-emitting diode microscopy can increase sensitivity for mycobacteria relative to acid-fast staining

Nonmicroscopic Techniques
- Sensitive, rapid, and easy-to-use techniques are needed to facilitate diagnosis in low-resource countries
- Molecular and immunologic detection kits for tuberculosis are commercially available but still suboptimal
  - Many new technologies are being developed
- Screening in HIV(+) or otherwise immune-suppressed people and in children is especially problematic

DIFFERENTIAL DIAGNOSIS

Other Infections
- Bacterial infections have similar cytologic features to many viral, fungal, and parasitic infections

Other Noninfectious Granulomas
- Sarcoidosis, rheumatoid nodules, and foreign body reactions may look similar to tuberculosis

Malignancy
- Reactive cells, epithelioid histiocytes, and necrotic debris may raise concern for malignancy

Oral Contaminant
- Most bacteria seen in lung specimens are oral contaminants with no clinical significance

DIAGNOSTIC CHECKLIST

Pathologic Interpretation Pearls
- Only small fraction of granulomas are due to tuberculosis
- Acid-fast staining is frequently negative in culture-positive mycobacterial disease

SELECTED REFERENCES

1. MacGregor-Fairlie M et al: Tuberculosis diagnostics: overcoming ancient challenges with modern solutions. Emerg Top Life Sci. 4(4):423-36, 2020
2. McHugh KE et al: The cytopathology of Actinomyces, Nocardia, and their mimickers. Diagn Cytopathol. 45(12):1105-15, 2017

Nocardia

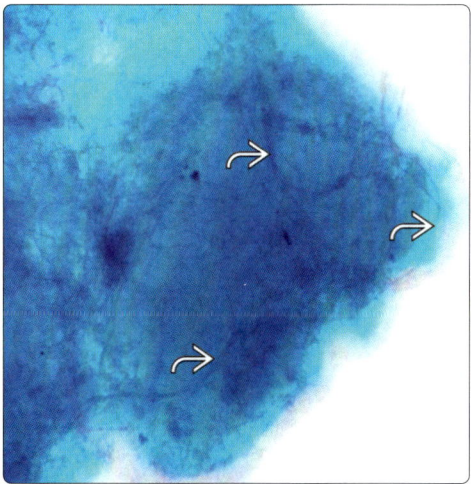

Oral Bacterial Contaminants

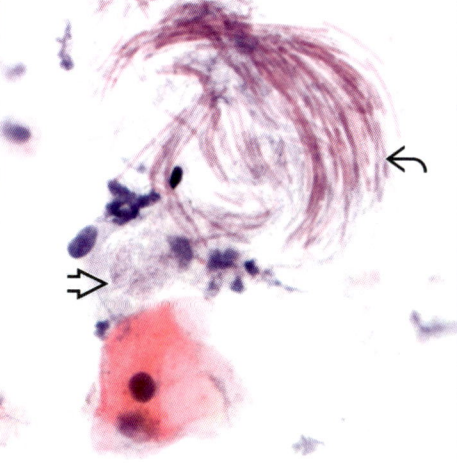

(Left) *ThinPrep bronchial brush specimen contains necrotic debris associated with filamentous Nocardia organisms ➡. (Right) Numerous bacterial rods ➡ as well as bacterial cocci ➡ can be seen adjacent to a squamous cell in this Pap-stained bronchial washing. These findings are consistent with oral origin.*

Sarcoidosis and Other Immune-Related Conditions

KEY FACTS

CLINICAL ISSUES
- Sarcoidosis is idiopathic granulomatous disease often involving lung and mediastinum
- Rheumatoid nodules may form in lung or pleura
- Eosinophilic pneumonia is diagnosed by presence of markedly increased eosinophils in right clinical setting
- Lung manifestations often reflect only 1 aspect of systemic disease

CYTOPATHOLOGY
- Multinucleated giant cells and epithelioid histiocyte aggregates are typical of sarcoidosis
  - Necrotic debris usually rare or absent
- Rheumatoid nodules may shed abundant necrotic debris, histiocytes, and giant cells
  - Histiocytes may have nuclear atypia or keratin-like orangophilic staining, raising concern for malignancy
- Eosinophilic pneumonia shows predominance of eosinophils and may have Charcot-Leyden crystals
- Giant cells may contain asteroid bodies, Schaumann bodies (lamellated calcifications around calcium oxalate), or Hamazaki-Wesenberg bodies (fungus-like giant lysosomes)
  - None of these are specific for sarcoidosis

ANCILLARY TESTS
- Fungal and mycobacterial stains to rule out organisms are essential in granulomatous diseases
- Serum angiotensin-converting enzyme level elevations support diagnosis of sarcoidosis

TOP DIFFERENTIAL DIAGNOSES
- Granulomatous inflammation due to infectious etiologies
- Other granulomatous responses, including foreign body reaction and response to tumors
- Clinical concern for malignancy often arises in context of sarcoidosis due to enlarged mediastinal nodes with high PET values
- Necrotic debris and bizarre cells in rheumatoid nodules may simulate malignancy

Granulomatous Inflammation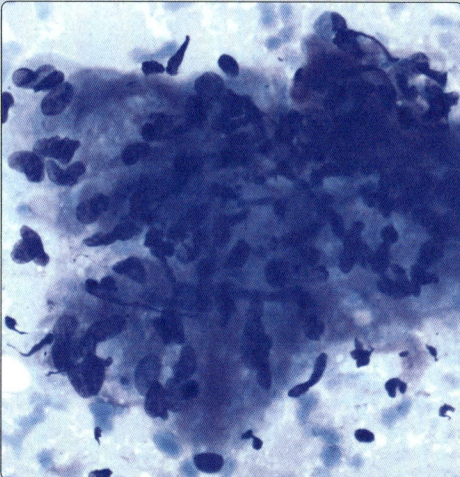

Giant Cell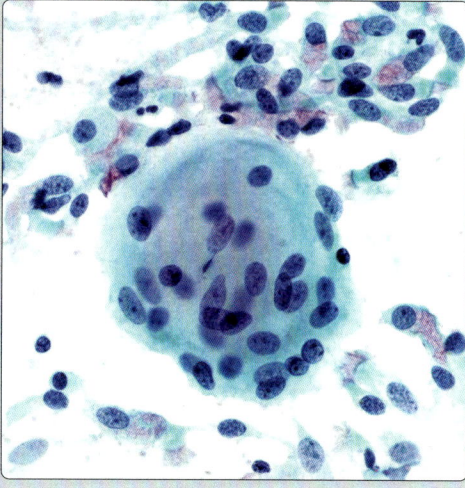

(Left) Aggregates of epithelioid histiocytes, seen here on a Diff-Quik stain, help to identify granulomatous inflammation. The lack of necrosis is compatible with the diagnosis of sarcoidosis. (Right) The possibility of sarcoidosis may be suggested only by the presence of occasional giant cells, seen here in a Pap-stained bronchial brushing.

Asteroid Body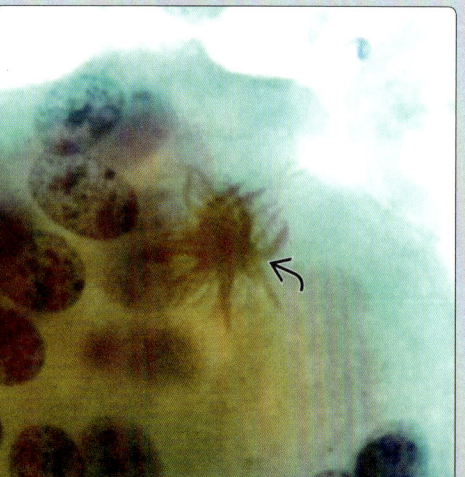

Nonnecrotizing Granulomas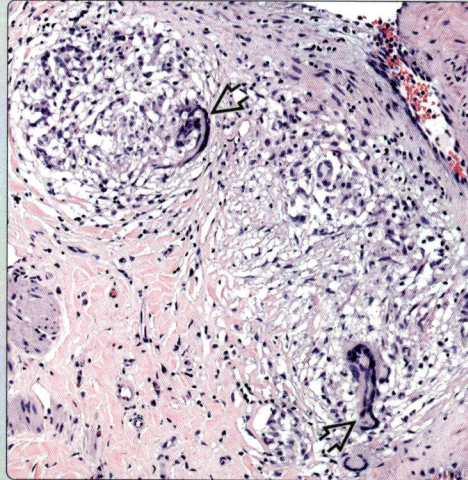

(Left) Inclusions within giant cells, such as the asteroid body ⇨ seen on this Pap stain, are common in sarcoidosis but not specific. These should not be confused with an organism or foreign material. (Right) H&E-stained histology section from a lung biopsy demonstrates the small, nonnecrotizing granulomas typical of sarcoidosis. Note also the associated giant cells ⇨.

Sarcoidosis and Other Immune-Related Conditions

CLINICAL ISSUES

Sarcoidosis
- Granulomatous disease of unknown etiology most often involving lung and mediastinum
- Diagnosis of exclusion requiring elimination of known infectious and other causes of granuloma formation
- Elevated angiotensin-converting enzyme levels in serum may aid diagnosis
- Sarcoid-like reaction to tumors, including lung carcinomas, may occur

Other Immune-Related Inflammatory Conditions
- Rheumatoid nodules may form in pleura or less commonly in lung parenchyma
  - Rheumatoid arthritis may also produce lung fibrosis
- Eosinophilic pneumonia is diagnosed by presence of markedly increased eosinophils in lavage specimens
  - May be acute, chronic, associated with vasculitis (Churg-Strauss disease) or secondary reaction
- Other immune-related diseases, such as hypersensitivity pneumonitis, Wegener granulomatosis, and Rosai-Dorfman disease, may involve lung but are very difficult to identify cytologically

CYTOPATHOLOGY

Cellularity
- Immune-related diseases often have increased cellularity due to inflammatory cells

Background
- Sarcoidosis usually does not have significant necrotic debris
- Necrotic debris is seen in many immune-related diseases, notably rheumatoid nodules

Cells
- Multinucleated giant cells and epithelioid histiocyte aggregates are typical of sarcoidosis
- Rheumatoid nodules also contain histiocytes and giant cells
- Numerous eosinophils characterize eosinophilic pneumonia

Nuclear Details
- Epithelioid histiocytes have elongated irregular nuclei with indistinct nucleoli
  - Hyperchromasia may be present

Cytoplasmic Details
- Giant cells may contain asteroid bodies, Schaumann bodies (lamellated calcifications around calcium oxalate), or Hamazaki-Wesenberg bodies (fungus-like giant lysosomes)
  - None of these are specific for sarcoidosis
- Epithelioid histiocytes may have degenerative orangeophilia of cytoplasm mimicking keratinization
  - This change is especially prevalent in rheumatoid nodules

DIFFERENTIAL DIAGNOSIS

Granulomatous Inflammation Due to Infectious Etiologies
- Fungal and mycobacterial stains &/or cultures or PCR are needed to rule out organisms

Other Granulomatous Responses
- Foreign bodies and tumors may incite giant cell reactions

Malignancy
- Sarcoidosis often produces enlarged mediastinal nodes with high PET values
- Necrotic debris and bizarre cells in rheumatoid nodules may simulate malignancy

DIAGNOSTIC CHECKLIST

Pathologic Interpretation Pearls
- Giant cells are primary cytologic manifestation of sarcoidosis but are not specific
- Marked increases in eosinophils may indicate eosinophilic pneumonia

SELECTED REFERENCES
1. Scano V et al: Role of EBUS-TBNA in non-neoplastic mediastinal lymphadenopathy: review of literature. Diagnostics (Basel). 12(2), 2022

Rheumatoid Nodule Debris and Histiocytes

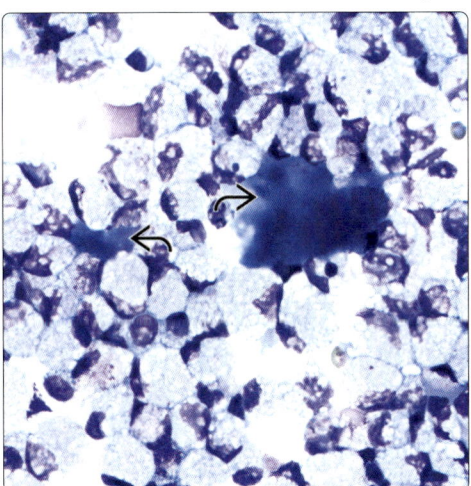

"Atypia" in Epithelioid Histiocyte

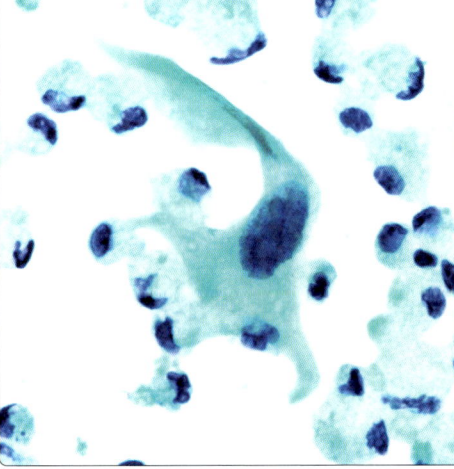

(Left) Rheumatoid nodules contain abundant amorphous debris ➔, such as the material seen here on Diff-Quik stain. Histiocytes, seen here with abundant vacuolated cytoplasm, are numerous and compose most of the cells in the specimen. **(Right)** Bizarre epithelioid histiocytes, such as the markedly enlarged cell with irregular cytoplasmic extensions seen here on Pap stain, may raise concern for malignancy in rheumatoid nodules.

Pulmonary Alveolar Proteinosis and Mimics

KEY FACTS

CLINICAL ISSUES
- Respiratory distress due to alveoli filled with proteinaceous material secondary to macrophage dysfunction or surfactant excess
- Usually autoimmune but also seen in association with immunosuppression, hematologic malignancies, inhalational exposures, congenital syndromes
- Bronchoalveolar lavage is treatment modality

IMAGING
- CT finding of crazy-paving patten with ground-glass opacities and thickened septa is distinctive

CYTOPATHOLOGY
- Globular homogeneous structures
- Abundant proteinaceous material in background
- Alveolar macrophages also contain proteinaceous debris in cytoplasmic vacuoles

MACROSCOPIC
- Lavage fluid is milky and settles into layers

ANCILLARY TESTS
- PAS-D
- Serum testing for GM-CSF autoantibody

TOP DIFFERENTIAL DIAGNOSES
- *Pneumocystis* pneumonia
  - "Foamy" alveolar casts with GMS-positive organisms
- Necrosis
  - Debris without distinct globules, associated with inflammatory or malignant cells
- Corpora amylacea
  - Usually few in number, weakly polarizable glycoprotein globules
- Amyloid
- Amiodarone toxicity

Globules and Granular Debris
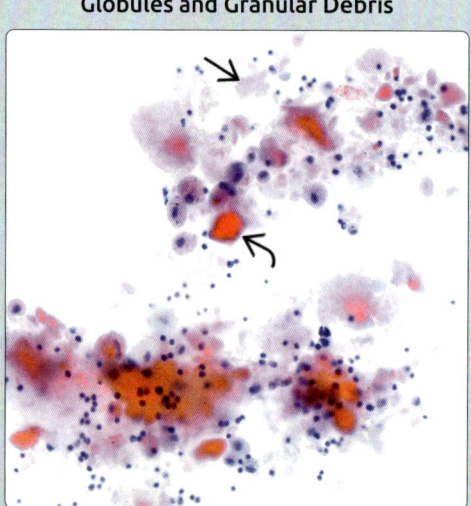

Globule Morphology
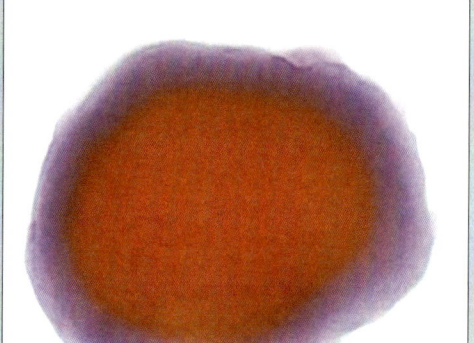

(Left) This Pap-stained lavage of pulmonary alveolar proteinosis contains characteristic large globules ⇒ and granular debris ➡. The globules are more specific and are the key to diagnosis. **(Right)** High-power examination of a globule shows typical 2-tone differential staining of the outer portion and core on Pap stain. The homogeneity of the material differentiates these globules from alveolar casts of Pneumocystis.

Cracking Artifact
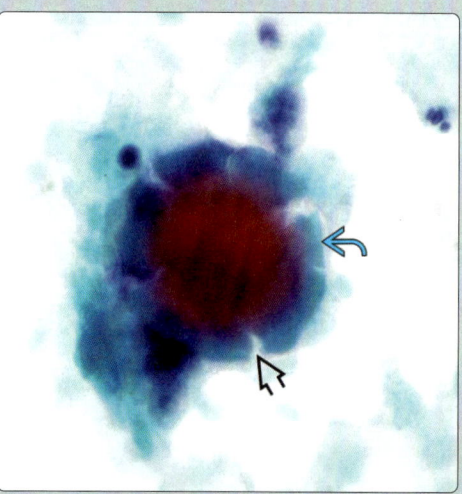

PAS Staining
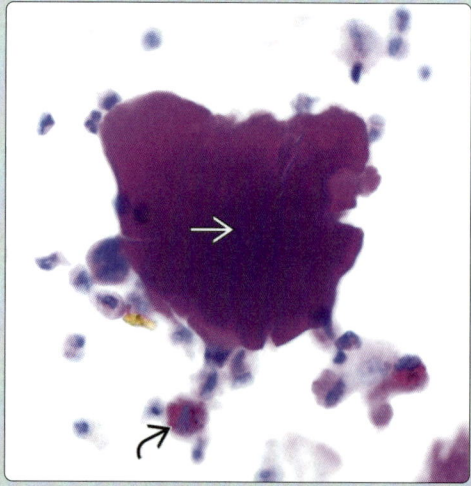

(Left) Another example of a globule from a ThinPrep specimen has sharply defined borders ⇒ and prominent "cracking" artifact ⇒ around the periphery due to alcohol fixation that homogenizes the proteinaceous material. **(Right)** PAS staining is strongly positive in the globules ➡, aiding in confirmation of the diagnosis. Also note the PAS-positive granules present within macrophages ⇒.

Pulmonary Alveolar Proteinosis and Mimics

TERMINOLOGY

Abbreviations
- Pulmonary alveolar proteinosis (PAP)

Definitions
- Nonneoplastic condition in which alveoli are filled with proteinaceous material

ETIOLOGY/PATHOGENESIS

Etiology
- Result of macrophage dysfunction or surfactant excess
- Usually autoimmune, due to formation of GM-CSF antibodies
- Can also be seen in association with immunosuppression, hematologic malignancies, inhalational exposures, rare congenital syndromes

CLINICAL ISSUES

Treatment
- Bronchoalveolar lavage
- Immune modulation with GM-CSF administration or rituximab

IMAGING

General Features
- CT finding of crazy-paving patten with ground-glass opacities and thickened septa is distinctive

CYTOPATHOLOGY

Background
- Proteinaceous material
  - Globular homogeneous structures
    - Alcohol fixation enhances this appearance
  - Scattered granular debris

Cells
- Alveolar macrophages also contain proteinaceous debris

MICROSCOPIC

Histologic Features
- Alveolar filling by granular proteinaceous material with preservation of alveolar architecture

DIFFERENTIAL DIAGNOSIS

Pneumocystis Pneumonia
- *Pneumocystis* casts have foamy appearance
- GMS-positive organisms

Necrosis
- No distinct globules; inflammatory or tumor cells

Corpora Amylacea
- Glycoprotein globules with faint concentric rings, positive for PAS, weakly polarizable, usually few in number

Amyloid
- Rarely forms distinct globules, positive for Congo red birefringence

Amiodarone Toxicity
- Lamellated inclusions in macrophages, lacks globules

DIAGNOSTIC CHECKLIST

Clinically Relevant Pathologic Features
- Gross appearance
  - Lavage fluid is milky
  - Settles into layers

Pathologic Interpretation Pearls
- PAS staining is diastase resistant and will highlight proteinaceous material

SELECTED REFERENCES
1. Jouneau S et al: Pulmonary alveolar proteinosis. Respirology. 25(8):816-26, 2020
2. Trapnell BC et al: Pulmonary alveolar proteinosis. Nat Rev Dis Primers. 5(1):16, 2019

Granular Debris
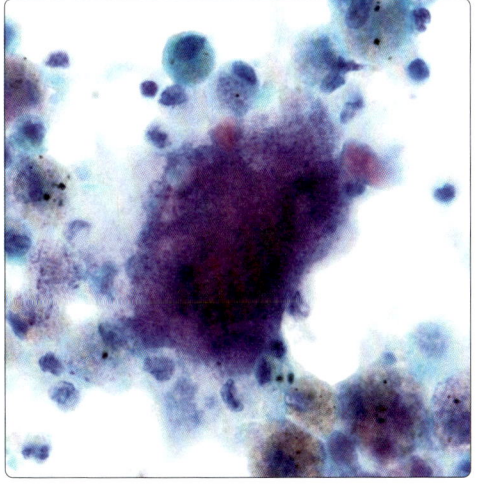

Stain Resistance in Globules
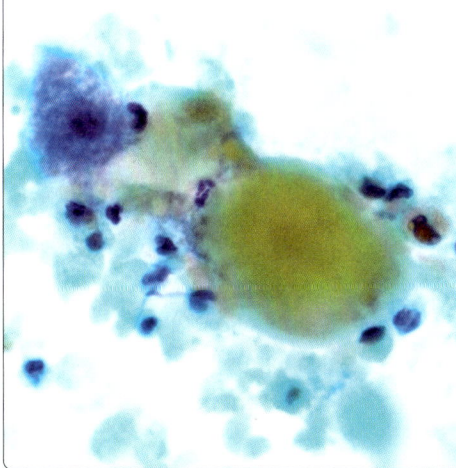

(Left) Granular proteinaceous debris, as seen in this Pap stain, is difficult to distinguish from necrotic debris and the alveolar casts of *Pneumocystis*. **(Right)** In some instances, the proteinaceous globules are resistant to Pap staining and may take on unusual colorations, such as this yellow hue.

Miscellaneous Findings, Including Contaminants

KEY FACTS

CLINICAL ISSUES

- Ferruginous bodies result from macrophage responses to indigestible inhaled foreign materials, including asbestos, silicates, carbon, or iron oxides
  - Large numbers of ferruginous bodies may be associated with pulmonary fibrosis, mesothelioma, or lung adenocarcinoma
- Aspiration pneumonia may be associated with plant matter, skeletal muscle, or lipid-laden macrophages
- Hemosiderin-laden macrophages are indicative of previous pulmonary hemorrhage and are common in lung transplant setting
- Charcot-Leyden crystals indicate marked elevation of eosinophils, such as in eosinophilic pneumonia

CYTOPATHOLOGY

- Asbestos bodies consist of iron-containing minerals surrounding asbestos fibers produced by macrophages
- Vegetable matter is distinguished from human cells and pathogens by refractile cell walls
- Lipid-laden macrophages have prominent vacuoles containing lipid material
- Hemosiderin-laden macrophages retain byproducts of hemoglobin metabolism within cytoplasm
- Ferruginous bodies and corpora amylacea are often surrounded by macrophages
- Charcot-Leyden crystals are associated with eosinophils
- Curschmann spirals result from inspissated mucus

TOP DIFFERENTIAL DIAGNOSES

- Asbestos body vs. pseudoasbestos ferruginous body
- Vegetable matter vs. pathogens
  - Plant fragments, pollen, or seeds may mimic fungal structures, parasites, or their eggs
- Vegetable matter vs. malignancy
  - Plant cells may raise concern for malignancy due to odd shapes, molding, or keratin-like orangeophilia

Asbestos Body

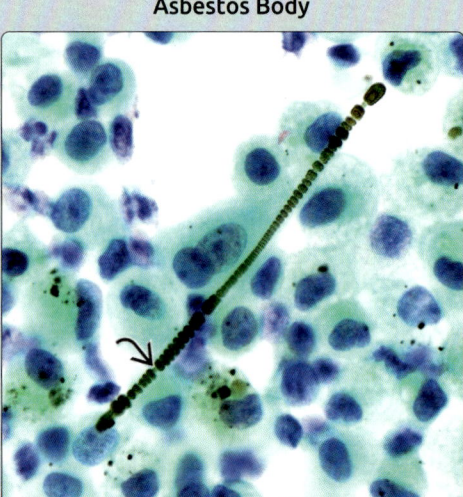

Plant Matter

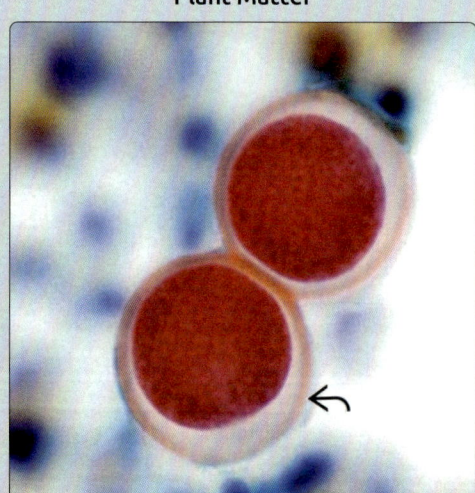

(Left) Asbestos bodies often show a beaded pattern with the clear asbestos fiber ➡ visible between mineral deposits. The color derives from iron, not the Pap stain. (Right) Plant matter shows distinctive refractile cell walls ➡ that do not take up Pap stain well. Aspiration or contamination can result in the presence of plant cells. Such cells can be confused with fungi, parasites, or even malignancy.

Lipid Vacuoles in Macrophages

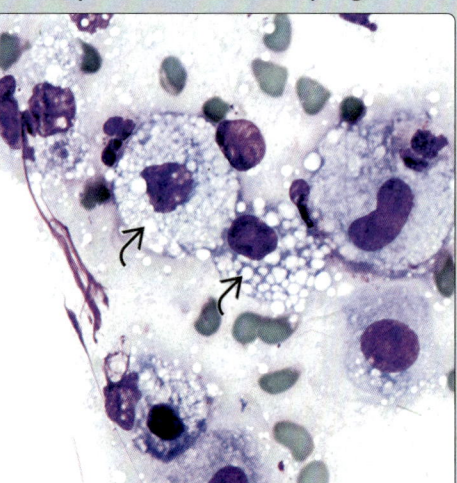

Hemosiderin-Laden Macrophages

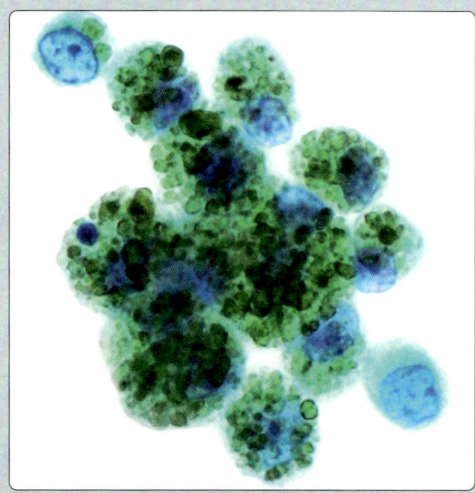

(Left) Macrophage cytoplasmic lipid vacuoles ➡ that are resistant to stains, including Diff-Quik, raise the possibility of a lipoid pneumonia. (Right) Large, coarse hemosiderin granules within macrophages are indicative of previous hemorrhage, as seen here in a ThinPrep. This finding is common in lung transplant patients due to bleeding before, during, or after the surgery.

Miscellaneous Findings, Including Contaminants

ETIOLOGY/PATHOGENESIS

Sources of Miscellaneous Findings
- These findings derive from exogenous materials (ferruginous bodies and aspirated plant matter), secretions (Curshmann spirals and corpora amylacea), inflammatory responses (lipid-laden and hemosiderin-laden macrophages and Charcot-Leyden crystals), and calcifications (microliths and psammoma bodies)

CLINICAL ISSUES

Ferruginous Body Exposures
- Ferruginous bodies result from macrophage responses to inhaled foreign materials
  - Asbestos bodies contain slender, colorless amphibole filament
  - Pseudoasbestos bodies may contain silicates, carbon, iron oxide, or other inhaled materials attributable to occupational exposure

Aspiration Pneumonia
- Food particles, including vegetable matter and skeletal muscle, may enter lung and induce acute inflammation and foreign body response

CYTOPATHOLOGY

Cells
- Ferruginous bodies and corpora amylacea are often surrounded by macrophages
- Charcot-Leyden crystals are associated with eosinophils

Cytoplasmic Details
- Lipid-laden macrophages will have increased cytoplasmic volume due to prominent vacuoles containing phagocytosed lipid material
- Hemosiderin-laden macrophages retain crystalline byproducts of hemoglobin metabolism within cytoplasm

MICROSCOPIC

Histologic Features
- Asbestos bodies may be associated with interstitial fibrosis

ANCILLARY TESTS

Identification of Asbestos Bodies
- Electron microscopy or x-ray diffraction analysis may be used as more precise method

DIFFERENTIAL DIAGNOSIS

Asbestos Bodies vs. Pseudoasbestos Bodies
- Careful examination of core material of ferruginous bodies is key to differentiating causes

Vegetable Matter vs. Pathogens
- Plant fragments, pollen, or seeds may mimic fungal structures, parasites, or their eggs

Vegetable Matter vs. Malignancy
- Plant cells may raise concern for malignancy due to odd shapes, molding, or keratin-like orangeophilia

SELECTED REFERENCES

1. Torous VF et al: Correlation between cytology Oil Red O staining and lung biopsy specimens: utility of the lipid-laden macrophage index. J Am Soc Cytopathol. 11(4):226-33, 2022
2. Abramson MJ et al: Occupational and environmental risk factors for idiopathic pulmonary fibrosis in Australia: case-control study. Thorax. 75(10):864-9, 2020
3. Walters GI: Occupational exposures and idiopathic pulmonary fibrosis. Curr Opin Allergy Clin Immunol. 20(2):103-11, 2020

Miscellaneous Findings in Lung Cytology and Their Significance

Finding	Description	Clinical Significance
Ferruginous body	Elongated concretion of iron, silica, and magnesium around foreign body, especially asbestos	In large numbers, indicates risk for asbestosis, mesothelioma, and lung carcinoma
Food particles	Vegetable matter with refractile cell walls and delicate internal structures, fragments of skeletal muscle	May indicate aspiration pneumonia but is often oral contaminant
Curschmann spiral	Spiral-shaped aggregates of mucus similar to overwound rope	Usually none, may be more frequent in association with mucus excess, such as in asthma
Charcot-Leyden crystals	Elongated diamond-shaped crystals formed from lysophospholipase of eosinophils	Indicates numerous activated eosinophils, such as in eosinophilic pneumonia
Corpora amylacea	Round, lamellated aggregates of glycoproteins with radial striations, lacking calcification	Incidental finding with no specific clinical significance
Microliths	Small calcified bodies with lamellations and radial striations	Rare autosomal recessive syndrome of pulmonary alveolar microlithiasis
Psammoma bodies	Lamellated calcifications, often associated with cells around periphery	Formed by malignancies, including adenocarcinoma with papillary structures
Lipid-laden macrophages	Macrophages with large vacuoles filled with lipid material demonstrable by Oil red O	Indicates lipoid pneumonia associated with aspiration or obstruction
Hemosiderin-laden macrophages	Macrophages containing chunky yellow-brown hemosiderin pigment	Results from pulmonary hemorrhage, frequently prominent in transplanted lungs

Adenocarcinoma

KEY FACTS

CLINICAL ISSUES
- Variable presentation: Incidental "coin" lesion to widespread metastasis
- Curable by surgery if low stage but poor prognosis for most patients

CYTOPATHOLOGY
- Prominent nucleoli are common
- Lepidic pattern carcinomas show nuclear grooves and pseudoinclusions
- Poorly differentiated carcinomas have marked anisonucleosis and pleomorphism
- Intracytoplasmic mucin is diagnostic
  - May be in small vacuoles or single large vacuole
- Abundant foamy cytoplasm is typical

ANCILLARY TESTS
- TTF-1 or napsin A to differentiate from squamous cell carcinoma or metastasis
  - Both are negative in ~ 20% of cases
- Molecular testing for mutation-specific chemotherapy
- PD-L1 for targeted immunotherapy

TOP DIFFERENTIAL DIAGNOSES
- Squamous cell carcinoma
  - If morphology and immunohistochemistry are inconclusive, diagnose as non-small cell carcinoma, not otherwise specified
- Carcinoma in situ and atypical adenomatous hyperplasia
  - Cannot be distinguished from lepidic pattern invasive adenocarcinoma by cytology alone
- Adenocarcinoma of extrathoracic origin
  - Clinical and radiologic correlation in conjunction with immunohistochemistry can resolve many, but not all, difficult cases
- Reactive changes
  - Well-differentiated adenocarcinoma and reactive changes have overlapping morphologic features

(Left) In this Pap stain, the comparison with the adjacent normal bronchial cells highlights the nuclear enlargement, clumpy chromatin, and jumbled architecture that is typically seen in adenocarcinoma. (Right) Adenocarcinoma typically shows moderate to marked nuclear pleomorphism, as seen in this Pap stain. Abundant foamy or vacuolated cytoplasm, as well as prominent nucleoli, are also frequently seen.

Nuclear Enlargement
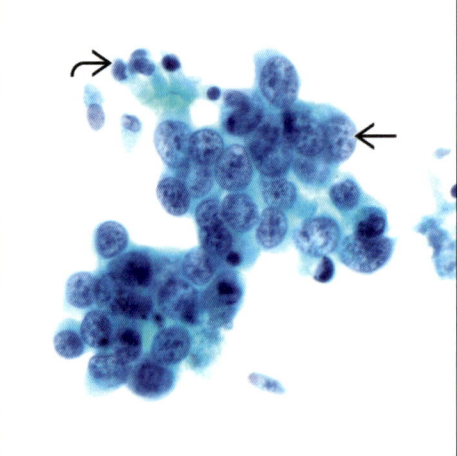

Nuclear Pleomorphism With Nucleoli
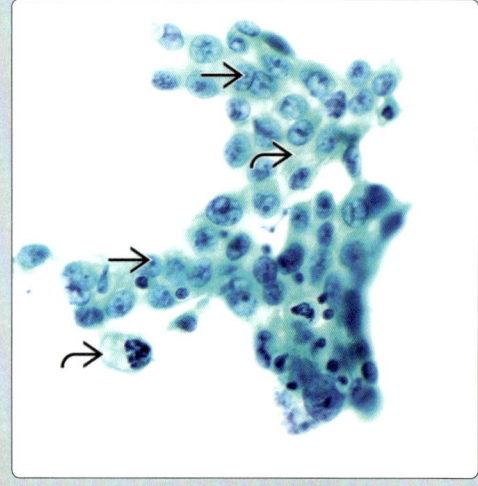

(Left) Two adenocarcinoma cells with markedly enlarged nuclei and cytoplasm relative to adjacent bronchial cells show a prominent vacuole with inspissated mucin and coarse chromatin in this Pap-stained smear. (Right) In some instances of adenocarcinoma, individual malignant cells may be prominent. Cytoplasmic vacuoles, as seen in this Pap stain, may impart a signet-ring appearance.

Marked Atypia
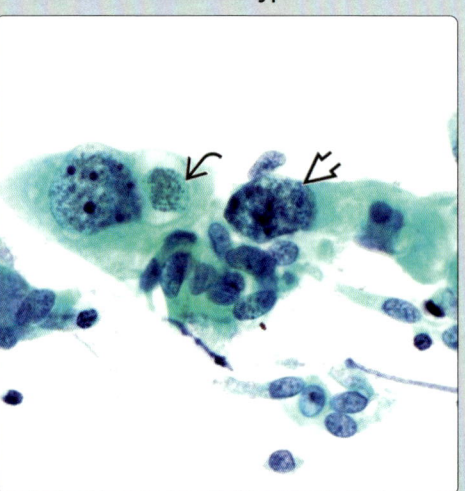

Prominent Individual Malignant Cells
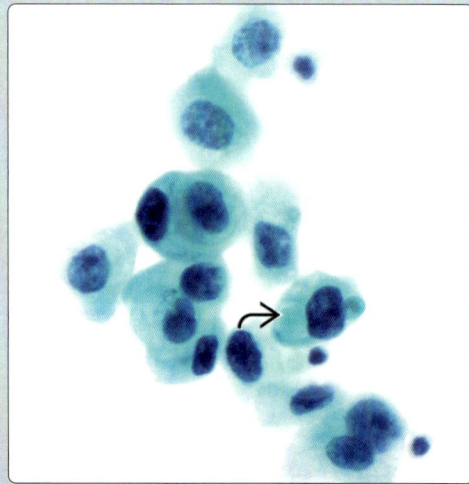

Adenocarcinoma

TERMINOLOGY

Definitions
- Malignant epithelial neoplasm with glandular differentiation

ETIOLOGY/PATHOGENESIS

Etiology
- Tumor probably originates from precursors to bronchial cells and pneumocytes
- Often associated with smoking but to lesser degree than other lung cancers
  - Most lung cancers in young people, and in those who have never smoked, are adenocarcinomas

CLINICAL ISSUES

Epidemiology
- Incidence
  - Lung carcinoma is #1 cause of cancer deaths worldwide (18% of all cancer deaths)
    - #1 cause of cancer death among both men (29%) and women (26%) in USA
    - Accounts for more cases than next 3 leading causes of cancer death (breast, prostate, and colon) combined
  - Adenocarcinoma comprises 1/2 of all lung cancers worldwide with highest percentage in East Asia

Presentation
- Variable: Incidental "coin" lesion to widespread metastasis

Treatment
- Surgical approaches
  - Surgery is indicated for localized tumors with limited metastasis
    - Most tumors present at advanced stage and are inoperable
  - Many patients are excluded because they cannot tolerate lost lung volume due to smoking-related chronic obstructive pulmonary disease
- Adjuvant therapy
  - Chemotherapy, radiation therapy, or both
  - New targeted therapies against *EGFR*, *ALK*, and *ROS1* mutations offer dramatic responses with few side effects, at least in short term

Prognosis
- Curable by surgery if low stage but poor prognosis for most patients

CYTOPATHOLOGY

Cellularity
- High cellularity is typical but may also be seen in some reactive processes

Pattern
- Patterns are highly variable and do not correlate well with histologic patterns in most cases
- Disaggregated signet-ring cells may be seen, rarely exclusively
- Frequent small, round clusters of cells may correspond to micropapillary pattern

Background
- Necrotic debris may be prominent
- Uncommon mucinous, colloid, or enteric adenocarcinomas may have abundant background mucin

Nuclear Details
- Prominent nucleoli are common
- Lepidic pattern adenocarcinomas have uniform nuclei with nuclear grooves and pseudoinclusions
- Poorly differentiated carcinomas have marked anisonucleosis and pleomorphism

Cytoplasmic Details
- Intracytoplasmic mucin is diagnostic
- Abundant foamy cytoplasm with numerous small vacuoles is common
- Cells may show single prominent vacuole, sometimes compressing nucleus into signet-ring shape
- Mucinous tumors have especially abundant apical cytoplasm filled with mucin
- Fetal-type adenocarcinoma has subnuclear glycogen vacuoles; squamoid morules may also be seen

MACROSCOPIC

General Features
- Typically peripheral but may be central

MICROSCOPIC

Histologic Features
- Invasive gland-forming or mucin-producing malignant cells
- Lepidic pattern adenocarcinoma may be mucinous or nonmucinous
  - May be in situ or minimally invasive, but complete histologic sampling is needed for confirmation
- Atypical adenomatous hyperplasia (AAH): Small lesion (< 0.5 cm) with uniformly atypical cells
  - Thought to be adenocarcinoma precursor
  - Rarely sampled by cytology due to small size and lack of symptoms

Predominant Pattern/Injury Type
- Multiple morphologic types are recognized by World Health Organization (WHO)
  - Common types include acinar, solid, and lepidic
  - Less common types include papillary, micropapillary, mucinous, colloid, enteric, and fetal

ANCILLARY TESTS

Immunohistochemistry
- TTF-1
  - Positive in ~ 80% of lung adenocarcinomas
  - Nuclear stain
  - Beware positive TTF-1 in neuroendocrine tumors and metastasis from thyroid or müllerian tract
- Napsin A
  - Also positive in ~ 80% of lung adenocarcinomas
  - Granular cytoplasmic staining
  - May be positive in cases that are TTF-1(-), but usually, both are positive or both are negative
- MOC31, Ber-EP4, mCEA, B72.3

Adenocarcinoma

- Numerous immunohistochemistry stains have been proposed to separate adenocarcinoma from epithelioid mesothelioma
- Not specific for adenocarcinoma of lung origin
- PD-L1
  - Staining used to determine eligibility for targeted immunotherapy
    – Cutoffs vary, but as little as 1% may make patients eligible; report percentage with membranous staining
    – 100 tumor cell minimum has been recommended for valid testing, but this is disputed
  - Limited data suggest that cell blocks are comparable to biopsy material in suitability for analysis, though evaluation of tumor-infiltrating lymphocytes may not be feasible in blocks
  - Distinguishing membranous positivity from nonspecific cytoplasmic staining is more difficult if smears are stained rather than cell blocks

Molecular Testing

- *EGFR* for targeted chemotherapy
  - *EGFR* mutations present in > 30% of adenocarcinomas in East Asians and ≤ 15% in other populations
  - Numerous activating gene mutations must be analyzed
  - Can be done by many different sequencing methods
  - Cell block is preferred, but smears may be used
  - *MET* amplification testing may be requested in patients with acquired resistance to *EGFR*-targeted therapy
- *ALK* for targeted chemotherapy
  - Translocation present in only ~ 4% of adenocarcinomas
  - Translocation involving *EML4* and *ALK*
  - Done by fluorescent in situ hybridization
  - Cell block is preferred, but smears may be used
- *ROS1* for targeted chemotherapy
  - Translocation present in 1-2% of adenocarcinomas
  - Homologous to *ALK*, with similar testing, and susceptible to same targeted agents
- *KRAS*
  - Most common mutation, not currently targetable; often tested because if present other mutations are excluded
  - Therapies under development targeting G12C mutation
- Other less common targetable mutations include *BRAF*, *ERBB2* (HER2), *MET*, *RET*, and *NTRK*
  - Multiplex molecular testing, such as whole-genome analysis, may eventually be needed to identify all relevant mutations in small cytology samples

DIFFERENTIAL DIAGNOSIS

Squamous Cell Carcinoma

- Clear-cut keratinization is diagnostic but often not present
- Immunohistochemistry positive for p40, diffuse p63, or CK5/6 supports squamous differentiation
- Combined adenosquamous carcinoma is rare

Non-Small Cell Carcinoma, Not Otherwise Specified

- Alternate cytology diagnosis for uncommon instances of morphology and immunocytochemistry ambiguous for adenocarcinoma vs. squamous cell carcinoma

Carcinoma In Situ and Atypical Adenomatous Hyperplasia

- Indistinguishable from well-differentiated invasive lepidic pattern adenocarcinoma by cytology

Mesothelioma

- Epithelioid mesothelioma can usually be separated by clinical presentation and immunohistochemistry panels

Salivary Gland-Type Tumors

- Shows characteristic features of salivary gland analogs
- Adenoid cystic carcinoma with basaloid cells and central matrix globules is most common

Pulmonary Blastoma

- Presence of morules and embryonic-type glandular structures

Adenocarcinoma of Extrathoracic Origin

- Immunohistochemistry positive for TTF-1 or napsin A strongly supports lung origin
  - TTF-1 can be positive in neuroendocrine, thyroid, and müllerian tumors
- Lung adenocarcinoma is typically CK7(+) and CK20(-)
  - Breast, pancreas, stomach, and other sources of metastasis may have same pattern
- Enteric adenocarcinomas may be indistinguishable from colorectal carcinoma
  - CK20 and CDX2 may be expressed by enteric adenocarcinoma of lung origin
- Lepidic pattern adenocarcinomas can have nuclear features reminiscent of papillary thyroid carcinoma
  - PAX8 and thyroglobulin can help identify thyroid origin

Reactive Changes

- Well-differentiated adenocarcinoma and reactive changes have overlapping morphologic features

DIAGNOSTIC CHECKLIST

Pathologic Interpretation Pearls

- Adenocarcinoma has highly variable cytologic features
- Common features include marked nuclear pleomorphism, prominent nucleoli, and foamy cytoplasm
- Mucin production is diagnostic
- Well-differentiated carcinomas, especially lepidic pattern, can be very difficult to distinguish from reactive changes
  - Term bronchioloalveolar carcinoma has been eliminated due to inconsistent application
  - Tumors previously characterized as bronchioloalveolar would now be considered lepidic pattern

SELECTED REFERENCES

1. VanderLaan PA et al: The rapidly evolving landscape of biomarker testing in non-small cell lung cancer. Cancer Cytopathol. 129(3):179-81, 2021
2. Roy-Chowdhuri S: Immunocytochemistry of cytology specimens for predictive biomarkers in lung cancer. Transl Lung Cancer Res. 9(3):898-905, 2020
3. Lindeman NI et al: Updated molecular testing guideline for the selection of lung cancer patients for treatment with targeted tyrosine kinase inhibitors: guideline from the College of American Pathologists, the International Association for the Study of Lung Cancer, and the Association for Molecular Pathology. Arch Pathol Lab Med. 142(3):321-46, 2018

Adenocarcinoma

Prominent Mucin Vacuoles

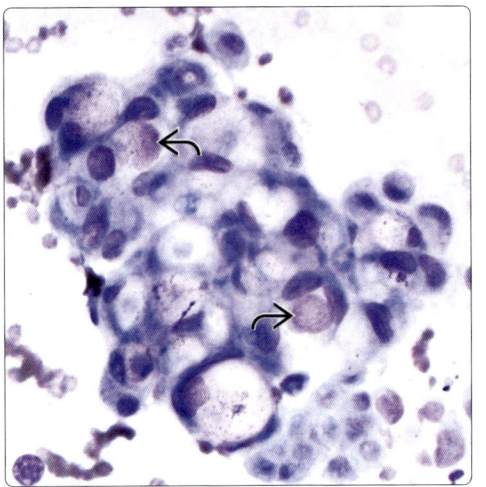

Lepidic Pattern Adenocarcinoma

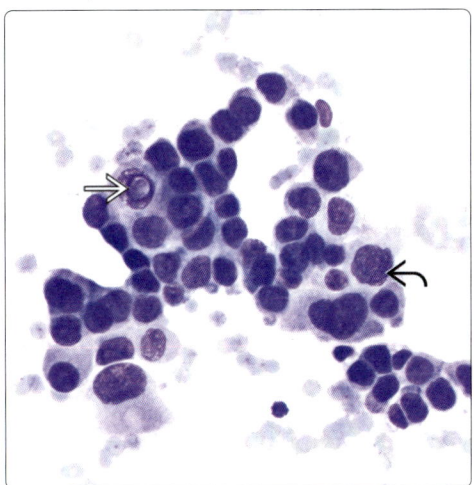

(Left) In some cases, prominent intracellular mucin within vacuoles of malignant cells ⇨ makes a confident diagnosis of adenocarcinoma possible with conventional stains alone, such as this Diff-Quik. **(Right)** Nuclear pseudoinclusions ⇨ and grooves ⇨, as seen in this Diff-Quik stain, often correspond to lepidic pattern adenocarcinoma. Here, the anisonucleosis aids recognition of malignancy, but some cases are very subtle.

Adenocarcinoma With Minimal Atypia

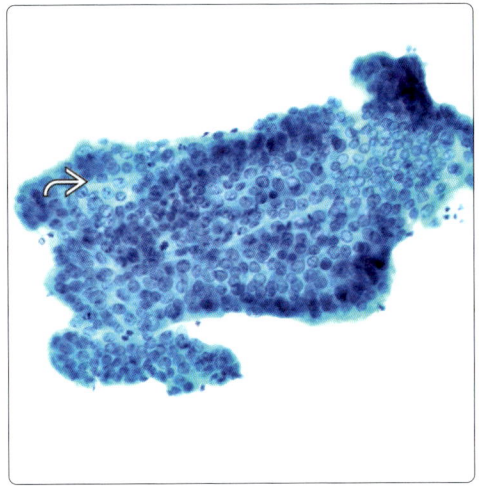

Marked Hypercellularity

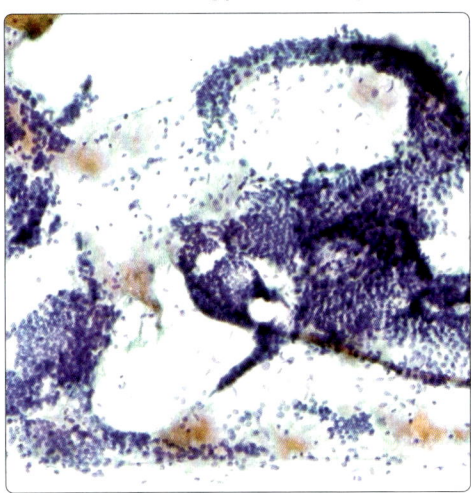

(Left) Some examples of adenocarcinoma show only minimal architectural disorder ⇨ and nuclear changes, making separation from a reactive process difficult, even in well-visualized, Pap-stained examples. **(Right)** Even in cases of adenocarcinoma with very bland cytology, extreme hypercellularity strongly suggests a neoplastic process. The large sheets of tumor cells in this Pap-stained smear suggest the diagnosis of lepidic-type adenocarcinoma.

Micropapillary Carcinoma

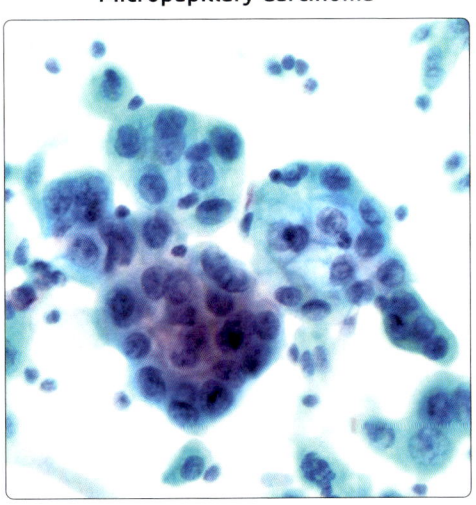

Mucinous Adenocarcinoma

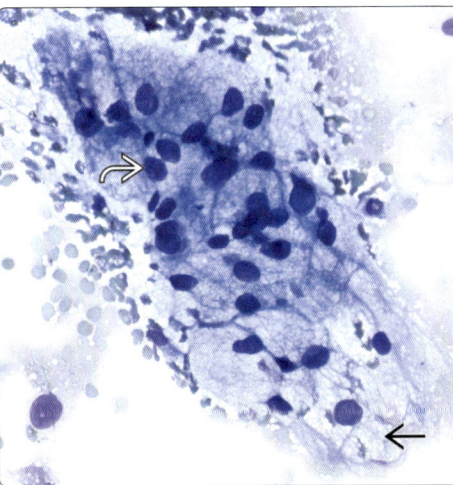

(Left) Micropapillary carcinoma shows small, round clusters of cells with marked nuclear pleomorphism in this Pap stain. These clusters are seen within lymphatic channels or surrounded by retraction artifact in histology. **(Right)** Diff-Quik-stained touch prep of a mucinous adenocarcinoma demonstrates the voluminous foamy cytoplasm ⇨ and relatively bland nuclei ⇨ typical of this variant.

Squamous Cell Carcinoma

KEY FACTS

TERMINOLOGY
- Malignant epithelial neoplasm with keratinization

CLINICAL ISSUES
- Poor prognosis
- Chemotherapy &/or radiation is often required
- Resection is indicated for low-stage tumors in patients who can tolerate loss of lung volume
- Diagnosis as squamous cell carcinoma eliminates many chemotherapy options available for adenocarcinoma or non-small cell carcinoma, not otherwise specified

CYTOPATHOLOGY
- "Hard" cytoplasm resulting from production of long-chain keratins is characteristic
- Orange G component of Pap stain is specific for keratinization
- Keratinization may produce robin's egg blue staining pattern on Diff-Quik stain
- Orangeophilic "tadpole" cells with elongated "tails" are very specific
- Necrosis, keratin debris, or foreign-body giant cells may be prominent
- Clumped or dark chromatin
- Pyknotic nuclei common in keratinizing cells

TOP DIFFERENTIAL DIAGNOSES
- Adenocarcinoma
  - Limited (2-stain) immunohistochemical panel is preferred to preserve cells for molecular testing
- Metastatic squamous cell carcinoma
  - p16 or HPV testing may be helpful if anogenital or oropharyngeal primary is suspected
- Reactive changes
  - Degenerating cells in setting of acute lung injury
- Benign squamous cells
  - Oral or bronchial squamous cells may show significant reactive atypia

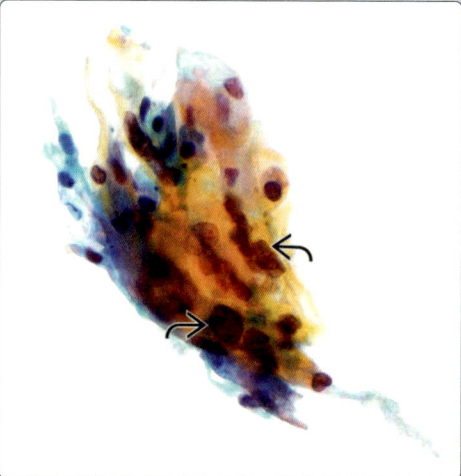

Keratinizing Squamous Cell Carcinoma

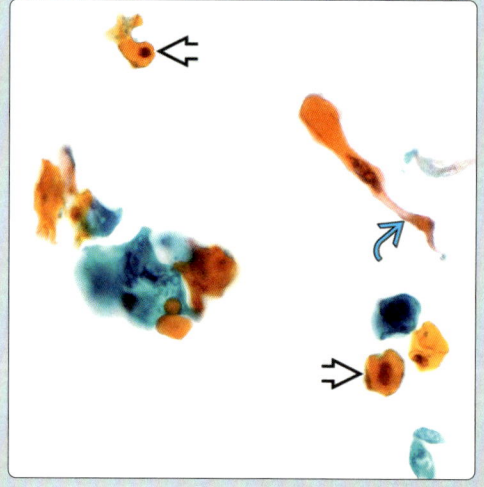

Individual Keratinized Malignant Cells

(Left) The combination of marked nuclear atypia ➔ and cytoplasmic keratinization, readily seen in Pap stains that contain orange G, is characteristic of squamous cell carcinoma. (Right) "Tadpole" cells with elongated cytoplasmic "tails" ➔ and individual small keratinizing cells with pyknotic nuclei ➔ are also helpful Pap stain findings.

Homogeneous Cytoplasm

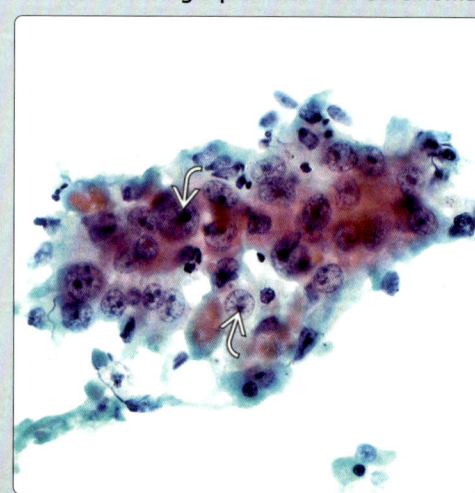

Nonkeratinizing Squamous Cell Carcinoma

(Left) In some instances, orangeophilia may not be as apparent, but "hard" homogeneous cytoplasm ➔ can still be appreciated on Pap stain. (Right) Nonkeratinizing squamous cell carcinoma frequently resembles adenocarcinoma with pleomorphic nuclei, clumpy chromatin, and prominent nucleoli ➔, as seen in this Pap stain.

Squamous Cell Carcinoma

CLINICAL ISSUES

Treatment
- Surgical approaches
  - Resection is indicated for low-stage tumors in patients who can tolerate loss of lung volume
- Adjuvant therapy
  - Chemotherapy &/or radiation

CYTOPATHOLOGY

Pattern
- Individual cells, clumps, sheets, or papillary structures

Background
- Necrosis, keratin debris, or foreign-body giant cells may be prominent

Nuclear Details
- Clumped or dark chromatin
- Pyknotic nuclei common in keratinizing cells

Cytoplasmic Details
- "Hard" cytoplasm resulting from production of long-chain keratins is characteristic
- Orange G component of Pap stain is specific for keratinization
- Keratinization may produce robin's egg blue staining pattern on Diff-Quik stain
- Orangeophilic "tadpole" cells with elongated "tails" are very specific

MACROSCOPIC

General Features
- Typically central but may be peripheral

MICROSCOPIC

Histologic Features
- Keratin pearls and intercellular bridges

ANCILLARY TESTS

Immunohistochemistry
- Expression of p40 (most specific), p63, or CK5/6 may help to distinguish from adenocarcinoma
  - If no definite keratinization is seen, but immunochemistry supports squamous differentiation, diagnose as non-small cell carcinoma, favor squamous cell carcinoma
- PD-L1 testing often needed for evaluation of possibility of treatment with PD-1 inhibitors

DIFFERENTIAL DIAGNOSIS

Adenocarcinoma
- Limited immunohistochemical panel (e.g., p40 and TTF-1) is preferred to allow for molecular testing

Small Cell Carcinoma
- Shows neuroendocrine differentiation (morphology and immunochemistry)

Metastatic Squamous Cell Carcinoma
- Testing for HPV by p16, in situ hybridization, or molecular methods can be helpful to favor anogenital or head and neck origin

Reactive Changes
- Reactive benign squamous cells or degenerating cells in acute respiratory distress syndrome

DIAGNOSTIC CHECKLIST

Pathologic Interpretation Pearls
- Unequivocal keratinization is diagnostic
- Diagnosis of squamous cell carcinoma should not be made lightly because it prevents molecular testing for mutations with targeted treatment

SELECTED REFERENCES

1. Sands JM et al: Next-generation sequencing informs diagnosis and identifies unexpected therapeutic targets in lung squamous cell carcinomas. Lung Cancer. 140:35-41, 2020

Focal Keratinization

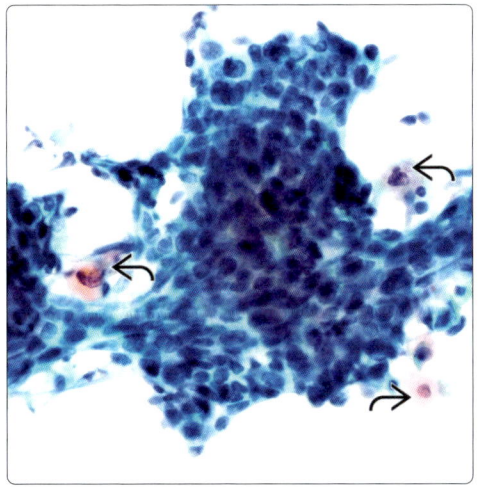

"Hard" Cytoplasm on Diff-Quik Stain

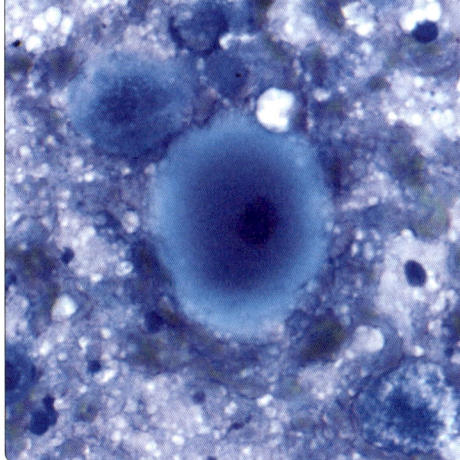

(Left) Not uncommonly, the Orange G component of the Pap stain highlights rare keratinizing cells ➔ in a tumor otherwise indistinguishable from adenocarcinoma. (Right) In Diff-Quik stains, keratinization takes the form of "hard" cytoplasm prominently seen here with an even, glassy consistency and a distinctive light blue tint. The nucleus is pyknotic, similar to how the nuclei often appear in orangeophilic cells on Pap stain. The adjacent cells are more degenerated.

Small Cell Carcinoma

KEY FACTS

TERMINOLOGY
- High-grade malignancy with scant cytoplasm and neuroendocrine differentiation

CLINICAL ISSUES
- Rapidly growing and metastasizing lung mass
- Very poor prognosis with life expectancy of months
- Chemotherapy and radiation; rarely surgery

CYTOPATHOLOGY
- Molding and crush artifact
- Large nuclei with salt and pepper chromatin
- Very scant cytoplasm
- Frequent mitosis and apoptosis
- Necrotic diathesis
- Usually high cellularity
- 2-3x size of background lymphocytes

ANCILLARY TESTS
- Neuroendocrine markers
- AE1/AE3 may be weak/focal or even negative

TOP DIFFERENTIAL DIAGNOSES
- Large cell neuroendocrine carcinoma
  - More abundant cytoplasm and prominent nucleoli
- Lymphoma
  - More dyscohesive with lymphoglandular bodies
- Metastasis
  - Small cell carcinoma can arise in other sites
  - Merkel cell carcinoma and small round blue cell sarcomas can look similar
- Non-small cell carcinoma
- Carcinoid or atypical carcinoid
  - Much less mitosis, apoptosis, necrosis; Ki-67 may help
- Reserve cell hyperplasia

Nuclear Molding

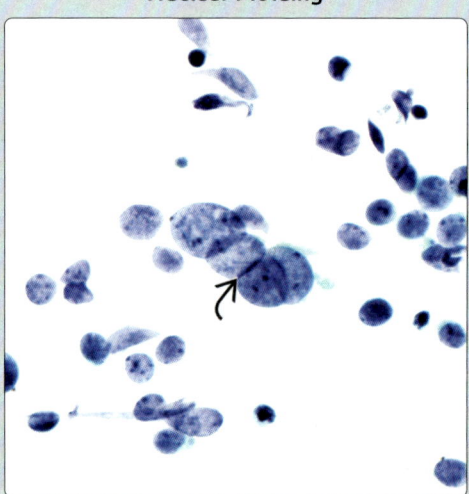

Prominent Apoptosis

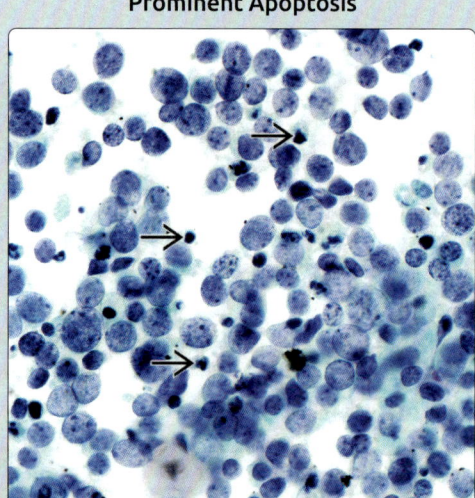

(Left) Small cell carcinoma often shows mutual compression of nuclei in adjacent cells known as molding ➡, seen best on a Pap stain. Although a few chromocenters are seen, the chromatin is predominantly distributed in a fine salt and pepper pattern. (Right) This Pap-stained example of small cell carcinoma shows numerous cells without recognizable cytoplasm as well as frequent apoptotic bodies ➡.

Hypercellularity

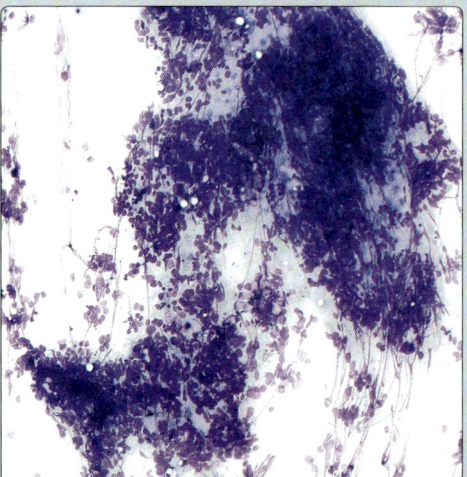

Rosette-Like Architecture

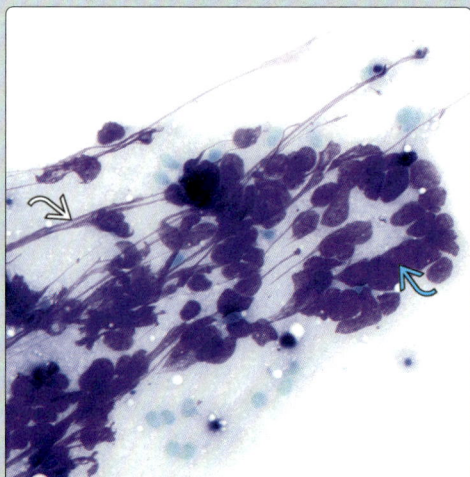

(Left) The typical low-power appearance on a Diff-Quik stain is that of a markedly hypercellular smear with high nuclear:cytoplasmic ratio cells, raising the differential of large cell lymphoma. The cohesiveness of the cells seen here favors carcinoma. (Right) On high power, rosette-like structures ➡ can occasionally be seen, as well as streaks of smeared nuclear material known as crush artifact ➡, highlighted by a Diff-Quik stain.

Small Cell Carcinoma

TERMINOLOGY

Definitions
- High-grade malignancy with scant cytoplasm and neuroendocrine differentiation

CLINICAL ISSUES

Presentation
- Rapidly growing and metastasizing lung mass

Treatment
- Chemotherapy and radiation; rarely surgery

CYTOPATHOLOGY

Pattern
- Molding with adjacent nuclei deforming one another; caterpillar appearance on sputum
- Crush artifact with smeared nuclear chromatin

Background
- Necrotic debris, apoptosis

Nuclear Details
- Intermittently dark and light salt and pepper chromatin evenly distributed in nucleus
- Nucleoli usually indistinct but may be present
- Frequent mitosis and pyknosis

Cytoplasmic Details
- Very scant cytoplasm

Cells
- 2-3x size of background lymphocytes

ANCILLARY TESTS

Immunohistochemistry
- Neuroendocrine markers: CD56 and synaptophysin are most useful
- Chromogranin is often negative due to scant cytoplasm
- INSM1 is promising new neuroendocrine marker with nuclear staining
- TTF-1 is usually positive
- AE1/AE3 may be weak/focal or even negative

Flow Cytometry
- CD56 and EpCAM

DIFFERENTIAL DIAGNOSIS

Large Cell Neuroendocrine Carcinoma
- More abundant cytoplasm and prominent nucleoli

Lymphoma
- More dyscohesive and has lymphoglandular bodies
- Distinct immunomarkers

Metastasis
- Small cell carcinoma of other organs, Merkel cell carcinoma, small round blue cell sarcomas
- TTF-1 is not lung specific in neuroendocrine carcinomas

Carcinoid or Atypical Carcinoid
- Lower grade; much less necrosis, apoptosis, and mitosis

Reserve Cell Hyperplasia
- Reactive change with few clusters of very small cells with high nuclear:cytoplasmic ratio

DIAGNOSTIC CHECKLIST

Pathologic Interpretation Pearls
- When malignant cells are few, they are easily missed due to their small size
- Be cautious if necrosis, mitosis, and apoptosis are not readily apparent

SELECTED REFERENCES
1. Sung S et al: Pulmonary small cell carcinoma: review, common and uncommon differentials, genomics and management. Diagn Cytopathol. 48(8):790-803, 2020
2. Doxtader EE et al: Insulinoma-associated protein 1 is a sensitive and specific marker of neuroendocrine lung neoplasms in cytology specimens. Cancer Cytopathol. 126(4):243-52, 2018

Biopsy Appearance
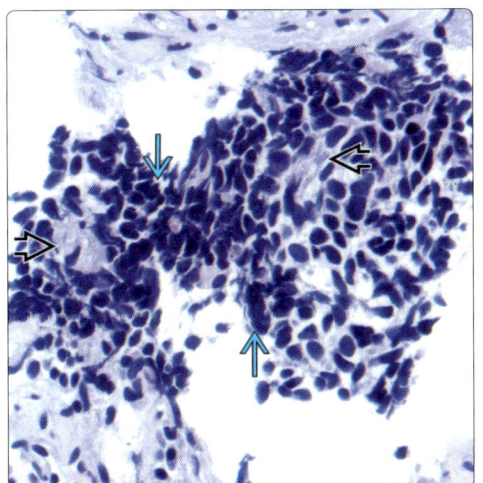

Synaptophysin Immunohistochemistry
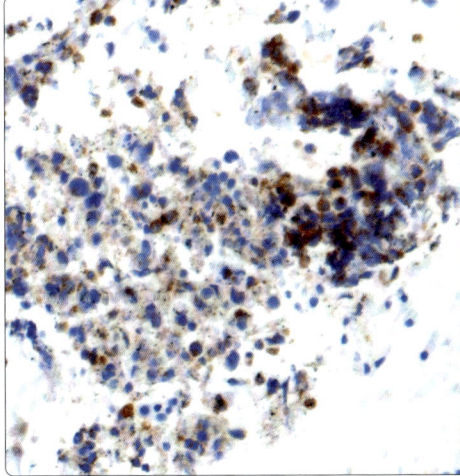

(Left) This nest of malignant cells within lung parenchyma in a core biopsy shows the same features typical of cytology specimens: Scant cytoplasm, nuclear molding ⇨, and even chromatin. Rosette-like structures ⇨ are also seen. The nuclei typically appear darker with H&E stain than Pap stain. (Right) This synaptophysin stain of a small biopsy shows typical granular and variable cytoplasmic staining. The relatively sparse neurosecretory granules of small cell carcinoma cause this staining pattern.

Large Cell Neuroendocrine Carcinoma

KEY FACTS

TERMINOLOGY
- High-grade malignancy with abundant cytoplasm and neuroendocrine differentiation

CLINICAL ISSUES
- Rapidly growing and metastasizing lung tumor
- Genomic testing may be helpful to aid in treatment decisions
- Poor prognosis but better than small cell carcinoma

CYTOPATHOLOGY
- High cellularity
- Necrotic debris
- Frequent mitosis
- Large nuclei with salt and pepper chromatin
- Prominent nucleoli
- Cytoplasm more abundant than in small cell carcinoma with less molding and crush artifact

MACROSCOPIC
- May be endobronchial or intraparenchymal tumor

ANCILLARY TESTS
- INSM1, synaptophysin, chromogranin positive
- TTF-1 often positive

TOP DIFFERENTIAL DIAGNOSES
- Small cell carcinoma
  - Less cytoplasm and indistinct nucleoli
- Typical or atypical carcinoid
  - Less mitotic activity and necrosis
- Non-small cell carcinoma
  - Lacks neuroendocrine nuclear features
  - Little or no staining for neuroendocrine markers (INSM1, synaptophysin, chromogranin)
- Metastatic neuroendocrine carcinoma
  - History is critical
  - TTF-1 and CDX2 may be helpful

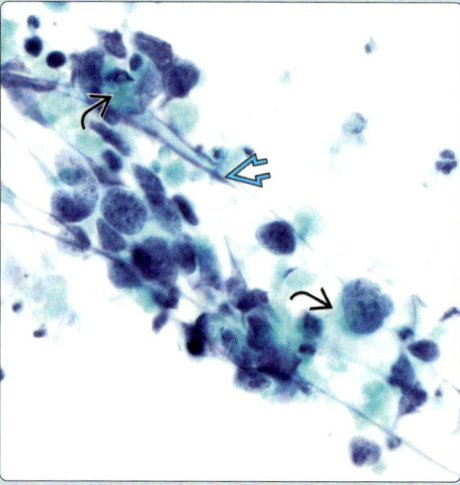

Large Cell Neuroendocrine Carcinoma on Pap Stain

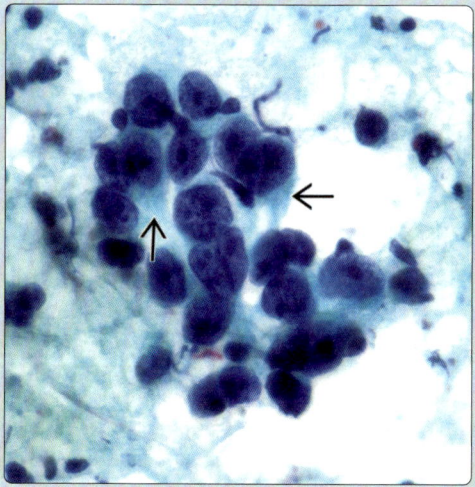

Prominent Nucleoli and Abundant Cytoplasm

(Left) This Pap-stained example of large cell neuroendocrine carcinoma shows the typical combination of small cell-like crush artifact ⇨ and non-small cell-like abundant cytoplasm ⇨. (Right) This aggregate of malignant cells from a large cell neuroendocrine carcinoma shows a combination of granular salt and pepper chromatin and prominent nucleoli that can be appreciated on Pap stain. Abundant cytoplasm ⇨ is also seen on some of the cells.

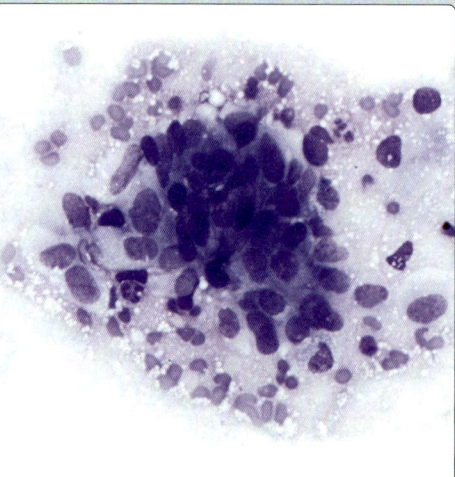

Lack of Nuclear Molding

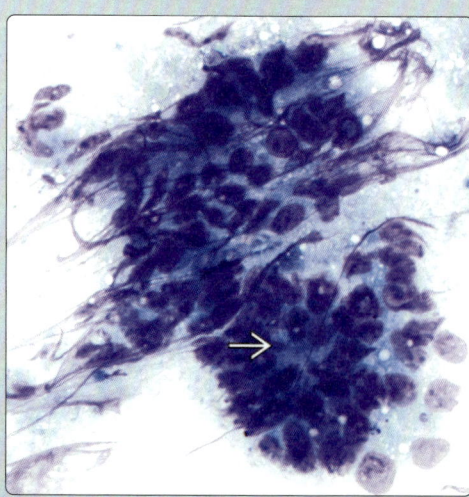

Rosette-Like Architecture

(Left) The nuclei resemble those of small cell carcinoma on Diff-Quik stain, but note the lack of molding despite tight clustering of cells and other nuclear contour irregularities. (Right) Rosette-like structures ⇨ are prominent in some cases of large cell neuroendocrine carcinoma, such as the one seen in this Diff-Quik-stained example.

Large Cell Neuroendocrine Carcinoma

TERMINOLOGY

Abbreviations
- Large cell neuroendocrine carcinoma (LCNEC)

Definitions
- High-grade malignancy with abundant cytoplasm and neuroendocrine differentiation

CLINICAL ISSUES

Presentation
- Rapidly growing and metastasizing lung tumor

Treatment
- Traditionally similar to small cell carcinoma but more likely to be resected if localized
- Genomic analysis may be helpful to decide on chemotherapy regimens and targeted therapy for LCNEC
  - Subsets may respond better to small cell-like vs. adenocarcinoma-like therapeutic approaches

CYTOPATHOLOGY

Cellularity
- High cellularity

Background
- Necrotic debris

Nuclear Details
- Large nuclei with salt and pepper chromatin
- Prominent nucleoli
- Frequent mitosis

Cytoplasmic Details
- More abundant than in small cell carcinoma with less molding and crush artifact

MICROSCOPIC

Histologic Features
- Abundant cytoplasm and prominent nucleoli
- Neuroendocrine markers must be positive
- > 10 mitotic figures per 10 HPF
- Comedo-like necrosis
- Organoid growth pattern resembling carcinoid

ANCILLARY TESTS

Immunohistochemistry
- INSM1, synaptophysin, chromogranin, CD56 positive
- TTF-1 often positive

DIFFERENTIAL DIAGNOSIS

Small Cell Carcinoma
- Less cytoplasm and indistinct nucleoli

Typical or Atypical Carcinoid
- Less mitotic activity and necrosis

Non-Small Cell Carcinoma
- Lacks salt and pepper chromatin
- Neuroendocrine markers (INSM1, synaptophysin, chromogranin) are absent or weak

Metastatic Neuroendocrine Carcinoma
- Clinical history of previous tumor of utmost importance
- Immunohistochemistry for TTF-1 and CDX2 may be helpful

DIAGNOSTIC CHECKLIST

Pathologic Interpretation Pearls
- Neuroendocrine appearance and immunohistochemistry are key to diagnosis of LCNEC
- Appears similar to small cell carcinoma but with more cytoplasm and obvious nucleoli

SELECTED REFERENCES

1. Yoshimura M et al: Molecular pathology of pulmonary large cell neuroendocrine carcinoma: novel concepts and treatments. Front Oncol. 11:671799, 2021
2. Baine MK et al: Multiple faces of pulmonary large cell neuroendocrine carcinoma: update with a focus on practical approach to diagnosis. Transl Lung Cancer Res. 9(3):860-78, 2020

Hypercellular Smear

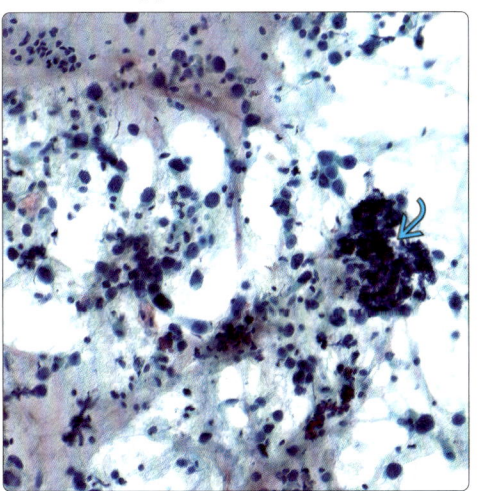

Anaplastic Giant Cell

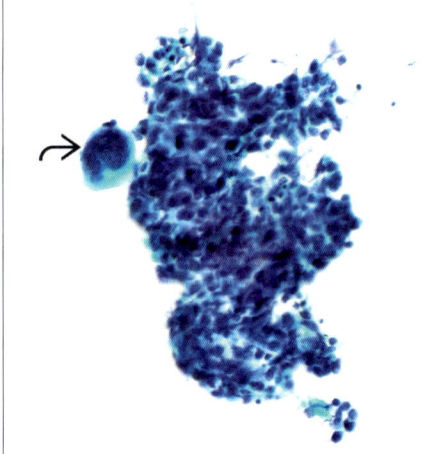

(Left) Large cell neuroendocrine carcinoma usually produces hypercellular smears with obviously malignant pleomorphic nuclei, as seen in the Pap-stained example. Focally, crush artifacts may make the tumor cells appear similar to small cell carcinoma ➔, but most of the cells have ample cytoplasm. (Right) Anaplastic giant cells ➔ are occasionally seen, as in this Pap-stained cluster, aiding diagnosis when present.

Carcinoid and Atypical Carcinoid

KEY FACTS

CLINICAL ISSUES
- Often incidental nodules
- May present with airway obstruction, paraneoplastic syndromes, or as part of syndrome of interstitial fibrosis and diffuse pulmonary neuroendocrine cell hyperplasia (DIPNECH)
- Surgical resection for attempted cure often possible
- Good prognosis

CYTOPATHOLOGY
- Typically plasmacytoid morphology but may be spindled or oncocytic
- Clumpy salt and pepper neuroendocrine chromatin
- Abundant cytoplasm but may not be apparent in some cytologic preparations
- Dispersed cells and aggregates that may show rosette-like, nested, trabecular, or pseudoglandular structures
- Nucleoli inconspicuous but sometimes more prominent in atypical carcinoid
- Mitotic activity scant in typical carcinoid but may be seen in atypical carcinoid

ANCILLARY TESTS
- Neuroendocrine markers key (INSM1, CD56, synaptophysin, chromogranin)
- Ki-67 in cell blocks may be useful to evaluate grade
- TTF-1 often positive but may be weak/focal

TOP DIFFERENTIAL DIAGNOSES
- High-grade neuroendocrine carcinomas may be mimicked by carcinoid tumors due to neuroendocrine chromatin, molding, and crush artifact
  - Look for necrosis and mitotic activity
- Bland carcinoid tumor cells may easily be dismissed as reactive bronchial cells or type II pneumocytes
  - High level of suspicion needed
- Metastatic neuroendocrine tumors from other sites may look identical
  - TTF-1 and CDX2 may be helpful

Typical Plasmacytoid Appearance

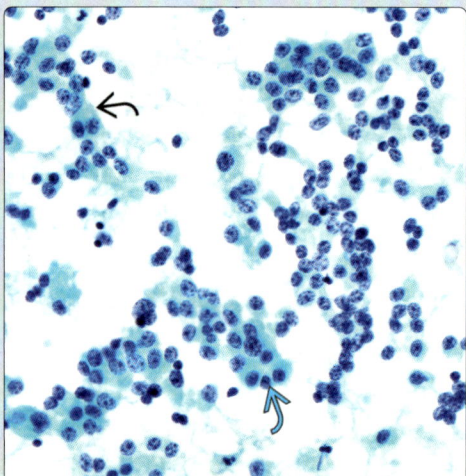

Rosette With Salt and Pepper Chromatin

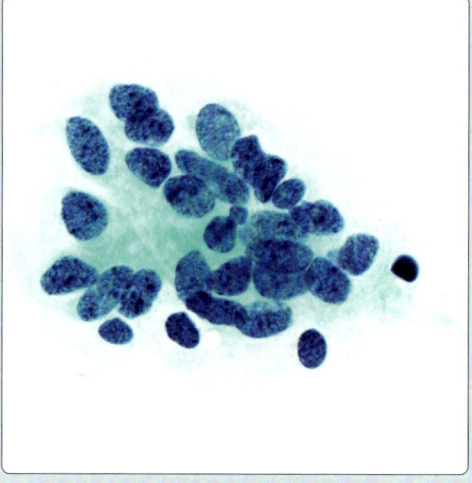

(Left) Carcinoid tumors typically show uniform neuroendocrine cells with abundant eccentric cytoplasm ⊞ retaining traces of organoid growth pattern ➔, as seen in this Pap stain. (Right) Pap-stained sample of carcinoid tumor shows a rosette structure with a central area of cytoplasm. The surrounding cell nuclei are elongated with clumpy salt and pepper chromatin.

Carcinoid Mimicking Small Cell Carcinoma

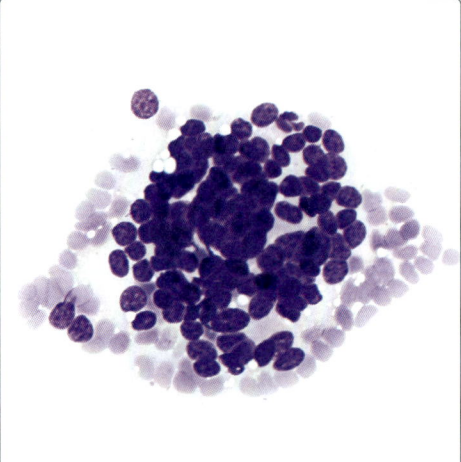

Carcinoid With Spindle Cell Morphology

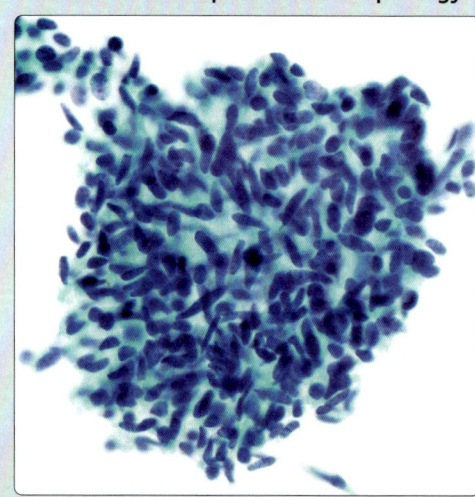

(Left) On Diff-Quik stain, the cytoplasm of carcinoid tumor cells may be less apparent, mimicking small cell carcinoma. Nuclear molding is relatively focal with less crush artifact, however. The lack of necrosis, apoptosis, or mitosis is also key to the recognition of the low-grade nature of these cells. (Right) Some carcinoid tumors have a prominent spindle cell component, as seen here in a ThinPrep specimen, that may lead to consideration of mesenchymal neoplasms.

Carcinoid and Atypical Carcinoid

TERMINOLOGY

Synonyms
- Low-grade and intermediate-grade neuroendocrine tumors of lung

CLINICAL ISSUES

Presentation
- Often incidental nodules, < 3 cm
- May present with airway obstruction, paraneoplastic syndromes, or as part of syndrome of interstitial fibrosis and diffuse pulmonary neuroendocrine cell hyperplasia (DIPNECH)
- Typically younger than patients with high-grade neuroendocrine tumors; not smoking related

CYTOPATHOLOGY

Pattern
- Dispersed cells and aggregates that may show rosette-like, nested, trabecular, or pseudoglandular structures

Background
- Usually clean, but necrosis may be seen in background of atypical carcinoma

Cells
- Usually plasmacytoid morphology but may be spindled or oncocytic

Nuclear Details
- Clumpy salt and pepper neuroendocrine chromatin
- Nucleoli inconspicuous but sometimes more prominent in atypical carcinoid
- Mitotic activity raises possibility of atypical carcinoid or high-grade neuroendocrine carcinoma

MICROSCOPIC

Histologic Features
- Distinctive organoid growth pattern
- Typical carcinoid has < 2 mitoses per 2 mm² and no necrosis (tumorlet if < 0.5 cm)
- Atypical carcinoid has 2-10 mitoses per 2 mm² or necrosis (usually punctate)

ANCILLARY TESTS

Immunohistochemistry
- Neuroendocrine markers (INSM1, CD56, synaptophysin, chromogranin) and proliferation marker Ki-67

DIFFERENTIAL DIAGNOSIS

High-Grade Neuroendocrine Carcinomas
- Carcinoid tumors may show molding and crush artifact resembling small cell carcinoma

Reactive Changes
- Bland tumor cells may mimic reactive bronchial cells

Metastatic Neuroendocrine Tumors
- TTF-1 and CDX2 immunohistochemistry may be helpful

DIAGNOSTIC CHECKLIST

Pathologic Interpretation Pearls
- Atypical carcinoid cannot be reliably separated from typical carcinoid by cytology alone
- Carcinoid tumors may show cytologic features concerning for high-grade neuroendocrine carcinomas but lack abundant mitosis, apoptosis, and necrosis
- Carcinoid tumors may be so bland as to not be recognized as neoplasm

SELECTED REFERENCES

1. Metovic J et al: Morphologic and molecular classification of lung neuroendocrine neoplasms. Virchows Arch. 478(1):5-19, 2021
2. Viswanathan K et al: Insulinoma-associated protein 1 is a sensitive and specific marker for lung neuroendocrine tumors in cytologic and surgical specimens. J Am Soc Cytopathol. 8(6):299-308, 2019
3. Hendifar AE et al: Neuroendocrine tumors of the lung: current challenges and advances in the diagnosis and management of well-differentiated disease. J Thorac Oncol. 12(3): 425-6, 2016

High Cellularity
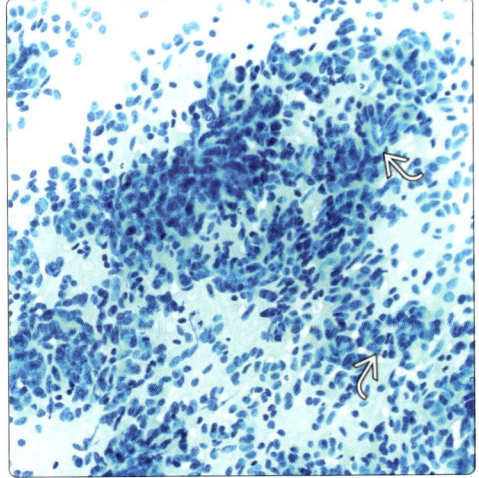

Biopsy Appearance
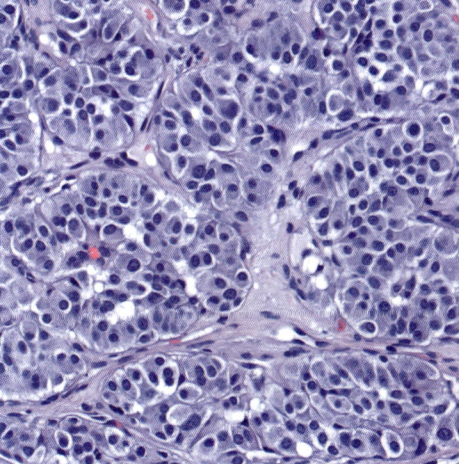

(Left) This Pap-stained FNA smear from a carcinoid tumor shows high cellularity with nuclei that vary from oval to spindle-like. Note the presence of subtle rosette-like structures ➡. *(Right)* This small biopsy of a carcinoid tumor stained with H&E shows nests of plasmacytoid tumor cells with abundant cytoplasm. Necrosis is absent, and mitoses are rare. This appearance is fairly easily recognized, but tumors with less cytoplasm and crush artifact may be more problematic.

Rare Benign and Low Malignant Potential Tumors

KEY FACTS

CLASSIFICATION

- Hamartoma is most common benign lung tumor
  - Results from overgrowth of mature mesenchymal elements
  - Contains entrapped epithelial elements that may raise concern for malignancy
- Pneumocytoma (sclerosing hemangioma) is benign tumor derived from pneumocytes (TTF-1 positive) that resembles vascular tumor histologically
- Solitary fibrous tumor is fibroblastic mesenchymal tumor (STAT6 positive) usually localized to pleura that may be multiple or malignant
- Clear cell (sugar) tumor is member of PEComa group (HMB-45 positive)
- Granular cell tumor is derived from Schwann cells (S100 positive), typically in bronchus
- Salivary gland analog tumors may arise primarily in lung from bronchial seromucinous glands

CLINICAL ISSUES

- Usually solitary, well-defined masses

CYTOPATHOLOGY

- Hamartoma consists of mixed benign stromal and glandular elements
- Pneumocytoma neoplastic cells form loose clusters surrounding stromal cores
- Solitary fibrous tumor features bland spindle cells with collagen in background
  - Uncommon malignant variants may have increased atypia
- Clear cell (sugar) tumor consists of bland cells with abundant finely vacuolated glycogen-rich cytoplasm
- Granular cell tumor consists of bland cells with abundant granular cytoplasm that is fragile and may be lost during preparation
- Salivary gland analog tumors look same as their counterparts in salivary glands

Solitary Fibrous Tumor

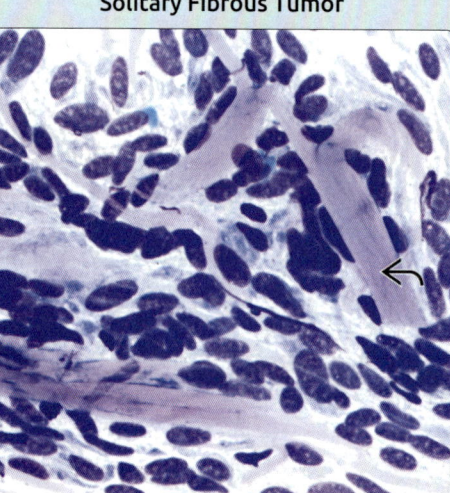

Clear Cell (Sugar) Tumor

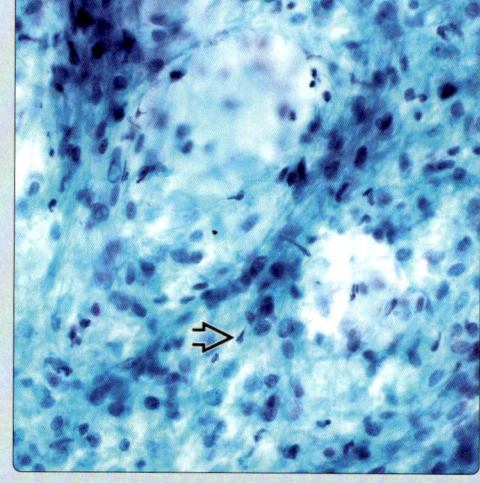

(Left) Solitary fibrous tumor consists of bland spindled cells with high nuclear:cytoplasmic ratio and fragmented collagen ➡ that is highlighted on this Diff-Quik stain. (Right) Clear cell (sugar) tumor is composed of cells with bland nuclei, abundant foamy cytoplasm, and transgressing vessels ➡ that are well visualized on this Pap stain.

Granular Cell Tumor

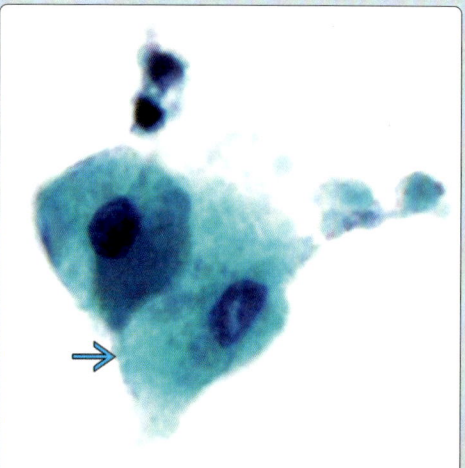

Pneumocytoma (Sclerosing Hemangioma)

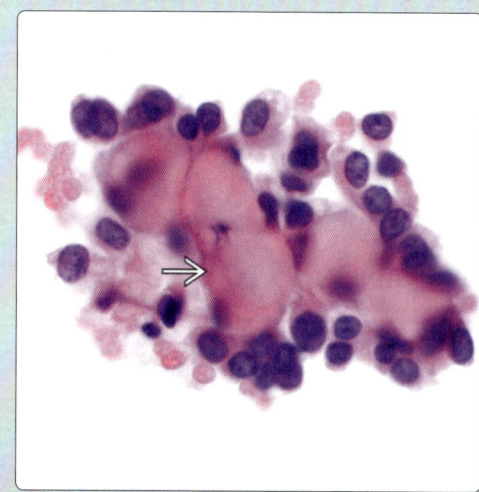

(Left) Granular cell tumor is characterized by abundant granular cytoplasm ➡, as seen in this ThinPrep example. (Right) The cells of pneumocytoma form loose clusters with fine chromatin, seen here in an H&E touch preparation. Collagenous stromal cores ➡ are a characteristic feature.

Rare Benign and Low Malignant Potential Tumors

CLASSIFICATION

Hamartoma
- Results from overgrowth of mature mesenchymal elements with entrapment of benign epithelium
- Most common benign lung tumor, presents as radiologic "popcorn" lobulated lesion
- Mixed fibrillary matrix highlighted by Diff-Quik and bland glandular elements

Pneumocytoma (Sclerosing Hemangioma)
- Arises from pneumocytes, though lesions resemble vascular tumors
- Incidental "coin" lesion, usually in women
- Loosely adherent cells around stromal cores with fine chromatin and nuclear pseudoinclusions
- TTF-1 positive

Solitary Fibrous Tumor
- Fibroblastic mesenchymal tumor often arising in pleura
- May be multiple despite name; may also be malignant
- Uniform bland spindle cells (except rare malignant variants) and ropy collagen
- STAT6, CD34, and BCL2 positive; S100 and cytokeratin negative

Clear Cell (Sugar) Tumor
- Arises from perivascular epithelioid cells (member of PEComa family)
- Sometimes associated with tuberous sclerosis, lymphangioleiomyomatosis, or angiomyolipoma
- Bland cells with finely vacuolated cytoplasm and transgressing vessels; naked nuclei may be numerous
- HMB-45 positive; PAS highlights cytoplasmic glycogen

Granular Cell Tumor
- Arises from Schwann cells, typically in bronchus, often with obstruction
- Polygonal epithelioid cells with granular cytoplasm and round nuclei
- S100 positive; PAS highlights granules

Salivary Gland Analog Tumors
- Arise from bronchial seromucinous glands
- Have same morphology and other characteristics as salivary gland counterparts

Other Tumors
- Papillomas, adenomas, and inflammatory myofibroblastic tumors are very difficult to diagnose cytologically due to bland cells
- Other cytologically distinctive tumors more commonly seen in other organs (but rarely in lung) include glomus tumor, giant cell tumor, lipoma, leiomyoma, and meningioma

CLINICAL ISSUES

Presentation
- Usually solitary, well-defined masses

DIFFERENTIAL DIAGNOSIS

Pneumocytoma (Sclerosing Hemangioma)
- Cells have similar appearance and staining pattern to well-differentiated adenocarcinoma

Clear Cell (Sugar) Tumor
- Closely resembles low Fuhrman grade metastatic renal cell carcinoma by cytology

DIAGNOSTIC CHECKLIST

Pathologic Interpretation Pearls
- Clinical and radiologic correlation is critical for correct diagnosis of these rare tumors
- Bland tumor cells may easily be missed among background normal lung cells in brushings and washings

SELECTED REFERENCES
1. Trabucco SMR et al: Pulmonary sclerosing pneumocytoma: a pre and intraoperative diagnostic challenge. Report of two cases and review of the literature. Medicina (Kaunas). 57(6):524, 2021
2. Finer EB et al: Granular cell tumor of the lung. Diagn Cytopathol. 47(4):345-6, 2019

Pulmonary Hamartoma
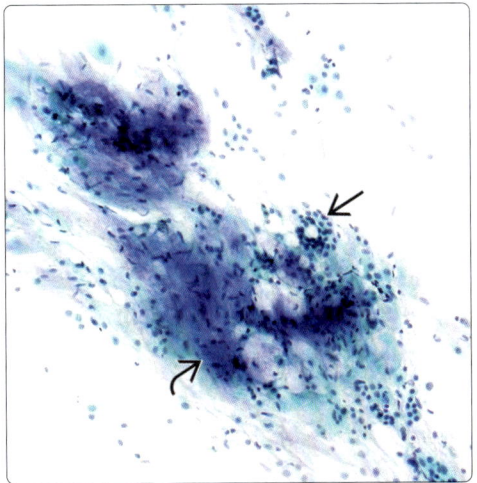

Hamartoma Fibrillary Stroma
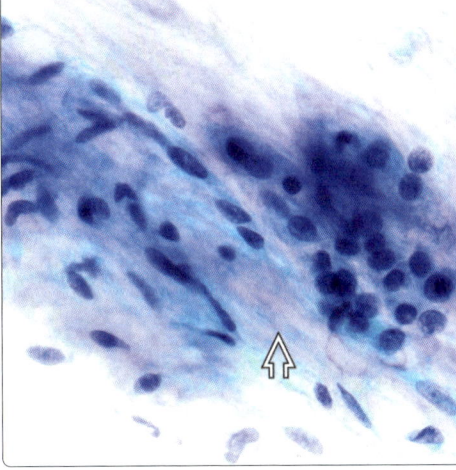

(Left) Aspiration of a pulmonary hamartoma will yield mixed benign mesenchymal ➡ and epithelial ➡ elements, as seen in this Pap stain. (Right) A closer view from the same case highlights the fibrillary appearance of the cartilaginous matrix ➡.

Rare Malignant Tumors

KEY FACTS

CLASSIFICATION
- Mesothelioma arises from pleural mesothelial cells and is asbestos and smoking related
- Salivary gland analog tumors identical to salivary gland primaries arise from bronchial seromucinous glands
  - Adenoid cystic carcinoma and mucoepidermoid carcinoma are most common
- Pulmonary blastoma typically arises in adulthood
- Pleuropulmonary blastoma arises in early childhood

CLINICAL ISSUES
- Consider mesothelioma for pleural-based tumors
- Salivary gland analog tumors may obstruct bronchus
- Pleuropulmonary blastoma is associated with congenital lung cysts

CYTOPATHOLOGY
- Epithelioid mesothelioma shows nuclear pleomorphism, prominent nucleoli, and vacuolated cytoplasm
- Ancillary studies, including immunohistochemistry and molecular genetic markers, are key
- Salivary gland analog tumors have same morphology as their counterparts in salivary glands
- Pulmonary blastoma contains both malignant epithelial elements and sarcomatoid elements
- Pleuropulmonary blastoma has predominant blastemic morphology with more mature sarcomatoid elements seen in some cases
- Sarcomatoid malignancies are difficult to diagnose by cytology alone
  - Primary sarcoma is rare, and sarcomatoid non-small cell carcinoma or metastasis must be excluded
  - Sarcomatoid mesothelioma is almost never diagnosed by cytology

TOP DIFFERENTIAL DIAGNOSES
- Lung carcinoma and metastasis must be considered before diagnosing these rare tumors

Biphasic Mesothelioma

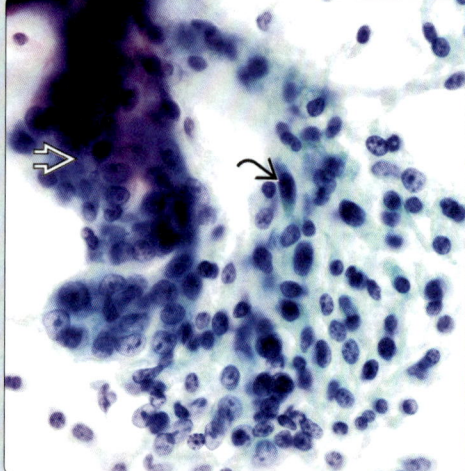

Intercellular Windows in Mesothelioma

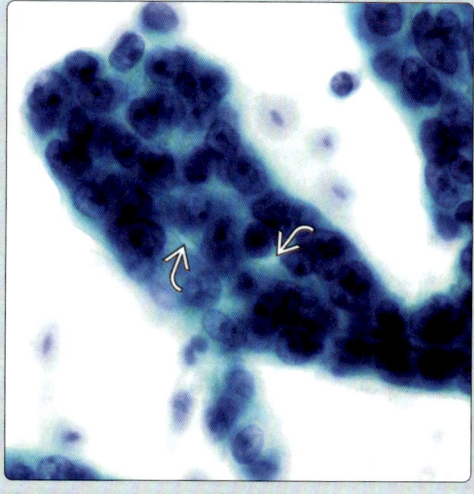

(Left) The spindle cell component of mesothelioma rarely appears in effusions but can be sampled by fine-needle aspiration ⇥, as seen in this Pap-stained example. An epithelioid component ⇥ is also present. *(Right)* A closer view of the epithelioid component from the same slide shows that features familiar from effusions, including windows ⇥, are retained.

Pulmonary Blastoma Biphasic Morphology

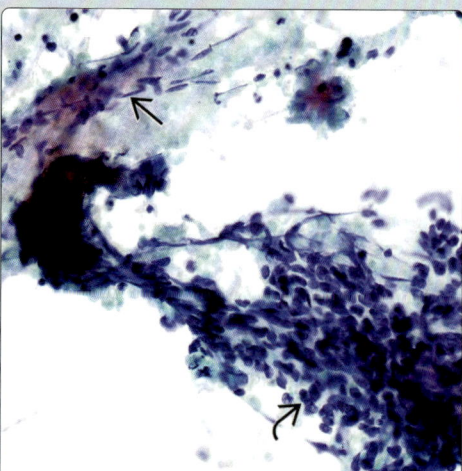

Malignant Features in Pulmonary Blastoma

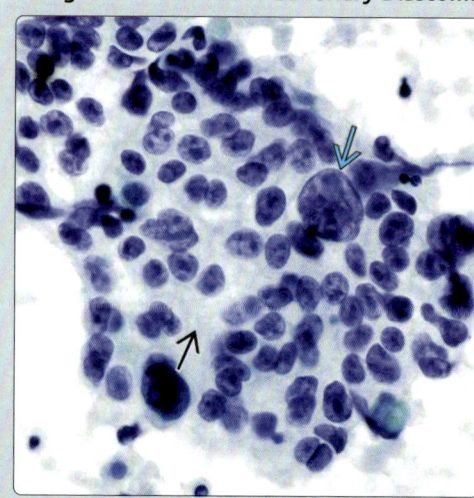

(Left) Biphasic morphology is also characteristic of pulmonary blastoma. In this Pap stain, mesenchymal ⇥ and glandular ⇥ components are visible. *(Right)* Another nearby cluster of glandular cells shows obviously malignant nuclear features ⇥ and abundant vacuolated cytoplasm ⇥.

Rare Malignant Tumors

CLASSIFICATION

Mesothelioma
- Pleura-based mass that arises from pleural mesothelial cells, usually in older adults
- Associated with asbestos exposure and smoking
- Characterized by malignant cells with pleomorphic nuclei, prominent nucleoli, and vacuolated cytoplasm
- Intercellular windows and hyaluronic acid in background may provide clues about diagnosis
- Although rarely seen in body fluids, spindle cell component may be present in fine-needle aspiration and small biopsy specimens

Salivary Gland Analog Tumors
- Arise from seromucinous glands of bronchus with same characteristics as their salivary gland counterparts
- Adenoid cystic carcinoma is most common, followed by mucoepidermoid carcinoma
- Epithelial-myoepithelial carcinoma and acinic cell carcinoma have also been reported

Pulmonary Blastoma
- Typically large, peripheral, well-circumscribed tumors, usually occurring in adults
- Loosely cohesive spindle cells and glandular cells with sub- and supranuclear glycogen vacuoles
- Sarcomatoid elements and morular nests may be seen

Pleuropulmonary Blastoma
- Occurs in very young children, typically associated with cystic lung lesions
- Undifferentiated blastemic small round blue cells and more differentiated spindle cells

Sarcoma
- Examples include malignant solitary fibrous tumor, synovial sarcoma, leiomyosarcoma, malignant peripheral nerve sheath tumor, angiosarcoma, and epithelioid hemangioendothelioma

ANCILLARY TESTS

Immunohistochemistry
- Panels, including calretinin and D2-40, may be very helpful if mesothelioma is suspected

DIFFERENTIAL DIAGNOSIS

Non-Small Cell Carcinoma
- Mesothelioma and pulmonary blastoma frequently resemble adenocarcinoma
- Sarcomatoid variants of non-small cell carcinomas are more common than true lung sarcomas

Metastasis
- May have spindle cell appearance resembling primary blastemic or sarcomatous malignancies
- Salivary gland-type primary carcinomas appear identical to metastases from salivary glands

DIAGNOSTIC CHECKLIST

Pathologic Interpretation Pearls
- Mesothelioma resembles non-small cell carcinoma; therefore, clinical/radiologic findings and ancillary testing are key to suggesting diagnosis
- Romanowsky stains highlight matrix of salivary gland-type tumors
- Consider sarcomatoid non-small cell carcinoma or metastasis before diagnosing rare primary blastemic or sarcomatous entities

SELECTED REFERENCES

1. Kunisaki SM et al: Pleuropulmonary blastoma in pediatric lung lesions. Pediatrics. 147(4)::e2020028357, 2021
2. Aldera AP et al: Endobronchial masses encountered on fine-needle aspiration biopsy: a focus on unusual entities. Diagn Cytopathol. 48(8):807-12, 2020
3. Doxtader EE et al: Primary salivary gland-type tumors of the tracheobronchial tree diagnosed by transbronchial fine needle aspiration: clinical and cytomorphologic features with histopathologic correlation. Diagn Cytopathol. 47(11):1168-76, 2019

Blastemic Cells in Pleuropulmonary Blastoma

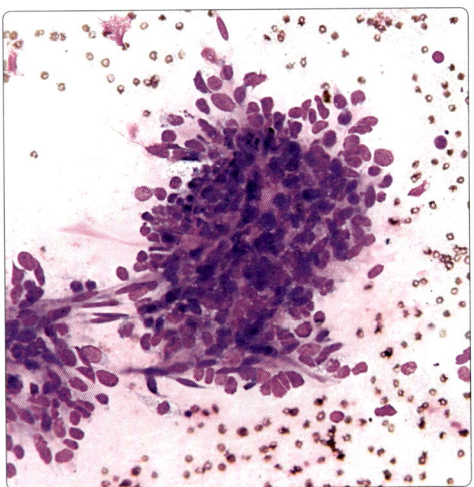

Spindle Cells in Pleuropulmonary Blastoma

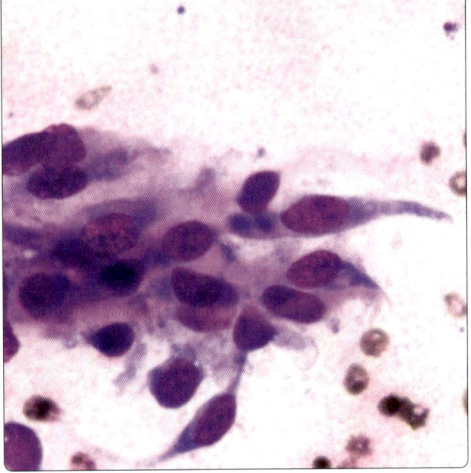

(Left) Diff-Quik-stained preparation from a pleuropulmonary blastoma shows blastemic cells that can be seen with scant cytoplasm and nuclear pleomorphism. (Right) The same pleuropulmonary blastoma case also contained more differentiated spindle cells with abundant cytoplasm.

NUT Carcinoma

KEY FACTS

ETIOLOGY/PATHOGENESIS
- Epithelial malignancy with rearrangement of *NUTM1* gene

CLINICAL ISSUES
- Rare, ~ 2.5% of small round blue cell tumors
- Most commonly presents in mediastinum or head and neck, often midline, but many other sites reported
- Typically young adults but wide age range
- Rapid onset of destructive malignant tumor, often with lymph node, bone, &/or pleural metastasis early in course

MICROSCOPIC
- Primitive, monotonous, undifferentiated cells; necrosis and acute inflammation are common
- Hypercellular and dyscohesive smears
- Round to oval nuclei; may be hypo- or hyperchromatic with prominent nucleoli
- Granular cytoplasm; may be stripped leaving bare nuclei, but nuclear molding is uncommon
- Abrupt foci of keratinization, when present, serves as clue to diagnosis

ANCILLARY TESTS
- NUT immunochemistry shows speckled nuclear positivity
- AE1/AE3, CK5/6, p63, p40 (+)
- CD34, synaptophysin, chromogranin, TTF-1, α-fetoprotein, CD99, FLI1 may be positive, potentially leading to misdiagnosis
- High Ki-67 index (usually > 80%)
- Break-apart FISH for NUT and *BRD4*
- PCR for *BRD4::NUTM1* [t(15;19)], *BRD3::NUTM1*, and other *NUTM1* variants

TOP DIFFERENTIAL DIAGNOSES
- Squamous cell carcinoma
- Germ cell tumors
- Neuroendocrine carcinoma
- Small round blue cell tumors

Dyscohesive Tumor Cells

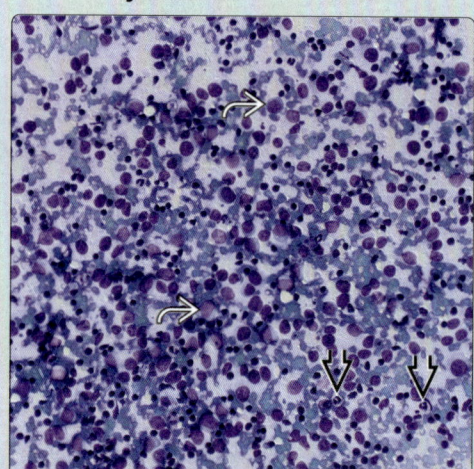

Primitive Malignant Cells

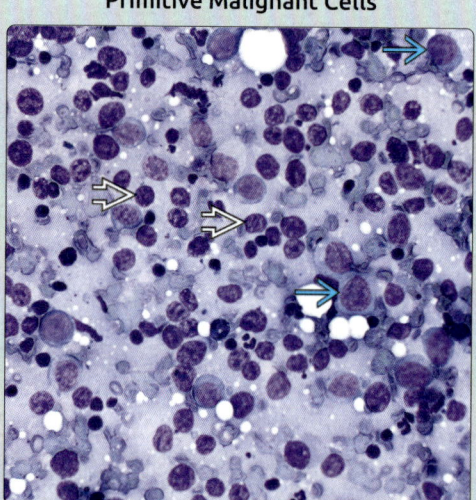

(Left) At low power, this Diff-Quik-stained smear of a NUT carcinoma metastatic to a lymph node shows dyscohesive tumor cells with scant pale cytoplasm ➡. Also note the presence of acute inflammation ➡. (Courtesy P. Wakely, MD.) (Right) At higher power, the same NUT carcinoma shows primitive oval to round nuclei with clumpy chromatin ➡. Note that the tumor cells are quite a bit larger than the background lymphocytes ➡. (Courtesy P. Wakely, MD.)

Frequent Mitosis

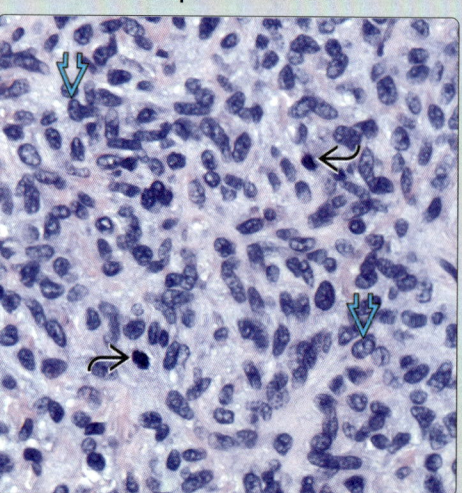

NUT Immunohistochemistry

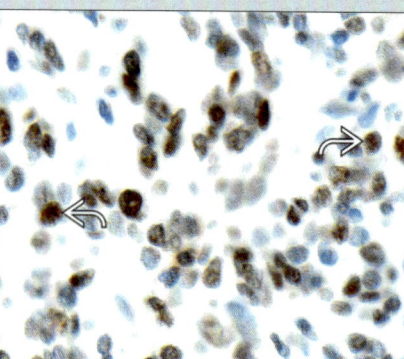

(Left) H&E-stained excision specimen shows a cellular tumor with ovoid monotonous nuclei and pale cytoplasm. Nucleoli are apparent ➡. No nuclear molding is seen. There is a high mitotic index ➡. (Right) NUT immunostain marks most of the tumor cell nuclei with a distinctive speckled pattern of inhomogeneous brown staining ➡. Nuclear positivity > 50% indicates a NUT-translocated tumor that can be confirmed by FISH or PCR.

SMARCA4-Deficient Undifferentiated Tumor

KEY FACTS

ETIOLOGY/PATHOGENESIS
- Poorly differentiated malignancy characterized by *SMARCA4* (BRG1) deficiency

CLINICAL ISSUES
- Strongly associated with smoking; mostly older men
- Most present at stage IV; poor prognosis

MICROSCOPIC
- Epithelioid loosely cohesive malignant cells
- Eccentric nuclei, usually monotonous but may be pleomorphic; vesicular chromatin and prominent nucleoli
- Rhabdoid cytoplasm may be seen; plasmacytoid and clear cell morphology may also be present
- High mitotic activity
- Various patterns in biopsies: Sheets, nodules, small, irregular nests
- May have fibrous or myxoid stroma
- Necrosis is common

ANCILLARY TESTS
- BRG1 loss detectable by immunochemistry
- Cytokeratins focal/weak (+), sometimes absent
- TTF-1, p40, claudin-4, SALL4, CD34 may be focally (+)
- Synaptophysin (+), sometimes strong/diffuse
- *SMARCA4* mutations can be detected by next-generation sequencing

TOP DIFFERENTIAL DIAGNOSES
- Non-small cell lung carcinoma
- Neuroendocrine carcinoma
- NUT carcinoma
- Mesothelioma
- Germ cell tumor
- Rhabdoid or epithelioid-appearing sarcoma or melanoma

DIAGNOSTIC CHECKLIST
- Consider BRG1/*SMARCA4* testing for undifferentiated thoracic tumors with weak or absent keratin staining

Undifferentiated Malignant Cells
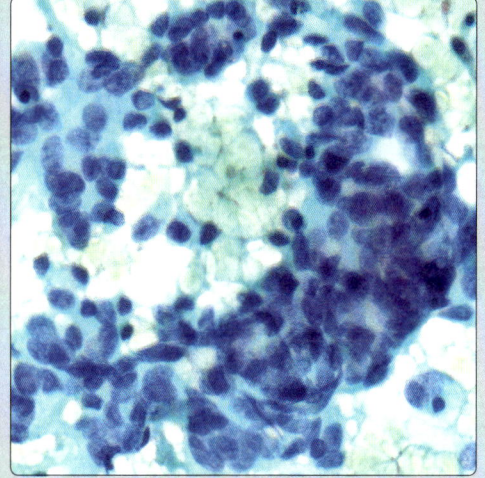

Prominent Nucleoli
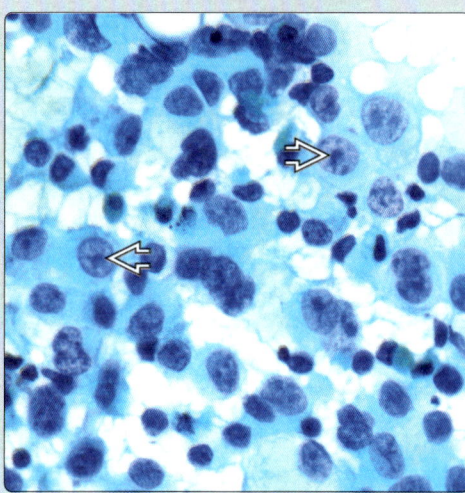

(Left) This Pap-stained FNA smear from a SMARCA4-deficient undifferentiated tumor (SD-UT) shows loosely cohesive tumor cells with surprisingly monotonous oval to round nuclei considering the primitive appearance of the cells. **(Right)** This Pap-stained example of SD-UT shows malignant cells with vesicular chromatin and prominent nucleoli ➨. The cytoplasm is voluminous and eccentric, imparting a vaguely plasmacytoid appearance.

Primitive-Appearing Cells
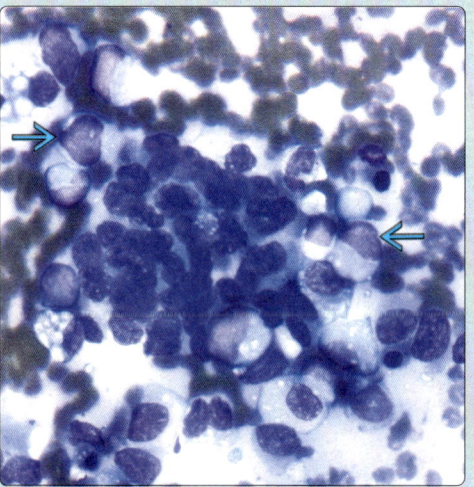

Rhabdoid Cells in Biopsy
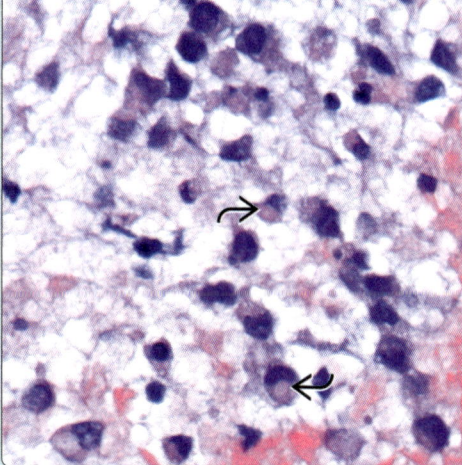

(Left) In this Diff-Quik stain of SD-UT, many of the malignant cells have a blast-like appearance with smooth chromatin ➨. Also note the eccentric, vacuolated cytoplasm. **(Right)** Disaggregated malignant cells from the edge of a small biopsy of SD-UT stained with H&E show focal rhabdoid morphology with prominent eosinophilic cytoplasmic inclusions ➨. This appearance should prompt consideration of this entity but may be absent or very focal.

Pulmonary Lymphoma

KEY FACTS

CLINICAL ISSUES
- Mucosa-associated lymphoid tissue (MALT) lymphoma accounts for most primary cases (70-80%)
  - Subtype of marginal zone B-cell lymphoma associated with chronic inflammation
- Diffuse large B-cell lymphoma may arise from MALT lymphoma or lymphomatoid granulomatosis
- Pulmonary lymphoma is often part of systemic disease
- Often mimics carcinoma radiologically and clinically

CYTOPATHOLOGY
- MALT lymphoma
  - Mixed population of lymphocytes resembling reactive proliferation
  - Monocytoid cells with prominent eccentric cytoplasm are present in many, but not all, cases
- Diffuse large B-cell lymphoma
  - Numerous large lymphocytes with polymorphous nuclei and scant cytoplasm
- Hodgkin lymphoma
  - Reed-Sternberg cells and variants with background mixed inflammatory cells

ANCILLARY TESTS
- Flow cytometry may be helpful to determine clonality and lineage in non-Hodgkin lymphomas

TOP DIFFERENTIAL DIAGNOSES
- Reactive lymphoid proliferations
  - Lymphocytic proliferation with prominent monocytoid cells should prompt consideration of MALT lymphoma
  - MALT lymphoma cannot be readily separated from reactive processes by cytology alone
  - Diagnosis of MALT lymphoma usually requires histology
  - Reed-Sternberg cells and many eosinophils aid in identification of Hodgkin lymphoma
- Small cell carcinoma
  - Large cell lymphomas may recapitulate many cytologic features of small cell carcinoma

Subtle Morphology of Mucosa-Associated Lymphoid Tissue Lymphoma

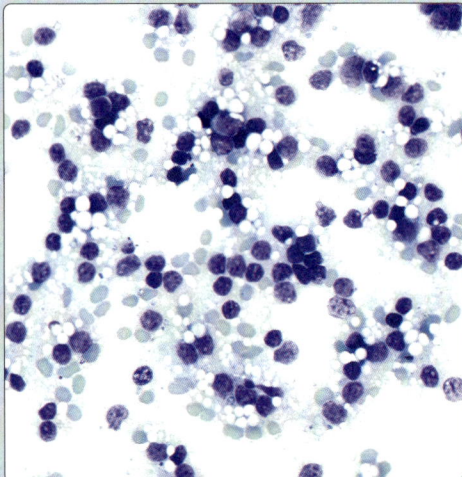

Monocytoid Cells in Mucosa-Associated Lymphoid Tissue Lymphoma

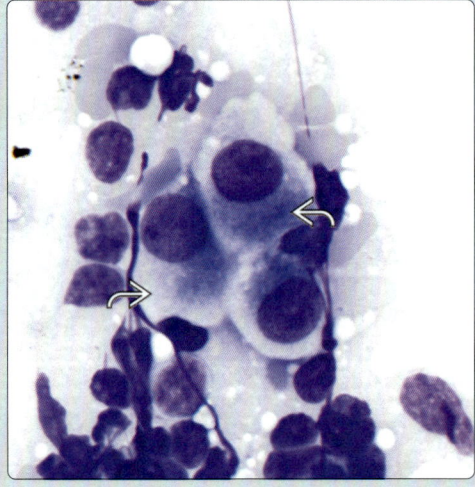

(Left) Low-power inspection of a Diff-Quik-stained pulmonary mucosa-associated lymphoid tissue (MALT) lymphoma shows a mixed population of lymphocytes not immediately suspicious for malignancy. **(Right)** Monocytoid cells ➡ with abundant cytoplasm, best appreciated on Diff-Quik stain, should raise suspicion of MALT lymphoma in the right clinical setting.

Diffuse Large B-Cell Lymphoma With Features Resembling Small Cell Carcinoma

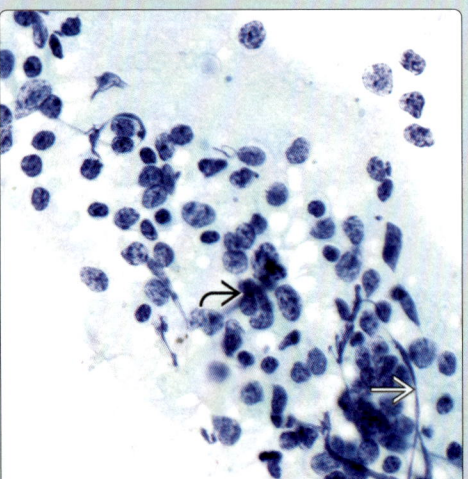

Prominent Nucleoli in Diffuse Large B-Cell Lymphoma Immunoblastic Cells

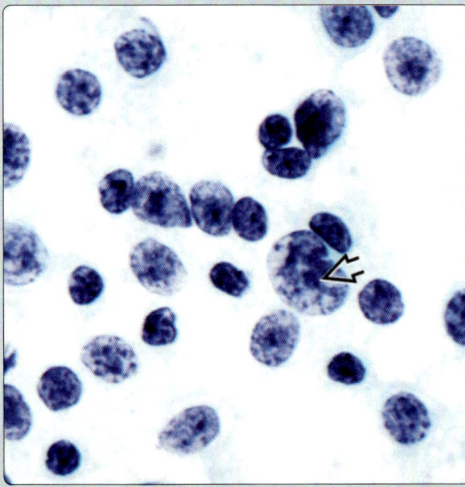

(Left) Diffuse large B-cell lymphoma consists of obviously malignant lymphocytes, as shown here on Pap stain. Molding ➡ and crush artifacts ➡ may be seen. **(Right)** Higher power examination with Pap stain shows prominent immunoblastic nucleoli ➡ that aid in differentiation from small cell carcinoma.

Pulmonary Lymphoma

CLINICAL ISSUES

Epidemiology
- Mucosa-associated lymphoid tissue (MALT) lymphoma accounts for most primary cases
  - Subtype of marginal zone B-cell lymphoma
  - Associated with chronic inflammation
  - Rare; < 1% of all lymphomas
  - a.k.a. bronchus-associated (BALT) lymphoma
- Diffuse large B-cell lymphoma
  - May evolve from MALT lymphoma or lymphomatoid granulomatosis, which is Epstein-Barr virus-driven lymphoproliferative disorder
  - Often part of systemic disease
- Others, including Hodgkin lymphoma, are usually component of systemic disease but can be primary

CYTOPATHOLOGY

Mucosa-Associated Lymphoid Tissue Lymphoma
- Mixed population of lymphocytes resembling reactive proliferation
  - Centrocytic, intermediate-sized lymphocytes with mild nuclear irregularities mixed with both small and large lymphocytes
- Monocytoid cells present in many, but not all, cases
  - Prominent eccentric cytoplasm on intermediate-sized lymphocytes
- Tingible body macrophages and plasma cells may be present

Diffuse Large B-Cell Lymphoma
- Numerous large lymphocytes with polymorphous nuclei and scant cytoplasm

Hodgkin Lymphoma
- Reed-Sternberg cells and variants with large irregular or multiple nuclei containing very prominent nucleoli
- Background mixed inflammatory cells, including prominent eosinophils

MICROSCOPIC

Histologic Features
- MALT lymphoma forms nodules concentrated around lymphatic channels with lymphoepithelial lesions
- Diffuse large B-cell lymphoma arising from lymphomatoid granulomatosis may show prominent angiodestructive infiltrates

ANCILLARY TESTS

Flow Cytometry
- May be helpful to determine clonality and lineage in non-Hodgkin lymphomas
- Can also aid in distinguishing large cell lymphoma from small cell carcinoma

DIFFERENTIAL DIAGNOSIS

Reactive Lymphoid Proliferations
- MALT lymphoma cannot be readily separated from reactive processes by cytology alone

Small Cell Carcinoma
- Large cell lymphomas may recapitulate many cytologic features of small cell carcinoma

DIAGNOSTIC CHECKLIST

Pathologic Interpretation Pearls
- Diagnosis of MALT lymphoma usually requires histology
- Lymphocytic proliferation with prominent monocytoid cells should prompt consideration of MALT lymphoma
- Large cell lymphoma and small cell carcinoma may appear similar but have distinctive immunoprofiles

SELECTED REFERENCES
1. He H et al: Clinicopathological characteristics and prognostic factors of primary pulmonary lymphoma. J Thorac Dis. 13(2):1106-17, 2021
2. Zhang MC et al: Clinical features and outcomes of pulmonary lymphoma: a single center experience of 180 cases. Lung Cancer. 132:39-44, 2019

Hodgkin Lymphoma
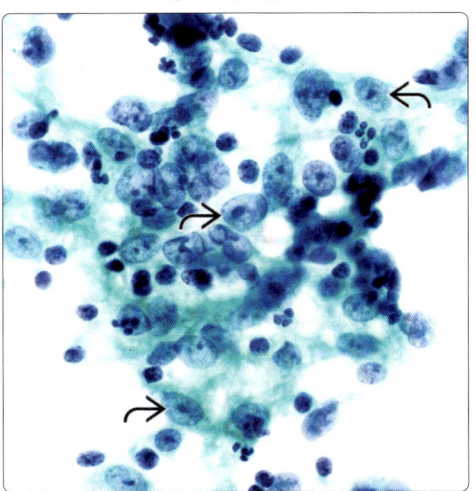

Reed-Sternberg Cell
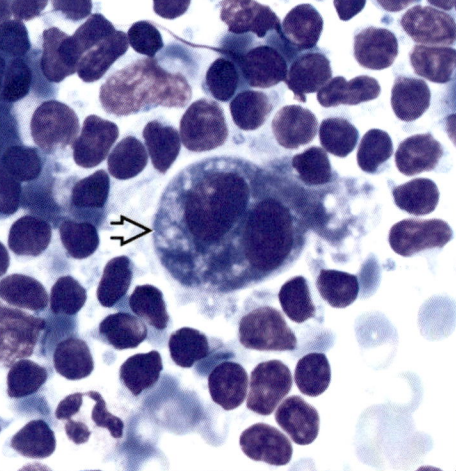

(Left) In this example of Hodgkin lymphoma involving the lung, numerous Reed-Sternberg variant cells ⇨ can be seen on Pap stain. *(Right)* In some cases of Hodgkin lymphoma, the presence of occasional classic Reed-Sternberg cells ⇨ in a mixed inflammatory background, as shown here on Diff-Quik stain, may be the only clue to diagnosis.

Pulmonary Metastasis

KEY FACTS

CLINICAL ISSUES
- Lung is one of most frequent sites of metastasis
- Metastases are most often of lung, breast, or gastrointestinal origin
- Multiple discrete tumors on radiology raises likelihood of metastasis
- History is critically important for correct diagnosis

CYTOPATHOLOGY
- Malignant cells have same morphology as originating tumor sites unless dedifferentiated
- Morphologic comparison with previous specimens from other sites is of great value
- Typically high cellularity
- Necrosis and debris are common

ANCILLARY TESTS
- Immunocytochemistry panels may aid in determining origin but must be interpreted with caution
- "Tissue of origin" or other gene panel molecular testing may be helpful in difficult cases

TOP DIFFERENTIAL DIAGNOSES
- Poorly differentiated primary vs. metastasis
  - Distinctive morphologic and immunocytochemical features may be lacking
- Primary vs. metastatic adenocarcinoma
  - Primary lung tumors may have enteric, mucinous, or signet-ring morphologies similar to metastases
  - Lung adenocarcinoma may express enteric markers typically associated with gastrointestinal origin
- Primary vs. metastatic squamous cell carcinoma
  - Lung squamous cell carcinomas lack distinctive features
  - HPV testing may be helpful to rule out some anogenital or head and neck primary sites
- Primary vs. metastatic neuroendocrine carcinoma
  - TTF-1 is often expressed in small cell carcinomas of extrapulmonary sites

Breast Carcinoma
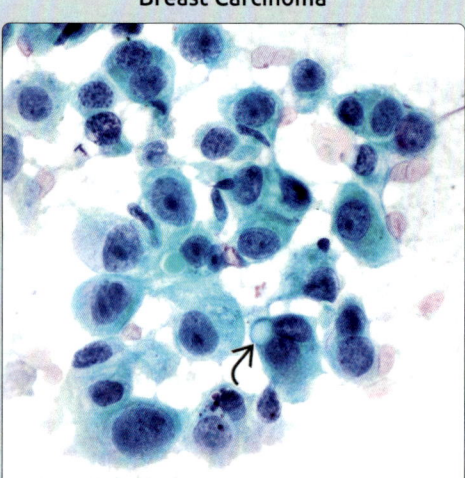

Colonic Adenocarcinoma
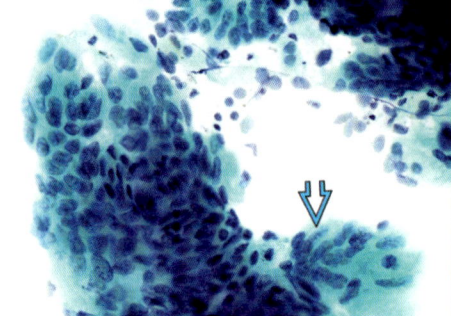

(Left) *In some instances, such as this Pap-stained metastatic breast carcinoma, distinctive features, such as dyscohesion and intracytoplasmic inclusions ⇨, may aid in correct identification.* **(Right)** *Colonic adenocarcinoma has a distinctive columnar morphology ⇨, seen here on Pap stain, but primary lung carcinoma with enteric differentiation could look the same as this metastasis and have the same immunocytochemistry profile.*

Pancreatic Adenocarcinoma
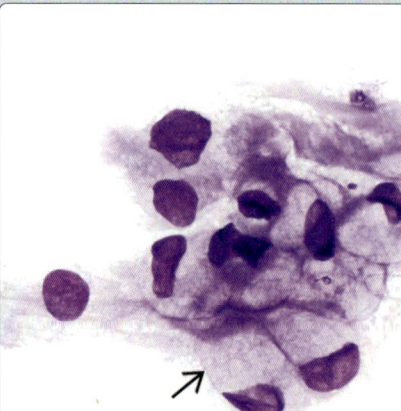

Melanoma
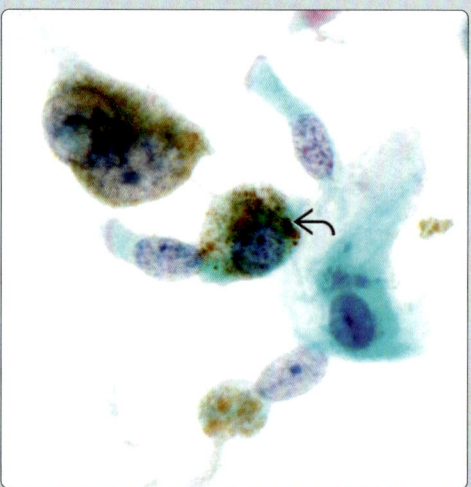

(Left) *Prominent mucin vacuoles ⇨, seen here on a Diff-Quik stain of metastatic pancreas carcinoma, may also be seen in primary mucinous lung carcinoma, making differentiation difficult.* **(Right)** *Melanoma is the most common noncarcinomatous metastatic tumor in the lung. Here, melanin production ⇨ is easily seen on Pap stain, but this helpful feature is usually absent.*

Pulmonary Metastasis

CLINICAL ISSUES

Presentation
- Awareness of presence of other prior or synchronous tumors is key

Natural History
- Lung is one of most frequent sites of metastasis
- Metastases are most often of lung, breast, or gastrointestinal origin

CYTOPATHOLOGY

Cellularity
- Typically high cellularity

Background
- Necrosis and debris are common in metastases

Cells
- Malignant cells have same morphology as originating tumor sites unless dedifferentiated

Cytology-Histology Correlation
- Morphologic comparison with previous specimens from other sites is of great value

MACROSCOPIC

General Features
- Presence of multiple discrete tumors raises question of metastasis

ANCILLARY TESTS

Immunohistochemistry
- Panels frequently aid in determining origin but are often not helpful or even confusing

Molecular Testing
- "Tissue of origin" or other gene panel molecular tests may be last resort in difficult cases

DIFFERENTIAL DIAGNOSIS

Poorly Differentiated Primary vs. Metastasis
- Distinctive morphologic and immunocytochemical features may be lacking

Primary vs. Metastatic Adenocarcinoma
- Primary lung tumors may have enteric, mucinous, or signet-ring morphologies similar to metastases
- Lung adenocarcinoma may express markers typically associated with gastrointestinal origin, such as CK20 and CDX2

Primary vs. Metastatic Squamous Cell Carcinoma
- Lung squamous cell carcinomas lack distinctive features
- HPV testing may be helpful to rule out some anogenital or head and neck primary sites

Primary vs. Metastatic Neuroendocrine Carcinoma
- TTF-1 is often expressed in small cell carcinomas of extrapulmonary sites

Papillary Carcinoma of Primary vs. Metastatic Origin
- Thyroid papillary carcinoma expresses TTF-1, but thyroglobulin can differentiate

Clear Cell Carcinoma of Primary vs. Metastatic Origin
- Renal cell carcinoma may express napsin A, but TTF-1 should be negative, and PAX8 should be positive

Lung Primary Carcinoma vs. Metastasis From Another Lung Tumor
- Intrapulmonary metastasis is common

Metastatic Melanoma or Sarcoma vs. Primary Origin
- Melanoma and many sarcomas may rarely originate in lung

SELECTED REFERENCES

1. Lee HW et al: Non-small cell carcinoma-not otherwise specified on cytology specimens in patients with solitary pulmonary lesion: primary lung cancer or metastatic cancer? J Cytol. 38(1):8-13, 2021
2. Vidarsdottir H et al: Immunohistochemical profiles in primary lung cancers and epithelial pulmonary metastases. Hum Pathol. 84:221-30, 2019

Urothelial Carcinoma

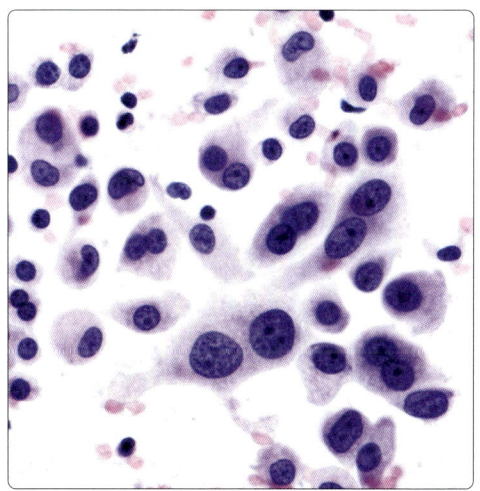

Prostatic Adenocarcinoma

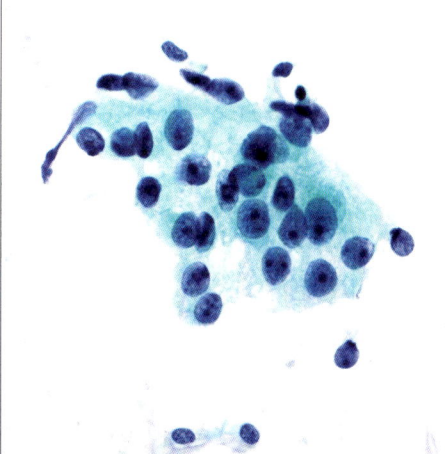

(Left) Many metastatic carcinomas, such as this urothelial carcinoma with squamoid morphology on Diff-Quik stain, may mimic primary tumors. Knowledge of previous malignancy or radiologically identified masses in other organs is key. (Right) Metastases, such as this Pap-stained prostatic carcinoma, may be extremely bland and difficult to identify as malignant without a thorough awareness of the history.

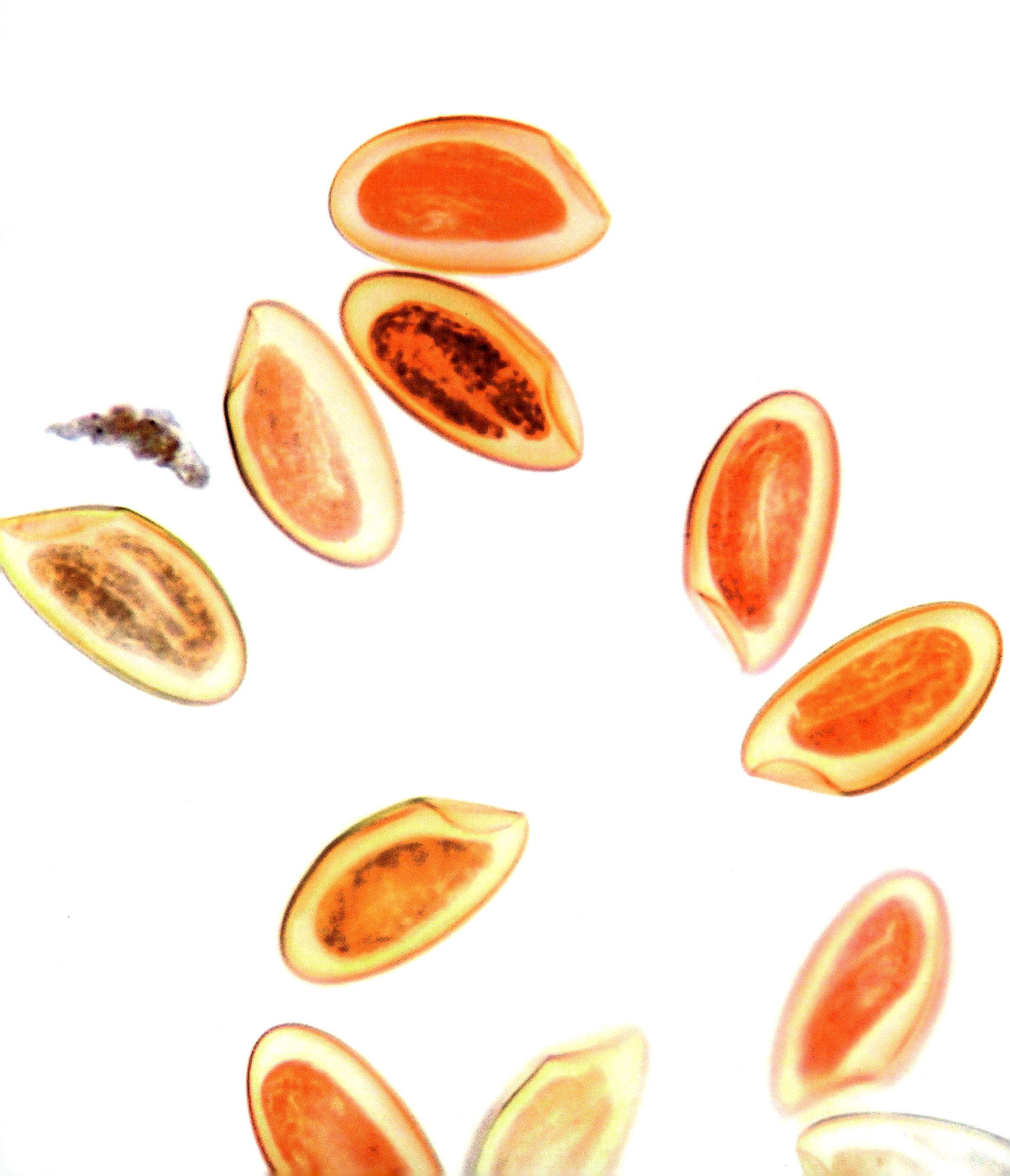

PART II
SECTION 2
Gastrointestinal Tract

Specimen Types in Gastrointestinal Cytology and Normal Cellular Components	146
Parasitic Infections	148
Viral Infections	150
Esophagitis and Barrett Esophagus	152
Esophageal Adenocarcinoma	154
Esophageal Squamous Cell Carcinoma	156
Gastritis and Intestinal Metaplasia	158
Gastric Adenocarcinoma	160
Gastric Lymphoma	162
Ampulla/Bile Duct/Pancreatic Duct Reactive Changes	164
Ampulla/Bile Duct/Pancreatic Duct Adenocarcinoma	166
Colorectal Adenoma/Carcinoma	168
Neuroendocrine Tumor/Carcinoma	170
Spindle Cell Neoplasms of Gastrointestinal Tract, Including Gastrointestinal Stromal Tumors	172

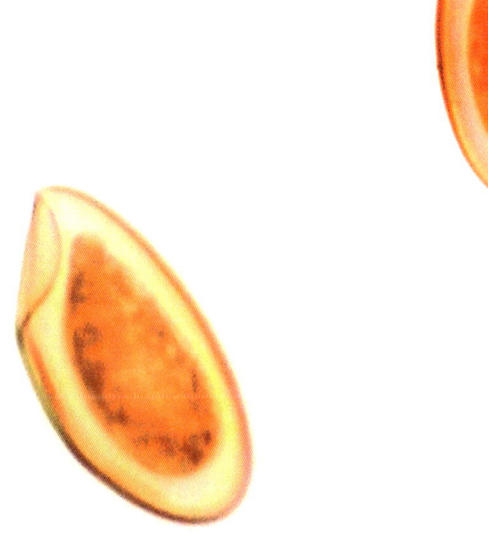
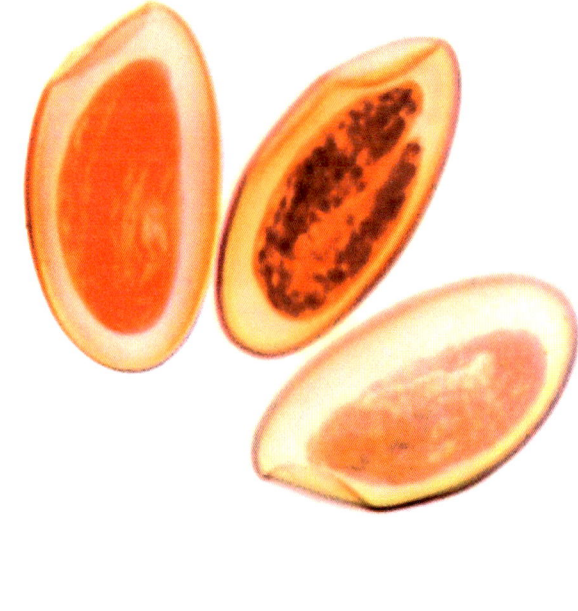

Specimen Types in Gastrointestinal Cytology and Normal Cellular Components

GASTROINTESTINAL CYTOLOGY

Clinical Indications

- Can be performed at time of endoscopy and complements tissue biopsy
- Benefits of cytologic sampling include
  - Less artifactual distortion of specimen
    - Cytologic samples are not subject to crush artifact (frequently occurs in small endoscopic biopsies)
    - Lesions composed of fragile cells (lymphoma, small cell carcinoma) may be better preserved in cytologic sample than in tissue biopsy
  - Less invasive procedure than tissue biopsy
  - Samples more surface area than tissue biopsy
  - Can sample lesions in deep/challenging locations or when bleeding due to ulcer or other reasons
- Cytology is preferred sampling method in some instances (diagnosis of candidal esophagitis, investigation of bile duct strictures, sampling of submucosal/intramural lesions)

TYPES OF GASTROINTESTINAL SPECIMENS

Brushing

- Taken at time of endoscopy
- Benefits
  - Samples wider surface area than tissue biopsy
  - Safer for patients with high risk of bleeding
  - More sensitive for detection of infectious agents than biopsy
  - Brushes can be used to sample stenotic lesions or lesions in areas that biopsy forceps cannot easily traverse (i.e., bile ducts)
  - Samples are amenable to processing using liquid-based preparations
- Limitations
  - Cannot sample predominantly infiltrative or submucosal/intramural lesions unless ulcerated
  - Difficult or impossible to diagnose invasion in malignancy

Washing

- Can be taken at time of endoscopy

Normal Esophageal Squamous Cells

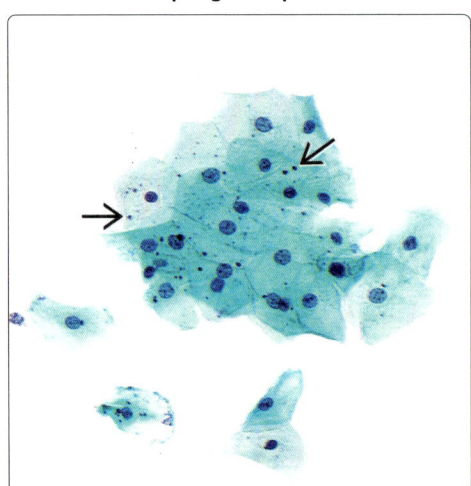

Normal Gastric Body Epithelium

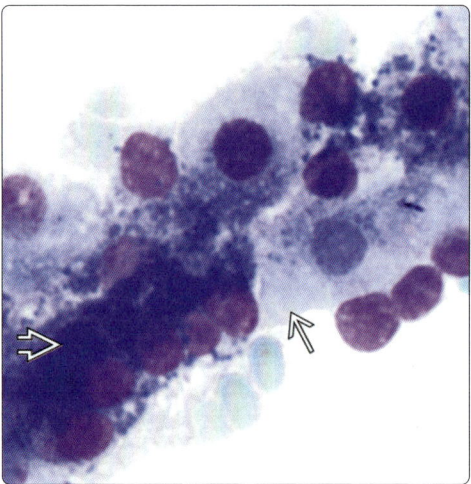

(Left) Pap-stained esophageal brushing shows normal superficial squamous epithelial cells. Scattered keratohyaline granules ➡ may be present. (Right) Normal gastric body type of epithelium as seen on Diff-Quik stain may be inadvertently aspirated during endoscopic ultrasound-guided FNA (EUS FNA) of pancreatic body and tail masses. The chief cells ➡ have a lighter clear cytoplasm compared to the darker purple granular cytoplasm of parietal cells ➡.

Normal Gastric Foveolar Epithelium

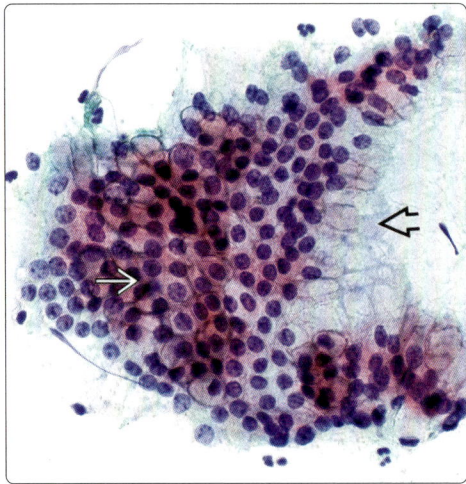

Common Bile Duct Epithelium

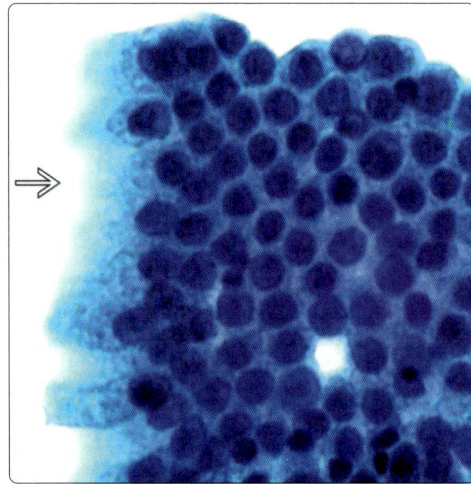

(Left) Pap stain of gastric brushing shows a sheet of benign foveolar cells with evenly spaced nuclei and apical mucin caps ➡. When en face, the epithelium has a uniform honeycomb distribution of nuclei ➡. (Right) Normal bile duct epithelium in a honeycomb pattern with distinct nuclei separated by an equal amount of spacing between cells is shown. The surface epithelium ➡ has low nuclear:cytoplasmic (N:C) ratios and abundant cytoplasm without any goblet cells or large mucin vacuoles.

Specimen Types in Gastrointestinal Cytology and Normal Cellular Components

- Benefits
  - Samples wide surface area
  - Can be used to sample stenotic lesions
  - Safer for patients with high risk of bleeding
- Limitations
  - Less useful for targeting discrete lesions
  - Cannot sample predominantly infiltrative or submucosal/intramural lesions unless ulcerated
  - Difficult or impossible to diagnose invasion in malignancy

Endoscopic Ultrasound-Guided FNA

- Benefits
  - Samples submucosal/intramural lesions often missed by forceps biopsy and brushing
  - Endoscopic ultrasound (EUS) is also used to assess depth of invasion of lesion (preoperative staging)
  - Immediate adequacy assessment results in fewer nondiagnostic samples and allows for appropriate specimen triage
    - Immediate feedback to endoscopist regarding quality of sample and need for additional passes
    - Material can be triaged for flow cytometry, cell block, or other ancillary studies
    - Can visualize lesion and needle in real time
- Limitations
  - Success of procedure is operator dependent
  - Familiarity with normal gastrointestinal tract contaminants important

NORMAL CELLULAR COMPONENTS

Esophagus

- Squamous epithelial cells
  - Small clusters and single cells
  - Intermediate squamous cells with slightly larger, paler nuclei and superficial squames with small, pyknotic nuclei; both have abundant cytoplasm with well-defined borders
- Glandular epithelial cells: From submucosal glands
  - Columnar cells with small, round basal nuclei and abundant foamy cytoplasm (usually not sampled)

Stomach

- Foveolar cells
  - Flat, orderly sheets of cells with evenly spaced nuclei or small strips of cells
  - Columnar cells with small, round, basally oriented nuclei with even chromatin, abundant foamy or vacuolated cytoplasm, and apical mucin cap
- Chief cells
  - Arranged in small, loose clusters or singly
  - Polygonal cells with small, round nuclei with even chromatin and granular basophilic cytoplasm (zymogen granules)
- Parietal cells
  - Arranged in small, loose clusters or singly
  - Pyramidal shape, larger nuclei, ± nucleoli, coarser chromatin, granular eosinophilic cytoplasm

Small Intestine and Colorectum

- Absorptive cells
  - Exfoliate in large, flat, well-defined, orderly sheets of cells with evenly spaced nuclei
  - Columnar cells with small, round, basally oriented nuclei with smooth chromatin, ± small nucleoli
    - Eosinophilic granular cytoplasm
    - Apical cytoplasmic density
- Goblet cells
  - Scattered among enterocytes; small basal nuclei with large cytoplasmic mucin vacuole

Pancreatic and Bile Ducts

- Ductal epithelial cells
  - Exfoliate in flat, orderly sheets with evenly spaced nuclei; rarely single cells
  - Columnar to cuboidal cells, basally oriented round nuclei with smooth chromatin, ± small nucleoli, foamy, vacuolated cytoplasm; ± goblet cells

SELECTED REFERENCES

1. Rana A et al: Endoscopic ultrasound-guided tissue acquisition: techniques and challenges. J Cytol. 36(1):1-7, 2019

Normal Duodenum

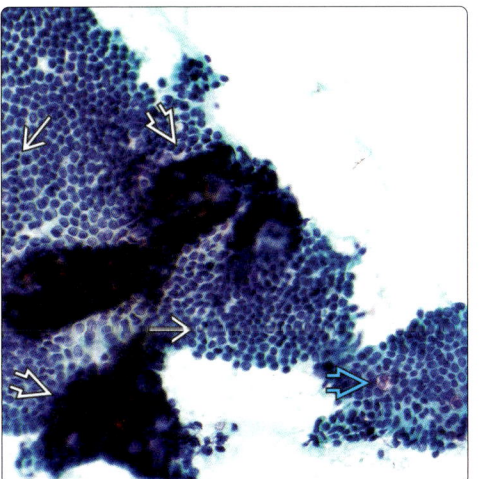

Intestinal Cells With Striated Border

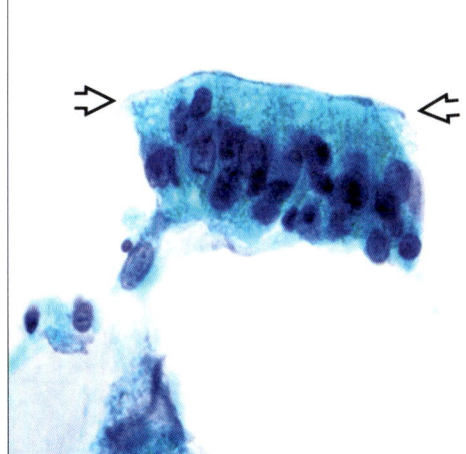

(Left) Pap-stained duodenal brushing shows a large cohesive sheet of enterocytes. Scattered goblet cells ⇨ are present. Rare intraepithelial lymphocytes ➔ may also be seen. Occasionally, intact or fragmented tubular glands ⇨ are identified. *(Right)* Pap-stained brushing shows a single strip of intestinal absorptive cells. The apical microvilli appear as a striated border ⇨.

Parasitic Infections

KEY FACTS

TERMINOLOGY

- *Giardia lamblia* (a.k.a. *Giardia duodenalis* or *Giardia intestinalis*): Protozoan, causes disease worldwide
  o Trophozoites found in duodenum
- *Strongyloides stercoralis*: Nematode, endemic to southeastern USA
  o Mature female organisms live within duodenal mucosa
  o In autoinfection, adult forms may invade bowel wall and perianal skin
- *Cryptosporidium* species: Protozoans; oocysts found in apical aspect of glandular epithelial cells of stomach, small and large bowel, and biliary tract
- *Entamoeba histolytica*: Ameba, usually contracted through contaminated water
- *Mycobacterium avium-intracellulare* (MAI): Atypical mycobacteria, ubiquitous in environment
- *Enterobius vermicularis* (a.k.a. pinworm): Nematode, most common helminth infectious organism in children in USA
  o Adult forms live in cecum and adjacent territory; eggs are deposited on perianal skin

CYTOPATHOLOGY

- *Giardia*: Pear-shaped trophozoites, 10-15 μm, binucleate; seen in endoscopic FNA or anal Pap specimens
  o *Giardia* cysts (11-12 μm, 4 nuclei, longitudinal fibrils) may also be seen on anal Pap
- *Strongyloides*: 2-3 mm, pointed tail, short buccal cavity; seen in respiratory specimens and anal Pap
- *Cryptosporidium*: Round, basophilic oocysts, 2-4 μm; GMS(+); acid fast; focus on apical aspect of cell to see
- *Entamoeba histolytica*: 60-100 μm; invasive forms ingest red blood cells; PAS(+)
- MAI: Pale, foamy macrophages full of organisms that appear as negative images on Diff-Quik; acid fast, PAS (+)
- *E. vermicularis*: Oblong egg (20 x 60 μm), flattened side, may be embryonated; rarely seen on Pap test

---

Giardia in Bile Duct Brushing

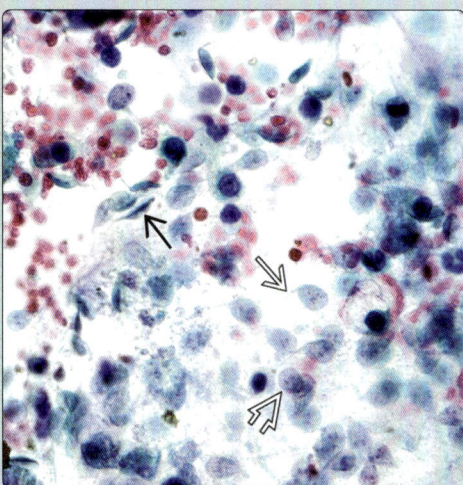

Giardia on Diff-Quik

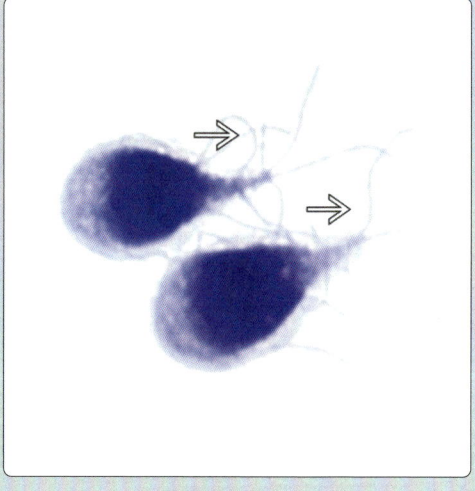

(Left) Pap-stained bile duct brushing with swarms of Giardia shows organisms on the edge ➡ with a crescentic appearance. Note the pear-shaped organisms with double nuclei ➡ and flagella ➡. (Right) This Diff-Quik-stained cytospin was prepared from formalin after the biopsies were removed. Note pear-shaped Giardia organisms with multiple flagella ➡. The nuclei may be difficult to see on Diff-Quik compared to a Pap stain.

Strongyloides

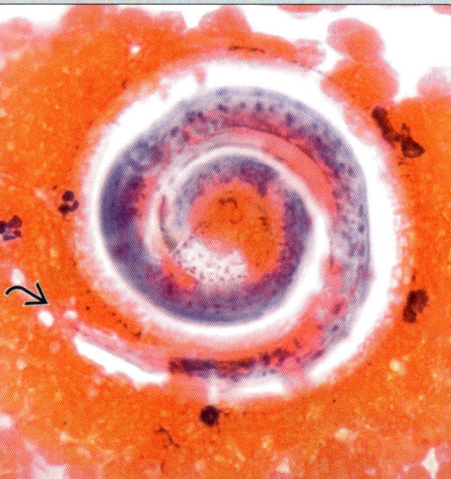

Enterobius vermicularis

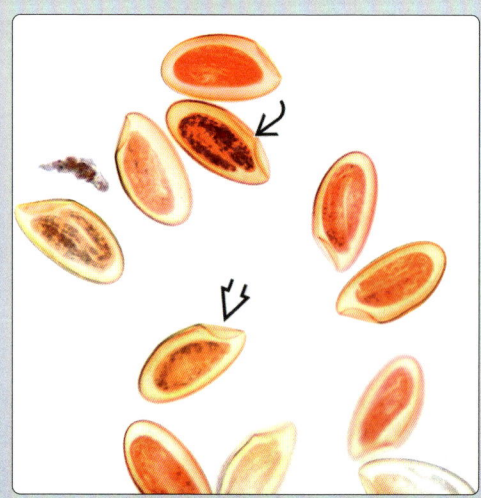

(Left) This Gram-stained colon washing shows a single Strongyloides larva. Note the characteristic pointed tail ➡. In some instances, especially if degenerating, the organisms may not stain well; it is important to consider that organisms may appear only as negative images. (Right) A conventional Pap test shows several eggs of Enterobius vermicularis. The oblong shape with 1 flattened side ➡ is characteristic. Some of the eggs are embryonated ➡.

Parasitic Infections

TERMINOLOGY

Definitions
- *Giardia lamblia* (a.k.a. *G. duodenalis* or *G. intestinalis*): Protozoan, causes disease worldwide
- *Strongyloides stercoralis*: Nematode, endemic to southeastern USA
- *Cryptosporidium* species: Protozoans; oocysts found in apical aspect of epithelial cells of stomach, small and large bowel, and biliary tract
- *Entamoeba histolytica*: Ameba, usually contracted via contaminated water
- *Mycobacterium avium-intracellulare* (MAI): Atypical mycobacteria, ubiquitous in environment
- *Enterobius vermicularis* (a.k.a. pinworm): Nematode, most common helminth infection in children in USA

ETIOLOGY/PATHOGENESIS

Infectious Agents
- *Giardia*: Trophozoites are infectious
- *Strongyloides*: Filariform larvae are infectious
- *Cryptosporidium*: *C. parvum* and *C. hominis* oocysts are infectious
- *E. histolytica*: Mature cysts are infectious
- MAI: Infects macrophages
- *E. vermicularis*: Egg is infective shortly after deposition

CYTOPATHOLOGY

Background
- *Giardia*: Pear-shaped trophozoites (10-15 µm) with 8 flagella, binucleate, prominent chromocenters
  - May be found incidentally on specimens from endoscopic FNA or on anal Pap tests
  - *Giardia* cysts (oval, 11-12 µm, 4 nuclei; longitudinal fibrils within cyst) may be seen on anal Pap test
- *Strongyloides*: Relatively large (2-3 mm), tail tapers to sharp point, short buccal cavity
  - May also appear in respiratory specimens and anal Pap tests
- *Cryptosporidium*: Round basophilic oocysts (2-4 µm) located in apical surface of GI epithelial cells; visible on Pap and Diff-Quik stains; GMS(+); acid fast on modified Kinyoun stain
  - Focus on plane with most apical aspect of cell
- *E. histolytica*: 60- to 100-µm trophozoites; look for ingested red blood cells in invasive forms; PAS(+)
- MAI: Rarely seen on brushings; pale, foamy macrophages stuffed with organisms; touch imprint cytology of tissue has been used in past
  - Appear as negative images on Diff-Quik within and outside of macrophages; acid fast, PAS (+)
- *E. vermicularis*: 20 x 60 µm, double-walled, oblong eggs, flattened on 1 side, may be embryonated; adult forms are larger (~ 1 cm); females have pointed posterior end

DIFFERENTIAL DIAGNOSIS

Giardia
- *Trichomonas*: Has only 1 nucleus, eosinophilic cytoplasmic granules; consider source

Strongyloides
- Hookworms (*Necator, Ancylostoma*): Longer buccal chamber, smaller genital primordium

Cryptosporidium
- Other coccidian protozoans (*Isospora, Cyclospora*)

E. histolytica
- Other amebae (*Escherichia coli, Dientamoeba fragilis*): Only invasive forms of *E. histolytica* will ingest red blood cells

MAI
- Other mycobacteria; *Tropheryma whipplei*

E. vermicularis
- *Trichuris trichiura*: Similar size egg, but has polar plugs
- Pollen: Lacks worm embryo

SELECTED REFERENCES
1. Terra SBSP et al: Incidental Giardia duodenalis cysts in exfoliative anal cytology: an immunocompetent adult female with prior squamous dysplasia. Diagn Cytopathol. 48(11):1141-3, 2020

Mycobacterium avium-intracellulare
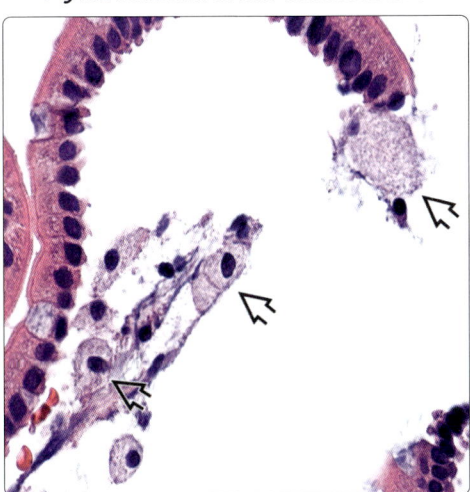

Mycobacterium avium-intracellulare on Acid-Fast Stain
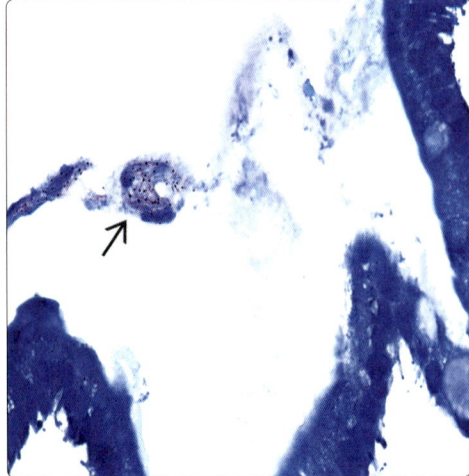

(Left) H&E-stained section shows a strip of benign epithelium and several macrophages with abundant pale cytoplasm due to intracellular organisms ⇨. (Right) Kinyoun stain highlights Mycobacterium avium-intracellulare within a macrophage ⇨.

Viral Infections

KEY FACTS

CLINICAL ISSUES
- Clinical history of immunosuppression; ulceration seen on endoscopy
- Symptoms vary with immune status of patient
- HSV esophagitis: Odynophagia, dysphagia, chest pain, fever; multiple discrete shallow ulcers in middistal esophagus
- CMV esophagitis: Odynophagia, dysphagia, multifocal erosion, or discrete ulceration
- HPV: Squamous papilloma, usually asymptomatic unless very large
- Adenovirus (AdV) gastritis, colitis: Epigastric pain, diarrhea, mucosal erosion/ulcer

CYTOPATHOLOGY
- HSV: Margination of chromatin, multinucleation, molding of nuclei; beware mononuclear infected cells
- CMV: Large infected cells with owl's eye inclusion may be exceedingly rare
- AdV: Amphophilic intranuclear inclusion, may be mistaken for CMV
- If liquid-based preparation is hypocellular, or if there is obscuring mucus or necrosis, consider making cytospins to better visualize cells of interest
- Differential diagnostic considerations
  - Chemotherapy, radiation, or ulcer may mimic viral changes
  - Cells with glycogenated nuclei or reactive changes may mimic koilocytes
  - HSV1, HSV2, and varicella zoster are cytomorphologically indistinguishable
  - In esophageal brushing, cells with viral cytopathic effect may represent contamination from oropharyngeal lesion

ANCILLARY TESTS
- Immunohistochemical stains can be performed on cytospins, thin-layer preparations, or cell blocks
- Viral culture and PCR also available

Herpes Viral Cowdry Type B Inclusion
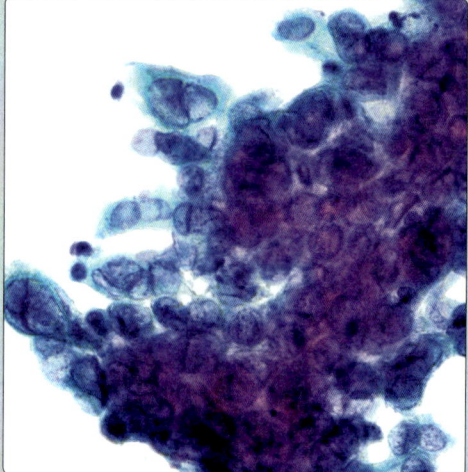

Herpes Viral Cytopathic Effect
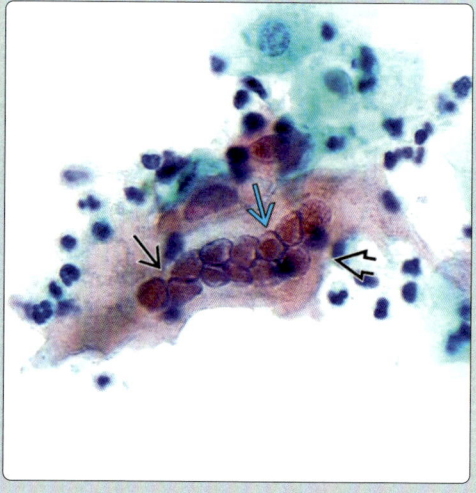

(Left) A large cluster of cells shows classic herpes simplex virus (HSV) viral cytopathic effect, the Cowdry type B nuclear inclusion. (Right) This Pap-stained esophageal brushing shows an HSV-infected squamous cell with the characteristic "3 Ms" of herpes viral cytopathic effect: Molding ⇨, multinucleation ⇨, and margination of chromatin ⇨.

Herpes Viral Cowdry Type A Inclusions
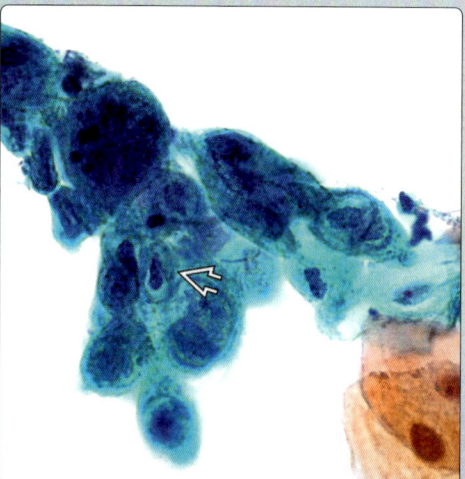

Cytomegalovirus Esophagitis
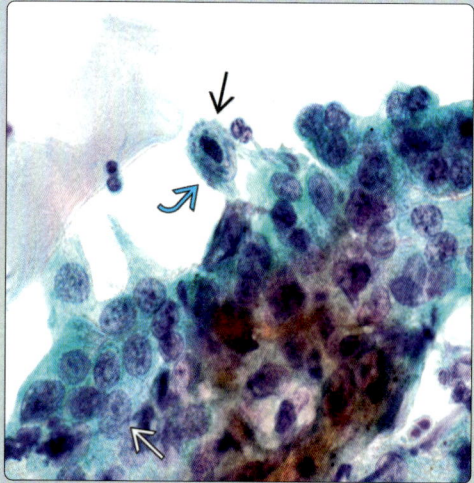

(Left) Herpesvirus-infected cells may also show Cowdry type A inclusions ⇨ similar to the inclusions seen in cytomegalovirus. (Right) Pap-stained esophageal brushing shows cytomegalovirus esophagitis. A single infected cell ⇨ has the characteristic intranuclear inclusion. Granular intracytoplasmic inclusions are also present ⇨. Background cells are benign with reactive features ⇨.

Viral Infections

TERMINOLOGY

Definitions
- Infection by herpes simplex virus (HSV)
  - Involves squamous epithelial cells
  - Most commonly seen in immunocompromised patients, but immunocompetent people may also be affected
- Infection by cytomegalovirus (CMV)
  - Can involve endothelial cells, fibroblasts, and glandular epithelium
- Infection by human papillomavirus (HPV)
  - Involves squamous epithelial cells
- Infection by adenovirus (AdV)
  - Involves glandular epithelial cells

CLINICAL ISSUES

Treatment
- HSV, CMV, AdV
  - Antiviral medications, supportive care

Prognosis
- Depends on immune status of patient

CYTOPATHOLOGY

Background
- HSV, CMV, AdV associated with ulceration: Acute inflammation, necrotic debris, and reactive cellular changes

Cells
- HSV has intranuclear inclusions only
  - "3 Ms": Molding of nuclei, margination of nuclear chromatin, and multinucleation
  - Mononuclear infected cells may also occur
  - Cowdry type B inclusions are most common with ground-glass nuclear change and margination of chromatin
  - Cowdry type A inclusions are also seen with dense inclusion surrounded by halo with margination of chromatin
- CMV has intranuclear and intracytoplasmic inclusions
  - Intranuclear inclusion: Cowdry type A; dense inclusion surrounded by halo (owl's eye)
  - Intracytoplasmic inclusions: Multiple, small, eosinophilic, and granular
  - Infected cells are very large (hence "megalovirus")
- HPV causes koilocytosis
- AdV has smudgy intranuclear inclusions, may be crescentic
  - Degenerative/reactive epithelial cells ± cytoplasmic vacuolization

ANCILLARY TESTS

Additional Diagnostic Modalities
- Immunocytochemistry, viral culture, PCR

DIFFERENTIAL DIAGNOSIS

Reactive Cytologic Atypia
- Chemotherapy, radiation, or ulcer may mimic viral changes
- Check for clinical history of radiotherapy &/or chemotherapy

Koilocytes
- Cells with glycogenated nuclei or reactive changes may mimic koilocytes

HSV1, HSV2, and Varicella-Zoster Virus
- Cytomorphologically indistinguishable

Oropharyngeal Lesions
- In esophageal brushing, cells with viral cytopathic effect may represent contamination from oropharyngeal lesion

SELECTED REFERENCES
1. Mostyka M et al: Clinicopathologic features of varicella zoster virus infection of the upper gastrointestinal tract. Am J Surg Pathol. 45(2):209-14, 2021
2. Hoversten P et al: Risk factors, endoscopic features, and clinical outcomes of cytomegalovirus esophagitis based on a 10-year analysis at a single center. Clin Gastroenterol Hepatol. 18(3):736-8, 2020
3. Hoversten P et al: Infections of the esophagus: an update on risk factors, diagnosis, and management. Dis Esophagus. 31(12), 2018

Cytomegalovirus Cytoplasmic Inclusions

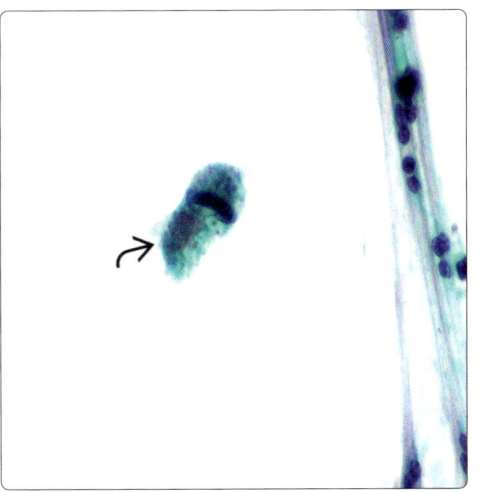

Human Papillomavirus Infection

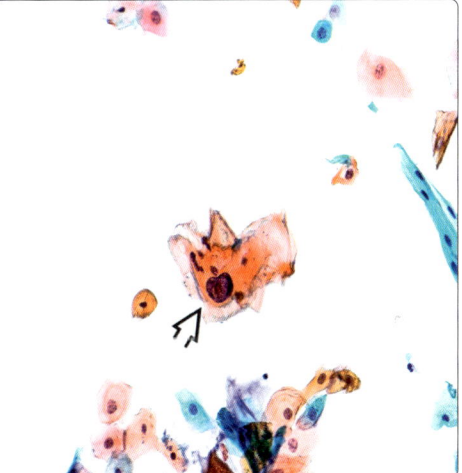

(Left) This cytomegalovirus-infected cell has prominent intracytoplasmic inclusions ➔ and the characteristic intranuclear inclusion, both easily visualized on Pap stain. *(Right)* A Pap-stained esophageal brushing with human papillomavirus effect is shown. This squamous cell has the large hyperchromatic nucleus ➔ characteristic of a koilocyte.

Esophagitis and Barrett Esophagus

KEY FACTS

CLINICAL ISSUES
- Endoscopic correlation is required
- Correlate with biopsy if available
  - Biopsy is usually preferred method of sampling

CYTOPATHOLOGY
- Barrett esophagus
  - True goblet cells: Mucin vacuoles ≥ 3x size of nucleus
  - Columnar cells: Delicate mucinous cytoplasm ± brush border (complete intestinal metaplasia)
  - Round to oval nuclei with smooth membranes, even chromatin, ± small nucleolus
  - Report presence or absence of dysplasia
- *Candida* esophagitis will show budding hyphae and yeast
- Viral esophagitis: Herpes most common with multinucleation, molding, and margination
- Reflux/erosive esophagitis shows large, flat, cohesive, orderly, streaming sheets of cells with well-defined borders
- Reactive atypia of epithelial cells may be marked; overlaps with low-grade dysplasia
  - Large nuclei, preserved N:C ratio
  - Even chromatin, smooth nuclear membranes, macronucleoli
  - Streaming of cell groups; flat with no 3D clusters
  - Inflammatory background ± necrosis
  - Mitotic figures but not atypical forms
  - Parabasal cells and reactive mesenchymal cells seen if ulcerated
  - No diffuse prominent atypia
  - No single intact atypical cells

TOP DIFFERENTIAL DIAGNOSES
- Normal foveolar epithelium: Look for true goblet cells; confirm sample is from area endoscopically compatible with Barrett esophagus
- Dysplasia: Look for 3D groups and individual cells with increased N:C ratio and coarse chromatin

Candida Esophagitis

Reflux Esophagitis: Reactive Changes

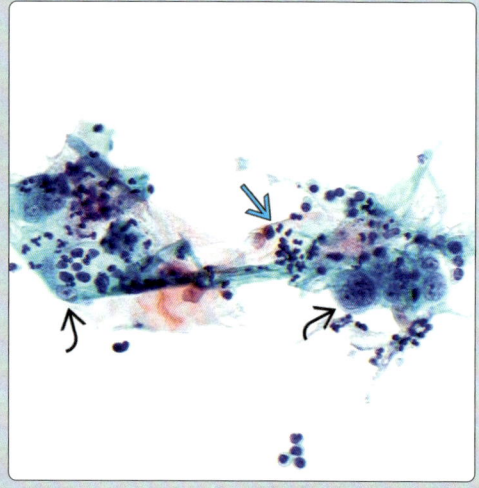

(Left) *Pap-stained esophageal brushing shows fungal yeast ➡ and pseudohyphae ➡ with reactive squamous cells ➡.* (Right) *This Pap-stained brushing of reflux esophagitis shows a spectrum of reactive changes. The nuclei are enlarged with prominent nucleoli ➡ but have round contours and relatively fine chromatin. Neutrophils ➡ are also present.*

Ulcerative Esophagitis

Ulcerative Esophagitis: Cell Block

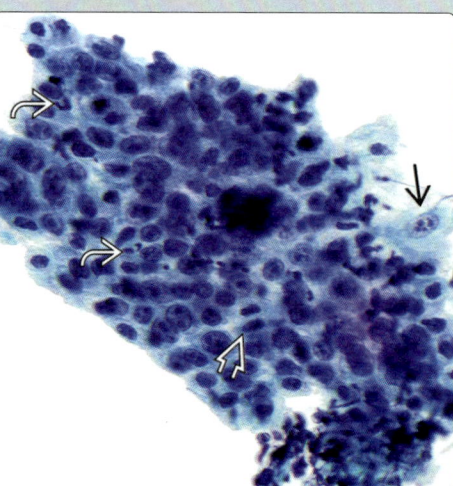
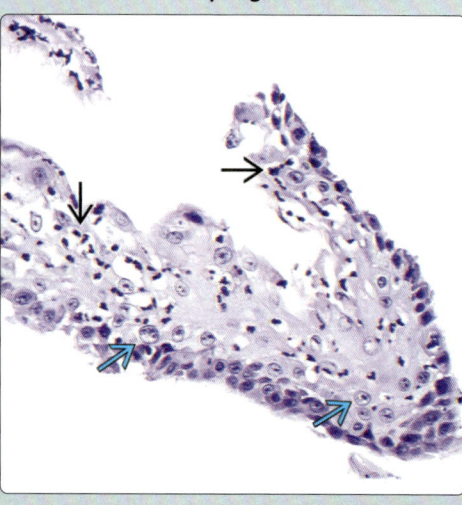

(Left) *Pap-stained brushing of an esophageal ulcer is shown. The cells are cohesive and arranged in a flat, streaming sheet. The nuclei are uniformly enlarged with prominent nucleoli ➡. There are scattered intraepithelial neutrophils ➡. Mitotic activity may be present ➡.* (Right) *H&E-stained cell block section from the same esophageal ulcer brushing is shown. The squamous cells have uniformly enlarged nuclei with prominent nucleoli and vesicular chromatin ➡. Intraepithelial neutrophils ➡ are easier to appreciate.*

Esophagitis and Barrett Esophagus

TERMINOLOGY

Definitions
- Barrett esophagus (BE): Clinicopathologic diagnosis
  - Columnar epithelium with goblet cells is found in area of BE (salmon-colored mucosa in tubular esophagus) on endoscopy
  - Goblet cells are required for diagnosis in USA

ETIOLOGY/PATHOGENESIS

Risk Factors
- BE: Gastroesophageal reflux disease (GERD), obesity, smoking, and alcohol
- Esophagitis: Reflux, infectious etiologies, and radiation therapy

CLINICAL ISSUES

Presentation
- Heartburn, dysphagia, cough; could be asymptomatic

Prognosis
- BE is precursor to esophageal adenocarcinoma
  - Estimated annual risk of progression: 0.5-1.0%

CYTOPATHOLOGY

Esophagitis
- Candidal esophagitis
  - Budding yeasts (10-12 μm), germ tubes, and pseudohyphae
- Viral esophagitis: Consider coinfections
- Reflux/erosive esophagitis
  - Large, flat, cohesive, orderly, streaming sheets of cells with well-defined borders
- Radiation/chemotherapy-related esophagitis
  - Karyomegaly with normal N:C ratio and polychromatic (2-tone) cytoplasm
  - Inflammatory/necrotic background, check for coexisting infection

Barrett Esophagus
- Medium to large, flat, cohesive, honeycomb sheets of columnar cells punctuated by goblet cells
  - Sheets of cells with sharp edges and cell polarity (basally oriented nucleus); uniform, evenly spaced nuclei without significant overlap
- Columnar cells: Delicate mucinous cytoplasm ± brush border (complete intestinal metaplasia); round to oval nuclei with smooth membranes, even chromatin, ± small nucleolus
- Goblet cells: Mucin vacuole ≥ 3x size of nucleus; nucleus compressed by vacuole
- Clean background unless esophagitis/ulceration is present with superimposed reactive atypia

DIFFERENTIAL DIAGNOSIS

Normal Foveolar Epithelium
- Look for true goblet cells; confirm sample is from area endoscopically compatible with BE

Barrett Esophagus With Dysplasia
- Cytology is not sensitive for detection of low-grade dysplasia in BE due to morphologic overlap with reactive atypia
- Small groups of less cohesive cells with loss of polarity
- Decreased cytoplasmic mucin; single atypical cells
- Elongated irregular nuclei, coarse chromatin
- Increased N:C ratio; pseudostratification

Recurrent Malignancy
- Many atypical cells with increased N:C ratio and hyperchromasia; if only rare atypical cells with near normal N:C ratio, favor radiation esophagitis

SELECTED REFERENCES

1. Pilonis ND et al: Use of a Cytosponge biomarker panel to prioritise endoscopic Barrett's oesophagus surveillance: a cross-sectional study followed by a real-world prospective pilot. Lancet Oncol. 23(2):270-278, 2022
2. Mohamed AA et al: Diagnosis and treatment of esophageal candidiasis: current updates. Can J Gastroenterol Hepatol. 2019:3585136, 2019

Barrett Esophagus

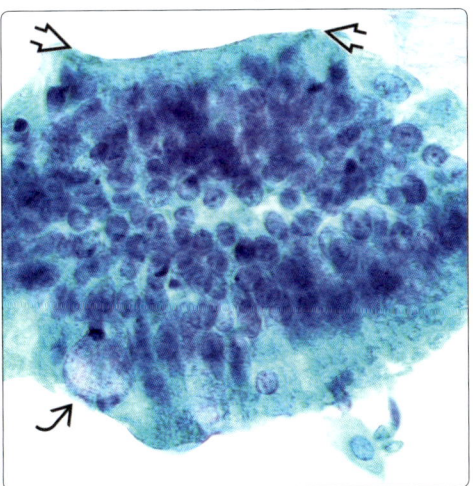

Radiation Esophagitis

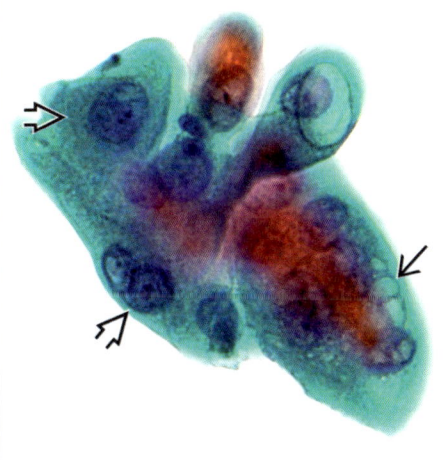

(Left) Pap-stained thin layer preparation shows a distinct goblet cell ➡, necessary to support the diagnosis of Barrett esophagus (BE) in the correct clinical and endoscopic setting. This example also features a brush border ➡ typical of complete intestinal metaplasia (not required for the diagnosis of BE but may be seen). *(Right)* Radiation esophagitis seen in a ThinPrep specimen shows cells with cytoplasmic vacuoles ➡ and a 2-tone cytoplasm. The nuclei are large with vesicular chromatin ➡, and the N:C ratio is nearly normal.

Esophageal Adenocarcinoma

KEY FACTS

ETIOLOGY/PATHOGENESIS
- Male sex, Barrett esophagus, gastroesophageal reflux disease, obesity, smoking, alcohol

CLINICAL ISSUES
- Dysphagia &/or retrosternal or epigastric pain

CYTOPATHOLOGY
- Adenocarcinoma usually arises in background of Barrett esophagus with high-grade dysplasia
- Adenocarcinoma
  - Increased nuclear:cytoplasmic ratio, coarse chromatin, irregular nuclear contours, pleomorphic nucleoli; 3D cell structures
  - Loss of polarity
  - Single intact malignant cells
  - Necrotic background
- Barrett esophagus with high-grade dysplasia
  - Elongated cells
  - Crowded pseudostratified strips
  - Less cohesive ± very rare single atypical cells
  - No 3D cell groups; no necrosis
- Differential diagnosis
  - Metastatic carcinoma
  - Ulcer with reactive atypia
    - Lacks 3D groups and overt features of malignancy
    - Rare cells with atypia
    - Streaming pattern with organization and polarity
  - Squamous cell carcinoma (poorly differentiated)
    - p40(+) on immunohistochemistry

ANCILLARY TESTS
- Cell block for immunostains to distinguish among poorly differentiated adenocarcinoma, squamous cell carcinoma, and metastatic tumor
- Immunostain for HER2 and FISH, if necessary, to assess for HER2 overexpression/amplification on cell block

Esophageal Adenocarcinoma
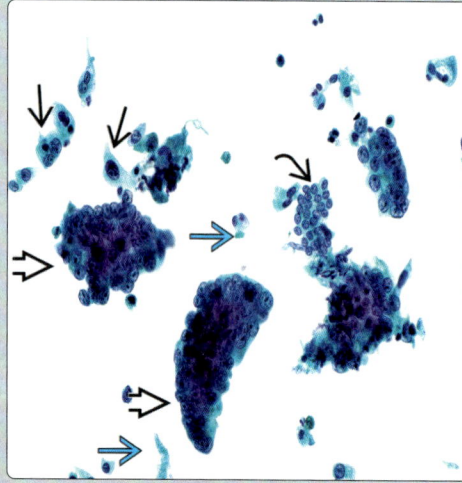

Adenocarcinoma With Dyshesive Cells
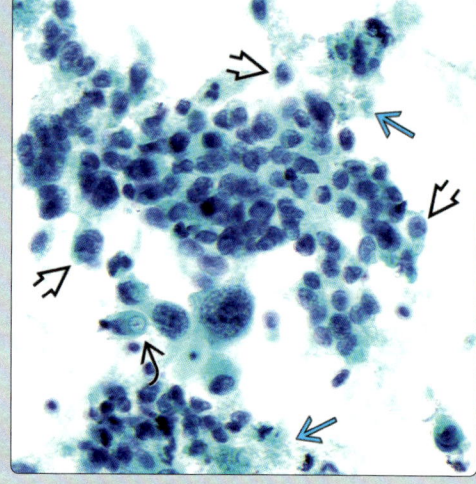

(Left) Pap-stained ThinPrep of an esophageal brushing shows 3D groups of tumor cells ⇨ and rare single malignant cells ⇨. A small sheet of benign columnar cells ⇨ is present for comparison. Note a subtle diathesis in the background ⇨, which can easily be missed on liquid-based preparations. (Right) Pap-stained FNA shows a disorganized, crowded group of malignant cells with nuclear overlap and dyshesive cells at the edges of the group ⇨. The diathesis ⇨ is easier to see on direct smears. Note the intracytoplasmic mucin vacuole ⇨.

Adenocarcinoma With Anisonucleosis
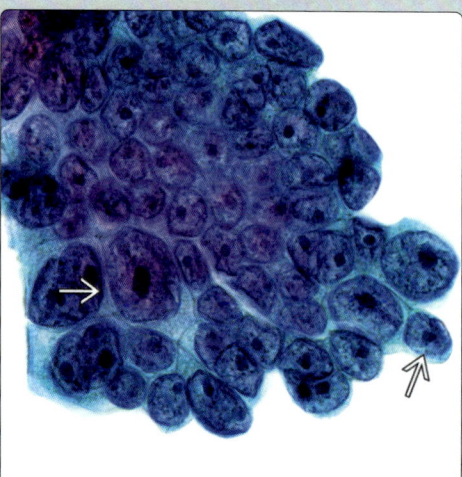

Esophageal Adenocarcinoma on Cell Block
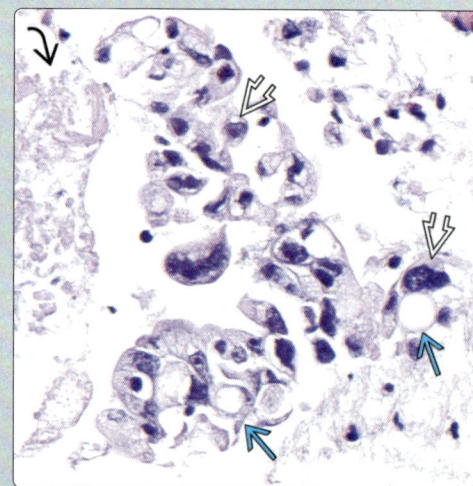

(Left) The tumor cells show nuclear crowding, variable nuclear size, and prominent nucleoli. Note the size difference between these 2 nuclei ⇨. (Right) H&E-stained cell block section from an EUS FNA of esophageal adenocarcinoma shows disorganized clusters of cells with large, irregular nuclei ⇨. Cytoplasmic mucin vacuoles ⇨ may be seen. Necrosis ⇨ is present in the background.

Esophageal Adenocarcinoma

TERMINOLOGY

Definitions
- Malignant epithelial tumor of esophagus with glandular differentiation
- Arises predominantly in lower 1/3 of esophagus in association with Barrett esophagus

CYTOPATHOLOGY

Cellularity
- High

Pattern
- 3D clusters of disorganized cells; small sheets of cells
- Loss of intercellular cohesion resulting in loose cell clusters and single intact malignant cells
- Loss of cell polarity with nuclear overlap and stratification
- May see gland or acinar formation

Background
- Necrotic, possibly bloody, cell debris

Cells
- Adenocarcinoma cells
- Background of Barrett esophagus with dysplasia may be seen
- Normal elements (squamous cells) may also be seen

Nuclear Details
- Enlarged nuclei with irregular contours and variable shapes
- Coarse and irregularly distributed chromatin with thick, irregular nuclear membrane
- 3x variation in nuclear size
- Pleomorphic macronucleoli, may be multiple

Cytoplasmic Details
- Intracytoplasmic mucin occasionally seen
- Cytoplasm usually decreased relative to size of nucleus

Cell Block Findings
- Acinar or glandular structures may be seen on cell block

ANCILLARY TESTS

Immunohistochemistry
- Immunostain for HER2 and FISH, if necessary, to assess for HER2 overexpression/amplification on cell block

Genetic Testing
- DNA ploidy analysis and FISH for 8q24 (*MYC*), 9p21 (*CDKN2A*), 17q12 (*ERBB2*), and 20q13 on esophageal brushing cytology is helpful for diagnosis of dysplasia and carcinoma in difficult cases

DIFFERENTIAL DIAGNOSIS

Barrett Esophagus With High-Grade Dysplasia
- Smaller groups of cells than seen with nondysplastic Barrett esophagus
- Cell groups retain some organization, polarity, and cohesion with rare (if any) intact single atypical cells
- Nuclear atypia with increased nuclear:cytoplasmic ratio and nuclear overlap but usually no pleomorphic nucleoli
- Elongated pseudostratified nuclei, hyperchromasia, irregular nuclear contours, coarse chromatin, decreased cytoplasmic mucin
- Lacks 3D structures and usually lacks necrotic background

Metastatic Carcinoma
- Clinical history, cell block, and immunostains are key

Ulcer With Reactive Atypia
- Lacks overt features of malignancy; no 3D cell groups
- Atypical cells are very rare; no diffuse atypia
- Cells with reactive atypia usually have streaming pattern with maintained organization

Poorly Differentiated Squamous Cell Carcinoma
- Cell block for p63 &/or p40 immunostains; both positive in squamous carcinoma

SELECTED REFERENCES
1. Bhutani N et al: Diagnostic utility of endoscopic brush cytology in upper gastrointestinal malignancies. Diagn Cytopathol. 49(3):418-23, 2021

High-Grade Dysplasia

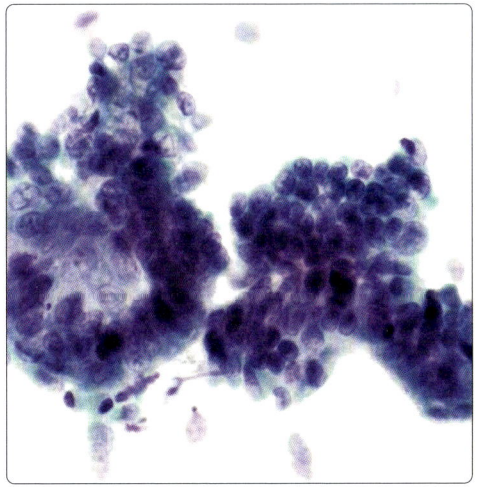

Single Intact Malignant Cell

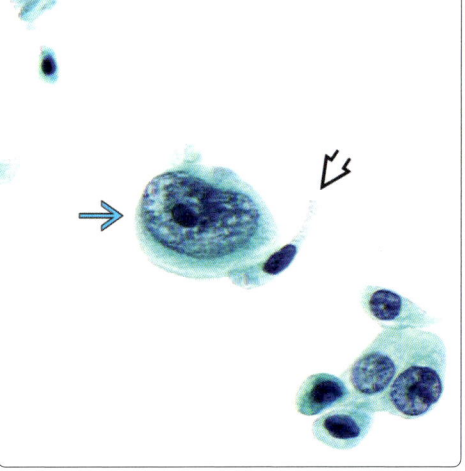

(Left) Pap-stained esophageal brushing with cohesive but crowded and disorganized cells with high-grade dysplasia is shown. The cells have decreased cytoplasmic mucin, nuclear overlap, and stratification. The background is clean, without diathesis. **(Right)** Pap stain shows a large single intact malignant cell ➡ with high nuclear:cytoplasmic ratio, large nucleus, and prominent nucleolus. Note the size difference between the tumor cell and the adjacent normal cell ➡.

Esophageal Squamous Cell Carcinoma

KEY FACTS

ETIOLOGY/PATHOGENESIS
- Male sex, tobacco, alcohol, thermal injury, human papillomavirus (HPV), achalasia, nutritional deficiency, ingestion of corrosives, Plummer-Vinson syndrome, tylosis, and celiac disease

CLINICAL ISSUES
- Squamous cell carcinoma (SqCa) usually occurs in mid or lower esophagus

CYTOPATHOLOGY
- Keratinizing SqCa: Pleomorphic keratinized cells, tadpole cells, ± keratin pearls, hyperchromatic nuclei
- Nonkeratinizing SqCa: Smaller cells with higher N:C ratio, scant cytoplasm
  o Dense/"hard" cytoplasm helpful if present focally
  o Random isolated keratinized cells, if present, also helpful
- Intercellular bridges, if present, are easier to find on cell block

ANCILLARY TESTS
- Cell block and immunostains if needed
  o p40(+)

TOP DIFFERENTIAL DIAGNOSES
- Squamous dysplasia
  o May be impossible to distinguish invasive SqCa from high-grade dysplasia on cytology alone, but necrotic background is clue for invasion; correlate with biopsy
- Poorly differentiated adenocarcinoma
- Reflux esophagitis
- Radiation esophagitis
- Malignant melanoma
  o Rare tumor, large nucleoli, should be considered in differential of poorly differentiated malignancy, melanoma markers (+)
- Lymphoma: Rare, consider in differential of poorly differentiated carcinoma

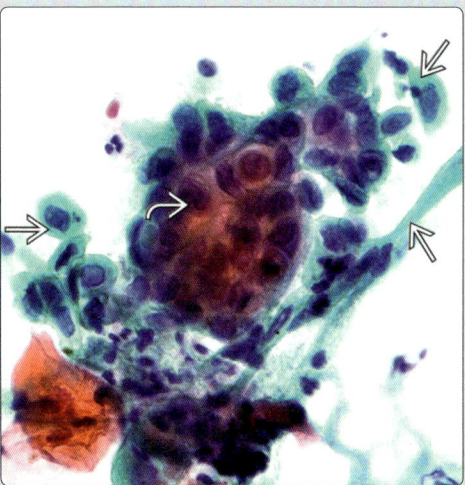

Squamous Cell Carcinoma

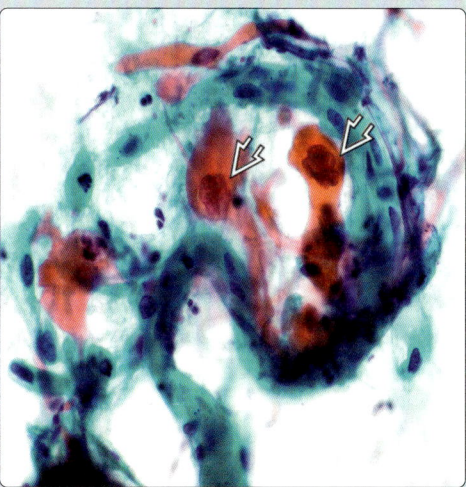

Keratinizing Squamous Cell Carcinoma

(Left) Pap-stained ThinPrep esophageal brushing shows a squamous cell carcinoma with varying degrees of squamous differentiation. Note the distinct single malignant cells with dense, hard cytoplasm ➡. The cells in the center of the cluster ➡ may be difficult to recognize as squamous. (Right) Pap-stained esophageal brushing shows bizarre cells of squamous cell carcinoma with densely keratinized cytoplasm. The nuclei are hyperchromatic with irregular contours ➡.

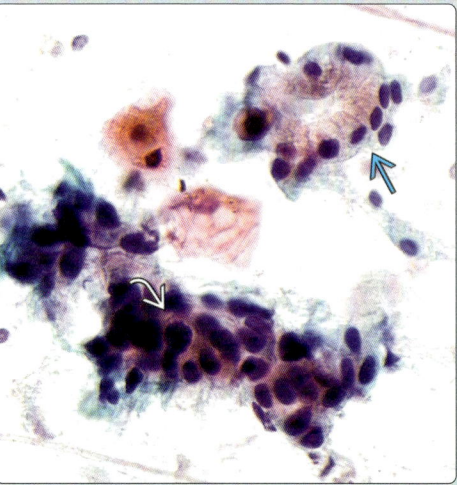

Poorly Differentiated Squamous Cell Carcinoma

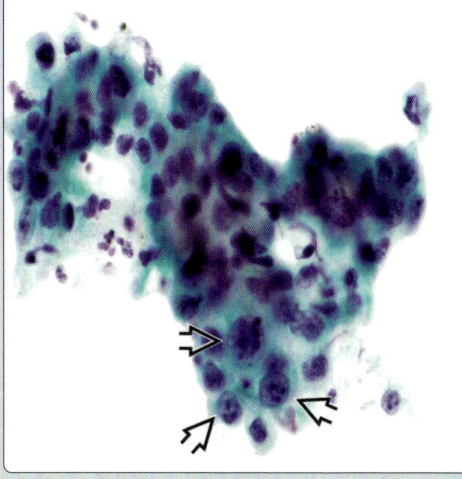

Poorly Differentiated Squamous Cell Carcinoma

(Left) Pap-stained esophageal brushing of a poorly differentiated squamous cell carcinoma shows a crowded sheet of cells with marked nuclear hyperchromasia and overlapping. A few cells in the center of the group have well-defined borders ➡. A small group of benign columnar cells ➡ is also present. (Right) Pap-stained thin-layer preparation of an esophageal brushing shows poorly differentiated squamous cell carcinoma with large hyperchromatic nuclei and prominent nucleoli ➡. The cell boundaries are indistinct.

Esophageal Squamous Cell Carcinoma

TERMINOLOGY

Abbreviations
- Squamous cell carcinoma (SqCa)

Definitions
- Malignant epithelial neoplasm with squamous cell differentiation; usually middle or lower 1/3 of esophagus

CLINICAL ISSUES

Presentation
- Difficulty swallowing

CYTOPATHOLOGY

Cellularity
- Usually high

Pattern
- Single cells and cells in loose clusters

Background
- Necrosis, inflammation

Cells
- SqCa may have keratinizing or nonkeratinizing cells, basaloid cells, spindle cells

Nuclear Details
- Keratinizing SqCa
  - Hyperchromatic nuclei, irregular chromatin, angular nuclear contours
- Nonkeratinizing SqCa
  - Nuclei may be larger with irregular contours and coarse, irregular chromatin, ± nucleoli
- Poorly differentiated SqCa
  - May have prominent pleomorphic nucleoli

Cytoplasmic Details
- Keratinizing SqCa
  - Orangeophilic cytoplasm, tadpole cells, refractile cytoplasmic rings around nucleus (reflects keratinization), ± keratin pearls, well-defined cytoplasmic edges
- Nonkeratinizing SqCa
  - Higher N:C ratios than keratinizing SqCa
  - Moderate amount of amphophilic cytoplasm on Pap

Adequacy Criteria
- Viable lesional tissue not obscured by necrosis

Cell Block Findings
- Intercellular bridges are easier to find on cell block

DIFFERENTIAL DIAGNOSIS

Reflux Esophagitis (Reactive Changes)
- Relatively focal and less severe atypia; may be difficult to distinguish from well-differentiated SqCa

Radiation Esophagitis
- Cells with near-normal N:C ratio and 2-tone cytoplasm; ± necrotic background

Poorly Differentiated Adenocarcinoma
- Cell block and immunostains: Adenocarcinoma is CK7(+); SqCa is p63 &/or p40 (+) (nuclear stain)

Spindle Cell Squamous Cell Carcinoma
- Biphasic tumor with nonkeratinizing spindled cells and sarcomatoid elements
  - Sarcomatoid elements are usually undifferentiated spindle cells, but specific differentiation has been reported

High-Grade Squamous Dysplasia
- Many features overlap with invasive carcinoma
  - Distinction may not be possible on cytology alone; correlate with biopsy

SELECTED REFERENCES

1. Zhang R et al: Endoscopic diagnosis and treatment of esophageal squamous cell carcinoma. Methods Mol Biol. 2129:47-62, 2020

Squamous Cell Carcinoma With Small Cells

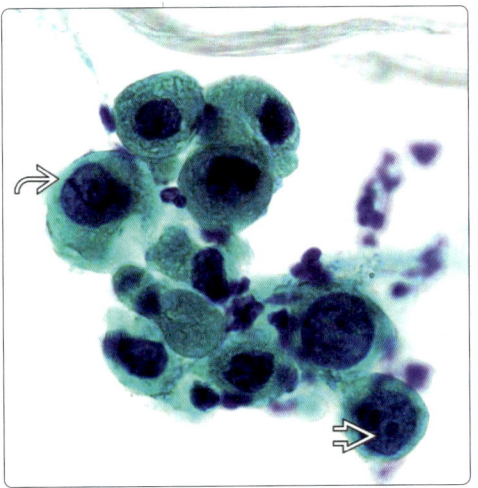

Squamous Cell Carcinoma in Cell Block

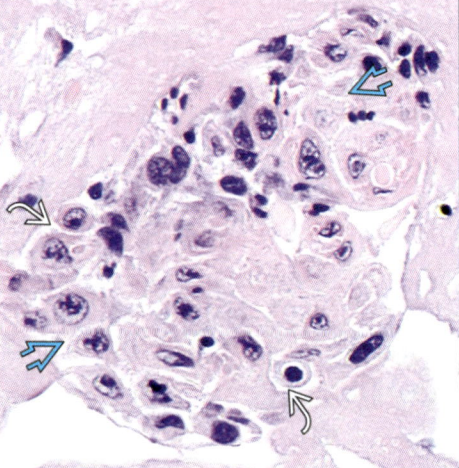

(Left) This squamous cell carcinoma has small cells with a high N:C ratio, dense cytoplasm, coarse chromatin, irregular nuclear contours ⇗, and occasional nucleoli ⇒. *(Right)* H&E-stained cell block section of squamous cell carcinoma shows a group of cohesive tumor cells with distinct cell borders ⇒ and intercellular bridges ⇒. The nuclei are enlarged and hyperchromatic with coarse chromatin.

Gastritis and Intestinal Metaplasia

KEY FACTS

TERMINOLOGY
- **Gastritis**: Mucosal injury resulting from imbalance between physiologic mucosal protection and causative noxious agents/mechanisms
- **Intestinal metaplasia (IM)**: Replacement of normal foveolar cells with specialized intestinal-type epithelium, including goblet cells and absorptive cells ± brush border

CYTOPATHOLOGY
- **Gastritis**: Reactive/reparative pattern with flat, cohesive, organized sheets of cells; ± nuclear streaming; ± inflammatory cells infiltrating cell sheets; few, if any, single atypical or only single cells
- Enlarged cells with preserved N:C ratio, prominent nucleoli, smooth nuclear membranes, mitotic activity but no atypical forms and no pleomorphism
- Marked reactive atypia may be difficult to distinguish from adenocarcinoma; can be problematic if picked up during EUS-guided pancreatic FNAs
- **Metaplastic goblet cells**: Sprinkled among absorptive cells, not in clusters or large groups; nucleus may be indented, even chromatin ± small nucleolus; clear mucin vacuole ≥ 3x size of nucleus
- If ulcerated, stromal cells with reactive atypia may be seen; parietal and chief cells are rarely seen

ANCILLARY TESTS
- Although *H. pylori* is visible on both Diff-Quik and Pap stains, immunostain, silver stain, and Alcian yellow stain may help to identify rare organisms

TOP DIFFERENTIAL DIAGNOSES
- **Adenocarcinoma**
  - Crowded, smaller dyshesive 3D cell groups, single intact malignant cells, necrotic background
- **High-grade dysplasia**
  - Dark nuclei with overlap and stratification; smaller crowded cell groups; few or no single atypical cells

Reactive Foveolar Cells in Gastritis
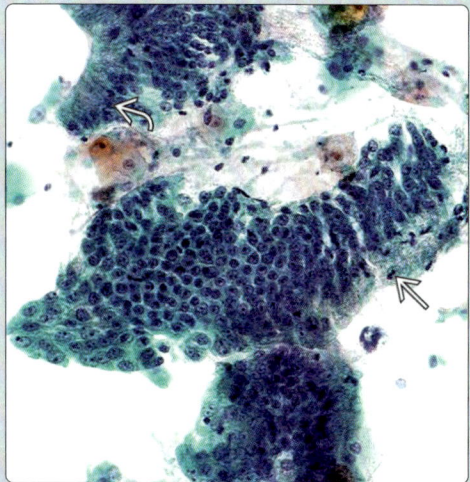

Reactive/Reparative Changes
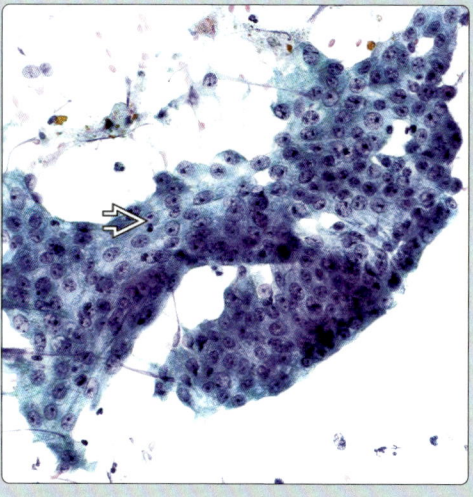

(Left) Pap-stained gastric brushing of gastritis shows reactive foveolar cells with enlarged nuclei and smooth nuclear contours. Cell polarity is maintained with basally oriented nuclei ➡. Scattered inflammatory cells infiltrate the sheets of cells ➡. *(Right)* Pap-stained gastric brushing of gastritis shows a flat sheet of enlarged cells with prominent nucleoli ➡ and a streaming pattern.

Intestinal Metaplasia With Goblet Cells
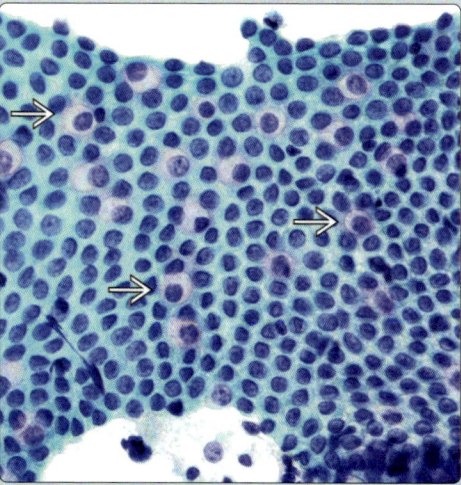

Helicobacter pylori on Pap Stain
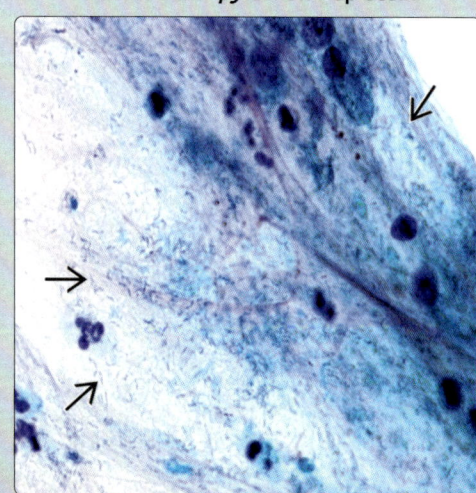

(Left) Pap-stained gastric brushing shows a sheet of foveolar cells with intestinal metaplasia. Here, the goblet cells have clear to eosinophilic mucinous cytoplasm ➡ and are sprinkled throughout this sheet of foveolar cells. *(Right)* Pap-stained gastric brushing shows numerous curved Helicobacter pylori ➡ within gastric mucus.

Gastritis and Intestinal Metaplasia

TERMINOLOGY

Abbreviations
- Intestinal metaplasia (IM)

ETIOLOGY/PATHOGENESIS

Gastritis
- *Helicobacter pylori:* Small (2- to 4-μm), curved, Gram-negative rod
- Chemotherapy/radiation therapy, high-dose NSAIDs, excess alcohol, iron pills, bisphosphonates, caustic agents
- Viral gastritis: Cytomegalovirus and herpes simplex virus are most common, usually among immunocompromised patients
- Ischemia, autoimmune, or Crohn disease
- Other infectious agents

Intestinal Metaplasia
- Occurs as response to injury, often associated with chronic atrophic gastritis &/or chronic *H. pylori* infection

CYTOPATHOLOGY

Cellularity
- Low to moderate

Pattern
- Gastritis has reactive/reparative pattern with flat, cohesive, organized sheets of cells; ± nuclear streaming; ± inflammatory cells infiltrating cell sheets; few, if any, single atypical cells
- Enlarged cells with preserved N:C ratio, prominent nucleoli, smooth nuclear membranes, mitotic activity but no atypical forms and no pleomorphism

Background
- Fibrin, acute inflammation, debris, degenerated cells
- ± granulomata; ± necrosis
- *H. pylori:* Extracellular, in gastric mucus
  - Seen on Diff-Quik and Pap stains

Cells
- Gastric foveolar cells: Round basal nucleus, fine chromatin, inconspicuous nuclei; columnar, pale, finely vacuolated mucinous cytoplasm; often loose cytoplasm; may see bare nuclei in background
- Metaplastic absorptive cells: Larger oval nucleus, less fine chromatin, small nucleolus; columnar, denser cytoplasm, ± apical brush border
- Metaplastic goblet cells: Sprinkled among absorptive cells, not in clusters or large groups; nucleus may be indented, even chromatin ± small nucleolus; clear mucin vacuole ≥ 3x size of nucleus
- If ulcerated, stromal cells with reactive atypia may be seen; parietal and chief cells are rarely seen

ANCILLARY TESTS

Special Stains, Immunocytochemistry
- *H. pylori:* Visible on Diff-Quik and Pap stains; also on immunostain, silver stain, and Alcian yellow stain
- Granulomatous inflammation: Acid fast and silver stains

DIFFERENTIAL DIAGNOSIS

Adenocarcinoma
- High N:C ratio, hyperchromasia, multiple &/or pleomorphic macronucleoli, irregular nuclear contours
- Crowded, smaller dyshesive 3D cell groups, single intact malignant cells, necrotic background

High-Grade Dysplasia
- Less severe atypia and disarray than adenocarcinoma
- Dark nuclei with overlap and stratification; smaller crowded cell groups; few or no single atypical cells

Pseudogoblet Cells
- Foveolar cells may be distended by mucin, but vacuole is usually < 3x size of nucleus

SELECTED REFERENCES
1. Weng CY et al: Helicobacter pylori eradication: exploring its impacts on the gastric mucosa. World J Gastroenterol. 27(31):5152-70, 2021

Gastric Ulcer Brushing
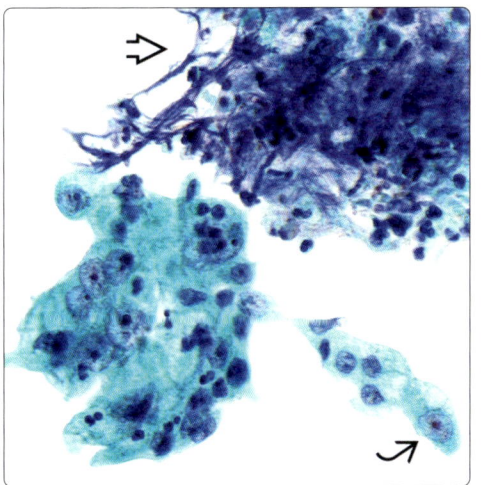

Fragment of Reactive Gastric Mucosa in Cell Block
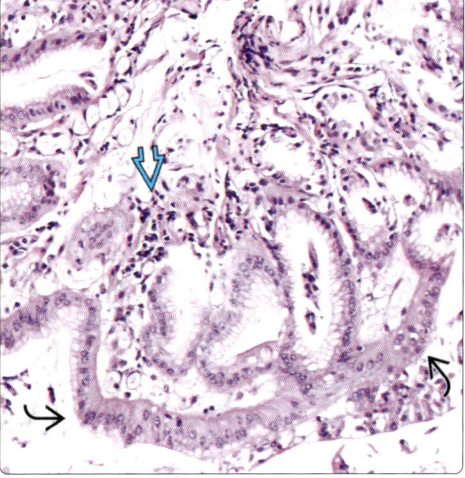

(Left) Pap-stained gastric ulcer brushing shows inflammatory debris ⇨ and foveolar cells with reactive changes. There are large nuclei with fine, even chromatin and distinct nucleoli ⇨. Note the preservation of near-normal N:C ratios. *(Right)* H&E-stained cell block section from gastric ulcer brushing shows an intact fragment of gastric mucosa. The epithelial cells have mild reactive changes, including enlarged nuclei with smooth contours and nucleoli ⇨. Scattered mixed inflammatory cells are seen in the lamina propria ⇨.

Gastric Adenocarcinoma

KEY FACTS

TERMINOLOGY
- Primary invasive epithelial gastric neoplasm
- Early adenocarcinomas: Limited to mucosa and submucosa, regardless of lymph node status
- Advanced adenocarcinomas: Invade muscularis propria and beyond
- Intestinal type: Papillary, tubular, and mucinous carcinomas
- Diffuse type: Poorly cohesive variants, including signet-ring cell carcinoma
- Mixed type: Mix of intestinal and diffuse types
- Indeterminate types: Undifferentiated, adenosquamous, medullary, squamous, hepatoid carcinomas

CYTOPATHOLOGY
- **Intestinal type**: Loose/disorganized 3D cell clusters; single malignant cells in background
  - Similar pattern as in other GI malignancies
- **Diffuse type**: Look for single cells; nuclei may be small and bland, resembling histiocytes
  - Signet-ring cells are characteristic but may also see high N:C ratio cells

ANCILLARY TESTS
- Immunostains to distinguish between carcinoma cells [CK(+)/CD68(-)] and histiocytes [CK(-)/CD68(+)]
- Cell block for HER2 immunochemistry and FISH, if needed

TOP DIFFERENTIAL DIAGNOSES
- **Gastric dysplasia**
  - More cohesive than carcinoma; fewer if any single intact atypical cells
- **Gastric lymphoma**: Immunochemistry is helpful
  - Lymphoma is CK(-) and CD45(+)
- **Ulcer/reactive atypia**
  - Flat cohesive sheets; no single atypical cells; ± necrotic background
- Correlate with endoscopic findings and biopsy

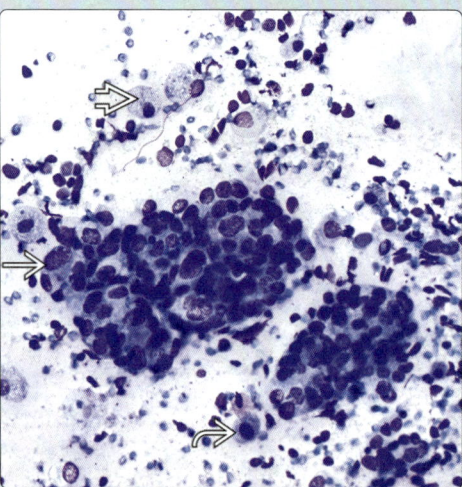

Gastric Adenocarcinoma: Intestinal Type

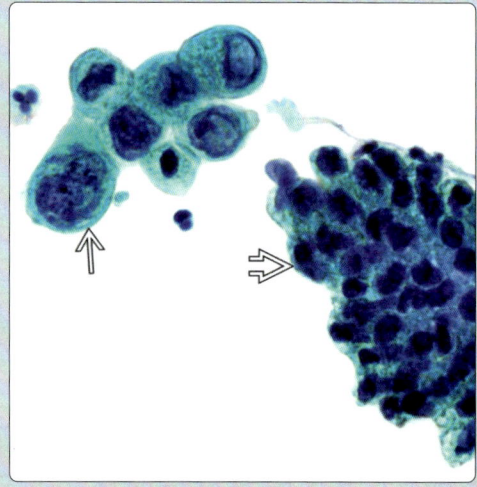

Contrast Between Adenocarcinoma and Benign Normal Cells

(Left) Diff-Quik-stained brushing shows disordered sheets with varying nuclear sizes and shapes ➡. The background is dirty with histiocytes ➡ and single intact malignant cells ➡. (Right) This Pap-stained gastric brushing on ThinPrep shows malignant cells ➡ that have large nuclei with irregular contours and an ↑ N:C ratio. They are much larger than the adjacent sheet of benign cells ➡.

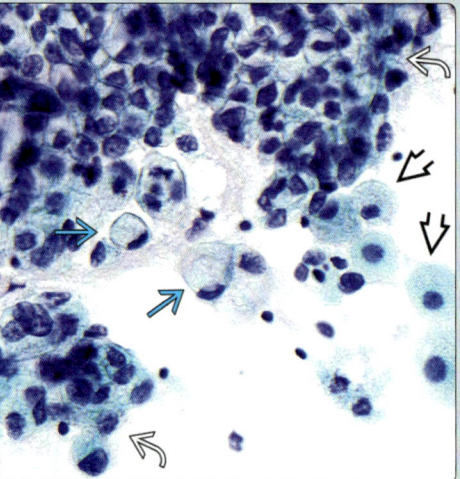

Adenocarcinoma With Signet-Ring Cells

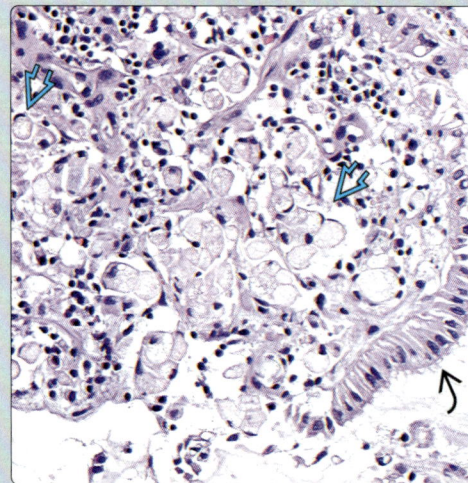

Poorly Cohesive Adenocarcinoma in Cell Block

(Left) Pap-stained FNA of a gastric mass shows adenocarcinoma with signet-ring cell ➡ features. Note the eosinophilic extracellular mucin and scattered macrophages ➡ in the background. The larger groups of cells show crowding and nuclear overlapping ➡. (Right) H&E-stained cell block section from gastric mass FNA shows an intact fragment of mucosa infiltrated by signet-ring cells ➡. The overlying foveolar epithelium ➡ is benign; therefore, a superficial brushing of this lesion could yield a false-negative result.

Gastric Adenocarcinoma

TERMINOLOGY

Definitions
- Primary invasive epithelial gastric neoplasm

ETIOLOGY/PATHOGENESIS

Infectious Agents
- *Helicobacter pylori* infection: Chronic inflammation → metaplasia → dysplasia → adenocarcinoma

Environmental Exposure
- Salt-cured and smoked foods, smoking

CYTOPATHOLOGY

Cellularity
- Intestinal type: High cellularity
- Diffuse type: Moderate to high cellularity; may not be ulcerated/mass-forming (i.e., linitis plastica pattern) and can be source of false-negatives if only brushing is performed

Pattern
- Intestinal type: Crowded disorganized 3D cell groups arranged in papillae, acini, sheets, strips of cells; single intact malignant cells
- Diffuse type: Disorganized 3D clusters of cells; single cell pattern may predominate

Background
- If ulcerated, necrotic debris may be present; ± tumor diathesis; ± extracellular mucin

Cells
- Intestinal type
  - Well differentiated: Tall columnar cells
  - Poorly differentiated: Cuboidal to oval cells
  - Round nuclei with fine or coarse chromatin; ± irregular nuclear contours; ≥ 1 nucleolus
  - Moderate to scant amount of delicate mucinous cytoplasm; ± apical brush border; high N:C ratio
- Diffuse type
  - More variable cell size and shape; less frequently ulcerated
    - Larger cells: Relatively abundant foamy cytoplasm; nuclei with prominent nucleoli
    - Smaller cells: Granular cytoplasm; nuclei with coarse, clumped cytoplasm; nuclei may be bland and confused with histiocytes
  - Targetoid cytoplasmic mucin or large signet-ring type cytoplasmic mucin vacuole
  - Hyperchromatic nucleus may be eccentric and compressed by mucin vacuole; if no mucin vacuole, high N:C ratio

ANCILLARY TESTS

Immunohistochemistry
- Cell block for HER2 immunochemistry and FISH, if needed

DIFFERENTIAL DIAGNOSIS

Ulcer/Reactive Atypia
- Cell sheets are more cohesive, flat, and organized
  - Few, if any, single intact atypical cells; ± necrotic background; usually low cellularity
  - Correlate with endoscopic findings and biopsy
- Abundant histiocytes in background may disguise or be mistaken for signet-ring cells: Histiocytes are CD68(+) and cytokeratin (-)

Gastric Dysplasia
- Cells are more cohesive with less severe atypia than seen in carcinoma; few, if any, single intact atypical cells; less cellular specimen

Gastric Lymphoma
- May mimic poorly differentiated adenocarcinoma
- Immunostains are helpful: Lymphoma is CD45(+) and cytokeratin (-)

SELECTED REFERENCES
1. Virgilio E et al: Prognostic role of intragastric cytopathology and microbiota in surgical patients with stomach cancer. J Cytol. 38(2):82-7, 2021

Gastric Adenocarcinoma

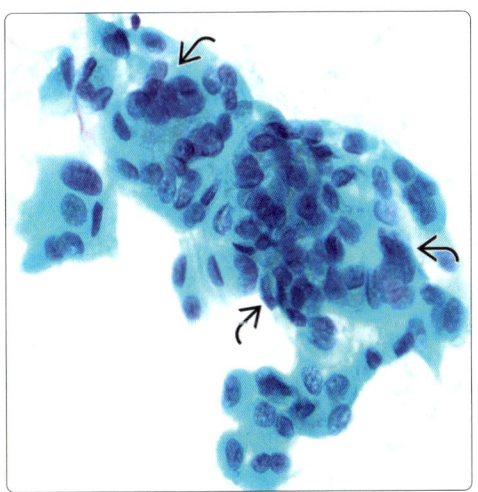

High Nuclear:Cytoplasmic Ratio Cells

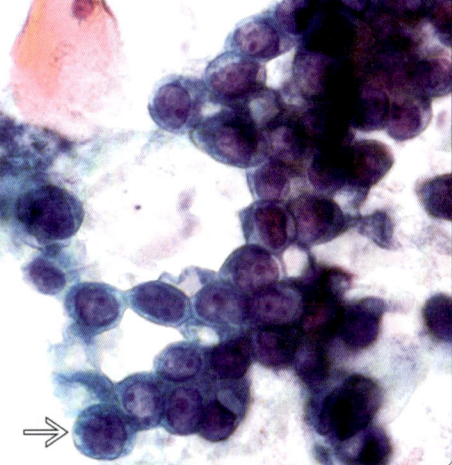

(Left) Pap-stained FNA of gastric adenocarcinoma has a syncytial cluster of disorganized cells with dark, large nuclei and prominent nuclear overlap ➦. (Right) Pap-stained gastric brushing smear shows a loose cluster of similarly sized malignant cells with high N:C ratios. The cytoplasm has fine mucin vacuoles ➡. Nuclear details of malignancy, such as irregular nuclear contours and prominent nucleoli, are seen.

Gastric Lymphoma

KEY FACTS

TERMINOLOGY
- Mucosa-associated lymphoid tissue (MALT) lymphoma (MALToma)
- Diffuse large B-cell lymphoma (DLBCL)

ETIOLOGY/PATHOGENESIS
- *Helicobacter pylori* infection: Stimulates T-cells to produce B-cell trophic cytokines that potentiate clonal expansion of B-cells

CLINICAL ISSUES
- 85% of all GI MALTomas are gastric
- 50% of primary gastric lymphomas are MALTomas
- *H. pylori* eradication therapy 1st-line treatment for GI MALToma; up to 80% regress with treatment

CYTOPATHOLOGY
- MALToma
  - Challenging diagnosis, usually not rendered on cytologic samples alone; correlate with biopsy
  - Composed of various types of predominantly small B lymphocytes; polymorphous population of centrocytes, monocytoid B-cells, plasma cells, and rare centroblasts
- DLBCL
  - Pleomorphic large cells, lymphoglandular bodies

ANCILLARY TESTS
- Currently no specific markers for MALToma, but flow cytometry can be helpful to prove clonality
- B-cells with CD20(+), coexpression of CD43 in 30-50%
- CD5, CD10, BCL6 (-)
- *API1::MALT1* fusion results from translocation t(11;18) in subset; associated with resistance to *H. Pylori* eradication therapy

TOP DIFFERENTIAL DIAGNOSES
- Distinction between MALToma and severe gastritis can be challenging
- DLBCL vs. poorly differentiated carcinoma
  - Immunochemistry and flow cytometry are helpful

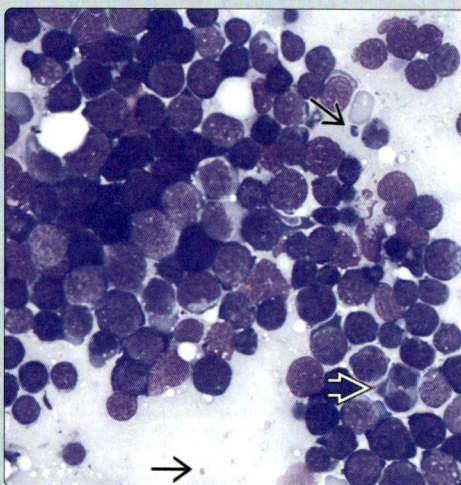

Diffuse Large B-Cell Lymphoma

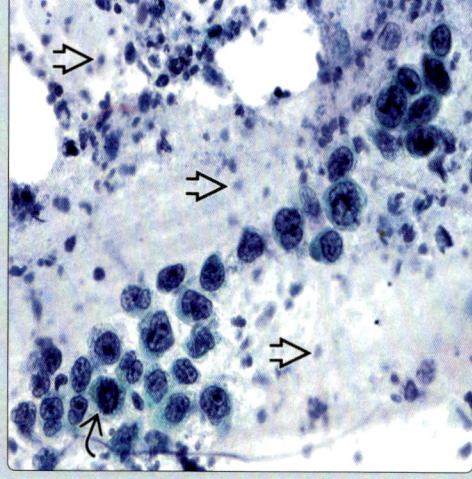

Diffuse Large B-Cell Lymphoma on Pap, High Power

(Left) Diff-Quik-stained FNA of gastric diffuse large B-cell lymphoma (DLBCL) shows a monotonous population of large lymphocytes with very scant basophilic cytoplasm. Lymphoglandular bodies ⇨ and atypical mitotic figures ⇨ may be seen. **(Right)** Pap-stained brushing of gastric DLBCL shows cells with scant cytoplasm, irregular nuclear contours, clumpy chromatin, and an atypical mitotic figure ⇨. Note lymphoglandular bodies ⇨.

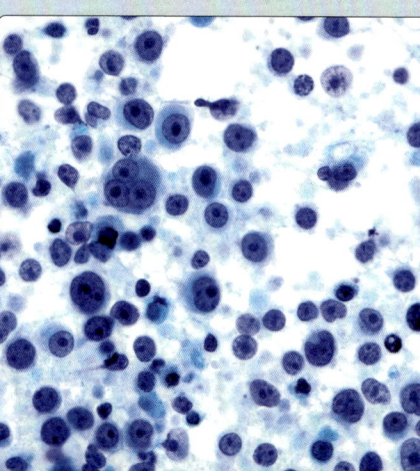

Diffuse Large B-Cell Lymphoma With Prominent Nucleoli

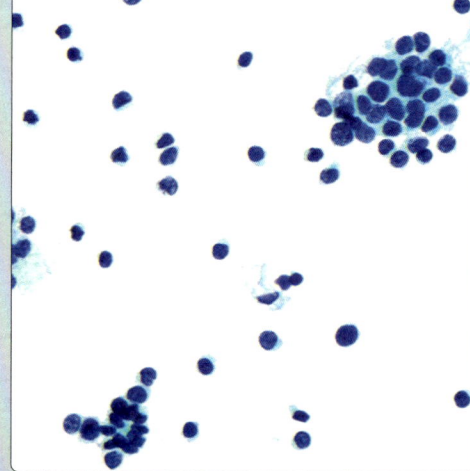

Mantle Cell Lymphoma

(Left) Pap-stained smear of DLBCL of the stomach with prominent nucleoli is shown. Ancillary testing for hematopathology markers by immunochemistry &/or flow cytometry is needed to confirm the diagnosis. **(Right)** Pap-stained thin layer preparation of transgastric EUS FNA of a periportal lymph node shows a monotonous population of small- to medium-sized lymphocytes. Immunochemical work-up was performed on the cell block to support the diagnosis of mantle cell lymphoma.

Gastric Lymphoma

TERMINOLOGY

Abbreviations
- Mucosa-associated lymphoid tissue (MALT) lymphoma (MALToma)
- Diffuse large B-cell lymphoma (DLBCL)

ETIOLOGY/PATHOGENESIS

Helicobacter pylori, Antigenic Stimulation
- H. pylori infection: Stimulates T cells to produce B-cell trophic cytokines in MALTomas

CYTOPATHOLOGY

Cellularity
- MALToma: Moderate to high
- DLBCL: Very high

Pattern
- MALToma: Dyshesive; neoplastic lymphocytes may infiltrate epithelial fragments
- DLBCL: Usually dyshesive; cell clustering may occur

Background
- MALToma: Lymphoglandular bodies (detached cytoplasmic fragments); if ulcerated, may see necrosis; H. pylori in gastric mucus
- DLBCL: Necrosis, lymphoglandular bodies; H. pylori is less frequently identified

Cells
- MALToma: Polymorphous population of small lymphocytes ± plasma cells
  - Centrocytes: Medium-sized lymphoid cells, cleaved nuclei, scant cytoplasm ± tiny nucleolus
  - Monocytoid B-cells: Similar to centrocytes but with relatively ample clear cytoplasm
  - Centroblasts: Larger with vesicular chromatin, 1-3 nucleoli, scant basophilic cytoplasm; should be rare
- DLBCL: Monomorphic large malignant lymphocytes with coarse chromatin and prominent &/or multiple nucleoli

Cell Block Findings
- MALToma: May be able to identify lymphoepithelial lesions if epithelial fragments are present

Cytology-Histology Correlation
- MALToma: Gastric glands infiltrated by small to medium neoplastic lymphocytes
- DLBCL: Destructive infiltrate of large lymphocytes with necrosis; less likely with H. pylori
- Lymphoepithelial lesions: ≥ 3 neoplastic lymphocytes causing epithelial damage; ± H. pylori

ANCILLARY TESTS

Flow Cytometry, Immunochemistry, Molecular (MALT)
- Currently no specific markers for MALToma but can be helpful to prove clonality
- B-cells, CD20(+) with expression of CD43 in 30-50%
- CD5, CD10, BCL6 (-)
- API1::MALT1 fusion results from translocation t(11;18)(q21;q21) in 26% and associated with resistance to H. pylori eradication therapy

DIFFERENTIAL DIAGNOSIS

Helicobacter pylori Gastritis
- Both gastritis and MALToma can show polymorphous lymphoid population; correlate with biopsy

Secondary Involvement of Stomach by Lymphoma
- Bulk of disease not located in stomach

Poorly Differentiated Carcinoma
- DLBCL may have prominent cell clustering, mimicking carcinoma; cytokeratin and CD45 on smears or cell block can distinguish

SELECTED REFERENCES
1. Alvarez-Lesmes J et al: Gastrointestinal tract lymphomas: a review of the most commonly encountered lymphomas. Arch Pathol Lab Med. 145(12):1585-96, 2021

MALToma With Reactive Epithelium

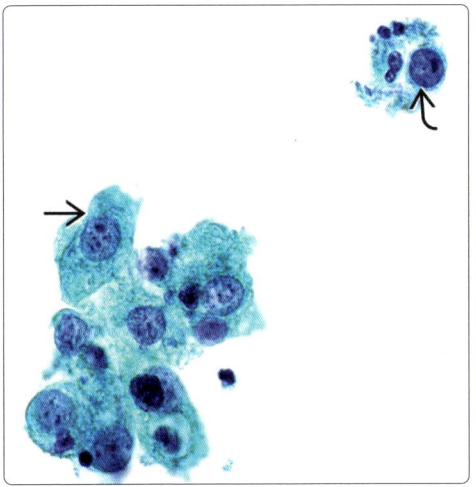

MALToma With Necrosis

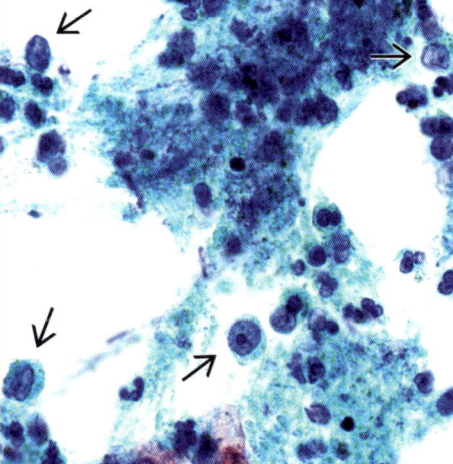

(Left) Pap-stained FNA of gastric lymphoma shows reactive epithelial cells ➡ and an atypical lymphocyte with a prominent nucleolus ➡. Biopsy showed mucosa-associated lymphoid tissue (MALT) lymphoma (MALToma). (Right) Pap-stained aspirate from a gastric MALToma shows polymorphous atypical lymphocytes ➡, necrosis, and acute inflammation. Biopsy and immunochemistry confirmed monoclonality.

Ampulla/Bile Duct/Pancreatic Duct Reactive Changes

KEY FACTS

CLINICAL ISSUES
- Often used to investigate etiology of strictures or obstruction of ducts
- Cytology useful in this setting as biopsy forceps may not pass through tight strictures
- Ampulla more easily accessible, so biopsy alone or biopsy with cytology performed more frequently than cytology alone
- Check for history of stent, which may cause striking reactive atypia
- For determination of patient care, correlation with clinical history, imaging, and endoscopic findings crucial
- Reactive epithelium may overlie invasive carcinoma (i.e., negative result may not be definitive)

CYTOPATHOLOGY
- Reactive cells may have nucleoli and mitotic figures, but N:C ratio preserved, and mitotic figures typical
- Cells arranged in flat, cohesive, streaming sheets with minimal nuclear crowding &/or overlap
- Nuclei may be enlarged but retain smooth contours and fine chromatin

ANCILLARY TESTS
- In difficult cases, especially in patients with stents and sclerosing cholangitis, reactive changes may be severe enough to be suspicious for adenocarcinoma
- FISH testing on liquid-based cytology is very useful with major therapeutic implications
- Next-generation sequencing platforms have recently shown comparable results to FISH testing

TOP DIFFERENTIAL DIAGNOSES
- Dysplasia of bile/pancreatic ducts
- Carcinoma of bile/pancreatic ducts
- Well-differentiated carcinomas are source of false-negative diagnoses

Reactive Bile Duct Epithelium
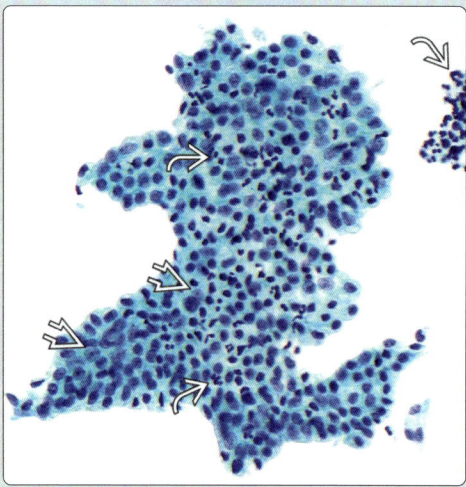

Normal Bile Duct Epithelium on Cell Block
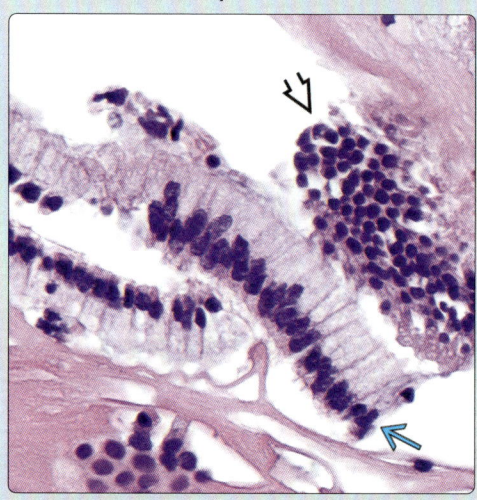

(Left) This Pap-stained bile duct brushing from a patient with a stent shows a flat cohesive sheet of cells infiltrated by neutrophils ➡. There is mild variation in nuclear size with even chromatin and small nucleoli ➡. Neutrophils are also present in the background. (Right) H&E stained cell block shows a section of normal bile duct epithelium. The honeycomb arrangement of nuclei is apparent when the epithelium is seen en face ➡. When seen on edge, the nuclei are basally located and round to oval ➡.

Normal and Reactive Bile Duct Epithelium
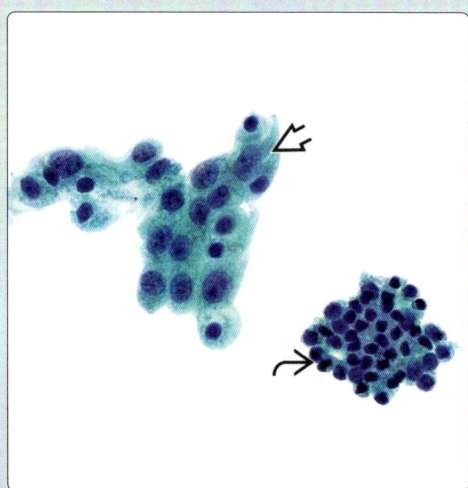

Normal and Atypical Bile Duct Cells
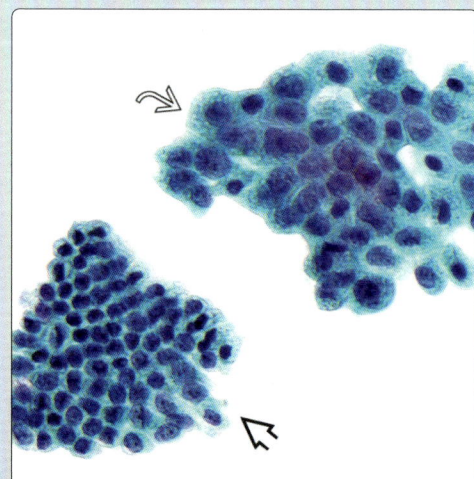

(Left) Pap-stained thin-layer preparation shows reactive ductal cells, which have nuclear enlargement with preservation of the N:C ratio ➡. Ductal cells without reactive changes ➡ are present for comparison. (Right) Pap-stained bile duct brushing shows a group of ductal cells with minimal reactive changes ➡ and a group with architectural disarray and nuclear enlargement ➡. FISH is a helpful tool to aid in risk stratification of atypical cases.

Ampulla/Bile Duct/Pancreatic Duct Reactive Changes

TERMINOLOGY

Definitions
- Benign epithelial changes of ampullary, bile duct, &/or pancreatic duct epithelium that occur in response to pathologic process

CYTOPATHOLOGY

Cellularity
- Low to moderate

Pattern
- Flat, cohesive sheets of evenly spaced ductal cells
  - Minimal to no crowding or nuclear overlap
  - Maintenance of cell polarity
- No 3D or true papillary structures

Background
- Bile/pancreatic duct brushing: ± bile pigment; ± inflammation; usually no necrosis
- Ampullary brushing: Gastric contaminants; gastrointestinal (i.e., nonneoplastic) mucin

Cells
- Pancreatic/bile duct brushing: Ductal cells (cells of bile duct & pancreatic duct morphologically identical) with well-defined cell borders arranged in flat sheets
- Ampulla brushing: Enterocytes, tall columnar cells with ample cytoplasm and basally oriented nucleus; ± apical brush border; cells arranged in strips and flat sheets

Nuclear Details
- Nuclear atypia may be seen, but relatively focal, with preservation of N:C ratio
- Some variation in nuclear size may occur, but not marked anisonucleosis (≥ 4x size variation among nuclei)
- Enlarged nuclei retain smooth membranes and fine chromatin; no hyperchromasia
- ± nucleoli, but no pleomorphic or macronucleoli
- ± scattered typical mitotic figures

Cytoplasmic Details
- Cytoplasm should be abundant; ± abundant mucin
- Squamous metaplasia may occur

Cell Block Findings
- Strips and sheets of well-organized, evenly spaced cells
- Nuclear enlargement and nucleoli, with normal N:C ratio

ANCILLARY TESTS

Biliary Cytology FISH Analysis and Next-Generation Sequencing
- In difficult cases, especially in patients with stents and sclerosing cholangitis, reactive changes may be severe enough to be suspicious for adenocarcinoma
- FISH testing on liquid-based cytology is very useful test with major therapeutic implications
  - FISH probe set (Mayo Clinic) targets 1q21 (*MCL1*), 7p12 (*EGFR*), 8q24 (*MYC*) and 9p21 (*CDKN2A*)
- Next-generation sequencing platforms have recently shown comparable results to FISH testing

DIFFERENTIAL DIAGNOSIS

Dysplasia of Bile/Pancreatic Ducts
- More cytologic and architectural atypia, coarser chromatin, nuclear membrane irregularities, distinct nucleoli; cells form smaller crowded clusters with some degree of nuclear overlap; ± single atypical cells

Carcinoma of Bile/Pancreatic Ducts
- Coarse chromatin, irregular nuclear contours, nuclear pleomorphism, macronucleoli
- Loose 3D clusters of cells; loss of cell polarity; nuclear crowding and overlap; necrotic background
- Single intact malignant cells

SELECTED REFERENCES
1. Harbhajanka A et al: Tiny but mighty: use of next generation sequencing on discarded cytocentrifuged bile duct brushing specimens to increase sensitivity of cytological diagnosis. Mod Pathol. 33(10):2019-2025, 2020

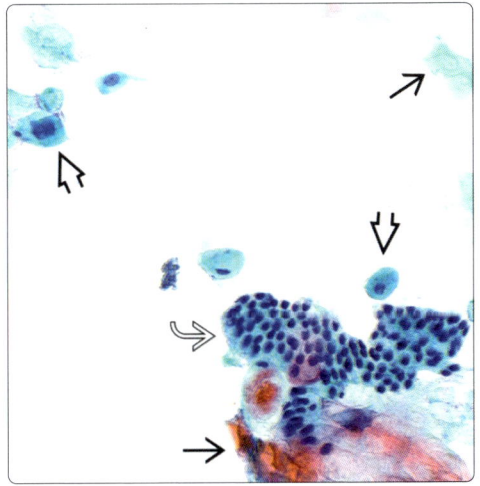

Biliary Aspirate With Squamous Metaplasia

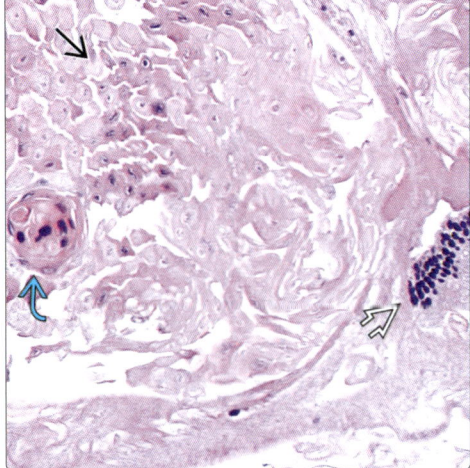

Biliary Aspirate With Squamous Metaplasia on Cell Block

(Left) Pap-stained biliary aspirate from a patient with a retained stent shows pronounced squamous metaplasia. A group of bland ductal cells ➡ is surrounded by squamous metaplastic cells ➡, some with keratinization ➡. *(Right)* H&E-stained cell block section from the same biliary aspirate with squamous metaplasia shows numerous squamous metaplastic cells ➡ and a squamous pearl ➡. A strip of benign ductal epithelium is also present ➡.

Ampulla/Bile Duct/Pancreatic Duct Adenocarcinoma

KEY FACTS

CLINICAL ISSUES
- Pancreatic ductal adenocarcinoma: Very nonspecific symptoms may result in delay in diagnosis
- Epigastric pain radiating to back, weight loss, painless jaundice
- Ampullary or bile duct adenocarcinoma: Patients usually present earlier due to signs/symptoms of biliary obstruction
- Primary sclerosing cholangitis and stents may cause marked reactive atypia

CYTOPATHOLOGY
- Crowded, 3D clusters of loosely cohesive malignant cells, necrosis, single intact malignant cells
- Nuclear molding, chromatin clumping, ↑ N:C ratio, irregular nuclear membranes, prominent nucleoli, and loss of cell cohesion are important features of malignancy
- Nuclear enlargement and pleomorphism (≥ 4x size difference among nuclei); macronucleoli
- Necrotic background and single intact atypical cells worrisome for malignancy
- High-grade dysplasia and invasive carcinoma may be morphologically indistinguishable
- Extensive necrosis may preclude accurate diagnosis
- Foamy or mucinous cytoplasm, loss of nuclear-cytoplasmic polarity; cytoplasm may be scant (due to ↑ N:C ratio); squamous metaplasia may occur
- Background often necrotic, hemorrhagic, ± mucin, ± bile
- Well-differentiated adenocarcinomas may show repair-like sheets with nuclear super crowding and subtle heterogeneity

ANCILLARY TESTS
- Pancreatobiliary-specific FISH probe set targets 1q21, 7p12, 8q24, and 9p21 to assess for losses or gains
- Polysomy most strongly linked to malignancy
- Next-generation sequencing has shown results comparable to FISH assay

Adenocarcinoma and Benign Ductal Cells
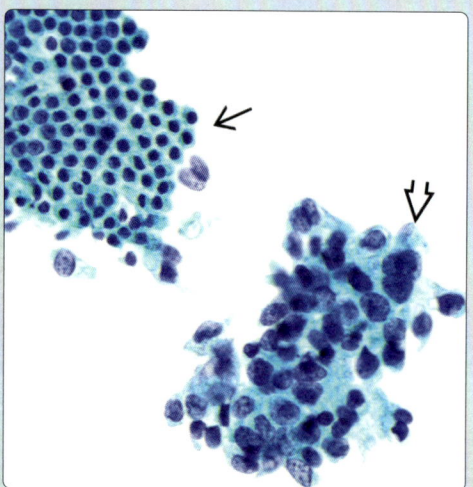

Adenocarcinoma With Anisonucleosis
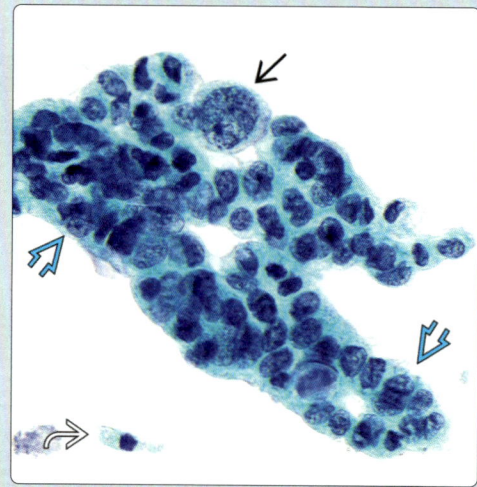

(Left) Pap-stained bile duct brushing shows a flat, cohesive sheet of benign ductal cells ➡ adjacent to a disorganized cluster of malignant cells with nuclear enlargement, hyperchromasia, and overlapping ➡. (Right) Pap-stained bile duct brushing shows a jumbled cluster of tumor cells. The largest nucleus ➡ is ≥ 4x larger than the other nuclei. The smaller nuclei show coarse chromatin and nuclear overlapping ➡. Note the single benign ductal cell for size comparison ➡.

Adenocarcinoma With Abundant Cytoplasm
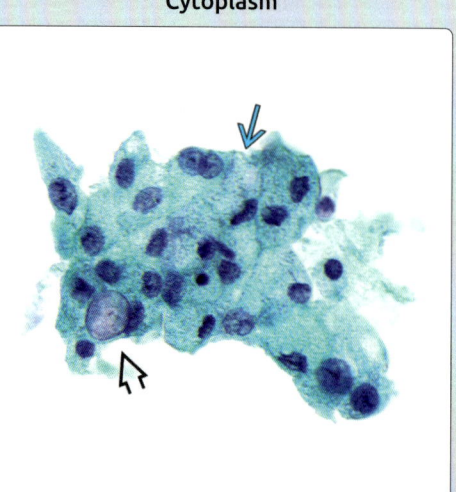

Adenocarcinoma on Cell Block
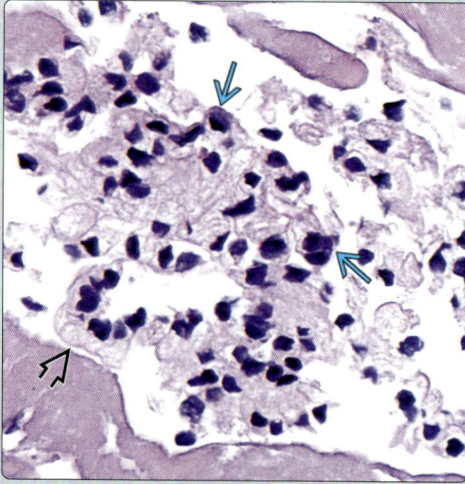

(Left) Pap-stained bile duct brushing shows adenocarcinoma with ample cytoplasm. There is loss of the normal honeycomb pattern, with haphazard spacing of nuclei. One cell shows an intracytoplasmic mucin vacuole ➡; others have abundant finely vacuolated cytoplasm ➡. (Right) H&E-stained cell block section of a well-differentiated adenocarcinoma shows abundant finely vacuolated mucinous cytoplasm ➡. The nuclei are hyperchromatic and angulated ➡ with loss of polarity.

Ampulla/Bile Duct/Pancreatic Duct Adenocarcinoma

TERMINOLOGY

Definitions
- Malignant epithelial neoplasm of pancreatic or bile ducts

ETIOLOGY/PATHOGENESIS

Pancreatic Duct Adenocarcinoma
- Smoking, *BRCA* mutation, chronic pancreatitis, family history/inherited syndromes (e.g., Peutz-Jeghers, Gardner syndromes)

Bile Duct Adenocarcinoma (Cholangiocarcinoma)
- Primary sclerosing cholangitis (PSC), choledochal cyst, anomalous union of ducts, parasitic infections (*Clonorchis sinensis*)

CYTOPATHOLOGY

Cellularity
- Moderate to high

Pattern
- Dyshesive/loose 3D cell clusters
- Loss of honeycomb pattern characteristic of benign ductal epithelium
- Single intact atypical cells

Background
- Often necrotic, hemorrhagic, ± mucin, ± bile

Cells
- Pancreatic or bile duct epithelial cells
- Enterocytes predominate in ampullary brushings

Nuclear Details
- Coarse, clumped, granular chromatin; ↑ N:C ratio; nuclear molding/indentation; nuclear enlargement and pleomorphism (≥ 4x size difference among nuclei); macronucleoli; irregular nuclear contours

Cytoplasmic Details
- Foamy or mucinous cytoplasm; loss of nuclear-cytoplasmic polarity; cytoplasm may be scant (due to ↑ N:C ratio); squamous metaplasia may occur

ANCILLARY TESTS

Fluorescence In Situ Hybridization
- In PSC patients monitored with serial biliary cytology, and in patients with cytologic features worrisome for dysplasia or malignancy, FISH is helpful tool
  - Pancreatobiliary-specific FISH probe set targets 1q21, 7p12, 8q24, and 9p21 to assess for losses or gains
    - More specific for detection of malignancy than UroVysion kit (targets chromosomes 3, 7, 17, and 9p21 to assess for polysomy)
  - Cytology with FISH has higher sensitivity for detection of malignancy in PSC patients than cytology alone
    - Polysomy is most suspicious feature for malignancy
- Next-generation sequencing shows similar performance

DIFFERENTIAL DIAGNOSIS

Reactive Atypia
- Near-normal N:C ratio; smooth nuclear membranes; smaller nucleoli; typical mitotic figures; ± inflammatory background; ± minimal nuclear overlap; good intercellular cohesion; no or very rare single atypical cells

Pancreatic/Bile Duct Intraepithelial Neoplasia
- High-grade dysplasia may be impossible to distinguish from invasive carcinoma (clinical correlation is key)
- Unless ulcerated, dysplasia lacks necrotic background

Metastatic Carcinoma
- Compare with prior malignancy; cell block and immunochemistry useful

SELECTED REFERENCES
1. Rosenbaum MW et al: Cytomorphologic characteristics of next-generation sequencing-positive bile duct brushing specimens. J Am Soc Cytopathol. 9(6):520-7, 2020

Adenocarcinoma, Foamy Gland Type

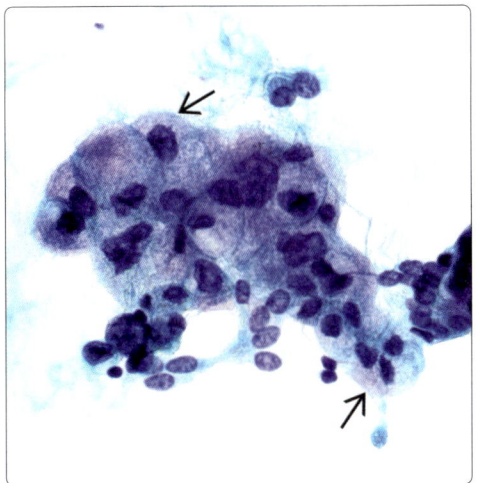

Adenocarcinoma, Drunken Honeycomb Pattern

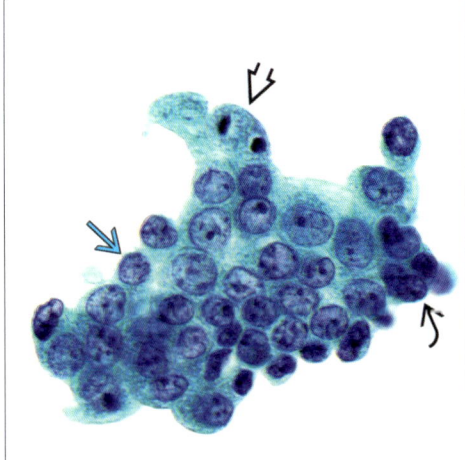

(Left) Pap-stained slide shows abundant finely vacuolated cytoplasm ➡ of cells with nuclear and architectural features of adenocarcinoma. **(Right)** Pap-stained bile duct brushing shows a group of malignant cells with nuclear crowding and overlapping. Note the variable distance between nuclei; some are more closely approximated ➡ while others have more space ➡. A mitotic figure is present ➡.

Colorectal Adenoma/Carcinoma

KEY FACTS

TERMINOLOGY
- Colorectal adenomas are proliferative dysplastic (premalignant) epithelial lesions that may show low- or high-grade dysplasia
- Colorectal carcinomas show invasion beyond muscularis mucosa, into at least submucosa, and arise from adenomas with high-grade dysplasia

CYTOPATHOLOGY
- Adenoma
  - High cellularity with usually clean background
  - Cohesive sheets and strips of cells with some architectural disarray
  - Colonic epithelial cells retain columnar configuration, elongated nuclei; fewer goblet cells
  - Long, slender fragments or papillary structures are clue to villous morphology
  - With progression along adenoma-carcinoma sequence, nuclei show more severe atypia
- Carcinoma
  - Cellular with background showing "dirty" necrosis, blood; subset may show abundant background mucin
  - Dyshesive clusters, single intact malignant cells
  - Malignant cells may be rounded or assume unusual shapes; tumor giant cells or signet-ring cells may be seen
  - Invasive carcinoma shows greater nuclear pleomorphism with more nuclear contour and chromatin pattern irregularities than nonneoplastic and dysplastic lesions
  - Loss of nuclear-cytoplasmic polarity, ↑ mitotic activity, single intact atypical cells, and necrosis are all features associated with, but not necessarily diagnostic of, malignancy
- Sampling of adenoma with high-grade dysplasia is potential source of false-positive diagnosis of invasive carcinoma
  - Distinction between adenoma and carcinoma may not always be possible
- Brushing may not adequately sample lesions that are predominantly infiltrative

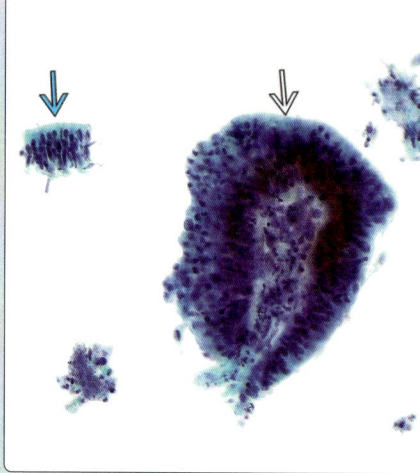

Adenoma, Papillary Frond

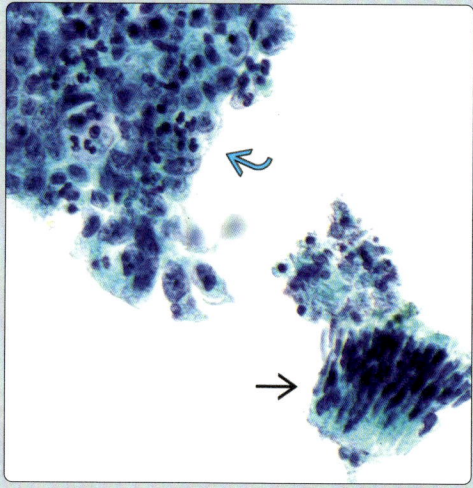

Adenoma and High-Grade Dysplasia

(Left) Papillary fragments ➡ may be seen in villous and tubulovillous adenomas. The nuclei and their configuration and polarization are similar to that seen in the adjacent strip ➡ on this Pap-stained brushing. *(Right)* This Pap-stained brushing of a colonic polyp shows a strip of adenomatous epithelium ➡ next to a disorganized cluster of cells with at least high-grade dysplasia ➡. The adenoma has well-organized pencillate nuclei, in contrast to the disorganized, crowded, and rounded nuclei of the higher grade lesion.

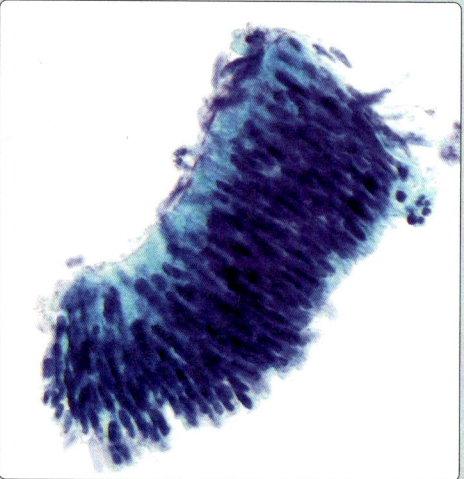

Nuclear Features of Tubular Adenoma

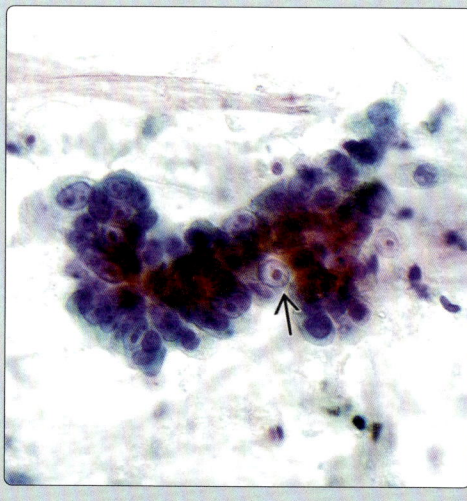

Nuclear Features of Adenocarcinoma

(Left) This Pap-stained brushing of a tubular adenoma highlights the marked nuclear crowding with maintenance of nuclear polarity typical of adenomas without high-grade dysplasia. The nuclei are elongated and hyperchromatic with dense, coarse chromatin. No nuclear rounding or nucleoli are present. *(Right)* This Pap-stained brushing of a colonic adenocarcinoma shows a jumbled cluster of rounded malignant cells with high N:C ratios and prominent eosinophilic nucleoli ➡.

Colorectal Adenoma/Carcinoma

CLINICAL ISSUES

Epidemiology
- Age
  - Prevalence ↑ with age: 20-30% by 50; 40-50% by 60
  - Nonsyndromic patients: Sharp ↑ of colorectal carcinoma at 40 years
    - CRC generally develops 1-2 decades later

Presentation
- Patients with small adenomas are usually asymptomatic, although larger adenomas may cause anemia or intussusception
- Patients with carcinomas may have lower gastrointestinal bleeding and anemia
  - Large tumors may cause obstruction

CYTOPATHOLOGY

Pattern
- Adenoma: Cohesive cellular sheets and strips of cells with some architectural disarray
- Carcinoma: Dyshesive cellular clusters, single intact malignant cells

Background
- Adenoma: Usually clean
- Carcinoma: "Dirty" necrosis, blood; mucinous carcinomas may show abundant background mucin

Cells
- Adenoma: Colonic epithelial cells retain columnar configuration, elongated nuclei; fewer goblet cells
- Carcinoma: Malignant cells may be rounded or assume unusual shapes; tumor giant cells may be seen; fewer goblet cells

Nuclear Details
- With progression along adenoma-carcinoma sequence, nuclei show more severe atypia, including
  - ↑ nuclear size, hyperchromasia, prominent &/or multiple nucleoli, coarse chromatin, irregular nuclear contours, rounded &/or pleomorphic nuclei
- Atypical mitotic figures may be seen

Cytoplasmic Details
- As dysplasia progresses, cytoplasm may have ↓ mucin content and cells have ↑ N:C ratio with loss of polarity
- Mucinous carcinomas may show signet-ring morphology with compressed nucleus and abundant cytoplasmic mucin

Cell Block Findings
- Strips or clusters of cells, necrotic background if ulcerated or invasive

Cytology-Histology Correlation
- Papillary fragments may be seen in villous adenomas

DIFFERENTIAL DIAGNOSIS

Reactive/Regenerative Changes
- Less severe and diffuse nuclear atypia
- Large cells with preserved N:C ratio
  - Nucleoli may be prominent, but chromatin is fine and nuclear membranes are smooth
- Cohesive, streaming flat sheets of cells
  - Rare, if any, single cells

Ulcer
- May see reactive stromal cells, fibrinopurulent debris, other reactive changes
- Less severe and diffuse nuclear atypia than adenoma/carcinoma; cells maintain near normal N:C ratio

Inflammatory Polyp
- Changes similar to ulcer with reactive stromal cells, inflammation, fibrinopurulent debris

SELECTED REFERENCES

1. Cheng S et al: Colonoscopic ultrasound-guided fine-needle aspiration using a curvilinear array transducer: a single-center retrospective cohort study. Dis Colon Rectum. 65(2):e80-84, 2022

Signet-Ring Cell Adenocarcinoma

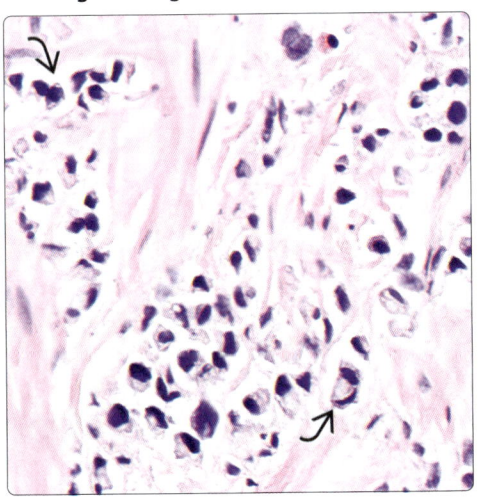

Signet-Ring Cell Adenocarcinoma

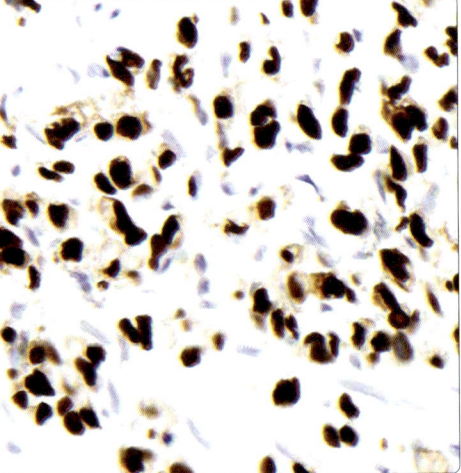

(Left) This H&E-stained transrectal EUS-guided fine needle biopsy of a perirectal tumor shows signet-ring cells infiltrating the perirectal tissue. Note the small, but hyperchromatic, tumor cells with intracytoplasmic mucin ➢. (Right) Immunostain for CDX2 shows positive nuclear staining in the tumor cells, confirming gastrointestinal origin.

Neuroendocrine Tumor/Carcinoma

KEY FACTS

TERMINOLOGY
- Neuroendocrine neoplasms, ranging from low to high grade, that may arise in esophagus, stomach, small intestine, and colorectum

CLINICAL ISSUES
- Most tumors are nonfunctioning
- Many tumors are submucosal and best sampled by endoscopic ultrasound-guided FNA
- If lesion ulcerated, brushing is option

CYTOPATHOLOGY
- Dispersed cell pattern, rosettes, loose clusters of cells with bland, monotonous nuclei, and finely stippled chromatin
- Necrosis, pleomorphism, prominent mitotic activity favor diagnosis of neuroendocrine carcinoma

ANCILLARY TESTS
- Immunostains for chromogranin, synaptophysin, and CD56 confirm neuroendocrine differentiation

- Ki-67 facilitates grading
- CD45(-) excludes lymphoma

TOP DIFFERENTIAL DIAGNOSES
- Lymphoma; poorly differentiated adenocarcinoma

GRADING
- WHO Grading system applies to tumors examined histologically; has been tried on cell blocks with varying results due to low cellularity
- Grade 1: Mitotic count < 2 per 2 mm² and Ki-67 index < 3%
- Grade 2: Mitotic count 2-20 per 2 mm² or Ki-67 index 3-20%
- Grade 3: Mitotic count > 20 per 2 mm² or Ki-67 index > 20%
- Mitotic count should be determined by counting area totaling 10 mm² and expressed as number of mitotic figures per 2 mm²
- Ki-67 index is reported as percent of positive tumor cells in areas of highest labeling (hot spots), recommendation is to count at least 500 tumor cells

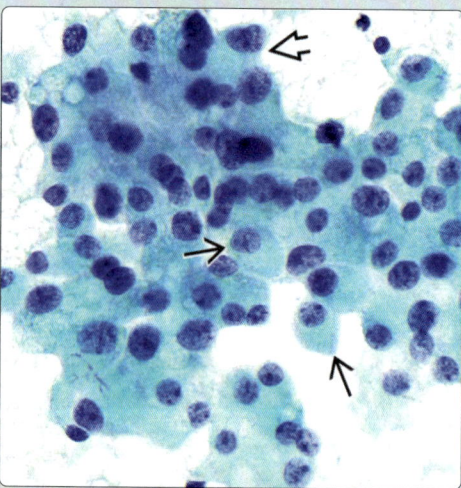

Neuroendocrine Tumor

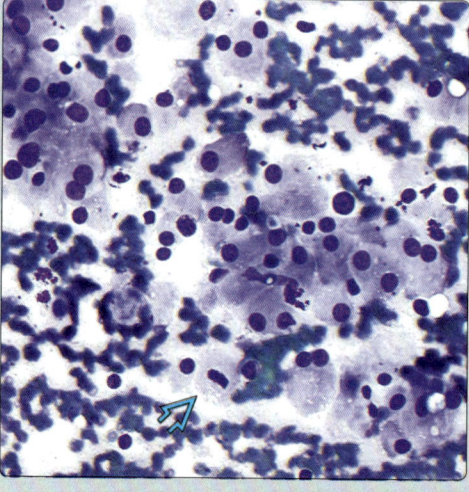

Neuroendocrine Tumor

(Left) This Pap-stained FNA of a duodenal neuroendocrine tumor (NET) shows a loosely cohesive group of monotonous cells with round nuclei and fine chromatin. Some cells have plasmacytoid ➡ morphology. Focal rosette formation ➡ is present. (Right) Diff-Quik-stained FNA of a duodenal NET shows bland plasmacytoid cells with round nuclei. Mitotic figures ➡ are rarely encountered. The resection specimen showed a grade 2 well-differentiated NET.

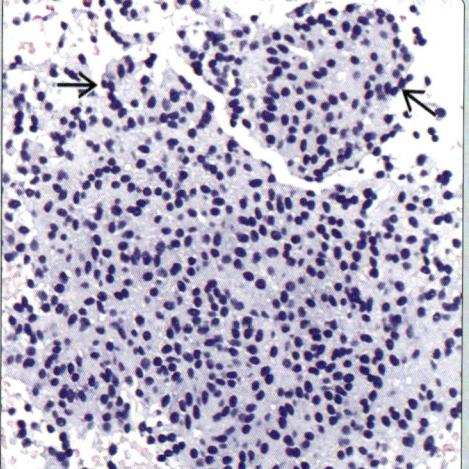

Neuroendocrine Tumor: Fine Needle Biopsy

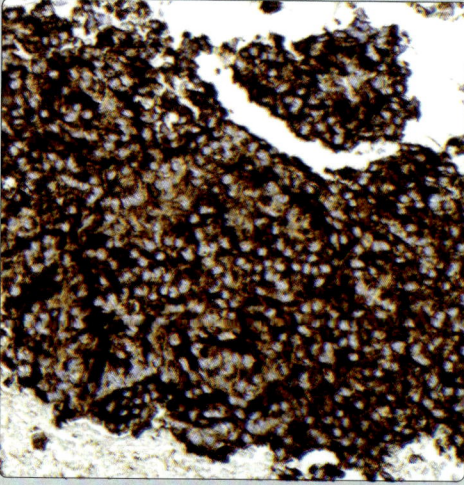

Neuroendocrine Tumor: Fine Needle Biopsy

(Left) H&E-stained section of an EUS-guided fine needle biopsy of a duodenal NET shows tumor cells with small, round nuclei. The tumor cells are arranged in rosettes ➡. (Right) Immunostain for chromogranin is performed on the same fine needle biopsy. Strong, diffuse positive staining supports neuroendocrine differentiation.

Neuroendocrine Tumor/Carcinoma

TERMINOLOGY

Abbreviations
- Neuroendocrine tumor (NET)
- Neuroendocrine carcinoma (NEC)

Synonyms
- Grade 1 (low grade, carcinoid), grade 2 (intermediate) and grade 3 (high grade) NETs: Well-differentiated NETs
- Large cell and small cell NECs: Poorly differentiated NECs, high-grade NECs

ETIOLOGY/PATHOGENESIS

Esophageal NET/NEC
- Very rare
- Usually NEC or mixed NEC with adenocarcinoma or squamous cell carcinoma

Gastric NET/NEC
- Enterochromaffin-like cell NETs most common
- Type I: Most common gastric NET; associated with autoimmune chronic atrophic gastritis
- Type II: Least common gastric NET; associated with multiple endocrine neoplasia type 1 (MEN1) and Zollinger-Ellison syndrome (ZES)
- Type III: Sporadic; not associated with autoimmune chronic atrophic gastritis, MEN1, or ZES

Small Bowel NET/NEC
- Majority nonsyndromic and sporadic
- Small bowel most common site of GI NETs

Colorectal NET/NEC
- Usually sporadic
- NEC may have associated adenocarcinoma

CYTOPATHOLOGY

Cellularity
- Hypercellular

Pattern
- Loose clusters, single cells, ± rosettes

Background
- NET and NEC: May have crushed cells in background
- NEC: Necrotic background

Cells
- NET: Monotonous round or spindled cells
- NEC: Apoptotic cells, ± pleomorphism

Nuclear Details
- NET: Finely stippled, even chromatin, smooth nuclear membranes
- NEC: Irregular, coarser chromatin, ± nucleoli, ± atypical mitoses

Cytoplasmic Details
- NET and NEC: Scant to moderate amount of delicate cytoplasm, often stripped

ANCILLARY TESTS

Immunohistochemistry
- Chromogranin, synaptophysin, and CD56 for neuroendocrine differentiation
- Ki-67 to assess proliferation

DIFFERENTIAL DIAGNOSIS

Lymphoma
- Single cell pattern; no clusters, rosettes, or true aggregates; CD45(+)

Poorly Differentiated Adenocarcinoma
- History and immunostains help determine primary site

SELECTED REFERENCES

1. Rindi G et al: Neuroendocrine neoplasia of the gastrointestinal tract revisited: towards precision medicine. Nat Rev Endocrinol. 16(10):590-607, 2020
2. Patel N et al: Neuroendocrine tumors of the gastrointestinal tract and pancreas. Surg Pathol Clin. 12(4):1021-44, 2019

Neuroendocrine Carcinoma

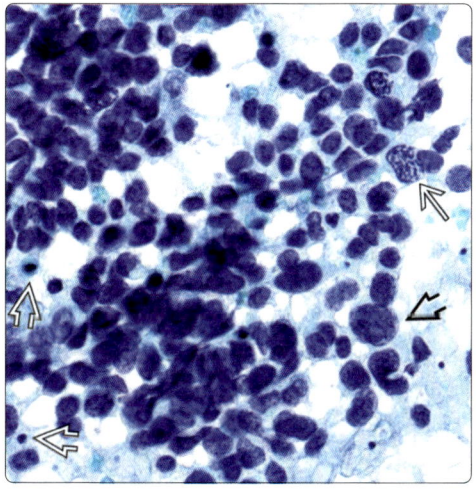

Large Cell Lymphoma

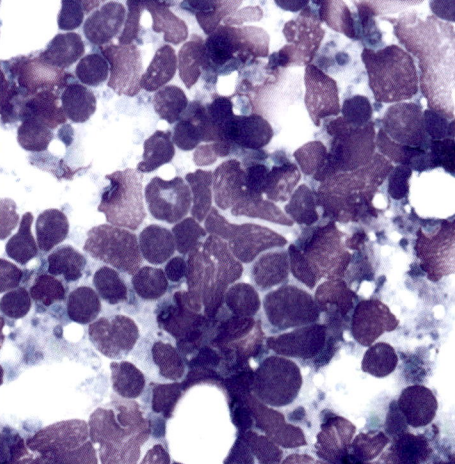

(Left) Pap-stained sample shows neuroendocrine carcinoma (NEC), small cell undifferentiated type, with nuclear pleomorphism ➡, mitosis ➡, and apoptosis ➡. (Right) Romanowsky-stained sample shows a high-grade lymphoma with large cells, which could be mistaken for NEC.

Spindle Cell Neoplasms of Gastrointestinal Tract, Including Gastrointestinal Stromal Tumors

TERMINOLOGY

Abbreviations
- Gastrointestinal stromal tumor (GIST)

Definitions
- GIST: Neoplasm arising from interstitial cells of Cajal; behavior depends on anatomic location, size, & mitotic activity
- Schwannoma: Neoplasm arising from Schwann cells of peripheral nerves; majority are benign, some associated with neurofibromatosis
- Leiomyoma: Neoplasm arising from smooth muscle cells; majority are benign

ETIOLOGY/PATHOGENESIS

GIST
- Associated with *KIT* or *PDGFRA* mutations
  - ~ 4,500 new cases/year in USA; median age: ~ 60 years; affects men & women equally
  - Stomach is most common site, followed by small bowel; rarely involves extraintestinal, duodenum, colon, rectum, & esophagus
  - ~ 20-25% of gastric GISTs are malignant; up to 40-50% of small bowel GISTs are malignant
  - Therapy: Tumors with *KIT* mutations → tyrosine kinase inhibitor imatinib (Gleevec); *KIT* exon 9 mutation → sunitinib malate (Sutent)
- ~ 10% have succinate dehydrogenase (SDH) deficiency
  - Mutation of SDH gene or other disruption in SDH pathway
  - Do not respond to imatinib (lack *KIT* mutations); more likely to have nodal metastasis
  - Usually younger patients; gastric tumors; epithelioid or mixed morphology

Schwannoma
- Most schwannomas are sporadic & benign
  - GI schwannomas usually arise within gastric muscularis propria; often have peripheral cuff of lymphoid tissue, this may not be appreciated on FNA

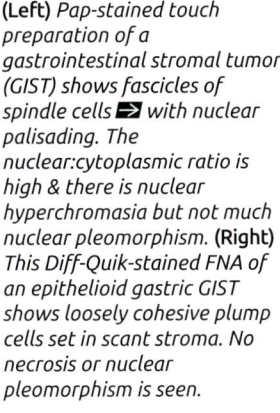

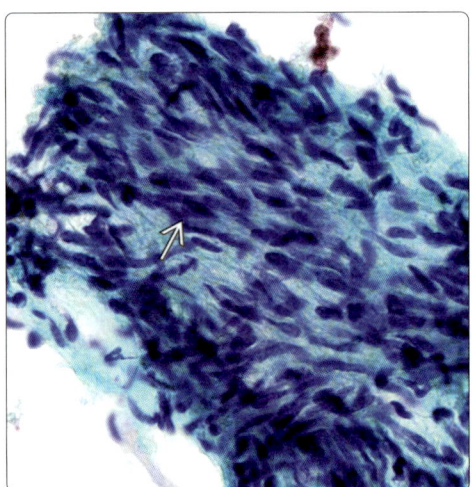

Spindle Cell Gastrointestinal Stromal Tumor

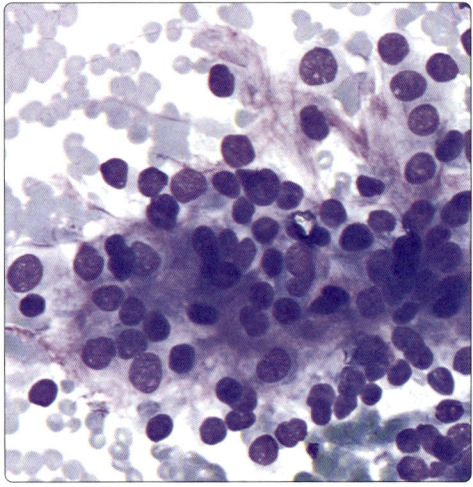

Epithelioid Gastrointestinal Stromal Tumor

(Left) Pap-stained touch preparation of a gastrointestinal stromal tumor (GIST) shows fascicles of spindle cells ➡ with nuclear palisading. The nuclear:cytoplasmic ratio is high & there is nuclear hyperchromasia but not much nuclear pleomorphism. (Right) This Diff-Quik-stained FNA of an epithelioid gastric GIST shows loosely cohesive plump cells set in scant stroma. No necrosis or nuclear pleomorphism is seen.

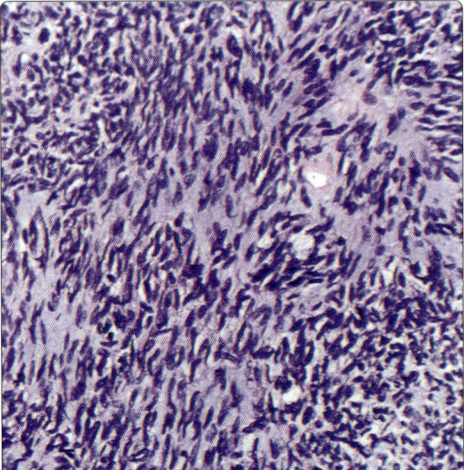

Cell Block of Spindle Cell Gastrointestinal Stromal Tumor

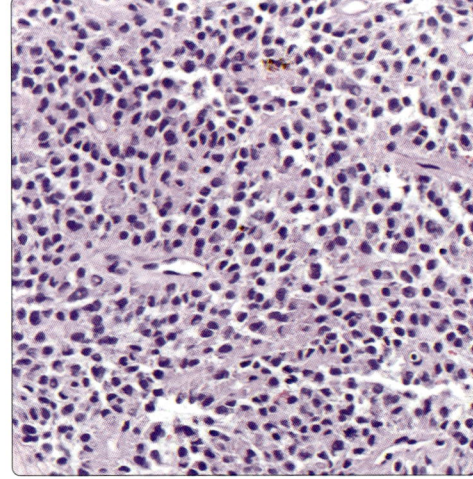

Cell Block of Epithelioid Gastrointestinal Stromal Tumor

(Left) H&E-stained cell block section from an EUS FNA of a gastric spindle cell GIST shows cohesive spindled cells arranged in fascicles with delicate eosinophilic cytoplasm. No mitosis or necrosis is seen. (Right) H&E-stained cell block section from an EUS FNA of a gastric epithelioid GIST shows round tumor cells arranged in sheets & loose clusters.

Spindle Cell Neoplasms of Gastrointestinal Tract, Including Gastrointestinal Stromal Tumors

Leiomyoma
- Benign neoplasms with smooth muscle differentiation
- More common in esophagus & colon; usually arise from muscularis mucosae

MICROSCOPIC

Cytopathology
- GIST
  - **Cellularity**: Intermediate to high
  - **Pattern**: Fairly cohesive & well-organized fascicles of spindled or epithelioid cells, few single cells
  - **Background**: Clean; if prior therapy or infarction, may see necrosis
  - **Cells**: Uniform, plump spindled or epithelioid cells with minimal if any atypia; no nuclear pleomorphism
  - **Nuclear details**: Oval elongated nuclei with blunted ends (spindle cell GIST) or rounded nuclei (epithelioid GIST); no nuclear pleomorphism, usually no conspicuous nucleoli
  - **Cytoplasmic details:** Spindle cell GIST: Scant inconspicuous fibrillary cytoplasm; epithelioid GIST: Moderate to abundant eosinophilic cytoplasm
  - **Cell block findings**: Cohesive fascicles of spindle cells or clusters of epithelioid cells
  - **IHC:** DOG1 & CD117 positivity confirms diagnosis; CD34 is frequently positive; loss of SDHB correlates with SDH deficiency
  - Increased mitotic activity & necrosis are worrisome features for malignancy, but these are best assessed on resection specimens since GIST can be large
- Schwannoma
  - **Cellularity**: Low to intermediate, tightly cohesive groups of well-organized spindle cells arranged in fascicles
  - **Background**: Clean; necrosis should not be seen; ± lymphoid aggregates usually seen at periphery of schwannoma
  - **Cells**: Spindle cells with inconspicuous fibrillary cytoplasm, indistinct cytoplasmic borders; few, if any, single cells
  - **Nuclear details**: Hyperchromatic spindle cells, some nuclei may have pointed or "fish hook" ends; no or minute nucleoli; ± intranuclear inclusions; ± random nuclear pleomorphism (ancient change); no mitotic activity
  - **Cytoplasmic details**: Scant fibrillary cytoplasm; mitotic activity & necrosis should be absent
  - **Cell block**: Antoni A (hypercellular, tightly packed, very organized cells) & Antoni B (hypocellular, less organized); ± hemosiderin deposition; ± Verocay bodies (tissue fragments with peripheral palisaded nuclei & central fibrillary area)
  - **IHC:** S100(+), strong & diffuse; nuclear SOX10(+) is also characteristic
- Leiomyoma
  - **Cellularity**: Low to intermediate; cohesive, bland spindle cells in fascicles
  - **Background**: Clean
  - **Cells**: Very bland spindle cells with moderate amount of eosinophilic cytoplasm
  - **Nuclear details**: Bland elongated nuclei with blunted ends; no nucleoli, no pleomorphism, few, if any, mitoses; smooth nuclear contours
  - **Cytoplasmic details**: Moderate amount of eosinophilic cytoplasm
  - **Cell block**: Fascicles of bland spindle cells, resembles normal smooth muscle
  - **IHC**: SMA, desmin, & h-caldesmon diffusely (+); S100 & CD117 (-)
  - In GI tract, differential diagnosis includes sampling of adjacent muscularis propria, so clinical & radiographic correlation is necessary
- Differential diagnosis
  - Leiomyosarcoma, solitary fibrous tumor, inflammatory fibroid polyp, desmoid tumor

SELECTED REFERENCES

1. Jin M et al: Mesenchymal neoplasms of the tubular gut and adjacent structures: experience with EUS-guided fine-needle aspiration cytopathology. J Am Soc Cytopathol. 9(6):528-39, 2020

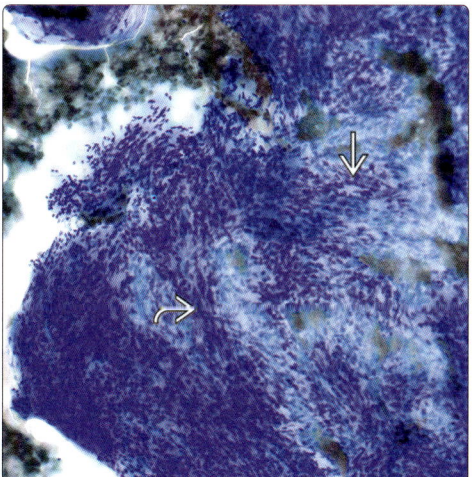

Spindle Cell Neoplasm of Wall of Gastrointestinal Tract

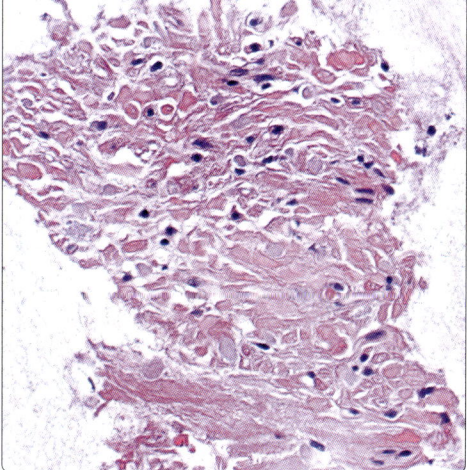

Leiomyoma

(Left) Diff-Quik-stained bundles of spindle cells ➡ with nuclear palisading & some open spaces ➡ are shown, likely corresponding to Verocay bodies. The tumor was strongly S100(+); DOG1 & desmin (-). These results support schwannoma. **(Right)** H&E-stained microbiopsy of an esophageal wall tumor without atypia or necrosis is shown. The tumor was strongly positive for desmin. Normal GI tract muscularis is also in the differential, but ultrasound confirmed the needle was in a mass lesion.

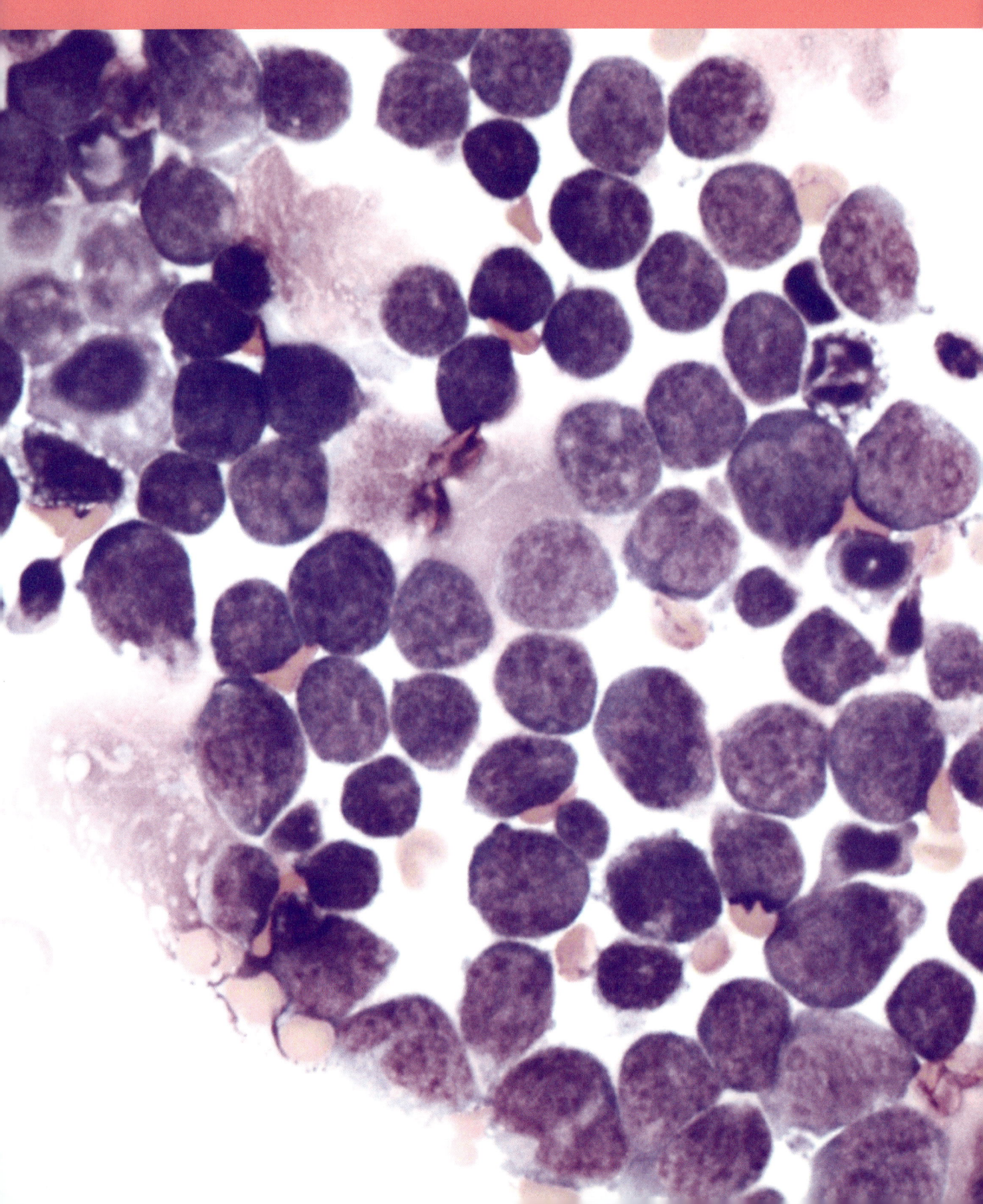

PART II
SECTION 3
Cerebrospinal Fluid

Normal Cerebrospinal Fluid and Contamination by Normal Elements	176
Infectious Meningitis	180
Aseptic and Mollaret Meningitis	182
Subarachnoid Hemorrhage	184
Neurodegenerative Diseases	186
Primary Brain Tumors	188
Leukemia and Lymphoma	190
Metastasis in Cerebrospinal Fluid	192

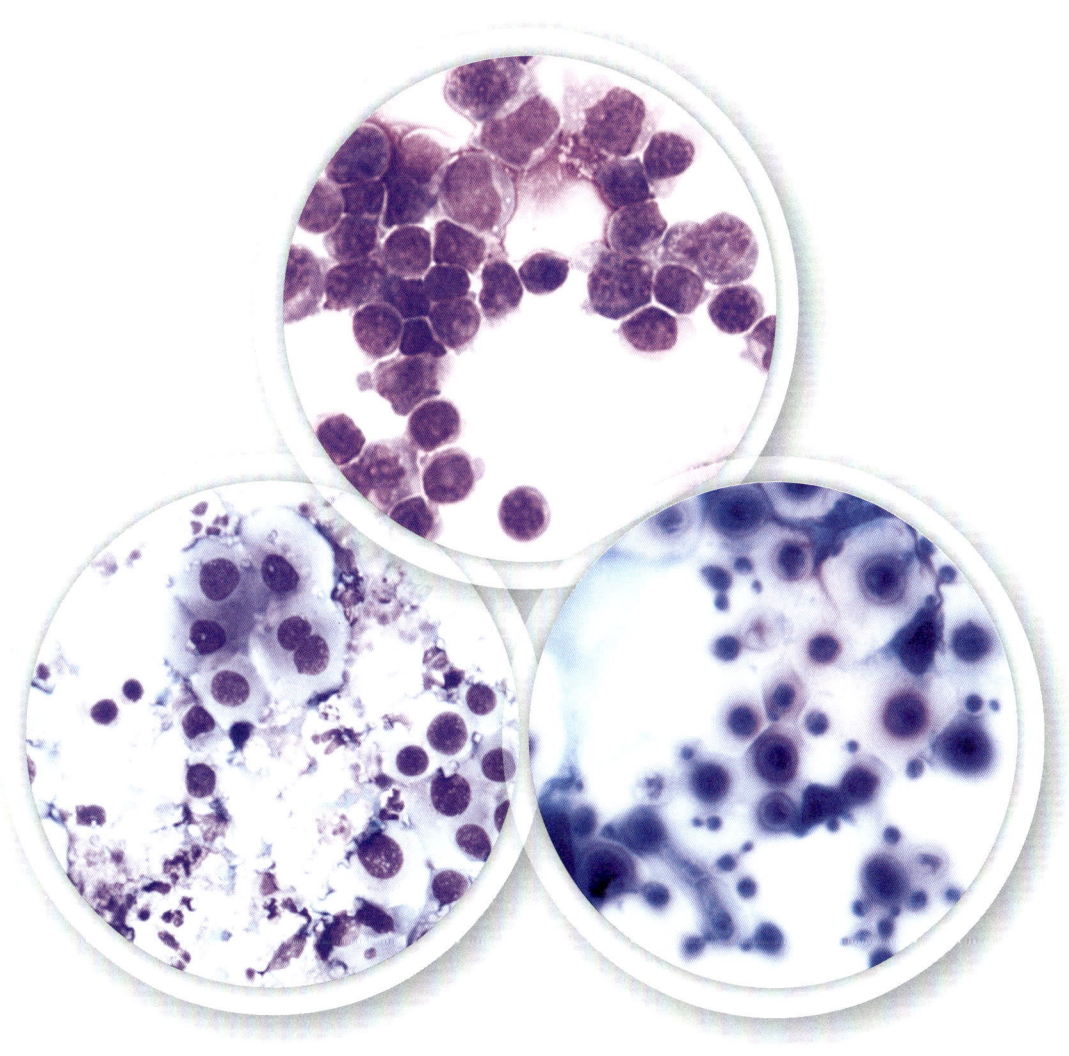

Normal Cerebrospinal Fluid and Contamination by Normal Elements

TERMINOLOGY

Abbreviations
- Cerebrospinal fluid (CSF)

CLINICAL IMPLICATIONS

Cytopathologic Examination of CSF
- Useful in diagnosis and posttherapeutic monitoring of
  - Tumors (space-occupying lesions)
    - Includes staging (e.g., medulloblastoma)
  - Neoplastic meningitis
  - Infections

Clinical Indication of Lumbar Puncture
- Urgent lumbar puncture (LP)
  - Cases of suspected CNS infection (i.e., meningitis, encephalitis)
  - Unexplained fever in infant or immunocompromised host
  - Possible subarachnoid hemorrhage in setting of negative CT scan (rare)
- Nonurgent LP
  - Evaluation of possible neuroimmunologic disorders (e.g., multiple sclerosis, Guillain-Barré syndrome)
  - Carcinomatous meningitis
  - CNS lymphoma/leukemia
- No indication for routine cases of dementia, ischemic strokes, or recurrent seizures

MACROSCOPIC

General Features
- Normal CSF is clear and colorless
- Total CSF volume: 90-150 mL (adults); 10-60 mL (children)
- ~ 500-600 mL/day is produced (adults)
- Protein concentration: 15-45 mg/dL (1/2-1/3 of serum)
- Glucose level: 50-80 mg/dL (60-80% of blood sugar)
- When tumor is primary diagnostic consideration, at least 3 mL, preferably > 5 mL, should be sent to cytologic examination
- CSF specimen should be processed as soon as possible in laboratory (ideally < 1 hour after LP)
- Source of CSF specimen obtained
  - LP (spinal tap)
    - Most common
  - Ventricle of brain
    - Fluid from ventriculoperitoneal shunt procedure
  - Cystic brain lesions or from cavity of previous surgery for brain tumor

MICROSCOPIC

General Features
- Normal CSF cells in adults
  - Only few small lymphocytes and monocytes
    - Lymphocytes generally have small, round nucleus and scant cytoplasm
    - Monocytes have irregular nuclei and more abundant cytoplasm
    - Under normal conditions, plasma cells are never seen
  - Acellular CSF cytology specimen is common and considered adequate for cytologic evaluation
  - Cell counts
    - Greater in neonates than in older people (10.17 ± 8.45 vs. 2.59 ± 8.45 cells/mm^3; monocyte vs. lymphocyte predominant, respectively)
  - Concentration techniques (such as centrifugation) frequently introduce artifacts
    - Nuclear contour irregularities may be increased

REPORTING CRITERIA

Terminology
- Negative for malignancy/benign
  - Including specific infections/infectious conditions
  - Acellular specimens are adequate/negative
- Atypical
  - Specify type of concerning cells to degree possible; use sparingly

(Left) *Diff-Quik-stained cytospin of cerebrospinal fluid (CSF) from a ventriculoperitoneal shunt (VPS) shows a small fragment of degenerated brain parenchyma (astrocytes ➡, probable microglia ➡).* (Right) *Diff-Quik-stained cytospin of a ventricular CSF specimen procured at craniotomy for glioblastoma shows a group of degenerated ependymal cells ➡ in a hemorrhagic background. The nuclei are slightly larger than those of neutrophils.*

Small Fragment of Brain Parenchyma

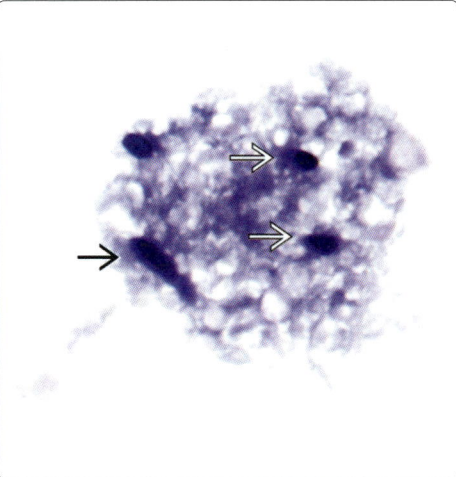

Group of Ependymal Cells

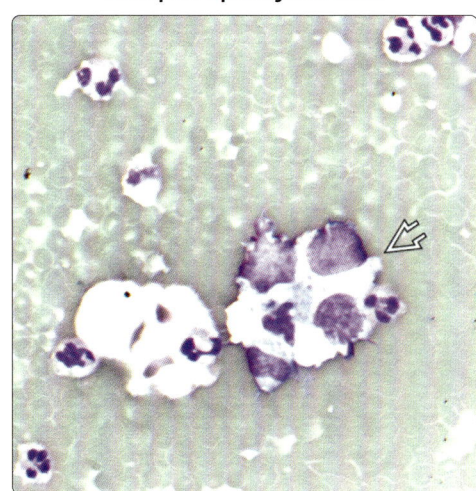

Normal Cerebrospinal Fluid and Contamination by Normal Elements

Immunochemistry for Differential Diagnosis of Benign Intracranial/Intraspinal Cells

	EMA	AE1/AE3	CD99	GFAP	Source of Cerebrospinal Fluid
Ependymal cells	(+); diffuse, cytoplasmic, dot-like	(-)	(+)	(+/-)	Ventricular fluid
Choroid plexus cells	(-)	(+)	(-/+)	(-)	Ventricular fluid
Pia-arachnoid cells	(+)	(-)	(-/+)	(-)	Lumbar puncture fluid

- o Usually specimen with rare cells of concern, may be helpful to prompt further work-up if malignancy was not high on differential
- Suspicious for malignancy
  - o Specify type of concerning cells
  - o Usually few cells but not sufficient for confident diagnosis of malignancy, often resolved by additional sampling
- Positive for malignancy
  - o Identify type with as much specificity as possible
  - o Ancillary studies often needed to confirm diagnosis, especially 1st time
- Nondiagnostic
  - o Specify if traumatic type or hematopoietic cell contamination

DIFFERENTIAL DIAGNOSIS

Benign Intracranial/Intraspinal Cells

- May be present in CSF
- Predominant cell types possibly seen, depend on sources of CSF specimen obtained
  - o Ventricular fluid and fluid from intracranial cavity secondary to previous neurosurgery
    - Ependymal cells, choroid plexus cells
    - Fragments of brain parenchyma
  - o LP specimen
    - Pia-arachnoid cells
    - Fibroblastic cells from paraspinal soft tissue
- Cytologic differential diagnosis
  - o Ependymal cells vs. choroid plexus cells
    - Cytologically indistinguishable in many instances
    - Small, loose clusters or cobblestone-like clusters of oval to columnar cells, resembling histiocytes with abundant cytoplasm and indistinct cell borders
    - Choroid plexus cells may have cilia
  - o Ependymal cells vs. pia-arachnoid cells
    - Cytologically very difficult to distinguish
    - Both types of cells show small, loose clusters of histiocyte-like cells
    - Source of CSF sample is important, and immunocytochemistry is helpful for differentiation
  - o Not confusing any of these benign cells with malignancy is of primary importance
- Immunocytochemical differential diagnosis
  - o Ependymal cells
    - EMA(+) (diffuse, cytoplasmic, or dot-like), CD99(+), GFAP(+/-)
  - o Choroid plexus cells
    - AE1/AE3(+), GFAP(-), EMA(-)
  - o Pia-arachnoid cells
    - EMA(+), CD99(-/+)

Extracranial/Extraspinal Contaminants

- Bone marrow cells (from vertebral bone by LP)
  - o Cytologically, hematopoietic elements are identified
  - o All 3 marrow elements may not be seen
  - o Cellularity may be very high
- Nucleus pulposus, anulus fibrosus, and cartilage endplate (from intervertebral disc/space by LP)
  - o Nucleus pulposus
    - Small fragments composed of mucoid/myxoid matrix with scattered small nuclei are seen
    - Variable degeneration is seen
  - o Anulus fibrosus
    - Fibrocartilage composed of fibrous matrix with scattered small nuclei
    - No apparent mucoid-rich areas are seen
    - Variable degeneration is noted
  - o Cartilage endplate (from vertebral body)
    - Hyaline cartilage characterized by cartilage cells with clearly visible perinuclear halo
- Anucleated squames/squamous cells from skin
  - o Differential diagnosis of anucleated squames/squamous cells in CSF
    - Ruptured teratomatous cysts (epidermoid/epidermal cysts)
    - Craniopharyngioma
    - Metastatic/invasive keratinizing squamous cell carcinomas (if atypia is present in squamous cells)
- Fibroblasts
  - o Commonly seen in LP specimens
  - o Deriving from paraspinal connective tissue or epidural/leptomeningeal tissue
  - o Single bland, spindle-shaped cells
  - o Cytologic distinction from arachnoid cells is difficult/impossible
- Starch granules
  - o Common contaminants, usually from glove powder
  - o Refractile particles often with cracked center
  - o Macrophages ingesting these particles may be seen
  - o Mimicking cryptococci
    - No capsule or budding is seen in starch granules

SELECTED REFERENCES

1. Wick M et al: Automated analysis of cerebrospinal fluid cells using commercially available blood cell analysis devices-a critical appraisal. Cells. 10(5), 2021
2. Rahimi J et al: Overview of cerebrospinal fluid cytology. Handb Clin Neurol. 145:563-71, 2017
3. Irani DN: Properties and composition of normal cerebrospinal fluid. In Irani DN et al: Cerebrospinal Fluid in Clinical Practice. 1st ed. Saunders, 2009
4. Sarnat HB: Histochemistry and immunocytochemistry of the developing ependyma and choroid plexus. Microsc Res Tech. 41(1):14-28, 1998

Normal Cerebrospinal Fluid and Contamination by Normal Elements

Ependymal Cell Sheet

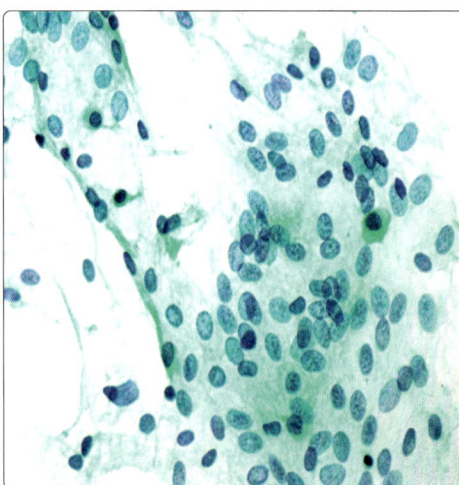

(Left) *Pap stain shows normal ependymal cells, which are seen in the CSF from a VPS. Note a sheet of epithelioid cells with fine nuclear chromatin.* **(Right)** *Immunocytochemistry for EMA shows intracytoplasmic dot-like positivity ⇨ in normal ependymal cells.*

EMA Dot-Like Pattern in Ependymal Cells

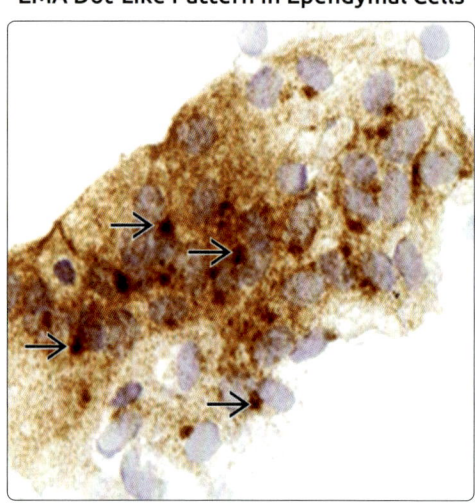

CD99 in Ependymal Cells

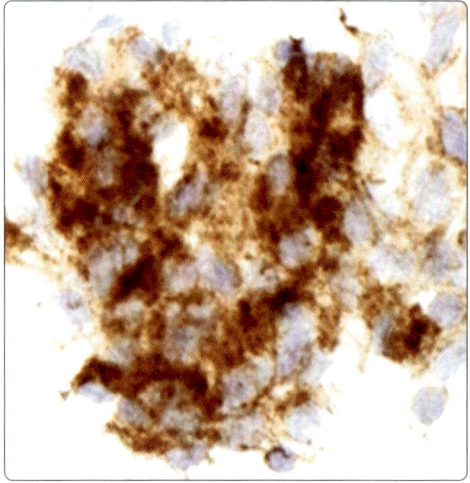

(Left) *Immunocytochemistry for CD99 shows cytoplasmic and membranous positivity in normal ependymal cells.* **(Right)** *Diff-Quik stain of normal choroid plexus cells in CSF from a VPS reveals a cluster of epithelioid cells with abundant cytoplasm. Intracytoplasmic vacuoles ⇨ of varying size are commonly seen.*

Choroid Plexus Cells With Vacuoles

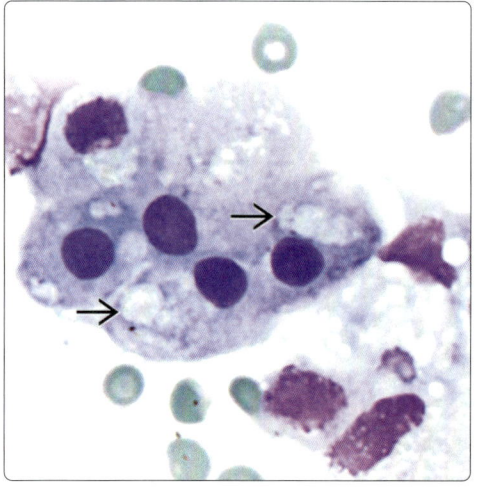

Choroid Plexus Cell Cluster

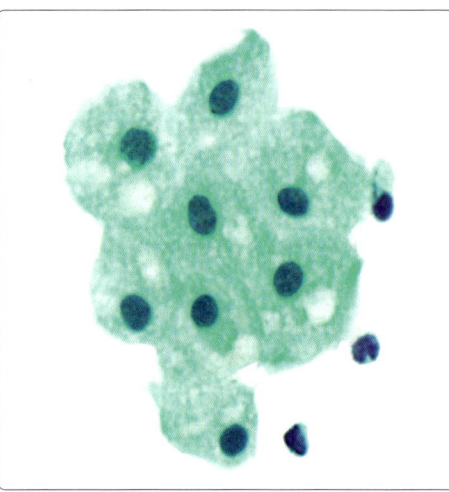

(Left) *Normal choroid plexus cells in CSF from a VPS are characterized by a cobblestone-like cluster of epithelioid cells with bland nuclei and abundant, somewhat granular cytoplasm as seen on this Pap stain.* **(Right)** *Immunocytochemistry for AE1/AE3 shows strong cytoplasmic positivity in normal choroid plexus cells.*

AE1/AE3 in Choroid Plexus Cells

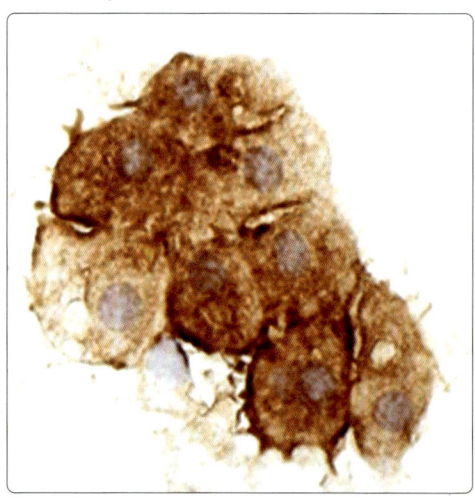

Normal Cerebrospinal Fluid and Contamination by Normal Elements

Pia-Arachnoid Cells, Loose Cluster

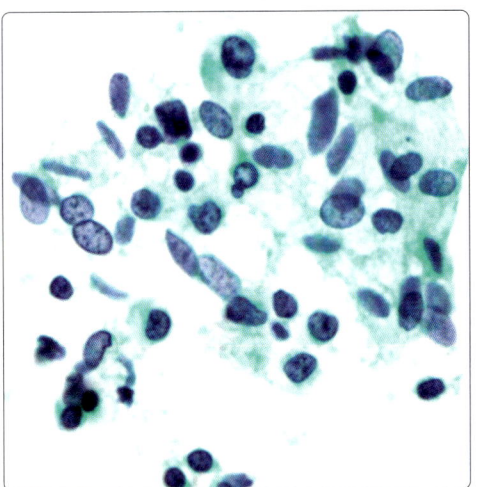

EMA in Pia-Arachnoid Cells

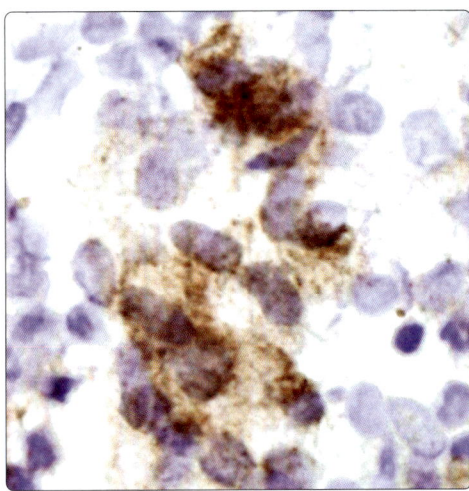

(Left) *Normal pia-arachnoid cells in CSF are seen as a loose cluster of spindled to epithelioid cells with bland cytologic features on Pap stain.* (Right) *Immunocytochemistry for EMA shows cytoplasmic positivity in normal pia-arachnoid cells.*

Brain Parenchyma With Capillaries

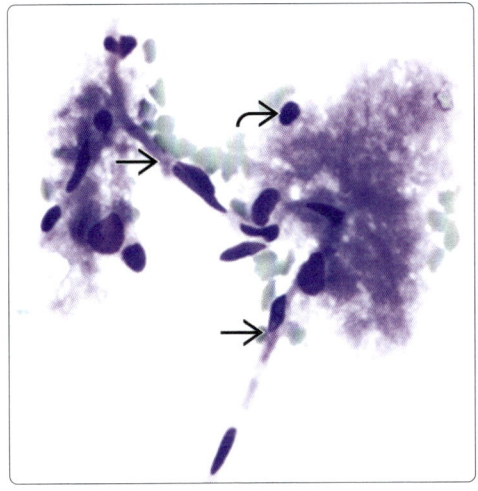

Brain Parenchyma With Microglia

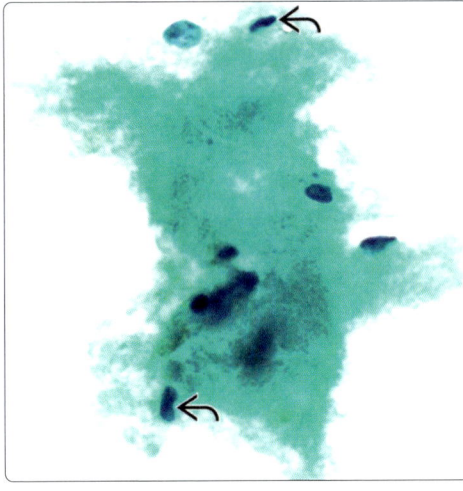

(Left) *Normal brain parenchyma seen in CSF from a VPS shows granular, fluffy material along with few capillaries ⇨ on this Diff-Quik stain. A glial cell (oligodendroglial cell) ⇨ is also seen.* (Right) *Normal brain parenchyma seen in CSF from a VPS shows an irregular fragment of granular, fluffy material on Pap stain. Few microglial cells are identified ⇨.*

Hematopoietic Cell Contaminants

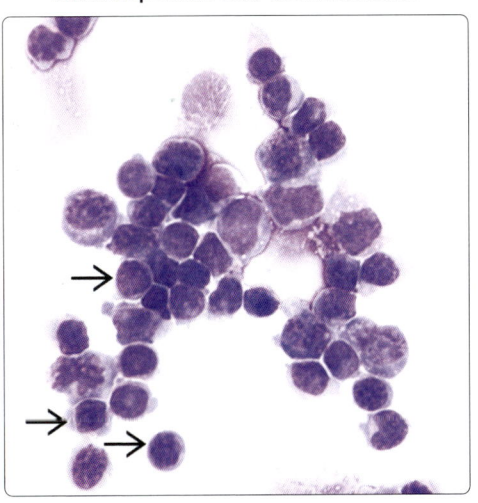

Nucleus Pulposus

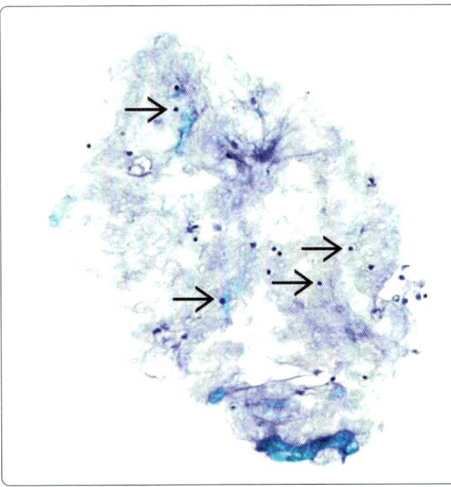

(Left) *High magnification of hematopoietic marrow elements (mainly erythroid precursor cells) ⇨ from vertebral bone marrow is shown on this Diff-Quik stain.* (Right) *Pap stain of nucleus pulposus from an intervertebral disc is shown. An abundant mucoid/myxoid matrix with multiple small nuclei ⇨ is seen.*

Infectious Meningitis

KEY FACTS

ETIOLOGY/PATHOGENESIS

- Most common causative organisms
  - Acute bacterial meningitis in immunocompetent adults: *Streptococcus pneumoniae*, *Neisseria meningitidis*, and *Haemophilus influenzae*
  - Acute fungal meningitis in immunocompromised patients: *Cryptococcus neoformans*, *Candida albicans*, and *Aspergillus fumigatus*

CYTOPATHOLOGY

- CSF pleocytosis (granulocyte, lymphocyte, or monocyte pleocytosis) is characteristic but nonspecific feature
- Some large infectious agents (e.g., *Cryptococcus*, *Candida*) can be identified cytologically
- Cryptococcal meningitis: Most common fungal organism observed in CSF
  - Refractile yeast forms 5-15 µm in diameter with narrow-based budding; mostly extracellular but can be engulfed by macrophages
- Herpes simplex virus (HSV) meningoencephalitis
  - Cytologic evidence of hemorrhage in CSF (e.g., red blood cells, hemosiderin-laden &/or lipid-laden macrophages)

ANCILLARY TESTS

- *Cryptococcus* organisms can be highlighted with GMS or PAS stains; mucicarmine stains capsule
- Microbiologic studies crucial for definitive diagnosis of infectious meningitis
- Cryptococcal antigen studies rapid and highly sensitive (~ 90%); culture also has high sensitivity
  - Uncommon capsule-deficient organisms may not be detected by antigen tests
- PCR testing most useful method for diagnosis of viral meningitis and is becoming primary for bacterial meningitis
- For lymphocytic pleocytosis, flow cytometric analysis may be required to exclude lymphoma/leukemia
- Elevated opening pressure, elevated CSF protein, and low CSF glucose indicate possibility of meningitis

Cryptococcus Yeast Forms

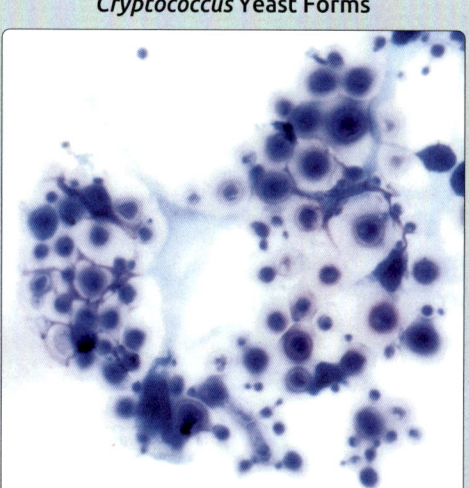

Cryptococcus in Macrophage

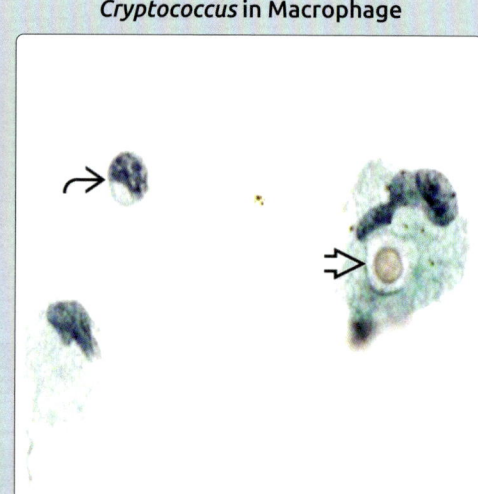

(Left) Diff-Quik-stained CSF specimen from a severely immunodeficient HIV patient shows remarkably large numbers of Cryptococcus yeast forms. Note the variability in the sizes of the individual organisms. (Right) In this case of cryptococcal meningitis, a Pap-stained CSF specimen shows a histiocyte phagocytosing a cryptococcal yeast with a mucopolysaccharide capsule ⇨. Note the size of the yeast relative to the lymphocyte ⇨.

Cryptococcus (High Magnification)

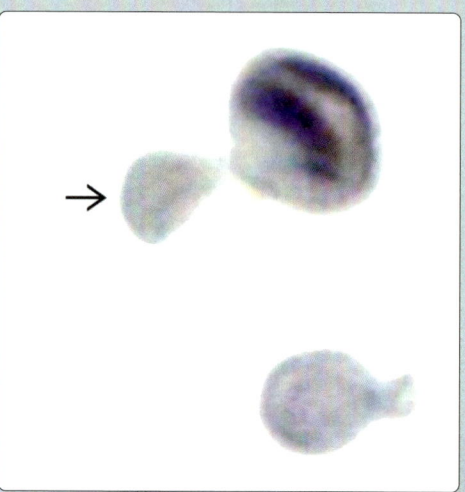

Acute Meningitis Due to *Candida*

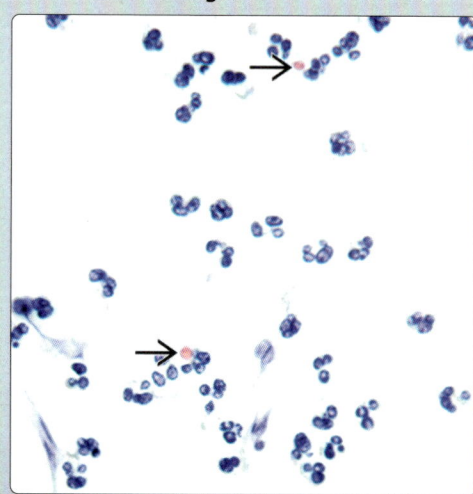

(Left) High-power view of a Pap-stained CSF specimen shows a budding yeast form ⇨ in this case of Cryptococcus meningitis. (Right) Pap stain of acute meningitis due to Candida species shows pleocytosis predominantly composed of neutrophils. Candida yeasts ⇨ are present.

Infectious Meningitis

TERMINOLOGY

Definitions
- Infectious meningitis: Leptomeningeal and subarachnoidal inflammation caused by infectious agents
  - Infectious meningoencephalitis: Underlying brain parenchymal inflammation extended from meningeal inflammation caused by infectious agents

ETIOLOGY/PATHOGENESIS

Infectious Agents
- Bacteria, fungi, viruses, parasites, and protozoa
  - Most common causative organisms
    - Acute bacterial meningitis in immunocompetent adults: *Streptococcus pneumoniae*, *Neisseria meningitidis*, and *Haemophilus influenzae*
    - Acute fungal meningitis in immunocompromised patients: *Cryptococcus neoformans*, *Candida albicans*, and *Aspergillus fumigatus*

CLINICAL ISSUES

Presentation
- Classic triad of symptoms: Neck stiffness, fever, and altered mental status; headache also common

Diagnostic Method
- Lumbar puncture to diagnose or exclude meningitis

CYTOPATHOLOGY

Cellularity
- CSF pleocytosis is characteristic

Pattern
- Granulocyte pleocytosis in CSF
  - Neutrophilic: Bacterial infections; early stage of meningitis caused by other infectious agents
  - Eosinophilic: Parasitic and mycotic infections
- Lymphocyte pleocytosis
  - Activated lymphocytes: Nonpurulent infections (e.g., virus, *Spirochaeta*)
  - Activated lymphocytes and plasma cells: Chronic infections
- Monocyte pleocytosis
  - Terminal phase of infections/inflammations with scavenger reaction

Background
- May be hemorrhagic &/or necrotic depending on severity of inflammation and of disruption of underlying brain parenchyma

Infection-Specific Findings
- Cryptococcal meningitis: Most common fungal organism observed in CSF
  - Microorganisms (5-15 μm in diameter) with narrow-based budding cytologically identified
- Herpes simplex virus (HSV) meningoencephalitis
  - Commonly involves temporal base
  - Cytologic evidence of hemorrhage in CSF (e.g., red blood cells, hemosiderin-laden &/or lipid-laden macrophages)

ANCILLARY TESTS

Viral Meningitis
- PCR test: Rapid, sensitive, and specific method of diagnosis for many viruses
- Flow cytometric analysis to exclude lymphoma/leukemia

Bacterial Meningitis
- PCR tests have high sensitivity and specificity, replacing staining and culture

Cryptococcal Meningitis
- Antigen assay and culture both ~ 90% sensitive

SELECTED REFERENCES
1. Shahan B et al: Cerebrospinal fluid analysis. Am Fam Physician. 103(7):422-8, 2021
2. Sood R et al: Cerebrospinal fluid pleocytosis in immunocompromised patients: can it be Cryptococcus. Diagn Cytopathol. 48(2):164-8, 2020

Reactive Lymphocytes and Histiocytes in Herpes Simplex Meningoencephalitis

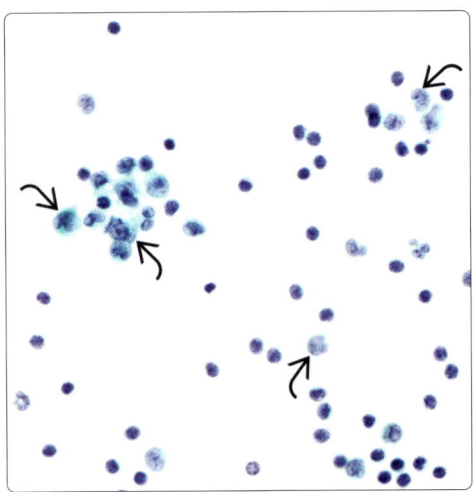

Neurosyphilis

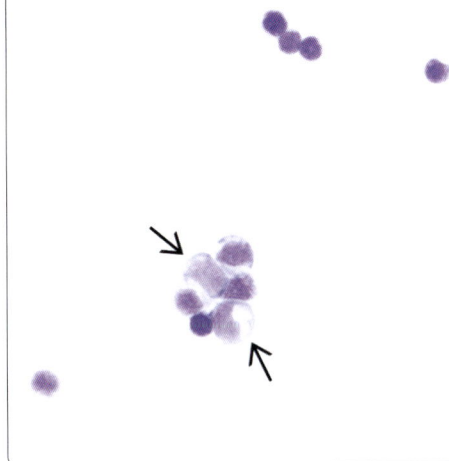

(Left) *Pap-stained CSF specimen from a patient with HSV meningoencephalitis shows lymphocytic pleocytosis with many histiocytes ➔. The findings are nonspecific; diagnosis of viral encephalitis needs to be verified by molecular methods.* **(Right)** *Diff-Quik-stained CSF cytospin from a patient with neurosyphilis shows lymphohistiocytic pleocytosis with few histiocytes ➔ (nonspecific finding). CSF is VDRL reactive.*

Aseptic and Mollaret Meningitis

KEY FACTS

TERMINOLOGY
- Aseptic meningitis: Not synonymous with viral meningitis but sometimes used interchangeably
  - Meningeal inflammation with negative routine bacterial cultures
- Mollaret meningitis: Recurrent episodes of meningitis of idiopathic etiology (original description)

ETIOLOGY/PATHOGENESIS
- Aseptic meningitis: Infection by variety of DNA or RNA viruses (especially enteroviruses) is most common cause
- Mollaret meningitis: Associated with herpes simplex virus type 2 in most cases

CYTOPATHOLOGY
- Aseptic meningitis: Neutrophilic leukocytosis, then lymphocytosis (early) and increased monocytes/histiocytes (late)
  - Later, increase in monocytes and macrophages is noted
  - Neutrophil predominance can persist even in later stage, mimicking bacterial meningitis
- Mollaret meningitis: Monocytic pleocytosis with Mollaret cells (footprints in sand appearance)
  - Degenerated monocytes ("ghost cells") can be seen

ANCILLARY TESTS
- Molecular testing for viruses may identify underlying cause
- Flow cytometric immunophenotyping of leukocytes is of great use to exclude lymphoma

TOP DIFFERENTIAL DIAGNOSES
- Lymphoma
  - Flow cytometric immunophenotyping is of help
- Bacterial (pyogenic) meningitis
  - Microbiological studies, including nucleic acid tests and biochemical tests of CSF, are very helpful
- Meningitis due to ruptured spinal dermoid/epidermoid cysts

Lymphocytosis in Aseptic Meningitis

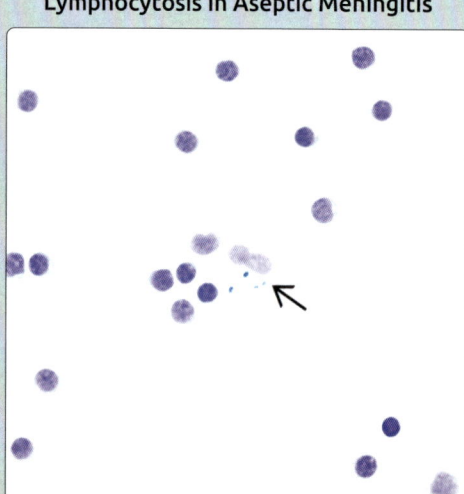

Lymphocyte Nuclear Irregularities in Aseptic Meningitis

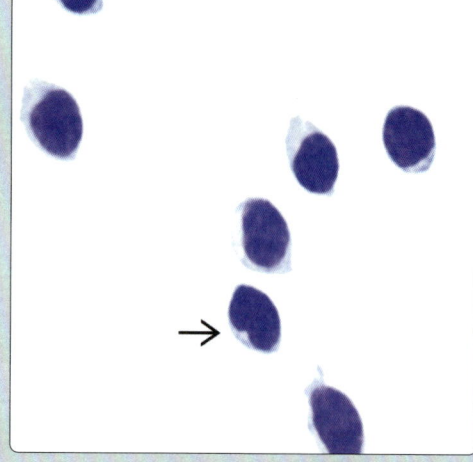

(Left) Diff-Quik stain shows pleocytosis composed predominantly of lymphocytes (i.e., lymphocytosis). A histiocyte phagocytizing debris is also present ➡. (Right) Diff-Quik stain (high-power view) shows abnormal nuclear lobation/indentation of some of the lymphocytes ➡. The changes are minor and not of the degree typical for lymphoma.

Monocytes and Histiocytes in Aseptic Meningitis

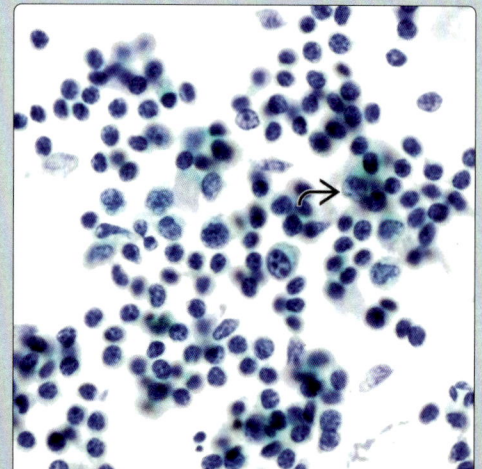

Lymphohistiocytic Infiltrates in Meninges

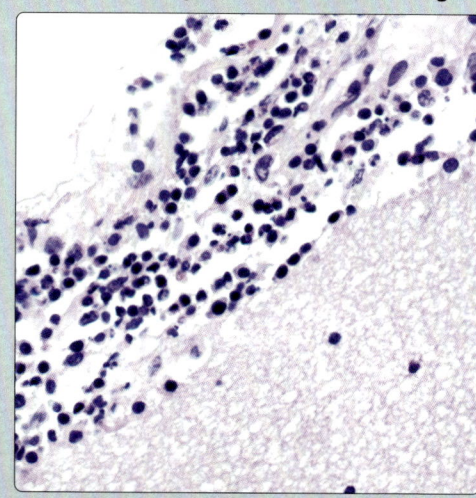

(Left) Pap stain reveals mixed inflammatory pleocytosis with scattered monocytes/histiocytes ➡. (Right) Histologic section (H&E stain) shows the leptomeninges filled with lymphohistiocytic infiltrates.

Aseptic and Mollaret Meningitis

TERMINOLOGY

Synonyms
- Aseptic meningitis: Not synonymous with viral meningitis but sometimes used interchangeably
- Mollaret meningitis: Benign, recurrent self-limiting aseptic meningitis

Definitions
- Aseptic meningitis: Meningeal inflammation with negative routine bacterial cultures
- Mollaret meningitis: Form of benign, recurrent, aseptic meningitis of idiopathic etiology (original description by Mollaret)

ETIOLOGY/PATHOGENESIS

Aseptic Meningitis
- Infection by variety of DNA or RNA viruses (especially enteroviruses) is most common cause

Mollaret Meningitis
- Associated with herpes simplex virus (HSV) type 2 in most cases
- Association with HSV type 1 and Epstein-Barr virus is also reported

CLINICAL ISSUES

Presentation
- Mollaret meningitis: Repeated episodes of fever, meningismus, and severe headaches separated by symptom-free intervals of weeks to months

CYTOPATHOLOGY

Aseptic Meningitis
- Neutrophilic leukocytosis in first 1-2 days, followed by lymphocytosis with activated lymphocytes and some plasma cells
  - Later, increase in monocytes and macrophages is noted
- Mitosis and abnormal nuclear lobation in lymphocytes and Russell bodies in plasma cells may be seen
- Neutrophil predominance can persist even in later stage (cytologically indistinguishable from bacterial meningitis)

Mollaret Meningitis
- CSF pleocytosis composed predominantly of monocytes, with variable numbers of neutrophils, lymphocytes, and plasma cells, is seen
  - Degenerated monocytes ("ghost cells") can be seen
- Mollaret cells are hallmark cells characterized by activated monocytes with abundant cytoplasm and multiple deep nuclear clefts, resembling footprints in sand
  - These cells are seen within 24 hours of onset of symptoms

DIFFERENTIAL DIAGNOSIS

Lymphoma (Meningeal Lymphomatosis)
- Atypical lymphocytic pleocytosis
- Small or indistinct nucleolus, regular perinucleolar area, smaller widely separated chromatin aggregates, and generally ample cytoplasm with perinuclear clearing favor reactive process
  - Flow cytometric immunophenotyping is of help

Bacterial Meningitis
- CSF cytologic distinction between bacterial and aseptic meningitis can be very difficult/impossible
- Microbiological studies, including nucleic acid tests and biochemical tests of CSF, are very helpful

Aseptic Recurrent Meningitis Caused by Spinal Dermoid/Epidermoid Cysts With Rupture
- Identifying squamous cells &/or squames in CSF is clue to diagnosis of dermoid/epidermoid cyst

SELECTED REFERENCES
1. Menon D et al: Mollaret's meningitis: CSF cytology to the rescue. Neurol India. 68(5):1229-31, 2020
2. Martínez-Girón R et al: Cerebrospinal fluid cytology in nonmalignant aseptic meningeal disorders. Diagn Cytopathol. 45(11):1020-9, 2017

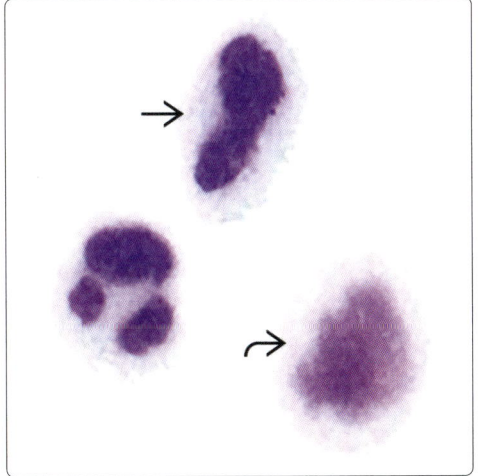

Mollaret Meningitis

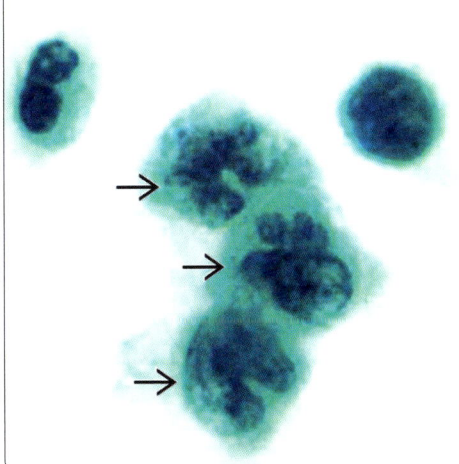

Mollaret Cell Nuclear Morphology

(Left) High-power Diff-Quik stain of Mollaret meningitis shows mixed inflammatory cells with a Mollaret cell ➡. A degenerated monocyte ("ghost cell") ➡ is also seen. (Right) Pap stain reveals Mollaret cells ➡ characterized by multiple deep nuclear clefts, depicting a so-called footprints in the sand appearance.

Subarachnoid Hemorrhage

KEY FACTS

TERMINOLOGY
- Definition: Extravasation of blood into subarachnoid space between pial and arachnoid membranes

ETIOLOGY/PATHOGENESIS
- Vast majority of nontraumatic subarachnoid hemorrhages are due to ruptured berry aneurysm

CLINICAL ISSUES
- Diagnosis requires high index of clinical suspicion with confirmatory radiology
- Lumbar puncture is performed to investigate aneurysmal sentinel leak too small to be detected by CT
- Signs and symptoms of sentinel leaks precede aneurysmal rupture by few hours to few months

CYTOPATHOLOGY
- Macrophages with intracytoplasmic halos, hemosiderin-laden and hematoidin-laden macrophages, and hemosiderin deposition are seen
  - Phagocytosis of RBCs > 4-6 hours after start of bleeding
  - Formation of halos requires 2-3 days
  - Hemosiderin pigments seen after 4-5 days
  - Hematoidin (orange-yellow crystals) in macrophage cytoplasm on ~ day 13
- Extracellular hematoidin seen as late as 6 months after hemorrhage
- Reactive meningothelial cells may be found

TOP DIFFERENTIAL DIAGNOSES
- Traumatic tap
  - CSF specimens of pathologic blood show poorly stained RBCs (degenerative change), erythrophagocytosis, and hemosiderin-laden macrophages
  - Traumatic tap has clear supernatant after centrifugation and shows well-preserved, intact RBCs like peripheral blood

Aneurysm (Gross Pathology)
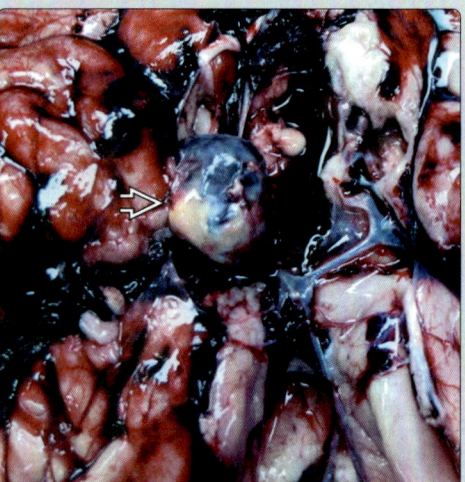

Hemorrhage Between Gyri
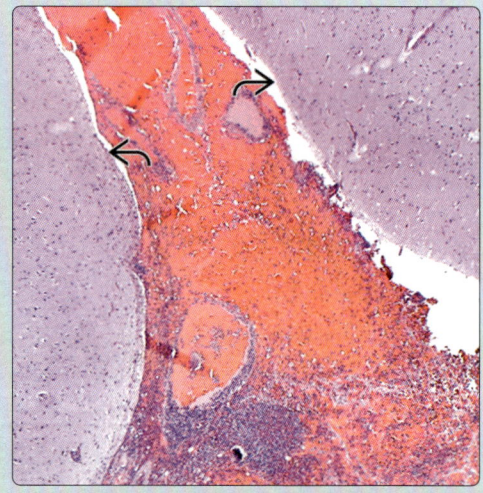

(Left) Base of the autopsied brain shows diffuse fresh subarachnoid hemorrhage, which is mostly washed to identify a 2.5-cm ruptured berry aneurysm ⇒. (Right) Histologic section of recent subarachnoid hemorrhage shows subarachnoid space between 2 gyri ⇒ that is filled with hemorrhage.

Hematoidin in Macrophages
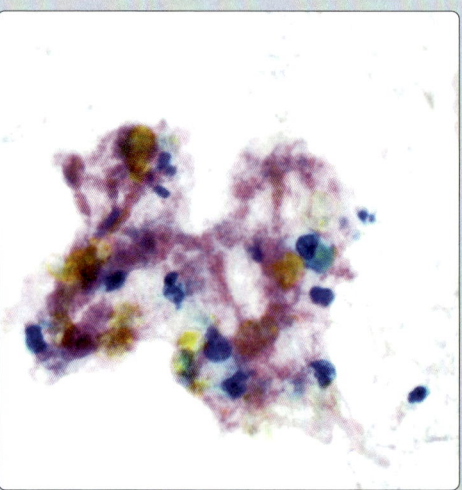

Macrophage With Intracytoplasmic Halos
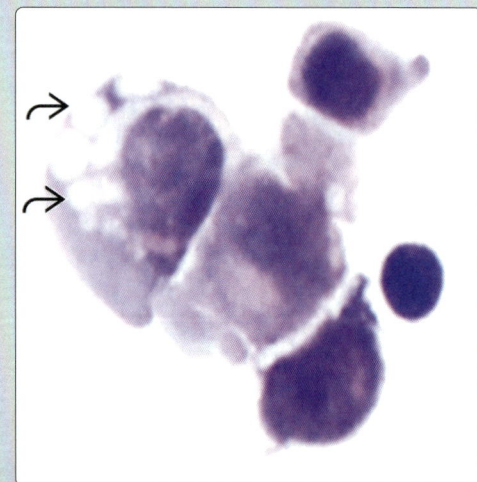

(Left) Pap-stained CSF specimen shows hematoidin pigments in a macrophage cytoplasm ~ 2 weeks after the hemorrhage occurred. (Right) Diff-Quik-stained CSF specimen shows a macrophage ⇒ with multiple intracytoplasmic halos. This feature is noted 2-3 days after the hemorrhage occurred.

Subarachnoid Hemorrhage

TERMINOLOGY

Abbreviations
- Subarachnoid hemorrhage (SAH)

Definitions
- Extravasation of blood into subarachnoid space between pial and arachnoid membranes

ETIOLOGY/PATHOGENESIS

Etiology
- Traumatic and nontraumatic
  - Vast majority of nontraumatic SAHs are due to ruptured berry aneurysm
    - Rupture of arteriovenous malformation is 2nd most identifiable cause
  - SAH may reflect secondary dissection of blood from intraparenchymal hemorrhage

CLINICAL ISSUES

Presentation
- Signs and symptoms of SAH range from subtle prodromal events (e.g., headache and dizziness) to classic presentation
  - Prodromal signs and symptoms
    - Usually result from sentinel leaks, mass effect of aneurysmal expansion, or emboli
  - Sentinel (a.k.a. warning) leaks
    - Reportedly occur in 30-50% of aneurysmal SAHs
    - Signs and symptoms precede aneurysm rupture by few hours to few months
- Classic presentation includes
  - Sudden onset of severe headache (classic feature)
  - Accompanying nausea or vomiting, symptoms of meningeal irritation, focal neurological deficits, or sudden loss of consciousness may also occur

Prognosis
- ~ 25% of patients die within 24 hours
- ~ 50% of affected individuals die in first 6 months

Diagnosis of SAH
- High index of clinical suspicion with confirmatory radiology (i.e., noncontrast CT) followed by lumbar puncture or CT angiography
- After diagnosis of SAH is established, further radiological studies (e.g., angiography) should be performed to identify source of hemorrhage
- Typical rationale for lumbar puncture: Exclude aneurysmal sentinel leak too small to be detected on CT scan

CYTOPATHOLOGY

Cells
- Reactive meningothelial cells may be found

Cytologic Pictures of SAH
- In obvious SAH cases, lumbar puncture is usually not performed
  - Lumbar puncture is performed for patients with subtle symptoms suggestive of minor SAH
- Phagocytosis of RBCs
  - > 4-6 hours after start of bleeding
- Digestion of phagocytosed RBCs
  - 2-3 days later
  - Formation of intracytoplasmic halos is seen in macrophages
- Hemosiderin pigments seen after 4-5 days
- Hematoidin (orange-yellow crystals) in macrophage cytoplasm on ~ day 13
- Extracellular hematoidin seen as late as 6 months after hemorrhage

DIFFERENTIAL DIAGNOSIS

Traumatic Tap
- Clear CSF supernatant after centrifugation
- Clot formation may be seen
- Microscopically, well-preserved, intact RBCs, such as peripheral blood, are seen
  - CSF specimens of pathologic bleed show poorly stained RBCs (degenerative change), erythrophagocytosis, and hemosiderin-laden macrophages

SELECTED REFERENCES

1. Wulff AB et al: Spectrophotometry of cerebrospinal fluid for xanthochromia is a sensitive and specific test for subarachnoid bleeding but adds little to computed tomography. Scand J Clin Lab Invest. 80(8):681-6, 2020
2. Müller-Jensen L et al: Cerebrospinal fluid cytology in subacute subarachnoid hemorrhage. Neurology. 95(15):699-700, 2020

Traumatic Tap vs. Pathologic Bleed

Feature	Traumatic Tap	Pathologic Bleed
Blood distribution (3-tube test)	Greatest in 1st tube, then decreases	Even distribution
Postcentrifuge inspection (at > 2,000 rpm for 5 minutes), unreliable < 12 hours after ictus	Clear supernatant	Xanthochromic (in UK, spectrophotometry*)
Clot formation	May clot (usually requires > 200,000 RBCs in sample)	Does not clot (because of defibrination)
Microscopic exam	Well-preserved RBCs, fresh blood	Poorly stained, degenerated RBCs ("crenated RBCs"); erythrophagocytosis; hemosiderin-laden macrophages

*CSF bilirubin, arising solely from in vivo conversion from liberated oxyhemoglobin, is tested by spectrophotometry.

Neurodegenerative Diseases

KEY FACTS

TERMINOLOGY

- Guillain-Barré syndrome (GBS) and chronic inflammatory demyelinating polyneuropathy (CIDP)
  - Peripheral polyneuropathies characterized by acute and chronic primary inflammatory demyelination, respectively
  - GBS: Postinfectious, immune-mediated disease targeting peripheral nerves
- Multiple sclerosis (MS)
  - Immune-mediated inflammatory demyelinating disease in CNS

CYTOPATHOLOGY

- Cytomorphologic features of GBS, CIDP, and MS are nonspecific
- CSF examination helps exclude other neurologic diseases with similar clinical features
- GBS and CIDP
  - Albuminocytologic dissociation in CSF (increased CSF protein without pleocytosis)
  - If significant pleocytosis is seen, consider other diagnoses (except HIV-associated GBS and CIDP)
- MS
  - Cellular reaction pattern
    - Lymphocytic in 2/3 of patients
    - Lymphocytic > > monocytic > mixed lymphomonocytic
  - Activated forms are seen in 10-30% of lymphocytic population and 10-40% of monocytic population
  - Plasma cells (including lymphoplasmacytes) are frequently seen
  - Lymphophages and mitotic figures may be seen
  - Neutrophils are usually not seen

ANCILLARY TESTS

- Oligoclonal immunoglobulin bands in CSF seen on electrophoresis of MS patients

Multiple Sclerosis: Lymphocytic Pleocytosis

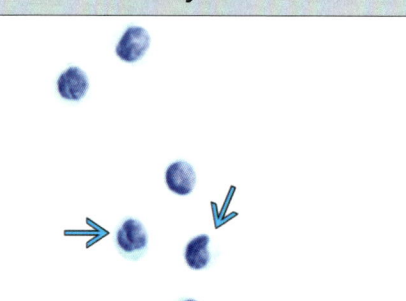

Multiple Sclerosis: Lymphocytes and Plasma Cells

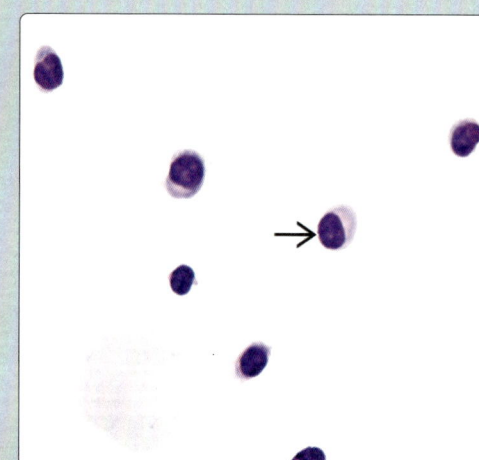

(Left) Pap-stained CSF cytospin from a multiple sclerosis (MS) patient shows lymphocytic pleocytosis with plasmacytoid cells ➡. Nuclear membrane irregularity ➡ is seen in some of the lymphocytes. (Right) Diff-Quik-stained CSF cytospin from an MS patient shows lymphocytic pleocytosis with plasma cells ➡. This is the most common cellular reaction noted in CSF of patients with this disease.

Multiple Sclerosis: Histology Features

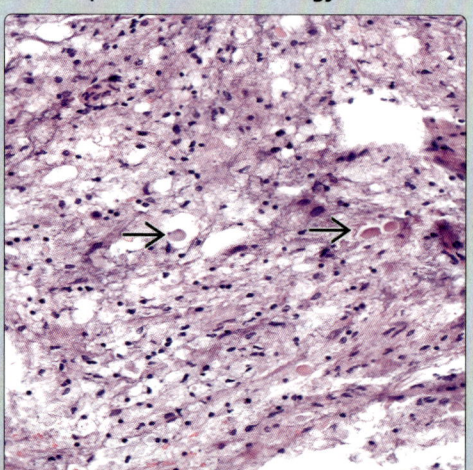

Multiple Sclerosis: Myelin Loss

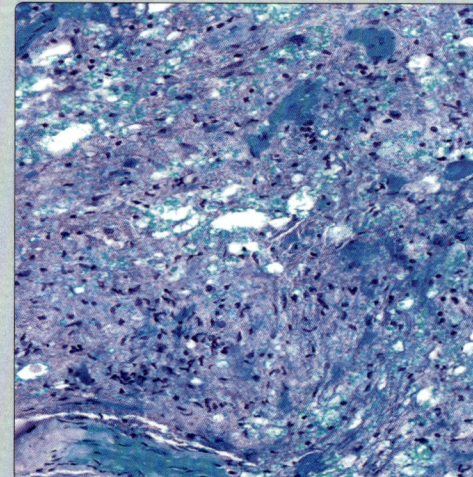

(Left) H&E-stained histologic section of MS shows white matter rarefaction with abundant foamy macrophages. Multiple axonal spheroids (representing axonal damage) ➡ are seen. (Right) Luxol fast blue-stained section of MS reveals diffuse loss of myelin, which is normally stained blue.

Neurodegenerative Diseases

TERMINOLOGY

Abbreviations
- Guillain-Barré syndrome (GBS)
- Chronic inflammatory demyelinating polyneuropathy (CIDP)
- Multiple sclerosis (MS)

Synonyms
- GBS is sometimes also referred to as acute inflammatory demyelinating polyneuropathy

Definitions
- GBS and CIDP
  - Peripheral polyneuropathies characterized by acute and chronic primary inflammatory demyelination, respectively
    - GBS: Postinfectious, immune-mediated disease targeting peripheral nerves
- MS
  - Immune-mediated inflammatory demyelinating disease in CNS

ETIOLOGY/PATHOGENESIS

Etiology
- GBS
  - Up to 2/3 of patients report antecedent bacterial and viral illness prior to onset of neurologic symptoms
  - In several studies, *Campylobacter jejuni* was most commonly isolated pathogen

CLINICAL ISSUES

Prognosis
- These diseases can be associated with significant morbidity

Clinical Differential Diagnosis
- GBS
  - West Nile encephalomyelitis
  - Nonpolio enterovirus encephalomyelitis
  - Lyme disease
  - HIV neuropathy
  - Neurosarcoidosis
- CIDP
  - Chronic acquired polyneuropathies
    - e.g., monoclonal gammopathies, diabetes, toxic neuropathies
  - Inherited neuropathies
    - e.g., Charcot-Marie-Tooth disease, transthyretin amyloid neuropathy
- MS
  - Postinfectious encephalomyelitis
  - Primary CNS vasculitis
  - Behçet disease
  - Progressive multifocal leukoencephalopathy
  - Neurosarcoidosis

CYTOPATHOLOGY

Cellularity
- MS: Mild pleocytosis is seen in nearly all patients

Pattern
- Nonspecific cytologic pattern

Background
- No necrosis or hemorrhage is seen

Cells
- Lymphocytes (including reactive lymphocytes), plasma cells, monocytes/histiocytes and (uncommonly) neutrophils

Cytologic Features of Multiple Sclerosis
- Cellular reaction pattern
  - Lymphocytic in 2/3 of patients
  - Lymphocytic >> monocytic > mixed lymphomonocytic
- Activated forms are seen in 10-30% of lymphocytic population and 10-40% of monocytic population
- No neutrophilic cellular reaction is observed
- Plasma cells (including lymphoplasmacytes) are frequently seen
- Foamy macrophages are sometimes seen
- Lymphophages and mitotic figures may be seen

Albuminocytologic Dissociation of CSF
- Characteristically seen in GBS and CIDP
- Defined as increase in proteins (frequently > 100 mg/dL) without increase in cell population
  - Exception: HIV-associated GBS and CIDP (mild lymphocytic pleocytosis is seen)
- GBS: Elevated CSF protein is seen in 50% of patients at presentation and in 90% on days 16-30

MICROSCOPIC

Histologic Features
- MS lesions show rarefied white matter due to loss of myelin with relative preservation of axons in CNS
  - Foamy macrophages are commonly seen
  - Loss of myelin is shown with Luxol fast blue stain
  - Preserved axons are highlighted with neurofilament protein immunostain
- CIDP is characterized by segmental demyelination and remyelination (onion bulb formation) in biopsied peripheral nerves
  - Sural nerve biopsy
    - Reduction in myelinated fiber density > demyelination > inflammation > onion bulb formation

ANCILLARY TESTS

Electrophoresis
- MS
  - Oligoclonal immunoglobulin bands in CSF

SELECTED REFERENCES

1. Berek K et al: Cerebrospinal fluid findings in 541 patients with clinically isolated syndrome and multiple sclerosis: a monocentric study. Front Immunol. 12:675307, 2021
2. Wurth S et al: Cerebrospinal fluid B cells and disease progression in multiple sclerosis - a longitudinal prospective study. PLoS One. 12(8):e0182462, 2017

Primary Brain Tumors

KEY FACTS

CLINICAL ISSUES
- Usually brain lesion has been detected radiologically prior to cytologic examination of CSF
- Adult brain tumors rarely appear in CSF; glioblastoma (GBM) is most frequent; ependymoma may also be seen
- In adults, except for tumors in pineal region (to check tumor markers), lumbar puncture is usually not performed for primary brain tumors
- CSF cytologic examination is important for pediatric brain tumors, especially medulloblastoma (MB), for clinical/therapeutic risk stratification

CYTOPATHOLOGY
- GBM: Medium to large tumor cells with hyperchromatic nuclei and variable amount of cytoplasm
- MB: Malignant small blue cells appear singly or arranged in small, cohesive groups
  - Mitotic activity can be seen
- Cells of primary brain tumors seen in CSF are usually degenerated
  - Glial cytoplasmic processes of glial tumors are usually not seen in CSF due to degeneration
- Presence of tumor cells in lumbar puncture CSF specimens generally implies leptomeningeal &/or ependymal involvement of tumor cells in glial tumors

TOP DIFFERENTIAL DIAGNOSES
- Metastatic malignant epithelial/epithelioid tumors
  - Primary brain tumors can exhibit epithelioid cytologic appearance
  - Based on cytomorphology alone, distinction between primary and secondary neoplasms is often very difficult or impossible
  - Immunocytochemistry is useful
  - Knowledge of prior malignancy, radiologic findings, and review of previous pathologic material are crucial

Glioblastoma
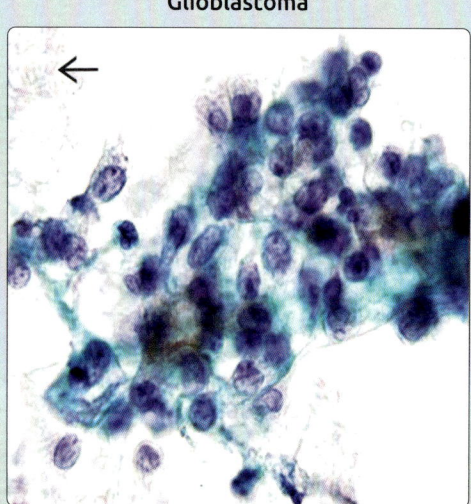

Medulloblastoma
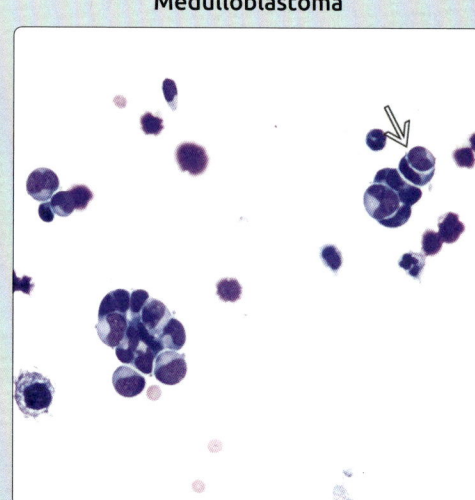

(Left) Pap stain of a ventricular fluid specimen in a patient with glioblastoma shows loosely cohesive atypical tumor cells with nuclear pleomorphism in a "dirty" background ➡. **(Right)** Diff-Quik stain of a medulloblastoma shows medium-sized atypical cells (but much larger than red blood cells) with hyperchromatic nuclei and a high nuclear:cytoplasmic ratio. Cell-in-cell phenomenon/structure is noted ➡.

Myxopapillary Ependymoma
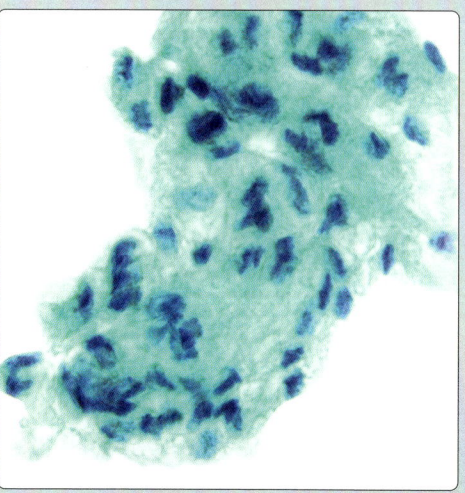

Choroid Plexus Carcinoma
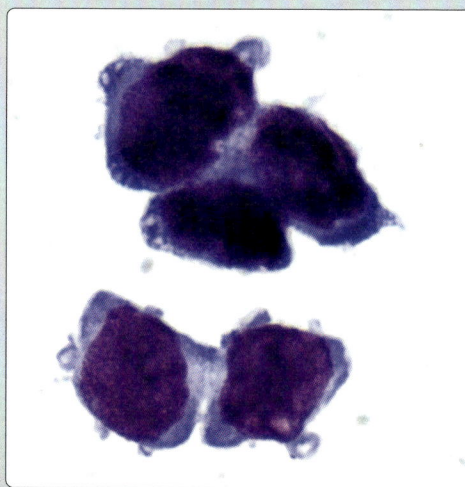

(Left) Pap-stained cluster of degenerative cells from a ruptured myxopapillary ependymoma shows fibrillary cytoplasm and mostly spindled nuclei. **(Right)** Diff-Quik stain of a choroid plexus carcinoma shows cohesive groups of large malignant cells with hyperchromatic nuclei and a high nuclear:cytoplasmic ratio.

Primary Brain Tumors

TERMINOLOGY

Abbreviations
- Glioblastoma (GBM), medulloblastoma (MB), atypical teratoid/rhabdoid tumor (AT/RT)

CLINICAL ISSUES

Potential Dissemination Through CSF
- Possible for any primary malignant brain tumors and some benign brain tumors
- In adults, identification of primary brain tumor cells in CSF is extremely rare
  - Adult CSF specimens: **GBMs** are most common
    - Less often, ependymomas
- In children, primary brain tumor cells are sometimes identified in CSF
  - Pediatric CSF specimens: **MBs** are most common
    - Rarely, AT/RTs, ependymomas, and choroid plexus carcinomas are seen
- WHO grade 1 brain tumors (e.g., pilocytic astrocytoma) can disseminate through CSF, although this is very rare

Clinical Utility of CSF Cytologic Examination
- In pediatric population, CSF cytology is used to determine presence or absence of CSF dissemination of primary brain tumors
  - MB: CSF cytologic findings are used for risk stratification (i.e., average-risk group vs. high-risk group)
    - Important for therapeutic management
- In adults, except for tumors in pineal region (to check tumor markers), lumbar puncture is usually **not** performed for primary brain tumors
  - Lumbar puncture may be performed if tumor has already been diagnosed as type that can commonly spread through CSF (e.g., ependymoma)
  - Most adult CSF specimens are from
    - Cystic tumor fluid (obtained at surgery)
    - Ventricular fluid (VF) (at ventriculoperitoneal shunting)
    - Fluid from intracranial cavity secondary to previous tumor resection

CYTOPATHOLOGY

Cellularity
- Lumbar puncture CSF specimens: Usually low tumor cellularity
- VF, fluid from intracranial cavity secondary to previous tumor resection, and fluid from cystic tumor: Variable cellularity (may be high)

Background
- Lumbar puncture CSF specimens, VF: Usually clean background
  - VF may contain few brain parenchymal fragments
- Fluid from intracranial cavity/fluid from cystic tumor: "Dirty" background with hemorrhage, necrotic debris, &/or brain parenchymal fragments

Cells
- Cells of primary brain tumors seen in CSF are usually degenerated
- Changes of chemoradiation therapy may be appreciated
- **GBM**: Medium to large tumor cells with hyperchromatic nuclei and variable amount of cytoplasm appear singly, or rarely, arranged in small, cohesive groups
- **MB**: Small to medium tumor cells with scant cytoplasm, hyperchromatic nuclei, and fine granular chromatin pattern; mitotic figures can be seen
  - Appear singly or arranged in small cohesive groups
  - Nuclear molding can be seen in tumor clusters
- **Other rare tumors**
  - Rhabdoid cells with eosinophilic cytoplasmic inclusion in AT/RT
  - Bland epithelioid cell groups in ependymoma

Cytoplasmic Details
- Glial cytoplasmic processes of glial tumors are usually not seen in CSF due to degeneration

Cytology-Histology Correlation
- Presence of tumor cells in lumbar puncture CSF specimens generally implies leptomeningeal &/or ependymal involvement of tumor cells in glial tumors

MICROSCOPIC

Histologic Features
- GBM
  - High-grade astrocytoma characterized by diffusely infiltrating atypical tumor cells with microvascular proliferation &/or tumor necrosis
  - Variety of histologic patterns (previously referred to as glioblastoma multiforme)
- MB
  - Classic type is characterized by densely packed, small, malignant blue cells with characteristic neuroblastic rosettes

DIFFERENTIAL DIAGNOSIS

Metastatic Malignant Epithelial/Epithelioid Tumors
- Primary brain tumors can exhibit epithelioid cytologic appearance
- Based on cytomorphology alone, distinction between primary and secondary neoplasms is often very difficult or impossible (e.g., metastatic small cell carcinoma vs. MB)
- Immunohistochemical studies on smears/cell block sections are helpful
- Knowledge of prior malignancy, radiologic findings, and review of previous pathologic material are crucial

DIAGNOSTIC CHECKLIST

Clinically Relevant Pathologic Features
- Cytologic identification of any large atypical cells in CSF of patient with history of primary brain tumor requires consideration of possibility of CSF dissemination

SELECTED REFERENCES

1. Birzu C et al: Leptomeningeal spread in glioblastoma: diagnostic and therapeutic challenges. Oncologist. 25(11):e1763-76, 2020
2. Ramkissoon LA et al: Genomic profiling of circulating tumor DNA from cerebrospinal fluid to guide clinical decision making for patients with primary and metastatic brain tumors. Front Neurol. 11:544680, 2020

Leukemia and Lymphoma

KEY FACTS

CLINICAL ISSUES

- Acute leukemia, Burkitt lymphoma, and lymphoblastic lymphoma patients at high risk of developing lymphomatous/leukemic meningitis
  - Cerebrospinal fluid cytology can be used to monitor therapeutic response
  - May be seen as either primary diagnosis or at time of relapse
  - Systemic lymphomas can involve leptomeninges in later stages

CYTOPATHOLOGY

- Cellular monotony, nuclear contour irregularity, pointed cytoplasmic borders, and more apoptotic and mitotic bodies favor lymphoma/leukemia
  - No single cytomorphologic parameter sufficient to detect neoplastic lymphocytes
- Cellularity may be sparse or abundant
- Lymphoglandular bodies usually absent
- Acute leukemia characterized by blasts with finer chromatin and more cellular uniformity than lymphomas
- Diffuse large B-cell lymphoma characterized by large, pleomorphic lymphocytes
- Other lymphomas may have very subtle morphologic features
  - Nuclear contour irregularities with prominent notches and protrusions may be clue to malignancy

ANCILLARY TESTS

- Flow cytometry very important given its high sensitivity
  - Sensitivity: 0.2% of total cell count for flow cytometry vs. 5% for cytology
- Flow cytometry also can be very useful to determine type of malignancy in 1st-time diagnoses

TOP DIFFERENTIAL DIAGNOSES

- Lymphocytic meningitis vs. mature B-cell lymphoma/leukemia

Diffuse Large B-Cell Lymphoma Nuclear Pleomorphism

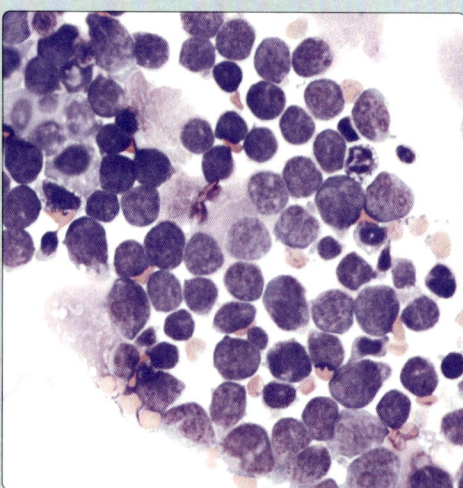

Acute Lymphoblastic Leukemia

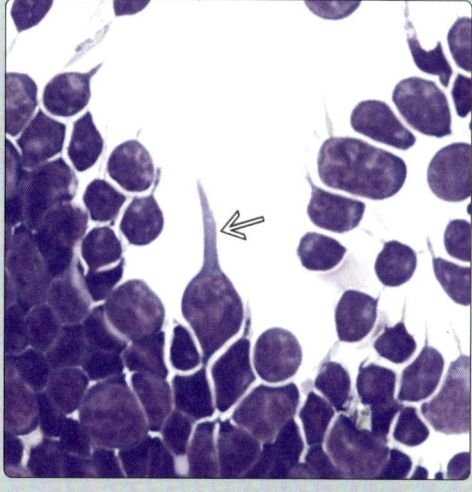

(Left) In this case of systemic diffuse large B-cell lymphoma with secondary involvement of leptomeninges, Diff-Quik-stained cytospin shows cellular, large atypical lymphoid cells with prominent nuclear pleomorphism. (Right) This cerebrospinal fluid (CSF) example of acute lymphoblastic leukemia stained with Diff-Quik on cytospin shows numerous blasts with a high nuclear:cytoplasmic ratio and irregular nuclei. Note the "hand mirror" morphology ➡.

Chronic Lymphocytic Leukemia

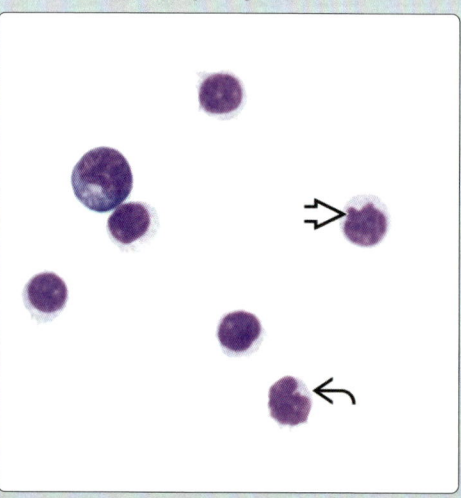

Adult T-Cell Leukemia

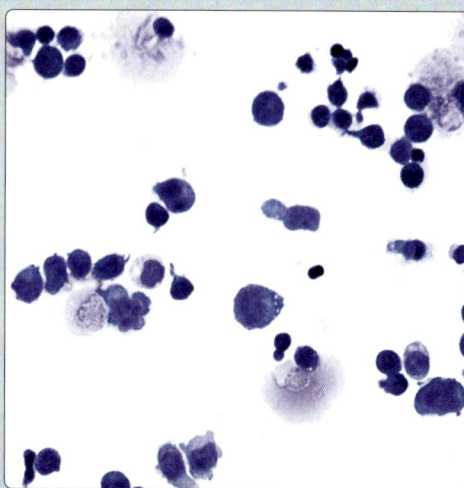

(Left) Diff-Quik-stained CSF specimen involved by chronic lymphocytic leukemia contains lymphocytes with nuclear notches ➡ and "noses" ➡. Such nuclear contour irregularities may lead to a suspicion of malignancy that can be confirmed by flow cytometry. (Right) In this example of adult T-cell leukemia, Giemsa-stained CSF cytospin smear shows many medium to large atypical lymphocytes with irregular/polylobulated nuclei.

Leukemia and Lymphoma

TERMINOLOGY

Abbreviations
- Diffuse large B-cell lymphoma (DLBCL)
- Acute myelogenous leukemia (AML)
- Acute lymphocytic leukemia (ALL)
- Chronic lymphocytic leukemia (CLL)

CLINICAL ISSUES

Presentation
- Lymphomatous/leukemic meningitis (LM)
  - May be seen at diagnosis or at relapse
  - Systemic lymphomas can involve leptomeninges in later stages

Lymphoma/Leukemia at Risk
- Patients with ALL, Burkitt lymphoma, lymphoblastic lymphoma, and AML at high risk for development of LM

CYTOPATHOLOGY

Cellularity
- Varies from sparse to abundant

Background
- Very few or absent lymphoglandular bodies

Cells
- Cellular monotony
- Most large cell lymphomas/leukemias show obvious cytologic atypia
  - Diagnosis usually straightforward

Nuclear Details
- Nuclear contour irregularity (including nuclear folds and notches)
  - Flower-like appearance reportedly occurs as frequently as in benign lymphocytosis
- Apoptotic and mitotic figures are more commonly seen

Cytoplasmic Details
- Pointed borders of cytoplasm (in contrast, round shape of whole cell is feature of benign lymphocytes)

ALL
- Larger than mature lymphocytes with scant cytoplasm
- Characteristic nuclear features include fine chromatin and visible nucleoli

CLL
- Rare in cerebrospinal fluid
  - Cytologic features of malignancy are less pronounced and can be confused with more common normal/reactive lymphocytes
- Since nonspecific meningeal reaction may be associated with lymphoma, polymorphous lymphoid population does not exclude diagnosis of CLL

ANCILLARY TESTS

Flow Cytometry
- Much more sensitive at detecting malignant cells
  - Sensitivity: 0.2% of total cell count for flow cytometry vs. 5% for cytology

DIFFERENTIAL DIAGNOSIS

Lymphocytic Meningitis
- Cellular monotony and nuclear contour irregularity favor neoplasm
- Flow cytometry helpful in this differential

SELECTED REFERENCES

1. Kim D et al: Standardizing a volume benchmark for cerebrospinal fluids for optimal diagnostic accuracy. Diagn Cytopathol. 49(2):258-66, 2021
2. Naydenov AV et al: Leptomeningeal carcinomatosis in chronic lymphocytic leukemia: a case report and review of the literature. Oncologist. 24(9):1237-45, 2019
3. Nam AS et al: Assessment of the utility of cytology and flow cytometry of cerebrospinal fluid samples in clinical practice. Acta Cytol. 62(2):130-6, 2018

Burkitt Lymphoma

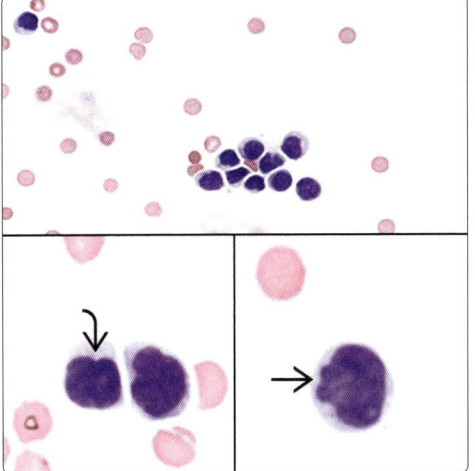

Acute Biphenotypic Leukemia

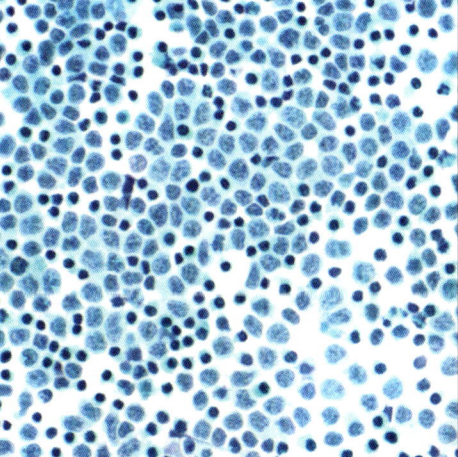

(Left) Composite image of Diff-Quik-stained CSF from a patient with Burkitt lymphoma shows an aggregate of atypical lymphocytes in the upper panel. In the lower panels, individual malignant cells show nuclear indentations ⮕ and protrusions ⮕. (Right) In this example of acute biphenotypic leukemia, numerous blast forms can be seen on Pap stain. The malignant cells are large with finer chromatin than mature lymphocytes.

Metastasis in Cerebrospinal Fluid

KEY FACTS

CLINICAL ISSUES
- Leptomeningeal carcinomatosis/metastasis has dismal prognosis with median survival of 20 weeks after diagnosis
- Breast and lung carcinomas comprise ~ 50% of all leptomeningeal metastases, excluding systemic lymphoma/leukemia
- Common initial presentations include cranial neuropathy and spinal cord dysfunction

CYTOPATHOLOGY
- Cells of metastatic carcinomas may be cytologically bland, but even those of small size are larger than transformed lymphocytes
- Metastatic breast carcinoma
  o Cells are usually single or in loose clusters or chains
  o Large, morular clusters like those seen in body cavity fluids are rare
  o Ductal carcinoma: Large cancer cells that may show peripheral cytoplasmic blebs or protrusions
  o Lobular carcinoma: Scattered cancer cells, sometimes with intracytoplasmic lumina or signet-ring-type mucin vacuoles
- Metastatic lung carcinoma
  o Adenocarcinoma: Large cancer cells with nucleoli
  o Small cell carcinoma: Often seen singly and also in clusters; sometimes arranged in short chains with nuclear molding; crush artifact may not be present

ANCILLARY TESTS
- Immunocytochemistry is not helpful to increase sensitivity
- May be of great value to identify primary site

TOP DIFFERENTIAL DIAGNOSES
- Reactive meningothelial cells
  o Reactive meningothelial cells can be identified as atypical epithelioid nests/clusters, mimicking bland-appearing cancer cell nests
  o Usually smaller than cancer cells and have no marked atypia or mitotic figures

Lung Adenocarcinoma, Pap Stain | Lung Adenocarcinoma: Diff-Quik Stain

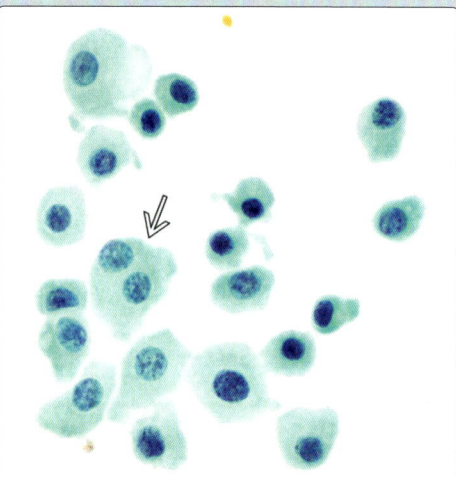
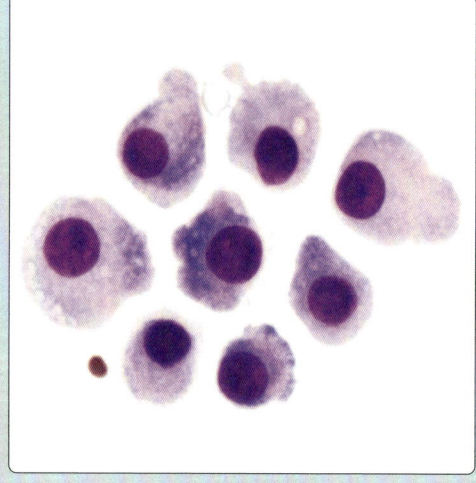

(Left) *Pap stain of metastatic lung adenocarcinoma shows large cancer cells with a binucleated cell ➡. Note the relatively bland appearance of metastatic carcinoma cells in the CSF setting.* (Right) *Diff-Quik stain from the same metastatic lung adenocarcinoma shows large malignant cells with eccentrically located nuclei and vacuolated cytoplasm.*

Renal Cell Carcinoma in CSF | Breast Carcinoma

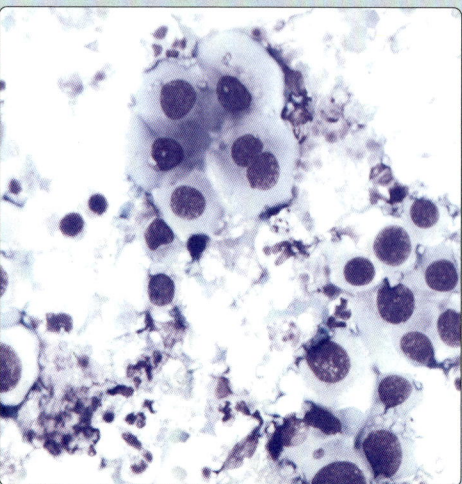
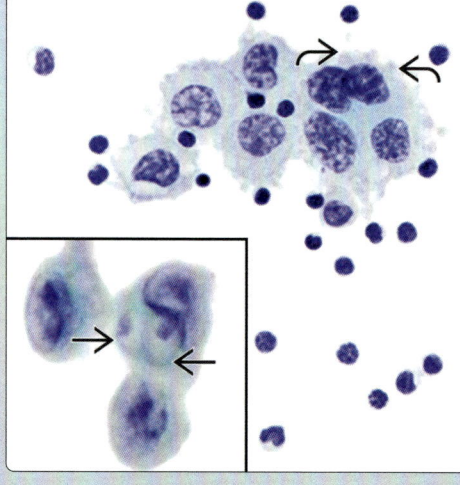

(Left) *Diff-Quik stained CSF from ventricle obtained at craniotomy in a patient with metastatic renal cell carcinoma in the brain shows multiple cohesive clusters of large atypical cells with abundant clear cytoplasm along with acute inflammation and debris.* (Right) *A cohesive cluster of large cells (ductal carcinoma) with peripheral cytoplasmic blebs ➡ is seen in this metastatic breast carcinoma. Inset shows intracytoplasmic lumina containing mucin ➡ characteristic of lobular carcinoma.*

Metastasis in Cerebrospinal Fluid

CLINICAL ISSUES

Presentation
- Common initial presentations include cranial neuropathy and spinal cord dysfunction

Prognosis
- Median survival: 20 weeks after diagnosis

Sites of Tumor Origin
- In order of frequency
  - Breast
  - Lung (adenocarcinoma > small cell carcinoma > > squamous cell carcinoma)
  - Skin (mostly melanoma)
  - Gastrointestinal tract
  - Genitourinary tract

CYTOPATHOLOGY

Cellularity
- Varies from scant to abundant

Pattern
- Metastatic breast carcinomas
  - Cells are usually single or form loose clusters
  - Tight balls and morulae of tumor cells are rare
  - Chains of cancer cells can be seen
  - Ductal carcinoma: Large, readily recognizable cancer cells that may show peripheral cytoplasmic blebs or protrusions
  - Lobular carcinoma: Scattered cancer cells (sometimes of signet-ring-type configuration)
    - Intracytoplasmic lumina containing mucin (target cells) may be seen
- Metastatic lung carcinomas
  - Adenocarcinoma: Large cancer cells with nucleoli
  - Small cell carcinoma: Often seen singly and also in clusters; sometimes arranged in short chains with nuclear molding; crush artifact may not be present

Background
- Varies from clear to necrotic &/or hemorrhagic
  - Necrosis &/or hemorrhage is usually seen in postsurgical specimens

Cells
- Tumor cells may be cytologically bland
- Cells of metastatic carcinomas, even of small size, are larger than transformed lymphocytes
- Degenerative features are commonly seen

Nuclear Details
- Mitotic figures may be present

Cytology-Histology Correlation
- Histologic examination (e.g., leptomeningeal biopsy) is usually not performed

ANCILLARY TESTS

Immunocytochemistry in Cerebrospinal Fluid Specimens
- Sensitivity in detection of malignant cells increases by < 2%
- Of great value in identifying primary site

DIFFERENTIAL DIAGNOSIS

Reactive Meningothelial Cells
- Reactive meningothelial cells can be identified as atypical epithelioid nests/clusters, mimicking bland-appearing cancer cell nests
- Usually, reactive meningothelial cells are smaller than cancer cells
- Presence of marked atypia &/or mitotic figures favors metastatic carcinoma

SELECTED REFERENCES

1. Le Rhun E et al: Prognostic validation and clinical implications of the EANO ESMO classification of leptomeningeal metastasis from solid tumors. Neuro Oncol. 23(7):1100-12, 2021
2. Pellerino A et al: Leptomeningeal metastases from solid tumors: recent advances in diagnosis and molecular approaches. Cancers (Basel). 13(12):2888, 2021

Small Cell Carcinoma
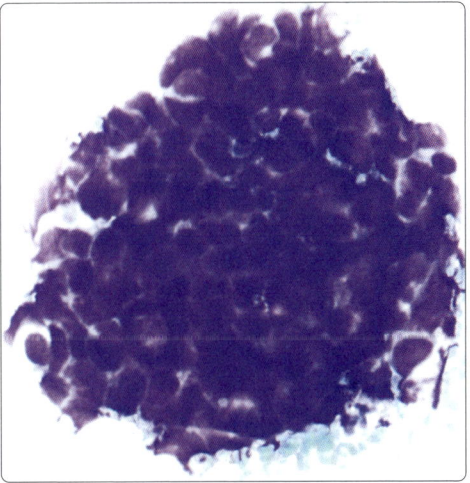

Small Cell Carcinoma (High Magnification)
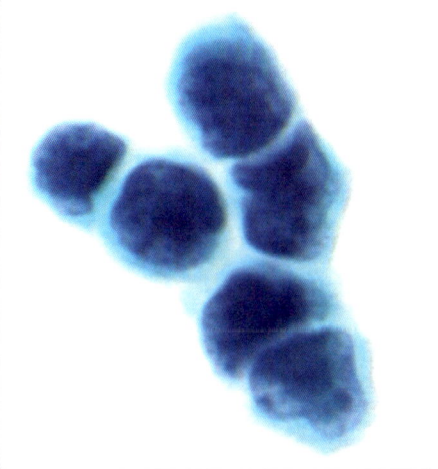

(Left) Diff-Quik-stained cytospin smear of metastatic pulmonary small cell carcinoma shows a tightly cohesive cluster of cells with a high nuclear:cytoplasmic ratio and nuclear molding. **(Right)** *Pap stain of metastatic small cell carcinoma from lung shows irregularly hyperchromatic nuclei with nuclear molding and a high nuclear:cytoplasmic ratio.*

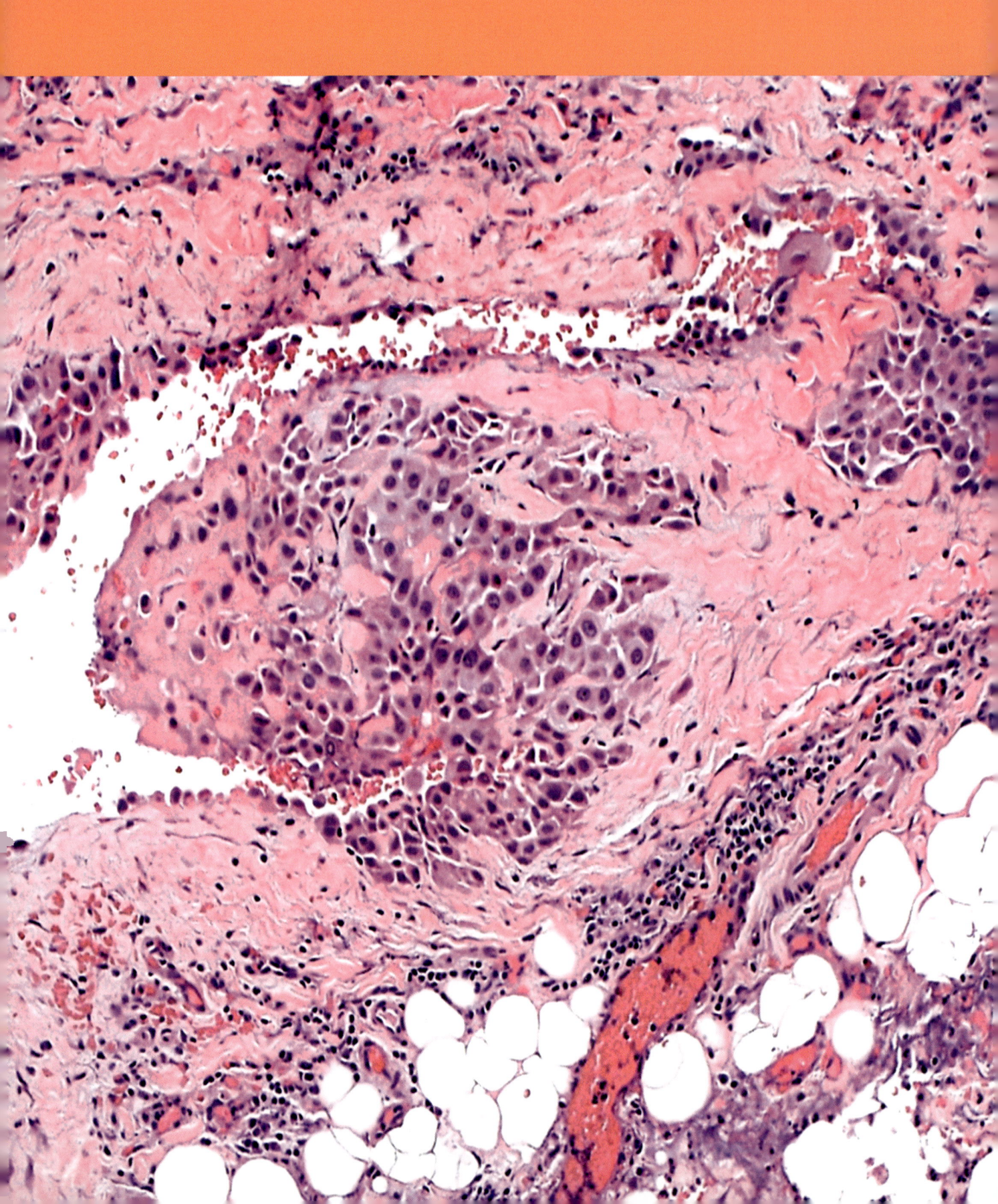

PART II
SECTION 4
Pleural, Peritoneal, Pericardial, and Pelvic Fluid and Washings

Normal Cellular Components, Reactive Mesothelial Proliferations, and Reporting Terminology	196
Infectious Conditions	200
Autoimmune Diseases	202
Malignant Effusion, Mesothelioma	204
Malignant Effusion, Carcinomas	208
Malignant Effusion, Sarcomas	212
Lymphoid Effusions and Lymphomas	214
Primary Effusion Lymphoma	216
Endometriosis and Endosalpingiosis	218
Ovarian Neoplasms	220
Immunocytochemistry, Histochemistry, and Other Ancillary Techniques	222

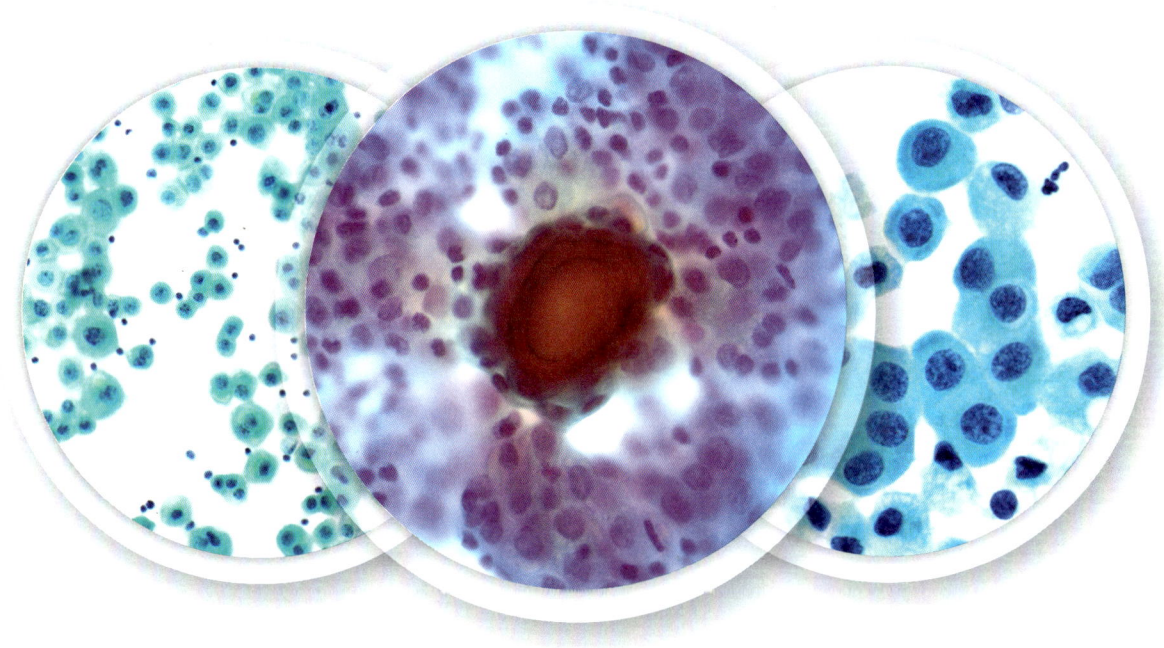

Normal Cellular Components, Reactive Mesothelial Proliferations, and Reporting Terminology

GENERAL PRINCIPLES

Pleural, Pericardial, and Peritoneal Cavities

- Lined by single layer of mesothelial cells and underlying loose fibroconnective tissue
- In normal conditions, serous cavities contain minimal amount of fluid for lubrication of surfaces
- Variety of conditions, including neoplastic and nonneoplastic, can result in accumulation of fluid or effusion
    - Reactive mesothelial hyperplasia often associated with infections, collagen vascular disease, drug reactions, pneumothorax, chest surgery, and trauma
    - Depending on physical, chemical, and microscopic characteristics of fluid, effusions can be subdivided into transudates and exudates
        - Distinction is important because most malignant effusions are exudates; therefore, cytologic evaluation of transudates is not as critical
    - Transudates: Result of intravascular pressure alteration
        - Attributable to heart failure, renal failure, or cirrhosis in most instances
        - Clear fluids with low specific gravity (< 1.015), low protein content (< 3 g/dL), and low lactate dehydrogenase (LDH) level (< serum LDH)
        - Have scant cellularity
    - Exudates: Result of mesothelium injury
        - Malignancy, infections, autoimmune disease, infarction, and trauma are major causes
        - Turbid fluids with greater specific gravity (> 1.015), high protein content (> 3g/dL), and high LDH level (> serum LDH)
        - Tend to have higher cellularity with numerous mesothelial cells, inflammatory cells, ± tumor cells

COLLECTION AND PROCESSING

Body Fluids

- Collected by aspiration of cavities or by pelvic washings at time of surgery
- Specimens are sent unfixed in heparinized bottles
- Specimens are processed immediately or refrigerated at 4 °C until time of slide preparation
- Specimens may be processed as direct smears, cytocentrifuge slides, thin-layer slides, or filter preparation
- Cell blocks can be prepared from fluid
    - Abundant fluid received in most specimens facilitates successful cell blocks
    - Cell block sections are useful to evaluate architecture and to perform immunocytochemical/special stains
    - Cell blocks may also be useful for molecular analysis, but often many benign cells are present, making analysis more difficult with false-negative results due to low percentage of malignant cells
- Fresh fluid can be submitted for flow cytometry, cytogenetics, or molecular analysis
    - Flow cytometry is unlikely to detect clonal population in absence of morphologic abnormality, high clinical suspicion, or history of lymphoma
- Peritoneal washings are often collected during staging of gynecologic or other nongynecologic peritoneal malignancies or to rule out malignancy
    - Peritoneal washings strip mesothelial surface, resulting in large sheets of cells that can be folded
    - Because these specimens are collected as part of surgical staging, correlation with concurrent surgical specimen is recommended
    - Rare benign or malignant endometrial cells can appear in these specimens due to artifactual intraoperative expulsion of cells via fallopian tubes

NORMAL CELLULAR COMPONENTS

Benign Effusions

- Contain variable numbers of mesothelial cells, histiocytes, lymphocytes, and red blood cells
- Mesothelial cells shed as single cells, sheets, or small clusters with scalloped periphery (< 10-15 cells per group)
- Reactive mesothelial hyperplasia can result in cellular sample with numerous single cells, papillary fragments, or 3D clusters
    - Psammoma bodies can be present

Normal Mesothelial Cells

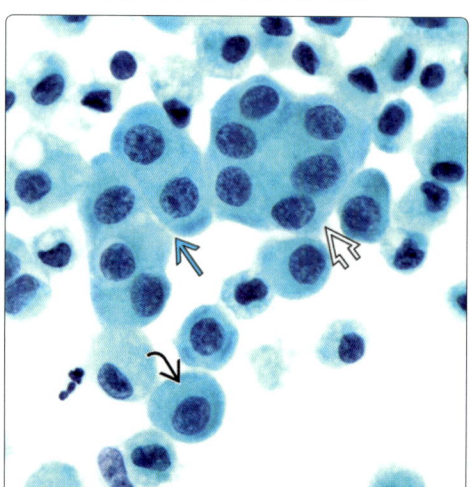

Diff-Quik Appearance of Mesothelial Cells

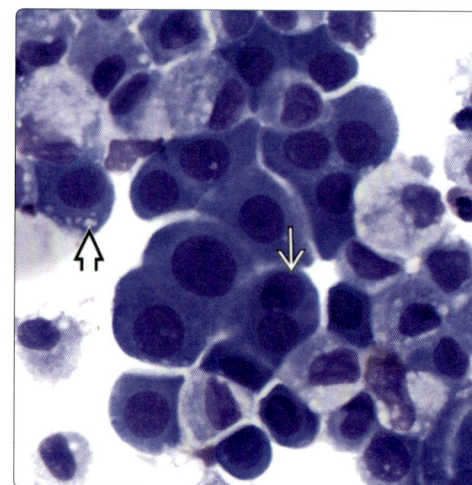

(Left) This cluster of Pap-stained mesothelial cells demonstrates several common features: A mix of clusters and individual cells, 2-tone cytoplasm ➡, peripheral lacy skirt ➡, and windows ➡. (Right) This image shows how the air-dried Diff-Quik stain highlights the large size of mesothelial cells relative to other cellular components, as well as the variation in nuclear size. Note the presence of prominent cytoplasmic vacuoles ➡ and binucleation ➡.

Normal Cellular Components, Reactive Mesothelial Proliferations, and Reporting Terminology

Cytomorphology of Mesothelial Cells
- Cuboidal to round cells with variable cell and nuclear size
- Abundant foamy, vacuolated, or dense cytoplasm with 2-tone appearance
- Peripheral clear outer rim ("lacy skirt") is result of long, slender microvilli
- Empty spaces between cells ("windows") also result from microvilli
- Occasionally, cell-within-cell arrangement ("hugging") may be seen
- Intracytoplasmic fluid-filled vacuoles that peripherally displace nucleus occur in small percentage of cells
- Binucleation or multinucleation are common
- Occasional multinucleated giant mesothelial cells can be seen in reactive conditions
- Nuclei are round to oval with fine chromatin and 1 or 2 nucleoli
- Nuclear membrane is smooth
- Occasional mitosis can be seen

Characteristics of Reactive Mesothelial Cells
- Highly cellular specimens with spectrum of normal to atypical cells
- 3D clusters, acinar groups, papillary fragments, and cell balls with cytologic features similar to background mesothelial cells
- Variation in nuclear size with increased nuclear:cytoplasmic ratio, irregular chromatin distribution, irregular nuclear contours, prominent nucleoli
  - Marked atypia of mesothelial cells can be seen in patients with uremia, dialysis, hepatitis, pancreatitis, and history of radiation/chemotherapy
  - It is important to take clinical history into consideration to avoid false-positive diagnosis

Cytomorphology of Other Normal Cellular Components
- Cytomorphology of histiocytes
  - Numerous histiocytes can be present in cases of cancer, tuberculosis, rheumatoid effusions, and embolism
  - Histiocytes do not form tight clusters, and no windows are seen between cells
  - Nucleus is folded or bean-shaped with granular chromatin
  - Cytoplasm can be foamy, granular, or vacuolated
- Cytomorphology of lymphocytes
  - Lymphocytic-rich effusions can be seen in cases of cancer, tuberculosis, and status post coronary artery bypass
  - Reactive T lymphocytes will be seen in any chronic effusion
  - T lymphocytes are small, often with irregular nuclear contours

DIFFERENTIAL DIAGNOSIS

Differential Diagnosis of Reactive Mesothelial Cells
- Metastatic malignancy
  - Has 2nd population of malignant cells
    - 2nd population of malignant cells may not be obvious in some cases that shed as single cells, such as lobular carcinomas, melanomas, sarcomas, and lymphomas
  - Correlation with clinical/radiologic findings and immunocytochemical stains are often required
    - International Mesothelioma Interest Group recommend ≥ 2 mesothelial (e.g., calretinin, D2-40) and ≥ 2 carcinoma markers (e.g., MOC-31, BER-EP4, claudin-4)
- Mesothelioma
  - Malignant mesothelioma effusions are usually very cellular, and high cellularity persists with repeated taps unless therapy has been initiated
  - Mesothelioma should be considered in cases with large clusters (> 15 cells per group) &/or marked cytologic atypia
  - It is necessary to correlate with clinical/radiologic findings (and surgical specimens when available) to avoid false-positive diagnosis

Differential Diagnosis of Lymphocyte-Rich Effusion
- Lymphoma
- Tuberculosis
- Immune-related conditions

INTERNATIONAL SYSTEM FOR SEROUS FLUID CYTOPATHOLOGY

Purpose and Origin
- Standardized diagnostic and reporting system produced by international collaborative effort in 2020
- Scant supporting studies at present; intended as baseline model to facilitate studies of its efficacy

Categories
- Nondiagnostic (ND)
  - Lack of mesothelial cells does not make specimen ND; pathologic process may still be identified in many cases
  - Acellular, hemorrhagic, or markedly degenerated samples may be ND
  - Minimum volume threshold is 50-75 mL
- Negative for malignancy (NFM)
  - Only benign cells present
- Atypia of undetermined significance (AUS)
  - Small numbers of cells with features making it difficult to exclude malignancy
  - Should be used sparingly in cases felt to be probably benign (ideally should have ~ 20% risk of malignancy)
- Suspicious for malignancy (SFM)
  - Likely malignant, but evidence falls short of confirmation (should have ~ 80% risk of malignancy)
  - Ancillary testing (immunochemistry, flow cytometry, genetic studies) can often be used to avoid this category
- Malignant-primary (MAL-P)
  - For definitive diagnosis of mesothelioma
- Malignant-secondary (MAL-S)
  - For diagnosis of carcinoma, lymphoma, melanoma, sarcoma, germ cell, or sex-cord stromal malignancy

SELECTED REFERENCES
1. Chandra A et al: The International System for Serous Fluid Cytopathology. Springer Nature, 2020
2. Pinto D et al: The International System for Reporting Serous Fluid Cytopathology-diagnostic categories and clinical management. J Am Soc Cytopathol. 9(6):469-77, 2020

Normal Cellular Components, Reactive Mesothelial Proliferations, and Reporting Terminology

Typical Appearance of Effusions

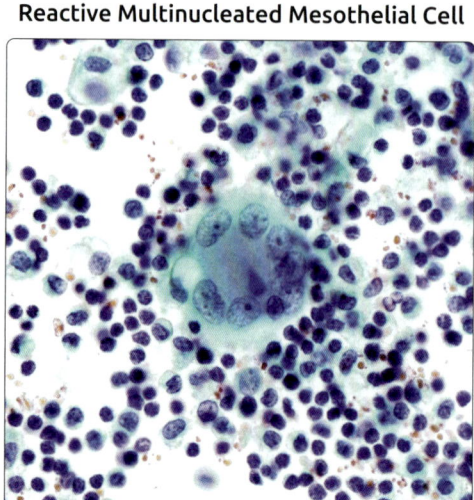

Reactive Multinucleated Mesothelial Cell

(Left) Pap stain shows a pleural effusion with mesothelial cells ⇨, histiocytes ⇨, and mixed acute and chronic inflammatory cells. Mesothelial cells have mild variation in cell and nuclear size. (Right) Pap stain of ascites in a patient with cirrhosis shows large multinucleated mesothelial cells and numerous T lymphocytes. Hepatocellular carcinoma rarely appears in fluids; in the setting of cirrhosis, almost all unusual cells are reactive in nature.

Reactive Nuclear Changes

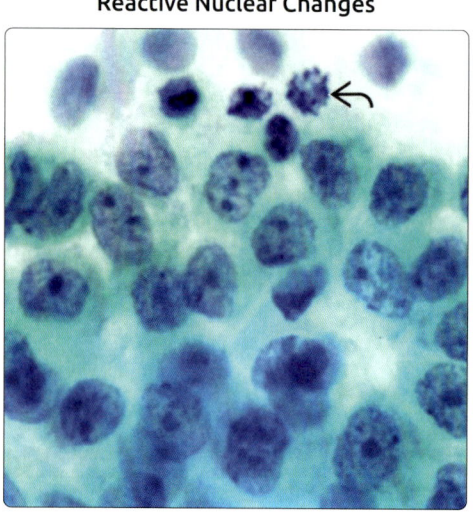

Acinar Mesothelial Structure

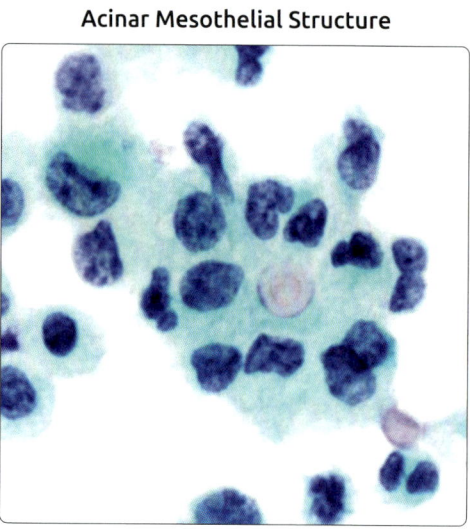

(Left) Pap stain of an effusion with sheets of reactive mesothelial cells demonstrates mild nuclear atypia, irregular nuclear membranes, prominent nucleoli, and occasional mitosis ⇨. (Right) Pap stain shows an effusion with reactive mesothelial cells forming an acinar structure, possibly raising concern for adenocarcinoma. However, the mesothelial cells forming the acinar structure have similar cytologic features to the background-dispersed mesothelial cells.

Large Fluid-Filled Vacuole

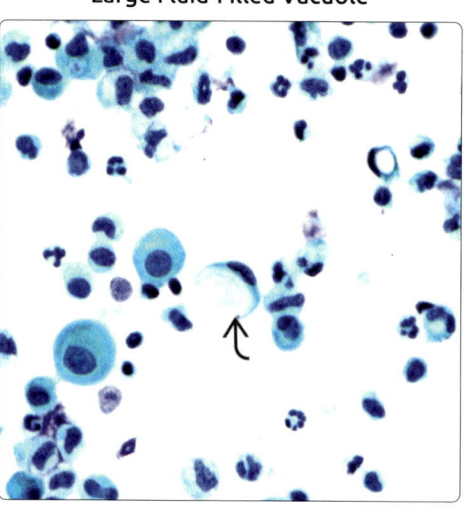

Psammoma Body

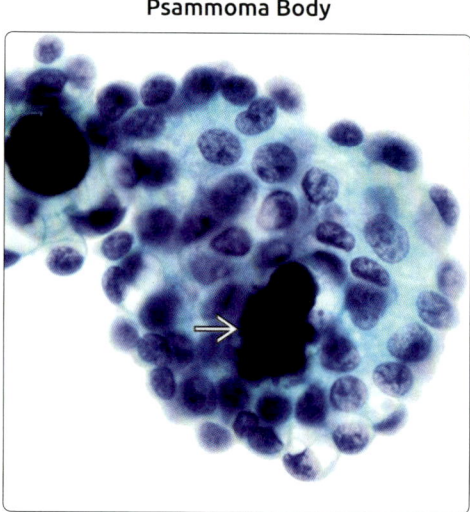

(Left) Pap stain shows an effusion with an occasional signet-ring-like cell ⇨. Benign mesothelial cells may imbibe fluid in their cytoplasm, displacing the nucleus. The nuclear features are similar to the surrounding benign mesothelial cells, helping to allay concern. (Right) Pap stain shows pleural effusion in a case of benign reactive mesothelial hyperplasia. A papillary group of benign mesothelial cells with associated psammoma body ⇨ is also shown.

Normal Cellular Components, Reactive Mesothelial Proliferations, and Reporting Terminology

Pelvic Wash Conventional Smear

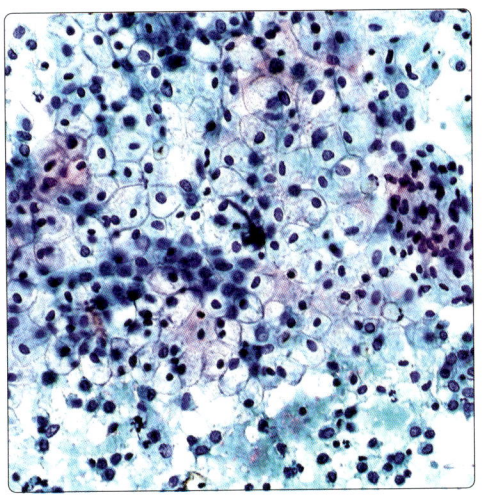

Large Sheets of Cells in Washing

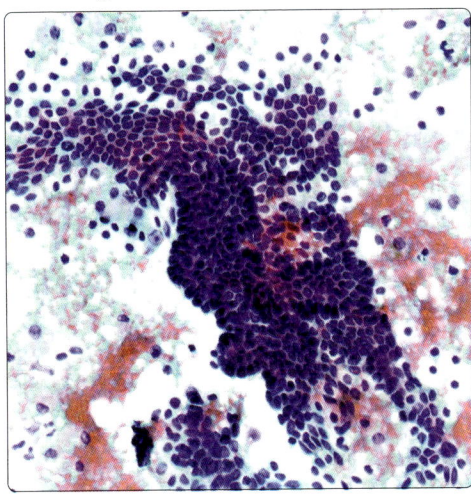

(Left) Pap stain of a pelvic wash shows directly obtained nonreactive mesothelial cells with very delicate clear cytoplasm, well-defined cell borders, and round to oval nuclei with fine chromatin. (Right) Pap stain of pelvic washing shows vigorous sampling resulting in a highly cellular specimen with large sheets that can be folded or rolled. Knowledge of how the sample is obtained and correlation with surgical specimen are necessary to avoid a false-positive diagnosis.

Mesothelial Sheet in ThinPrep

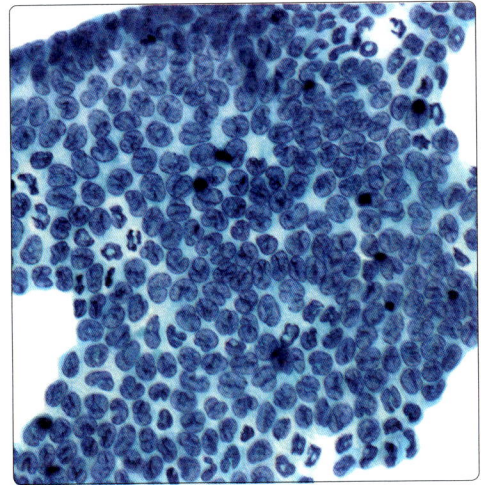

Collagen Ball

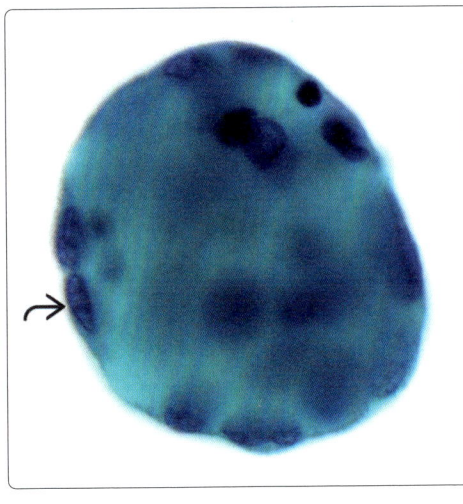

(Left) Peritoneal washings prepared by the ThinPrep method may show considerable nuclear contour irregularities in benign mesothelial cells. The regular order and flatness of the sheet of mesothelial cells are reassuring features. (Right) This collagen ball from a ThinPrep of a peritoneal washing demonstrates the homogeneous core of collagenous material surrounded by flattened mesothelial cells on the outer surface ➥.

Reactive Hyperplasia in Cell Block

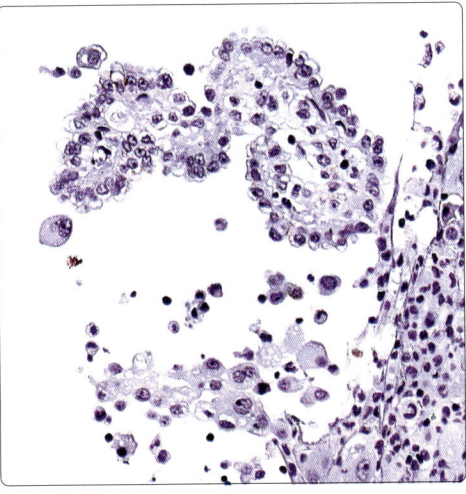

D2-40 Staining of Reactive Hyperplasia

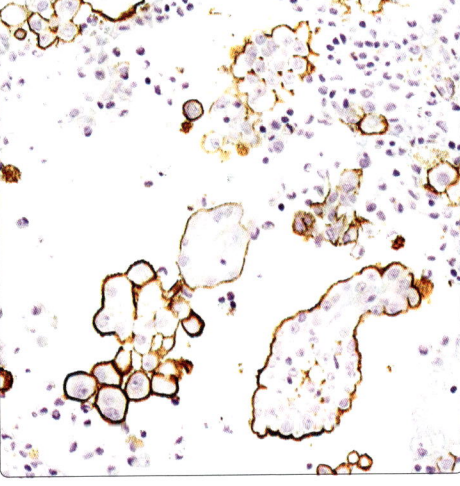

(Left) A cell block in a case of reactive mesothelial hyperplasia shows a papillary arrangement that raises suspicion for carcinoma. Negative staining for Moc-31, monoclonal CEA, and other carcinoma markers supports mesothelial origin. (Right) D2-40 immunocytochemical stain performed on a cell block demonstrates positive membranous staining of reactive mesothelial cells. D2-40 is helpful to rule out carcinoma but will not discriminate between reactive and malignant mesothelial cells.

Infectious Conditions

KEY FACTS

CLINICAL ISSUES
- Infectious effusions are most commonly parapneumonic effusions associated with bacterial pneumonia
- Tuberculosis is most common cause of pleural effusions in resource-limited countries but is rare in USA
- Viruses may also cause effusions, including COVID-19

CYTOPATHOLOGY
- Most infectious effusions are bacterial in origin and have nonspecific mixed inflammation with predominance of neutrophils
- Effusions with numerous neutrophils are often associated with bacterial pneumonia, inflammation/injury to bowel with peritonitis, or spontaneous bacterial peritonitis associated with cirrhosis
- Eosinophil-rich infectious effusions can be caused by parasitic infections, fungal infections, or pulmonary tuberculosis
- Lymphocyte-rich infectious effusions can be caused by viral infections or pulmonary tuberculosis
- Special stains, immunohistochemical stains, or molecular testing to determine specific viral signatures or etiology can be performed on cell block

TOP DIFFERENTIAL DIAGNOSES
- Effusions with nonspecific inflammatory background can be caused by neoplasms, pulmonary emboli, metabolic or autoimmune diseases, and others
- Eosinophilic effusions are only rarely associated with parasites; usually idiopathic or associated with pneumothorax or previous sampling

DIAGNOSTIC CHECKLIST
- Most infectious effusions are secondary to bacterial infections and therefore cannot be definitively diagnosed by cytology alone
- Rarely, specifically identifiable fungal organisms may be found in effusions

Cryptococcal Effusion
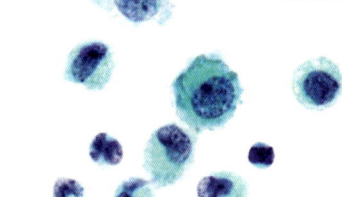

Mucicarmine Highlighting *Cryptococcus*
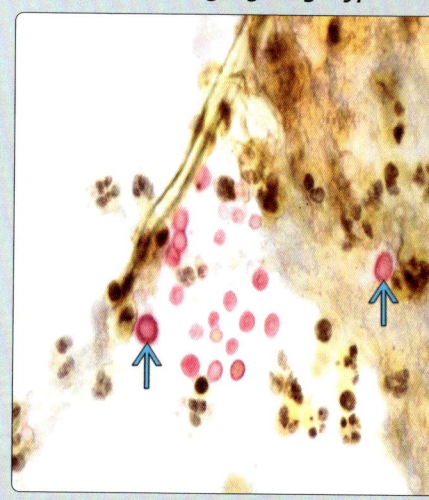

(Left) Pap stain shows Cryptococcus neoformans ➡ in the pleural fluid of an immunocompromised patient with disseminated disease. The organisms are refractile, aiding in identification during screening. (Right) Mucicarmine stain highlights the thick, mucin-positive capsule ➡ of Cryptococcus. This stain is more specific than GMS or PAS when Cryptococcus is suspected but will fail to detect capsule-deficient variants.

GMS-Positive Fungus
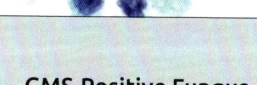
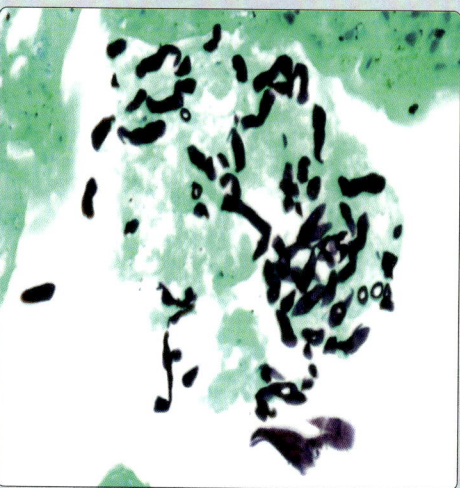

Coccidioides Spherule
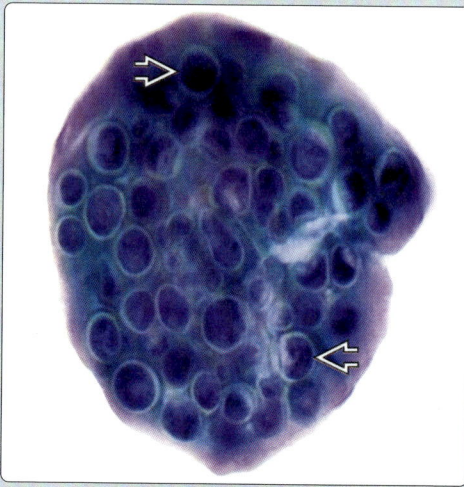

(Left) GMS stain performed on a cell block from an effusion specimen can highlight fungal elements, such as these hyphal forms. Fungi may be difficult to appreciate with conventional cytologic staining alone. (Right) Pap stain shows Coccidioides immitis in a severely immunocompromised patient with disseminated pulmonary infection and effusion. Note the large spherule filled with numerous endospores ➡.

Infectious Conditions

CLINICAL ISSUES

Epidemiology
- Most infectious effusions are caused by bacterial organisms
  - ~ 40% of patients with pneumonia develop effusions
- Tuberculosis is most common cause of pleural effusions in resource-limited countries
  - However, it is rare in USA
- Fungal organisms identified in fluids include *Candida* species, *Cryptococcus neoformans*, *Coccidioides immitis*, *Blastomyces dermatitidis*, and *Aspergillus niger*
- Viruses may also cause effusions
  - Effusion-causing viruses recognizable in cytology specimens include Herpesvirus and Cytomegalovirus
  - Patients with severe/critical COVID-19 pneumonia can present with pleural (28%) and pericardial (16%) effusions

Laboratory Tests
- Microbiology cultures or molecular studies are usually needed for specific diagnosis of etiology

Prognosis
- Most respond well to appropriate antibiotic treatment

CYTOPATHOLOGY

Cellularity
- Moderate to highly cellular

Pattern
- Dispersed cells or small clusters of inflammatory cells, histiocytes, and mesothelial cells

Background
- Blood, cellular debris, or necrotic background

Cells
- Effusions with numerous neutrophils are often associated with bacterial pneumonia, inflammation/injury to bowel with peritonitis, or spontaneous bacterial peritonitis secondary to cirrhosis
- Eosinophil-rich infectious effusions can be caused by parasitic infections, fungal infections, or pulmonary tuberculosis
- Lymphocyte-rich infectious effusions can be caused by viral infections or pulmonary tuberculosis

Nuclear Details
- Reactive mesothelial cells with nuclear size variation, multinucleation, coarse chromatin, and prominent nucleoli
  - Rarely, intranuclear viral inclusions can be seen

Cytoplasmic Details
- Mesothelial cells have cytoplasmic vacuoles, and phagocytic histiocytes contain cellular debris and intracellular organisms

Cell Block Findings
- Special stains, immunohistochemical stains, or molecular testing to determine specific viral signatures or etiology can be performed on cell block

DIFFERENTIAL DIAGNOSIS

Effusions With Mixed Inflammation
- Malignant effusion, autoimmune or metabolic disease

Eosinophilic Effusions
- Idiopathic origin, pneumothorax, pulmonary infarct, Hodgkin disease, or drug reactions

Lymphocyte-Rich Effusions
- Cirrhosis, heart failure, renal failure, or lymphoma

DIAGNOSTIC CHECKLIST

Pathologic Interpretation Pearls
- Most infectious effusions are secondary to bacteria
  - Therefore, etiologic diagnosis requires clinical/radiologic and culture correlation

SELECTED REFERENCES
1. Chong WH et al: The incidence of pleural effusion in COVID-19 pneumonia: state-of-the-art review. Heart Lung. 50(4):481-90, 2021

Actinomyces Associated With Chest Tube
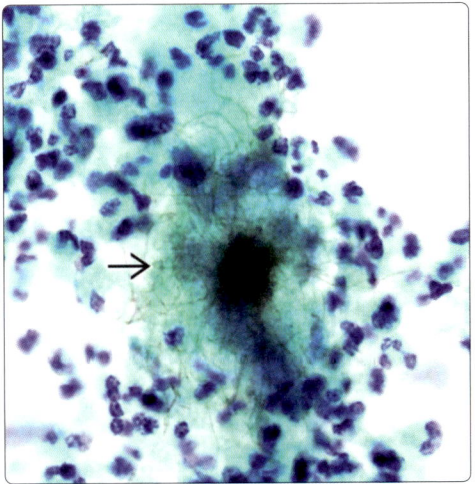

PAS Highlighting *Actinomyces*
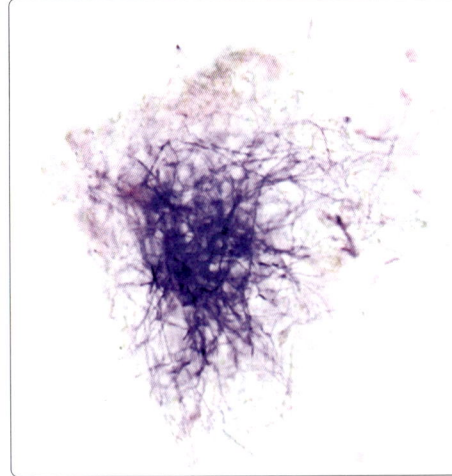

(Left) Pap stain shows filamentous clusters ➡ of Actinomyces organisms identified in pleural fluid extracted from a patient with an infected chest tube. *(Right)* PAS special stain highlights the bacterial filaments. Actinomyces must be carefully differentiated from Nocardia and fungal organisms, including Candida.

Autoimmune Diseases

KEY FACTS

CLINICAL ISSUES

- < 5% of rheumatoid arthritis (RA) patients develop pleural disease
  - More common in male patients with longstanding articular disease and subcutaneous rheumatoid nodules
- 30-50% of patients with systemic lupus erythematosus (SLE) develop pleural effusions
  - May be unilateral or bilateral, associated with immune-mediated pleuritis, drug reactions, or infections
  - Pericardial effusions may also occur

CYTOPATHOLOGY

- RA effusions
  - Seen in minority of patients (< 5%) with established rheumatoid disease
  - Spindled, epithelioid, or multinucleated macrophages
  - Mixed inflammation and granular material in background
  - Often have aggregates of clumped granular material on cell block
- SLE effusions
  - More common, seen in up to 50% of patients
  - Have nonspecific cytologic findings with lymphocytes, neutrophils, and lupus erythematosus (LE) cells (seen in only ~ 25%)
  - LE cells contain cytoplasmic hematoxylin body that indents nucleus into crescent-like shape

TOP DIFFERENTIAL DIAGNOSES

- Infections with necrotizing granulomas
- Trauma/infarct
- Metabolic diseases
- Malignancies with nonspecific inflammation

DIAGNOSTIC CHECKLIST

- Cytologic findings are pathognomonic of RA
- SLE effusions are nonspecific
  - Presence of LE cells is not diagnostic of lupus

Lupus Erythematosus Cell

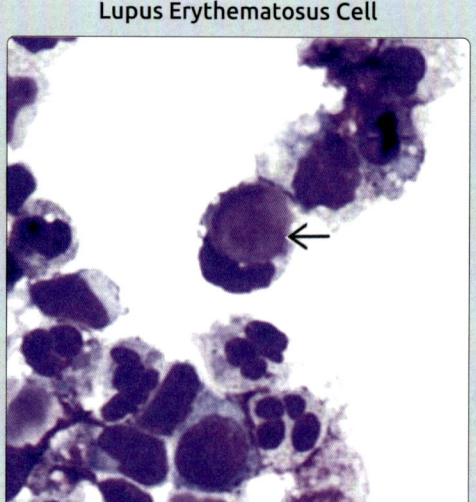

Hematoxylin Bodies

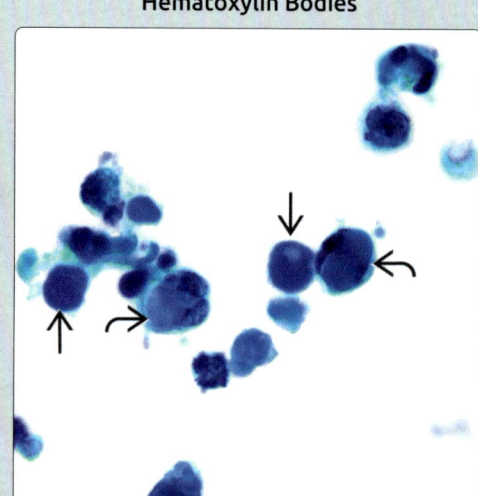

(Left) Diff-Quik stain shows pleural effusion on a patient with systemic lupus erythematosus (SLE). Note a lupus erythematosus (LE) cell with a large magenta intracytoplasmic inclusion that pushes the nucleus to the side ⊇. (Right) Florid examples of LE in fluids may have numerous homogenized aggregates of nuclear material, known as hematoxylin bodies, not only within LE cells ⊇, but also in the background ⊇, as shown by this Pap-stained example.

Rheumatoid Effusion

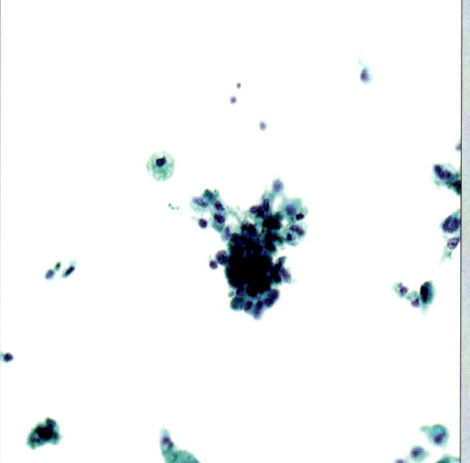

Granular Debris and Histiocytes

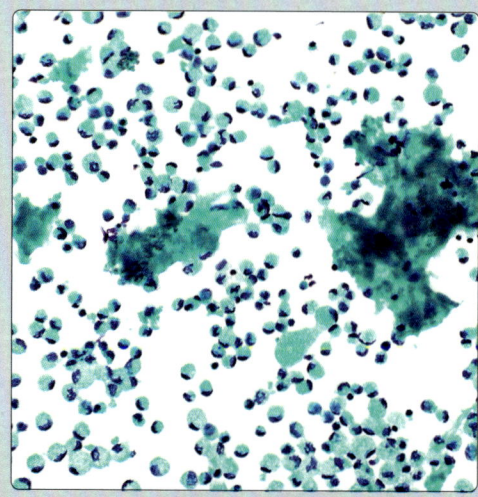

(Left) Pap stain of a pleural effusion in a patient with rheumatoid arthritis contains few multinucleated giant cells and spindled histiocytes. (Right) Pap stain of a rheumatoid effusion shows abundant acellular granular material and background of numerous foamy macrophages.

Autoimmune Diseases

TERMINOLOGY

Definitions
- Effusions resulting from immunologically mediated inflammation of serosa
- Rheumatoid arthritis (RA) and systemic lupus erythematosus (SLE)
  - Most common autoimmune diseases that cause effusions

CLINICAL ISSUES

Prognosis
- < 5% of RA patients develop pleural disease
  - More common in male patients with longstanding articular disease and subcutaneous rheumatoid nodules
- 30-50% of patients with SLE develop pleural effusions
  - Unilateral or bilateral
    - Can present with pericardial effusions
  - Effusions can be due to
    - Immune-mediated pleuritis
    - Drug-induced lupus pleuritis
    - Other complications, such as infections

CYTOPATHOLOGY

Pattern
- Macrophages
- Rare or absent mesothelial cells

Background
- RA effusions
  - Abundant amorphous coarsely granular debris
- SLE effusions
  - Pseudochylous effusions with cholesterol crystals

Cells
- RA effusions
  - Spindled, epithelioid, or multinucleated macrophages that may appear atypical
  - Lymphocytes and neutrophils admixed with amorphous granular material
- SLE effusions
  - Lymphocytes, neutrophils, and lupus erythematosus (LE) cells (seen in ~ 25% of SLE effusions)

Cytoplasmic Details
- LE cells are neutrophils or macrophages, which contain intracytoplasmic degenerated nuclear material forming hematoxylin body that indents nucleus

Cell Block Findings
- RA effusions often have large aggregates of clumped granular material on cell block

DIFFERENTIAL DIAGNOSIS

Rheumatoid Arthritis Effusions
- Infections with necrotizing granulomas
- Lupus-like syndrome secondary to treatment
- SLE effusion

Systemic Lupus Erythematosus Effusions
- Lupus pleuritis
  - Diagnosis is established using American Rheumatism Association criteria
- RA effusions
- Lupus-like syndrome secondary to treatment

DIAGNOSTIC CHECKLIST

Pathologic Interpretation Pearls
- Cytologic findings are pathognomonic of RA
- SLE effusions are nonspecific
  - Presence of LE cells is not diagnostic of SLE

SELECTED REFERENCES

1. Depascale R et al: Diagnosis and management of lung involvement in systemic lupus erythematosus and Sjögren's syndrome: a literature review. Ther Adv Musculoskelet Dis. 13:1759720X211040696, 2021
2. Ip H et al: Multidisciplinary approach to connective tissue disease (CTD) related pleural effusions: a four-year retrospective evaluation. BMC Pulm Med. 19(1):161, 2019

Rheumatoid Effusion Cell Block

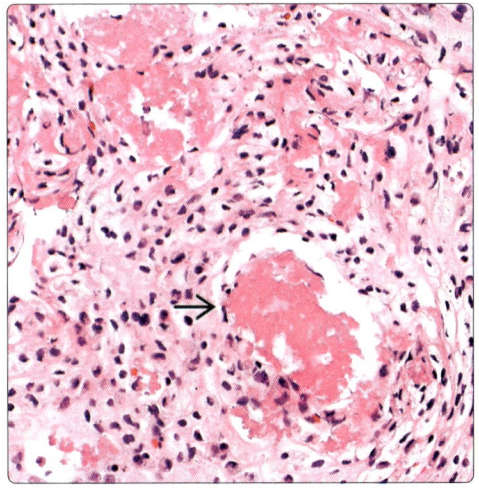

CD68 in Rheumatoid Effusion

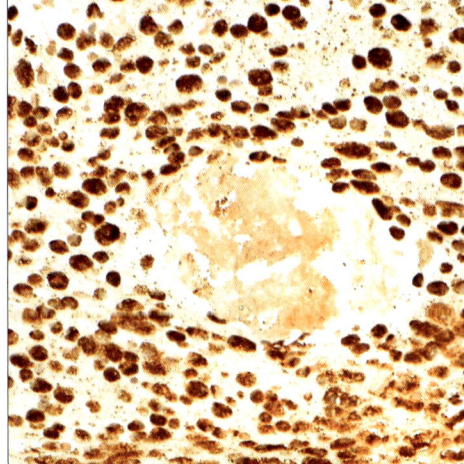

(Left) H&E-stained cell block performed on pleural effusion of a rheumatoid arthritis patient shows aggregates of acellular granular material ➔ with numerous epithelioid histiocytes. (Right) CD68 immunocytochemical stain performed on a cell block of a rheumatoid effusion demonstrates diffuse positive staining of numerous epithelioid histiocytes.

Malignant Effusion, Mesothelioma

KEY FACTS

CLINICAL ISSUES

- Diffuse malignant mesothelioma (DMM) accounts for 1-4% of malignant pleural effusions and < 1% of malignant peritoneal effusions
- Most commonly seen in older male patients with prior asbestos exposure
- Bloody or honey-colored and voluminous effusions
- Grows on pleural surfaces as masses or multiple nodules that eventually encase lung

CYTOPATHOLOGY

- Diagnosis can be achieved in up to 80% of cases if cytologic findings are combined with biopsy and history
- Cells often have deceptively bland cytologic features that recapitulate normal mesothelial cells
- Epithelial DMM has round to oval nuclei with irregular/coarse chromatin and prominent nucleoli
- Cytoplasm of epithelial DMM can be vacuolated or dense with peripheral halo

TOP DIFFERENTIAL DIAGNOSES

- Reactive mesothelial cells
  - DMM effusions often have larger clusters or morulae
  - Malignant cells conserve normal nuclear:cytoplasmic ratio, but cytomegaly and some atypia are often present
  - Loss of immunostaining for BAP1 or MTAP (or 9p21 deletion as alternative to MTAP) support malignancy; significant minority of mesotheliomas cannot be confirmed by these tests
  - Distinction may require histology in some cases
- Adenocarcinoma
  - DMM effusions show morphologic continuum of cells, whereas adenocarcinomas contain dual population
  - Clusters of DMM cells have scalloped borders, whereas in adenocarcinomas, clusters of malignant cells have smooth cell borders
  - Panel of immunocytochemical stains that includes ≥ 2 markers each for mesothelial cells and carcinoma cells is often required

Numerous Large Clusters

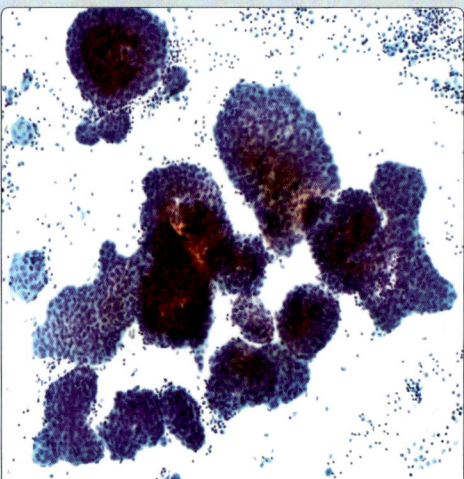

Scalloped Borders

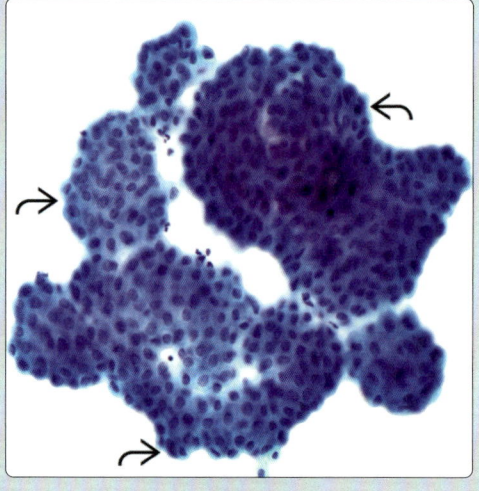

(Left) Pap stain of a pleural effusion shows a highly cellular specimen with numerous large clusters of diffuse malignant mesothelioma (DMM) cells. Each cluster or morula contains hundreds of cells. (Right) Pap stain of pleural effusion of DMM shows a large cluster of cells with scalloped borders ➡ and a branching irregular pattern. Effusions containing many large clusters are almost always malignant.

2-Tone Cytoplasm and Windows

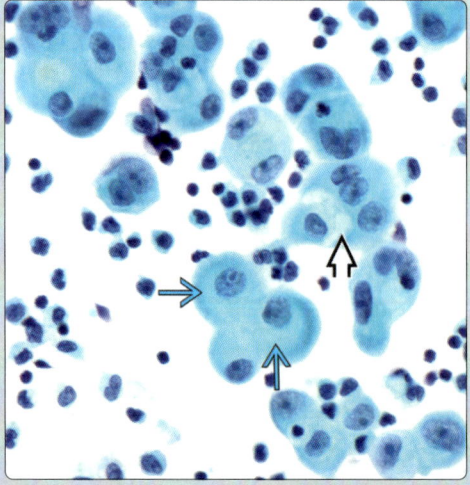

Negative BAP1 in Malignant Mesothelioma

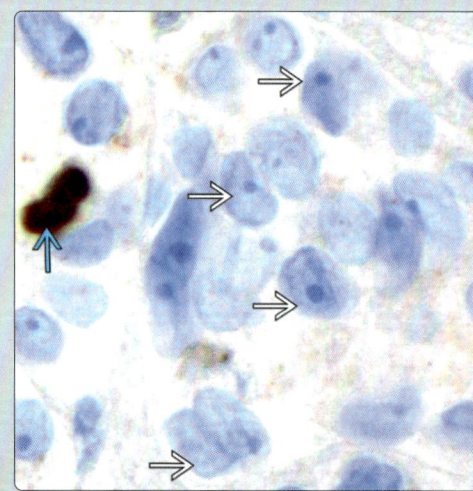

(Left) Some examples of mesothelioma do not have large morular clusters but instead contain individual cells and small groups. This Pap-stained example shows large malignant cells that retain the 2-tone cytoplasm ➡ and windows ➡ characteristic of mesothelial cells. Frequent multinucleation and nuclear pleomorphism raise suspicion for malignancy. (Right) Cell block shows negative BAP1 stain in the tumor cell nuclei ➡. The nucleus of a polymorphonuclear leukocyte stains positive ➡, serving as an internal control.

Malignant Effusion, Mesothelioma

TERMINOLOGY

Abbreviations
- Diffuse malignant mesothelioma (DMM)

CLINICAL ISSUES

Epidemiology
- DMM is rare primary serosal malignancy most commonly seen in older male patients with prior asbestos exposure
- DMM accounts for 1-4% of malignant pleural effusions and < 1% of malignant peritoneal effusions

Presentation
- Most patients present decades after initial asbestos exposure with pleuritic pain and shortness of breath
- In cases of DMM, bloody or honey-colored and voluminous pleural effusions often occur
- Grossly, DMM grows on pleural surfaces as masses or multiple nodules that eventually encase lung
- Localized malignant mesothelioma is rare variant presenting as single nodule
- Mesothelioma in situ has recently been recognized as diagnostic entity; presents as unexplained recurrent effusions
- Well-differentiated papillary mesothelioma is usually incidental peritoneal lesion found in women

Prognosis
- DMM is aggressive tumor, and most patients die of disease within 2 years of diagnosis
- Localized malignant mesothelioma may be cured if completely excised
  - Well-differentiated papillary mesothelioma is benign disease

CYTOPATHOLOGY

Cellularity
- Effusions caused by DMM are highly cellular
- Cellularity persists with multiple taps as opposed to reactive conditions

Pattern
- Large clusters with scalloped borders, 3D morular groups, or numerous single cells

Cells
- Cells of epithelial DMM often have deceptively bland cytologic features that recapitulate normal mesothelial cells, but usually, some cytomegaly is appreciable
- Only epithelial components are seen in body cavity fluids
- Squamoid orangeophilic cells with pyknotic nuclei may be seen in some cases
- Signet-ring-like cells or cells with marked nuclear atypia may mimic adenocarcinoma

Nuclear Details
- Epithelial DMM has round to oval nuclei with irregular/coarse chromatin and prominent nucleoli
- Binucleation and multinucleation can be seen
- Nuclear atypia is mild to moderate in most cases, but significant minority may have high nuclear grade

Cytoplasmic Details
- Cytoplasm of epithelial DMM can be vacuolated or dense with peripheral halo
- In most cases of DMM, cells have abundant cytoplasm, thus retaining normal nuclear:cytoplasmic ratio
- Slender microvilli can be appreciated in some cases

ANCILLARY TESTS

Immunohistochemistry
- Loss of BAP1 &/or MTAP staining has high specificity for mesothelioma

In Situ Hybridization
- Cytogenetic analysis by FISH demonstrates clonal deletions; 9p21 deletion with loss of p16 is most useful

DIFFERENTIAL DIAGNOSIS

Benign Reactive Mesothelial Hyperplasia
- DMM effusions tend to be more cellular, and cellularity persists after multiple taps
- Malignant cells are usually larger and, in some cases, more atypical, than reactive mesothelial cells
- Immunocytochemistry for BAP1/MTAP alongside FISH testing for loss of p16 has shown excellent specificity in diagnosis of DMM and may facilitate early identification of DMM or mesothelioma in situ

Adenocarcinoma
- Can diffusely infiltrate serosal surfaces with similar histologic and cytologic pattern as DMM
- DMM effusions show morphologic continuum of cells, while adenocarcinomas contain dual population
- Clusters of DMM cells have scalloped borders, whereas in adenocarcinomas, clusters of malignant cells have smooth cell borders
- DMM cells can have dense or vacuolated cytoplasm and retain slit-like separation (windows) between cells
- Morphology alone is usually not sufficient to make definite diagnosis; therefore, panel of immunocytochemical stains is needed
  - Stains for DMM include calretinin, D2-40, HEG1, CK5/6, mesothelin, thrombomodulin, HBME-1, WT1
  - Stains for adenocarcinomas include claudin-4, MOC-31, BER-EP4, B72.3, mCEA
  - International Mesothelioma Interest Group recommends at least 2 mesothelial and 2 carcinoma markers

REPORTING

International System Category
- Malignant-primary (MAL-P)

SELECTED REFERENCES

1. Chevrier M et al: Testing for BAP1 loss and CDKN2A/p16 homozygous deletion improves the accurate diagnosis of mesothelial proliferations in effusion cytology. Cancer Cytopathol. 128(12):939-47, 2020
2. Siddiqui MT et al: Proceedings of the American Society of Cytopathology companion session at the 2019 United States and Canadian Academy of Pathology Annual meeting, part 2: effusion cytology with focus on theranostics and diagnosis of malignant mesothelioma. J Am Soc Cytopathol. 8(6):352-61, 2019

Malignant Effusion, Mesothelioma

(Left) Pap stain of DMM shows malignant cells retaining some of the characteristics of mesothelial cells, including long, slender microvilli ⇨. **(Right)** Pap stain of pleural effusion demonstrates single cells and cohesive clusters of cells with mildly atypical cytologic features. This example contains a core of hyaline collagenous material ⇨.

Microvilli
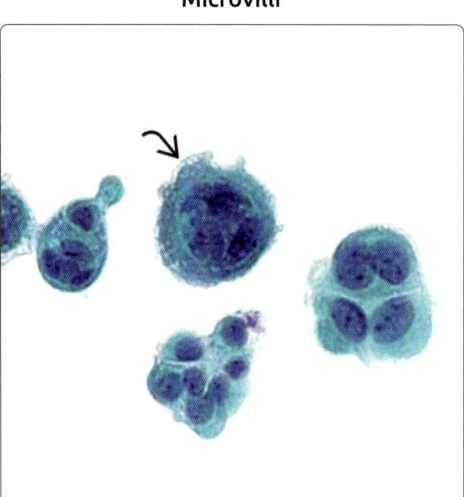

Hyaline Core in Morular Clusters
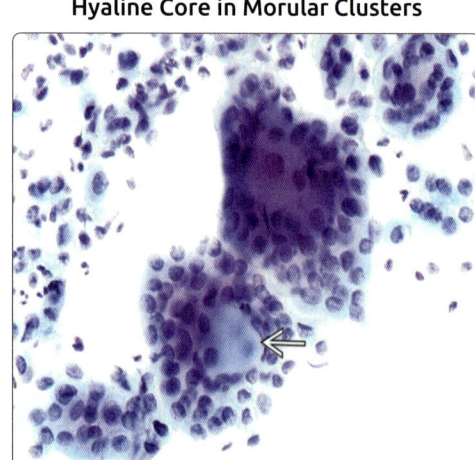

(Left) Pap stain of pleural effusion with low-grade DMM shows small clusters with mild nuclear atypia that retain characteristics of benign mesothelial cells. Cases with this morphology are difficult to diagnose by cytology. **(Right)** Pap stain shows pleural effusion with a low-grade DMM. This is a high cellularity specimen with single cell pattern. The cells have bland cytologic features with preserved nuclear:cytoplasmic ratio. However, cytomegaly ⇨ can be appreciated when compared with benign mesothelial cells ⇨.

Mild Atypia
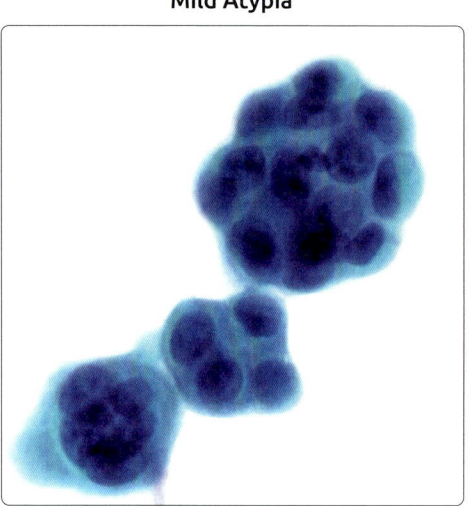

Cytomegaly
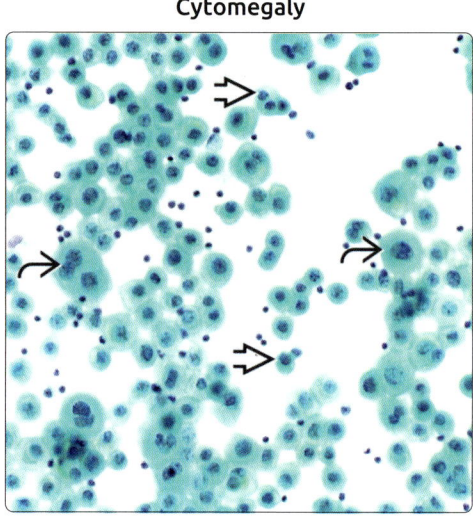

(Left) A minority of epithelioid DMM may have marked nuclear pleomorphism with prominent nucleoli ⇨, consistent with a high-grade malignancy. In this example, the 2-tone cytoplasm typical of mesothelial cells can be seen in the Pap stain ⇨, favoring mesothelial origin. **(Right)** Some high-grade DMMs have markedly atypical and multilobated nuclei ⇨. The Pap stain highlights the coarse chromatin in this example. Immunocytochemistry can confirm that the atypical cells are of mesothelial origin.

Large Nucleoli
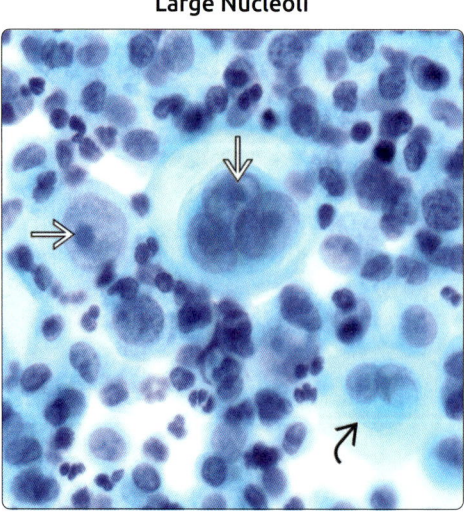

Coarse Chromatin
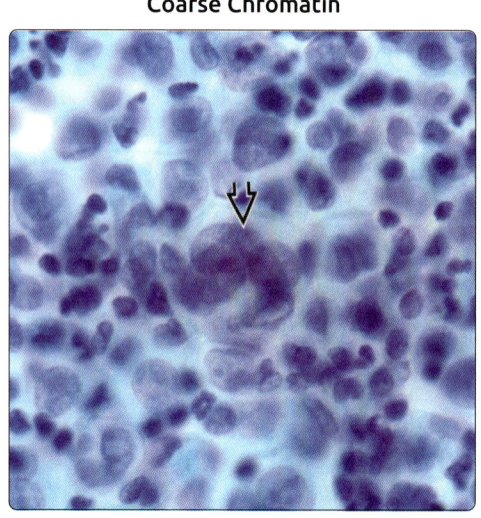

Malignant Effusion, Mesothelioma

Parakeratotic-Like Cells

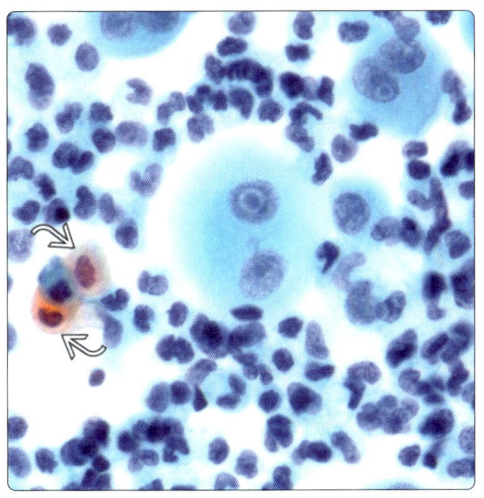

Psammoma Body

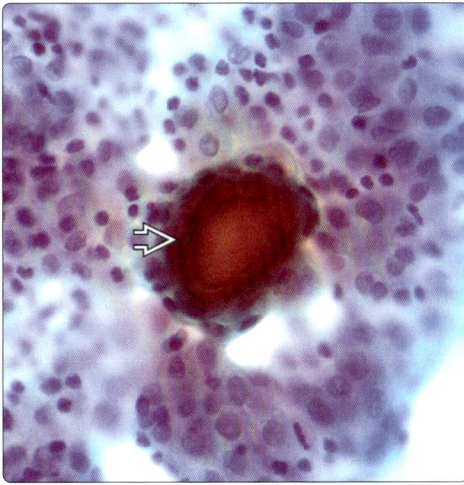

(Left) Some examples of mesothelioma contain small parakeratotic-like cells ➡ with orangeophilic cytoplasm and pyknotic nuclei. In this Pap-stained cytospin, these cells are seen in the vicinity of large, atypical mesothelial cells with an inflammatory background. (Right) This example of a peritoneal DMM with papillary architecture in the corresponding biopsy showed psammoma bodies ➡ in the Pap-stained ascites fluid. Note the large clusters of surrounding malignant cells with nuclear contour irregularities.

Collagenous Core on Cell Block

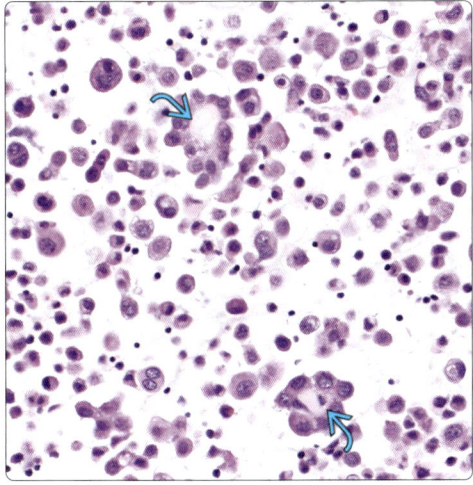

Bland Mesothelial Clusters on Cell Block

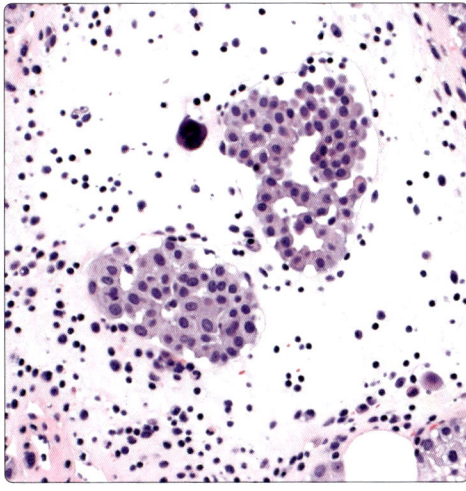

(Left) H&E-stained cell block shows pleural DMM. There is a single population of malignant cells with variable degree of atypia. Some of the clusters of malignant cells surround a collagenous core ➡. (Right) H&E-stained cell block of a low-grade DMM shows a single population of cells with bland cytologic features. A panel of immunostains, including 2 mesothelial and 2 carcinoma markers, is useful to confirm mesothelial origin. BAP1 stain and MTAP stain/9p21 FISH help to distinguish such cells from a reactive process.

Surface Mesothelial Hyperplasia

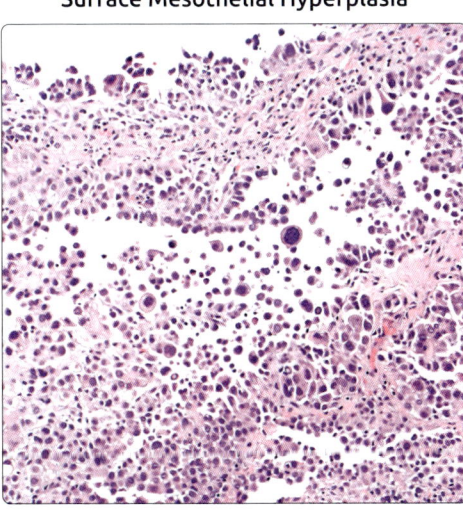

Invasion Amid Collagen Bundles

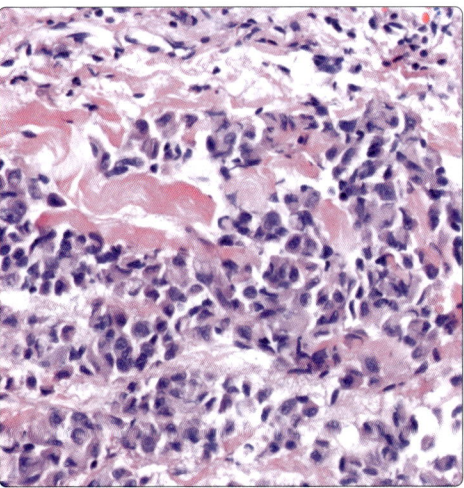

(Left) Marked mesothelial hyperplasia along the pleural surface is often seen in mesothelioma, as in this H&E-stained section, but benign mesothelial hyperplasia can have a similar appearance. (Right) High-power H&E image demonstrates the subtle infiltrative pattern without desmoplasia, typical of mesothelioma. Pancytokeratin stains are often used to highlight the malignant cells in difficult cases. Invasion is diagnostic of DMM.

Malignant Effusion, Carcinomas

KEY FACTS

CLINICAL ISSUES
- ~ 30% of all body fluids are malignant effusions
- Carcinomas account for great majority of malignant effusions in adult patients
- Diagnosis of malignancy in body fluid is indicative of high-stage tumor
  - Grim prognosis
- Cytology is cost-effective and accurate method for detecting malignancy in effusion with overall sensitivity of 58-71% and specificity close to 100%

CYTOPATHOLOGY
- Malignant effusions are usually highly cellular
- Key feature is presence of dual population of tumor cells with background mesothelial and inflammatory cells
- Some carcinomas, especially lobular breast carcinoma and gastric carcinoma, can produce uniform population of single malignant cells with subtle morphology
- Adenocarcinomas exfoliate as large cohesive clusters or spheres with smooth cell borders, papillary fragments, or dispersed single cells
- Squamous cell carcinomas present as single cells, sheets, or cohesive clusters
- Small cell carcinomas exfoliate as single cells, short chains, or small tight clusters of tumor cells
- Architecture and nuclear features on cytology preparations correlate with cell block findings and, in most cases, with histology of primary neoplasm

TOP DIFFERENTIAL DIAGNOSES
- Benign effusions secondary to infections, therapy effect, trauma, or metabolic disorders have reactive mesothelial cells with atypia worrisome for malignancy
- Differential diagnosis with malignant mesotheliomas requires panel of immunohistochemical stains
- Poorly differentiated carcinomas can shed in dispersed single cell pattern resembling large cell lymphomas

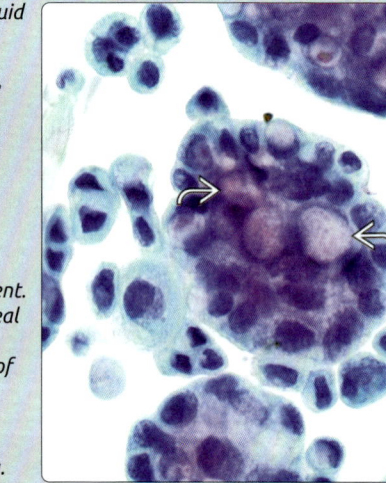

Typical Adenocarcinoma

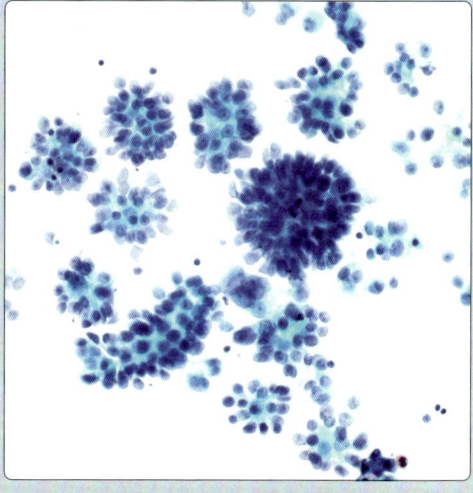

Papillary Serous Carcinoma of Peritoneum

(Left) Pap stain of pleural fluid shows metastatic lung adenocarcinoma. Most metastatic carcinomas have obvious malignant features, including a high nuclear:cytoplasmic ratio, nuclear pleomorphism, hyperchromatic irregular nucleus, and prominent nucleoli. Intracytoplasmic mucin vacuoles ➡ are evident. *(Right)* Pap stain of peritoneal fluid shows metastatic papillary serous carcinoma of the ovary. The tumor exfoliates as papillary fragments and cell clusters with variable nuclear atypia.

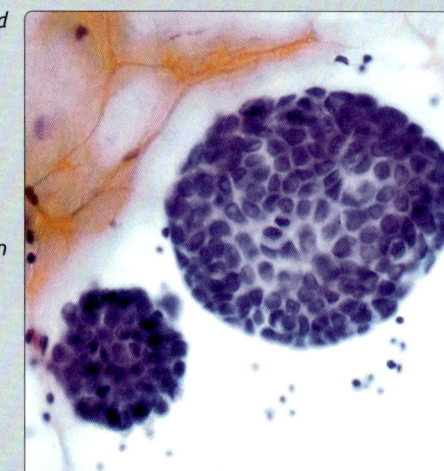

Breast Carcinoma "Cannon Balls"

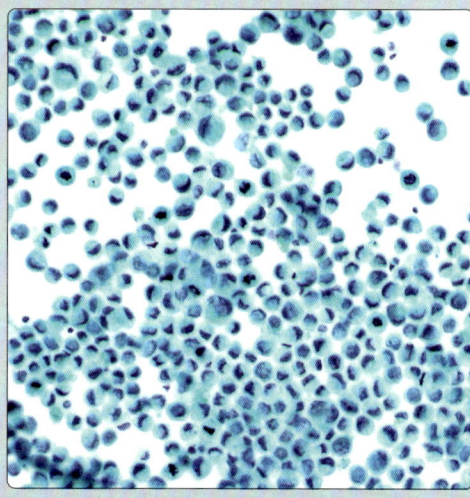

Single Cell Malignant Population

(Left) Pap stain of pleural fluid shows dense spherical groups or morulae of metastatic ductal adenocarcinoma. Clusters and spheres of metastatic adenocarcinoma have smooth cell borders. *(Right)* Pap-stained gastric carcinoma composed of individual malignant cells is an exception to the "2 cell populations" rule. Here, all of the cells are malignant, and background mesothelial cells are inconspicuous.

Malignant Effusion, Carcinomas

CLINICAL ISSUES

Presentation
- ~ 30% of all body fluids are malignant effusions
- Carcinomas account for great majority of malignant effusions in adult patients
- Most patients have known primary neoplasm or multiple primary tumors
  - Malignant effusion is 1st manifestation of occult primary in up to 17% of patients
- Cytology is cost effective and accurate method for detecting malignancy in effusion
  - Sensitivity for diagnosing malignancy: 73% in recent review of literature
  - Specificity of cytologic diagnosis is almost 100%
    - Rate of false-positive diagnosis is < 1%
    - Most occur in cases with marked mesothelial atypia
- Adenocarcinomas account for 60-65% of pleural and pericardial malignant effusions and 80% of peritoneal malignant effusions
  - Breast cancer: Most common primary in malignant pleural/pericardial effusions in females
  - Lung cancer: Most common primary in malignant pleural/pericardial effusions in males and 2nd most common in females
- Squamous cell carcinomas account for 2-4% of all malignant effusions
  - Most are poorly differentiated carcinomas from lung, cervix, or esophagus
- Small cell carcinomas account for 4% of pericardial and 2-9% of malignant pleural effusions

Prognosis
- Diagnosis of malignancy in body fluid is indicative of high-stage tumor with poor prognosis
- Median survival for patients with positive effusion is < 6 months

CYTOPATHOLOGY

Cellularity
- Malignant effusions are usually highly cellular
  - Cellularity persists in repeated taps

Pattern
- Adenocarcinomas exfoliate as large, cohesive clusters or spheres with smooth cell borders, papillary fragments, or dispersed single cells
- Squamous cell carcinomas present as single cells, sheets, or cohesive clusters
- Small cell carcinomas exfoliate as single cells, short chains, or small, tight clusters of tumor cells

Background
- Variable amount of inflammatory cells ± necrotic debris
  - Background mucin and foamy macrophages in cases of pseudomyxoma peritonei
  - Psammoma bodies can be seen in carcinomas with papillary architecture (i.e., ovarian serous carcinoma, lung, thyroid, mesotheliomas)
    - Psammoma bodies are not diagnostic of malignancy, as they can also be seen in endosalpingiosis or mesothelial hyperplasia
  - Squamous and small cell carcinomas often have karyorrhectic debris
    - Anucleated squamous cells are often present in squamous cell carcinomas

Cells
- Most cases display obvious malignant features with pleomorphic cells and high nuclear:cytoplasmic ratio
  - Breast carcinoma, ductal type: Dense spherical groups/morulae, clusters, or single cells
    - Lobular carcinoma: Single cells, short chains, or clusters of small hyperchromatic cells with high nuclear:cytoplasmic ratio and intracytoplasmic mucin droplets
    - Immunohistochemical (IHC) stains for diagnosis/biomarkers: GATA3, GCDFP-15, mammaglobin, ER, PR, and HER2/neu
  - Lung carcinoma: Variable architecture, including papillary groups, clusters, sheets, and single cells
    - Most are high-grade adenocarcinomas with obvious malignant features
    - IHC markers include TTF-1, NAPSIN-A, and CK7
  - Gastrointestinal adenocarcinomas: Often show intestinal morphology and prominent mucin vacuoles
    - Gastric adenocarcinomas: Single malignant cells are most characteristic
    - Colon adenocarcinoma: Clusters of columnar cells with elongated nuclei and necrosis
    - Pancreatic adenocarcinomas: High-grade adenocarcinomas with pleomorphic single cells and clusters; squamous differentiation can be present
    - Pseudomyxoma peritonei: Extracellular mucin and few columnar cells with cytoplasmic mucin (most are of appendiceal origin)
  - Serous neoplasms of müllerian origin: Most are high grade with papillary fragments and pleomorphic cells
    - Low-grade serous carcinomas: Papillary fragments and clusters of cells with subtle cytologic atypia
  - Squamous cell carcinomas: Usually poorly differentiated
    - Sheets, clusters, or single cells with dense cytoplasm and hyperchromatic nucleus
    - ± anucleated squamous cells and necrotic debris
  - Small cell carcinomas: Single cells, tight clusters, or short chains
    - High nuclear:cytoplasmic ratio, scant cytoplasm, stippled chromatin, and nuclear molding
  - Others include renal cell, urothelial, and endometrioid with morphology similar to primary tumors

Nuclear Details
- In most cases, tumor cells have large nucleus with nuclear contour irregularity, coarse chromatin, and prominent nucleoli
  - Nuclear abnormalities are more subtle in lobular carcinoma, gastric carcinoma, and low-grade serous carcinomas
- Squamous cell carcinomas: Pyknotic irregular nucleus
- Small cell carcinomas: High nuclear:cytoplasmic ratio, stippled chromatin, and nuclear molding

Malignant Effusion, Carcinomas

Cytoplasmic Details
- Adenocarcinomas often have cytoplasmic vacuolization
  - Lobular carcinomas of breast: Intracytoplasmic mucin droplets
  - Signet-ring adenocarcinomas: Large intracytoplasmic vacuoles that displace/distort nucleus
- Squamous cell carcinomas: Dense cytoplasm that can be orangeophilic depending on degree of keratinization
- Small cell carcinomas: Scant cytoplasm with high nuclear:cytoplasmic ratio

Cell Block Findings
- Malignant cells on cell block form tight clusters, papillae, or acini sometimes situated in empty space or lacunae

Cytology-Histology Correlation
- Architecture and nuclear features on cytology preparations correlate with cell block findings and, in most cases, with histology of primary neoplasm

DIFFERENTIAL DIAGNOSIS

Carcinoma vs. Benign Reactive Effusion
- Most malignant effusions are caused by high-grade carcinomas with obvious 2nd population of tumor cells
  - 2nd population of tumor cells is not evident in many cases of lobular carcinoma of breast and gastric carcinoma
- Benign effusions have mesothelial cells with variable reactive changes, inflammatory cells, and histocytes
  - Marked reactive atypia can be seen in setting of pulmonary infarction, tuberculosis, chemotherapy, acute pancreatitis, cirrhosis, and patients on renal dialysis
    - Correlation of cytomorphologic features with clinical history and radiologic findings is essential to avoid false-positive diagnosis
  - Panel of IHC stains is used when morphology is equivocal
    - Panel of IHC stains should include ≥ 2 mesothelial and carcinoma markers

Carcinoma vs. Malignant Mesothelioma
- In malignant mesothelioma, morphologic spectrum between malignant and reactive benign mesothelial cells is seen
  - Clusters of mesothelioma cells often have scalloped cell border, whereas adenocarcinoma clusters have smooth cell border
  - Malignant mesothelioma cells have abundant, dense cytoplasm with peripheral lucent zone ("lacy skirt") and windows between cells
  - Differential diagnosis cannot depend on morphology alone; it requires confirmation by panel of IHC stains with both mesothelial markers and carcinoma markers
    - Based on sensitivity and specificity, best overall carcinoma markers include Claudin-4, MOC-31, and BER-EP4

Carcinoma vs. Melanoma
- Most patients with malignant effusions associated with melanoma have known history of cutaneous or extracutaneous melanoma
  - However, ~ 5% of patients present with metastatic disease with no known primary
- Metastatic melanoma exfoliates as single round cell with large prominent nucleolus
  - ± intranuclear pseudoinclusion and cytoplasmic pigmentation
  - Cell clusters are uncommon
  - IHC stains for melanoma include S100, HMB-45, and melanin

Carcinoma vs. Non-Hodgkin Lymphoma
- Poorly differentiated carcinomas can shed in dispersed single cell pattern resembling large cell lymphomas
- Artifactual crowding in cases of lymphomas can mimic cluster formation
- Karyorrhexis is prominent feature in many lymphomas and is uncommon in other malignant effusions
- Panel of IHC stains (e.g., CD45, keratins) can be helpful

Carcinoma vs. Small Round Cell Sarcomas
- Sarcomas metastasize to serosal surface late in course of disease
  - Most patients have well-documented diagnosis
- Small round cell sarcomas (Ewing sarcoma, primitive neuroectodermal tumor, neuroblastoma, embryonal rhabdomyosarcoma) exfoliate as single dispersed cells that can mimic carcinomas
  - It is necessary to correlate with history and clinical findings
  - IHC (e.g., CD99, FLI-1, desmin, myogenin) is useful

Carcinoma vs. Germ Cell Tumors
- Very rare; seen in setting of advanced disease
- Seminoma/dysgerminoma and nonseminomatous germ cell tumors resemble carcinoma morphologically
- IHC (e.g., SALL4, OCT4, HCG) can be helpful, depending on type of germ cell tumor

Small Cell Carcinoma vs. Lymphoma
- Small cell carcinoma cells have tendency to form small clusters and chains
  - Have more pronounced nuclear irregularity with nuclear molding
- Small cell carcinomas are immunoreactive for CK7, TTF-1, and CD56

DIAGNOSTIC CHECKLIST

Pathologic Interpretation Pearls
- Malignant effusions contain dual population of cells, including background mesothelial, inflammatory cells, and foreign population of carcinoma cells

REPORTING

International System Category
- Included in malignant-secondary (MAL-S)

SELECTED REFERENCES
1. Dorry M et al: Pleural effusions associated with squamous cell lung carcinoma have a low diagnostic yield and a poor prognosis. Transl Lung Cancer Res. 10(6):2500-8, 2021
2. Chandra A et al: The International System for Serous Fluid Cytopathology. Springer, 2020

Malignant Effusion, Carcinomas

Signet-Ring Cell
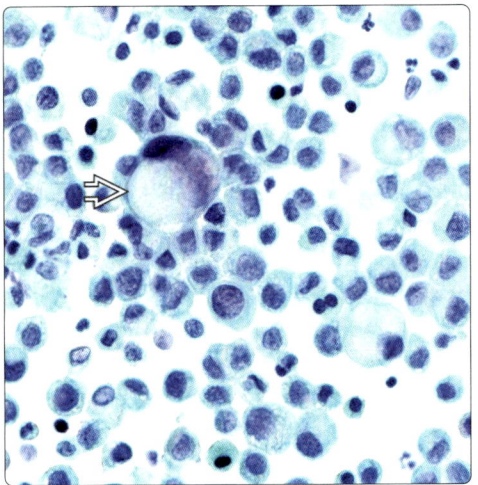

Lobular Breast Carcinoma
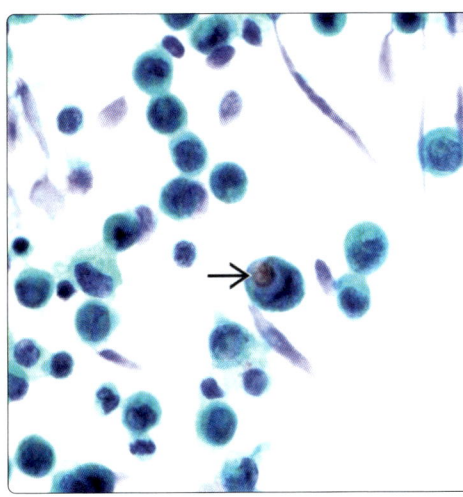

(Left) Pap stain of peritoneal fluid shows metastatic gastric adenocarcinoma with numerous single malignant cells, some with significant nuclear pleomorphism and signet-ring morphology. Signet-ring cells have large mucin vacuoles that displace and indent the nucleus ⇨. (Right) Pap stain of pleural fluid shows metastatic lobular carcinoma. Note the dispersed single cell pattern. The tumor cells are small with mild nuclear atypia and an occasional intracytoplasmic mucin droplet ⇨.

Keratinizing Squamous Cell Carcinoma
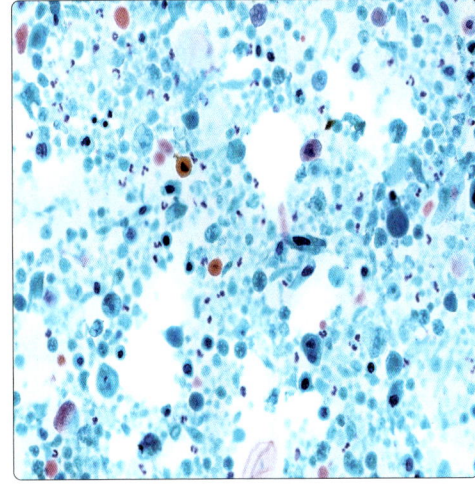

Small Cell Carcinoma
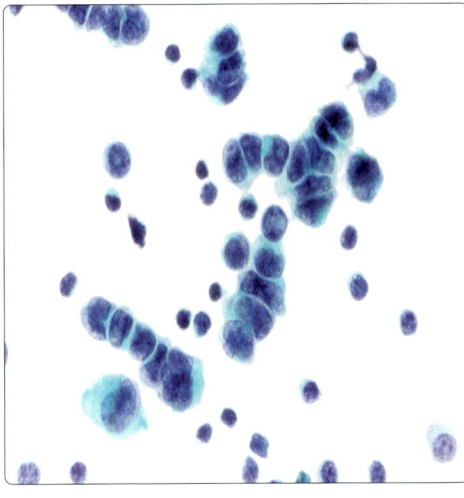

(Left) Pap stain of pleural fluid in metastatic squamous cell carcinoma is characterized by single tumor cells with dense cyanophilic to orangeophilic cytoplasm and hyperchromatic nucleus. Numerous anucleated necrotic tumor cells are present. (Right) Pap stain of a malignant pleural effusion shows small cell carcinoma of the lung with a high nuclear:cytoplasmic ratio, stippled chromatin, and nuclear molding. Chains of malignant cells are variably referred to as "caterpillars," "vertebral columns," or "stacks of coins."

Intestinal-Type Adenocarcinoma
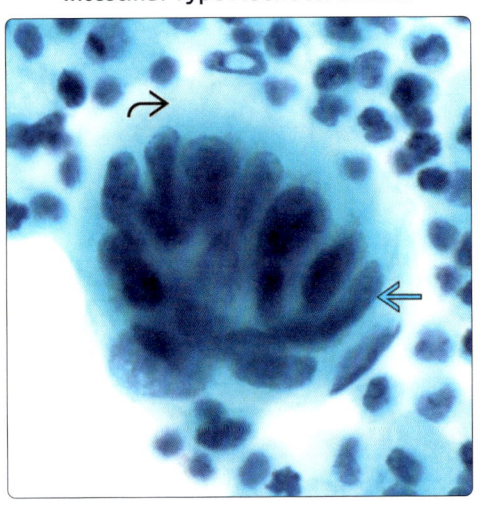

MOC-31 Membranous Staining
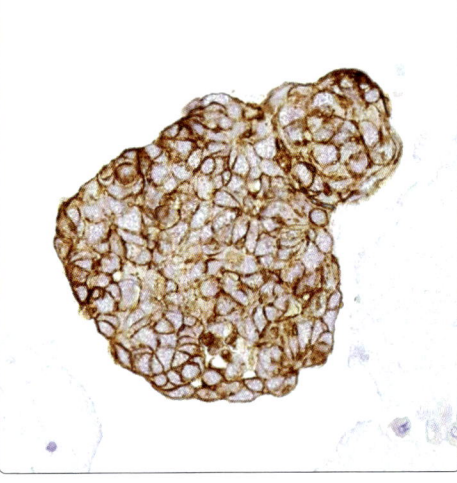

(Left) Morphology and immunocytochemistry of metastatic adenocarcinoma from gastrointestinal sites is often nonspecific, but in some instances, such as this Pap-stained metastatic colon carcinoma, intestinal differentiation can be suspected because of elongate nuclei ⇨ and abundant, apical cytoplasm ⇨. (Right) MOC-31, one of the most robust and versatile adenocarcinoma immunostains, has a distinctive membranous pattern. BER-EP4, another EpCam marker, also shows similar membranous staining.

Malignant Effusion, Sarcomas

KEY FACTS

CLASSIFICATION
- Malignant-secondary (MAL-S) in international system

CLINICAL ISSUES
- Most sarcomas of body cavity fluids are metastases
- Sarcomas account for small minority of malignant effusions
- Diagnosis is usually made in setting of known primary
- Primary serosal sarcomas include synovial sarcomas, vascular sarcomas, and malignant solitary fibrous tumor
- Leiomyosarcoma or well-differentiated liposarcoma may involve peritoneal fluids
- Pediatric small round blue cell tumors with tendency to be seen in fluids include desmoplastic small round cell tumor and rhabdomyosarcoma

CYTOPATHOLOGY
- Most cases exhibit scant cellularity
- Sarcoma cells usually exfoliate as single cells or loose clusters
- Often bloody &/or abundant proteinaceous debris
- Due to suspension in fluid, cells tend to "round up," obscuring morphology
- Morphology of tumor cells in fluids can differ from that of original tumor
- Cytomorphology is usually not sufficiently distinctive for specific diagnosis without ancillary studies, though in many cases, malignancy can be established

ANCILLARY TESTS
- Immunocytochemistry is often very helpful to differentiate from more common mimics
- Cytogenetics and other molecular tests may also be helpful to determine definitive diagnosis

TOP DIFFERENTIAL DIAGNOSES
- Melanoma
- Poorly differentiated carcinoma
- Malignant mesothelioma
- Lymphoma

Angiosarcoma
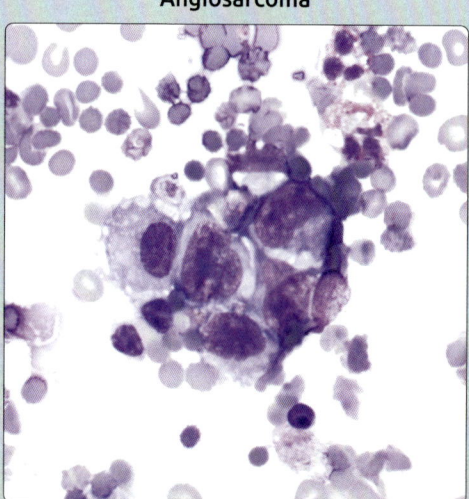

Undifferentiated Pleomorphic Sarcoma
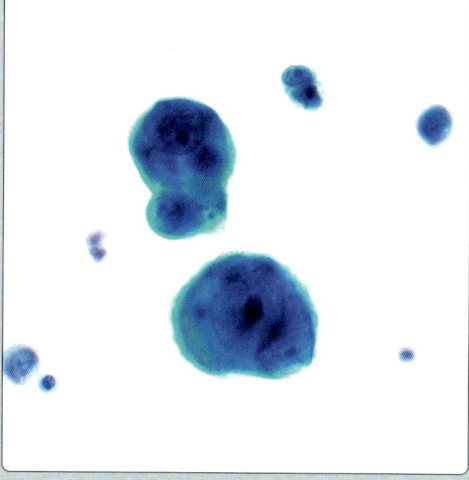

(Left) Many sarcomas have an epithelioid appearance in fluids, such as this Diff-Quik-stained pleural fluid showing malignant cells, consistent with history of metastatic angiosarcoma. Clinical correlation and ancillary tests are necessary for diagnosis. **(Right)** Pap stain of pleural fluid in a case of metastatic undifferentiated pleomorphic sarcoma shows markedly atypical, obviously malignant tumor cells, but features specific for sarcoma are not appreciated. (Courtesy J. Zhang, MD.)

Alveolar Rhabdomyosarcoma
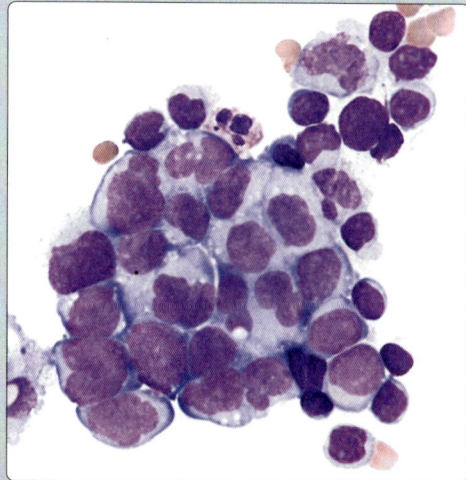

Desmoplastic Small Round Cell Tumor
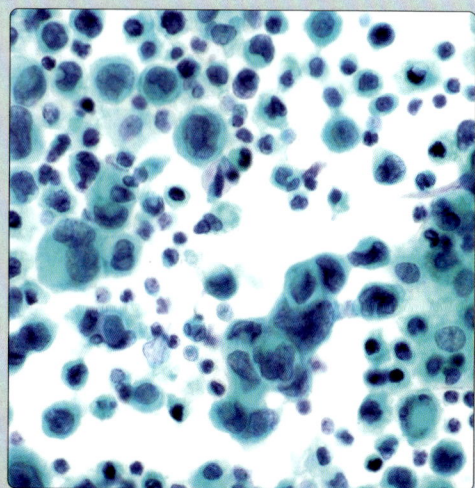

(Left) Diff-Quik-stained pleural fluid of alveolar rhabdomyosarcoma shows loose cohesive clusters of tumor cells. The differential diagnosis must include small round blue cell tumors, including acute lymphoblastic lymphoma. (Courtesy N. Quintanilla, MD.) **(Right)** Pap stain shows peritoneal fluid in a patient with desmoplastic small round cell tumor. Differential includes small round blue cell sarcomas, large cell lymphoma, melanoma, and poorly differentiated carcinomas.

Malignant Effusion, Sarcomas

CLINICAL ISSUES

Presentation
- Mesenchymal tumors of pleura, pericardium, and peritoneum are relatively rare
  - Vast majority are benign
- Primary sarcomas are exceedingly rare; most sarcomas are metastases
  - Synovial sarcomas, vascular sarcomas, and malignant solitary fibrous tumors may arise from pleura or other serosal surfaces
    - Present with pain and symptomatic effusions
    - Circumscribed mass or may grow diffusely over serosal surface, simulating diffuse malignant mesothelioma (DMM)
    - Hemorrhagic effusions
  - Leiomyosarcomas and well-differentiated liposarcomas may arise retroperitoneally and involve peritoneal fluids
  - Pediatric small round blue cell sarcomas, including desmoplastic small round cell tumor and rhabdomyosarcoma, may involve fluids
- Sarcomas account for small minority of malignant effusions, and diagnosis is usually made in setting of known primary

Prognosis
- Effusion is poor prognostic indicator for sarcomas, especially if malignant cells are identified

CYTOPATHOLOGY

Cellularity
- Most cases exhibit scant cellularity

Pattern
- Sarcoma cells exfoliate as single cells or loose clusters

Background
- Bloody &/or proteinaceous background

Cells
- Depending on type of sarcoma, cells can range from large and pleomorphic to small and uniform
  - Spindle cell morphology is rarely preserved in fluids

Nuclear Details
- In most cases, sarcomas in fluids have round to oval nuclei
- High-grade sarcomas may show more obvious pleomorphism and prominent nucleoli

Cytoplasmic Details
- Abundant and vacuolated in epithelioid sarcomas and liposarcoma
- Scant in pediatric small round blue cell sarcomas

Cytology-Histology Correlation
- Morphology of tumor cells in fluids can exhibit variety of morphologic features that differ from those of original tumor
  - Therefore, accuracy of diagnosis improves when correlated with clinical information and prior or concurrent surgical material
  - Sarcomas, such as epithelioid hemangioendothelioma (EHE), share morphologic features with more common tumors, such as adenocarcinoma and mesothelioma

DIFFERENTIAL DIAGNOSIS

Malignant Melanoma
- Melanomas, like sarcomas, often exfoliate as single cells with binucleation; however, melanoma cells have eccentric nuclei with prominent round nucleoli

Poorly Differentiated Carcinoma
- Can present as single cells but often have some clustering of malignant cells

Malignant Mesothelioma
- Correlation with clinical findings and immunocytochemical stains are usually necessary to differentiate sarcomatous mesothelioma from sarcomas

Lymphoma
- History is usually known or ancillary testing for diagnosis

SELECTED REFERENCES
1. Wang J et al: Cytologic presentation and clinicopathologic correlation of Mullerian carcinosarcoma on serous fluid samples. J Am Soc Cytopathol. 11(4):210-17, 2022

Characteristics of Sarcomas in Body Cavity Fluids

Sarcoma Type	Clinical Features	Cytomorphology
Angiosarcoma	May arise as primary tumor of serous linings	Marked nuclear atypia, epithelioid appearance
Epithelioid hemangioendothelioma	May arise as primary tumor of serous linings	Bland nuclei, epithelioid appearance
Synovial sarcoma	May arise as primary tumor of pleura	Oval cells with irregular nuclear contours
Malignant solitary fibrous tumor	Usually pleural primary	Oval cells with variable pleomorphism
Leiomyosarcoma	May have uterine or retroperitoneal primary	Large single cells with pleomorphic nuclei
Well-differentiated liposarcoma	May have retroperitoneal primary	Large single cells with vacuolated cytoplasm
Desmoplastic small round cell tumor	Child or young adult, pelvis or retroperitoneum	Small round blue cells, may aggregate
Embryonal rhabdomyosarcoma	Pediatric tumor, pelvis or retroperitoneum	Small round blue cells, may be elongate
Alveolar rhabdomyosarcoma	Pediatric tumor, usually metastatic	Small round blue cells with eccentric nuclei
Undifferentiated pleomorphic sarcoma	Metastatic disease, usually known history	Markedly atypical and pleomorphic nuclei

Lymphoid Effusions and Lymphomas

KEY FACTS

CLINICAL ISSUES

- Benign lymphoid effusions often have no obvious cause
  - Tuberculosis is frequent cause in developing countries
  - Lymphoid-rich reactive effusions contain mainly small mature T lymphocytes
- 10-15% of malignant effusions are caused by lymphomas
  - More common in pleural effusions
- Exact classification of lymphomas in fluids is based on flow cytometry, immunocytochemistry, and correlation of previous biopsy
  - Some degree of cytologic subclassification can be achieved based on cell size and nuclear features

CYTOPATHOLOGY

- Low-grade B-cell lymphomas show monomorphic population of small lymphocytes not readily distinguishable from reactive T cells
- Diffuse large B-cell lymphoma: Large immunoblasts or centroblasts
- Lymphoblastic lymphoma: Small- to medium-sized cells with smooth or irregular nuclear membrane, fine chromatin, scant cytoplasm, and inconspicuous nucleoli
- Burkitt lymphoma: Small- to medium-sized cells with noncleaved nuclei, prominent nucleoli, and scant to moderate vacuolated cytoplasm
- Hodgkin disease effusions: Reed-Sternberg cells or mononuclear variants, often with mixed inflammatory background

TOP DIFFERENTIAL DIAGNOSES

- Benign lymphocytic effusions overlap morphologically with chronic lymphocytic leukemia and other low-grade lymphomas
  - Clinical history/suspicion is key; flow cytometry can help to rule out lymphoma when there is high index of suspicion
- Small round blue cell tumors, melanoma, and some dyscohesive carcinomas are in differential for large cell lymphomas

Diffuse Large B-Cell Lymphoma
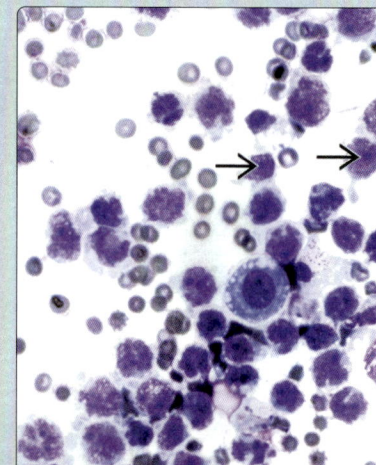

Chronic Lymphocytic Leukemia/Lymphoma
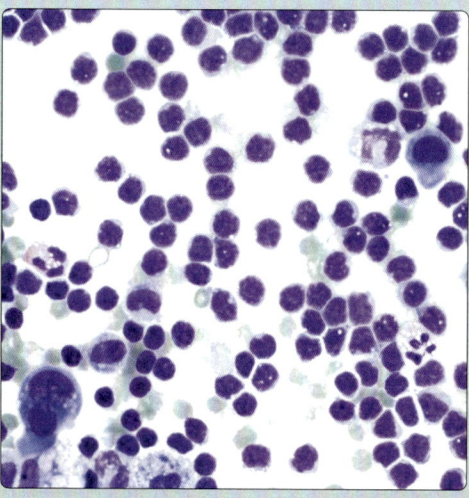

(Left) Diff-Quik stain of a pleural effusion with diffuse large B-cell lymphoma shows large malignant cells with round nuclei, clumpy chromatin, and prominent nucleoli ➡. (Right) Diff-Quik shows pleural fluid with chronic lymphocytic leukemia characterized by a uniform population of small mature lymphocytes with scant cytoplasm and clumped chromatin. Differential diagnosis includes benign lymphocyte-rich effusions.

Burkitt Lymphoma
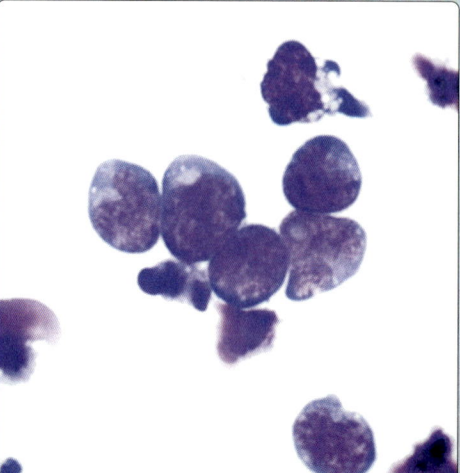

T-Lymphoblastic Leukemia/Lymphoma
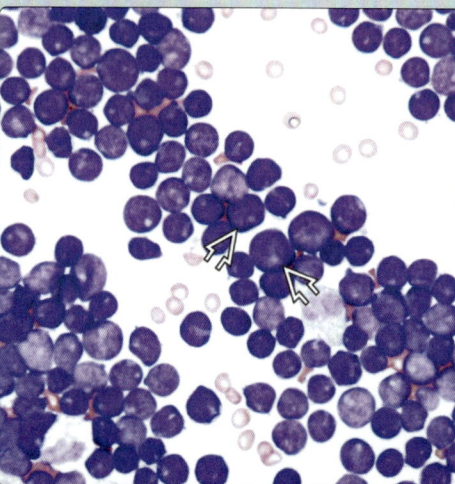

(Left) Diff-Quik stain shows ascites in Burkitt lymphoma characterized by medium-sized cells with cytoplasmic vacuolization, clumped chromatin, and nucleoli. (Right) Diff-Quik-stained cytospin of pleural effusion in a case of T-lymphoblastic leukemia/lymphoma demonstrates cells with high nuclear:cytoplasmic ratio, fine chromatin, and scant dark cytoplasm ➡.

Lymphoid Effusions and Lymphomas

CLINICAL ISSUES

Presentation
- Benign lymphoid-rich effusions can be seen in patients with tuberculosis, status post coronary artery bypass, or in situations with no obvious underlying cause
  - Tuberculosis is most common cause of pleural effusion in developing countries
  - Lymphoid-rich effusions contain small, mature T lymphocytes
- In adult patients, 10-15% of all malignant effusions are caused by lymphomas
  - Most represent secondary involvement of serosal surfaces as part of disseminated disease
- Hodgkin disease (HD) effusions are caused by spread from mediastinal lymphadenopathy or thoracic duct obstruction
- Non-Hodgkin lymphoma (NHL) effusions are usually caused by direct pleural/pulmonary involvement
- Patients with NHL pleural effusions present with shortness of breath, mediastinal tumors, lymphadenopathy, and extranodal solid tumors
- Exact classification of lymphomas in fluids is based on flow cytometry, immunocytochemistry, and correlation of previous biopsy
  - Some degree of cytologic subclassification can be achieved based on cell size and nuclear features
- Leukemic effusions are more common in pediatric population

Prognosis
- Effusions due to lymphomas reduce overall survival and predict disease relapse after chemotherapy

CYTOPATHOLOGY

Cellularity
- Highly cellular cytologic preparations

Pattern
- Dyscohesive lymphoid cells with background of scant reactive mesothelial cells

Background
- Karyorrhectic debris is usually present in lymphomas but is rarely seen in benign lymphocytic effusions

Cells
- Chronic lymphocytic leukemia/small lymphocytic leukemia (CLL/SLL): Monomorphic population of small lymphocytes not readily distinguishable from reactive lymphoid cells
  - Low-grade lymphomas in general are difficult to separate from benign T cells by morphology alone
  - Flow cytometry has low yield in patients with many small lymphocytes but no clinical suspicion or history of lymphoma
- Diffuse large B-cell lymphoma: Large immunoblasts or centroblasts with variable amounts of cytoplasm
- Lymphoblastic lymphoma: Small- to medium-sized cells with smooth or irregular nuclear membrane, fine chromatin, scant cytoplasm, and inconspicuous nucleoli
- Burkitt lymphoma: Small- to medium-sized cells with noncleaved nuclei, prominent nucleoli, and scant to moderate vacuolated cytoplasm
- HD effusions: Reed-Sternberg cells or mononuclear variants, often with mixed inflammatory background

DIFFERENTIAL DIAGNOSIS

Benign Lymphocytic Effusion
- CLL/SLL and other low-grade NHL may look similar

Small Round Blue Cell Tumors
- Pediatric sarcomas may resemble NHL

Melanoma, Small Cell Carcinoma, and Poorly Differentiated Carcinomas
- Can shed in noncohesive pattern resembling lymphomas

SELECTED REFERENCES

1. Li J et al: Serous effusions diagnostic accuracy for hematopoietic malignancies: a cyto-histological correlation. Front Med (Lausanne). 7:615080, 2020
2. Patel T et al: The value of cytology in diagnosis of serous effusions in malignant lymphomas: An experience of a tertiary care center. Diagn Cytopathol. 47(8):776-82, 2019

High-Grade B-Cell Lymphoma

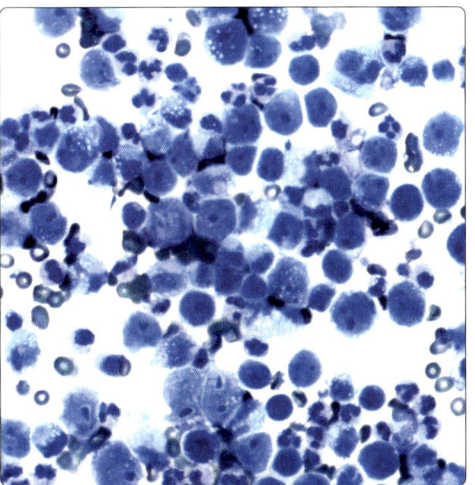

ThinPrep of Diffuse Large B-Cell Lymphoma

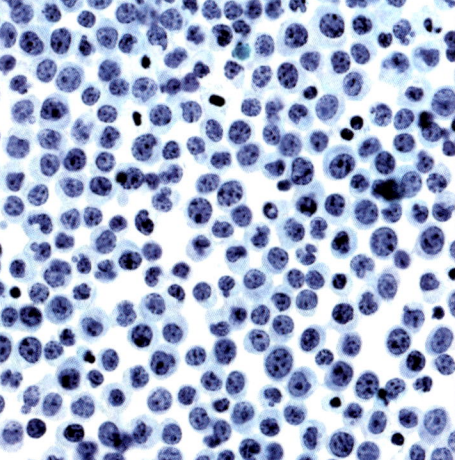

(Left) Diff-Quik stain shows the marked nuclear pleomorphism characteristic of large cell lymphomas seen in body cavity fluids, such as this double-hit lymphoma with rearrangements of MYC and BCL2. (Right) Although the Diff-Quik stain more closely resembles the Wright stain used in hematopathology, facilitating diagnosis in many cases, the Pap stain, such as in this ThinPrep, offers superior nuclear detail, here highlighting the marked chromatin clumping in an example of diffuse large B-cell lymphoma.

Primary Effusion Lymphoma

KEY FACTS

CLINICAL ISSUES
- Presentation as lymphomatous growth in pleural, peritoneal, &/or pericardial effusions
- Usually no obvious mass lesions
- Poor prognosis
- Associated with HIV or other immune deficiency; 4% of all HIV-related lymphomas

CYTOPATHOLOGY
- Variable, ranging from immunoblastic to anaplastic to plasmablastic
- Medium- to large-sized atypical cells, many with irregular nuclear contours, prominent nucleoli, and abundant cytoplasm (± vacuolated)

ANCILLARY TESTS
- HHV-8(+) is essential for diagnosis
- Plasma cell-associated markers (+)
- Cytoplasmic Ig λ-light chain (+/-)
- CD30(+), CD45/LCA(+/-)
- EBER(+) in ~ 80% of cases
- Pan-B-cell markers (-)

TOP DIFFERENTIAL DIAGNOSES
- Large B-cell lymphoma
- Plasmablastic lymphoma/myeloma
- Burkitt lymphoma
- HHV-8-unrelated primary effusion lymphoma (PEL)-like lymphoma
- Melanoma; poorly differentiated carcinoma

DIAGNOSTIC CHECKLIST
- Diagnosis is usually based on cytologic examination of body fluids
- Many lymphomas, mostly aggressive types, can present with neoplastic serous effusion
- PEL is associated with immunodeficiency and has evidence of HHV-8 infection

Large Atypical Lymphocytes

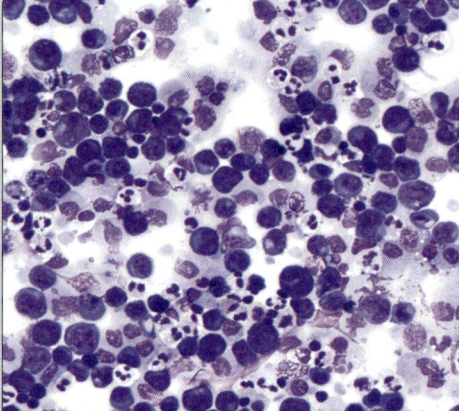

Irregular Nuclei

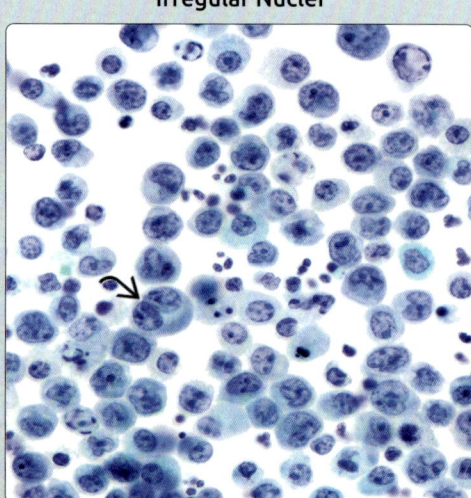

(Left) Diff-Quik-stained slide of pleural fluid shows a dispersed population of large atypical cells admixed with neutrophils. **(Right)** Pap-stained slides show neoplastic cells, occasionally binucleated ➡, with irregular nuclei, prominent nucleoli, and moderately abundant cytoplasm.

Mitosis and Apoptosis

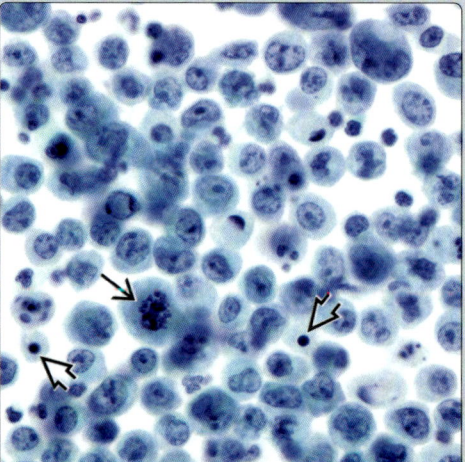

Vacuolated Cytoplasm

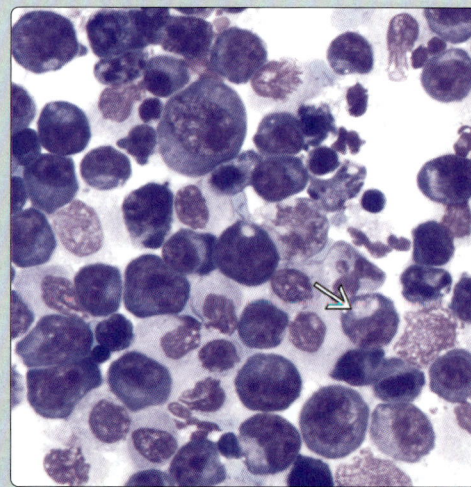

(Left) Pap-stained slides show neoplastic cells with marked nuclear contour irregularities and clumpy chromatin. Note the mitotic figure ➡ and apoptotic bodies ➡ in the background. **(Right)** Diff-Quik-stained slide demonstrates basophilic cytoplasm with occasional vacuoles ➡ or perinuclear hofs.

Primary Effusion Lymphoma

TERMINOLOGY

Definitions
- Primary effusion lymphoma (PEL) is human herpesvirus 8 (HHV-8)-associated large B-cell neoplasm most often involving pleural, peritoneal, or pericardial cavities
  - Rare PEL-like lymphomas not associated with HHV-8 have been reported
- HHV-8(+) lymphomas indistinguishable from PEL rarely present as solid tumor mass
  - These tumors are designated as extracavitary or solid variants of PEL

CLINICAL ISSUES

Presentation
- Usually no distinct extracavitary tumor masses &/or organomegaly
- Symptoms commonly result from massive malignant effusion
- Systemic dissemination can occur during course of disease
- Associated with HIV infection or other severe, acquired immunodeficiencies

CYTOPATHOLOGY

Cells
- Cytomorphologic appearances ranging from immunoblastic to anaplastic and exhibiting frequent plasmablastic differentiation
- Medium- to large-sized atypical cells, many with irregular nuclear contours, prominent nucleoli, and abundant cytoplasm (± vacuolated)

ANCILLARY TESTS

Immunohistochemistry
- HHV-8(+) is essential for diagnosis
- Plasma cell-associated markers (+)
- Cytoplasmic Ig λ-light chain (+/-)
- CD30(+), CD45/LCA(+/-)

Flow Cytometry
- CD45/LCA(+), CD19(-), CD20(-), CD22(-), CD10(-), FMC-7(-)
- Surface Ig light-chain expression is rare
- Aberrant T-cell markers are positive in subset of cases

In Situ Hybridization
- EBER(+) in ~ 80% of cases

Genetic Testing
- Monoclonal *IGH* gene rearrangements
- Monoclonal T-cell receptor rearrangements in subset
- Usually complex karyotype

DIFFERENTIAL DIAGNOSIS

Large B-Cell Lymphoma
- HHV-8(-), pan-B-cell markers (+)

Plasmablastic Lymphoma
- Associated with HIV(+) and EBV(+), HHV-8(-)

Plasmablastic Plasma Cell Myeloma
- Presence of atypical but more mature plasma cells, EBER(-)

Burkitt Lymphoma
- *MYC*-associated translocations in almost all cases

Primary Effusion Lymphoma-Like Lymphoma
- HHV-8(-), usually HIV(-), usually pan-B-cell antigen (+)

Melanoma
- S100(+), HMB-45(+), Melan-A (+)

Poorly Differentiated Carcinoma
- Cytokeratin (+), CD38(-), IRF-4/MUM1(-)

SELECTED REFERENCES
1. Hu Z et al: Primary effusion lymphoma: a clinicopathological study of 70 cases. Cancers (Basel). 13(4), 2021
2. Rossi G et al: Human herpesvirus-8-positive primary effusion lymphoma in HIV-negative patients: single institution case series with a multidisciplinary characterization. Cancer Cytopathol. 129(1):62-74, 2021
3. Shimada K et al: Biology and management of primary effusion lymphoma. Blood. 132(18):1879-88, 2018

Marked Nuclear Pleomorphism
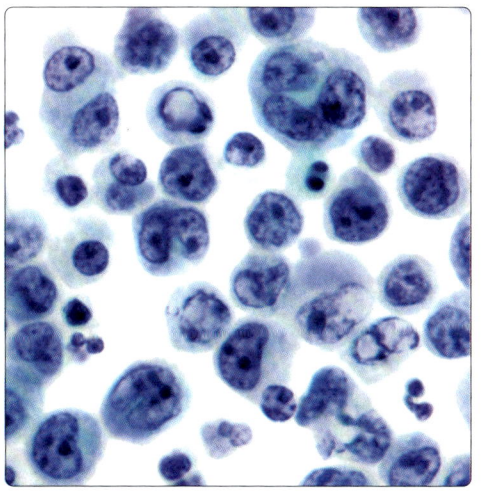

HHV-8 Immunostain
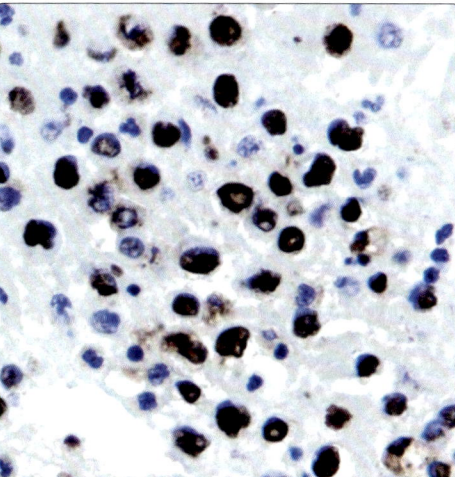

(Left) Primary effusion lymphoma shows neoplastic cells with pleomorphic nuclei often containing prominent nucleoli. Binucleated and multinucleated tumor cells are also present. *(Right)* Immunostaining performed on a cell block section shows that the tumor cells are positive for human herpesvirus 8 (HHV-8), the causative virus.

Endometriosis and Endosalpingiosis

KEY FACTS

CLINICAL ISSUES
- Can be identified in pelvic washes performed at time of gynecologic surgery
- Endometriosis is most often seen in peritoneal cavity and is rare in thoracic cavity
- Necessary to recognize features, as they can be source of false-positive diagnosis
- Procedures with intrauterine mechanical manipulation can dislodge benign or malignant müllerian epithelium into pelvic cavity

CYTOPATHOLOGY
- Endometriosis
  - Glandular cells surrounding stromal cells
  - Epithelial cells are often vacuolated and have small, oval to round, bland, uniform nuclei with small nucleoli
  - Stromal cells have spindled nuclei and often show degenerative changes
  - Hemosiderophages ± bloody background may be seen
- Endosalpingiosis
  - Papillary/tubular structures with cuboidal/low columnar cells
  - Glandular cells have scant basophilic cytoplasm ± cilia and have eccentric oval nuclei with fine chromatin and small nucleoli
  - Psammoma bodies can be seen

TOP DIFFERENTIAL DIAGNOSES
- Reactive mesothelial cells/mesothelioma
  - Immunocytochemistry is helpful; PAX8 for müllerian origin vs. D2-40 and calretinin for mesothelial cells
- Endometrioid adenocarcinoma
  - Greater atypia
  - Correlation with surgical pathology material is key
- Borderline and low-grade serous epithelial neoplasms
  - Usually more atypia in neoplasms
  - May be impossible to confidently differentiate endometriosis or endosalpingiosis in some cases

Endometriosis With Glands and Stroma
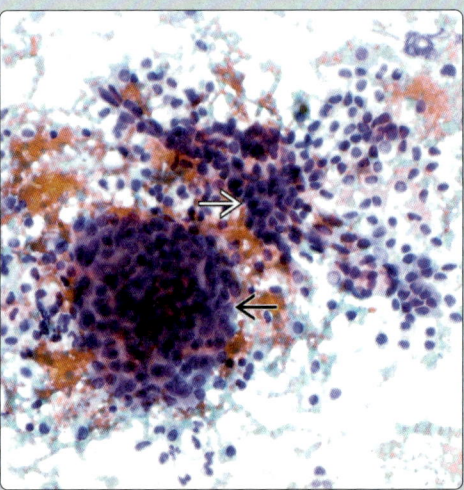

Endometriosis in ThinPrep
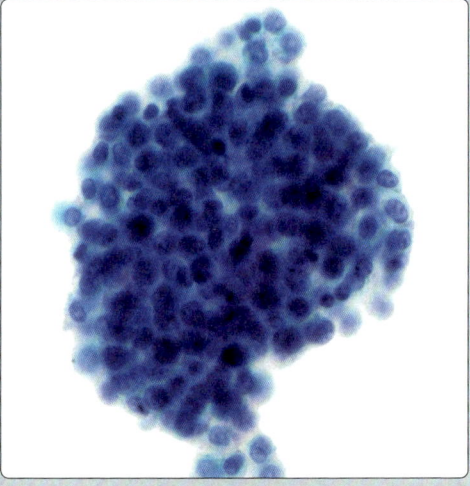

(Left) Pap-stained smear of a pelvic wash in a patient with ovarian endometriosis shows groups of bland-appearing glandular cells ➡ and spindled stromal cells ➡ in a bloody background. (Right) This example of endometriosis identified in a ThinPrep prepared from pelvic washings shows the similarity of the cell groups to the endometrial cells seen in cervicovaginal Pap tests.

Endosalpingiosis With Cilia
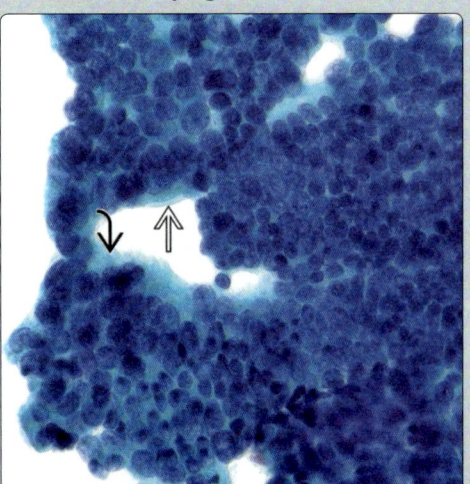

Endosalpingiosis With Atypia
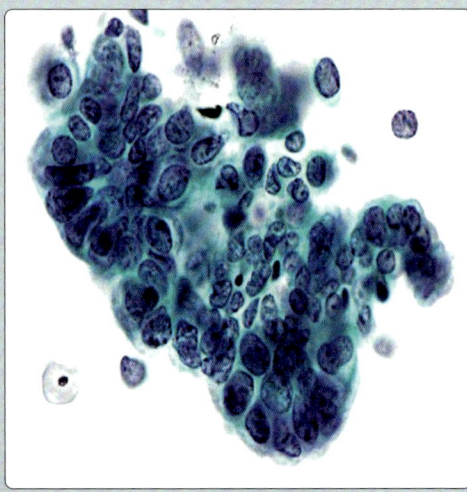

(Left) ThinPrep of a pelvic washing shows a large aggregate of tubal-type cells with complex architecture. There is anisonucleosis and dark chromatin present, but the abundant apical cytoplasm ➡ and cilia ➡ help to confirm a benign diagnosis. (Right) Pap stain of pelvic wash in a patient with ovarian cystadenofibroma and endosalpingiosis shows presence of mild nuclear atypia and overlap, which can mimic a low-grade serous neoplasm.

Endometriosis and Endosalpingiosis

CLINICAL ISSUES

Epidemiology
- Age
  - Predominantly seen in women of reproductive age

Presentation
- Can be identified in pelvic washes (PW) performed at time of gynecologic surgery
  - Necessary to recognize features, as they can be source of false-positive diagnosis
  - Procedures with intrauterine mechanical manipulation can dislodge benign or malignant müllerian epithelium into pelvic cavity
    - These contaminants may include benign tubal epithelium, benign endometrium, or endometrial carcinoma
- Pelvic endometriosis causes dysmenorrhea, pain, and infertility
- Pleural cavity endometriosis causes cough, shortness of breath, pleuritic pain, and hemorrhage

CYTOPATHOLOGY

Cellularity
- Low to moderate cellularity

Pattern
- Endometriosis: Small cohesive clusters of glandular/stromal cells
- Endosalpingiosis: Papillary/tubular structures often with psammoma bodies

Background
- Endometriosis: Hemosiderophages (seen in ~ 1/3 of patients), reactive mesothelial cells, ± bloody background

Cells
- Endometriosis: Clusters of round glandular cells and spindled stromal cells, often with degenerative changes
- Endosalpingiosis: Papillary/tubular structures with cuboidal to low columnar cells arranged in orderly fashion

Nuclear Details
- Endometriosis: Glandular cells have oval to round monotonous nuclei with small nucleoli
  - Stromal cells have spindle-shaped nuclei with degenerative changes
- Endosalpingiosis: Eccentric oval nuclei with fine chromatin and small nucleoli

Cytoplasmic Details
- Endometriosis: Cytoplasm of glandular cells is often vacuolated
  - Stromal cells have scant indistinct cytoplasm
- Endosalpingiosis: Scant basophilic cytoplasm ± cilia

Cell Block Findings
- Endometriosis: Fragments containing endometrial glands/stroma and hemosiderophages
- Endosalpingiosis: Small papillary or tubular structures of columnar/cuboidal cells are often ciliated
- Nonneoplastic müllerian epithelia, such as endometriosis and endosalpingiosis, express PAX8 on immunohistochemical stain

Cytology-Histology Correlation
- It is necessary to correlate with corresponding surgical specimens
  - However, in many cases, surgical specimens have no apparent endometriosis/endosalpingiosis of peritoneal surface

DIFFERENTIAL DIAGNOSIS

Reactive Mesothelial Cells
- Reactive mesothelial cells can mimic endosalpingiosis or endometriosis with reactive changes
- Immunohistochemical panels that include mesothelial and epithelial markers can be helpful
  - PAX8 immunohistochemical stain is highly sensitive/specific marker for müllerian epithelium

Endometrioid Adenocarcinoma
- Sheds as cohesive clusters or single cells with more cytologic atypia
  - Necessary to correlate with corresponding surgical specimen

Borderline and Low-Grade Serous Neoplasms
- Serous borderline neoplasms have complex papillary fragments, small uniform cells with high nuclear:cytoplasmic ratio, and inconspicuous nucleoli
  - Positive PW in cases of serous borderline neoplasms can represent shedding from primary ovarian tumor or be indicative of peritoneal implants
- Low-grade serous carcinomas have papillae or clusters of glandular cells, often with more atypia and few mitosis
- However, endometriosis and endosalpingiosis may exhibit atypical/reactive changes that are indistinguishable from borderline or low-grade serous neoplasms

Mesothelioma and Mesothelial Hyperplasia
- Mesotheliomas shed as highly cellular clusters with variable degree of cytologic atypia
- Immunohistochemical studies will lead to correct interpretation

DIAGNOSTIC CHECKLIST

Pathologic Interpretation Pearls
- In hypercellular specimens &/or in cases with atypical reactive features, correlation with surgical specimen is needed to ensure adequate diagnosis
- It is also necessary to take into account type of intraoperative surgical techniques at time of collection
  - Intrauterine mechanical manipulation during laparoscopy may be source of dislodged/displaced müllerian epithelium in PW

SELECTED REFERENCES

1. Chan-Tiopianco M et al: Clinical presentation and management of endometriosis-related hemorrhagic ascites: a case report and systematic review of the literature. Cureus. 13(6):e15828, 2021
2. Wang P et al: Endometriosis-related pleural effusion: a case report and a PRISMA-compliant systematic review. Front Med (Lausanne). 8:631048, 2021

Ovarian Neoplasms

KEY FACTS

CLINICAL ISSUES
- Cytologic examination of ascitic fluid or pelvic washings is part of staging of ovarian carcinomas
  - Most patients present with advanced disease and malignant ascites
- Most common cause of malignant peritoneal effusions in women, comprising 30-35% of positive effusions

CYTOPATHOLOGY
- Moderate to highly cellular effusions
- Cohesive clusters, some of which have papillary architecture, &/or single malignant cells
- High-grade serous carcinomas have pleomorphic, large, irregular nuclei with prominent nucleoli
- Low-grade serous carcinomas have more uniform cells with slight nuclear enlargement and relatively uniform nucleoli
- Large cytoplasmic vacuoles are seen in most serous, clear cell, and mucinous neoplasms
- Psammoma bodies may be present in cases of serous neoplasms but are not diagnostic
- Other ovarian tumors, such as germ cell or sex cord-stromal tumors, rarely cause malignant effusions

TOP DIFFERENTIAL DIAGNOSES
- High-grade serous vs. low-grade serous carcinoma
  - Staining pattern with p53 and p16 may aid in distinction
  - Important because high grade receives neoadjuvant therapy with interval debulking to decrease morbidity whereas low grade goes directly to debulking
- Borderline and low-grade serous carcinomas vs. reactive mesothelial hyperplasia
  - Correlation with clinical history and surgical pathology usually resolves issue
- High-grade ovarian carcinomas vs. other nongynecologic metastatic carcinomas
  - PAX8 is highly sensitive and specific marker of müllerian neoplasms

High-Grade Serous Carcinoma
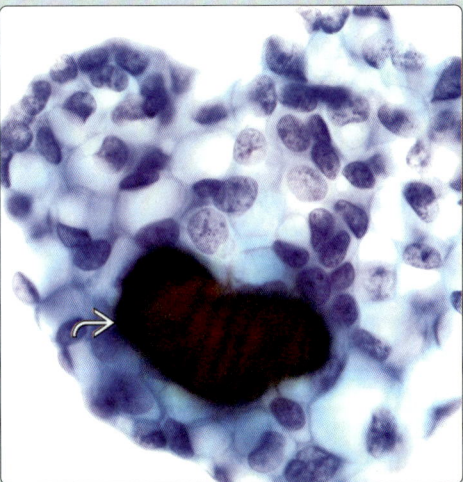

Low-Grade Serous Carcinoma
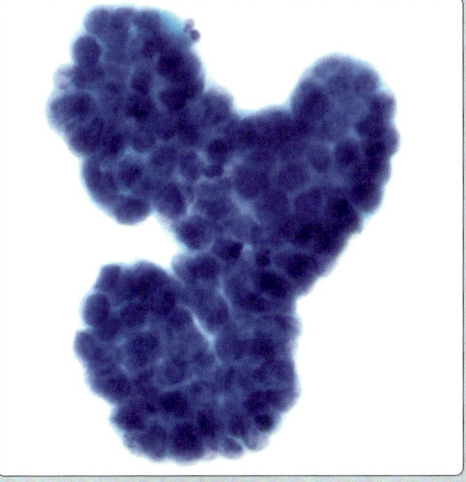

(Left) Pap stain of ascites with high-grade serous carcinoma, characterized by large pleomorphic tumor cells with clear vacuolated cytoplasm, shows a psammoma body ➢. **(Right)** Pap stain of pelvic wash of a low-grade serous carcinoma shows neoplastic cells that form tight papillary clusters with slight nuclear atypia. Borderline serous neoplasms can show similar cytologic features.

Papillary Clusters in Serous Carcinoma
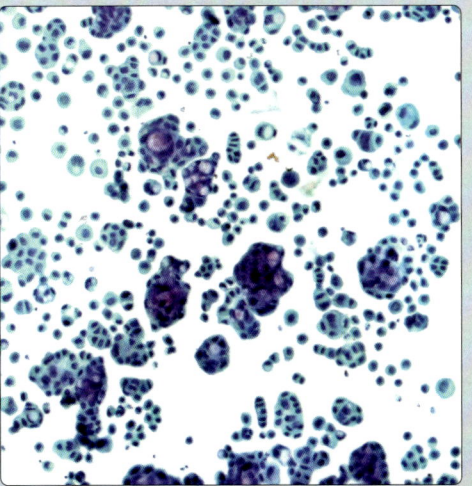

Clear Cell Carcinoma
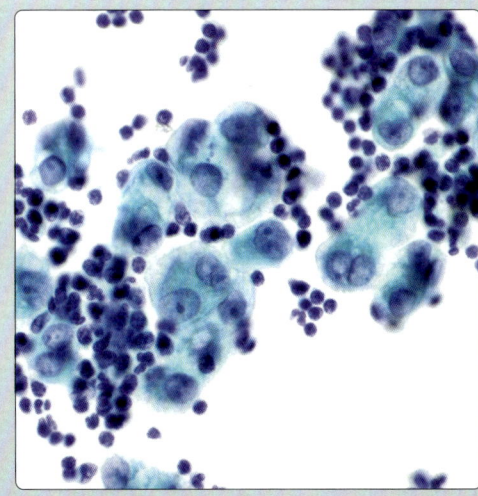

(Left) On low-power examination of peritoneal fluids, knobby clusters of cells corresponding to papillae are striking in many cases of both low- and high-grade papillary carcinoma, as exemplified by this Pap-stained high-grade serous carcinoma with serosal involvement. **(Right)** Pap stain of ascites in a case of clear cell carcinoma shows tumor cells with irregular nuclei, vesicular chromatin, prominent nucleoli, and vacuolated cytoplasm.

Ovarian Neoplasms

CLINICAL ISSUES

Epidemiology
- Most common cause of malignant peritoneal effusions in women, comprising 30-35% of positive effusions

Prognosis
- Cytologic examination of ascitic fluid or pelvic washings is part of ovarian surface carcinoma staging
  - Positive peritoneal cytology is seen in many cases due to advanced stage/surface involvement at presentation

CYTOPATHOLOGY

Cellularity
- Moderate to highly cellular effusions

Pattern
- Cohesive clusters, some of which have papillary architecture, &/or single malignant cells

Background
- Psammoma bodies may be present in cases of serous neoplasms but are not diagnostic
- Mucinous background can be present in cases of mucinous carcinoma involving peritoneum

Nuclear Details
- High-grade serous carcinomas have pleomorphic, large, irregular nuclei with prominent nucleoli
- Low-grade serous carcinomas have more uniform cells with slight nuclear enlargement and relatively uniform nucleoli

Cytoplasmic Details
- Large cytoplasmic vacuoles are seen in most serous, clear cell, and mucinous neoplasms

Cytology-Histology Correlation
- Low-grade serous carcinomas and serous borderline tumors have implants composed of papillae lined by cells with minimal cytologic atypia and occasional mitosis
  - Cytology specimens can contain small clusters or papillae with similar low-grade cytologic features
- High-grade serous carcinomas have complex papillae with cellular stratification, marked atypia, and mitosis
  - Cytology specimens contain clusters and single highly pleomorphic tumor cells
- Endosalpingiosis usually exhibit fewer tubular or small branching papillary structures, ± psammoma bodies
- Most cases of pseudomyxoma peritonei are associated with primary appendiceal mucinous tumors
  - Rarely associated with ovarian mucinous tumors
- Other ovarian tumors, such as germ cell or sex cord-stromal tumors, rarely cause malignant effusions

DIFFERENTIAL DIAGNOSIS

High-Grade Serous Carcinoma vs. Low-Grade Serous Carcinoma
- High-grade serous carcinomas often display significant nuclear atypia; low-grade serous neoplasms contain small clusters and papillae with mild to moderate atypia; psammoma bodies are frequently present
- In high-grade serous carcinoma, most common p53 staining pattern is diffuse strong staining (overexpression) or null type (complete absence); low-grade serous carcinomas generally show wild-type immunoreactivity
- Strong diffuse p16 expression is seen in cases of high-grade serous carcinoma; low-grade serous neoplasms have variable patchy staining

Reactive Mesothelial Hyperplasia and Mesothelioma
- Have cytologic features similar to those of borderline serous neoplasms and low-grade serous carcinomas

Other Nongynecologic Metastatic Carcinomas
- Clinical correlation is essential to select appropriate immunostains to determine site of origin
  - PAX8 is highly sensitive and specific müllerian marker

SELECTED REFERENCES
1. Ren S et al: Gynecologic serous carcinoma: an immunohistochemical analysis of malignant body fluid specimens. Arch Pathol Lab Med. 143(6):677-82, 2019

Mucinous Carcinoma

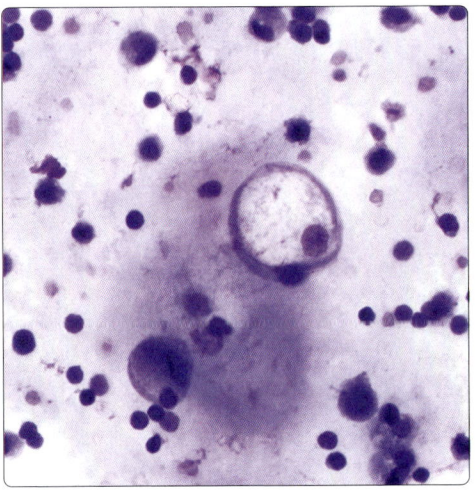

Granulosa Cell Tumor

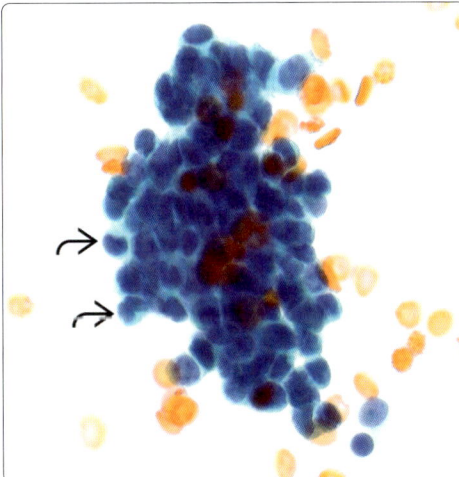

(Left) Diff-Quik stain of ascites in a case of mucinous carcinoma reveals abundant background mucin and few relatively bland tumor cells. (Right) This washing from a granulosa cell tumor with peritoneal spread shows cohesive clusters of high nucleus:cytoplasmic ratio cells. On Pap stain, the characteristic nuclear contour irregularities ⊵ can be clearly seen.

Immunocytochemistry, Histochemistry, and Other Ancillary Techniques

TERMINOLOGY

Abbreviations
- Immunocytochemistry (ICC)
- Immunohistochemistry (IHC)
- In situ hybridization (ISH)
- Polymerase chain reaction (PCR)
- Flow cytometry (FC)

USE OF ANCILLARY STUDIES IN BODY FLUID SPECIMENS

Cell Block Preparations
- If malignancy suspected, histochemical, ICC, and other ancillary techniques can be performed on cell blocks to increase diagnostic accuracy
- Histochemical stains and ICC can be done on cell blocks because multiple duplicate slides can be obtained
  - Other tests that can be performed on cell block include ISH and PCR
  - In addition, cell blocks show architectural features of tissue fragments, which can be compared with histopathologic sections
- Sensitivity increases to 83-85% when ≥ 2 preparation methods utilized (e.g., cytocentrifuge and cell block)
- Traditionally, cell blocks prepared from cell pellet using plasma thrombin clot or HistoGel method
- ICC and molecular testing can also be performed utilizing Cellient cell blocks
  - Alcohol fixation in Cellient requires specific validation

INDICATIONS FOR HISTOCHEMICAL STAINS IN BODY FLUIDS

Reactive Mesothelial Cells/Mesotheliomas From Adenocarcinoma
- Reactive mesothelial cells can have significant cytologic atypia and thus mimic carcinomas
  - Atypical features with intracytoplasmic vacuoles
  - Simulate signet-ring adenocarcinoma
- Malignant mesotheliomas can present as 3D clusters and papillary groups that simulate carcinomas
- Histochemical stains that aid in DDx include mucicarmine stain and PAS with diastase

Detection of Infectious Organisms
- Gomori methenamine silver, mucicarmine, Kinyoun and Fite acid-fast stains are some histochemical stains that can be used to detect fungal or mycobacterial organisms
- ICC stains and molecular testing can be utilized to detect viral organisms

INDICATIONS FOR IHC STAINS IN BODY FLUIDS

Reactive Mesothelial Cells/Mesotheliomas From Adenocarcinoma
- Highly cellular specimens with atypical cytologic features can mimic adenocarcinoma
  - If malignancy suspected, cell block prepared to perform panel of ICC stains
    - ICC most widely used ancillary method and has been shown to increase overall diagnostic accuracy
  - Necessary to correlate cytomorphology with clinical history and radiologic findings to select most appropriate ICC stains
  - Recommended to include 2 mesothelial and 2 carcinoma markers in panel
  - Some ICC expressed in both mesothelial and epithelial cells
    - CK7, AE1/AE3, and EMA expressed in both benign or malignant mesothelial cells and lung adenocarcinomas
    - AE1/AE3, CK5/6, and EMA positive in both mesothelioma/reactive mesothelial cells and squamous cell carcinomas of lung
    - WT1 and mesothelin expressed in peritoneal mesothelial cells and serous neoplasms of ovary
    - These overlaps in expression limit utility of these common markers in body fluids

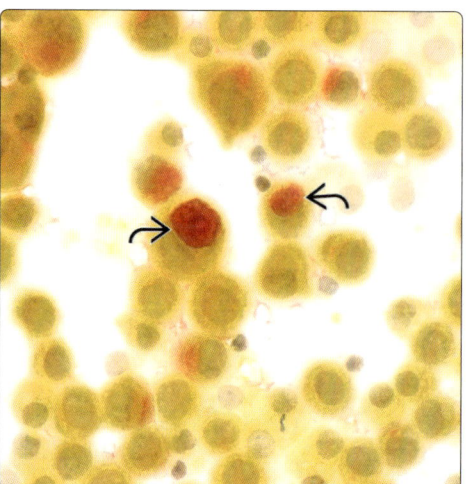

Mucicarmine-Positive Breast Carcinoma

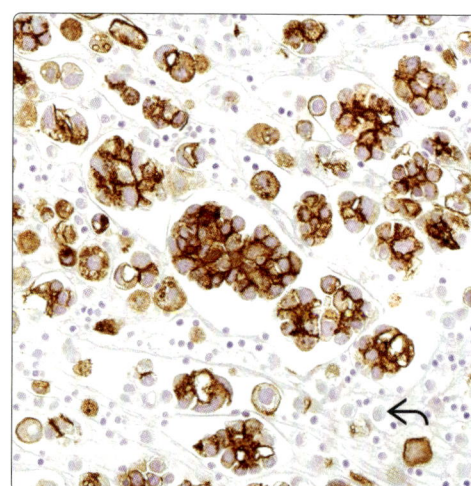

MOC-31 Positive Breast Carcinoma

(Left) Mucicarmine stain highlights the mucin vacuoles ➠ in a lobular breast carcinoma with signet-ring morphology. (Right) MOC-31 stained cell block shows malignant pleural effusion in a patient with metastatic breast carcinoma. Background mesothelial cells ➠ and inflammatory cells are negative.

Immunocytochemistry, Histochemistry, and Other Ancillary Techniques

Differential Stains for Mesotheliomas and Adenocarcinomas

Stain	Adenocarcinoma	Mesothelioma/Reactive Mesothelial Cells
PAS with diastase	(+) highlights neutral mucin	(-)
Alcian blue/hyaluronidase	(+) highlights neutral mucin	(-)
Mucicarmine	(+) highlights neutral mucin	(+/-) weak focal staining

ICC Staining Patterns for Benign or Malignant Mesothelial Cells vs. Adenocarcinoma

ICC Stain	Adenocarcinoma	Mesothelioma/Reactive Mesothelium
Claudin-4	(+) membranous	(-)
MOC-31	(+) membranous	(-)
BER-EP4	(+) membranous	(-)
mCEA	(+) cytoplasmic	(-)
LEU-M1	(+) cytoplasmic	(-)
B72.3	(+) cytoplasmic	(-)
Calretinin	(-)	(+) nuclear and cytoplasmic
D2-40	(-)	(+) membranous
HBME-1	(-)	(+) membranous
HEG1	(-) (+ in serous carcinoma of ovary)	(+) membranous (-/+ in reactive mesothelium)
WT1	(-) (+ in serous carcinoma of ovary)	(+) nuclear
Mesothelin	(-) (+ in serous carcinoma of ovary)	(+) membranous

ICC = immunocytochemistry.

Determine Primary Site of Malignancy

- ICC stains helpful in determining possible primary site, especially in patients with occult primary and patients with history of multiple primary malignancies
- Consider cytomorphology, site of effusion, sex, and clinical history in order to perform most specific markers
- General adenocarcinoma markers coupled with more specific markers often helpful
  ○ Adenocarcinomas of lung: TTF-1, Napsin-A
  ○ Squamous cell carcinomas: p40, p63, p16 in HPV-driven squamous cell carcinomas of anogenital or oropharyngeal origin
    – MOC-31, BER-EP4, and mCEA often positive in squamous cell carcinomas as well as adenocarcinomas
  ○ Small cell carcinomas: CD56, TTF-1, synaptophysin
    – Napsin-A negative in cases of pulmonary small cell carcinomas
  ○ Breast carcinomas: GATA3, BRST-2, mammaglobin
    – ER, PR, and HER2/neu can be used for diagnosis, prognostic/therapeutic considerations
    – GATA3 more sensitive than ER, mammaglobin, or GCDFP-15 in detecting metastatic breast cancer, and GATA3 may be used as 1st-line marker in limited ICC panel
  ○ Ovarian or peritoneal primary: PAX8, CA125, WT1
    – WT1 also positive in mesothelial cells
  ○ Colon: CK20, CDX2, villin
  ○ Upper gastrointestinal (esophagus, stomach, and pancreaticobiliary): CDX2 &/or CK20 may be positive in minority of cases
    – Often, most specific marker positive in these tumors is CK7, making confident identification difficult in body fluids
  ○ Renal cell carcinoma: PAX8, PAX2, CD10, RCC
  ○ Melanoma: S100, Melan-A, HMB-45, SOX10
  ○ ICC stains that can be used for diagnosis of lymphoma include CD45, pan-B and T-cell ICC, and others depending of cytomorphology

INDICATIONS FOR USE OF FLOW CYTOMETRY IN BODY FLUIDS

Lymphoma vs. Reactive Lymphocytic Effusion

- FC is rapid and sensitive method of detecting monoclonal B-cell population or aberrant T-cell antigen expression
- Other ancillary techniques utilized in differential diagnosis of lymphomas include cytogenetics, molecular genetics, and ISH
- FC unlikely to identify new malignancies in cases with morphologically normal lymphocytes and no clinical suspicion of lymphoma
- Mere presence of numerous lymphocytes does not require FC work-up

Reactive Effusions vs. Metastatic Carcinomas

- FC immunophenotyping being explored as rapid, reproducible, and sensitive method for detection of cellular antigens, such as cytokeratin and BER-EP4

SELECTED REFERENCES

1. Vojtek M et al: Claudin-4 immunohistochemistry is a useful pan-carcinoma marker for serous effusion specimens. Cytopathology. 30(6):614-9, 2019

Immunocytochemistry, Histochemistry, and Other Ancillary Techniques

Acid-Fast Stain Highlighting Mycobacteria

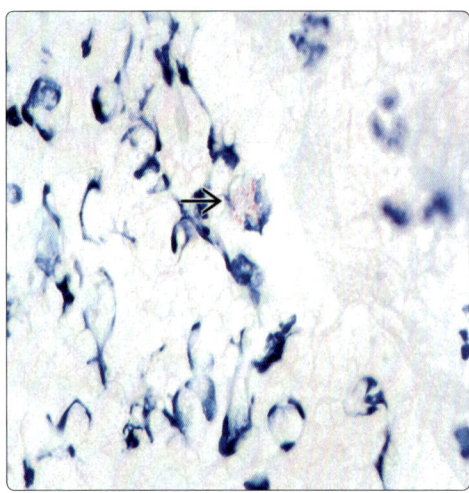

GMS-Positive Fungus in Pleural Fluid

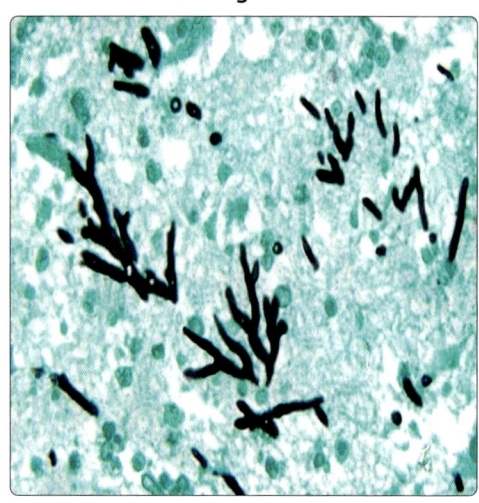

(Left) Kinyoun acid-fast special stain performed on cytospin preparation of pleural effusion in a patient with pleural tuberculosis shows positive staining of acid-fast bacilli ➡. Tuberculosis is the most common cause of pleural effusions in resource-limited countries. **(Right)** GMS special stain of a pleural effusion highlights numerous fungal organisms morphologically resembling Aspergillus.

Calretinin in Mesothelioma

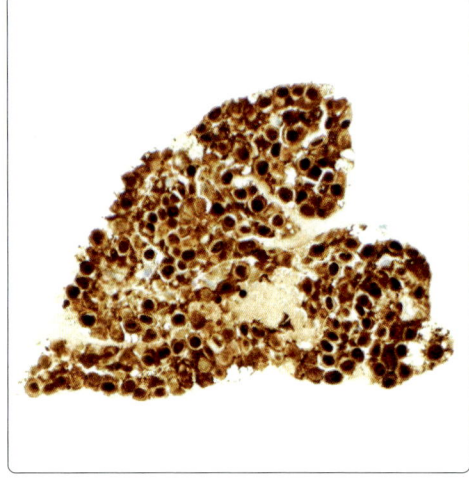

CK5/6 in Mesothelioma

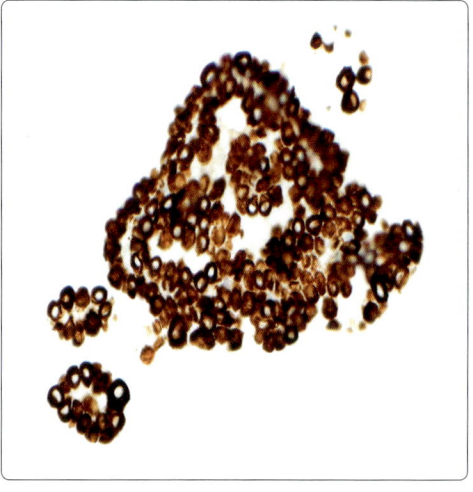

(Left) Calretinin immunocytochemical (ICC) stain was performed in a case of malignant mesothelioma in a pleural effusion. Epithelial mesothelioma shows positive cytoplasmic and nuclear staining with calretinin antibody. **(Right)** CK5/6 ICC in a case of an epithelial mesothelioma shows strong, diffuse staining. Lung adenocarcinomas are generally negative; however, squamous cell carcinomas are immunopositive for CK5/6.

D2-40 in Mesothelioma

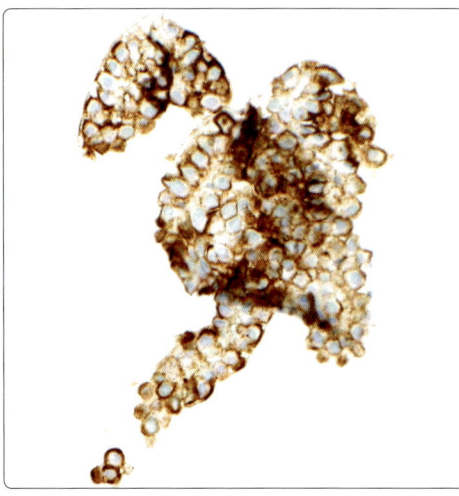

D2-40 in Reactive Mesothelial Cells

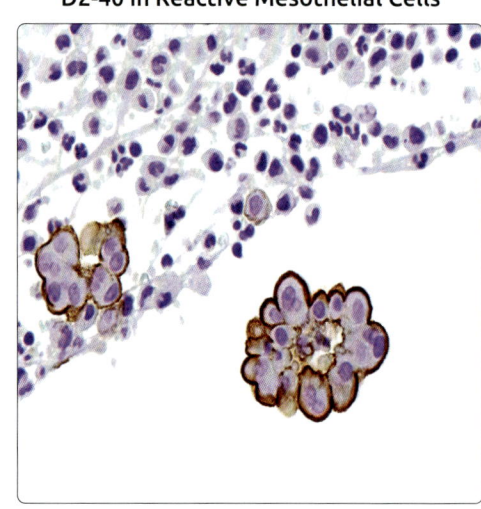

(Left) D2-40 ICC in a case of epithelial mesothelioma shows membranous staining. D2-40 stains both benign and malignant mesothelial cells. However, the presence of large irregular clusters, as seen in this case, is highly suspicious for malignant mesothelioma. **(Right)** D2-40 ICC stain demonstrates a positive membranous stain in small clusters of reactive benign mesothelial cells. The background inflammatory cells are negative.

Immunocytochemistry, Histochemistry, and Other Ancillary Techniques

BER-EP4 in Breast Adenocarcinoma

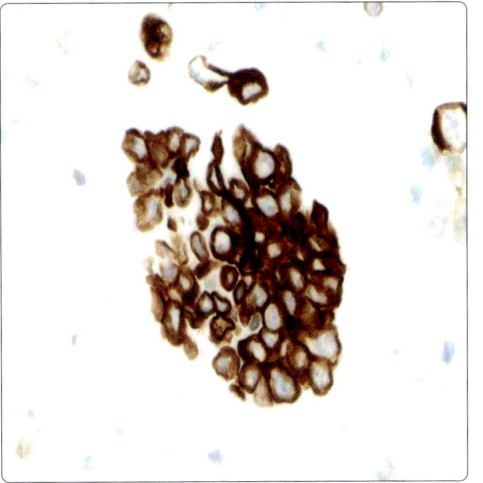

Monoclonal CEA for Lung Adenocarcinoma

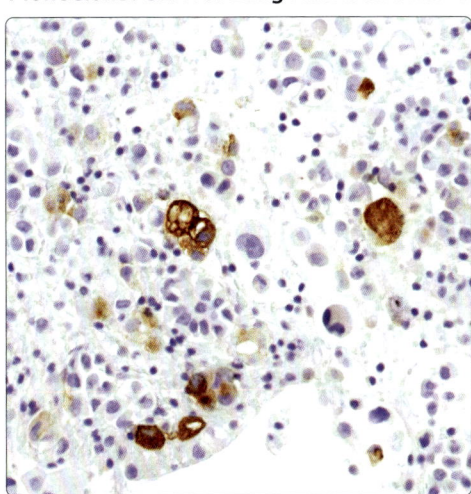

(Left) BER-EP4 shows membranous staining similar to MOC-31, another antibody directed against the same target epitope: EpCAM. Both stains provide crisp staining of target malignant clusters, such as this breast cancer. (Right) In many cases, adenocarcinoma markers are patchy, such as this mCEA that is only staining a subset of the malignant cells. Careful review of ICC is needed, especially in cases with few cells of concern present in the cell block.

ER-Positive Breast Carcinoma

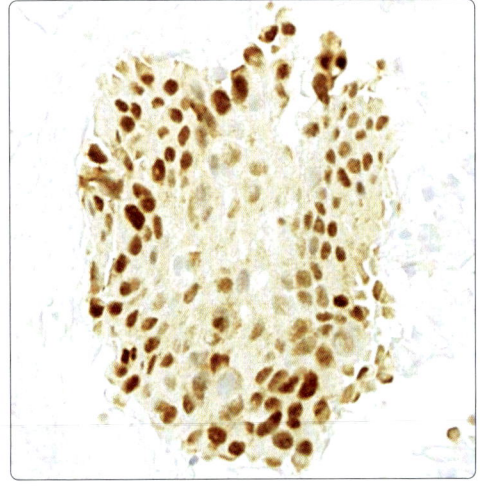

HER2-Positive Breast Carcinoma

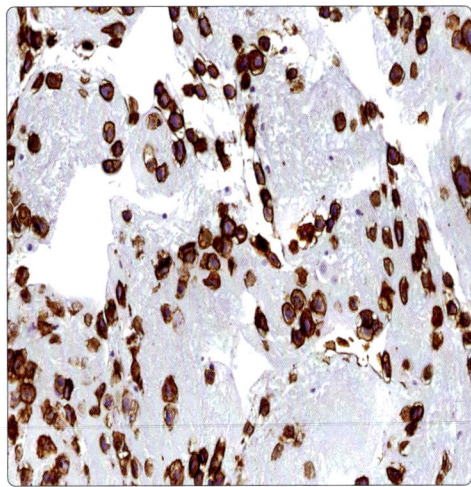

(Left) ER ICC in a case of metastatic breast carcinoma in a pleural effusion shows diffuse positive nuclear staining. ICC stains, such as ER, PR, and HER2/neu, can aid in the differential diagnosis of primary site and as prognostic/therapeutic biomarkers. (Right) ICC for HER2/neu shows a diffuse positive membrane stain (score: 3+). Results of ER, PR, and HER2/neu ICC have important prognostic and therapeutic implications. Attention to fixation times is needed for cell blocks used for prognostic markers.

TTF-1 in Lung Adenocarcinoma

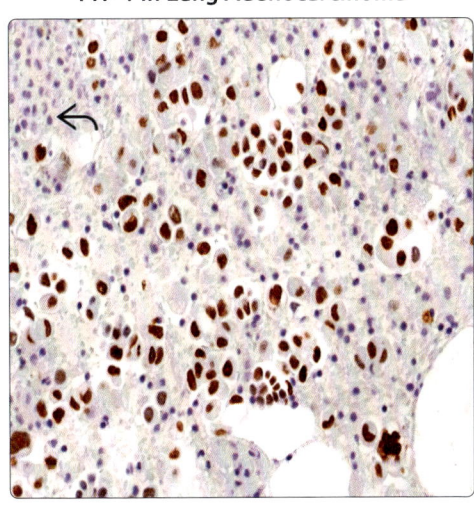

PAX8 in Ovarian Serous Carcinoma

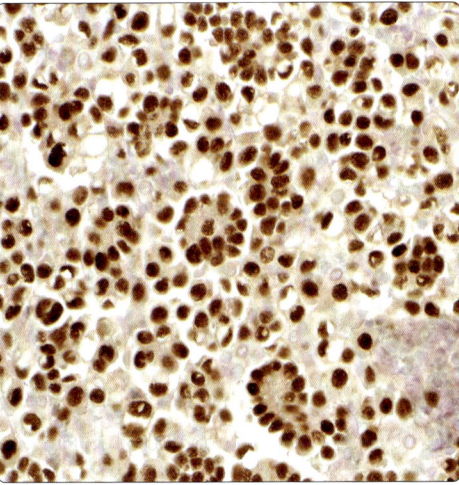

(Left) TTF-1 ICC stain in a case of metastatic pulmonary adenocarcinoma demonstrates an intense positive nuclear stain. The background mesothelial and inflammatory cells are immunonegative ⮕. (Right) Positive nuclear staining for PAX8 in a case of metastatic ovarian serous carcinoma is shown. ICC staining for PAX8 is sensitive and specific for tumors of müllerian origin and renal carcinomas.

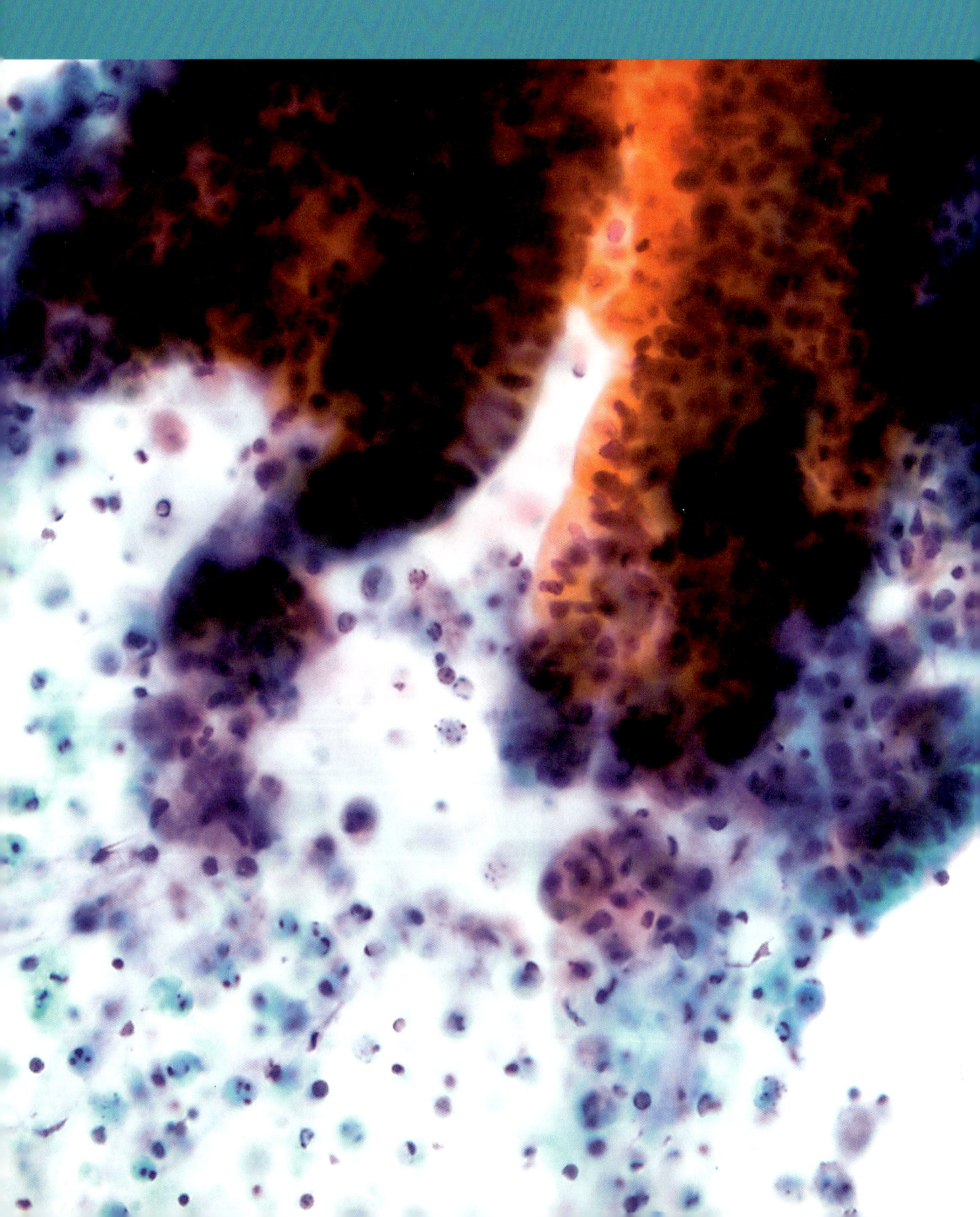

PART II
SECTION 5
Urinary Cytology

Normal Urinary Cytology, Specimen Types, and Reporting Terminology	228
Ileal Conduit Specimens	232
Noninfectious Benign Conditions	234
Infectious Benign Conditions	236
Reactive Urothelial Changes	238
Low-Grade Urothelial Lesions	240
Atypical Urothelial Cells	241
High-Grade Urothelial Dysplasia/Carcinoma/Carcinoma In Situ	242
Squamous Cell Carcinoma of Urinary Bladder	244
Adenocarcinoma of Urinary Bladder	246
Other Malignancies in Urinary Cytology	248
Renal Pelvic Cytology	250
Ancillary Testing, UroVysion, and Others	252

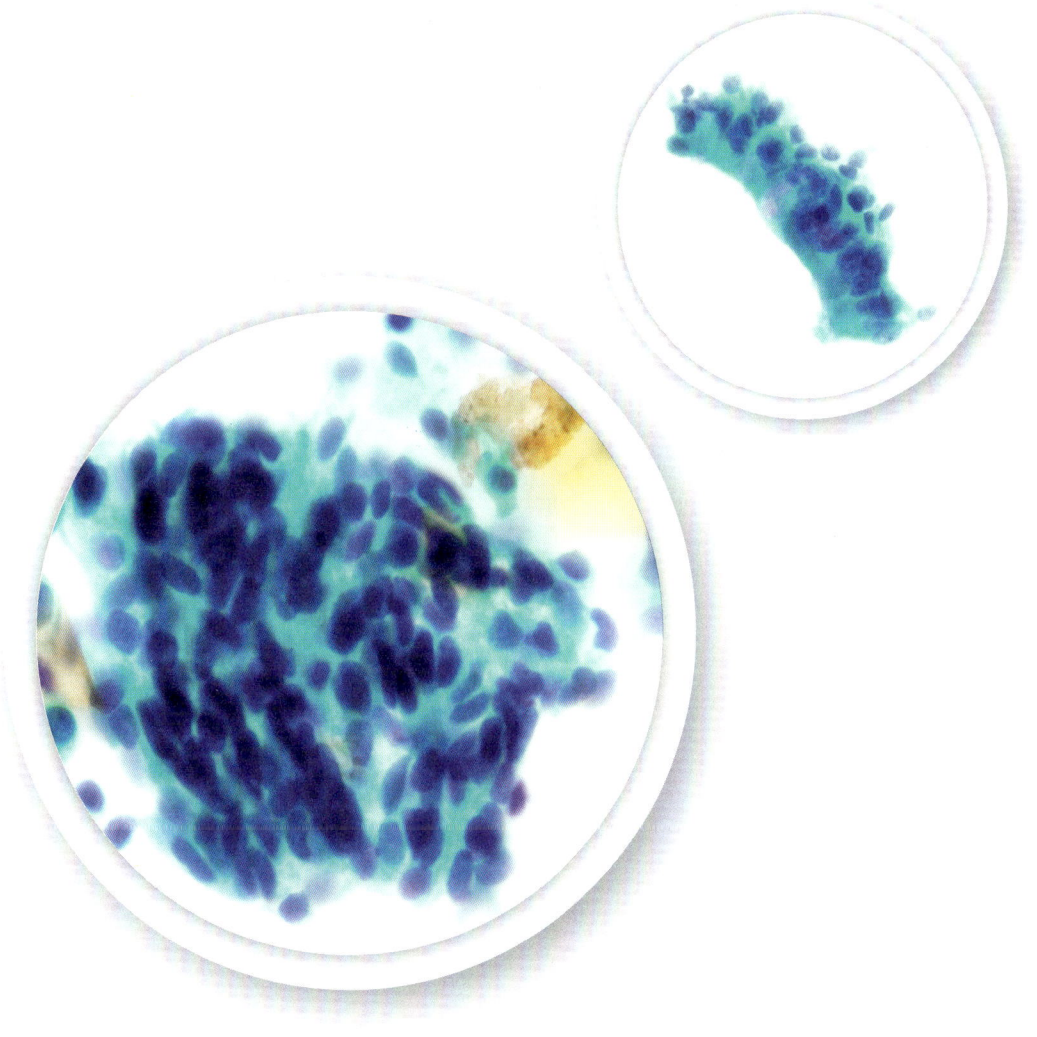

Normal Urinary Cytology, Specimen Types, and Reporting Terminology

SPECIMEN TYPES

Voided (Clean Catch)
- Recommended for screening
- Easiest to obtain
- Late morning or early afternoon collection preferred
  - 1st/early morning and collection bag specimens contain degenerative cells from prolonged exposure in urine
- Remember, specimen also includes urethral sampling/origin of cells
- Usually 1 specimen is sufficient
- Cytology has < 50% sensitivity for bladder tumors overall but performs better for high-grade tumors
  - High specificity for high-grade urothelial carcinoma (HGUC) (~ 95%)
  - Sensitivity rises to ~ 70% when low-grade tumors are excluded
- Ancillary studies can be performed to enhance screening but are costly

Catheterization
- Avoids contamination from external male genitalia and female cervical/vaginal/vulvar contamination
- More likely to be cellular &/or contain clusters of urothelial cells than clean-catch specimens
- Often shows marked degenerative changes if collected from indwelling catheters

Urinary Bladder Wash (Barbotage)
- Preferred when there is high clinical suspicion of malignancy
- Useful to follow patients with known history of urothelial neoplasm
- Samples large surface area
- More cellular than voided urine specimens
- Ancillary studies can be used to aid in assessment of residual/recurrent disease
- Directed washings of upper tracts may be performed, although cellularity and sensitivity are typically lower

Normal Findings in Instrumented Urine
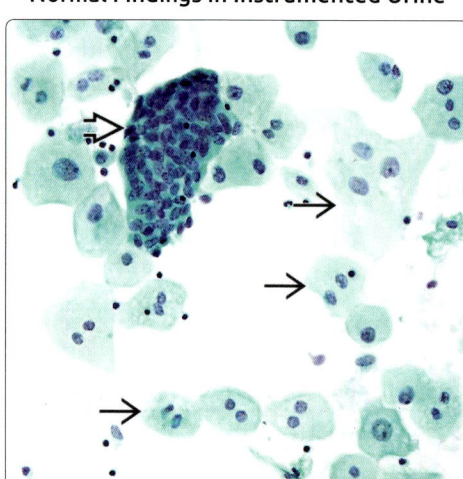

Umbrella Cell
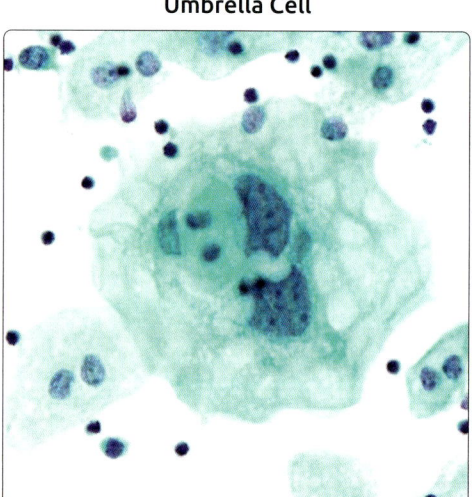

(Left) A cluster of tightly cohesive basal-type urothelial cells ⇨ is present in a background of numerous umbrella cells ⇨ on a Pap stain of a postcatheterization bladder specimen. (Right) Umbrella cells can become quite large with bizarre nuclei, as shown in this Pap stain. However, the overall nuclear:cytoplasmic ratio is low.

Intermediate and Umbrella Cells
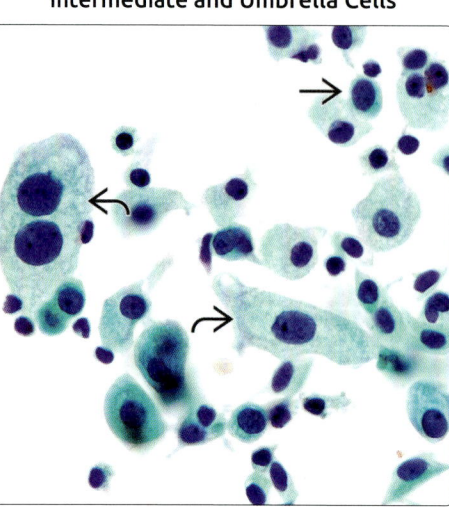

Renal Tubular Cells
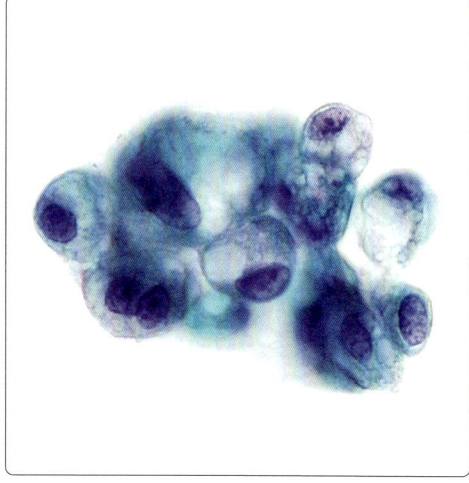

(Left) Pap-stained washing sample contains a mixture of umbrella cells ⇨ and intermediate cells ⇨ in a background of inflammation. Although the cells have variable appearances, the abundant cytoplasm and bland nuclei are the key features. (Right) These reactive/degenerative renal tubular cells on Pap stain show numerous intracytoplasmic vacuoles. However, the nuclei are bland with fine chromatin and smooth nuclear borders.

Normal Urinary Cytology, Specimen Types, and Reporting Terminology

Ileal Conduit Specimens
- Patients do not have functioning urinary bladder usually due to cystectomy for prior urothelial carcinoma
- Examined cytologically to rule out upper tract urothelial lesions

CYTOLOGIC FEATURES
Basal Urothelial Cells
- Small cells
- High nuclear:cytoplasmic (N:C) ratio
- Hyperchromatic, uniform, round nuclei
- Smooth chromatin and inconspicuous nucleoli
- Usually in groups but may occur singly

Intermediate Urothelial Cells
- Intermediate size
- Cuboidal or pyramidal shape
- Finely dispersed, smooth chromatin and inconspicuous nucleoli
- Fair amount of associated cytoplasm
- May be present singly or in loose clusters

Superficial Umbrella Cells
- Often most numerous cell type
- Very large size
- Large nuclei, frequently bi- or multinucleated
- Abundant, often vacuolated cytoplasm
- Nuclei can show bizarre sizes and shapes, but cells continue to show overall low N:C ratio
- Usually occur as single cells

Squamous Cells
- May represent cervicovaginal/genitourinary contamination in clean-catch specimens
- Squamous metaplasia can occur in trigone area of urinary bladder, especially in women
- May also represent urethral origin in clean-catch specimens

Glandular Cells
- Cystitis cystica/glandularis
- Glandular/intestinal metaplasia
- Urachal remnants
- Endometrial/müllerian cells
- Prostatic/seminal vesicle origin
- Ileal conduit specimens

Renal Tubular Cells
- Usually poorly preserved
- Small, dark nuclei
- Abundant, often granular cytoplasm
- Reactive changes include slight nuclear atypia (enlarged nuclei, pleomorphism, hyperchromasia, and nucleoli)
  - Fairly abundant granular or vacuolated cytoplasm may be seen
- More often present in cases of renal injury or disease

Spermatozoa
- Small, round head with elongated tail

Crystals
- Uric acid most common

Corpora Amylacea
- Rounded, blue-green structures; may be fragmented

Inflammation
- Neutrophils or lymphocytes usually

Contaminants
- Pollen
- Lubricant

DIAGNOSTIC CHECKLIST
Pathologic Interpretation Pearls
- Urologists can see low-grade urothelial neoplasms (LGUNs) at time of cystoscopy, as cystoscope magnifies to ~ 1 mm
- Urologists cannot reliably see flat urothelial lesions (e.g., carcinoma in situ)
- Low-grade neoplasms have low risk of progression to invasive disease
- Carcinoma in situ shows high risk of progression
- Therefore, cytologists play important role in identifying presence or absence of high-grade lesions, especially carcinoma in situ, in these urologic specimens
- All specimen types may be processed by liquid-based modalities or cytospins
- Residual material may be used to for cell block or for ancillary testing (UroVysion FISH and others)

PARIS SYSTEM FOR REPORTING URINARY CYTOLOGY
Basics
- 2nd edition published in 2022 based on work of international consensus group
- Establishes universal standard for urinary cytology terminology
- Emphasizes role of cytology in identification of high-grade lesions
  - Low-grade papillary lesions are responsibility of urologists to identify

Adequacy
- Voided urine: All specimens should be examined
  - Volumes < 30 mL unsatisfactory if also scant cellularity and no abnormal cells
- Instrumented urine: Adequacy based on cellularity but based on limited data so far
  - Satisfactory: 2,600 cells
    - Corresponds to at least 20 urothelial cells per 10 consecutive HPF in ThinPrep
    - 2,600 cells corresponds to 47 urothelial cells per 10 HPF in SurePath
  - Satisfactory but less than optimal: 10-20 cells per 10 HPF (ThinPrep)
  - Unsatisfactory: < 10 cells per 10 HPF (ThinPrep)
    - Also obscuring lubricant, inflammatory cells, or red cells
    - Use unsatisfactory rather than atypical urothelial cells (AUC) if there is extensive artifact-related "atypia"

Negative for High-Grade Urothelial Carcinoma
- Benign urothelial, glandular, or squamous cells
  - Includes tissue fragments, sheets, and clusters

Normal Urinary Cytology, Specimen Types, and Reporting Terminology

– Benign urothelial tissue fragments refer to benign-appearing cells in papillary-like arrangements but without true fibrovascular cores
– Such fragments in voided urine have traditionally caused much consternation due to concern over missing low-grade papillary urothelial neoplasms
– Paris System unequivocally includes such findings in negative category, even though some may correspond to low-grade carcinoma on follow-up
- Changes related to known benign processes
  o Lithiasis
  o Viral cytopathic effect (polyomavirus/BK virus "decoy cells")
  o Treatment effects
    – Radiation
    – Chemotherapy
    – Bacille Calmette-Guérin immunotherapy with granulomatous response

Atypical Urothelial Cells

- Mild to moderate cytologic atypia
- Major feature: Nonsuperficial, nondegenerated urothelial cells with increased N:C ratio > 0.5 (> 50%)
  o Must be present for interpretation of AUC
- 1 of 3 minor criteria also required [if > 1 present, consider suspicious for HGUC (SHGUC) or HGUC]
  o Nuclear hyperchromasia (relative to normal superficial urothelial cells)
    – Should not be as pronounced as SHGUC or HGUC
    – Normal basal and intermediate cells in instrumented urine may have high N:C ratio and mild hyperchromasia; these should be placed in negative category
  o Irregular nuclear membranes
    – Irregular nuclear shape and variably thickened chromatinic rim but usually still round, not oval
  o Irregular, coarse, clumped chromatin
- AUC may be appropriate choice if there is extensive degenerative change but otherwise concerning for HGUC
- Eccentric nuclei, loss of nuclear polarity may be present in AUC
  o Consider also glandular cells, renal tubular cells
  o Other features are needed for interpretation of AUC
- Nuclear enlargement relative to intermediate or basal urothelial cells is often seen in AUC
  o Subset may have cell shrinkage, however, so nuclear enlargement is not necessary criterion
- Most cases have few cells of concern
  o No upper limit in Paris System
  o More cells of concern corresponds to higher risk on follow-up
- Reporting rates for AUC category are not well established
  o Pre-Paris System studies have wide range of "atypical": 2-31%
    – Follow-up rates of HGUC range: 8.3-37.5%
    – Rates of malignancy are inversely proportional to "atypical" rate
  o Follow-up studies are needed to determine consensus upper limit for AUC use in practice

Suspicious for High-Grade Urothelial Carcinoma

- Reflects presence of urothelial cells with severe atypia that falls short of HGUC diagnosis but is beyond AUC category
- As practical matter, SHGUC is used in cases with too few abnormal cells for definitive diagnosis of HGUC
- Criteria: Nonsuperficial, nondegenerated urothelial cells showing
  o Increased N:C ratio > 0.7 (> 70%)
    – Lower ratios of 0.5-0.7 may be acceptable if other features are present, especially if voided urine or known history of HGUC
  o Moderate to severe hyperchromasia
  o In addition, 1 of 2 following features
    – Irregular clumpy chromatin
    – Markedly irregular nuclear membranes
- 5-10 cells with these features should be present; > 10 cells should be in HGUC category
  o More cellular instrumented urine specimens are more likely to be properly assigned to SHGUC category if number of cells is closer to 10
- Cells of interest are usually seen as single cells, but clusters may occur
- Nuclear size is usually at least 2x normal intermediate or basal urothelial cell nuclei, but this is not mandatory
- Features that may be present but are not required
  o Eccentric nuclear location
  o Necrotic background
  o Pleomorphism
  o Mitoses
  o Apoptotic bodies
  o Prominent nucleoli
- SHGUC should not be rendered on degenerated cells
- Follow-up malignancy rates for SHGUC only slightly lower (59-94%) than HGUC (76-100%) using Paris criteria

High-Grade Urothelial Carcinoma

- Criteria: Minimum of 5-10 malignant cells needed; at least 10 cells in instrumented specimen
  o N:C ratio: > 0.7 (> 70%)
  o Moderate to severe hyperchromasia
  o Markedly irregular nuclear membranes
  o Coarse/clumped chromatin
- Other notable cytologic features not required for diagnosis
  o Cellular pleomorphism
  o Marked variation in cellular sizes and shapes
  o Scant, pale, or dense cytoplasm
  o Prominent nucleoli
  o Mitoses
  o Necrotic debris
  o Inflammation
- HGUC with squamous differentiation: Malignant squamous cells with keratinization &/or intercellular bridges admixed with malignant cells showing typical HGUC features
  o Nuclei in malignant squamous cells may be elongated/spindle-shaped
  o Keratin flakes and necrosis may be observed in background
- HGUC with glandular differentiation: Malignant cells with true gland formation admixed with malignant cells showing typical HGUC features

Normal Urinary Cytology, Specimen Types, and Reporting Terminology

Morphologic Criteria for Paris System Categories

Category	Nuclear: Cytoplasmic Ratio (1)	Nuclear Chromasia (2)	Chromatinic Rim/Nuclear Membrane (3)	Chromatin Quality (4)	Mandatory (Major) Features	Minor Features	Number of Cells
Atypical urothelial cells	> 0.5	Similar to umbrella cells (normal) or dark/very dark (minor feature)	Fine and even (normal) or uneven shape and thickness (minor feature)	Finely granular (normal) or coarsely clumped (minor feature)	1	2-4 (at least 1 minor feature must be 2nd feature identified in cells of interest)	Usually few (but no defined limit)
Suspicious for high-grade urothelial carcinoma	> 0.7	Very dark	Uneven shape and thickness	Coarsely clumped	1 and 2	3, 4 (at least 1 of these must be 3rd feature identified in cells of interest)	Very few (< 5-10 cells)
High-grade urothelial carcinoma	> 0.7	Very dark	Uneven shape and thickness	Coarsely clumped	1 and 2	3, 4 (at least 1 of these must be 3rd feature identified in cells of interest)	Numerous (> 5-10 cells)

Modified from Barkan et al: J Am Soc Cytopathol. 5(3):177-88, 2016.

Relative Risk of Paris System Categories, Based on Studies to Date

Category	Risk of High-Grade Malignancy	Management
Unsatisfactory/nondiagnostic	0-16%	Repeat cytology, cystoscopy in 3 months if increased clinical suspicion
Negative for high-grade urothelial carcinoma	8-24%	Clinical follow-up as needed
Low-grade urothelial neoplasm	0-44%	Need cystoscopy and biopsy to further evaluate grade and stage
Atypical urothelial cells	24-53%	Clinical follow-up as needed; potential use of ancillary testing
Suspicious for high-grade urothelial carcinoma	59-94%	More aggressive follow-up, cystoscopy, biopsy
High-grade urothelial carcinoma	76-100%	More aggressive follow-up, cystoscopy, biopsy, staging
Other malignancy	76-100%	More aggressive follow-up, cystoscopy, biopsy, staging

Wojcik et al: Risk of high-grade malignancy percentages: The Paris System for Reporting Urinary Cytology. 2nd ed. Springer. 253, 2022

- Rates of reporting HGUC will vary with patient population sampled
- Positive predictive value and specificity for HGUC should be very high

Low-Grade Urothelial Neoplasm
- Combined cytologic term encompassing low-grade papillary urothelial carcinoma, papillary urothelial neoplasm of low malignant potential, urothelial proliferation of unknown malignant potential, urothelial papilloma, and flat low-grade intraurothelial dysplasia
- Criteria: 3D cellular papillary clusters with fibrovascular cores, including capillaries, without high-grade cytologic features
  - Cell blocks may be useful to identify fibrovascular cores in select case
- Subsumed under negative for HGUC in Paris 2nd edition; no longer separate category
- Features previously used as criteria for low-grade lesions
  - 3D cell clusters without fibrovascular cores
  - Increased numbers of monotonous single cells
  - Cytoplasmic homogeneity
  - Nuclear border irregularity (without other features concerning for HGUC)
  - Increased N:C ratio (without other features concerning for HGUC)
- Occasional specimens may be very cellular and composed predominantly of cercariform individual cells
  - May be acceptable to include comment that LGUN is considered but still in negative category

Other Malignancies
- Squamous cell carcinoma
  - 2nd most common primary malignancy (2-5%; higher in regions with *Schistosoma hematobium*)
- Adenocarcinoma
  - 3rd most common primary malignancy (0.5-2.5%)
- Small cell carcinoma
- Sarcomas (leiomyosarcoma, angiosarcoma, others)
- Hematologic malignancies (lymphoma, plasma cell myeloma)
- Melanoma

SELECTED REFERENCES
1. Wojcik EM et al: The Paris System for Reporting Urinary Cytology. 2nd ed. Springer, 2022
2. Pastorello RG et al: Experience on the use of the Paris System for reporting urinary cytopathology: review of the published literature. J Am Soc Cytopathol. 10(1):79-87, 2021
3. Rohra P et al: Effect of the Paris System for reporting urinary cytology with histologic follow-up. Diagn Cytopathol. 49(6):691-9, 2021

Ileal Conduit Specimens

KEY FACTS

TERMINOLOGY
- Ileal conduit refers to a small portion of ileum transformed into urine reservoir at time of cystectomy for urothelial carcinoma

CLINICAL ISSUES
- Because urothelial carcinoma can be multicentric disease, ileal conduit specimens may be submitted to exclude de novo carcinoma of ureters or renal pelvis or recurrence of initial carcinoma

CYTOPATHOLOGY
- Hypercellular
- Epithelial cells from small intestine may appear columnar or more rounded if degenerated
  o May see goblet cells distended by mucin
- "Dirty" background containing karyorrhectic debris, bacteria, macrophages, and inflammatory cells
  o Often cleaner on liquid-based preparations
- Large sheets of glandular cells may be seen on cytospins
- Intestinal epithelial clusters and luminal debris on cell blocks

TOP DIFFERENTIAL DIAGNOSES
- Recurrent urothelial carcinoma
  o Often interpreted as atypical due to degeneration

DIAGNOSTIC CHECKLIST
- Hypercellular, mixed population of small intestinal columnar cells (± goblet cells), debris, bacteria, macrophages, and inflammatory cells
  o Looks like contaminated specimen if history is not provided
- On liquid-based preparations, mostly single columnar cells are seen; "dirty" background removed by filter
- Degenerated nonneoplastic intestinal epithelial cells may simulate degenerated malignant urothelial cells
  o Need to find viable malignant cells to make diagnosis of recurrence

Typical Cytospin Appearance
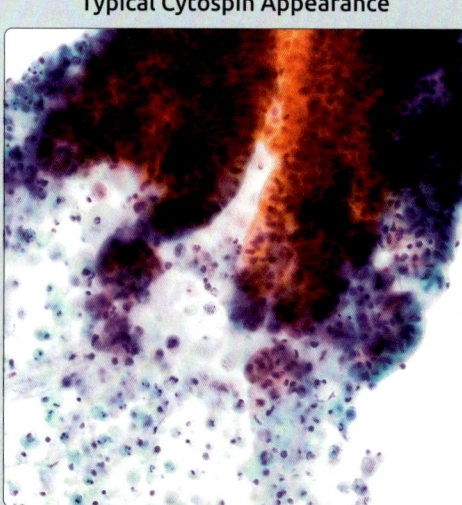

Typical ThinPrep Appearance
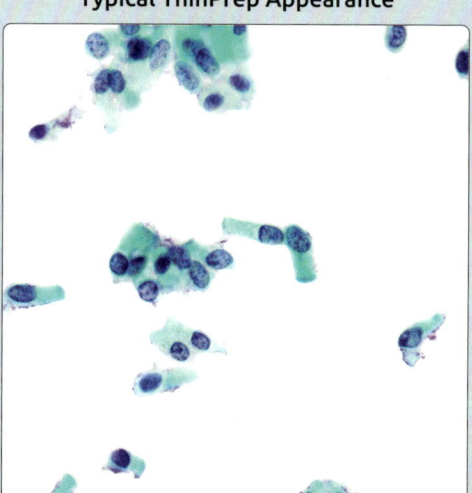

(Left) Cohesive sheets of small intestinal columnar cells are shown at upper right and a "dirty" background of macrophages, cellular debris, and inflammatory cells are present at lower left of this Pap stain. (Right) On liquid-based preparations, such as this ThinPrep, columnar cells are often dyshesive. The background debris and inflammatory cells are usually removed by the filter.

Columnar Architecture With Goblet Cells
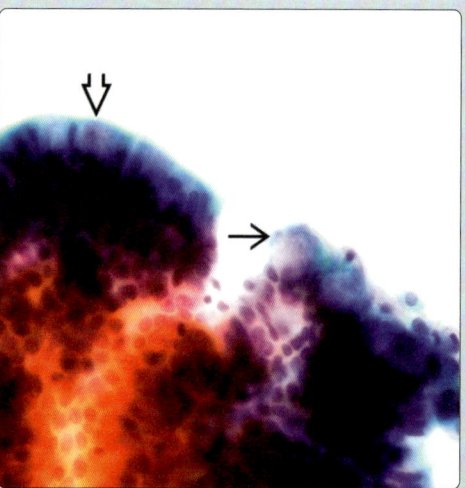

Background Findings
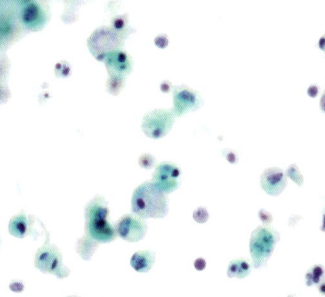

(Left) Higher power of Pap-stained cytospin shows the columnar nature of small intestinal mucosa ⮕ with rare goblet cells ⮕. (Right) A background of macrophages, mixed inflammation, and cellular debris is shown on Pap stain. Occasionally, no epithelial cells may be included, and this may be the only material in the specimen.

Ileal Conduit Specimens

TERMINOLOGY

Synonyms
- Ileal pouch, Indiana pouch, urinary diversion

Definitions
- At time of cystectomy for urothelial carcinoma, small portion of ileum is resected and transformed into urine reservoir

CLINICAL ISSUES

Presentation
- Prior cystectomy often not mentioned on requisition; correlation with clinical history is key

Prognosis
- Because urothelial carcinoma can be multicentric disease, ileal conduit specimens may be submitted to exclude de novo carcinoma of ureters or renal pelvis or recurrence of initial carcinoma

CYTOPATHOLOGY

Cellularity
- Hypercellular

Pattern
- Epithelial cells from small intestine may present as single columnar or round cells in liquid-based preparations and are often seen in cohesive sheets on cytospin

Background
- "Dirty," containing karyorrhectic debris, bacteria, macrophages, and inflammatory cells on cytospin; clean on liquid-based preparations

Cells
- Mixed population consisting of epithelial cells from small intestine, bacteria, macrophages, and inflammatory cells on cytospin; often just epithelial cells on liquid-based preparations

Nuclear Details
- Hypochromatic; may be dark and hyperchromatic secondary to degeneration

Cytoplasmic Details
- Pale; may see goblet cells distended by mucin

Cell Block Findings
- Intestinal epithelium and luminal debris

MICROSCOPIC

Histologic Features
- Over time, normal villous architecture of ileum is replaced by flattened mucosa, which is direct result of chronic irritation of mucosa by urine
  - Secondary infection can occur

DIFFERENTIAL DIAGNOSIS

Recurrent Urothelial Carcinoma
- May be difficult to find viable malignant cells, which should show hyperchromatic, irregular nuclei, and high N:C ratios

DIAGNOSTIC CHECKLIST

Pathologic Interpretation Pearls
- Hypercellular, mixed population of small intestinal epithelial cells (± goblet cells), debris, bacteria, macrophages, and inflammatory cells
  - Looks like contaminated specimen if history is not provided
- Degenerated nonneoplastic intestinal epithelial cells may simulate degenerated malignant cells
  - Need to find viable malignant cells to make diagnosis of recurrence

SELECTED REFERENCES

1. Rodríguez-Serrano A et al: Prognostic value of urinary cytology for detecting urothelial carcinoma recurrence after radical cystectomy. Actas Urol Esp (Engl Ed). 45(6):466-72, 2021

Macrophages and Debris
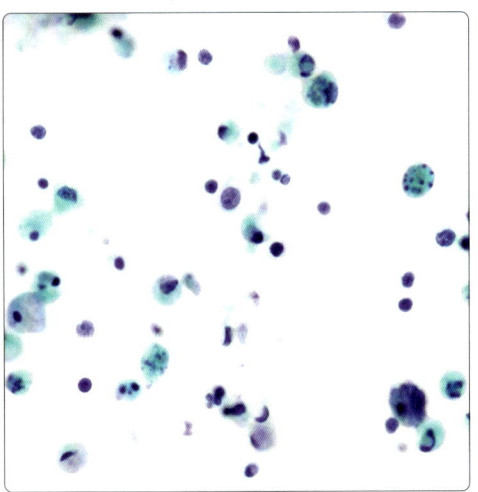

Columnar Cells From Intestinal Lining
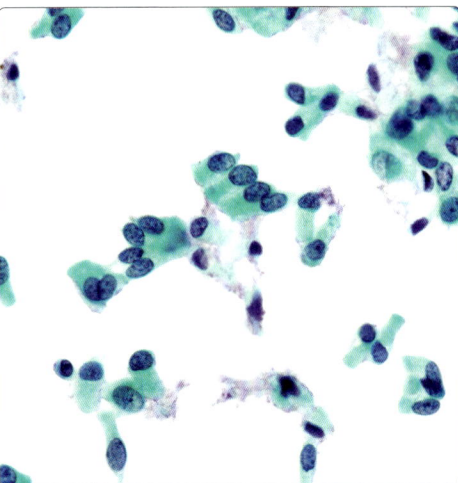

(Left) The background of cytospin preparations is often "dirty" with macrophages, bacteria, cellular debris, and inflammatory cells, as seen in this Pap stain. (Right) In liquid-based preparations, mostly dyshesive small intestinal columnar cells are present, as shown in this Pap stain.

Noninfectious Benign Conditions

KEY FACTS

CYTOPATHOLOGY

- In general, these benign lesions rarely shed into urine and are typically scant when present
- Cystitis glandularis
  - Single cells or cohesive clusters of hyperchromatic columnar cells, ± goblet cells
  - Columnar cells of cystitis glandularis are often hyperchromatic but not coarsely granular and have regular nuclear membranes and lower nuclear:cytoplasmic ratios
- Endometriosis
  - Endometriosis shows endometrial glands &/or stroma in tight hyperchromatic cell groups, similar to those seen on gynecologic Pap test
  - Less commonly, ciliated tubal-type or endocervical-like glandular cells may also be seen (known as müllerianosis)
- Nephrogenic adenoma (metaplasia)
  - Bland renal tubular-type cells with cuboidal, hobnail, or flat appearance
  - Tubuloglandular or papillary architecture
- Pseudosarcomatous myofibroblastic proliferations
  - Spindled or epithelioid cells with abundant cytoplasm and variable nuclear features
- Follicular and eosinophilic cystitis
  - Follicular and eosinophilic cystitis inflammatory conditions may show abundant lymphocytes and eosinophils, respectively
- Bacille Calmette-Guérin (BCG) therapy
  - Cases of prior BCG therapy may show increased numbers of lymphocytes; granulomas are rarely seen

TOP DIFFERENTIAL DIAGNOSES

- Cystitis glandularis, endometriosis, and nephrogenic adenoma are more uniform and less cellular than adenocarcinoma
- Pseudosarcomatous myofibroblastic proliferations may resemble carcinoma or sarcoma but should have more abundant cytoplasm, paler nuclei, and lower cellularity

Cystitis Glandularis
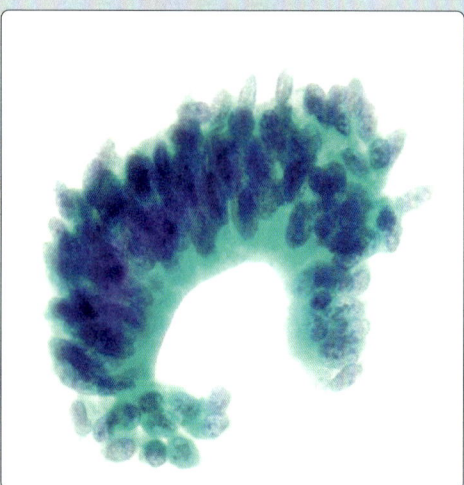

Benign Glandular Cells in ThinPrep
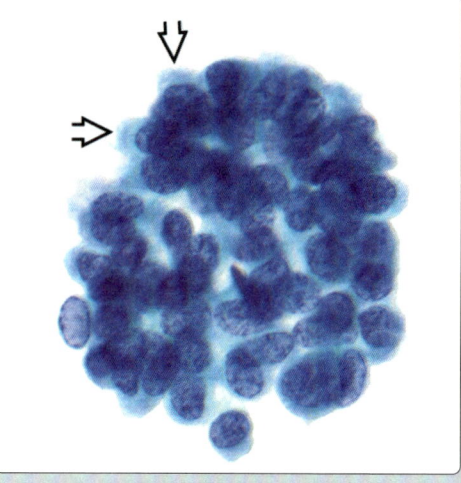

(Left) Pap stain demonstrates cystitis glandularis with elongated hyperchromatic columnar cells and apical cytoplasm, resembling benign intestinal mucosa. (Right) This ThinPrep of a voided urine specimen contained clusters of bland, uniform glandular cells. The apical cytoplasm ⇒ is less distinct in the liquid-based preparation but can still be clearly seen on close examination.

Nephrogenic Adenoma
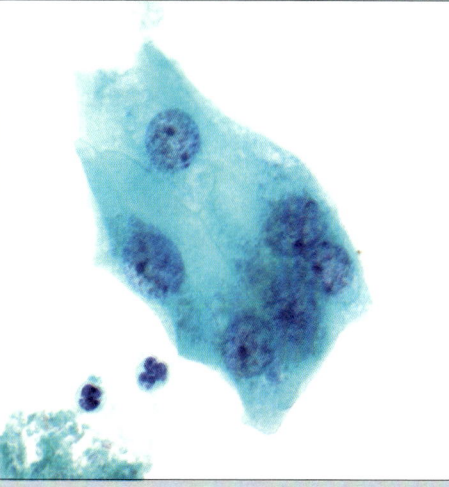

Pseudosarcomatous Myofibroblastic Lesion
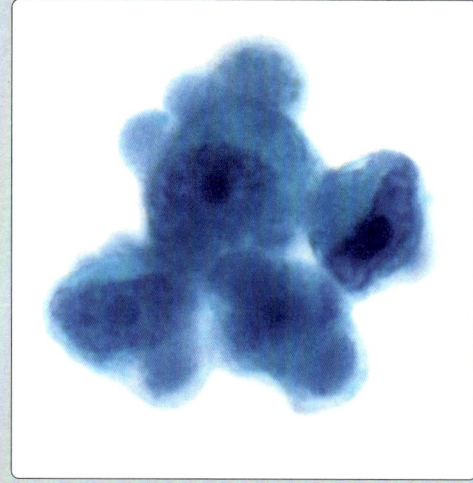

(Left) This cluster of cells from a ThinPrep of voided urine from a patient with a papillary nephrogenic adenoma of the bladder shows unusual but obviously benign cells with voluminous cytoplasm and uniform nuclei with pale chromatin. (Right) Cells from a pseudosarcomatous myofibroblastic lesion may appear bizarre due to degeneration with clumpy chromatin and prominent nucleoli on a Pap stain. These cells can be epithelioid or spindle-shaped. Abundant cytoplasm is a clue to the benign nature of the cells.

Noninfectious Benign Conditions

CLINICAL ISSUES

Prognosis
- Generally excellent prognosis

CYTOPATHOLOGY

Cellularity
- In general, benign nonurothelial lesions are usually present below mucosal surface in rests within lamina propria or in bladder wall
  - Unless there is mucosal ulcer, they rarely shed into urine
  - Therefore, diagnostic cells for these conditions are usually few

Cystitis Glandularis
- Single cells or cohesive clusters of hyperchromatic columnar cells, ± goblet cells
- Columnar cells of cystitis glandularis are often hyperchromatic but not coarsely granular and have regular nuclear membranes and lower nuclear:cytoplasmic ratios

Endometriosis
- Endometriosis shows endometrial glands &/or stroma in tight hyperchromatic cell groups, similar to those seen on gynecologic Pap test
- Endometrial cells are hyperchromatic and small with high nuclear:cytoplasmic ratios
- Less commonly, ciliated tubal-type or endocervical-like glandular cells may also be seen
  - Known as müllerianosis when mixed elements are seen

Nephrogenic Adenoma (Metaplasia)
- Renal tubular epithelium in areas of urothelial injury
- Cells may be cuboidal, hobnail, or flat with tubuloglandular or papillary architecture
- Uniform nuclei, sometimes with nucleoli

Pseudosarcomatous Myofibroblastic Proliferations
- a.k.a. postoperative spindle cell nodule, pseudosarcomatous fibromyxoid tumor, and inflammatory pseudotumor
- Spindle cells that may appear epithelioid in some cases; should have abundant cytoplasm
- Nuclei may be hyperchromatic, hypochromatic, or vesicular with prominent nucleoli
- Cells may appear bizarre due to degeneration in urine specimens

Follicular and Eosinophilic Cystitis
- Follicular and eosinophilic cystitis inflammatory conditions may show abundant lymphocytes and eosinophils, respectively

Bacille Calmette-Guérin (BCG) Therapy
- Cases of prior BCG therapy may show increased numbers of lymphocytes
- Granulomas are rarely seen

DIFFERENTIAL DIAGNOSIS

Urothelial Carcinoma
- Nephrogenic adenoma or pseudosarcomatous myofibroblastic proliferations may mimic malignancy; awareness of history and cystoscopic findings is key
- Enlarged, hyperchromatic nuclei and high nuclear:cytoplasmic ratios favor malignancy

Adenocarcinoma
- Usually more cellular and more atypical than cystitis glandularis, endometriosis, or nephrogenic adenoma
- PAX8(+) in endometriosis and nephrogenic adenoma

DIAGNOSTIC CHECKLIST

Pathologic Interpretation Pearls
- Clinical history is often helpful to avoid overdiagnosis
- These lesions may be difficult to identify precisely, but recognition of their benign nature is usually sufficient

SELECTED REFERENCES
1. Samaratunga H et al: Tumour-like lesions of the urinary bladder. Pathology. 53(1):44-55, 2021
2. Kryvenko ON et al: Mimickers of urothelial neoplasia. Ann Diagn Pathol. 38:11-9, 2019

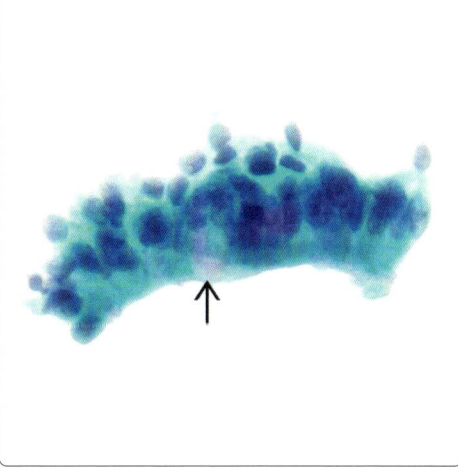

Large Cluster of Glandular Cells | **Goblet Cell in Cystitis Glandularis**

(Left) This Pap-stained cytospin from a bladder washing of a patient with cystitis glandularis shows a large cluster of cells with uniform and evenly spaced nuclei. A low-grade papillary urothelial neoplasm could be considered in the differential, but the columnar cell morphology with a rim of apical cytoplasm is distinctive. (Right) This fragment of intestinal-type mucosa from cystitis glandularis contains a goblet cell ➡ that stains a distinctive pink color on the Pap stain.

Infectious Benign Conditions

KEY FACTS

CYTOPATHOLOGY
- Polyomavirus (BK virus) produces decoy cells that mimic urothelial carcinoma
  - Nuclei are prominent and very dark, often with peripheral net-like chromatin condensation and cytoplasmic comet tail on one side
- Herpesvirus exhibits multinucleation, margination of chromatin, and molding of nuclei
- Cytomegalovirus (CMV) shows large basophilic or eosinophilic nuclear inclusion surrounded by clear halo
- Human papillomavirus (HPV) demonstrates features as described in gynecologic specimens
  - Both low-grade and high-grade changes can be seen

TOP DIFFERENTIAL DIAGNOSES
- Urothelial carcinoma
  - Both urothelial carcinoma and polyomavirus demonstrate enlarged, dark nuclei
  - Carcinoma shows more nuclear membrane irregularity and coarsely granular chromatin
  - Nuclei of virally infected cells are more homogeneous and glassy or smudgy
- Degenerative changes
  - Degeneration of cell nuclei can produce appearance similar to polyomavirus
  - Immunocytochemistry for polyomavirus can be used if needed

DIAGNOSTIC CHECKLIST
- Immunocytochemistry or special stains for microorganisms can be performed on cell block material
- Urine cytology can be used to screen for presence of polyomavirus in renal transplants
- Presence of HPV-infected cells, or even cells suggestive of high-grade squamous intraepithelial lesion from cervicovaginal source, may be seen in clean-catch specimens; referral to gynecologist is indicated

Polyomavirus Decoy Cells
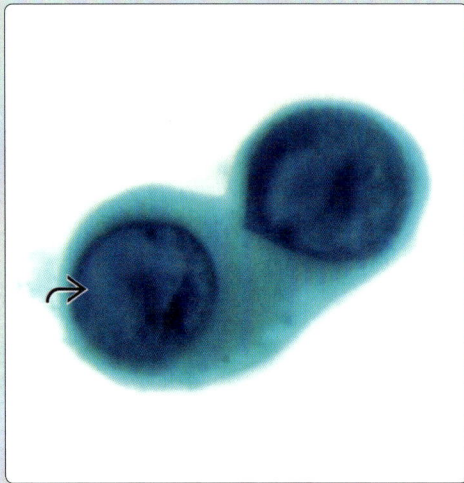

Polyomavirus Net-Like Chromatin
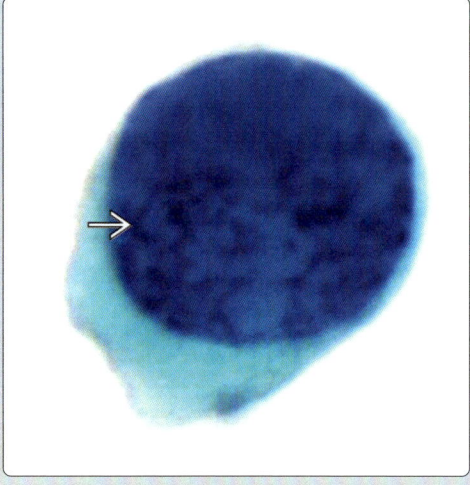

(Left) Two Pap-stained polyomavirus-infected cells show the characteristic dark nuclei with "glassy" or "smudgy" chromatin ➡. Although the cells resemble urothelial carcinoma on low power, careful examination usually makes their viral origin obvious. (Right) Careful examination of decoy cells at high power often reveals the presence of peripheral chromatin in a mesh pattern resembling a net or chain-link fence ➡, as seen in this ThinPrep example.

Herpesvirus
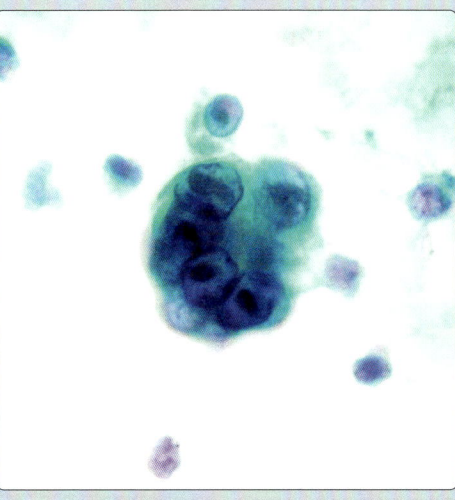

High-Grade Squamous Intraepithelial Lesion
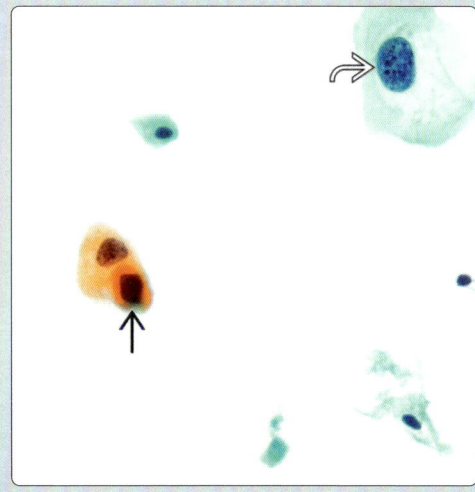

(Left) A Pap stain of herpesvirus shows multinucleation and margination of the chromatin and some nuclear molding. Nuclear inclusions are also seen in this example. (Right) Pap stain shows an atypical squamous cell with a dark, irregular nucleus and high nuclear:cytoplasmic ratio ➡ in a background of cells that show features of a low-grade squamous intraepithelial lesion (note the enlarged squamous cell nucleus ➡). The finding of HSIL warrants referral to a gynecologist.

Infectious Benign Conditions

TERMINOLOGY

Abbreviations
- Cytomegalovirus (CMV)
- Human papillomavirus (HPV)

Synonyms
- Polyomavirus = BK virus

CLINICAL ISSUES

Site
- Polyomavirus may derive from urothelium or renal cells
- Many infections may represent contamination from gynecologic or even anal sources in clean-catch specimens

CYTOPATHOLOGY

Nuclear Details
- Nuclei of virally infected cells are generally large
- Polyomavirus nuclei are dark and basophilic; called decoy cells because they mimic urothelial carcinoma
  - Unlike coarsely granular chromatin of urothelial carcinoma, viral inclusion imparts homogeneous, smudgy look to nucleus
  - Net-like peripheral condensations of chromatin can sometimes be seen
- Herpesvirus produces classic nuclear M triad: Multinucleation, margination of chromatin, and molding
- CMV shows large basophilic or eosinophilic nuclear inclusion surrounded by clear halo
- HPV demonstrates features as described in gynecologic specimens
  - Presence of HPV may be secondary to lesions of lower urinary tract or may represent contamination from gynecologic source

Cytoplasmic Details
- Polyomavirus may induce "comet cell" configuration with cytoplasmic tail on one side
- Cytoplasm of CMV-infected cells can show granules
- Perinuclear cytoplasmic halos may be seen in HPV

Nonviral Infections
- Pseudohyphae and yeast forms of *Candida* can be seen in association with inflammation &/or reactive urothelial cells
  - Often, *Candida* is seen in clean-catch urine specimens and may represent gynecologic contamination
- Pear-shaped *Trichomonas* also often represents contamination or coinfection
  - Eccentric nucleus, eosinophilic cytoplasmic granules, and flagellum are visible if organism is well preserved

DIFFERENTIAL DIAGNOSIS

Urothelial Carcinoma
- Both urothelial carcinoma and polyomavirus demonstrate enlarged, dark nuclei
- Carcinoma shows more nuclear membrane irregularity and coarsely granular chromatin
- Nuclei of virally infected cells are more homogeneous and glassy or smudgy
- If needed, immunocytochemistry for polyomavirus can be attempted on cell block for confirmation

DIAGNOSTIC CHECKLIST

Pathologic Interpretation Pearls
- Immunocytochemistry or special stains for microorganisms can be performed on cell block material
- Viral inclusions impart glassy or smudgy look to nuclei
- Presence of HPV-infected cells or even cells suggestive of high-grade squamous intraepithelial lesion from cervicovaginal source may be seen in clean-catch specimens
  - Referral to gynecologist should be suggested
- Urine cytology can be used to screen for presence of polyomavirus in renal transplants

SELECTED REFERENCES
1. Alwahaibi NY et al: Decoy cells versus plasma real-time polymerase chain reaction for the detection of polyomaviruses in renal transplant patients: a single institutional experience. J Cytol. 37(1):30-3, 2020
2. Xing J et al: Diagnostic utility of urine cytology in early detection of polyomavirus in transplant patients. J Am Soc Cytopathol. 6(1):28-32, 2017

Candida

Variation of Appearance in Polyomavirus

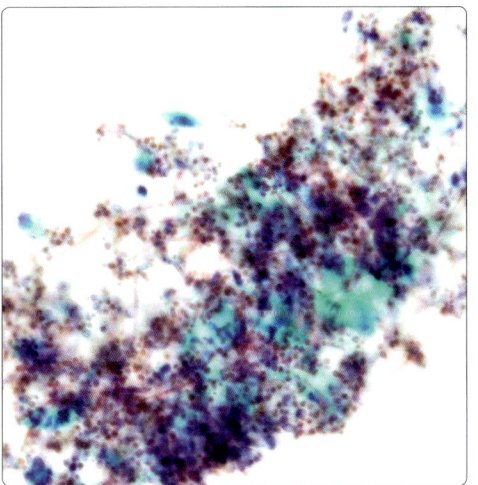
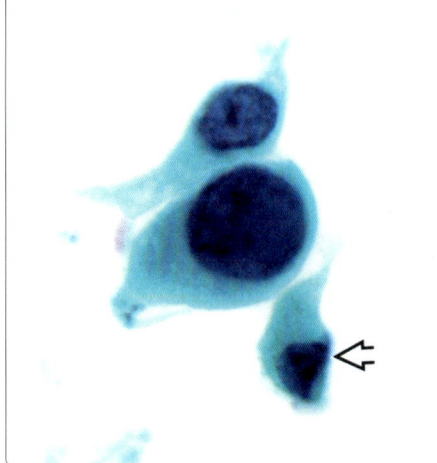

(Left) *Numerous pseudohyphae and yeast forms of Candida are present on Pap stain. Candida may represent a true urinary tract infection or a contaminant and is often associated with reactive changes in epithelial cells.* **(Right)** *These 3 Pap-stained cells in a case of florid polyomavirus infection demonstrate a range of changes with degeneration giving one cell an irregular nucleus ⇒ that might be concerning for carcinoma in another context.*

Reactive Urothelial Changes

KEY FACTS

ETIOLOGY/PATHOGENESIS
- Stones, instrumentation, &/or radiation/chemotherapy

CYTOPATHOLOGY
- Stones and instrumentation
  - Urothelial cells are arranged in tight papillary-like groups (often large and numerous)
  - Usually round nuclei, centrally placed with minimal pleomorphism
  - Minimal nuclear membrane irregularity
  - Fine, even chromatin, but there can be some hyperchromasia
  - Normal-sized nuclei, but nuclear:cytoplasmic (N:C) ratio can be increased, though usually < 0.5
- Radiation and chemotherapy
  - Normocellular or hypocellular specimens with rare affected cells scattered amongst normal urothelium
  - Cells affected by radiation/chemotherapy appear as single cells or in small groups
  - Nucleomegaly, but because overall cell size is increased as well, there is no increased N:C ratio
  - Coarse chromatin and prominent nucleoli may be seen
  - Cytoplasmic vacuoles are common
  - Polychromasia may occur

TOP DIFFERENTIAL DIAGNOSES
- High-grade urothelial carcinoma (HGUC)
  - Demonstrates more single cells, higher N:C ratios (> 0.7), more nuclear hyperchromasia, and greater degree of nuclear membrane and chromatin irregularity

DIAGNOSTIC CHECKLIST
- Similar features in stones/instrumentation/low-grade neoplasms
  - Role of cytologists is exclusion of high-grade urothelial carcinoma
  - Paris System classifies hypercellular specimens of both reactive and low-grade neoplastic origin as negative for HGUC

Urolithiasis Hypercellularity

Numerous Clusters in Urolithiasis

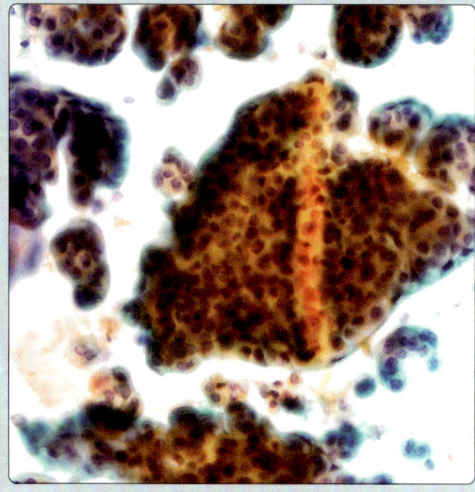

(Left) This Pap-stained urine specimen from a patient with urolithiasis shows high cellularity. The urothelial cells often appear in large cohesive papillary-like clusters that lack true fibrovascular cores. (Right) Numerous papillary-like clusters are present on Pap stain. No atypical single cells with high nuclear:cytoplasmic (N:C) ratios are seen in the background.

Bland Nuclei

Abundant Cytoplasm

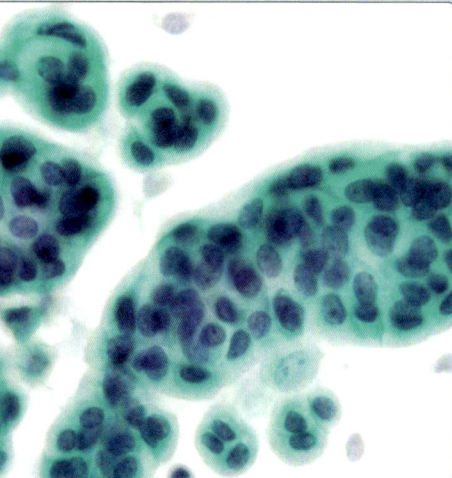
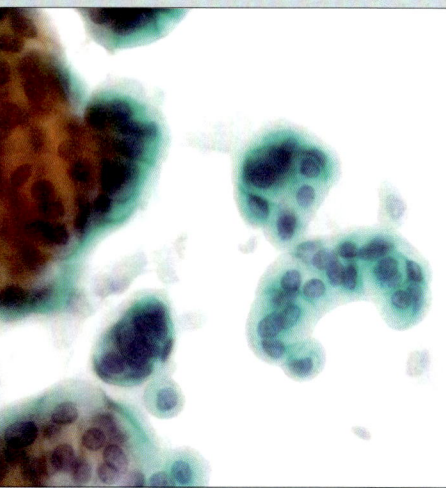

(Left) The nuclei within the clusters are centrally placed and show bland, even chromatin on this Pap stain. (Right) There is no clumpy chromatin or irregularity of nuclear membranes on this Pap stain. Ample cytoplasm is seen with an N:C ratio < 0.5. The individual cells in the background have similar features.

Reactive Urothelial Changes

ETIOLOGY/PATHOGENESIS

Most Common Causes
- Stones, instrumentation, &/or radiation/chemotherapy

CYTOPATHOLOGY

Background
- Normal urothelium

Cells
- Most cells seen are urothelial in origin, though radiation may involve some stromal cells if there is ulcer

Stones and Instrumentation
- High cellularity
- Urothelial cells are arranged in tight papillary-like groups (often large and numerous)
  - These lack fibrovascular cores
- Usually round nuclei, centrally placed with minimal pleomorphism
- Minimal nuclear membrane irregularity
- Fine, even chromatin, but there can be some hyperchromasia
- Normal-sized nuclei, but nuclear:cytoplasmic (N:C) ratio can be increased
  - N:C ratio should be < 0.5 in most instances
- Nucleoli can be prominent
- Squamous metaplastic cells may be seen

Radiation and Chemotherapy
- Normocellular or hypocellular specimens with rare affected cells scattered amongst normal urothelium
- Cells affected by radiation/chemotherapy appear as single cells or in small groups
  - Bizarre arrangements of cell groups are sometimes present
- Nucleomegaly, but because overall cell size is increased as well, there is no increased N:C ratio
- Chromatin can be coarse
  - Some membrane irregularity may be present
- Nucleoli can be prominent
- Multinucleation may occur
- Can demonstrate cytoplasmic vacuoles, often degenerative
- Polychromasia may be present

DIFFERENTIAL DIAGNOSIS

High-Grade Urothelial Carcinoma
- Demonstrates more single cells, higher N:C ratios, more nuclear hyperchromasia, and greater degree of nuclear membrane and chromatin irregularity
- Smaller cells with higher N:C ratios than bizarre cells produced by radiation/chemotherapy
- History of radiation/chemotherapy is helpful to avoid overinterpretation of reactive changes

Low-Grade Papillary Urothelial Neoplasm
- Generally, stones, instrumentation, and low-grade papillary urothelial neoplasms all show similar features
  - All should be called negative for high-grade urothelial carcinoma
  - Presence of true fibrovascular cores is only reliable indicator of papillary neoplasm

DIAGNOSTIC CHECKLIST

Pathologic Interpretation Pearls
- Features secondary to stones or instrumentation overlap with features of low-grade papillary urothelial neoplasms
  - In Paris System, this is less problematic than in past because both are in negative for high-grade urothelial carcinoma category
- Large atypical cells with abundant cytoplasm should prompt investigation of history to rule out radiation change before rendering interpretation of atypical

SELECTED REFERENCES
1. McLoughlin LC et al: The prognostic value of urinary cytology after trimodal therapy (TMT) for muscle-invasive bladder cancer. Urol Oncol. ePub, 2022
2. Bakkar R et al: Impact of the Paris System for reporting urine cytopathology on predictive values of the equivocal diagnostic categories and interobserver agreement. Cytojournal. 16:21, 2019

Radiation Changes
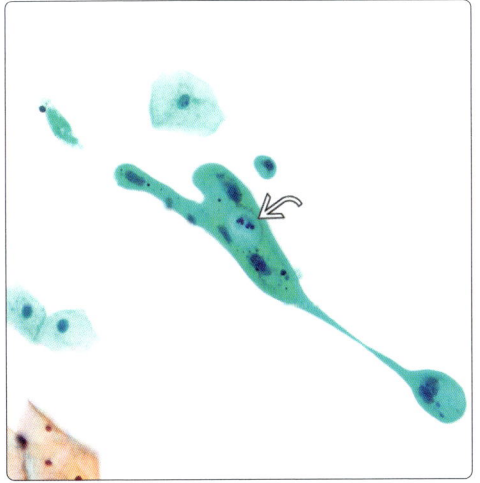

Chemotherapy Changes
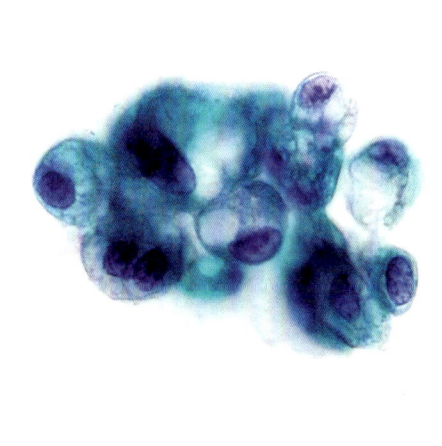

(Left) Radiation can produce bizarre cell shapes. There is nuclear hyperchromasia but a low N:C ratio. A cytoplasmic vacuole ➡ is present in this Pap stain. (Right) These Pap-stained urothelial cells from a patient undergoing chemotherapy show numerous cytoplasmic vacuoles. The nuclei are somewhat irregular, but overall, the appearance of the cells is benign with a low N:C ratio.

Low-Grade Urothelial Lesions

KEY FACTS

TERMINOLOGY
- Includes low-grade papillary urothelial carcinoma, papillary urothelial neoplasm of low malignant potential, urothelial papilloma, and low-grade dysplasia

CLINICAL ISSUES
- Low-grade lesions can be seen by cystoscopy, making identification by cytologists unnecessary
- Good prognosis, rarely progresses to high-grade lesion

CYTOPATHOLOGY
- Visualization of true fibrovascular core is needed for diagnosis
- Numerous, tightly cohesive papillary groups are present, often with irregular contours at periphery
- Single cells may be present, but nuclear criteria for high-grade carcinoma are absent
- Monotonous cells with increased N:C ratios
- Cercariform cells with eccentric nuclei and elongated cytoplasm may be seen
- Fine, even chromatin with, at most, mild hyperchromasia
- Nuclear membrane irregularity may be increased
- Often high cellularity, especially on washings, but can be normocellular

TOP DIFFERENTIAL DIAGNOSES
- High-grade urothelial carcinoma
  - Higher N:C ratio (> 0.7), darker hyperchromasia, greater nuclear membrane irregularity, coarse clumpy chromatin
- Urolithiasis/instrumentation
  - Numerous papillary clusters of urothelial cells showing minimal nuclear pleomorphism, fine, even chromatin, and minimal nuclear membrane irregularity

DIAGNOSTIC CHECKLIST
- Possible low-grade lesions without fibrovascular cores should be classified as negative; however, comment may be included, raising possibility of low-grade neoplasm

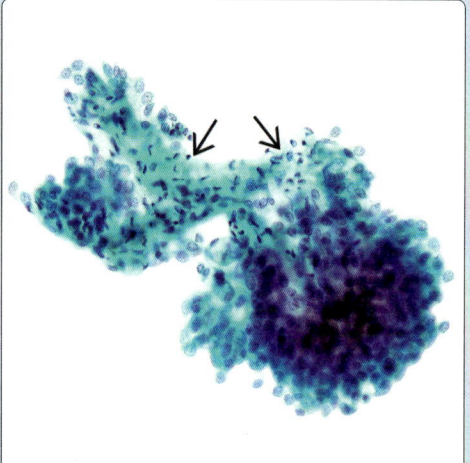

Low-Grade Urothelial Neoplasm

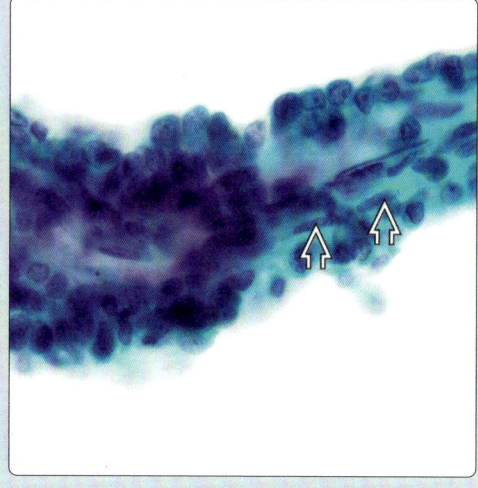

Fibrovascular Core

(Left) *This cluster of urothelial cells qualifies for a diagnosis of low-grade urothelial neoplasm due to the presence of true fibrovascular cores ➡ that confirm that the fragment derives from a papillary lesion.* (Right) *This cluster of urothelial cells from a ThinPrep specimen has a central fibrovascular core. Numerous endothelial cells ➡ are seen, confirming the presence of a vessel. Also note the increased N:C ratio and mild nuclear contour irregularities of the urothelial cells.*

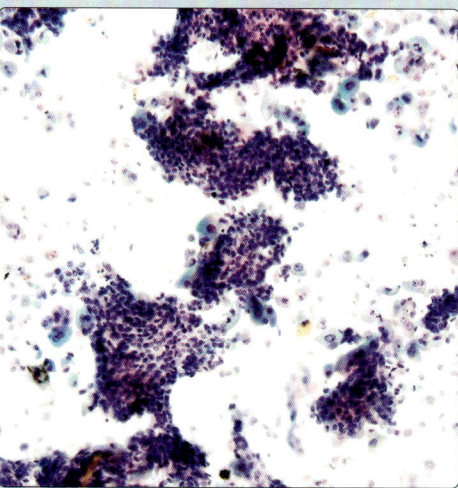

Large, Irregular Clusters

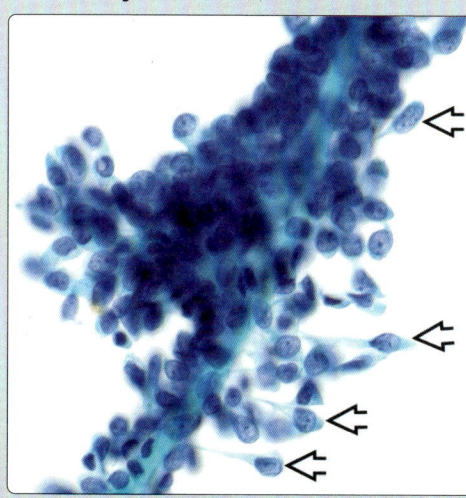

Loosely Attached Cercariform Cells

(Left) *The presence of numerous large, irregular clusters of urothelial cells, such as those seen in this Pap-stained cytospin, suggests the possibility of a low-grade urothelial neoplasm. However, in the absence of fibrovascular cores, such a specimen should be called negative.* (Right) *This ThinPrep prepared from a renal pelvis brushing of a low-grade papillary urothelial carcinoma shows cercariform cells ➡ with elongated cytoplasmic processes and mildly pleomorphic nuclei attached to a central fibrovascular core.*

Atypical Urothelial Cells

KEY FACTS

TERMINOLOGY
- Atypical urothelial cells (AUC) is interpretive category of Paris System for reporting urinary cytology
- By definition, AUC requires increased N:C ratio (≥ 0.5) due to nuclear enlargement + at least 1 of following
  - Nuclear hyperchromasia
  - Irregular nuclear membranes
  - Irregular, coarse, clumped chromatin

CLINICAL ISSUES
- AUC will precede diagnosis of high-grade urothelial carcinoma (HGUC) in 1/4-1/2 of cases
- Many AUC correspond to benign reactive changes

MICROSCOPIC
- High N:C ratio, at least 0.5, attributable to nuclear enlargement
- Additional nuclear changes that may or may not be present (≥ 1 required)
  - Increased chromatin content resulting in dark staining
  - Contour irregularities with variably thickened rim
  - Coarse, clumpy, asymmetric chromatin
- Degenerative changes may contribute to diagnostic uncertainty, leading to AUC interpretation

ANCILLARY TESTS
- UroVysion FISH testing is most common triage test

TOP DIFFERENTIAL DIAGNOSES
- HGUC or suspicious for HGUC
  - If N:C ratio exceeds 0.7 and all nuclear features are present, 1 of these interpretations should be used
- Reactive changes
  - Many AUC will turn out to be of reactive origin
- Degenerative changes
  - Degeneration, in and of itself, does not constitute atypia

Atypia in Inflammatory Background

Rare Atypical Cells

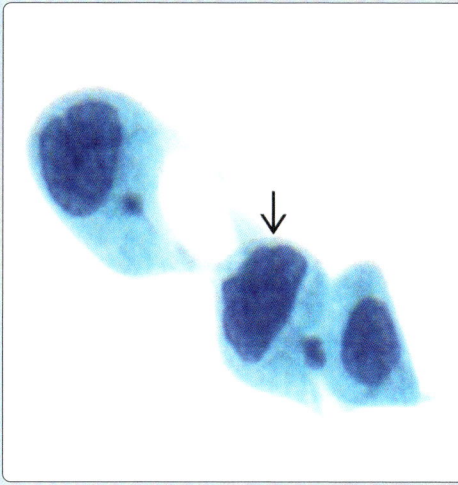

(Left) These atypical urothelial cells in a Pap-stained cytospin are in an acute inflammatory context. The nuclei are large and irregular with clumpy chromatin with at least 1 cell appearing to have an N:C ratio of 0.5 ➡. The findings are concerning for high-grade urothelial carcinoma (HGUC), but no cells have an N:C ratio approaching 0.7. (Right) This ThinPrep urine specimen contains only rare atypical cells. The nuclei are markedly irregular. The cell in the center ➡ has an N:C ratio of ~ 0.5, but none approach 0.7.

Atypical Cells in Cluster

Atypia in Context of Degeneration

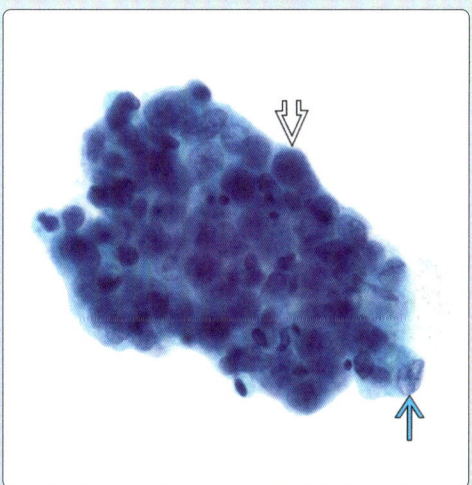
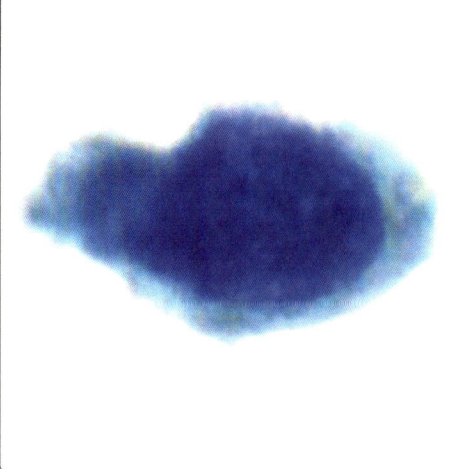

(Left) This group of atypical cells in a Pap test shows nuclear enlargement ➡ and nuclear contour irregularities ➡ in cells at the periphery. The N:C ratio is difficult to assess in this context, but some cells appear to be 0.5-0.7. (Right) This cell in a Pap-stained cytospin shows a very large, dark, irregular nucleus with an N:C ratio approaching 0.7. However, the chromatin appears smudgy, and the cytoplasm is ragged, indicating degeneration. In such cases, atypical urothelial cells are an appropriate interpretation.

High-Grade Urothelial Dysplasia/Carcinoma/Carcinoma In Situ

KEY FACTS

TERMINOLOGY
- Paris System cytologic category of high-grade urothelial carcinoma (HGUC) incorporates invasive carcinoma, high-grade papillary carcinoma, and carcinoma in situ

CLINICAL ISSUES
- 7th most common cancer worldwide
- More common in males, Whites, and smokers
- Usually presents after 60 years of age

CYTOPATHOLOGY
- Increased nuclear:cytoplasmic ratio (> 0.7)
- Nuclear hyperchromasia, irregular nuclear membranes, and coarsely granular chromatin should also be present
- Pleomorphism, nucleoli, and mitoses may be present
- Single cells and loosely cohesive clusters
- Typically high cellularity (at least 5-10 malignant cells needed for diagnosis)

TOP DIFFERENTIAL DIAGNOSES
- Low-grade urothelial lesions
  - Less pleomorphism, finer chromatin, less nuclear membrane irregularity, few/no single atypical cells, more papillary clusters
- Reactive/radiation/chemotherapy effect
  - Cells often have cytoplasmic and nuclear vacuolization
  - Often bizarre nuclear shapes with multinucleation
- Polyomavirus
  - "Decoy" cells are hyperchromatic but with smudgy or glassy look to nuclei
- Atypical urothelial cells or suspicious for HGUC
  - Atypical urothelial cells have lower nuclear:cytoplasmic ratio (> 0.5) and fewer/less-developed nuclear features
  - Suspicious for HGUC has similar criteria but lower cellularity (< 5-10 cells of interest)

Typical High-Grade Urothelial Carcinoma
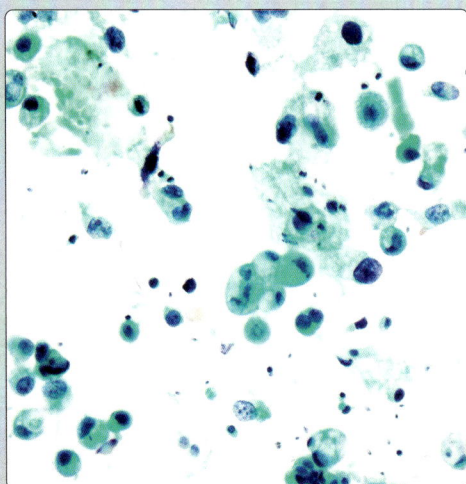

High-Grade Urothelial Carcinoma Cluster
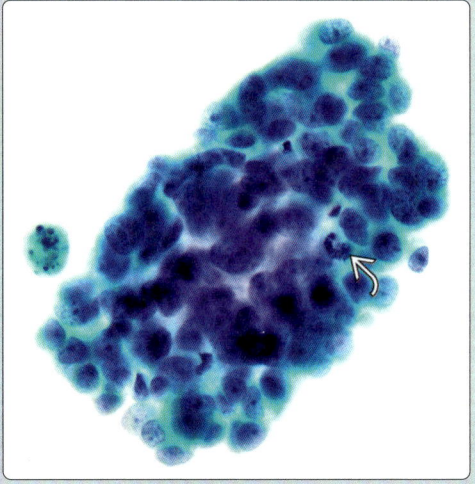

(Left) The presence of numerous, single, markedly atypical and pleomorphic cells, as seen in this Pap-stained slide, is a feature of malignancy and is not seen in low-grade lesions. Almost all of these cells are malignant. **(Right)** Pap-stained cluster of malignant cells shows nuclear hyperchromasia, irregular nuclear membranes, coarsely clumped chromatin, and high nuclear:cytoplasmic ratios (> 0.7). Prominent nucleoli are also seen. A mitotic figure is present ➡.

High-Power View of Nuclear Features
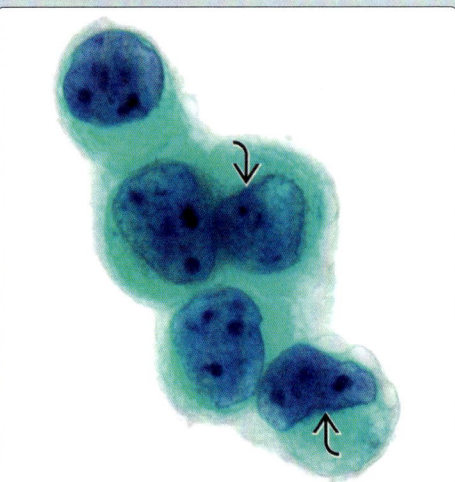

Hypo- and Hyperchromatic Nuclei
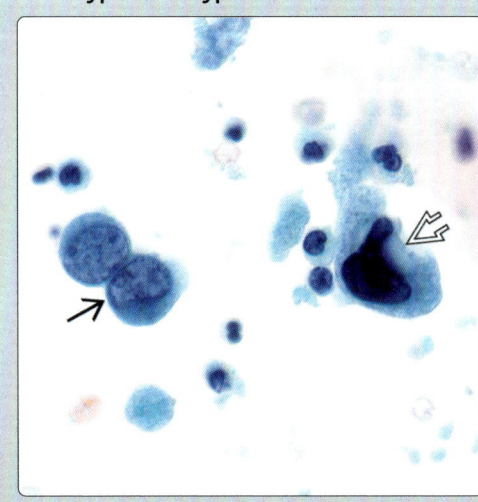

(Left) On this Pap stain under oil immersion, these malignant cells show irregular nuclear membranes and unevenly distributed clumpy chromatin. Note focal thickening of the nuclear membranes ➡. **(Right)** In this Pap-stained cytospin, malignant cells with hypochromatic nuclei that are large and irregular with high nuclear:cytoplasmic ratio are seen on the left ➡. Another malignant cell with nuclear hyperchromasia and a nucleus with a boomerang-like shape is seen on the right ➡.

High-Grade Urothelial Dysplasia/Carcinoma/Carcinoma In Situ

TERMINOLOGY

Abbreviations
- Paris System cytologic category of high-grade urothelial carcinoma (HGUC) incorporates invasive carcinoma, high-grade papillary carcinoma, and carcinoma in situ

CLINICAL ISSUES

Epidemiology
- Incidence
  - 7th most common cancer worldwide
  - More common in males, Whites, and smokers
    - Associated with schistosomiasis or occupational exposures in certain populations
- Age
  - Usually presents after 60 years

Treatment
- Various forms of intravesical therapy
  - Bacillus Calmette-Guérin is most common
- Cystectomy for muscle-invasive carcinoma

CYTOPATHOLOGY

Cellularity
- Typically high cellularity

Pattern
- Single cells and loosely cohesive clusters

Background
- Invasive tumors may show necrotic debris

Nuclear Details
- Increased nuclear:cytoplasmic ratio (> 0.7)
  - While in most cases, malignant cells meeting this criteria will be numerous, in some cases, only a few cells will meet this benchmark
- Hyperchromasia, irregular nuclear membranes, and coarsely granular chromatin should be present
- Pleomorphism, nucleoli, and mitoses may be present but are not morphologic criteria key to diagnosis
- Hypochromatic nuclei may be seen in some cases, which are usually but not always in minority of malignant cells

Cytoplasmic Details
- Cytoplasm is generally homogeneous

ANCILLARY TESTS

Immunohistochemistry
- hTERT staining shows promise as alternative method for morphologic detection of urothelial carcinoma

In Situ Hybridization
- UroVysion FISH analysis detects chromosomal aberrations commonly associated with urothelial carcinoma

DIFFERENTIAL DIAGNOSIS

Low-Grade Urothelial Lesions
- Less pleomorphism, finer chromatin, less nuclear membrane irregularity, few/no single atypical cells, more papillary clusters

Reactive/Radiation/Chemotherapy Effect
- Cells often have intracytoplasmic and nuclear vacuolization
- Often bizarre nuclear shapes with multinucleation

Polyomavirus
- "Decoy" cells are hyperchromatic but with smudgy or glassy look to nuclei

Atypical Urothelial Cells or Suspicious for High-Grade Urothelial Carcinoma
- If less well-developed features &/or lower cellularity, consider indeterminate categories

SELECTED REFERENCES
1. Wojcik EM et al: We'll always have Paris: the Paris System for reporting urinary cytology 2022. J Am Soc Cytopathol. 11(2):62-6, 2022
2. Renshaw AA et al: High-grade urothelial carcinoma with hypochromatic chromatin in urine cytology. J Am Soc Cytopathol. 10(1):25-8, 2021

Marked Pleomorphism
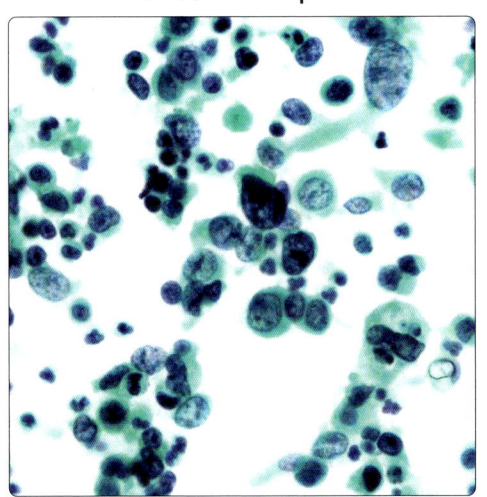

Clumpy Chromatin
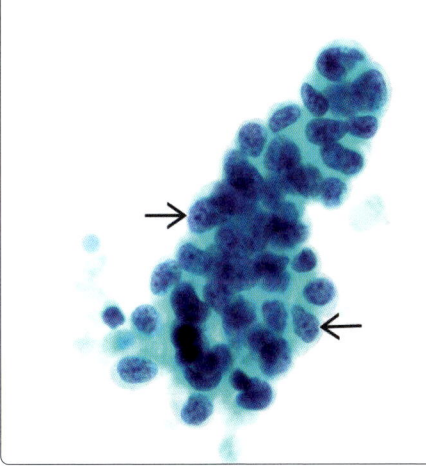

(Left) On this Pap stain, the malignant nuclei demonstrate marked pleomorphism, hyperchromasia, and membrane irregularity. (Right) These cells depict the coarsely granular chromatin ⮕ classically described as a feature of malignancy. Note the nuclear pleomorphism and the presence of nuclear:cytoplasmic ratios > 0.7 in some of the cells.

Squamous Cell Carcinoma of Urinary Bladder

KEY FACTS

TERMINOLOGY
- Definition: Malignant epithelial neoplasm of bladder with pure squamous cell phenotype

ETIOLOGY/PATHOGENESIS
- Chronic inflammatory conditions with squamous metaplasia are risk factors
  - Schistosoma infection is principal risk factor in endemic areas
  - Other risk factors include stones, chronic indwelling catheters, neurogenic bladder, and chronic cyclophosphamide treatment
- Associated with tobacco smoking

CLINICAL ISSUES
- Varies with geographic region (incidence higher in areas of endemic schistosomiasis)
  - 5% of bladder tumors in USA
  - 75% of bladder tumors in Egypt and Sudan
- Radical cystectomy is standard therapy, often in conjunction with radiation

CYTOPATHOLOGY
- Hyperchromasia and pleomorphism
- Irregular, often sharply angulated nuclear shapes
- May show prominent nucleoli
- Most squamous carcinomas are keratinizing, so cytoplasm is often orangeophilic and dense
- Similar in appearance to keratinizing squamous cell carcinoma of other sites

TOP DIFFERENTIAL DIAGNOSES
- Invasive urothelial carcinoma
  - Urothelial carcinoma with focal squamous differentiation is much more common except in areas with endemic schistosomiasis
- Secondary squamous cell carcinoma
  - Consider anal or cervical primary; HPV testing may be helpful

Orangeophilic Cytoplasm
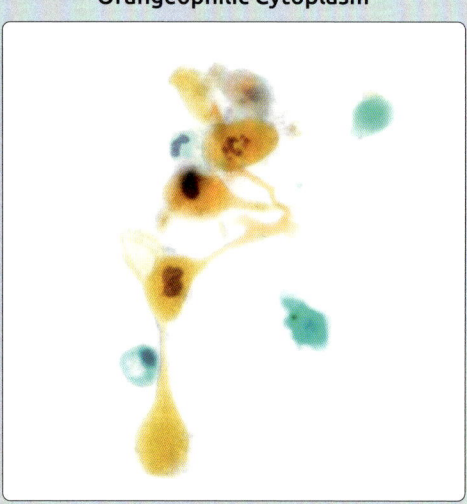

Nuclear Pleomorphism
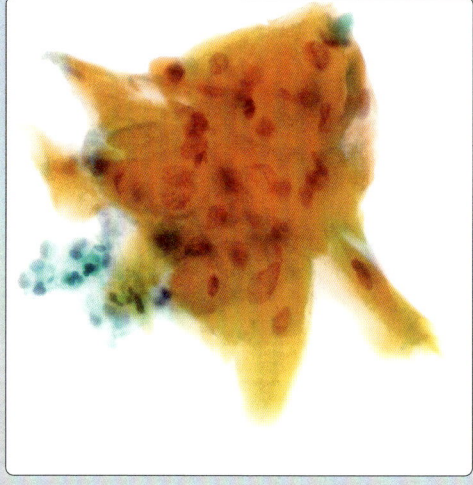

(Left) Pap-stained cells show hyperchromasia and angular nuclear membranes. The cytoplasm is densely orangeophilic. (Right) Cells on this Pap stain of squamous cell carcinoma (SqCa) demonstrate pleomorphism, nuclear overlapping, and irregular nuclear membranes.

Angulated Nucleus
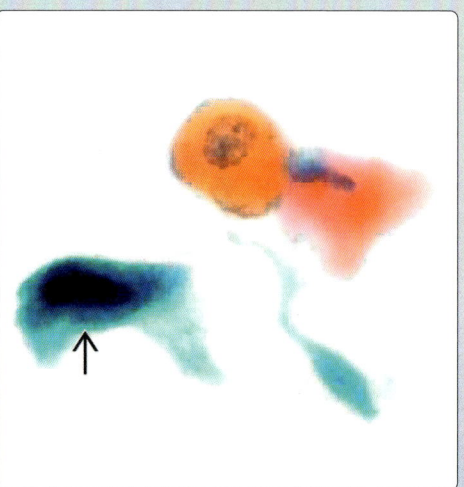

Abundant Cytoplasm
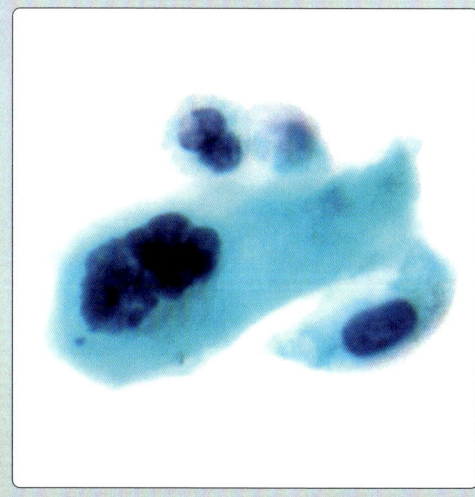

(Left) This markedly atypical nonkeratinized cell ➡ shows nuclear hyperchromasia with sharp angulation of the nucleus on Pap stain. (Right) SqCa cell shows very abundant cytoplasm, but still can be recognized as malignant due to the markedly atypical nuclear features. SqCa of the bladder often do not show the high nuclear:cytoplasmic ratios typical of urothelial carcinomas.

Squamous Cell Carcinoma of Urinary Bladder

TERMINOLOGY

Abbreviations
- Squamous cell carcinoma (SqCa)

Definitions
- Malignant epithelial neoplasm of bladder with pure squamous cell phenotype

ETIOLOGY/PATHOGENESIS

Developmental Anomaly
- Bladder exstrophy

Environmental Exposure
- Associated with tobacco smoking

Infectious Agents
- Chronic inflammatory conditions with squamous metaplasia are risk factors
- Strongly associated with schistosomal infection
  o Other chronic bladder infections are also associated with increased risk
- HPV association is probably very rare

CLINICAL ISSUES

Epidemiology
- Incidence
  o Varies by geographic region (incidence higher in areas with endemic schistosomiasis)
    – 5% of bladder tumors in USA
    – 75% in Egypt/Sudan (bladder cancer represents 1/3 of all cancers in Egypt)

Treatment
- Surgical approaches
  o Radical cystectomy is standard therapy
- Adjuvant therapy
  o Often have neoadjuvant or adjuvant radiation

Prognosis
- Poor prognosis

CYTOPATHOLOGY

Nuclear Details
- Hyperchromasia and pleomorphism
- Irregular, often sharply angulated shapes
- May show prominent nucleoli

Cytoplasmic Details
- Most SqCa is keratinizing, so cytoplasm is often orangeophilic and dense

DIFFERENTIAL DIAGNOSIS

Invasive Urothelial Carcinoma With Squamous Differentiation
- Associated component of urothelial carcinoma

Keratinizing Squamous Metaplasia
- No overtly malignant features

Direct Extension of Squamous Cell Carcinoma From Adjacent Organs
- May be morphologically identical to primary vesical SqCa
- Consider cervical or anal primary

DIAGNOSTIC CHECKLIST

Pathologic Interpretation Pearls
- Poorly differentiated urothelial carcinoma can show squamous differentiation, so carcinoma must be of pure squamous cytology to classify as primary SqCa
- Direct extension of SqCa or contamination from gynecologic source will show similar features; clinical history is key; HPV testing may be helpful

SELECTED REFERENCES

1. Collins K et al: Prevalence of high-risk human papillomavirus in primary squamous cell carcinoma of urinary bladder. Pathol Res Pract. 216(9):153084, 2020

Squamous Carcinoma Without Orangophilia

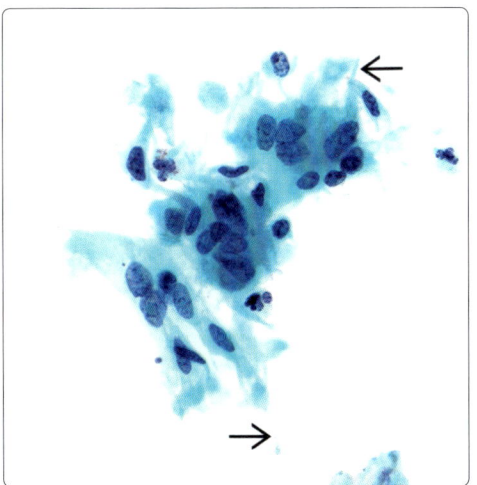

Urothelial Carcinoma With Squamous Differentiation

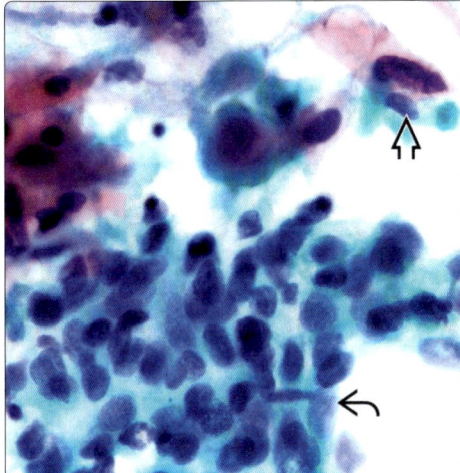

(Left) This example of SqCa of the bladder shows typical dense cytoplasm with slender cytoplasmic extensions ⟶ but lacks staining with the Orange G component of the Pap stain, making appreciation of the squamous differentiation more difficult. (Right) Pap stain shows conventional urothelial carcinoma ⟶ with focal squamous differentiation ⟶. This would not qualify as SqCa.

Adenocarcinoma of Urinary Bladder

KEY FACTS

ETIOLOGY/PATHOGENESIS
- Associated with exstrophy, metaplasia, nonfunctioning bladder, chronic irritation, obstruction, endometriosis, *Schistosoma haematobium*

CLINICAL ISSUES
- Rare primary bladder neoplasm (< 2% of bladder malignancies)

IMAGING
- Lesion arising in dome may represent urachal carcinoma

CYTOPATHOLOGY
- Vesicular chromatin with prominent nucleoli
- Vacuolated cytoplasm
  - May contain intracytoplasmic mucin vacuoles
- Malignant cells may have glandular pattern or be individual signet-ring cells
- Background mucin may be prominent

MICROSCOPIC
- Bladder adenocarcinoma may have enteric, colloid, signet-ring, hepatoid, mixed, or other nonspecific morphologies
- Very rare clear cell adenocarcinoma resembles müllerian counterpart

TOP DIFFERENTIAL DIAGNOSES
- Direct invasion by prostatic adenocarcinoma
- Direct invasion or metastatic colorectal adenocarcinoma
- Metastatic adenocarcinoma from other sites (kidney, ovary, breast, lung, stomach)
- Urothelial carcinoma with glandular differentiation
- Cystitis glandularis

DIAGNOSTIC CHECKLIST
- Primary adenocarcinoma of bladder is extremely rare
- Possibility of origin from distant or contiguous anatomic site should be carefully considered before diagnosis is rendered

Adenocarcinoma Cluster and Single Cell
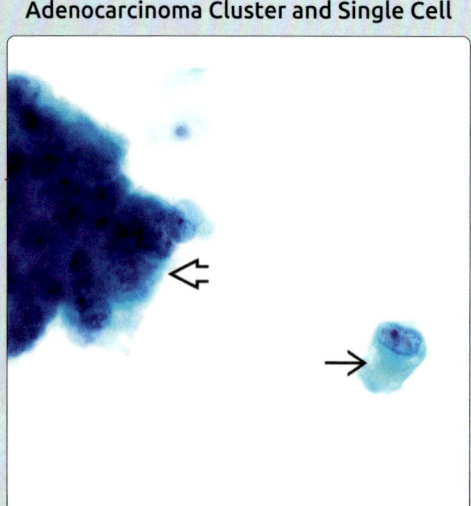

Prominent Nucleoli
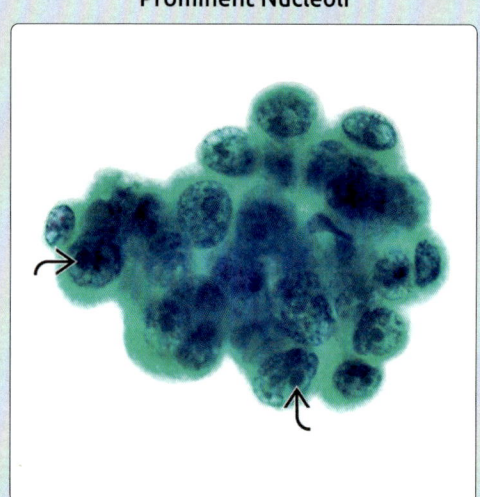

(Left) Adenocarcinoma may be present as single cells or in cohesive clusters ➡, as seen in this Pap-stained slide. The single cell shows some cytoplasmic vacuolization ➡. (Right) These urothelial adenocarcinoma cells demonstrate vesicular chromatin with prominent nucleoli ➡ on Pap stain.

Adenocarcinoma Cells
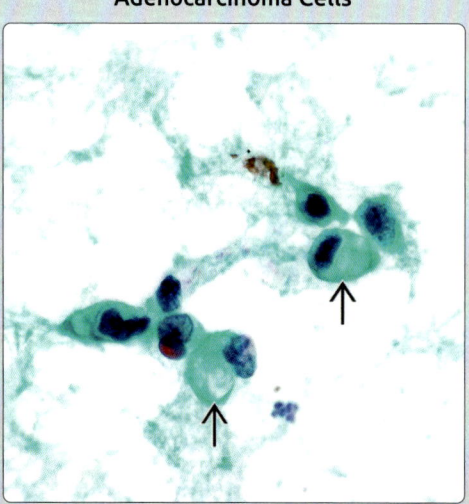

Mucin Vacuole
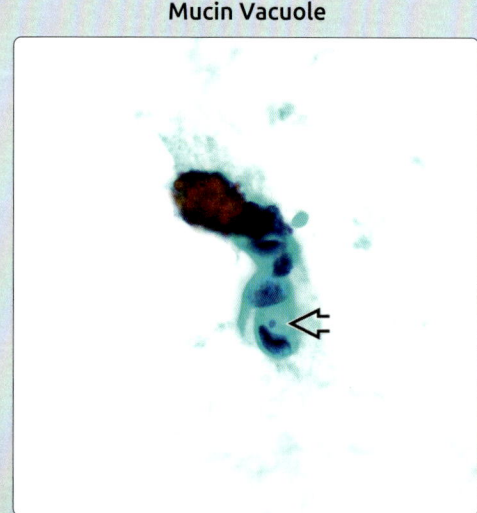

(Left) Urothelial adenocarcinoma shows individual cells with vacuolated cytoplasm ➡ and markedly irregular, pleomorphic nuclei on Pap stain. Note also the background debris. (Right) Adenocarcinoma cell on Pap stain shows a prominent intracytoplasmic mucin vacuole ➡ imparting a signet-ring cell appearance.

Adenocarcinoma of Urinary Bladder

TERMINOLOGY

Definitions
- Primary gland-forming carcinoma of urinary bladder not associated with urothelial or squamous carcinoma component

ETIOLOGY/PATHOGENESIS

Developmental and Acquired
- Exstrophy, metaplasia, nonfunctioning bladder, chronic irritation, obstruction, endometriosis, *Schistosoma haematobium*

CLINICAL ISSUES

Epidemiology
- Incidence
  - Rare primary bladder neoplasm (< 2% of bladder malignancies)

Presentation
- Hematuria is most common, also dysuria
  - Rarely mucusuria

CYTOPATHOLOGY

Pattern
- Malignant cells may have glandular pattern or be individual signet-ring cells

Background
- Mucin may be prominent, especially in colloid carcinoma variants

Nuclear Details
- Vesicular chromatin with prominent nucleoli

Cytoplasmic Details
- Vacuolated cytoplasm
  - May contain intracytoplasmic mucin vacuoles

MICROSCOPIC

Histologic Features
- Bladder adenocarcinoma may have enteric, colloid, signet-ring, hepatoid, mixed, or other nonspecific morphologies
- Very rare clear cell adenocarcinoma resembles müllerian counterpart

DIFFERENTIAL DIAGNOSIS

Direct Invasion by Prostatic Adenocarcinoma
- More common than primary adenocarcinoma
- Monomorphic round nuclei with prominent nucleoli suggest prostate origin
- Often expresses *NKX3.1*, PSA, and PAP
  - Primary bladder adenocarcinoma may express PAP

Direct Invasion or Metastatic Colorectal Adenocarcinoma
- May be cytologically indistinguishable from bladder primary
- Immunocytochemistry also overlaps: CK20 and CDX2 are often positive in primary bladder adenocarcinoma
- Colonoscopy is often required for more definitive distinction

Other Metastatic Adenocarcinoma
- Gastric signet-ring cell and ovarian serous and clear cell carcinomas may be indistinguishable morphologically

Extensive Cystitis Glandularis
- Distinguished by bland nuclear features

Invasive Urothelial Carcinoma With Glandular Differentiation
- Identifiable component of typical urothelial carcinoma rules out adenocarcinoma

SELECTED REFERENCES
1. Manini C et al: Unusual faces of bladder cancer. Cancers (Basel). 12(12), 2020
2. Lin X et al: Importance of identification of prostatic adenocarcinoma in urine cytology. J Am Soc Cytopathol. 7(5):268-73, 2018

High-Grade Prostatic Adenocarcinoma

Bland Prostatic Adenocarcinoma

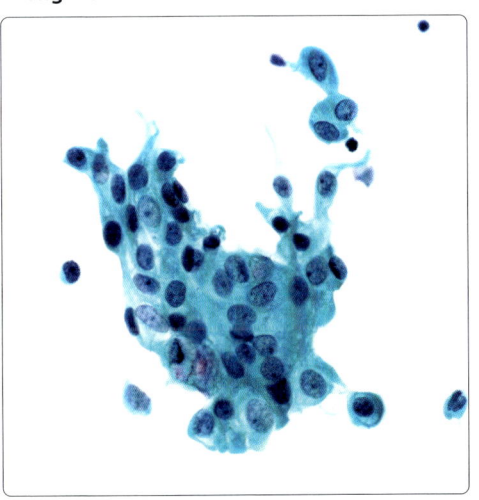
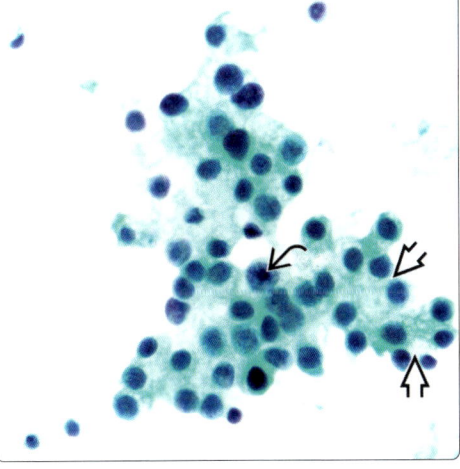

(Left) Gleason 4+5 prostatic adenocarcinoma invasive into the bladder, seen on Pap stain, demonstrates the degree to which extrinsic malignancies can mimic primary adenocarcinoma. History and immunocytochemistry are key to diagnosis. *(Right)* Pap stain of prostatic adenocarcinoma in a urine specimen shows little nuclear pleomorphism but prominent nucleoli ➡. An acinar pattern ➡ can be appreciated. Cells such as these can easily be misinterpreted as benign.

Other Malignancies in Urinary Cytology

KEY FACTS

CLINICAL ISSUES
- Primary small cell carcinoma is rare (< 1% of all bladder malignancies)
- Urinary tract may also be involved by metastasis (breast, lung, melanoma) or direct extension (kidney, prostate, ovary, cervix, large bowel)
- Renal cell carcinoma seldom appears in urine despite proximity to urinary tract

CYTOPATHOLOGY
- Small cell carcinoma: Cohesive, hyperchromatic nuclei with molding; high nuclear:cytoplasmic ratio
- Kidney: Open chromatin, prominent nucleoli, little pleomorphism, vacuolated cytoplasm
- Melanoma: Often vesicular chromatin with prominent nucleoli; pigment is characteristic but not always present
- Extrinsic adenocarcinoma: Variable appearance depending on type but often prominent nucleoli and vacuolated cytoplasm

TOP DIFFERENTIAL DIAGNOSES
- Small cell carcinoma: Resembles small cell carcinoma of other sites; necrosis present; neuroendocrine markers and sometimes TTF-1 (+)
- Renal cell carcinoma: May be associated with capillaries; PAX8(+)
- Prostate adenocarcinoma: Monotonous bland nuclei, prominent nucleoli, acinar formation; PSA and PAP (+)
- Colorectal adenocarcinoma: Round or elongated, cigar-shaped, hyperchromatic nuclei; necrosis; CDX2 and villin (+), CK7(-); CK20(+) in both colorectal and urothelial carcinomas
- Melanoma: Often dyshesive; melanin pigment may be absent; nuclei may show typical features of melanomas elsewhere; S100, HMB-45, and Melan-A (+)

DIAGNOSTIC CHECKLIST
- Clinical and radiologic correlation is key to correctly identifying these rare nonurothelial tumors

Small Cell Carcinoma of Bladder
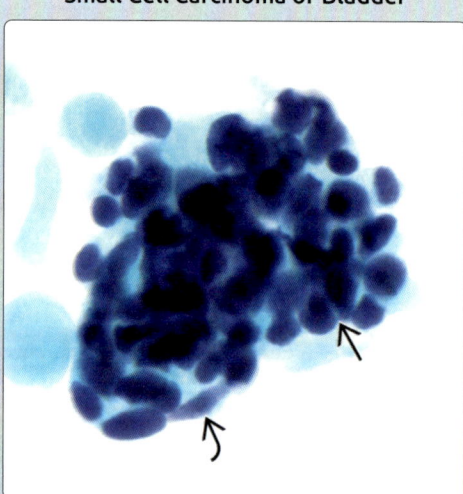

Small Cell Carcinoma at Low Power
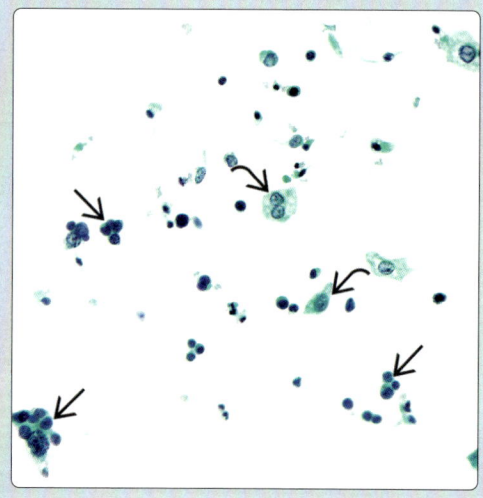

(Left) Cluster of small cell carcinoma cells on a ThinPrep demonstrates marked hyperchromasia and scant cytoplasm. Nuclear molding ⇨ and carrot-shaped nuclei ⇨ can be appreciated. *(Right)* Small hyperchromatic cells from a small cell carcinoma ⇨ of the bladder are seen scattered between non-neoplastic urothelial cells ⇨ in this Pap stain.

Prostate Carcinoma in ThinPrep of Urine
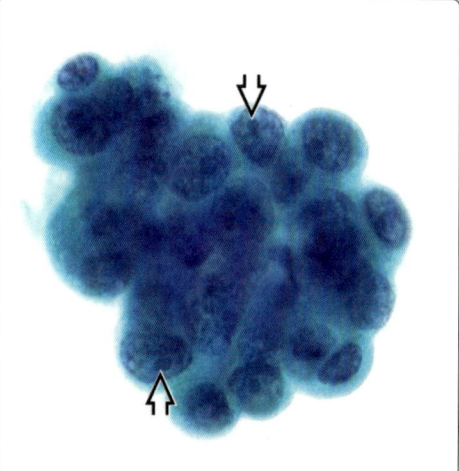

Prostate Carcinoma in Cytospin
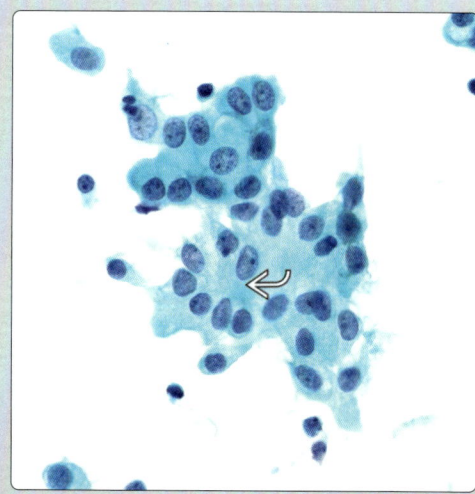

(Left) This cluster of malignant cells in a ThinPrep from a voided urine of a patient with prostatic adenocarcinoma involving the urethra shows cells with clumpy chromatin, prominent nucleoli ⇨, and vacuolated cytoplasm. *(Right)* This cluster of prostatic adenocarcinoma cells that shed into the urine shows acinar architecture ⇨, abundant cytoplasm, and nuclei with prominent nucleoli and little nuclear pleomorphism, all seen distinctly in this Pap-stained cytospin preparation.

Other Malignancies in Urinary Cytology

CLINICAL ISSUES

Presentation
- Primary small cell carcinoma is rare (< 1% of all bladder malignancies)
- Urinary tract may also be involved by metastasis (breast, lung, melanoma) or direct extension (kidney, prostate, ovary, cervix, large bowel)
- Renal cell carcinoma seldom appears in urine despite proximity to urinary tract

CYTOPATHOLOGY

Nuclear Details
- Small cell carcinoma: Cohesive, hyperchromatic nuclei with molding; high nuclear:cytoplasmic ratio
- Kidney: Open chromatin, prominent nucleoli, little pleomorphism
- Melanoma: Often vesicular chromatin with prominent nucleoli
- Extrinsic adenocarcinoma: Variable appearance depending on type but often prominent nucleoli

Cytoplasmic Details
- Melanoma: Pigment may be present
- Adenocarcinomas in general demonstrate finely vacuolated or foamy cytoplasm

Cell Block Findings
- Perform cell blocks for immunohistochemical staining

DIFFERENTIAL DIAGNOSIS

Urothelial Carcinoma
- Much more common, must be ruled out before diagnosis of one of these rare tumors

Small Cell Carcinoma
- May coexist with typical urothelial carcinoma
- Resembles small cell carcinoma of other sites
- Abundant necrosis in background

Renal Cell Carcinoma
- Open chromatin; nucleoli may be prominent
- Fine, wispy, or vacuolated cytoplasm
- May be associated with transgressing capillaries

Prostate Adenocarcinoma
- Often little nuclear pleomorphism
- Prominent nucleoli, acinar formation
- PSA and PAP (+)

Colorectal Adenocarcinoma
- Round or elongated, hyperchromatic nuclei; necrosis

Breast Adenocarcinoma
- Cohesive or dyshesive; may show little pleomorphism with bland, small, plasmacytoid nuclei
- May show intracytoplasmic mucin

Pulmonary Adenocarcinoma
- Nuclear pleomorphism, prominent nucleoli

Ovarian Adenocarcinoma
- Often highly pleomorphic nuclei, prominent nucleoli, vacuolated cytoplasm, psammoma bodies

Cervical Squamous Cell Carcinoma
- Often poorly differentiated

Melanoma
- Often dyshesive
- Melanin pigment may be absent
- Nuclei may show typical features of melanomas elsewhere

Lymphoma
- Dyshesive cells, high nuclear:cytoplasmic ratio

SELECTED REFERENCES

1. AbdullGaffar B et al: The value of intercluster single cell streaks, triplet signet ring cells, and a two-cell population in urine small cell neuroendocrine carcinoma. Cytopathology. 32(5):700-4, 2021
2. Lin X et al: Importance of identification of prostatic adenocarcinoma in urine cytology. J Am Soc Cytopathol. 7(5):268-73, 2018

Renal Cell Carcinoma in Voided Urine

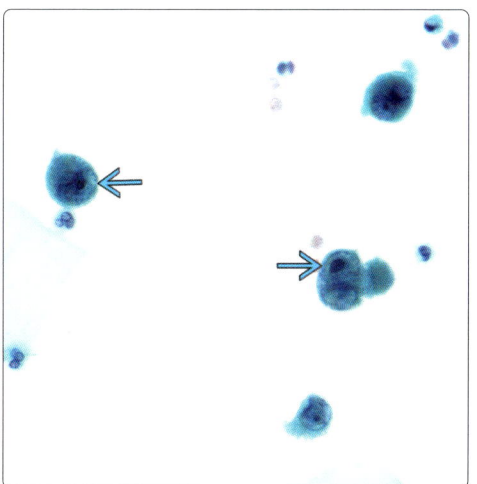

Renal Cell Carcinoma With Vessels

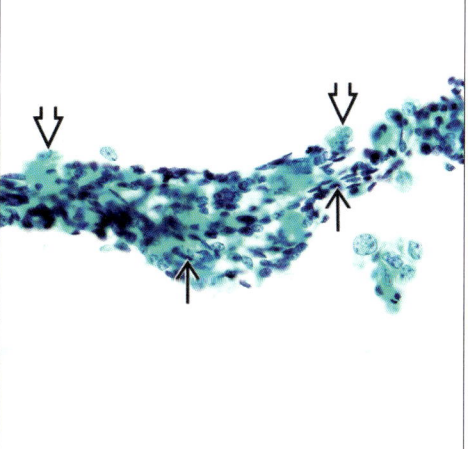

(Left) In this Pap-stained voided urine specimen, degenerated cells derived from a renal cell carcinoma can be seen, an uncommon finding even in patients with a kidney mass. Note the prominent nucleoli in large nuclei ➡ and vacuolated cytoplasm. (Right) Rounded tumor cells ➡ intimately associated with small, elongated endothelial cells ➡ suggest renal cell carcinoma on this Pap stain of a renal pelvis brushing.

Renal Pelvic Cytology

KEY FACTS

CLINICAL ISSUES

- Useful for investigation of filling defects seen on pyelogram
  o Both stones and tumors can cause filling defects
  o Surveillance of low-grade lesions of renal pelvis
- Ureteropyeloscopic brushings and washings allow sampling of lesions deep in renal pelvis or in calyceal system (areas not easily accessed with biopsy forceps)
  o Allows urologist to localize lesions and sample appropriate areas
- Bilateral washings may be performed with normal side serving as control for comparison

MICROSCOPIC

- Samples from renal pelvis often show greater baseline atypia than seen in other specimens from urinary tract
- Urothelial cells often smaller with slightly higher nuclear:cytoplasmic (N:C) ratio
- Brushings and washings of renal pelvis often more cellular than bladder washings
- Entities encountered in renal pelvis
  o Instrumentation/stone/reactive atypia
    – Cohesive clusters with smooth contours, ± papillary-like architecture
    – Minimal nuclear membrane irregularities, smooth, evenly distributed chromatin; may have prominent nucleoli
  o Low-grade urothelial neoplasms
    – Fibrovascular cores needed for identification
  o High-grade urothelial carcinoma
    – Diagnosed using same criteria as in bladder
    – At least 10 cells meeting criteria needed for positive diagnosis because all renal pelvis specimens instrumented
  o Renal cell carcinoma

ANCILLARY TESTS

- FISH or other genetic testing may be useful in indeterminate specimens, similar to bladder washings

Atypical Cells in Renal Pelvis Washing

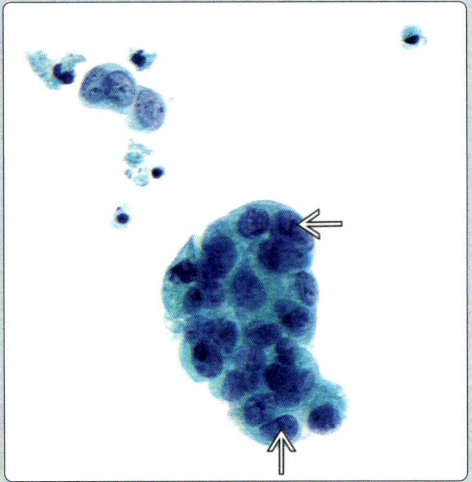

Cell Block of Renal Pelvis Mass

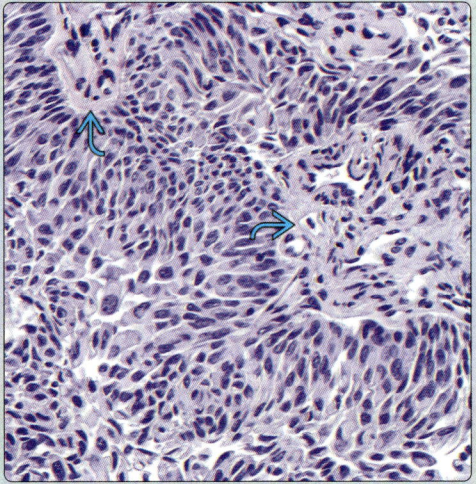

(Left) Pap-stained thin layer preparation of renal pelvis washing shows clusters of atypical urothelial cells with hyperchromatic nuclei and occasional prominent nucleoli ⇨. (Right) Corresponding cell block shows fibrovascular cores ⇨ as well as high grade cytologic features. The cell block helps to confirm the diagnosis of high grade urothelial carcinoma.

Urothelial Cell Cluster With Atypia

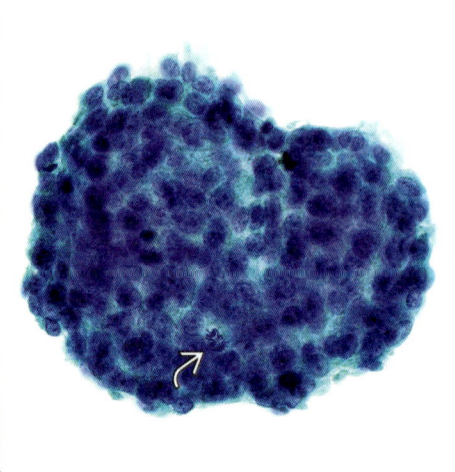

Fibrovascular Core on Cell Block

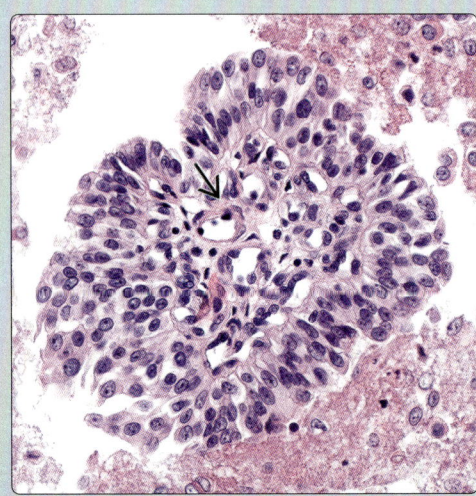

(Left) Pap-stained renal pelvis brushing shows a disorganized cluster of urothelial cells with an irregular border and mitotic activity ⇨. The findings are concerning for low-grade urothelial neoplasm, but that diagnosis requires a fibrovascular core. (Right) H&E-stained cell block section shows a papilla with a fibrovascular core ⇨, which is diagnostic for low-grade urothelial neoplasm. Cell blocks can be useful to confirm papillary cores in specimens with concerning filling defects.

Renal Pelvic Cytology

CLINICAL ISSUES

Indications
- Investigation of filling defects seen on pyelogram
  - Both stones and tumors can cause filling defects
- Surveillance of low-grade lesions of renal pelvis
- Surveillance of patients with history of urothelial neoplasia
  - Patients with history of urothelial carcinoma of bladder or ureter may be followed with repeat cytology

Methods for Sampling Renal Pelvis
- Ureteropyeloscopic brushings and washings
  - Allows sampling deep in renal pelvis or in calyceal system (areas not easily accessed with biopsy forceps)
  - Allows urologist to localize lesions and sample appropriate areas
  - Bilateral washings may be performed with normal side serving as control for comparison
- Percutaneous biopsy
  - May be performed under fluoroscopic guidance

MICROSCOPIC

Cytologic Features
- Increased baseline atypia
  - Samples from renal pelvis often show greater baseline atypia than seen in other specimens from urinary tract
  - Urothelial cells often smaller with slightly higher nuclear:cytoplasmic (N:C) ratio
- Increased cellularity
  - Brushings and washings of renal pelvis often more cellular than bladder washings

Entities Encountered in Renal Pelvis
- Instrumentation/stone/reactive atypia
  - Cohesive clusters with smooth contours, ± papillary-like architecture
  - Minimal nuclear membrane irregularities, smooth, evenly distributed chromatin; may have prominent nucleoli
  - Clusters may have peripheral collar of cytoplasm
  - Correlate with history of stones, instrumentation
- Low-grade urothelial neoplasms (LGUN)
  - More cellular specimen, but without high-grade nuclei
  - Cell clusters more frequent than reactive conditions
  - Not possible to distinguish from reactive atypia without fibrovascular cores, a rare finding
- High-grade urothelial carcinoma (HGUC)
  - Very cellular specimen, disorganized cell clusters, single intact atypical cells; at least 10 cells needed
  - High N:C ratio (> 0.7), irregular nuclei with coarse/clumped and hyperchromatic chromatin
  - Cells tend to have smaller nuclei and total diameter with less cytoplasm but should still meet Paris System criteria
  - Cellular changes not fully meeting criteria may be classified as "atypical urothelial cells" or "suspicious for HGUC," as in bladder
  - Due to lack of nonsurgical treatment options, interpretation should aim to maximize specificity; err on the side of "atypical" or "suspicious" rather than HGUC
  - Urothelial carcinoma may show squamous and glandular differentiation
- Renal cell carcinoma
  - May involve renal pelvis
  - Enlarged eccentric nuclei with prominent nucleoli and irregular chromatin
  - Delicate vacuolated cytoplasm may be stripped, leaving bare nuclei
  - Malignant cells dangling from delicate blood vessels
  - Hemorrhage and necrosis may be seen
- Squamous cell carcinoma
- Adenocarcinoma

ANCILLARY TESTS

Genetic Testing
- FISH or other genetic testing may be useful in indeterminate specimens, similar to bladder washings

SELECTED REFERENCES
1. McIntire PJ et al: High-grade urothelial carcinoma in urine cytology: different spaces - different faces, highlighting morphologic variance. J Am Soc Cytopathol. 10(1):36-40, 2021

Upper Tract High-Grade Urothelial Carcinoma

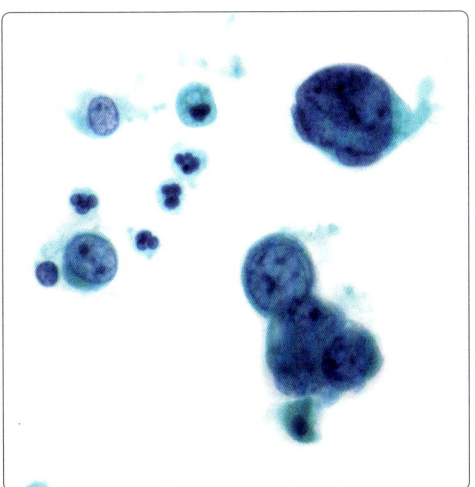

Stone-Related Urothelial Cell Cluster

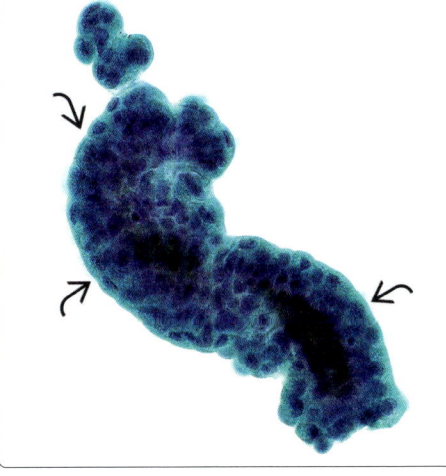

(Left) These cells from a ThinPrep of an upper tract washing show marked nuclear pleomorphism and atypia with a high nuclear:cytoplasmic ratio. Upper tract malignant cells tend to have less cytoplasm than malignant cells from the bladder. (Right) Pap-stained renal pelvis brush from a patient with stones shows a cluster of urothelial cells with a well-defined peripheral collar of cytoplasm ⮕. Stones may produce filling defects and papillary-like clusters with reactive atypia, mimicking low-grade urothelial neoplasms.

Ancillary Testing, UroVysion, and Others

UROVYSION

Background
- Genetic alterations are associated with bladder cancer
  - Most frequent involve chromosomes 1, 3, 5, 7, 9, 11, 17
- Test uses FISH probes to visualize chromosomal copy numbers (3, 7, and 17) and 9p21 deletion
- FDA-approved test for
  - Monitoring for tumor recurrence in patients with history of bladder cancer
  - Evaluation of hematuria patients suspected of having bladder cancer

Type of Analysis
- Multicolor FISH probe (Abbott Molecular)
  - Contains 4 probes that simultaneously evaluate on per cell basis
    - Centromeric 3 (CEP 3): Red signal
    - Centromeric 7 (CEP 5): Green signal
    - Centromeric 17 (CEP 17): Aqua signal
    - Locus-specific 9p21 (LSI 9p21): Gold signal
- Procedure
  - Slide preparations/methods: Cytospin, ThinPrep, filter, drop method
  - Fixation of slide in FISH fixative
  - Pretreatment (unleash DNA from bound proteins)
  - Denaturation and hybridization (unwind double helices to allow binding of probe to DNA)
  - Post wash, counterstain, and coverslip
  - Score slide and photograph
  - Requires technical expertise, extensive sampling, handling and preparation, and special equipment

Equipment
- Epifluorescence microscope and 4 filters

FISH Results (per Manufacturer)
- Positive FISH result based on 25 morphologically abnormal cells
  - ≥ 4 cells with polysomy (≥ 3 copies of ≥ 2 chromosomes) or ≥ 12 cells with homozygous 9p21 deletion
- Negative FISH result: Criteria for positive result not met in satisfactory specimen
- Unsatisfactory specimen
  - < 25 well-preserved, nonoverlapping epithelial cells for evaluation

Sensitivity and Specificity
- Highly variable in different studies: Sensitivity reported from 8-100% and specificity from 29-100%
- Factors affecting test results
  - False-negatives
    - Low-grade papillary neoplasms may be diploid
    - Neoplastic cells may not shed in urine or are sparse
    - Voided urine may contain primarily mature squamous cells
    - Poorly preserved cells not amenable for analysis
  - False-positives
    - Scored umbrella cells, which are often tetraploid and found in bladder washings
    - Split signals, especially in degenerated specimens
    - Polyomavirus-infected cells
    - Other malignancies may be FISH positive, not specific
  - Other factors
    - Abundant bacteria hampering signal counting due to autofluorescence
    - Abundant acute inflammatory cells obscuring epithelial cells
    - Excessive lubricant may interfere with signal counting
- Most effective when used in high-risk populations, including patients with atypical or suspicious cytology

IMMUNOCYT/UCYT+

Background
- Test designed to detect changes at cellular level
  - 3 monoclonal antibodies to specific antigens in tumors of transitional epithelium
- ImmunoCyt/uCyt+ test is used in conjunction with cytology
- FDA-approved test for surveillance of recurrent bladder cancer

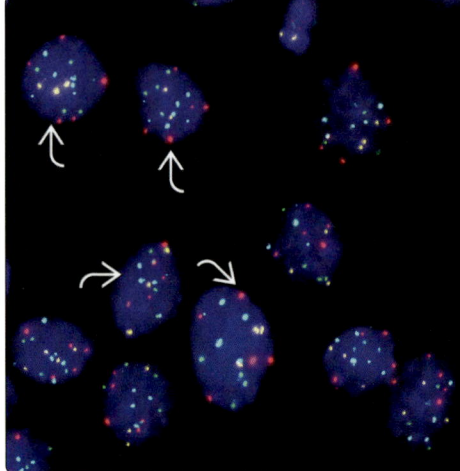

Normal FISH | Aneuploid-Positive FISH

(Left) FISH on urine cytospin shows diploid cells with 2 signals for centromeres 3 (red), 7 (green), 17 (aqua), and locus-specific 9p21 (gold); 25 such cells would be a negative FISH result. [Courtesy A. Khanna, CT (ASCP).] (Right) FISH shows aneuploid cells ➡ with > 2 signals for centromeres 3 (red), 7 (green), &/or 17 (aqua). ≥ 4 such cells out of 25 analyzed cells would be a positive FISH result. [Courtesy A. Khanna, CT (ASCP).]

Ancillary Testing, UroVysion, and Others

Type of Analysis

- Immunocytologic fluorescent assay that contains 3 monoclonal antibodies (Scimedx)
  - M344: Antibody to mucin-like antigen on exfoliated tumor cells, green fluorescein label
  - LDQ10: Antibody to mucin-like antigen on exfoliated tumor cells, green fluorescein label
  - 19A211: Antibody to high molecular weight glycosylated form of carcinoembryonic antigen, Texas red label
- Procedure
  - Cells fixed on slides and analyzed by fluorescence microscope equipped with appropriate filters
  - Requires technical expertise, extensive sampling handling, and preparation as well as special equipment
- Results
  - Positive score: If single red or green cell is observed
  - Negative score: If no red or green cell is observed
    - Must contain minimum of 500 cells for valid scoring

Equipment

- Fluorescence microscope and appropriate filters

Sensitivity and Specificity

- Sensitivity: 81-89%
  - Higher in detecting low-grade tumors than cytology
- Specificity: 61-85.9%

NUCLEAR MATRIX PROTEIN 22

Background

- Nuclear matrix proteins (NMPs)
  - Part of structural framework of nucleus
  - Involved in DNA replication, RNA transcription, and regulation of gene expression
  - Released in urine following apoptosis of urothelial cells
  - Elevated in urothelial carcinoma
- Test designed to detect NMPs in urine
- FDA-approved test for surveillance of recurrent cancer
- Urinary cytology results are not considered

Type of Analysis

- NMP22 BladderChek (Alere)
  - Qualitative, point-of-care test
  - Cartridge detects elevated levels of NMP-22 in urine

Sensitivity and Specificity

- More sensitive but less specific than cytology
- Factors affecting test results
  - Urinary tract infections, urolithiasis, history of bladder interposition, other malignancies, intravesical therapies, and cystoscopy may cause false-positive results

BTA TEST

Background

- Detects human complement factor H-related protein (hCFHrp) in urine
  - Similar to human complement factor
  - May have role in helping tumor cells evade host's immune defense
- FDA-approved tests for surveillance of recurrent cancer
- Urinary cytology results are not considered

Type of Analysis

- 2 tests commercially available
  - BTA stat (Polymedco): Qualitative, point-of-care test
  - BTA TRAK (Polymedco): Enzyme-linked immunosorbent type of qualitative assay

Sensitivity and Specificity

- More sensitive but less specific than cytology
- Factors affecting test results
  - Inflammation, hematuria, recent instrumentation, calculi, BCG therapy, antiinflammatory drugs, and nicotine can increase hCFHrp levels and cause false-positive results

NEWER TESTS

Genetic Tests

- Many recently developed tests analyze DNA, mRNA, miRNA, or lncRNA to detect genes of interest
  - *FGFR3* and *TERT* genes are common targets, but also many others depending on specific test
  - Some target methylation or microsatellite instability
- Commercial mRNA tests include CxBladder Detect and Xpert Bladder Cancer Monitor
- Potential to replace cytology for screening, at least in some circumstances

Nongenetic Targets

- Vesicle concentration or contents may be analyzed
- Proteins including urinary midkine protein may also be targeted

SENSITIVITY IMPROVEMENT CONSIDERATIONS

Low-Grade Papillary Neoplasms

- In Paris System, almost all low-grade papillary neoplasms will be called negative
  - These tests may be able to detect some low-grade lesions "missed" by cytology but not all
  - Clinical utility of finding such low-grade lesions is questionable

High-Grade Urothelial Carcinoma

- Increased sensitivity would be most useful in setting of screening for hematuria or monitoring for recurrence
  - Existing ancillary tests are limited by significant numbers of false-positives and false-negatives
  - Decades of research have not found markers obviously superior to cytology when all factors, including cost of increased follow-up, are considered
- Triage of equivocal cytology results is important application for FISH

SELECTED REFERENCES

1. Charpentier M et al: Noninvasive urine-based tests to diagnose or detect recurrence of bladder cancer. Cancers (Basel). 13(7), 2021
2. Ng K et al: Urinary biomarkers in bladder cancer: a review of the current landscape and future directions. Urol Oncol. 39(1):41-51, 2021
3. Dimashkieh H et al: Evaluation of UroVysion and cytology for bladder cancer detection: a study of 1835 paired urine samples with clinical and histologic correlation. Cancer Cytopathol. 121(10):591-7, 2013

PART III
Fine-Needle Aspiration, Superficial

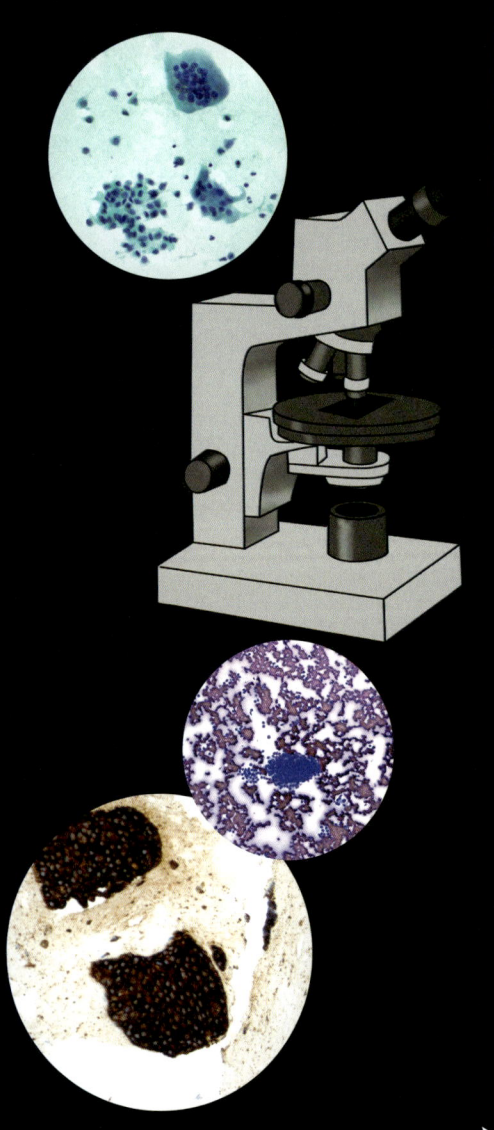

Fine-needle aspiration cytology

1844: F. Rynd
Invents hollow needle

1853: J. Paget
Breast FNA for cancer diagnosis

1883: H. Leyden
Diagnosis of bacterial pneumonia by lung puncture

1912: H. Hirschfeld
Diagnosis of cutaneous lymphomas and other tumors by FNA

1922: J. Ewing
Introduction of FNA in New York

1930: R. Ferguson
Evaluation of prostate gland by FNA

1934: A. Pavlowsky's monograph on FNA in mediastinal disorders; H. Martin and E. Ellis establish FNA at Memorial Sloan Kettering Cancer Center in New York

2nd half of the 20th century
S. Franzen, J. Zajicek, T. Lowhagen: Perfect, publish, and popularize FNA as diagnostic procedure

1992: P. Vilmann
First EUS-FNA of pancreas

1996 (breast): Reporting terminology conference at National Cancer Institute in Bethesda, Maryland

2002: Development of tru-cut biopsy needle for EUS procedures

2007 (thyroid): Reporting terminology conference at National Cancer Institute

2011 onward: Development of core needle biopsies for EUS and EBUS procedures by various manufacturers

**PART III
SECTION 1**
Overview

Superficial Aspiration Technique · 256

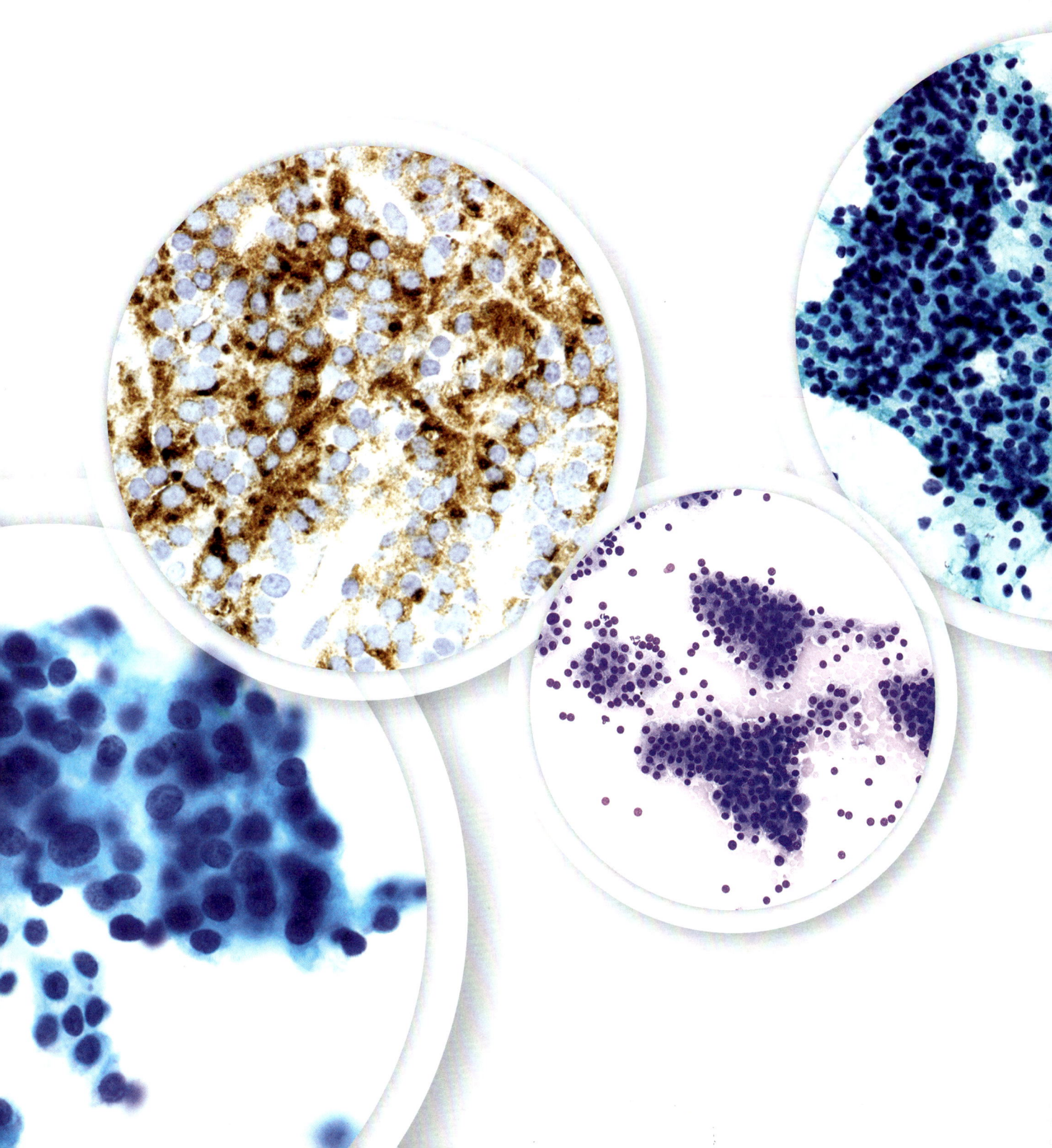

Superficial Aspiration Technique

BEFORE PROCEDURE

Examination and Patient Consent

- Obtain history and examine site to be aspirated
- Fully discuss procedure and answer all questions, which ameliorates apprehension and often obviates use of anesthetic
- Risk of bleeding is minimized by use of fine needle and application of pressure after needle removal
- Risk of infection is minimized by using sterile technique

SUPPLIES FOR PROCEDURE

Required

- Needles, usually 25 gauge or 27 gauge, 5/8 in in length
  - Consider larger gauge (21) for fat pad aspirates
  - May use 1.5 in for deeper lesions
- Syringe, usually 10 mL with Luer lock tip
- Betadine &/or alcohol
- Sterile gloves
- Sterile gauze
- Slides (plus slides optimal for possible immunocytochemical applications)
  - Consider frosted slides for aspirates containing fatty tissue
- Alcohol spray fixative
- Cell preservative solution
  - For flow cytometry (RPMI) or cell block (RPMI, formalin, or CytoLyt)
  - Special medium for molecular testing when indicated
- Culture tubes (routine, fungus, and TB)
- Slide tray
- Marker for labeling of slide with patient identifiers
- Diff-Quik stain for immediate adequacy assessment/rapid on-site evaluation (ROSE)
- Microscope

Optional

- Topical or local anesthetic, ice packs
- Handle or "gun" to contain syringe
- Bandage (usually not required with small-gauge needles but may be necessary to protect clothing, etc.)

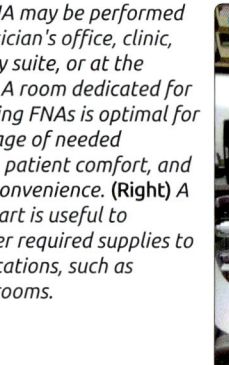

(Left) FNA may be performed in a physician's office, clinic, radiology suite, or at the bedside. A room dedicated for performing FNAs is optimal for the storage of needed supplies, patient comfort, and overall convenience. (Right) A mobile cart is useful to maneuver required supplies to other locations, such as patient rooms.

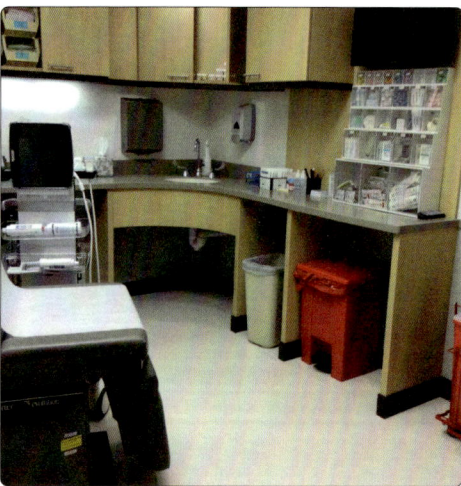

Fine-Needle Aspiration Clinic

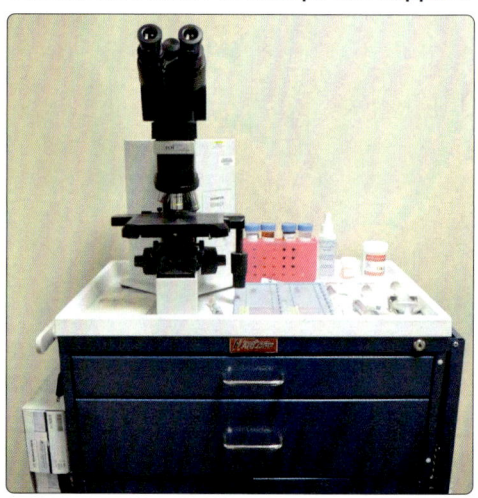

Mobile Cart With Microscope and Supplies

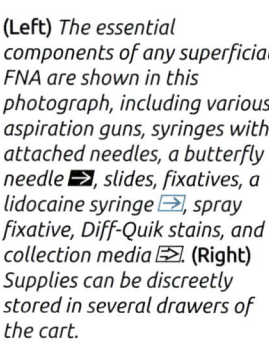

(Left) The essential components of any superficial FNA are shown in this photograph, including various aspiration guns, syringes with attached needles, a butterfly needle ➡, slides, fixatives, a lidocaine syringe ➡, spray fixative, Diff-Quik stains, and collection media ➡. (Right) Supplies can be discreetly stored in several drawers of the cart.

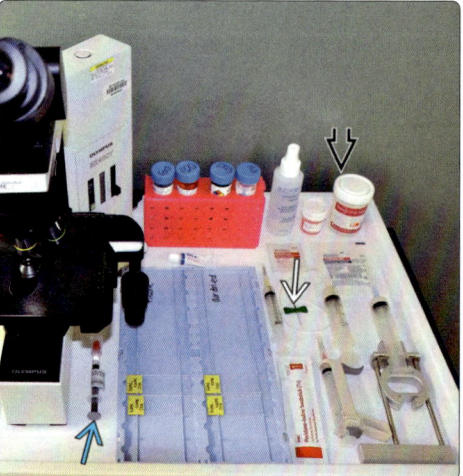

Layout of Mobile Aspiration Cart

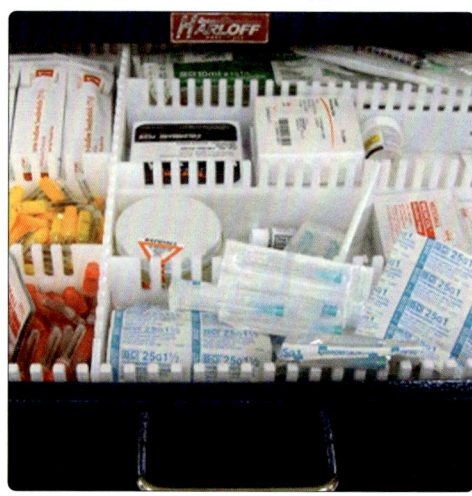

Fine-Needle Aspiration Supplies Drawer

Superficial Aspiration Technique

ASPIRATION TECHNIQUE

Basic Fine-Needle Aspiration Technique

- After obtaining consent, determine optimal position of patient to access lesion with consideration for patient comfort
  - Avoid traversing skeletal muscle and vascular areas as much as possible
- Sterilize skin/mucosa with Betadine &/or alcohol
  - Supplement with anesthetics as needed
    - In some sites, such as oral cavity, topical anesthetic spray is preferred
- Immobilize lesion between 2 fingers or fingertips
  - Use caution, particularly in intraoral aspirates
    - Consider bite guard or use of visual instead of tactile assistance
- Using quick motion, enter skin at angle best determined to access lesion
  - Deep lesions are often best accessed at 90° angle
  - Small amount of air should already be in syringe to assist with displacement of material obtained onto slides
  - Syringe may be placed in various holders for operator comfort
  - In certain situations, butterfly needle may be preferred
- Move needle in back-and-forth, side-to-side cutting motion in fan-like pattern for 5-10 seconds while pulling back on trigger to aspirate material into hub of needle; avoid fan-like motion in thyroid
  - Use tactile sensation to confirm needle is in lesion
  - If large amount of fresh blood is observed in needle hub, discontinue procedure immediately
  - Motion > 10 seconds increases likelihood of excessive clotting
- Release trigger, remove needle, and apply sterile pressure over area for ~ 1 minute or until cessation of bleeding
  - Use of low-dose anticoagulants does not preclude aspiration (adjust procedure by decreasing length of time under skin and applying pressure after procedure for greater duration)
  - Use ice pack with firm pressure between passes if needed to control bleeding
    - Keep ice pack at site post procedure for ~ 2 hours if patient is on anticoagulants and bleeds easily during procedure
- Express aspirated material using plunger onto slide labeled with ≥ 2 patient identifiers and carefully smear material across slide
  - One slide is air dried and stained using Diff-Quik methodology
  - Corresponding opposite slide is alcohol fixed for Pap or rapid Pap methodology
  - Rapidity in this step is essential to eliminate as much air-drying artifact (on Pap slide) and clotting as possible
  - Aspirating small amount of air into syringe before procedure obviates alternative of (after having performed procedure) removing needle, pulling air into syringe, and then reapplying needle to express material onto slide (1st is faster and safer)
  - Gently (gravity assisted) place one slide on top of another, and move each in opposite directions to smear material across 2 slides
    - Any increased pressure may cause rupture of delicate cells
  - In cases of abundant aspirated material, such as cyst, place needle onto slide and allow only 1 or 2 drops onto slide
- Rinse remainder of aspirate in various collection media
  - RPMI for flow cytometry or cell block (fluid should be turbid)
  - CytoLyt or formalin for cell block
  - Culture bottles for microbiologic studies
- Additional passes as needed to complete procedure based on adequacy assessment
  - Usually 3-4 passes are required

French Technique (Capillary Action, No Aspiration)

- Useful when operator needs better/finer control of needle in tight spaces where addition of syringe is too cumbersome or in cellular lesions
- Connect needle to syringe and remove plunger before aspiration
- Basic FNA technique is followed except that needle is used in cutting motion only
  - No supplemental suction (negative pressure) is applied during procedure
- Material is expressed onto slides as above by inserting plunger post procedure

Butterfly Technique

- Useful in areas, such as oral cavity, without enough space to optimally move needle with attached syringe
- Main drawback of this technique is that it requires 2 operators: One to move butterfly needle back and forth and another to provide suction

Abdominal Fat Pad Aspiration

- Use larger needle between 18-21 gauges
- More aggressive sampling using aspiration gun until drop of fat is visible in syringe
- Consider using combination of frosted or charged slides for smears
- Cut cell block slides at 7-10 μm for Congo red stains

COMPLICATIONS

All Are Uncommonly Encountered

- Hematomas
  - Minimize with immediate cessation of procedure once fresh blood is visualized in needle hub
  - Apply ice pack and pressure
- Dizziness/fainting
  - Use Trendelenburg position
- Pneumothorax
  - Possible in chest wall, axillary, supraclavicular locations
  - Avoid deep penetration as much as possible
- Needle tract seeding/tissue alterations
  - Rare with small-gauge needles and experienced operators

SELECTED REFERENCES

1. Voskuil RT et al: The utility of fine-needle aspiration: how FNA has affected our musculoskeletal oncology practice. J Am Soc Cytopathol. 9(6):596-601, 2020

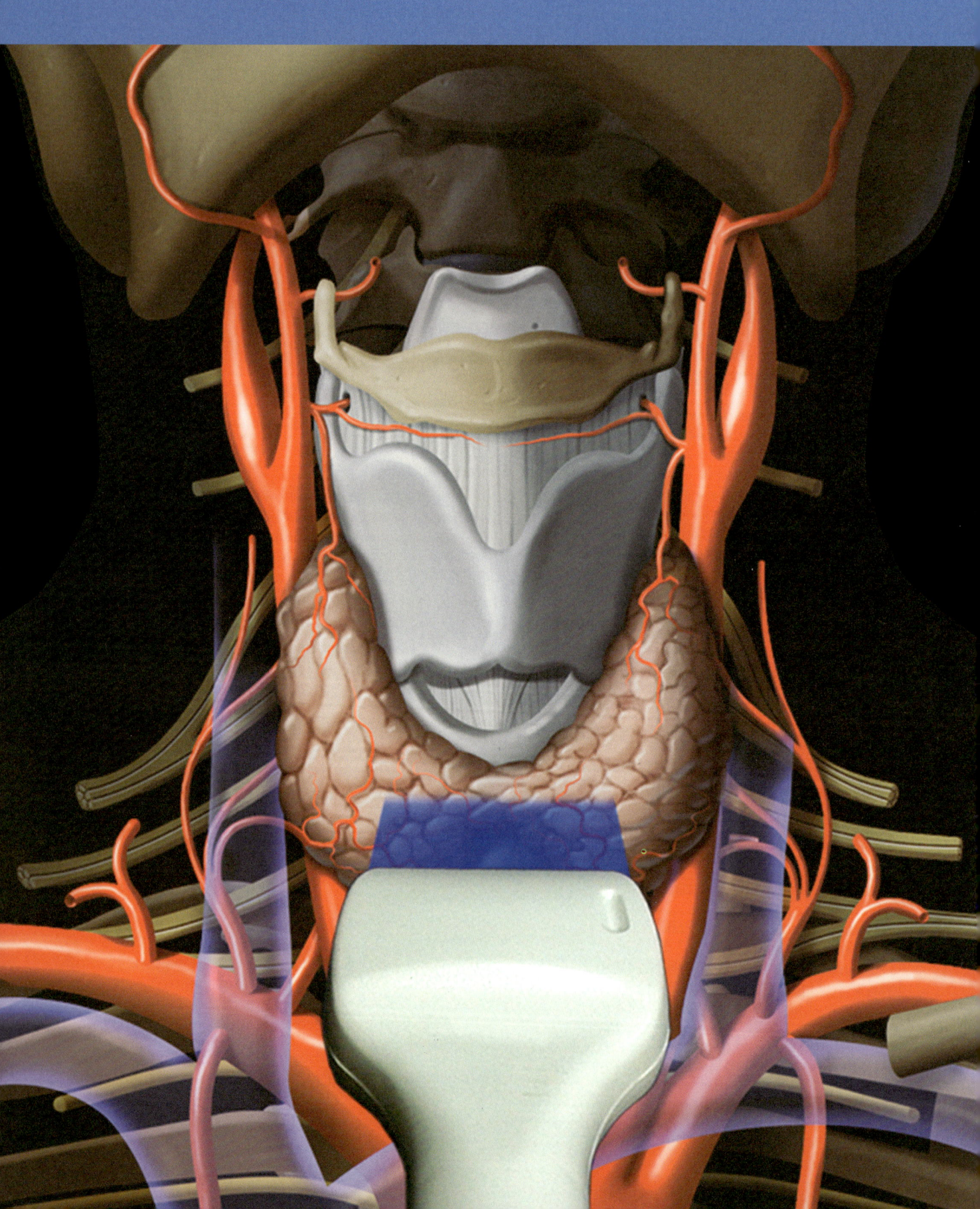

PART III
SECTION 2
Thyroid Gland

Ultrasound-Guided Thyroid Fine-Needle Aspiration	260
Thyroid Fine-Needle Aspiration Reporting Terminology and Specimen Adequacy	266
Adenomatous (Benign Follicular) Nodule	268
Chronic Lymphocytic/Hashimoto Thyroiditis	270
Granulomatous Thyroiditis	272
Graves Disease/Diffuse Toxic Goiter	274
Pigmented Thyroid Lesions and Crystals	275
Atypia of Undetermined Significance/Follicular Lesion of Undetermined Significance	276
Follicular Neoplasm/Suspicious for a Follicular Neoplasm	280
Follicular Neoplasm, Oncocytic (Hürthle Cell) Type	284
Papillary Thyroid Carcinoma, Classic Subtype	286
Papillary Thyroid Carcinoma Subtypes	290
Medullary Thyroid Carcinoma	298
Poorly Differentiated Thyroid Carcinoma	302
Anaplastic Thyroid Carcinoma	304
Thyroid Lymphoma	306
Metastatic Carcinoma to Thyroid	308
Other Nonneoplastic and Neoplastic Thyroid Lesions Encountered on Thyroid FNA	310

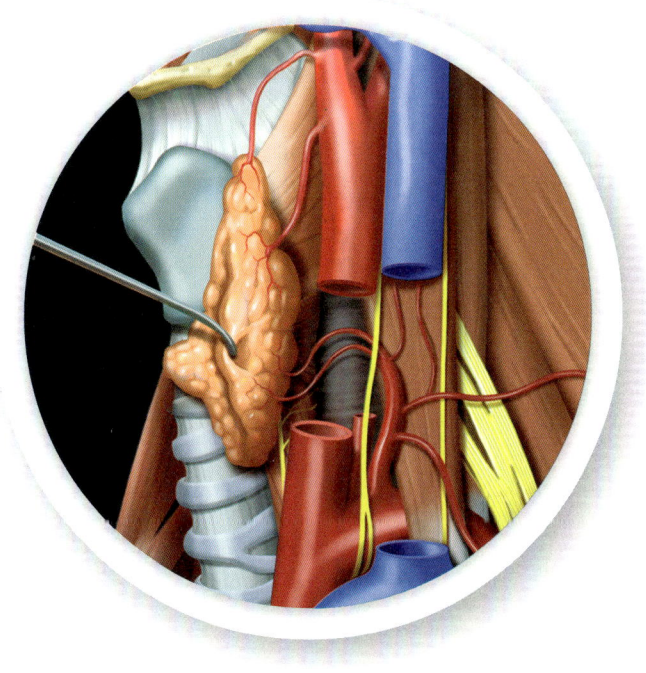

Ultrasound-Guided Thyroid Fine-Needle Aspiration

TERMINOLOGY

Ultrasound Principles and Definitions

- Ultrasound (US) is primary imaging modality for assessing thyroid nodules
- Echogenicity refers to brightness of tissues
  - **Hyperechoic**: More echogenic (brighter) than surrounding structures
  - **Isoechoic**: Same echogenicity as surrounding structures
  - **Hypoechoic**: Less echogenic (darker) than surrounding structures
  - **Anechoic**: No echoes within lesion (appears black)
    - Anechoic structures are usually simple cysts
- **Posterior shadowing**
  - Certain structures, such as large calcifications and gas, are very bright reflectors and do not allow sound beams to travel further
  - Tissues deep to these bright reflectors appear black or gray (shadowed)
- **Enhanced through-transmission**
  - When US beam travels through fluid (e.g., simple cyst), there is no tissue to reflect sound beam back, so it appears anechoic (black)
  - Because sound beam is not attenuated as it travels through cyst, it is stronger when it hits tissues beyond cyst, making them appear brighter (enhanced through-transmission)
- **Comet-tail artifact**
  - When US beam hits small crystalline structure, it may cause reverberation
  - Appears as small, bright echo with progressively smaller echoes posteriorly
    - Creates inverted triangle or comet shape
  - Colloid commonly creates comet-tail artifacts
- **Transducer types**
  - Higher frequency (7-15 MHz) linear transducers have better resolution but poorer penetration
    - Used to evaluate superficial structures
    - Ideally suited for thyroid gland
  - Lower frequency (2-6 MHz) vector transducers have better penetration but poorer resolution
    - Used to evaluate and biopsy deeper structures, such as liver and retroperitoneum

ANATOMY

Thyroid Gland

- H- or U-shaped gland in cervical neck, anterior and lateral to trachea with 2 lateral lobes connected by isthmus
  - Each lobe measures ~ 4 cm in height, often asymmetric
  - 40% of people have pyramidal lobe ascending from isthmus area toward hyoid bone
- Need to be aware of complex surrounding anatomy when planning biopsy
  - Posteromedially are tracheoesophageal grooves
    - Contains esophagus, paratracheal lymph nodes, recurrent laryngeal nerve, parathyroid glands
  - Posterolaterally are carotid sheaths
    - Contains common carotid artery, internal jugular vein, vagus nerve
  - Anterolaterally are sternocleidomastoid and infrahyoid strap muscles
- Arterial supply
  - Superior thyroid arteries arise from 1st anterior branch of external carotid artery
  - Inferior thyroid arteries arise from thyrocervical trunk, branch of subclavian artery

ULTRASOUND

Normal Thyroid Gland

- Thyroid parenchyma is homogeneous and mildly hyperechoic compared with adjacent muscles
- Both longitudinal and transverse scans, including adjacent lymph nodes, are required for comprehensive evaluation
- Document and characterize any lesions, specifically in relationship to trachea, major vessels in carotid sheath, and extrathyroidal extension

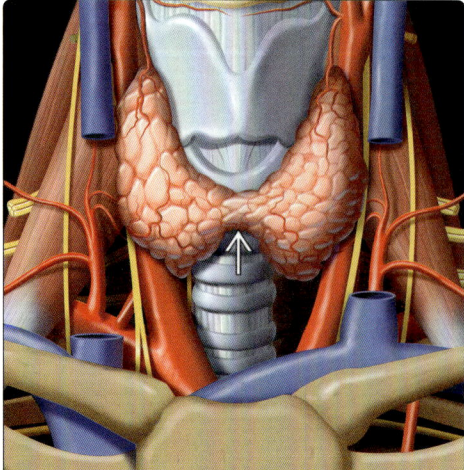

Thyroid Shape and Location

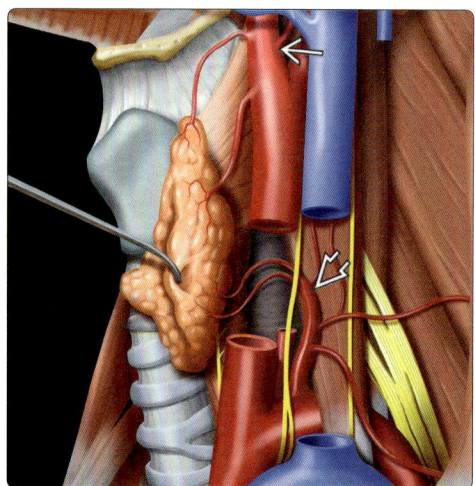

Thyroid Blood Supply

(Left) Frontal graphic of the neck with the strap muscles removed shows the H-shaped thyroid gland overlying the trachea. The thin isthmus ➡ attaches the 2 lobes. (Right) Lateral graphic shows the blood supply to the thyroid gland with 2 superior thyroidal arteries from the external carotid artery ➡ and 2 inferior thyroidal arteries from the thyrocervical trunk ➡, a branch of the subclavian artery.

Ultrasound-Guided Thyroid Fine-Needle Aspiration

Nodules
- Thyroid nodules are common and often incidentally found on physical exam or imaging procedures being done for other reasons
- Important to know which features are associated with carcinoma and therefore warrant biopsy
- **Suspicious sonographic features**
  - Solid nodules with lobular or irregular borders
  - Nodule appears hypoechoic when compared with normal thyroid
  - Presence of microcalcifications
    - Punctate, nonshadowing, echogenic foci
  - Nodule taller than wide
  - Adenopathy: Suspicious lymph node has loss of normal, echogenic, fatty hilum
- **Sonographic features favoring benignancy**
  - Purely cystic nodule
  - Spongiform appearance: Abundant colloid creates small cysts in lesion making it appear sponge-like
  - Calcifications with linear, comet-tail appearance
  - Nodule is isoechoic or hyperechoic compared with normal thyroid
- Both benign and malignant lesions may show increased vascular flow, so color Doppler is not good discriminator regarding need for biopsy

BIOPSY

Patient Selection
- Guidelines vary but all include decision algorithm using sonographic features and nodule size
- 2 most commonly used guidelines are from American College of Radiology (ACR) and American Thyroid Association (ATA)
- **ACR Thyroid Imaging, Reporting and Data System (TI-RADS)** committee formed to standardize lexicon and biopsy recommendations based on imaging appearance
  - Nodules are scored on 5 categories: Composition, echogenicity, shape, margin, and echogenic foci
  - Points from each category are added together to determine classification
    - **TI-RADS 1 (TR1)**: 0 points, benign; no FNA
    - **TR2**: 2 points, not suspicious; no FNA
    - **TR3**: 3 points, mildly suspicious
      - FNA if ≥ 2.5 cm
      - Follow if ≥ 1.5 cm
    - **TR4**: 4-6 points, moderately suspicious
      - FNA if ≥ 1.5 cm
      - Follow if ≥ 1.0 cm
    - **TR5**: ≥ 7 points, highly suspicious
      - FNA if ≥ 1.0 cm
      - Follow if ≥ 0.5 cm

General Considerations
- May either palpate nodule or use US guidance
  - US guidance improves diagnostic yield
    - Direct visualization allows targeting of most suspicious area
    - Particularly helpful if nodule has both cystic and solid components
  - US guidance helps avoid important surrounding structures (e.g., carotid artery, recurrent laryngeal nerve)
- Always perform FNA with cytopathologist present
  - Ensures correct slide preparation
  - Fewer unsatisfactory biopsies
    - Examination by cytopathologist at time of biopsy allows determination of when adequate amount of tissue has been obtained

Ultrasound-Guided FNA
- Place patient supine with pillow under neck
  - This extends neck, making more room for transducer
- Use small footprint high-frequency transducer
  - "Hockey stick" transducers are ideal for thyroid
- Mark area for biopsy
- Sterilize skin with Betadine or other sterilizing agent
  - Sterile draping is not generally done
- May anesthetize skin with 1% lidocaine
  - Give patient option
    - Lidocaine burns and is often more uncomfortable than small needle used for biopsy
  - Anesthetize only superficial structures
    - Do not infiltrate lidocaine into thyroid nodule as it may affect aspirate
- Use small (generally 25-gauge) FNA needles
- Biopsy techniques
  - French technique
    - Needle only, without syringe
    - Hold needle near hub for better control
    - Capillary action only, no aspiration
  - 10-cc syringe without suction
    - Syringe is often easier to handle than needle alone
    - Attach syringe to needle and pull plunger back so there is 2-3 cc of air in syringe
    - This creates negative pressure in needle assisting in aspiration
    - With air already in syringe, it is easier to express aspirate onto slide
  - 10-cc syringe with suction
    - If inadequate results with either of previous techniques, may use suction while performing biopsy
    - Usually not necessary
    - More likely to get blood in hub
  - 22-gauge core biopsy may be performed if FNA material is deemed inadequate for diagnosis by cytopathologist
- Use direct US guidance during biopsy
  - Target most suspicious area of nodule (e.g., microcalcifications)
  - Hold needle and transducer in same plane visualizing entire shaft of needle while entering nodule
  - Once needle is appropriately placed, begin biopsy using short rapid cutting motion while continuing to directly observe under US
    - Continue biopsying for ~ 10 seconds
  - Pass sample to cytopathologist for appropriate slide preparation
  - 3-4 passes are generally required
    - Make sure entire lesion is sampled
    - Cytopathologist determines when adequate tissue has been obtained

Ultrasound-Guided Thyroid Fine-Needle Aspiration

American College of Radiology TI-RADS

Category	Feature	Points
Composition (choose 1)	Cystic or almost completely cystic	0
	Spongiform	0
	Mixed cystic and solid	1
	Solid or almost completely solid	2
Echogenicity (choose 1)	Anechoic	0
	Hyperechoic or isoechoic	1
	Hypoechoic	2
	Very hypoechoic	3
Shape (choose 1)	Wider than tall	0
	Taller than wide	3
Margin (choose 1)	Smooth	0
	Ill defined	0
	Lobulated or irregular	2
	Extrathyroid extension	3
Echogenic foci (choose all that apply)	None or large comet-tail artifacts	0
	Macrocalcifications	1
	Peripheral (rim) calcifications	2
	Punctate echogenic foci	3

Points are added together for total TI-RADS score. Three or more points generally require biopsy depending on size of nodule.

Tessler FN et al: ACR Thyroid Imaging, Reporting and Data System (TI-RADS): white paper of the ACR TI-RADS committee. J Am Coll Radiol. 14(5):587-95, 2017.

American Thyroid Association Guidelines Task Force

Sonographic Pattern	Ultrasound Features	Estimated Risk of Malignancy	FNA Size Cutoff (Largest Dimension)
High suspicion	Solid hypoechoic nodule or solid hypoechoic, component of partially cystic nodule with 1 or more of following features: Irregular margins (infiltrative, microlobulated), microcalcifications, taller than wide, rim calcifications with small extrusive soft tissue component, evidence of extrathyroidal extension	> 70-90%	Recommend FNA at ≥ 1 cm
Intermediate suspicion	Hypoechoic solid nodule with smooth margins **without** microcalcifications, extrathyroidal extension, or taller than wide shape	10-20%	Recommend FNA at ≥ 1 cm
Low suspicion	Isoechoic or hyperechoic solid nodule, or partially cystic nodule with eccentric solid areas, **without** microcalcification, irregular margin or extrathyroidal extension, or taller than wide shape.	5-10%	Recommend FNA at ≥ 1.5 cm
Very low suspicion	Spongiform or partially cystic nodules **without** any other suspicious features	< 3%	Consider FNA at ≥ 2 cm (observation without FNA is also reasonable option)

Haugen BR et al: 2015 American Thyroid Association management guidelines for adult patients with thyroid nodules and differentiated thyroid cancer. Thyroid. 26(1):1-133, 2016.

SELECTED REFERENCES

1. Belovarac B et al: Evaluation of ACR TI-RADS cytologically indeterminate thyroid nodules and molecular profiles: a single-institutional experience. J Am Soc Cytopathol. 11(3):165-72, 2022
2. Darouassi Y et al: The impact of the ultrasound classification on the rate of thyroid surgery indications: a 577 cases series. J Ultrasound. ePub, 2022
3. Strieder DL et al: Using an ultrasonography risk stratification system to enhance the thyroid fine needle aspiration performance. Eur J Radiol. 150:110244, 2022
4. Merhav G et al: Validation of TIRADS ACR risk assessment of thyroid nodules in comparison to the ATA guidelines. J Clin Imaging Sci. 11:37, 2021
5. Xia R et al: Do ACR TI-RADS scores demonstrate unique thyroid molecular profiles? Ultrasonography. 41(3):480-92, 2020

Ultrasound-Guided Thyroid Fine-Needle Aspiration

Midline Transducer Positioning

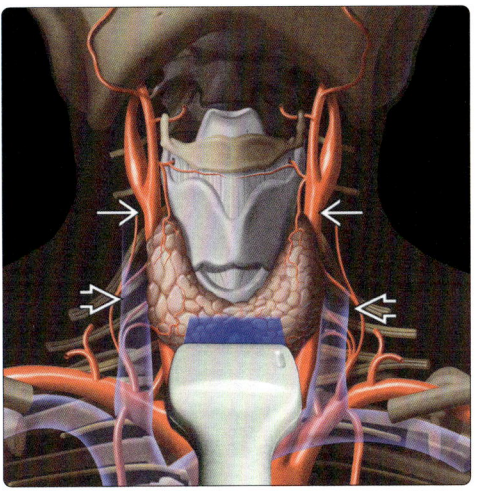

Midline Ultrasound of Thyroid

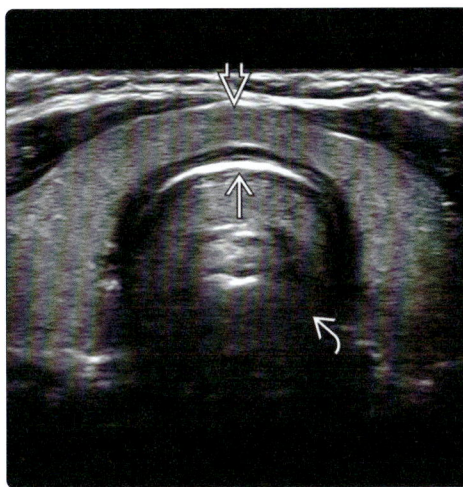

(Left) Graphic shows the ultrasound transducer placed on the isthmus of the thyroid gland. Note that the carotid arteries ➡ run along the lateral margin slightly posterior to the gland. The jugular veins ➡ (partially ghosted in this graphic) run lateral to the carotid arteries. (Right) Ultrasound from the same plane shows the thin isthmus ➡ connecting the 2 lobes of the gland. Air within the trachea creates a bright reflection ➡ with posterior shadowing behind it ➡.

Transverse Lateral Transducer Positioning

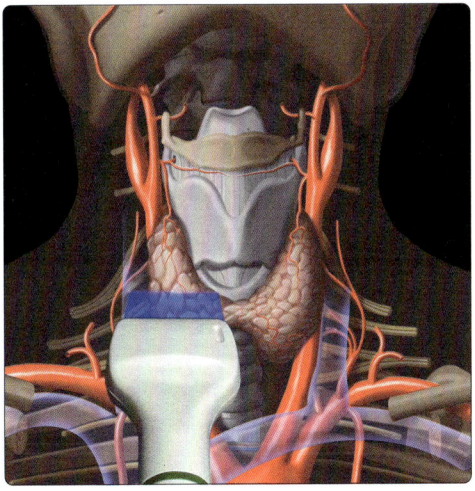

Transverse Ultrasound of Right Lobe

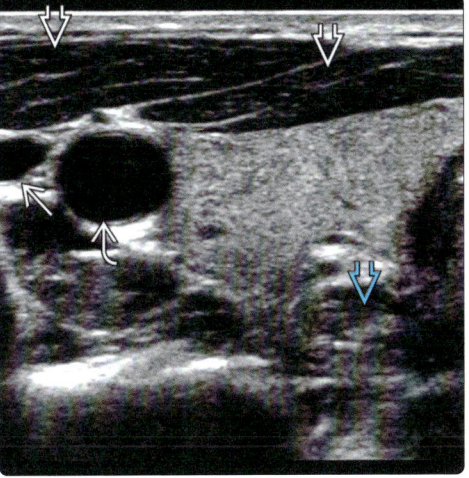

(Left) Graphic shows the ultrasound transducer positioned transversely on the right lobe of the thyroid gland. (Right) Transverse ultrasound of the right lobe shows the hypoechoic, overlying strap muscles ➡, the carotid artery ➡, and the jugular vein ➡. The esophagus ➡ can sometimes be visualized posterior to the gland and should not be mistaken for a nodule. The parathyroid glands are also located posterior to the thyroid but are usually not seen unless enlarged.

Longitudinal Lateral Transducer Positioning

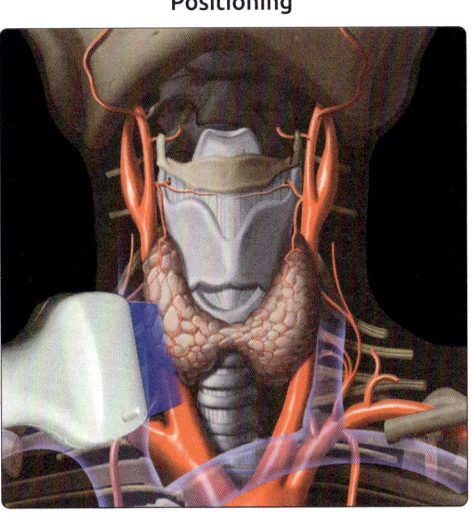

Longitudinal Doppler Ultrasound of Right Lobe

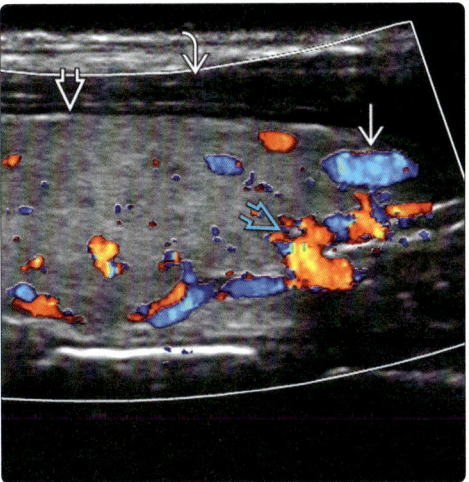

(Left) Graphic shows the ultrasound transducer positioned along the long axis of the right lower lobe of the thyroid. (Right) Longitudinal color Doppler ultrasound in the same plane shows the almond shape of the lobe. The thyroid capsule ➡ clearly delineates the homogeneous, hyperechoic thyroid from the overlying hypoechoic strap muscles ➡. The thyroid is a very vascular organ. Both the inferior thyroidal artery ➡ and vein ➡ are seen.

Ultrasound-Guided Thyroid Fine-Needle Aspiration

Typical Features of Colloid Cyst

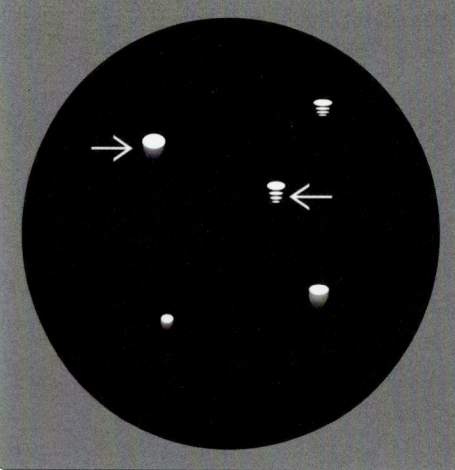

(Left) Graphic shows an anechoic (black) cyst with bright echoes within it. These have an inverted triangle shape ➡ (comet-tail artifact). This pattern is classically seen in a colloid cyst.

Ultrasound of Colloid Cyst

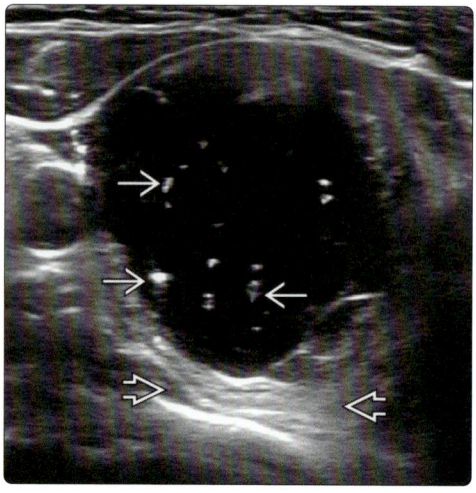

(Right) Ultrasound of a colloid cyst shows multiple floating bright echoes with comet-tail artifacts ➡. The cyst is otherwise anechoic with the tissues behind it appearing brighter ➡ (enhanced through-transmission). This should be recognized as a benign lesion, and no biopsy is required.

Suspicious Pattern of Calcifications

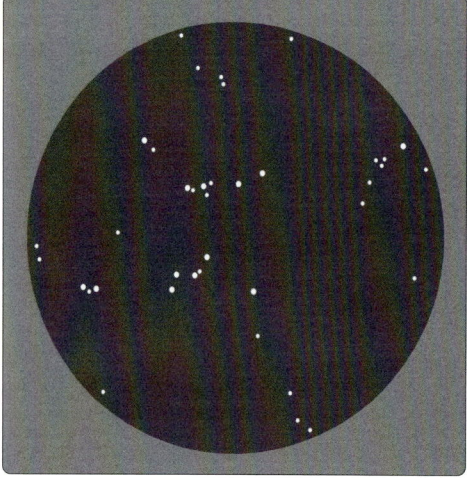

(Left) This graphic shows punctate, echogenic foci (microcalcifications) scattered throughout a solid nodule. This is a highly suspicious pattern.

Ultrasound Findings Suspicious for Papillary Carcinoma

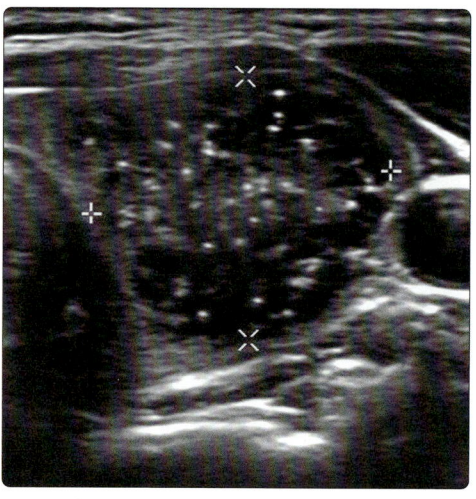

(Right) Ultrasound shows a large, hypoechoic solid nodule (cursors) with multiple scattered microcalcifications throughout the lesion. These features are highly suspicious, and the lesion requires biopsy regardless of patient history. FNA showed papillary carcinoma.

Benign Spongiform Nodule

(Left) This nodule ➡ in the right lobe of the thyroid has multiple small cysts, giving it a lacy or spongiform appearance (carotid artery ➡). This is a common benign appearance and does not require biopsy.

Cyst With Small Solid Component

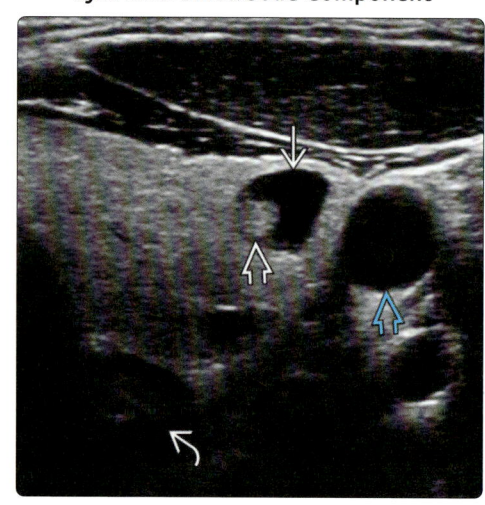

(Right) This cystic nodule ➡ has a small solid component ➡, which is isoechoic to the adjacent normal thyroid. It is small (6 mm) and has no suspicious features and does not warrant biopsy. The esophagus ➡ is seen in this image and should not be confused with a nodule. The carotid artery ➡ is also seen.

Ultrasound-Guided Thyroid Fine-Needle Aspiration

French Technique for Ultrasound-Guided FNA

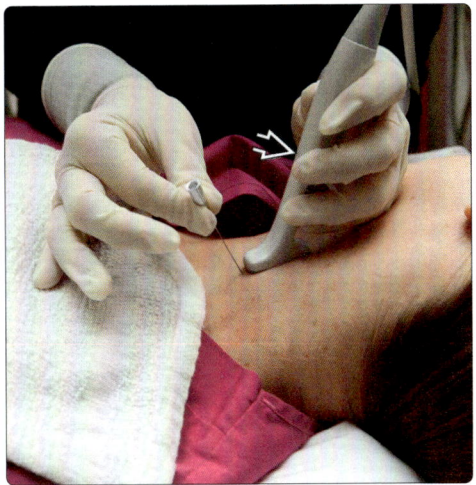

Ultrasound-Guided FNA Using Syringe

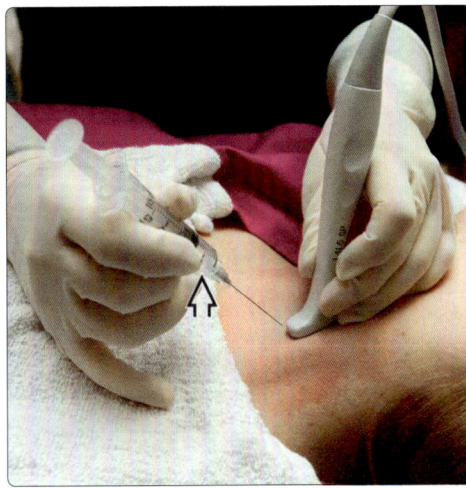

(Left) Ultrasound-guided biopsy should use a high-frequency, small footprint ("hockey stick") transducer ➡. This is the French technique, which uses the capillary action of the needle alone. **(Right)** Biopsy can also be performed with a syringe on the needle. If the plunger is pulled back 2-3 cc ➡ after the needle is attached, it creates negative pressure aiding in aspiration. Active aspiration can be performed but is usually not required and is more likely to contaminate the sample with blood.

Hypoechoic Nodule, Taller Than Wide

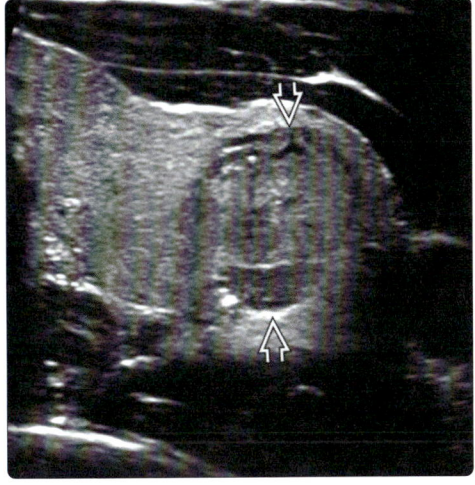

Ultrasound Guidance of Needle for Thorough Nodule Sampling

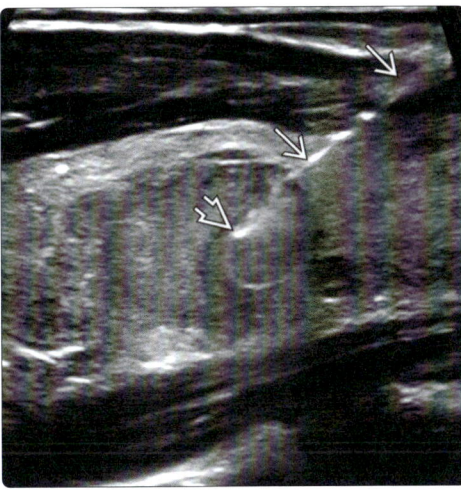

(Left) Ultrasound of the left lobe of the thyroid gland shows a 2.5-cm solid nodule ➡. It is mildly hypoechoic compared with the surrounding normal thyroid parenchyma, and it is taller than wide. The size and appearance of this nodule require a biopsy. **(Right)** Ultrasound from the biopsy shows the length of the needle ➡ with the tip ➡ in the nodule. Using direct ultrasound guidance ensures that the entire nodule is sampled. The FNA showed papillary carcinoma.

Color Doppler Ultrasound

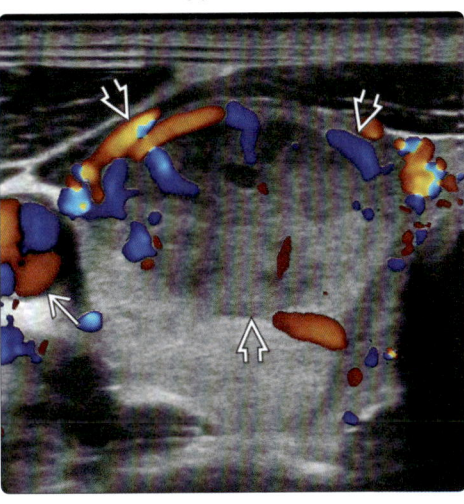

Use of Ultrasound Guidance to Avoid Carotid Artery

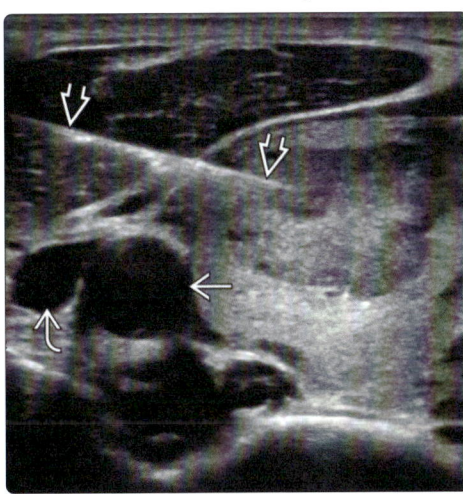

(Left) Color Doppler ultrasound shows increased flow within a thyroid nodule ➡. Note that it is immediately adjacent to the carotid artery ➡. Most solid nodules have increased flow so Doppler cannot differentiate benign from malignant, and it is not part of the risk stratification criteria. **(Right)** Ultrasound during the biopsy shows the course of the needle ➡. Note that a very shallow, oblique angle was taken to avoid the carotid artery ➡ and jugular vein ➡. FNA showed benign nodule with follicular cells and abundant colloid.

Thyroid Fine-Needle Aspiration
Reporting Terminology and Specimen Adequacy

TERMINOLOGY

Definitions

- Criteria for adequacy
  - Adequate thyroid FNA biopsy contains ≥ 6 groups of well-visualized follicular cells with ≥ 10 cells per group (well-stained cells without any air drying or other factors that obstruct visualization)
  - Currently same adequacy criteria for liquid-based preparations, though recent publications suggest lower number may be adequate without affecting sensitivity or specificity
- Exceptions
  - Atypia: If any cytologic or architectural atypia, classify specimen as atypia of undetermined significance (AUS)
  - Colloid nodules: Benign nodules that have abundant thick colloid and follicular cells; may be compressed and atrophic, hence, may never reach required 6/10 rule
  - Solid nodules with inflammation, including lymphocytic/Hashimoto thyroiditis, granulomatous thyroiditis, or abscess

The Bethesda System for Reporting Thyroid Cytology

- Nondiagnostic (ND)
  - Cyst fluid only
    - Cyst fluid ± histiocytes but lacking 6 groups with 10 cells or thick colloid
    - Risk of malignancy is very low if simple cyst, < 3 cm, and in proper clinical setting (ultrasound evidence)
    - Since pathologist may not know clinical scenario, there is small chance of intracystic papillary carcinoma
    - Hence, best to report as ND, cystic contents only
  - Virtually acellular specimen
    - Specimen with < 6 groups with 10 cells
      - Lower threshold being considered, as most end up being benign on follow-up
  - Other
    - Material not representative of thyroid (e.g., muscle or trachea)
    - Specimen obscured by blood, artifact, ultrasound gel, or poor fixation/staining, which makes accurate interpretation difficult

Nondiagnostic, Foreign Material

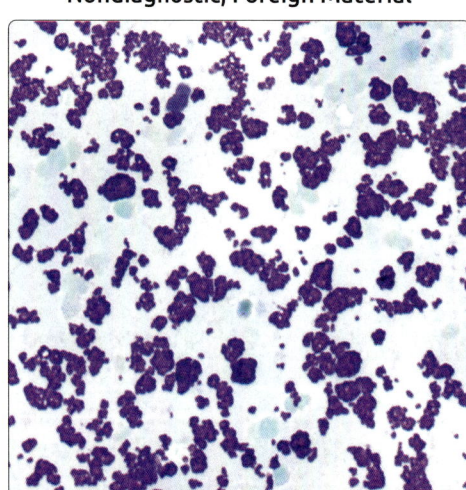

Nondiagnostic, Cyst Contents Only

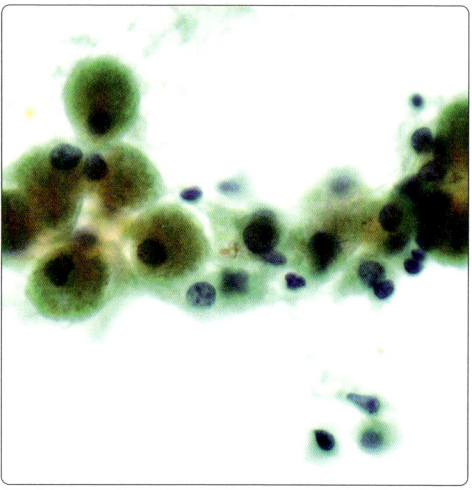

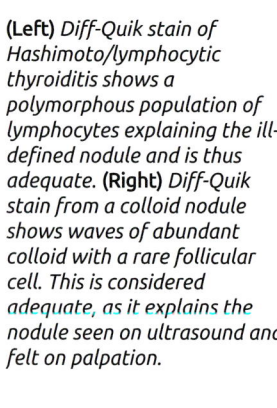

(Left) Diff-Quik-stained smear shows foreign material (most likely ultrasound gel) with absence of colloid or follicular cells or other cellular elements. **(Right)** Pap stain of an aspirate diagnosed as having only cystic contents is characterized by hemosiderin-laden macrophages and some watery colloid but no follicular cells.

Lymphocytic Thyroiditis, Adequate

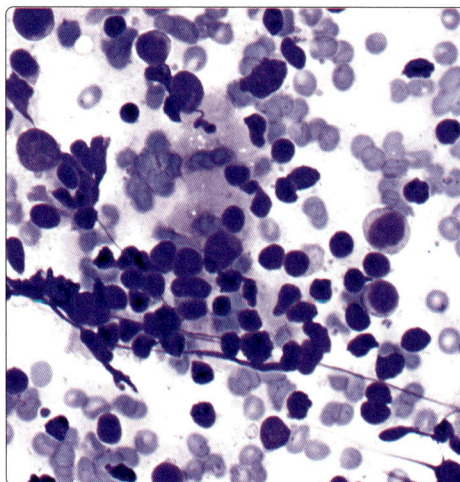

Colloid Nodule, Adequate

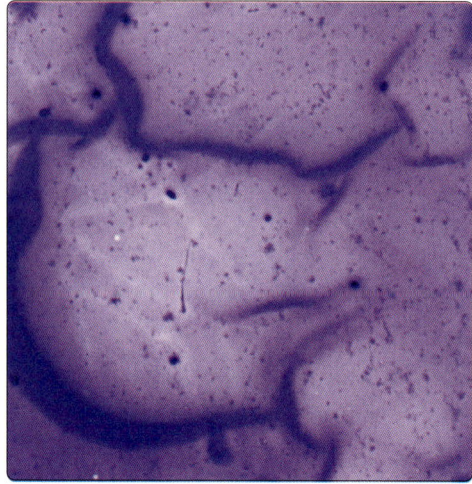

(Left) Diff-Quik stain of Hashimoto/lymphocytic thyroiditis shows a polymorphous population of lymphocytes explaining the ill-defined nodule and is thus adequate. **(Right)** Diff-Quik stain from a colloid nodule shows waves of abundant colloid with a rare follicular cell. This is considered adequate, as it explains the nodule seen on ultrasound and felt on palpation.

Thyroid Fine-Needle Aspiration Reporting Terminology and Specimen Adequacy

TBSRTC, BTA/RCP, Italian System, ROM and Clinical Algorithms

BTA/RCP Terminology (ROM%)	Italian	TBSRTC 2023 (Category Number)	ROM TBSRTC 2017 (%)	ROM TBSRTC With NIFTP as Benign (%)(2017)	Suggested Usual Management	Optional Note
Thy1, Thy1c (cystic) (12%)	TIR1 ND, TIR1c ND cystic	Nondiagnostic (ND) (I)	5-10%	5-10%	Reaspirate with US guidance	N/A
Thy2, nonneoplastic (NN) Thy2c NN, cystic (5%)	TIR2 non-malignant	Benign (II)	0-3%	0-3%	Clinical and ultrasound follow-up	N/A
Thy3a neoplasm possible (atypia) (25%)	TIR3A low-risk IDL	AUS (III) (low and high risk)	~10-30%	6-18%	Repeat FNA, molecular testing or lobectomy	N/A
Thy3f neoplasm possible (follicular) (31%)	TIR3B high-risk IDL	FN, including oncocytic (IV)	25-40%	10-40%	Molecular testing, lobectomy	Follow-up may show follicular adenoma/carcinoma, FVPTC, or recently described NIFTP, which is indolent
Thy4 suspicious of malignancy (79%)	TIR4 suspicious	Suspicious for malignancy (V)	50-75%	45-60%	Near-total thyroidectomy or lobectomy*	Specify if concerned about FVPTC and NIFTP vs. other thyroid malignancies
Thy5 malignant (98%)	TIR5 malignant	Malignant (VI)	97-99%	94-96%	Near-total thyroidectomy or lobectomy*	~3-4% of malignant cases may turn out to be NIFTP (especially if follicular patterned)

ROM = risk of malignancy; FVPTC = follicular variant of papillary thyroid carcinoma; NIFTP = noninvasive follicular thyroid neoplasm with papillary-like nuclear features; HCT = Hürthle cell type; IDL = indeterminate lesion; TBSRTC = The Bethesda System for Reporting Thyroid Cytology; BTA-RTC = British Thyroid Association-Royal College of Physicians (BTA-RCP). *Some studies suggest molecular testing to determine type/extent of surgery

Table modified from Ali et al: The Bethesda System for Reporting Thyroid Cytopathology. Springer, 2018; ROM in various categories of the UK RCP Thy terminology for thyroid FNA cytology from: Poller et al, Cancer Cytopathol. 128(1):36-42, 2020.

- **Benign**
  - Consistent with benign follicular/adenomatous or colloid nodule
  - Consistent with lymphocytic/Hashimoto thyroiditis (in proper clinical setting)
  - Consistent with granulomatous thyroiditis
  - Other benign conditions
- **AUS**
  - Architectural &/or nuclear atypia; could be in compromised &/or paucicellular specimen
  - "FLUS/follicular lesion of undetermined significance" terminology likely to be discontinued in 2023 version, and AUS divided into high risk and low risk based on follow-up and molecular testing risk stratification findings
- **Follicular neoplasm (FN)**
  - Specify if oncocytic (Hürthle cell) type
  - "Suspicious for" FN terminology to be discontinued in 2023 update
- **Suspicious for malignancy (SM)**
  - Suspicious for papillary carcinoma
    - May include follicular variant of papillary thyroid carcinoma (FVPTC) or noninvasive follicular thyroid neoplasm with papillary-like nuclear features (NIFTP) (specify if concerned about these)
  - Suspicious for medullary carcinoma
  - Suspicious for metastatic carcinoma
  - Suspicious for lymphoma
  - Suspicious for other malignancy (specify)
- **Malignant/positive for malignancy**
  - Papillary thyroid carcinoma (consider adding note if possible FVPTC, NIFTP)
  - Medullary thyroid carcinoma
  - Poorly differentiated carcinoma
  - Undifferentiated/anaplastic carcinoma
  - Lymphoma; metastatic carcinoma
  - Other malignant process

Molecular Testing for Thyroid Fine-Needle Aspirations, Guidelines

- American Thyroid Association has guidelines on use of molecular testing in various thyroid reporting categories
- Type of molecular testing varies by availability, regulatory framework, and resource settings

SELECTED REFERENCES

1. Onken AM et al: Combined molecular and histologic end points inform cancer risk estimates for thyroid nodules classified as atypia of undetermined significance. Cancer Cytopathol. 129(12):947-55, 2021
2. Poller DN et al: Risk of malignancy in the various categories of the UK Royal College of Pathologists Thy terminology for thyroid FNA cytology: a systematic review and meta-analysis. Cancer Cytopathol. 128(1):36-42, 2020
3. Ali SZ et al: The Bethesda System for Reporting Thyroid Cytopathology: Definitions, Criteria and Explanatory Notes. Springer, 2018

Adenomatous (Benign Follicular) Nodule

KEY FACTS

TERMINOLOGY
- Adenomatous hyperplasia, nodular goiter, colloid nodule, adenomatoid nodule, benign follicular nodule (Bethesda terminology)

ETIOLOGY/PATHOGENESIS
- Iodine deficiency, goitrogenous diet
- Hereditary in subset
- Pathogenesis for most cases is unknown

CLINICAL ISSUES
- Palpable, asymmetric thyroid nodules
- Rare: Hoarseness, dysphagia, and disfigurement
- Peak in 5th-6th decades; F > M

CYTOPATHOLOGY
- Usually low cellularity with abundant colloid; can be variable
- Background: Usually watery and thin colloid, which forms film-like coating with waves
  - Lysed red blood cells, hemosiderin-laden macrophages, multinucleated giant cells, cholesterol clefts, and regenerative papillary structures may be seen in nodules with cystic degeneration
  - Dense colloid has refractile quality and shows cracks
- Large, flat sheets of evenly spaced follicular cells
- Macro- and microfollicles (characterized by small follicles with 10-15 cells)
  - Up to 50% microfollicles may be seen in some cases
- Reactive/regenerative/symplastic changes may be present
- Abundant granular cytoplasmic changes (oncocytic/Hürtheloid) often seen
- Colloid nodules have thick colloid but paucicellular

TOP DIFFERENTIAL DIAGNOSES
- Follicular neoplasm: More cellular, > 50% microfollicular architecture, less colloid, less nuclear variability
- Papillary thyroid carcinoma: Characteristic nuclear features

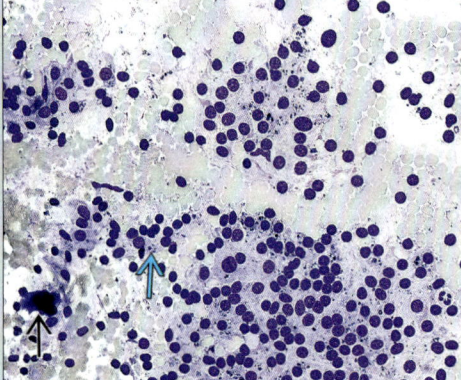

Adenomatous (Benign Follicular) Nodule

(Left) Diff-Quik-stained smear of an adenomatous nodule shows follicles of varying sizes, watery colloid, blood, and scant, dense colloid ➡. Also note the intracytoplasmic hemosiderin granules ➡.

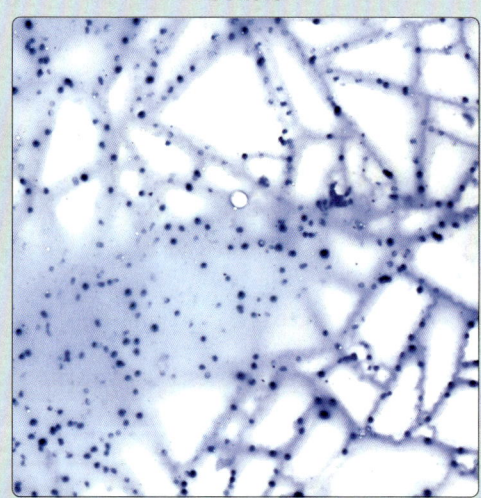

Colloid

(Right) Diff-Quik-stained smear shows abundant watery colloid in an adenomatous nodule. Sometimes, colloid cracks in a geometric pattern and falls off of the slide.

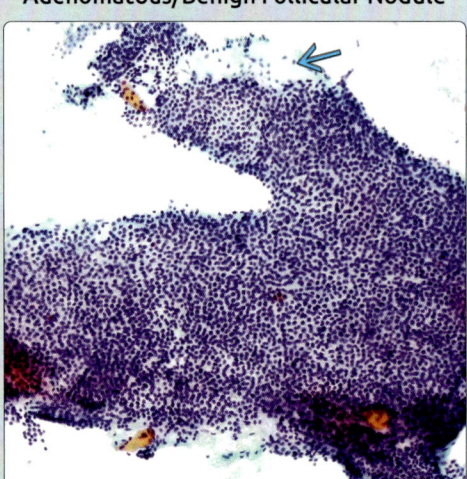

Adenomatous/Benign Follicular Nodule

(Left) Pap-stained smear at low magnification shows a macrofollicle with small, dark, evenly spaced nuclei in a background of watery colloid ➡.

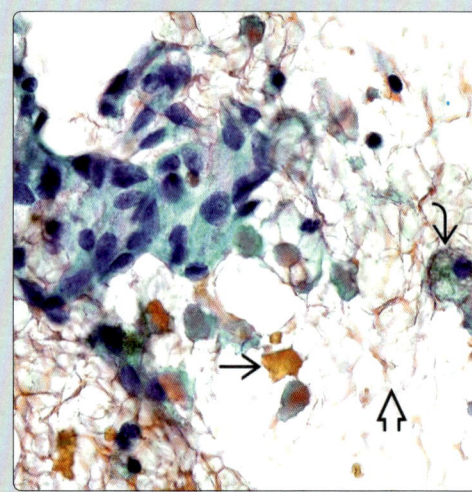

Cyst-Related Reactive Change

(Right) Pap-stained smear shows an adenomatous nodule with cystic degeneration and reactive atypia. There are hemosiderin-laden macrophages ➡, dense colloid ➡, and watery colloid ➡ in the background.

Adenomatous (Benign Follicular) Nodule

TERMINOLOGY

Synonyms
- Adenomatous hyperplasia, nodular goiter, colloid nodule, adenomatoid nodule, benign follicular nodule (Bethesda terminology)

CLINICAL ISSUES

Epidemiology
- Incidence
  - Palpable nodules in 5-7% of adult population
  - Ultrasound-detected nodules in up to 50% of adults

Presentation
- Usually multiple asymmetric nodules
- Sudden enlargement or pain due to intranodular bleeding
- Rare: Tracheal obstruction, neck disfigurement, or hoarseness due to enlarged gland

Treatment
- Clinical follow-up for most cases
- American Thyroid Association management guidelines based on size and sonographic risk pattern of nodule

Prognosis
- Implied risk of malignancy 0-3% (Bethesda System category II)

Image Findings
- Ultrasonography: Hypoechoic or hyperechoic nodules

CYTOPATHOLOGY

Cellularity
- Usually low cellularity with abundant colloid
  - Cellularity can vary from low to high
  - Colloid nodules show very low cellularity with abundant colloid

Pattern
- Large, flat sheets of evenly spaced follicular cells in honeycomb arrangement
- Macro- and microfollicles (characterized by small follicles with 10-15 cells)
- Up to 50% microfollicles may be seen in some cases

Background
- Colloid: Usually watery and thin colloid, which forms film-like coating with waves

Cells
- Bland, uniform cells
- Mild atypia may be seen in nodules with cystic degeneration

Nuclear Details
- Round to oval nuclei with smooth nuclear membrane, granular chromatin, inconspicuous nucleoli
- Reactive follicular cells may have prominent nucleoli
- Nuclear size variability common

Cytoplasmic Details
- Pale and delicate
- May have abundant granular cytoplasm in cells with Hürtheloid changes

Adequacy Criteria
- At least 6 groups of well-preserved, well-visualized cells with 6-10 cells in each group

DIAGNOSTIC CHECKLIST

Pathologic Interpretation Pearls
- In air-dried smears, watery colloid can result in rouleaux formation of red blood cells
- Differential diagnosis of colloid: Serum (in bloody smears), skeletal muscle (for hard colloid)

SELECTED REFERENCES
1. Kobaly K et al: Contemporary management of thyroid nodules. Annu Rev Med. 73:517-28, 2022
2. Nagasaki K et al: A Japanese family with DICER1 syndrome found in childhood-onset multinodular goitre. Horm Res Paediatr. 93(7-8):477-82, 2020
3. Ali SZ et al: The Bethesda System for Reporting Thyroid Cytopathology: Definitions, Criteria and Explanatory Notes. Springer, 2017

Varying Follicle Sizes

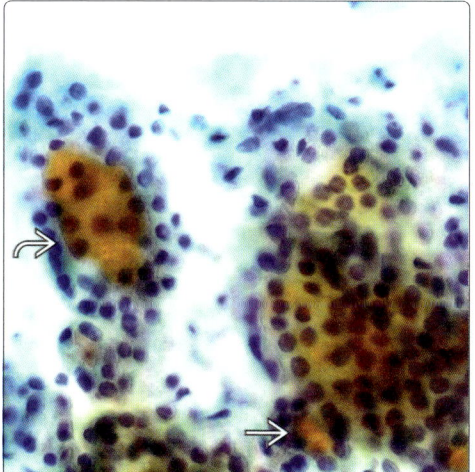

Symplastic Changes in Benign Follicular/Adenomatous Nodule

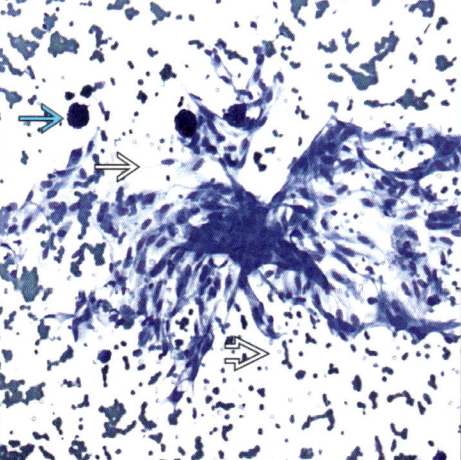

(Left) Pap-stained section shows varying follicular sizes. Both microfollicles ➡ and macrofollicles ➡ are seen with central colloid within the follicles, which stains orange. *(Right)* Symplastic changes are characterized by pulled-out cytoplasm imparting a spindle cell appearance ➡. The hemosiderin-laden macrophages ➡ in the background are indicative of recent hemorrhage and cystic degeneration. The pale blue hue to the background and rouleaux formation ➡ point to watery colloid.

Chronic Lymphocytic/Hashimoto Thyroiditis

KEY FACTS

ETIOLOGY/PATHOGENESIS
- Autoimmune disease, IgG4-related disease, infection, excess iodine intake
- Subtypes include classic type, fibrous variant, and IgG4 related

CLINICAL ISSUES
- Female predominance (10:1); 30-60 years of age in classic type
  - Fibrous and IgG4 types may be equal in male and female patients
- Antithyroid antibodies present in 90% of cases
  - Increased serum IgG4 in IgG4 variant
- Prognosis generally good, but there is increased risk of lymphoma and papillary carcinoma
- Flow cytometry may show abnormal κ:λ ratio
  - Should not be misdiagnosed as lymphoma

CYTOPATHOLOGY
- Cellular aspirate with Hürthle cells, lymphocytes, plasma cells, macrophages, and giant cells
  - Fibrous and atrophic variants are hypocellular, and lymphocytes may be very scant
  - Does not require minimum of 6 follicular cell clusters to be considered adequate
- Numerous reactive Hürthle cells may raise concern for neoplastic process
  - Rarely Hürthle cells with grooves, intranuclear holes, and cytologic atypia
  - Lymphocytes infiltrate Hürthle cells, unlike in true Hürthle cell neoplasm

TOP DIFFERENTIAL DIAGNOSES
- Hürthle cell neoplasm, papillary thyroid carcinoma (PTC), lymphoma, Riedel thyroiditis, Graves disease
- Open chromatin and rare nuclear "holes" or grooves may be seen and are pitfall for overdiagnosis as PTC

Mixed Lymphoid Population With Scant Colloid

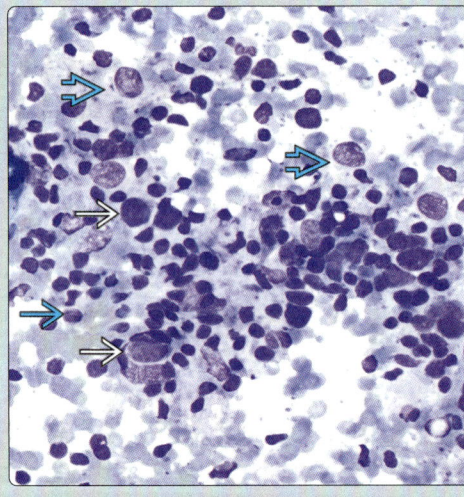

Lymphocytic Thyroiditis With Abundant Hürthle Cells

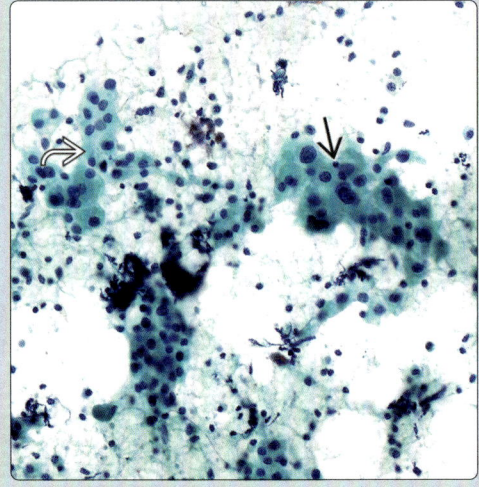

(Left) Diff-Quik-stained smear from Hashimoto/lymphocytic thyroiditis shows a polymorphous population of large ⇨ and small lymphocytes ⇨ and tingible body macrophages ⇨. (Right) Pap-stained low-power image shows Hürthle/oncocytic ⇨ cells with abundant granular cytoplasm in a background of variably sized lymphocytes. Note the infiltration of lymphocytes into the groups of oncocytic cells ⇨.

Giant Cell

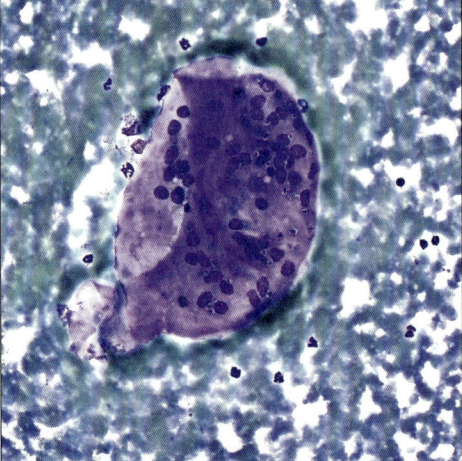

Plasma Cells in Lymphocytic Thyroiditis

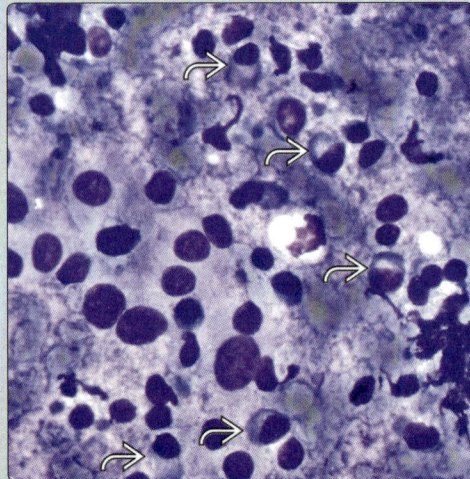

(Left) Multinucleated giant cells may be seen in lymphocytic thyroiditis, as seen on this Diff-Quik-stained smear. (Right) A predominance of plasma cells ⇨ should raise concern for IgG4 variant, and serum IgG4 levels should be investigated.

Chronic Lymphocytic/Hashimoto Thyroiditis

TERMINOLOGY

Definitions
- Autoimmune disease characterized by diffuse lymphoplasmacytic infiltration of thyroid gland

ETIOLOGY/PATHOGENESIS

Autoimmune
- Elevated circulating antithyroid antibodies
- HLA proteins on follicular cells
- May be part of IgG4-related systemic disease

Possible Environmental/Exogenous Factors
- Excess iodine intake
- Viral and bacterial infections

CLINICAL ISSUES

Presentation
- Gradual thyroid failure, transient hyperthyroidism
- Compression of trachea or recurrent laryngeal nerve
- May be associated with other autoimmune diseases
- Rare: Hashimoto encephalopathy

Laboratory Tests
- Antithyroid peroxidase antibodies in 90% of patients
- Antithyroglobulin antibody in > 60% of patients
- Elevated IgG4 in IgG4 variants

CYTOPATHOLOGY

Cellularity
- Cellular aspirate
  - Abundant lymphocytes
  - Sheets, small groups, or individual Hürthle cells
- Fibrous and atrophic variants are hypocellular

Cells
- Oncocytes/Hürthle cells in background of scant to absent colloid
- Abundant polymorphous T-cell-rich mature lymphocytes, plasma cells, multinucleated giant cells, and tingible body macrophages

Nuclear Details
- Hürthle cells: Enlarged nuclei with prominent nucleoli
  - Sometimes may have pyknotic nuclei
  - May have reactive atypia

Cytoplasmic Details
- Hürthle cells: Abundant granular cytoplasm

Adequacy Criteria
- Abundant lymphoid cells and variable number of Hürthle cells (does not require minimum of 6 follicular cell clusters to be considered adequate)

ANCILLARY TESTS

Flow Cytometry
- Only if clinically or morphologically suspicious or older patient
- Flow cytometry may show abnormal κ:λ ratio

DIFFERENTIAL DIAGNOSIS

Neoplasms
- Hürthle cell proliferation mimics Hürthle cell neoplasm
- Hürthle cells with nuclear grooves and holes mimic papillary thyroid carcinoma (PTC) (true PTC has nuclear changes in several clusters)
- Mucosa-associated lymphoid tissue (MALT) lymphoma
- Warthin-like PTC

Other Thyroiditides
- Riedel thyroiditis, Graves disease

SELECTED REFERENCES
1. Cho YY et al: Malignancy rate of Bethesda class III thyroid nodules based on the presence of chronic lymphocytic thyroiditis in surgical patients. Front Endocrinol (Lausanne). 12:745395, 2021

Hürthle Cell Nodule
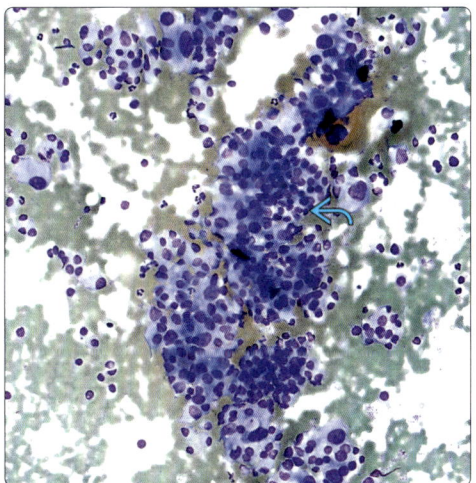

Hürthle Cell With Nuclear Groove
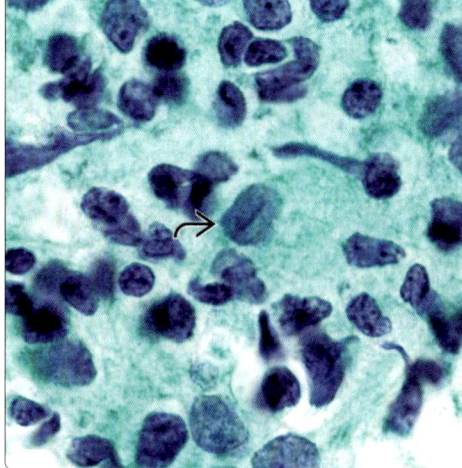

(Left) Diff-Quik stain demonstrates Hürthle cell nodule/proliferation in Hashimoto thyroiditis. Paucity of background lymphocytes is a major pitfall in overdiagnosis of Hürthle cell neoplasm. Presence of lymphocytes ➡ infiltrating Hürthle cell clusters is a helpful clue to differentiate this from a neoplasm. (Right) Pap stain illustrates a Hürthle cell with a nuclear groove ➡ mimicking papillary thyroid carcinoma (PTC). True PTC usually shows characteristic nuclear features in several cell clusters.

Granulomatous Thyroiditis

KEY FACTS

CLINICAL ISSUES
- Accounts for < 3% of all thyroid disease
- Most common in 2nd-5th decades
- 3-6x more common in females than in males
- Etiologies: Subacute (de Quervain) thyroiditis (COVID-19, other viruses), infectious agents (fungi, TB), sarcoidosis

CYTOPATHOLOGY
- Varies with etiology and stage of disease
- Subacute (de Quervain) thyroiditis
  - Early disease: Acute inflammatory cells with microabscesses
  - Late phase: Follicular cells, mixed inflammation, granulomas, multinucleated giant cells, and foamy macrophages
  - Careful search for organisms should be made
  - Tissue should be submitted for fungal, bacterial, and mycobacterial cultures
- Fungal thyroiditis
  - Fungal organisms may be seen on routine Pap or Diff-Quik slides but best seen on GMS or PAS stains
- Mycobacterial thyroiditis
  - Necrosis within granulomas
  - Need confirmation by culture or special stains
- Cell block can be used for special stains

TOP DIFFERENTIAL DIAGNOSES
- Lymphocytic thyroiditis
- Papillary carcinoma (due to presence of giant cells)

DIAGNOSTIC CHECKLIST
- Subacute (de Quervain) thyroiditis most common cause of granulomatous thyroiditis
- Due to high iodine content, rich blood supply, and lymphatic drainage, thyroid gland resistant to infection
- Although infection extremely rare, if mixed inflammation or granulomas are seen, tissue should be submitted for microbiology cultures and special stains

Granulomatous Thyroiditis
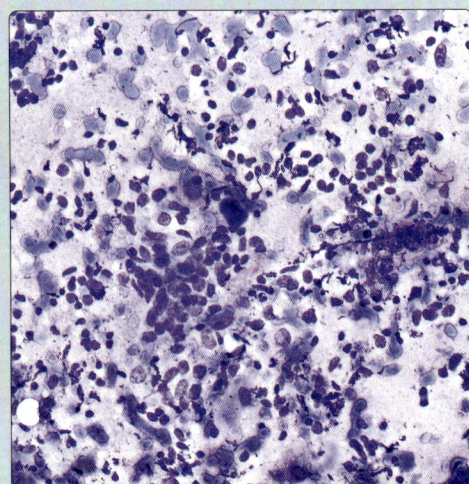

Giant Cell in Granulomatous Thyroiditis
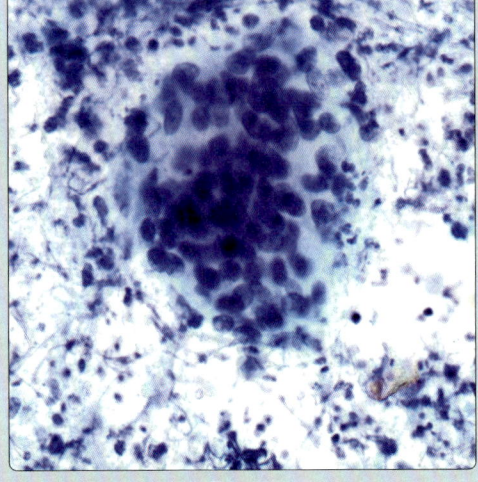

(Left) Diff-Quik-stained slide shows granulomatous thyroiditis (GT). Chronic inflammation in the background may mimic lymphocytic thyroiditis. (Right) Pap-stained high-power image of GT illustrates multinucleated giant cells in a background of necrosis and acute and chronic inflammation. Multinucleated cells may have up to 50 nuclei per cell.

Granuloma
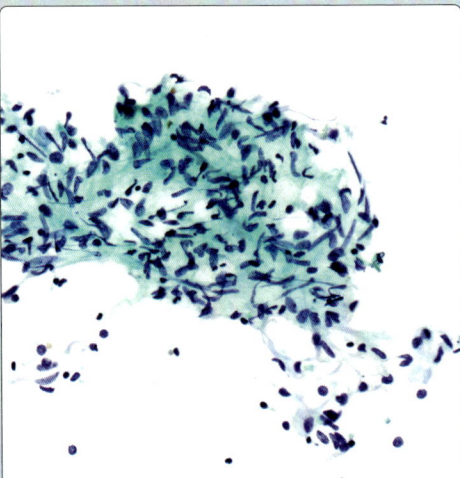

Granulomatous Thyroiditis Histology
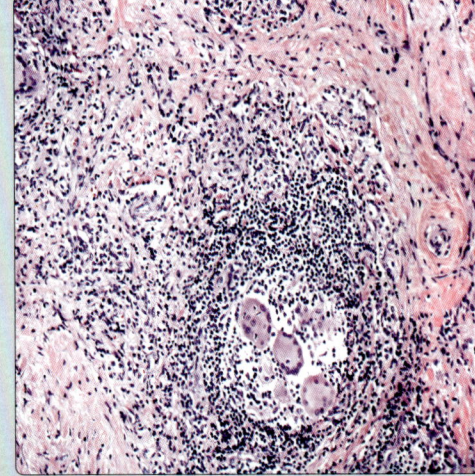

(Left) Pap-stained smear shows a well-formed, nonnecrotizing granuloma in a case of de Quervain thyroiditis. The histiocytes have haphazard elongate nuclei and syncytial cytoplasm. (Right) H&E-stained section of the subsequent thyroidectomy shows well-formed granulomas, chronic inflammation, and multinucleated giant cells.

Granulomatous Thyroiditis

TERMINOLOGY

Synonyms
- Subacute/de Quervain thyroiditis

ETIOLOGY/PATHOGENESIS

Subacute Thyroiditis
- Circulating antibodies to various viruses, including measles, influenza, adenovirus, and mumps
- Transient thyroid antibodies have been reported
- Genetics: Association between granulomatous thyroiditis (GT) and *HLA-B35*
- COVID-19-related subacute thyroiditis: mRNA encoding for ACE-2 receptor expressed in thyroid follicular cells, making them potential target for SARS-CoV-2 entry

Infectious Agents
- **Fungal infection**: *Blastomyces, Cryptococcus, Aspergillus, Histoplasma, Mucor*
- **Tuberculosis**: Mycobacterial infection

Others
- **Sarcoidosis**: Part of systemic disease or primary

CLINICAL ISSUES

Presentation
- **Subacute (de Quervain) thyroiditis)**
  o Incidence: < 3% of all thyroid disease, F:M = 3-6:1; mean age: 45 years
  o **Clinical presentation**
    – Symmetrically enlarged, tender, and hard gland
    – History of prior viral infection
    – Pain aggravated by swallowing or neck movement
    – Malaise, fatigue, fever, chills, anorexia, myalgia
    – Laboratory findings: Initial thyrotoxicosis, elevated erythrocyte sedimentation rate and C-reactive protein, followed by hypothyroid phase
    – Diagnosis based on clinical findings; tissue diagnosis rarely needed
    – Prognosis: Complete resolution in few months
    – Treatment: Corticosteroids &/or analgesics
- **Granulomatous infection**
  o Very uncommon, can occur at any age and sex
  o Most common in immunocompromised patients

CYTOPATHOLOGY

Cellularity
- Cytology varies with disease progression and etiology
  o Aspirates may be acellular with advanced fibrosis
- Subacute (de Quervain) thyroiditis
  o Early disease: Acute inflammatory cells with microabscesses (rarely biopsied)
  o Later phase: Mixed inflammation and granulomas
- Fungal thyroiditis
  o Inflammatory cells and granulomas
  o Fungal organisms may be seen on routine Pap or Diff-Quik slides but best seen on GMS or PAS stains
- Mycobacterial thyroiditis
  o Necrosis within granulomas
  o Need confirmation by culture or special stains

Cells
- Follicular cells admixed with inflammatory cells
  o Neutrophils, lymphocytes, epithelioid histiocytes, multinucleated giant cells (up to 50 nuclei per cell), and foamy macrophages

DIFFERENTIAL DIAGNOSIS

Other Thyroiditides
- Lymphocytes and giant cells can be misdiagnosed as lymphocytic thyroiditis

Neoplasms
- Giant cells may raise concern for papillary carcinoma

SELECTED REFERENCES
1. Abreu R et al: Subacute (de Quervain) thyroiditis during the COVID-19 pandemic. Cancer Cytopathol. 129(11):844-6, 2021

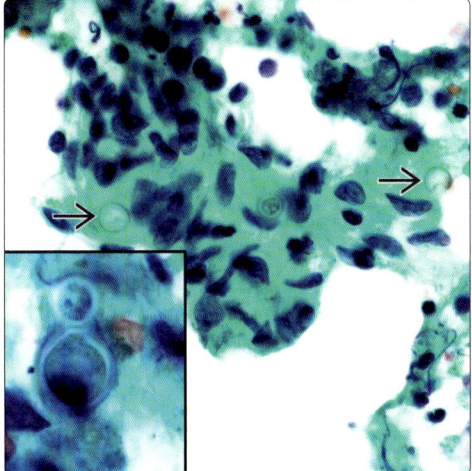

Blastomycosis

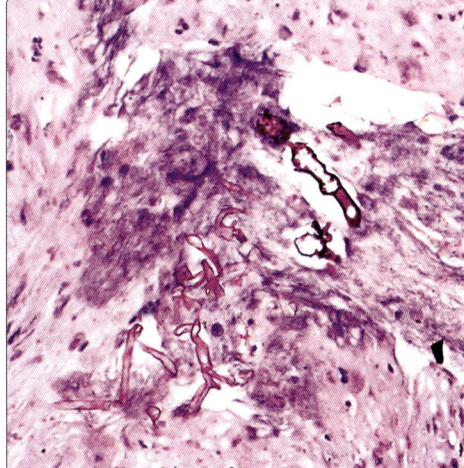

Mucor in Cell Block

(Left) Pap-stained smear of thyroid FNA shows fungal spores ➡ in a well-formed granuloma. Inset illustrates broad-based budding yeasts with thick-walled refractile capsules, consistent with blastomycosis. *(Right)* PAS stain, performed on cell block, shows fungal hyphae morphologically consistent with the Mucor/Rhizopus family

Graves Disease/Diffuse Toxic Goiter

KEY FACTS

TERMINOLOGY
- Autoimmune disease characterized by diffuse goiter, thyrotoxicosis, infiltrative ophthalmopathy, &, occasionally, infiltrative dermatopathology

CLINICAL ISSUES
- Most common cause of hyperthyroidism in USA
- Most common cause of spontaneous hyperthyroidism in patients younger than 40 years
- TSHR antibody is most specific for Graves disease but may also be seen in other thyroiditides, such as Hashimoto thyroiditis (HT)
- Strongly associated with haplotypes HLA-B8 & HLA-DR3

CYTOPATHOLOGY
- Low to moderately cellular specimen
- Scant, watery, pale colloid on Pap stain
- Sheets of follicular cells with peripherally located nuclei & marginal vacuoles adjacent to nuclei
- Follicular cells in sheets or microfollicles
- Oncocytic changes may be present in up to 1/2 of cytologic specimens
- Posttreatment specimens can demonstrate atypia & low nuclear:cytoplasmic ratios
- Lymphocytes may be present in specimen

TOP DIFFERENTIAL DIAGNOSES
- **Papillary thyroid carcinoma (PTC)**: Graves disease may have papillary structures with fibrovascular cores & psammoma bodies but lacks nuclear features of PTC
  - Inflammatory response may cause adherence to skeletal muscle mimicking invasive PTC
- **HT**: Distinction from early HT may be difficult clinically as it may present initially with hyperthyroid symptoms
- **Toxic multinodular goiter**: Nodularity, majority of gland with follicles having abundant colloid & characteristic antibody panel is absent

Marginal Cytoplasmic Vacuoles
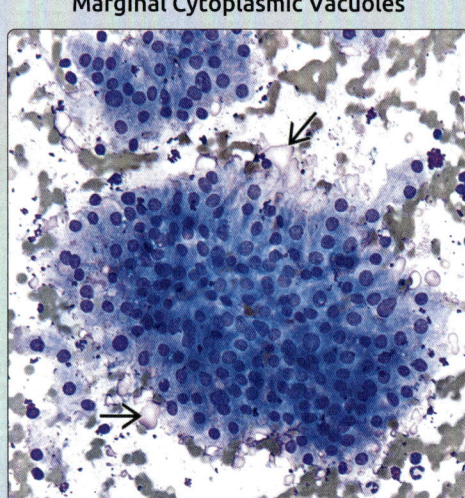

Papillary-Like Projections in Graves Disease
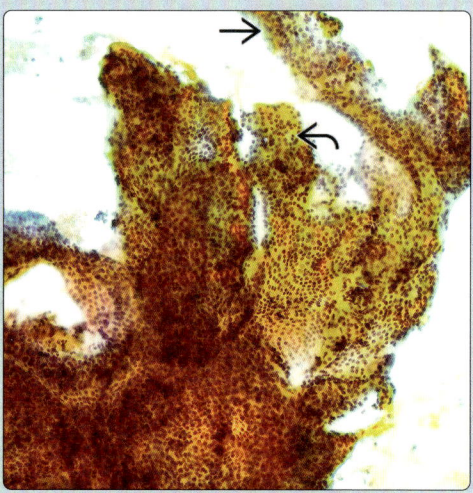

(Left) Diff-Quik-stained sheet of benign follicular cells shows marginal cytoplasmic vacuoles with magenta-pink frayed edges ⇨, the so-called flame cells seen in Graves disease. (Courtesy S. Ali, MD.) (Right) Pap stain shows benign follicular cells with hyperplastic papillary-like projections ⇨ and focal microfollicles ⇨.

Histology of Papillary-Like Projections
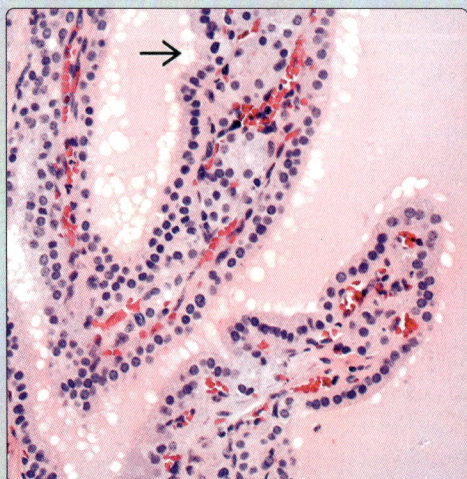

Posttreatment Atypia
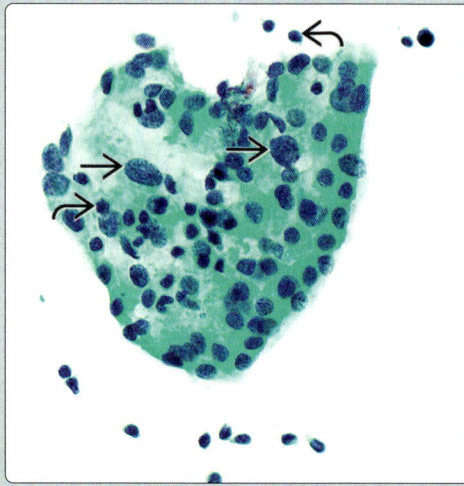

(Left) H&E-stained cell block shows complex papillary hyperplasia with follicular lumina with scalloped colloid ⇨ often seen in Graves disease. (Right) Pap-stained posttreatment aspirate of Graves disease shows oncocytic (Hürthle) cells with atypia ⇨, albeit with a low nuclear:cytoplasmic ratio, and scattered lymphocytes ⇨.

Pigmented Thyroid Lesions and Crystals

KEY FACTS

TERMINOLOGY
- Intrathyroidal deposition of endogenous or exogenous material, including iron, lipofuscin, degradation products of minocycline, and crystals

CYTOPATHOLOGY
- **Hemosiderin**: Can be found in macrophages, follicular cells, and stromal fragments in adenomatous nodules as well as neoplasms
  - Coarse, brown to yellow, refractile pigment on Pap
  - Iron stain (Prussian blue) demonstrates deposits
- **Lipofuscin**: Pigment in follicular epithelial cells
  - Intracytoplasmic, yellow to light brown, granular-appearing pigment on Pap stain
  - PAS-positive, diastase-sensitive intracytoplasmic material
  - Lipid (Sudan IV) and lipofuscin stains may be helpful
  - Iron stains negative
- **Minocycline**: Identified in cytoplasm of follicular cells as granular and black or within follicular lumina as large black deposits mixed with colloid
  - Positive with PAS, lipid, and lipofuscin stains
  - May be positive on Fontana-Masson and negative on iron stains
- **Calcifications**: Psammoma bodies
  - Concentric laminations: Seen in papillary carcinoma as well as benign conditions
- **Crystals**: Usually within colloid, calcium oxalate on analysis
  - No association with any disease or entity but more common in benign conditions
- **Melanin**: Very rare in thyroid aspirates
  - Powdery cytoplasmic brown pigment on Pap stain and blue on Diff-Quik stain
  - Seen in medullary carcinoma, melanocytic variant, or widely metastatic malignant melanoma
- **Foreign material**: Teflon due to vocal cord injection
  - Usually within giant cells

Hemosiderin
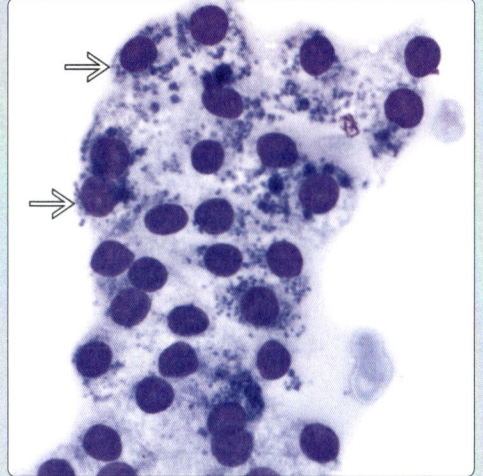

Calcium Oxalate Crystals
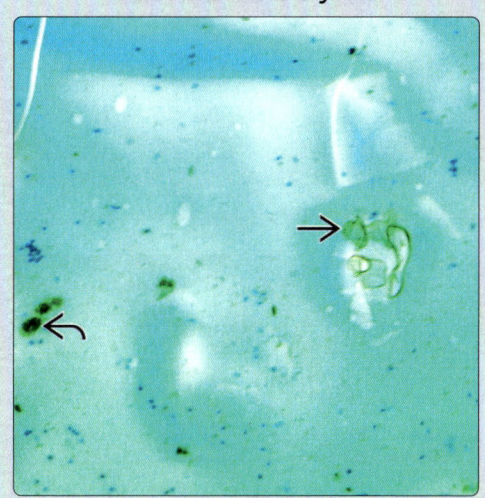

(Left) Diff-Quik stain shows the blue granules ➡ of hemosiderin in the cytoplasm of benign follicular cells from an adenomatous nodule with cystic degeneration. **(Right)** Pap stain of a colloid nodule shows refractile (and polarizable) calcium oxalate crystals ➡ and hemosiderin ➡ in a sea of colloid.

Minocycline Crystals
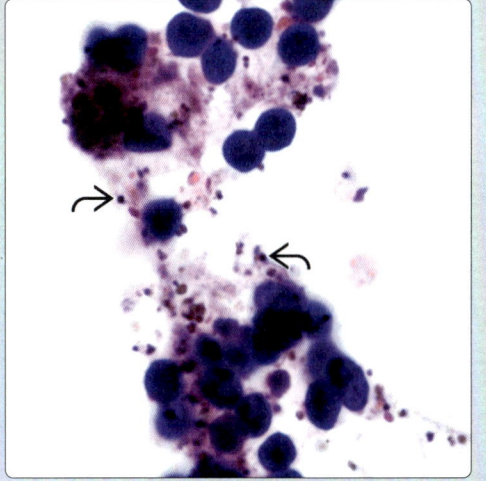

Teflon Granuloma
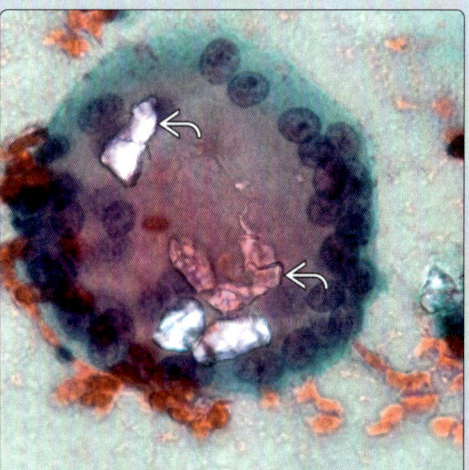

(Left) H&E-stained touch prep shows dark brown to black minocycline crystals ➡ in the cytoplasm of follicular cells. **(Right)** Pap stain shows refractile crystals ➡ in a giant cell in a case of Teflon granuloma from previous vocal cord injection.

Atypia of Undetermined Significance/Follicular Lesion of Undetermined Significance

TERMINOLOGY

Synonyms
- Atypia of undetermined significance (AUS)
- Follicular lesion of undetermined significance (FLUS)
- These terms are intended to be interchangeable; use of both in same laboratory to imply cytologic vs. architectural atypia is not recommended and can be confusing
- Based on publications since introduction of this terminology, 2023 update is considering eliminating FLUS and dividing AUS into low- and high-risk types
  o Exact nomenclature to be decided
  o High-risk types of AUS are those with nuclear atypia or mixed nuclear and architectural atypia
  o Low-risk types are those with concerning architectural or oncocytic features but not nuclear atypia

Definitions
- Specimen that contains cells of follicular, lymphoid, or other origin
- Contains architectural or nuclear atypia that is more than would be expected in benign nodule but that falls short of being suspicious for malignancy or follicular or oncocytic (Hürthle cell) neoplasm
  – Could be focal in otherwise benign specimen or due to compromised specimen, either from low cellularity or from artifacts, such as air drying, blood, or ultrasound gel
- Different possible scenarios resulting in AUS/FLUS diagnosis can be generally divided into following main categories
  o Cytologic atypia
  o Architectural atypia
  o Cytologic and architectural atypia
  o Compromised specimen due to artifacts, etc.
  o Oncocytic (Hürthle cell) aspirates
  o Atypia not otherwise specified
  o Atypical lymphoid cells (rule out lymphoma)

Nuclear Atypia in Lymphocytic Thyroiditis

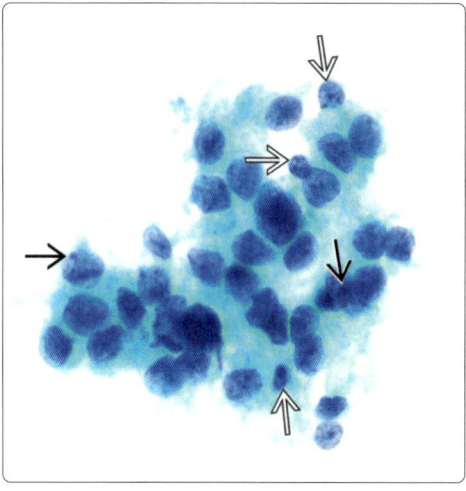

AUS, Focal Nuclear Atypia in Benign Nodule

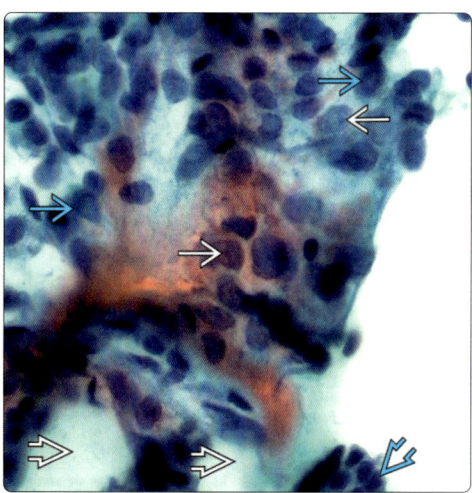

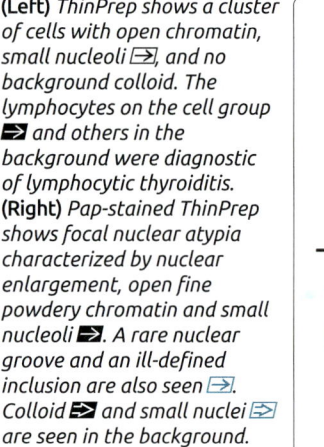

(Left) ThinPrep shows a cluster of cells with open chromatin, small nucleoli ➡, and no background colloid. The lymphocytes on the cell group ➡ and others in the background were diagnostic of lymphocytic thyroiditis. (Right) Pap-stained ThinPrep shows focal nuclear atypia characterized by nuclear enlargement, open fine powdery chromatin and small nucleoli ➡. A rare nuclear groove and an ill-defined inclusion are also seen ➡. Colloid ➡ and small nuclei ➡ are seen in the background.

Uniform Architectural and Nuclear Atypia

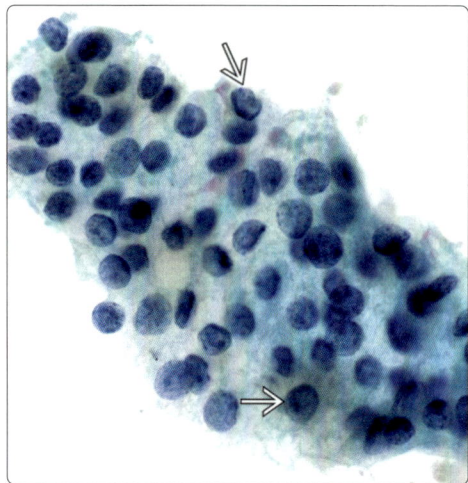

Compromised Specimen With Clotting

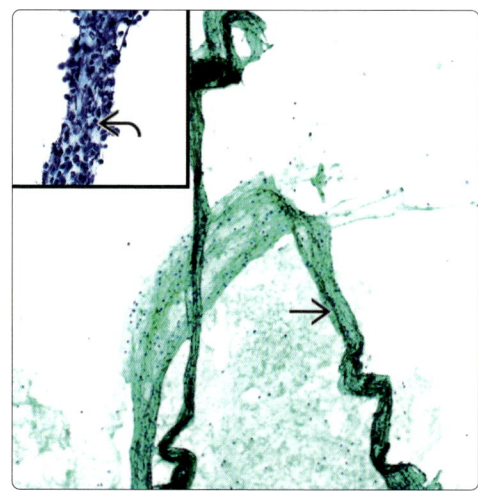

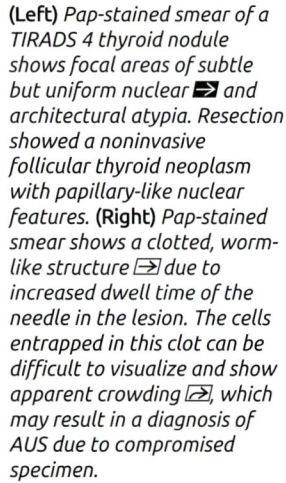

(Left) Pap-stained smear of a TIRADS 4 thyroid nodule shows focal areas of subtle but uniform nuclear ➡ and architectural atypia. Resection showed a noninvasive follicular thyroid neoplasm with papillary-like nuclear features. (Right) Pap-stained smear shows a clotted, worm-like structure ➡ due to increased dwell time of the needle in the lesion. The cells entrapped in this clot can be difficult to visualize and show apparent crowding ➡, which may result in a diagnosis of AUS due to compromised specimen.

Atypia of Undetermined Significance/Follicular Lesion of Undetermined Significance

DIFFERENT SCENARIOS AND CRITERIA FOR AUS/FLUS DIAGNOSIS

Cytologic Atypia (Higher Risk of Malignancy)

- Focal cytologic atypia [focal nuclear features of papillary thyroid carcinoma (PTC)]
  - Pale nuclear chromatin, oval nuclei, intranuclear cytoplasmic inclusions, nuclear contour irregularity; limited to very rare groups of cells in otherwise benign sample
  - These could be in background of Hashimoto thyroiditis or multinodular goiter
- Extensive but mild cytologic atypia
  - Most cells have mildly enlarged, slightly pale nuclei with limited contour irregularity and absent intranuclear cytoplasmic inclusions
- Cyst contents and atypical cyst lining cells
  - Atypia in cyst lining cells beyond what is normally expected in cyst aspirations or cystic nodules
  - Minor component of cells with nuclear elongation, grooves, cleared/powdery chromatin, raising concern for papillary carcinoma but not sufficient for diagnosis of "suspicious for malignancy"
- Histiocytoid cells (concern for cystic papillary carcinoma)
  - Larger than usual for true histiocytes, either isolated or in microfollicles or clusters
  - Round nuclei, high N:C ratio, and glassy/hard cytoplasm (compared to true histiocytes)
  - Absence of hemosiderin in cytoplasm (unlike histiocytes)
  - Large discrete vacuolization of cytoplasm (unlike fine vacuoles of histiocytes)
  - Staining of cytospins or cell block may help (CD68 and cytokeratin)

Architectural Atypia (Lower Risk of Malignancy)

- Scant cellularity with rare clusters of microfollicles/trabeculae
  - Cellularity too low for diagnosis of follicular neoplasm/suspicious for follicular neoplasm
  - However, architecture cannot be ignored, precluding diagnosis as nondiagnostic specimen
- Cellular specimen with focal prominence of microfollicles
  - Cellular specimen, but proportion of microfollicles not sufficient for diagnosis of follicular neoplasm, though more than what would be expected with adenomatous nodule
  - Benign adenomatous nodule findings on most passes, but 1 pass shows microfollicular pattern

Cytologic and Architectural Atypia (Higher Risk of Malignancy)

- Mild but diffuse cytologic and architectural atypia [may be seen with follicular subtype of papillary carcinoma (FSPTC) or noninvasive follicular thyroid neoplasm with papillary-like nuclear features (NIFTP)]

Oncocytic (Hürthle Cell) Aspirates (Lower Risk of Malignancy)

- Predominance of oncocytic (Hürthle) cells
  - In setting that suggests lymphocytic/Hashimoto thyroiditis or adenomatous nodule from multinodular goiter
  - Clinically lymphocytic thyroiditis but lymphocytes are absent and only Hürthle cells present
  - Clinically multinodular goiter, but aspirate yields predominant population of oncocytic cells
  - Predominant or exclusive population of Hürthle/oncocytic cells in sparsely cellular specimen with scant colloid but insufficient for definitive diagnosis of Hürthle cell neoplasm

Atypia, Not Otherwise Specified

- Rare/minor population of follicular cells with nuclear enlargement accompanied by nucleoli
- These changes could be from radioactive iodine, carbimazole, or others, but history may not be available
- Psammoma bodies in absence of nuclear features of PTC
  - Lamellar bodies of inspissated colloid may be mistaken for psammoma bodies
  - Small globules of thick colloid in liquid-based preparations may also mimic psammoma bodies
  - Positive predictive value (PPV) for psammoma bodies in thyroid aspirates is ~ 50%; hence, in absence of other features of PTC, best to interpret as AUS/FLUS
- Atypical cells of uncertain origin, raising possibility of other epithelial or mesenchymal processes but without availability of history or ancillary diagnostic studies
- Other instances of atypia not described above
  - Remember, AUS/FLUS is diagnosis of last resort

Atypical or Monotonous Lymphoid Infiltrate

- Could be in background of Hashimoto and would require immunophenotyping by flow cytometry for definitive diagnosis
- In absence of sufficient changes for diagnosis of "suspicious for lymphoma," these could be classified as "atypical lymphoid cells" with repeat aspirate for flow cytometry

Preparation Artifact Notes

- By themselves, preparation artifacts and hypocellularity do not warrant AUS/FLUS diagnosis, provided there is no atypia and changes are only focal in otherwise obviously benign case
- However, there are scenarios where AUS/FLUS diagnosis can be made (after acknowledging compromised nature of specimen)
  - Air-drying artifact that hinders adequate evaluation of cellular and nuclear atypia
  - Clotting artifact resulting in apparent cellular crowding
  - Excessive blood, obscuring cells and architectural evaluation
- Excessive ultrasound gel, obscuring architectural or nuclear evaluation, is best interpreted as nondiagnostic unless worrisome atypia

REPORTING CRITERIA

Reporting Rates

- At time of 2007 Bethesda conference, reporting rates for AUS/FLUS were expected to be between 2-7%
  - Unfortunately, indiscriminate use of this AUS/FLUS category has resulted in rates as high as 22%
  - Maximum reporting rate of 10% is more realistic benchmark

Atypia of Undetermined Significance/Follicular Lesion of Undetermined Significance

Comparison of Commercial Molecular Tests for Indeterminate Thyroid Nodules (USA) (AUS and FN Categories, Based on Clinical Validation Studies)

	Afirma GSC	ThyGeNEXT & ThyraMIR	ThysoSeq v3
Sample size in validation study	190	178	247
NIFTP and cancer prevelance	24%	30%	28%
Benign call rate	54%	46%	61%
NPV and PPV	96%, 47%	95%, 52%*	97%, 66%
Sensitivity and specificity	91%, 68%	93%, 62%*	94%, 82%

AUS = atypia of undetermined significance; FN = follicular neoplasm; GSC = gene sequencing classifier; NPV = negative predictive value; PPV = positive predictive value.

*Only results with high probability of cancer or NIFTP considered positive test results, and those with low probablilty of cancer on ThyGeNEXT and ThyraMIR considered negative.

Abbreviated from: Molecular tests for risk-stratifying cytologically indeterminate thyroid nodules: an overview of commercially available testing platforms in the United States by Nishino M et al: J. Mol. Pathol. 2,135-46, 2021.

- Malignant outcomes at time of meeting were expected to be between 5-15%
  - Actual outcomes have varied widely
  - 2017 version of Bethesda has revised risk of malignancy (ROM) based on data published since 2007 as well as considering newer indolent entity of NIFTP, which cannot be diagnosed cytologically
  - Some NIFTP cases will be diagnosed in AUS/FLUS category pushing down ROM

Reporting Notes
- Interpretation of AUS/FLUS implies that specimen is adequate
- Narrative comments as to cytologic vs. architectural atypia are encouraged
- Avoid using phases associated with malignancy (nuclear pseudoinclusions, rule out papillary carcinoma) that may prompt surgery

Management of AUS/FLUS
- Repeat FNA under ultrasound guidance
  - Manage based on repeat diagnosis
    - ~ 10-30% of repeat FNAs result in AUS/FLUS diagnosis
  - If repeat AUS or worse, consider lobectomy
  - ROM in AUS/FLUS category varies with type of atypia
    - AUS due to cytologic atypia has mean ROM of 47%
    - AUS/FLUS due to Hürthle cell/oncocytic atypia has ROM of 5%
- Reflex molecular testing per guidelines (preferred approach)
  - Molecular-derived ROM calculation may be better option for clinical decision making and comparison
- For management decision, combination of cytologic, molecular, sonographic, clinical, and patient preference should be taken into consideration

Notes on Molecular Testing
- Reflex molecular testing from residual in CytoLyt vial or collecting in specialized media for commercially available molecular testing at time of FNA (1st time or repeat) is preferred option
- Different testing algorithms are available commercially for triage or can be laboratory-developed test with appropriate validation
- "Rule out" test like Afirma gene expression classifier (GEC) is best suited when prevalence of malignancy is low; newer gene sequencing classifier (GSC) is also rule in test
  - Benign/negative result on GEC results in ROM dropping from 24% to 5%, thus justifying observation over surgery
  - ~ 50% of GEC tests in AUS/FLUS are negative/benign
  - GSC has higher benign call rate and higher ROM for suspicious result
  - AUS/FLUS cases due to Hürthle/oncocytic changes tend to perform poorly with false suspicious results on GEC (only 15% ROM on subsequent resection)
  - Addition of GSC by Afirma has resolved issue with oncocytic specimens

Performance Measures
- AUS:malignant ratio can be calculated for lab as well as individual pathologist
- Can be used as performance measure and for benchmarking
- Based on studies, higher AUS rate = lower rate of malignancy on follow-up, implying imprecision/overinterpretation
- Recommend ratio between 1 and 3
  - If ratio is > 3, overuse of AUS; if < 1, may be underdiagnosing malignancy as suspicious
- No national benchmarking numbers are available yet

SELECTED REFERENCES
1. Kim TH et al: The evolution of "atypia" in thyroid fine-needle aspiration specimens. Diagn Cytopathol. 50(4):146-53, 2022
2. Livhits MJ et al: Effectiveness of molecular testing techniques for diagnosis of indeterminate thyroid nodules: a randomized clinical trial. JAMA Oncol. 7(1):70-7, 2021
3. Nishino M et al: Molecular tests for risk-stratifying cytologically indeterminate thyroid nodules: an overview of commercially available testing platforms in the United States. J Mol Pathol 2(2):135-46, 2021
4. Onken AM et al: Combined molecular and histologic end points inform cancer risk estimates for thyroid nodules classified as atypia of undetermined significance. Cancer Cytopathol. 129(12):947-55, 2021
5. Ohori NP et al: Molecular-derived estimation of risk of malignancy for indeterminate thyroid cytology diagnoses. J Am Soc Cytopathol. 9(4):213-20, 2020

Atypia of Undetermined Significance/Follicular Lesion of Undetermined Significance

Histiocytoid and Squamoid Cell Cluster

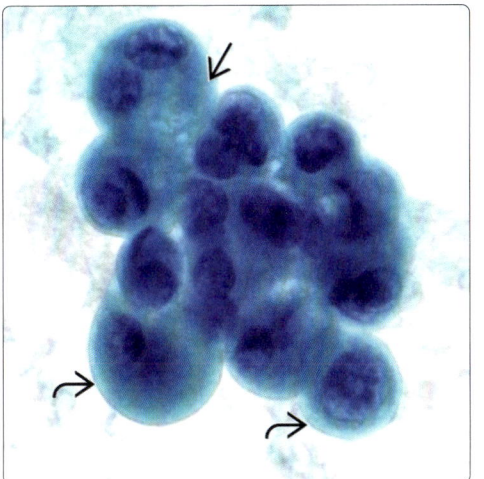

Atypical Oncocytic but Degenerated Cells

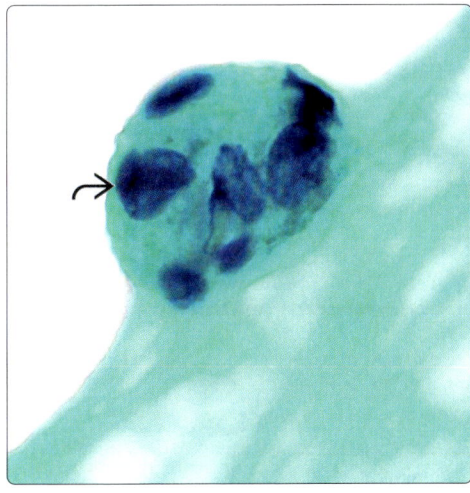

(Left) *Rare cluster of atypical Pap-stained cells shows high nuclear:cytoplasmic ratio and cytoplasm that varies from delicate with vacuoles ➡ (histiocytoid) to hard and squamoid ➡ in an otherwise bloody/acellular aspirate from a cystic nodule. Resection proved cystic papillary carcinoma.* (Right) *Pap stain shows a rare microfollicle of atypical hürthleoid cells with smudged, irregular nuclei ➡ in a paucicellular clotted specimen that was interpreted as AUS.*

AUS: Architectural and Nuclear Atypia

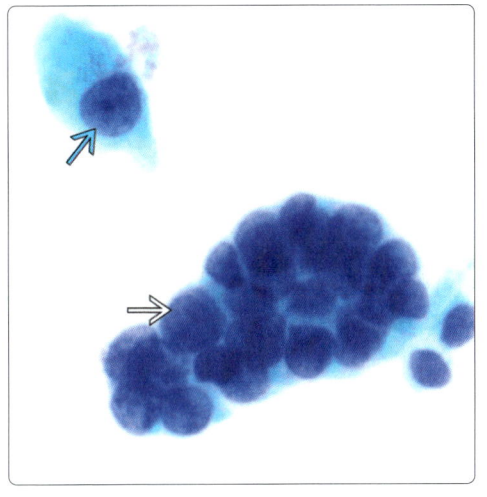

Psammoma Body in Otherwise Acellular Aspirate

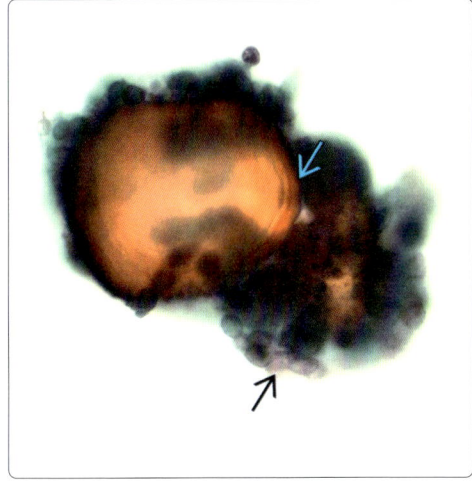

(Left) *ThinPrep of a hypocellular TIRADS 4 aspirate shows a single microfollicular-patterned cluster with open powdery chromatin ➡ but absent other features of papillary thyroid carcinoma (PTC). Note the squamoid cell ➡ with a nucleolus.* (Right) *Pap smear of cystic thyroid nodule shows a single psammoma body ➡ with small attached degenerated cells ➡ interpreted as AUS. Note the characteristic concentric lamellations. Follow-up proved intracystic PTC.*

Repair-Like Sheet With Atypia

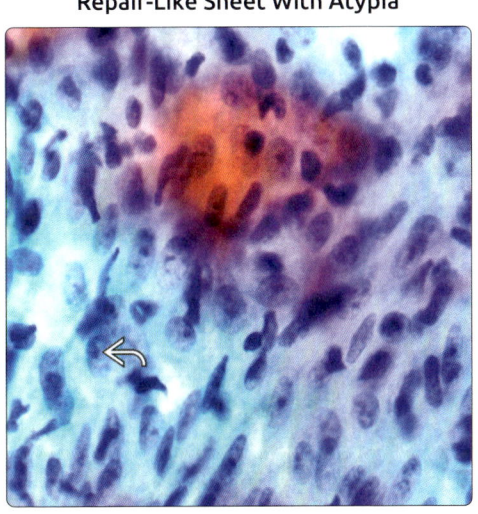

Atypical Lymphoid Cells

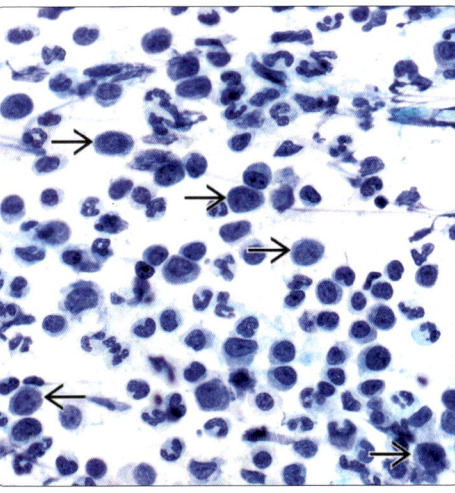

(Left) *Pap stain shows a large sheet of repair-like cells with open chromatin and nucleoli ➡ as well as some atypia. Changes were considered to be beyond the usual symplastic/repair-like changes from a nodule with cystic degeneration and hence interpreted as AUS.* (Right) *Pap stain of Hashimoto thyroiditis from an older patient shows a population of larger blast-like cells ➡, raising concern for lymphoma. Immunophenotyping by flow can resolve the issue if sufficient specimen is available.*

Follicular Neoplasm/Suspicious for a Follicular Neoplasm

TERMINOLOGY

Abbreviations
- Follicular neoplasm (FN), suspicious for (SFN) (Thyroid Bethesda System/TBS 2008 and 2018)
- FN preferred terminology

Definitions
- FN/SFN is defined as cellular aspirate consisting of follicular cells, most of which are arranged in microfollicles, characterized by altered architectural pattern with significant cell crowding &/or microfollicle formation
- If specimen is sparsely cellular but consists only of rare microfollicles, then it can be assigned to atypia of undetermined significance/follicular lesion of undetermined significance (AUS/FLUS) category
- Cases with features suspicious for papillary thyroid carcinoma (PTC) are excluded from this category and are best reported as suspicious for malignancy/malignant
- Cases with only subtle nuclear features of PTC (mild nuclear changes, ↑ nuclear size, chromatin clearing, nuclear irregularity) can be classified as FN/SFN as long as true papillae and intranuclear cytoplasmic inclusions are absent
  - Comment can be added in report about invasive follicular subtype of PTC (FSPTC) or its indolent counterpart, noninvasive follicular thyroid neoplasm with papillary-like nuclear features (NIFTP)
- Lab should decide on preferred terminology (FN or SFN) and not use them interchangeably; SFN most likely will be dropped in 2023 update
- Risk of malignancy (ROM): 25-40%

CYTOPATHOLOGY

Cellularity and Pattern
- Moderate to marked cellularity
- Microfollicular or, rarely, trabecular pattern and dispersed isolated cells
  - Microfollicle defined as crowded or flat groups of < 15 follicular cells, arranged in circle that is at least 2/3 complete; usually uniform in size; distinct from spherules

Crowded Microfollicular Pattern
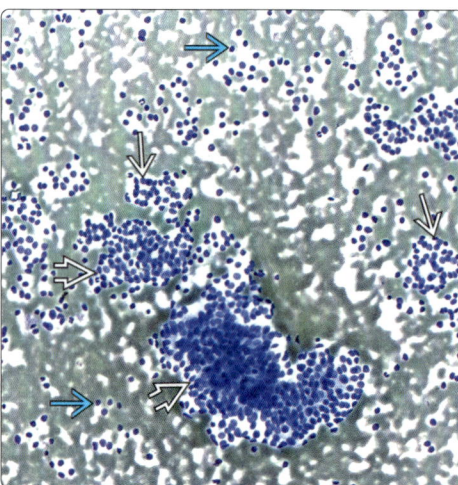

Cellular Microfollicular Pattern
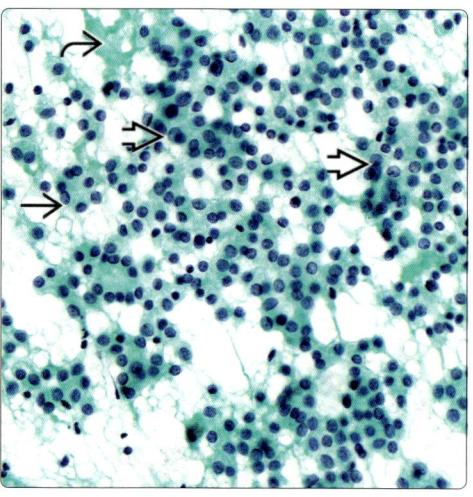

(Left) Diff-Quik stain of a solitary, well-circumscribed nodule shows microfollicles ➡ and trabeculae ➡ with nuclear crowding. Dispersed nuclei are seen in the background ➡, which lacks watery colloid. Interpreted as follicular neoplasm (FN), resection showed follicular adenoma. (Right) Pap stain of thyroid FNA smear shows microfollicles ➡ and trailing dense colloid from within a follicle ➡. There is a lack of watery colloid, and the nuclei show focal crowding ➡. Resection diagnosis was follicular adenoma.

Trabecular Pattern With Microfollicles
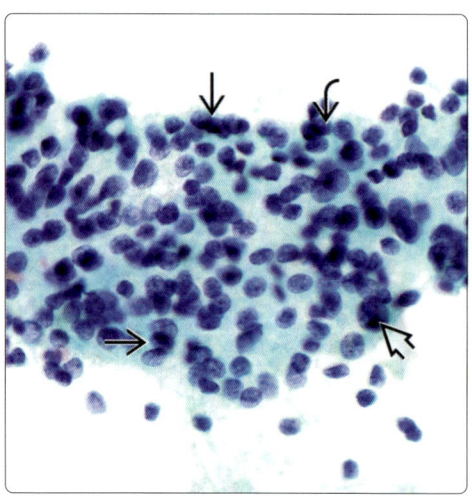

Collection of Microfollicles on ThinPrep
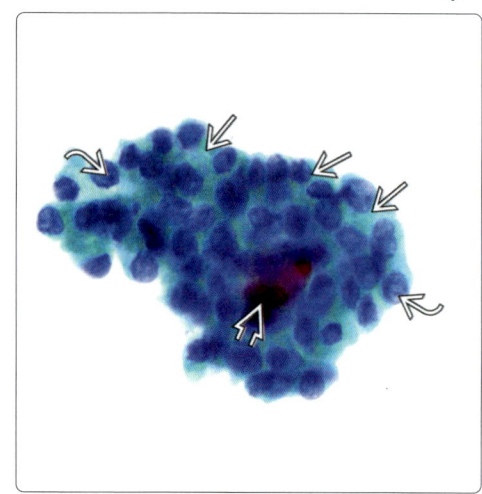

(Left) Pap-stained smear of thyroid aspirate shows a trabecular pattern formed by compressed microfollicles ➡. There is nuclear crowding and overlapping ➡. Colloid is scant and abrupt and enlarged nuclei of endocrine atypia are seen ➡. (Right) Pap stain shows a collection of microfollicles ➡ with retained colloid in the center of one of the follicles ➡. The nuclear chromatin is powdery with rare tiny nucleoli ➡ concerning for papillary thyroid carcinoma (PTC); however, features of PTC are not well developed.

Follicular Neoplasm/Suspicious for a Follicular Neoplasm

- Clusters of crowded follicular cells in ribbon-like pattern are referred to as trabeculae

Background
- Usually lacks watery colloid
- Dense, round colloid may be present in center of microfollicles or separated from follicles in process of smearing
- Rarely, watery colloid and few macrofollicles

Cells
- Cells forming microfollicles are normal or slightly enlarged, uniform, with scant or moderate amount of cytoplasm

Nuclear Details
- Nuclei are round, mildly hyperchromatic with evenly distributed chromatin and small/inconspicuous nucleoli
- Rarely, some nuclear atypia characterized by nuclear enlargement, variation in size, and prominent nucleoli
- Rarely, enlarged nuclei with contour irregularity and mild/focal chromatin clearing (subtle features suggesting FSPTC or NIFTP)

Cytoplasmic Details
- Scant to moderate; occasionally oncocytic or clear

Cell Block Findings
- Can be useful for immunohistochemistry or molecular studies

Liquid-Based Cytology
- Most findings similar to those of smears except cellularity can be variable
- Better nuclear details with conspicuous nucleoli
- Dense round follicular colloid is better seen

Cytology-Histology Correlation
- Resection usually shows either cellular adenomatous nodule, follicular adenoma (FA), follicular carcinoma (FC), FSPTC, or NIFTP

FOLLICULAR ADENOMA

Incidence
- Most present in 5th-6th decades; F:M = 4-5:1

Presentation
- Slow growing, incidentally discovered on palpation or ultrasound
- Solitary, well delineated, round to oval, usually 1-3 cm; can have hemorrhage and cystic degeneration
- Bleeding in mass can result in sudden pain, tenderness, and increase in size

Image Findings
- Isoechoic on ultrasound (usually) but can be hypo- or hyperechoic

Histology
- Well-defined, usually thin capsule
- Architecture varies, may present as solid (embryonal), trabecular, microfollicular, normofollicular, macrofollicular, insular, and papillary patterns
- Nuclei are basal and evenly spaced
- Isolated bizarre atypical cells may be seen
- Cytoplasm can be clear, eosinophilic, amphophilic, or oncocytoid (due to abnormal mitochondria accumulation)
- Many variants described (oncocytic/Hürthle, toxic, lipoadenoma, signet-ring, atypical)

Genetics
- Activating point mutations of RAS genes (specifically *NRAS* and *HRAS*) in ~ 30% of cases
- If *PAX8::PPARγ* rearrangement is detected, then look for vascular/capsular invasion, as it is most likely FC

FOLLICULAR CARCINOMA

Incidence
- ~ 0.8/100,000 persons per year
- 5th and 6th decades, F:M = 2-2.5:1

Presentation
- Usually asymptomatic, solitary, slowly enlarging thyroid mass
- Distant metastasis in up to 20% (lungs and bone)

Prognosis
- 20-year survival rate: 97% for minimally invasive, 50% for widely invasive

Histology
- Encapsulated, round to oval solitary tumor with thicker and more irregular capsule compared with FA
- Capsular or vascular invasion required for diagnosis of carcinoma
  - Hence, distinction between FA and FC cannot be made on FNA unless widely invasive or metastatic
- Microfollicular, solid, cystic, trabecular, and insular patterns possible, but usually 1 pattern predominates
- Histology and variants similar to FA

Genetics
- Loss of heterozygosity (LOH) is characteristic
- *PPARγ* gene found in up to 50%; RAS abnormal in up to 50% (not carcinoma specific)
  - Activating mutations in codon 61 of *NRAS* and *HRAS* genes are most common
  - Translocation t(2;3)(q13;p25) leads to fusion of *PAX8* and *PPARγ* (*PAX8::PPARγ* rearrangement)
- *GRIM19* gene mutations in oncocytic tumors

DIFFERENTIAL DIAGNOSIS

Follicular Variant of Papillary Thyroid Carcinoma
- Usually presents as microfollicular pattern
  - Macrofollicular variant is very rare
- Nuclear chromatin is more open and may show grooves and intranuclear cytoplasmic inclusions similar to papillary carcinoma
- *BRAF* V600E mutation on molecular testing in some cases

Noninvasive Follicular Thyroid Neoplasm With Papillary-Like Nuclear Features
- Recently described entity with excellent prognosis characterized by well-circumscribed tumor without vascular or capsular invasion
- Lacks psammoma bodies or insular architecture, ≤ 1% papillary fronds

Follicular Neoplasm/Suspicious for a Follicular Neoplasm

Cytologic Differences Between AN, SFN, FSPTC, and NIFTP

Criterion	Benign AN	FN/SFN	FSPTC	NIFTP
Cellularity	Variable	Usually cellular	Usually cellular	Variable but usually cellular
Colloid	Abundant, watery	In follicles, rarely watery	Usually scant but can be watery	Scant and dense
Cells	Macro- and microfollicles, honeycombed sheets with no nuclear crowding or overlapping	Microfollicular pattern (max: 15 cells)	Microfollicular (rarely macrofollicular)	Microfollicular
Nuclei	Dark, small, condensed chromatin, size of lymphocyte	Nuclear overlap or crowding in microfollicles, larger than AN; dark, granular chromatin with small nucleoli	Oval, pale chromatin with grooves or INCI, size > AN or SFN; 2-3 small, marginated nucleoli	Oval, pale chromatin with grooves; rare or ill-developed INCI; lacks papillae or psammoma bodies
Degeneration	Frequent	May be seen	Uncommon	Uncommon
Clinical	Multiple nodules	Usually single	Usually single	Single, encapsulated, noninvasive
Molecular	N/A	*NRAS* and *HRAS* in 30%; *PAX8::PARγ* in up to 50% of follicular carcinoma	*BRAF* V600E, *RAS* up to 70%	*RAS* up to 60%, *BRAF* K601E, *THADA* ~ 30%, *PAX8::PPARG* up to 40%

AN = adenomatous nodule; INCI = intranuclear cytoplasmic inclusions; SFN = suspicious for follicular neoplasm; FSPTC = invasive follicular subtype of papillary thyroid carcinoma; NIFTP = noninvasive follicular thyroid neoplasm with papillary-like nuclear features.

Positive Predictive Value of Cytologic Diagnosis of SFN and SFNHCT

Study (1st Author and Year)	SFN	SFNHCT
TBSRTC estimate (2007)	15-30%	20-45%
TBSRTC estimate (2018)	25-40%; with NIFTP considered benign, 10-40%	10-40%

NIFTP = noninvasive follicular thyroid neoplasm with papillary-like nuclear features; SFNHCT = suspicious for follicular neoplasm, Hürthle cell (oncocytic) type; TBSRTC = The Bethesda System for Reporting Thyroid Cytology.

- Histologic diagnosis, cannot accurately diagnose on cytology
- Cytologically looks like FSPTC and usually interpreted as FN/SFN, AUS/FLUS, or suspicious for PTC in most cases, thus altering ROM of these 3 categories
- Molecular testing shows *RAS* and *BRAF* V601K mutations

Adenomatous Nodule(s)
- Usually multinodular and with mixed macro- and microfollicular pattern
- Size varies from few millimeters to several centimeters
- Can have up to 50% microfollicles; hence, may be interpreted as FN
- Usually less cellular and more colloid than FA or FC

Parathyroid Adenoma/Carcinoma
- Microfollicular pattern without thick or thin colloid
- Usually history of hyperparathyroidism/hypercalcemia
- Rarely intrathyroidal and asymptomatic and may be mistaken for FN
- Parathormone positive, thyroglobulin negative

Hashimoto Thyroiditis
- Can have microfollicular pattern but usually not dominant
- Lymphocytes infiltrating microfollicles should be clue to Hashimoto thyroiditis (HT)
- Can be problematic if burnt-out HT with few lymphocytes

Other Clear Cell Tumors
- e.g., renal cell carcinoma (RCC)
  - History and immunohistochemistry can help
  - Thyroglobulin and TTF-1(-) in tumor cells of RCC

Medullary Carcinoma
- Rarely has follicular pattern
- Characteristic salt and pepper chromatin
- Calcitonin, CEA, chromogranin, and synaptophysin positive

Poorly Differentiated Thyroid Carcinoma
- Thought to arise from preexisting follicular or papillary carcinoma; characterized by rapid growth in longstanding nodule
- Necrosis &/or mitosis should suggest this entity
- Definitive diagnosis on histology upon resection

SELECTED REFERENCES
1. Marina M et al: Combination of ultrasound and molecular testing in malignancy risk estimate of Bethesda category IV thyroid nodules: results from a single-institution prospective study. J Endocrinol Invest. 44(12):2635-43, 2021

Follicular Neoplasm/Suspicious for a Follicular Neoplasm

FN With Subtle Features of FSPTC or NIFTP

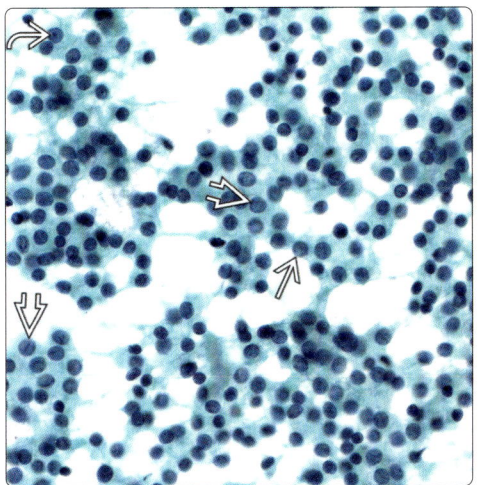

Parathyroid Adenoma With Crowded Microfollicles and Lack of Colloid

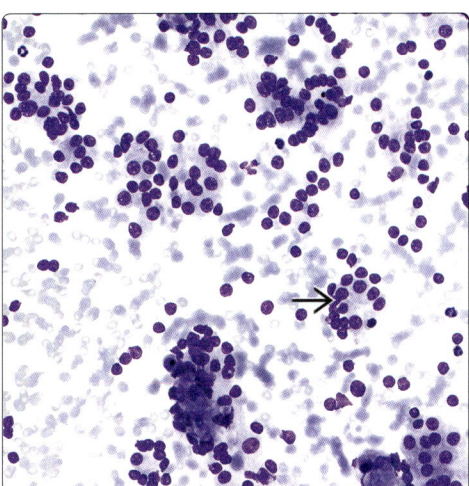

(Left) Pap-stained cellular smear with a crowded microfollicular pattern from a well-circumscribed nodule shows areas of fine, powdery chromatin ➡, nuclear grooves ➡, and micronucleoli ➡ but lacking overt papillae, intranuclear cytoplasmic inclusions, or psammoma bodies. (Right) Diff-Quik-stained thyroid aspirate shows a solitary nodule with a microfollicular pattern ➡ with a lack of watery or dense colloid in this case of intrathyroidal parathyroid adenoma.

Microfollicles With Dense Luminal Colloid

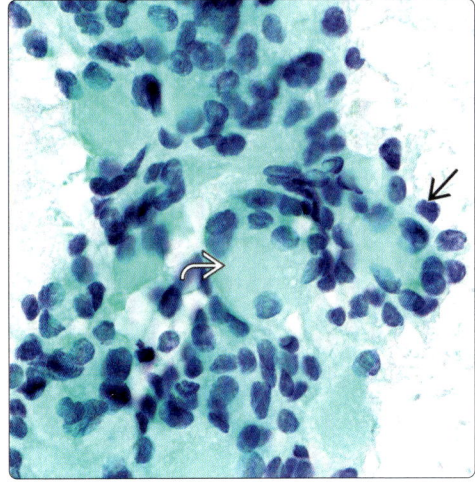

Follicular and Insular Carcinoma

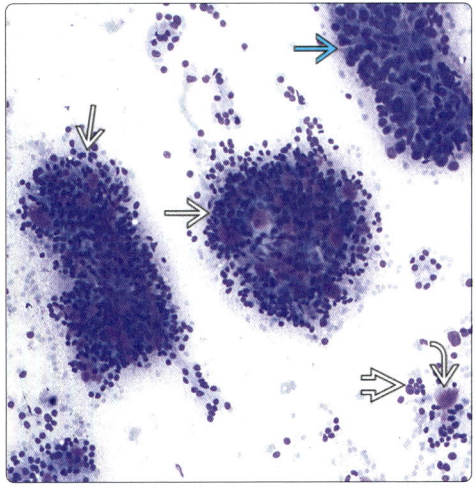

(Left) Pap stain shows microfollicular complex with waxy, green central colloid ➡ surrounded by follicular cells ➡ from a thyroid aspiration of follicular carcinoma. (Right) Diff-Quik stain of follicular carcinoma shows crowded microfollicular complexes ➡ with dense central colloid. There is a 3rd hypercellular, insular configuration of cells, which are more atypical ➡, larger, and clearly malignant. Other isolated microfollicles ➡ with trailing, dense colloid are also seen ➡.

Microfollicles and Flares in Graves Disease

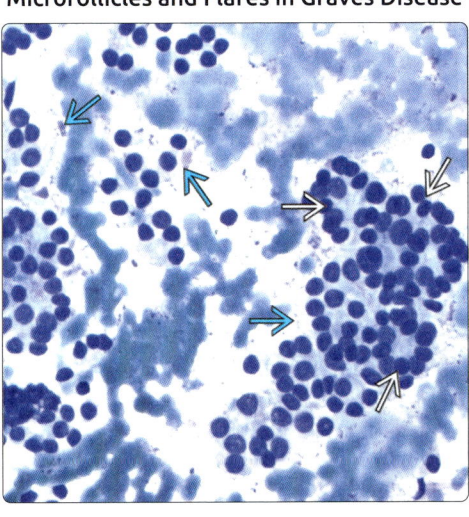

Hashimoto Thyroiditis With Microfollicle and Lymphocytes

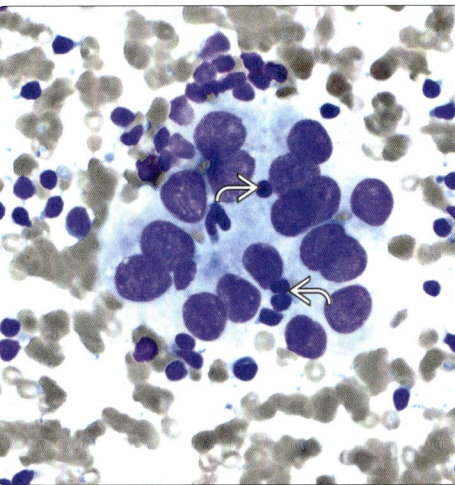

(Left) Diff-Quik stained smear of a dominant nodule from a patient with Graves disease shows a microfollicular pattern ➡ and flares ➡ characteristic of Graves disease. (Right) Diff-Quik stain shows a microfollicle with open chromatin and infiltrating lymphocytes ➡, which are hallmark features for the diagnosis of Hashimoto thyroiditis.

Follicular Neoplasm, Oncocytic (Hürthle Cell) Type

KEY FACTS

TERMINOLOGY
- Cellular aspirate composed almost entirely of oncocytic cells, excluding oncocytes with features of papillary thyroid carcinoma (PTC)

CLINICAL ISSUES
- 3-15% of thyroid neoplasms; F:M = 3:1
- Implied risk of malignancy: 10-40% (per 2017 Bethesda Guidelines for reporting thyroid cytopathology)
- Treatment is lobectomy
- Most nodules diagnosed as SFNOCT are hyperplastic or benign adenomas

CYTOPATHOLOGY
- Cellular smears with > 75% oncocytic cells
- Crowded groups, small clusters, or dyscohesive cells
- Transgressing vessels when seen suggest neoplasm
- Polygonal cells with abundant granular cytoplasm, large round nuclei, and prominent nucleoli
- Blue or gray-pink cytoplasm on Diff-Quik, green on Pap
- Large, central or eccentric, dark round nuclei with binucleation
- Large cells with > 2x variability in size: Large cell dysplasia
- Small cells with high N:C ratio: Small cell dysplasia
- Prominent nucleoli and anisonucleosis common
- Absent or scant colloid, absent lymphocytes (excluding blood elements)

ANCILLARY TESTS
- Thyroglobulin (+), HMWK(+), TTF-1(+), CK5/6(+)
- *RAS* mutations most prevalent and mostly associated with benign lesions and NIFTP

TOP DIFFERENTIAL DIAGNOSES
- Adenomatous nodules with oncocytic cell hyperplasia, PTC, medullary carcinoma, lymphocytic thyroiditis, and parathyroid neoplasia
- Sparsely cellular nodules consisting of oncocytic cells only best interpreted as AUS/FLUS with explanatory note

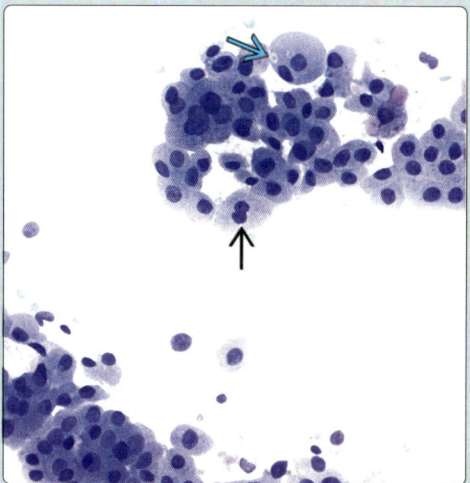

Intracytoplasmic Lumina in Oncocytic Cells

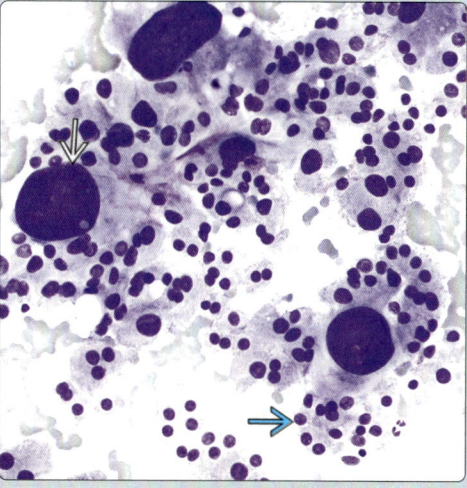

Small and Large Cell Dysplasia

(Left) Oncocytic cells with abundant granular cytoplasm containing intracytoplasmic lumina ⇒ are shown. There is binucleation ⇒ with prominent nucleoli and absence of background colloid. (Right) Diff-Quik stain shows oncocytic (Hürthle) cells with small cell dysplasia ⇒ and large cell dysplasia with > 2x nuclear size variation ⇒ in a case interpreted as suspicious for follicular neoplasm, oncocytic (Hürthle cell) type.

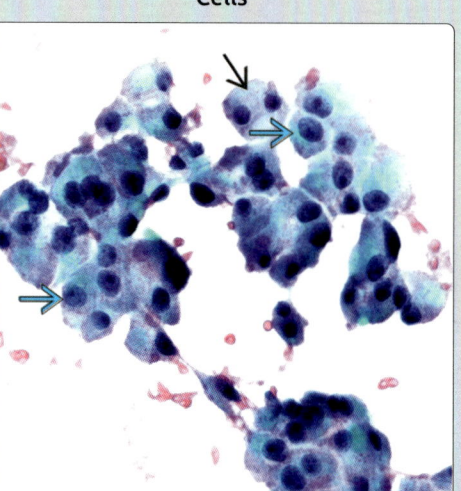

3D Microfollicular Groups of Oncocytic Cells

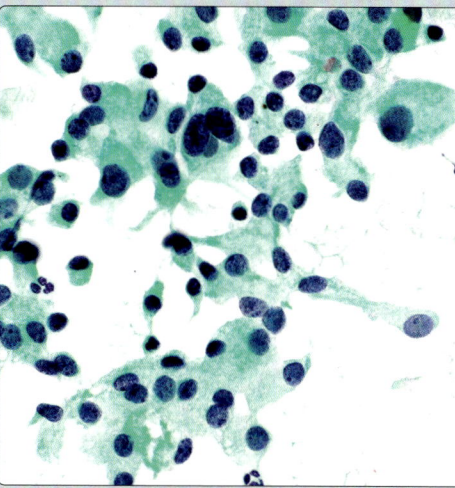

Oncocytic Medullary Carcinoma

(Left) Pap stain of oncocytic (Hürthle cell) nodule shows 3D groups of oncocytic cells with microfollicular architecture. The cells have blue-green cytoplasm and eccentric nuclei with prominent nucleoli ⇒ and binucleation ⇒. (Right) Pap stain shows dyscohesive cells in oncocytic medullary thyroid carcinoma (MTC). Cytoplasmic processes, coarse chromatin, and binucleation warrant additional studies to rule out MTC. The large nucleoli of a true oncocytic neoplasm are absent.

Follicular Neoplasm, Oncocytic (Hürthle Cell) Type

TERMINOLOGY

Abbreviations
- Follicular neoplasm, oncocytic (Hürthle cell) type (FNOCT), suspicious for FNOCT (SFNOCT)

Definitions
- Cellular aspirate composed almost entirely (≥ 75%) of oncocytic (Hürthle) cells, excluding oncocytes with features of papillary thyroid carcinoma (PTC)

ETIOLOGY/PATHOGENESIS

Hürthle Cell Changes
- Metaplastic changes due to intracytoplasmic accumulation of altered mitochondria
- Can occur in reactive or neoplastic processes

CLINICAL ISSUES

Epidemiology
- Incidence
  - 3-10% of thyroid neoplasms; F:M = 3:1

Prognosis
- Implied risk of malignancy: 10-40% (per 2017 Bethesda Guidelines for reporting thyroid cytopathology)

CYTOPATHOLOGY

Pattern
- Cellular smears with > 75% oncocytic cells
- Crowded sheets, 3D groups, small clusters, or single dyscohesive cells
- Transgressing vessels when seen support neoplasm
- Absent or scant colloid, absent lymphocytes

Cells
- Size variability is common: Polygonal or round cells with abundant granular cytoplasm and well-defined cell borders; blue or gray-pink on Diff-Quik, green on Pap stain
- Large cells with > 2x variability in size: Large cell dysplasia
- Small cells with high N:C ratio: Small cell dysplasia

Nuclear Details
- Large, central or eccentric, dark round nuclei with binucleation
- Prominent nucleoli and anisonucleosis common

ANCILLARY TESTS

Molecular testing
- Alterations in mitochondrial DNA or *GRIM19* (NDUFA13) gene; copy number variations in 1/3
- Afirma (genomic sequencing classifier) shows sensitivity and specificity for Hürthle cell neoplasm (adenoma and carcinoma) of 89% and 59%, respectively
- Thyroseq (multigene next-generation sequencing) shows sensitivity and specificity for Hürthle cell neoplasm of 93% and 69%, respectively

DIFFERENTIAL DIAGNOSIS

Adenomatous Nodule (Goiter) With Oncocytic Hyperplasia
- Usually mixed cellularity: Flat sheets of oncocytic cells; follicular cells, some with reactive atypia; moderate to abundant colloid

Lymphocytic/Hashimoto Thyroiditis
- Lymphocytes or plasma cells infiltrating Hürthle cells

Medullary Thyroid Carcinoma
- Lacks macronucleoli, calcitonin (+), CEA(+), thyroglobulin (-)

Oncocytic Papillary Thyroid Carcinoma
- Nuclear groove/inclusion in Hürthle cells mimic PTC

Metastatic Oncocytic Malignancies
- Cytomorphologic features of oncocytic malignancies from other sites can mimic FNOCT very closely

SELECTED REFERENCES
1. Doerfler WR et al: Molecular alterations in Hürthle cell nodules and preoperative cancer risk. Endocr Relat Cancer. 28(5):301-9, 2021

Oncocytic Cells With Reactive Changes

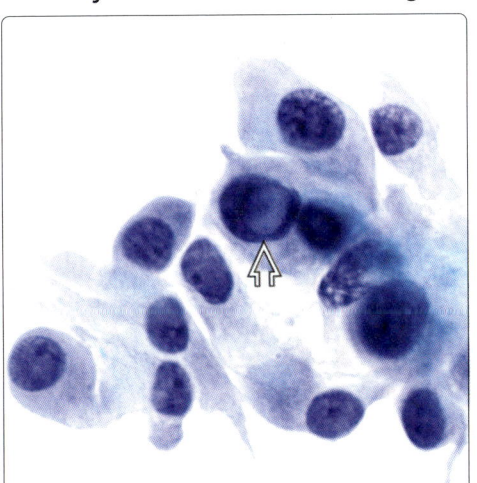

Transgressing Vessels and Oncocytic Cells

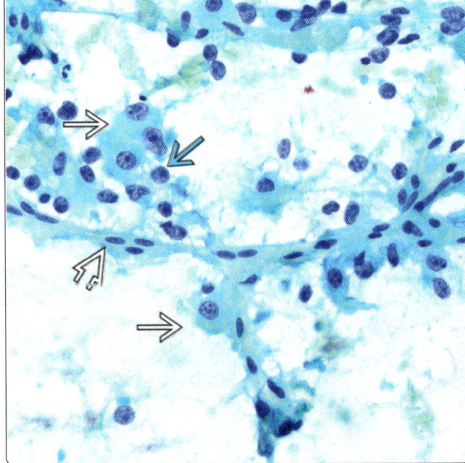

(Left) Pap stain shows oncocytic cells with reactive changes. Marked size variability and nuclear pseudoinclusion ➡ mimic papillary carcinoma. *(Right)* Pap stain of solitary large thyroid nodule in patient with known history of metastatic hepatocellular carcinoma is shown. The cells have abundant granular cytoplasm ➡, large, abnormal nuclei with nucleoli ➡, and transgressing vessels ➡ as in Hürthle cell neoplasms. Cells were TTF-1(-) and Arginase (+), consistent with hepatocellular carcinoma.

Papillary Thyroid Carcinoma, Classic Subtype

KEY FACTS

ETIOLOGY/PATHOGENESIS
- Radiation, somatic rearrangements, genetics

CLINICAL ISSUES
- Most common endocrine malignancy
- F:M = 2-4:1
- Prognosis is excellent (10-year survival rate > 90%)
- Some genetic and morphologic subtypes are more aggressive
  - Subclassification on cytology is usually not possible and has minimal management impact

CYTOPATHOLOGY
- Pattern: Cellular smears or liquid-based preparations
- Cells arranged in groups, syncytial sheets, papillary tissue fragments, and avascular papillary fronds
- Oval nuclei with irregular membrane, nuclear grooves, nuclear overlap, fine, powdery chromatin, psammoma bodies
- Intranuclear inclusions, multinucleated giant cells, dense squamoid cytoplasm, thick colloid
- Follicular variant may have abundant watery colloid
- Limit diagnosis of papillary thyroid carcinoma (PTC) to cases with multiple diagnostic features, such as papillary architecture, psammoma bodies, or numerous inclusions, to avoid overdiagnosis

ANCILLARY TESTS
- Can be performed on paraffin blocks, CytoLyt, cells scraped from smears
  - Propriety media offered by commercial labs performing testing
- *BRAF* V600E mutation is present in ~ 50% of PTC, classic variant cases
  - Varies in subtypes

TOP DIFFERENTIAL DIAGNOSES
- Papillary hyperplasia, Hashimoto thyroiditis, medullary carcinoma, oncocytic (Hürthle cell) neoplasm

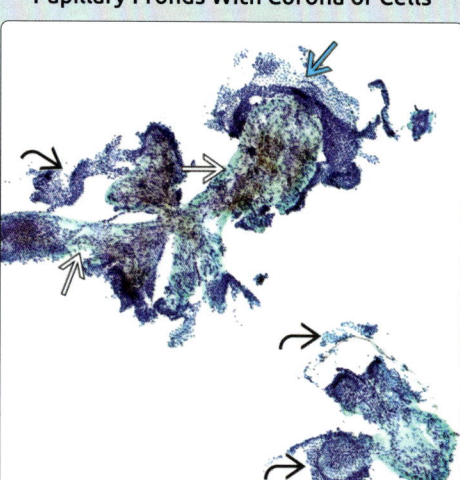

Papillary Fronds With Corona of Cells

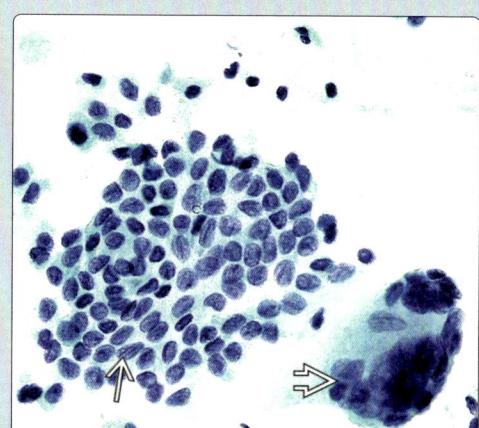

Nuclear Grooves and Giant Cells

(Left) *Pap stain shows classic papillary thyroid carcinoma (PTC) with fibrovascular cores ➡ and a corona of cells ➡. The cells can easily detach from the cores, resulting in large and small sheets being smeared on the slide ➡. Note the absence of watery colloid in background. The avascular sheets have a swirling pattern of nuclei.* (Right) *Pap stain of PTC shows a multinucleated giant cell ➡ and a syncytial group of cells with elongated nuclei. Nuclear grooves ➡ are present in most of the cells in this cluster.*

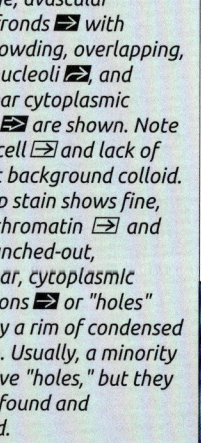

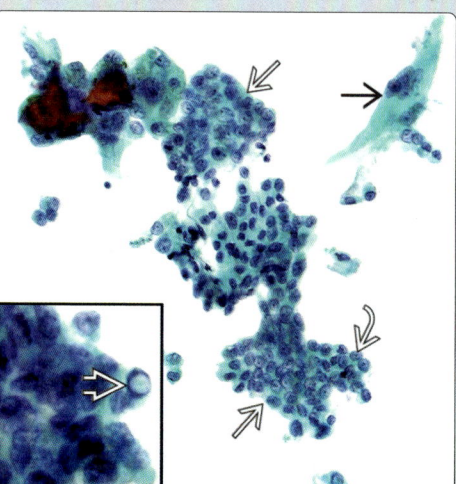

Papillary Thyroid Carcinoma on ThinPrep

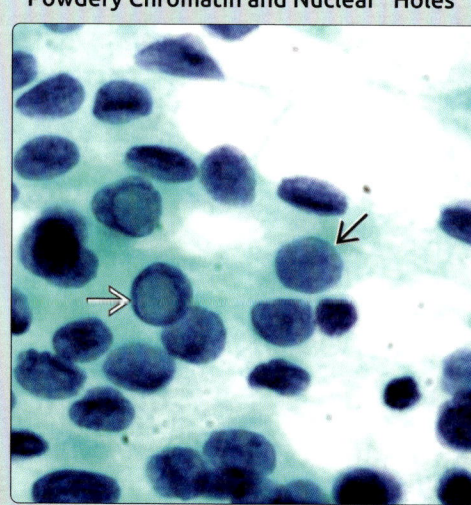

Powdery Chromatin and Nuclear "Holes"

(Left) *Large, avascular papillary fronds ➡ with nuclear crowding, overlapping, grooves, nucleoli ➡, and intranuclear cytoplasmic inclusions ➡ are shown. Note the giant cell ➡ and lack of significant background colloid.* (Right) *Pap stain shows fine, powdery chromatin ➡ and sharply punched-out, intranuclear, cytoplasmic invaginations ➡ or "holes" outlined by a rim of condensed chromatin. Usually, a minority of cells have "holes," but they are easily found and recognized.*

Papillary Thyroid Carcinoma, Classic Subtype

TERMINOLOGY

Abbreviations
- Papillary thyroid carcinoma (PTC)

ETIOLOGY/PATHOGENESIS

Environmental Exposure
- Radiation exposure
- Iodine excess

Preexisting Benign Thyroid Disease
- Association with lymphocytic thyroiditis, goiter, and Graves disease is controversial

Somatic Mutations and Rearrangements
- *BRAF* mutations
- *RET/PTC* rearrangement
- *RAS* mutation

Familial Syndromes
- Familial PTC syndromes (familial nonmedullary thyroid carcinoma syndromes)
  o Carney complex
  o Werner syndrome
- Multiple endocrine neoplasia 2A
  o *RET* germline mutation
- PTEN hamartoma tumor syndrome

CLINICAL ISSUES

Epidemiology
- Incidence
  o Most common endocrine malignancy, type of thyroid cancer, and pediatric thyroid malignancy
    – Usually multifocal and more aggressive in children
  o Incidence is increasing worldwide
- Age
  o 1st peak: 20-30 years; 2nd peak: 55-60 years
    – Rare before 15 years
- Sex
  o F:M = 2-4:1
    – In children and in patients > 50 years of age, female preponderance is less pronounced
- Ethnicity
  o Occurs more often in White than in Black populations

Presentation
- May present as palpable thyroid mass
- May present with enlarged cervical lymph nodes
- Incidental finding during routine physical exam or head and neck ultrasonography

Treatment
- Total or near-total thyroidectomy if high-risk patient and tumor > 4 cm (per American Thyroid Association guidelines, depends on size, and metastasis, extrathyroidal extension)
- Lymph node resection if lymph node metastasis is present
- Radioactive iodine ablation after thyroidectomy

Prognosis
- Excellent: 10-year survival rate > 90%
- Poor prognostic factors: Older age, male sex, extrathyroid extension, and tumor > 4 cm
- Tumors with infiltrative borders have worse prognosis than encapsulated tumors
- *RET/NCOA4* and *TERT* (+) papillary carcinomas tend to have slightly worse prognosis
- *BRAF* status may influence management
- Distant metastasis to lung, bone, or other organs is rare, associated with poor prognosis

IMAGING

Ultrasonographic Findings
- Hypo- or isoechoic nodule with ill-defined borders
- Useful for guiding FNA biopsies
- Determination of size and whether solid or cystic

CT Findings
- Preferred for evaluating extent of suspected tracheal or mediastinal involvement

CYTOPATHOLOGY

Pattern
- Cellular aspirates, arranged in groups, syncytial sheets, papillary tissue fragments, and avascular papillary fronds

Background
- Scant, thick, and ropy/"bubblegum" colloid
- Histiocytes, blood, and hemosiderin-laden macrophages may be present in large tumors with cystic changes
- Psammoma bodies are present in < 1/2 of all cases
  o Round, deep purple with concentric laminations
  o May be only evidence of metastasis to lymph nodes

Cells
- Polygonal, cuboidal, flattened, columnar, oncocytic, or hobnailed
  o Usually 2-3x larger than normal follicular cells
  o Nuclear:cytoplasmic ratio is increased
- Multinucleated giant cells may be present

Nuclear Details
- Large nuclei with irregular nuclear membranes
  o Nuclei may be oval, elongated, crescent-shaped, asymmetric, angulated, or convoluted
- Fine, powdery, and pale chromatin
- Intranuclear pseudoinclusions
  o Pale-staining, well-demarcated vacuoles resulting from intranuclear invaginations of cytoplasm
  o Usually easily recognizable in tumor cells in classic subtype
- Nuclear grooves due to infolding of nuclear membrane
  o Discrete, longitudinal groove through long axis of nucleus, resembling coffee beans
  o Nuclear grooves are present in majority of cells
- Small peripherally located nucleoli may be present
- Nuclei are crowded and frequently overlap
- Only diagnose PTC if nuclear features are prominent and pseudoinclusions are readily identified
  o This will minimize overdiagnosis of noninvasive follicular thyroid neoplasm with papillary-like nuclear features (NIFTP)

Papillary Thyroid Carcinoma, Classic Subtype

Cytoplasmic Details
- Lightly eosinophilic and delicate but can also be clear
- Eosinophilic and granular in oncocytic and tall cell variants
- Oncocytic/squamoid cytoplasm is common

Liquid-Based Cytology (ThinPrep and SurePath)
- Usually cellular
- Intranuclear inclusions are enhanced, nucleoli easily seen
- Other nuclear features are more difficult to recognize

Cell Block Findings
- Can be used for additional studies

MACROSCOPIC

General Features
- Grossly, can be solitary; however, multifocality is common (up to 65%)
- Solid or cystic; encapsulated or infiltrative

Size
- From microscopic up to 10 cm; mean: 1-3 cm
- Occult PTC/microcarcinoma: < 1 cm in greatest dimension

ANCILLARY TESTS

Immunohistochemistry
- TTF-1 (nuclear), thyroglobulin (cytoplasmic), galectin-3 (cytoplasmic), HBME-1 (membranous), BRAF V600E
  - IHC not needed for diagnosis

Genetic Testing
- Can be performed on paraffin blocks, CytoLyt, cells scraped from smears
- RET/PTC
  - Intrachromosomal inversion or translocation
- BRAF
  - BRAF V600E mutation is present in ~ 50% of classic subtype of PTC cases
  - Frequency varies among different subtypes of PTC
  - Uncommon in radiation-induced cases
- NTRK
  - Present in 10% of PTC cases, tend to have focal or subtle nuclear features
    - Seen in ~ 3% of post-Chernobyl cases
- TERT, EML4 e13::ALK e20
  - Indicates aggressive behavior
  - Global DNA hypomethylation

DIFFERENTIAL DIAGNOSIS

Papillary Hyperplasia
- Cells lining papillae do **not** have features of PTC
- Can be seen in hyperplastic nodules or Graves disease

Follicular Lesion (Adenomatous Nodule and Follicular Neoplasm)
- Nuclear clearing may be seen in less well-preserved areas of follicular lesions but lack characteristic nuclear features of PTC in majority of cells
- Follicular variant of PTC may have abundant watery colloid and less pronounced nuclear features, which may lead to false-negative diagnosis on cytology or histology

Noninvasive Follicular Thyroid Neoplasm With Papillary-Like Nuclei
- Microfollicles with minimal or no tendency to form papillae, subtle nuclear features, watery colloid, and absence of psammoma bodies

Hashimoto Thyroiditis
- Nuclei are typically uniform and round
- Lymphocytic infiltrate in oncocytic (Hürthle cell) groups
- Usually lack nuclear grooves and inclusions seen in PTC
- Be cautious when diagnosing PTC in Hashimoto thyroiditis

Medullary Thyroid Carcinoma
- Polygonal or spindle-shaped cells with granular cytoplasm and eccentric, round to oval nuclei with fine chromatin
- May have intranuclear inclusions, but nuclear features of PTC are not seen in majority of cells
- Calcitonin positive

Hyalinizing Trabecular Tumor
- Elongated cells with longitudinal nuclear grooves and many pseudoinclusions and psammoma bodies
- Cells are radially oriented around hyaline stromal material
- Rare; cytology difficult to differentiate from that of PTC
- RET/PTC1 rearrangements reported
  - No BRAF or RAS mutations

DIAGNOSTIC CHECKLIST

Pathologic Interpretation Pearls
- Diagnosis of PTC relies heavily on characteristic nuclear features
- Per new Bethesda guidelines, positive predictive value (PPV) for PTC diagnosis on cytology is 94-96% (post introduction of NIFTP)
- Multiple diagnostic features/criteria must be present in majority of cells for definitive diagnosis
- If only few diagnostic features are present, case should be diagnosed as suspicious for PTC, which has PPV of 45-60%
  - These cases are managed by lobectomy
- If only few diagnostic features are present, these may represent indolent NIFTP and are best managed by lobectomy
  - Better to call suspicious for carcinoma on cytology or, if follicular patterned, as follicular neoplasm
- In lesion with cystic changes, look very carefully for cytologic features of PTC
- Intranuclear inclusions can also be seen in medullary carcinoma, oncocytic (Hürthle cell) neoplasms, hyalinizing trabecular tumor, and antithyroid therapy

SELECTED REFERENCES

1. Baloch ZW et al: Overview of the 2022 WHO Classification of Thyroid Neoplasms. Endocr Pathol. 33(1):27-63, 2022
2. Park J et al: Dissection of molecular and histological subtypes of papillary thyroid cancer using alternative splicing profiles. Exp Mol Med. 54(3):263-72, 2022
3. Anand N et al: Diagnostic efficacy of BRAFV600E immunocytochemistry in thyroid aspirates in Bethesda category IV and papillary thyroid carcinoma. J Cytol. 38(3):113-9, 2021
4. Abi-Raad R et al: Fine-needle aspiration cytomorphology of papillary thyroid carcinoma with NTRK gene rearrangement from a case series with predominantly indeterminate cytology. Cancer Cytopathol. 128(11):803-11, 2020

Papillary Thyroid Carcinoma, Classic Subtype

Papillary Fronds on Low Magnification

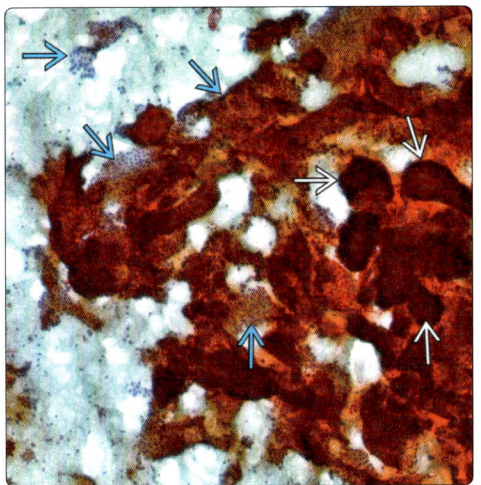

Papillae With Fibrovascular Cores

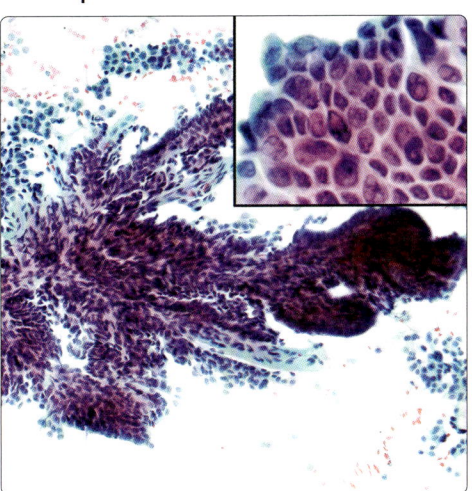

(Left) Pap-stained smear shows a large tissue fragment of papillary carcinoma. The intact papillary fronds ➡ with fibrovascular cores, as well as the larger avascular fronds ➡ with sheet-like configuration, are seen on low magnification. (Right) Pap stain of PTC demonstrates papillae with delicate, branching vascular cores at low magnification. High-power view (inset) illustrates characteristic nuclear features of PTC.

Psammoma Body and Nuclear Features

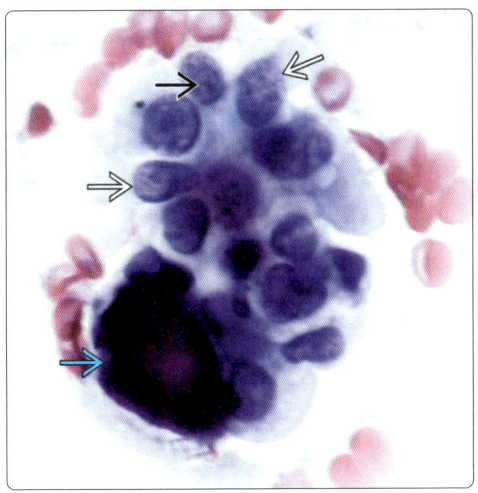

Syncytium of Nuclei With Papillary Thyroid Carcinoma Features

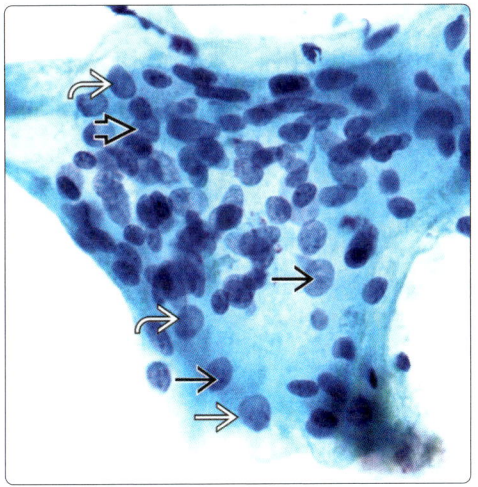

(Left) Pap-stained smear shows a cluster of cells with powdery chromatin ➡, small nucleoli ➡, and a psammoma body ➡. < 50% of PTCs show psammoma bodies. (Right) Pap-stained FNA shows a syncytium of nuclei entrapped in colloid. The nuclei have fine, powdery chromatin ➡, small nucleoli ➡, and grooves ➡. The intranuclear cytoplasmic inclusions ➡ are not well developed or distinct.

Repair-Like Features in Papillary Carcinoma

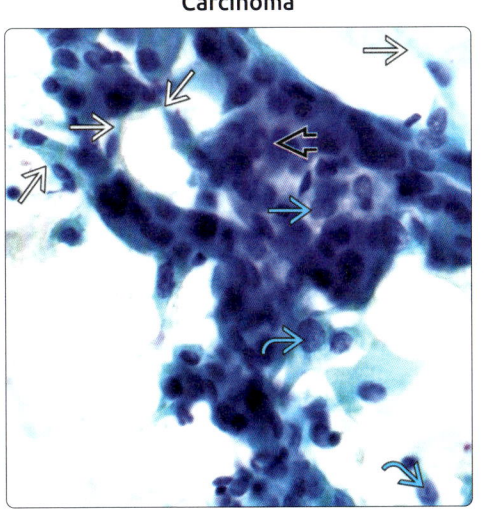

Papillae in Graves Disease

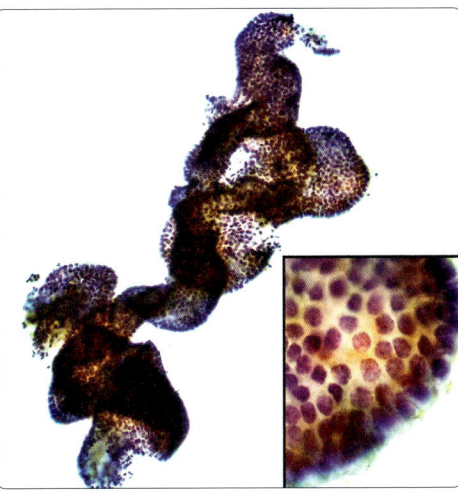

(Left) Pap-stained FNA shows a repair-like arrangement of the cells with pulled-out cytoplasm ➡. Note the nuclear features with intranuclear cytoplasmic inclusions ➡, powdery chromatin ➡, and small nucleoli ➡. (Right) Papillae are not pathognomonic for PTC. This Pap stain illustrates papillary structures in Graves disease. High-power inset shows round, uniform nuclei without nuclear irregularity or intranuclear inclusions.

Papillary Thyroid Carcinoma Subtypes

TERMINOLOGY

Abbreviations
- Papillary thyroid carcinoma (PTC)
- Follicular variant of PTC (FVPTC)
- Noninvasive follicular thyroid neoplasm with papillary-like nuclear features (NIFTP)

FVPTC AND NIFTP

General Features
- ~ 30% of all thyroid cancers; F:M = 4:1; age 20-80 years, mean: 46 years
- Cytologically, it is not possible to distinguish NIFTP from invasive FVPTC; distinction based on surgical resection and complete pathologic evaluation
- In 2022 WHO classification, NIFTP is considered low-risk follicular cell-derived neoplasm with excellent prognosis
- **Histologically**, both are characterized by irregularly shaped, small- to medium-sized follicles with hypereosinophilic colloid on H&E stain
  - Nuclear overlap and crowding, powdery nuclear chromatin with nucleoli
  - Papillae and psammoma bodies rare or absent
  - Intranuclear cytoplasmic inclusions rare/not as abundant as classic or other subtypes
- FVPTC is malignant neoplasm; 2 types: Infiltrative and encapsulated with capsular/vascular invasion

Cytology
- Cytologically cannot distinguish invasive FVPTC from NIFTP
  - Usually cellular samples with microfollicles and syncytial-like fragments containing microfollicular pattern
  - Branching staghorn-shaped sheets of cells are helpful clues on low-power scanning, if present
  - Colloid typically thick and within follicles or trailing follicles
  - Pale nuclei with open, powdery chromatin with micronucleoli and nuclear grooves
  - Intranuclear cytoplasmic inclusions are found in fewer cells compared to usual papillary carcinoma
  - Psammoma bodies and papillary fibrovascular forms are rare or absent
  - Multinucleated giant cells and cystic changes are uncommon
  - Cytologic diagnosis of "malignant" should not be made in absence of fibrovascular cores/papillary fronds, psammoma bodies, many intranuclear cytoplasmic inclusions
    - Best to designate such cases as "suspicious for malignancy" or in "follicular neoplasm" category; rarely in AUS if hypocellular
    - Molecular testing helps with surgical planning
    - Managed with hemithyroidectomy; further management based on findings in resected specimen
    - Based on published literature, most are cytologically reported in follicular neoplasm (TBS IV), suspicious (TBS V) or AUS (TBS III) categories
- **Molecular testing**
  - Infiltrative FVPTC: *BRAF* V600E, *RET*::PTC fusion, *NTRK* fusion, *ALK* fusion
    - Encapsulated FVPTC: *RAS* mutations (like follicular carcinoma)
  - NIFTP: *RAS* mutations, *PAX8*::*PPARG* fusion, *BRAF* K601E, *EIF1AX*, *THADA* fusion

CYSTIC SUBTYPE

General Features and Cytology
- ~ 10% of PTC are cystic
- Thin, watery, brown or clear cyst fluid on aspiration; need to aspirate wall or residual area once cyst is drained
- **Palpation-guided FNAs** yield abundant hemosiderin-laden macrophages and degenerating atypical follicular cells in cyst fluid
- Atypical histiocytoid cells: Hypervacuolated, histiocyte-like follicular cells with some features of PTC
- Sometimes only few groups of cells with subtle features of PTC are present
  - In cystic lesion, close examination of rare follicular cells is very important

Follicular Variant of PTC on ThinPrep

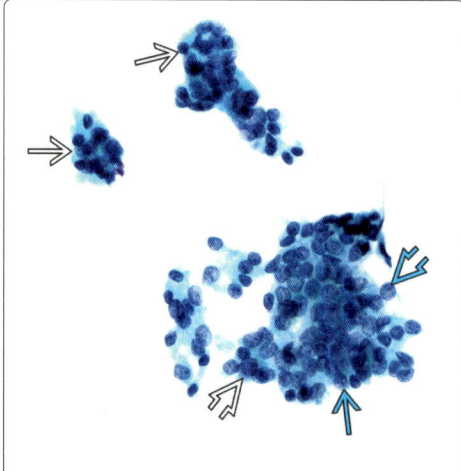

Papillary Carcinoma, Cystic Subtype

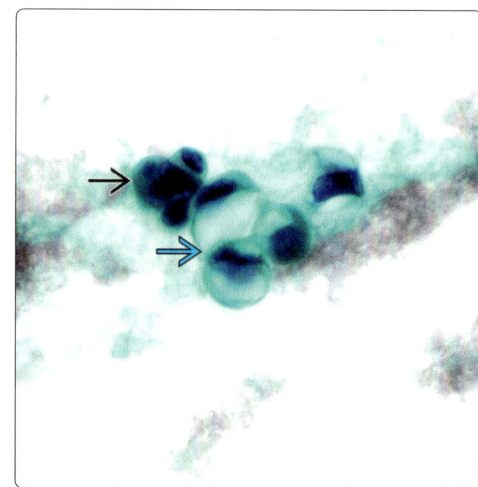

(Left) ThinPrep shows a collection of tight microfollicles ➡ and a jigsaw puzzle-like larger sheet that also shows internal microfollicles ➡. There is nuclear overlap and powdery, open chromatin. Grooves ➡ and small nucleoli ➡ are seen. (Right) This Pap-stained smear shows a hypervacuolated cluster ➡ of cells with enlarged irregular nuclei and fine chromatin. Some cells are degenerated ➡. Note the bloody background. Since there were only a few degenerated clusters, this case was interpreted as AUS.

Papillary Thyroid Carcinoma Subtypes

- o May be underdiagnosed as cyst contents or atypia of undetermined significance
- **US-guided FNAs** with aspiration of solid/mural nodule once cyst is drained is ideal for cystic PTC
  - o Well-sampled, intramural nodule is more cellular and may contain papillae, clusters of isolated tumor cells, or sheets with swirls or cartwheel arrangement of tumor cells with nuclear features of PTC

TALL CELL SUBTYPE

General Features
- Most common aggressive subtype, usually in older patients
- 5-19% of PTCs; M > F; average age: 55 years
- *BRAF* V600E mutation in up to 90% of cases
- *TP53* mutation in ~ 60% of cases, *TERT* promoter mutation in 30% of cases

Cytology
- Papillary clusters or dyscohesive single cells
- Tall or polygonal cells with granular, eosinophilic/oncocytic cytoplasm
- Low nuclear:cytoplasmic ratio
  - o Cell height is 3x cell width, basal round/oval nuclei
- Cytoplasmic tail is common, fewer psammoma bodies compared to classic PTC
- Most abundant nuclear pseudoinclusions, often multiple in single nucleus resulting in "soap bubble" nuclei
- Pleomorphism, cellular atypia, and mitoses more common than in conventional PTC

COLUMNAR CELL SUBTYPE

General Features
- Rare, aggressive variant (0.15-0.2% of PTC cases); F:M = 2:1
- Extrathyroid extension and metastasis are common
- Compared to classic PTC, tall cell (TC), columnar cell (CC), and hobnail (HN) subtypes, have more aggressive clinicopathologic features
- Based on American Thyroid Association risk stratification scheme, TC, CC, HN subtypes have intermediate risk of structural recurrence

Cytology
- 3D clusters of pseudostratified columnar cells with high nuclear:cytoplasmic ratio
- Hyperchromatic, oval to elongated nuclei with coarse chromatin (instead of pale nuclei of PTC)
- Characteristic PTC nuclear features are rare
- TTF-1, thyroglobulin (+)
- According to some studies, columnar variant may be CDX2(+) in ~ 50% of cases
- Molecular: 50% harbor *BRAF* V600E mutations, *BRAF* fusions, loss of *CDKN2A*, and copy number alterations (recurrent gain of chromosome 1q)
- *RAS*, *TERT* promoter, and *TP53* are rare molecular alterations in this subtype

Differential Diagnosis
- Metastatic colon or endometrial carcinoma or benign respiratory epithelium

HOBNAIL SUBTYPE

General Features
- < 2% of PTC, more aggressive behavior
- Can be seen in combination with other more aggressive subtypes, such as TC subtype

Cytology
- Papillary and micropapillary architecture without fibrovascular cores and areas of cellular dyscohesiveness
- Cuboidal, oval, or teardrop-shaped cells with abundant eosinophilic cytoplasm
- Nuclei are apically placed, producing bulge that leads to HN appearance, a.k.a. "comet" cells
  - o ≥ 30% HN cells
- Characteristic PTC nuclear features are usually present
- Multiple intranuclear cytoplasmic inclusions within same nucleus results in soap bubble nuclear appearance
- **Molecular**: *BRAF* mutation common, up to 80% of cases
  - o *TP53*, *TERT* promoter, *PIK3CA*
  - o Rarely *RET* rearrangements, molecular *CTNNB1*, *EGFR*, *ATK1*, *ATM*, *ARID2*, *NOTCH1*

DIFFUSE SCLEROSING SUBTYPE

General Features
- Rare, aggressive variant; < 6% of all PTC; younger age; F > M
- Diffuse involvement of thyroid lobes without dominant nodule, often with extrathyroid extension and lymph node metastasis
- 30-75% of cases associated with Hashimoto thyroiditis
- Higher incidence of lymph node and lung metastasis at presentation
- Mortality similar to classic PTC
- **US**: Can mimic Hashimoto on US
  - o Widespread microcalcifications result in characteristic snowstorm appearance on US

Cytology
- Most cases with lymphocytic background, which may be mistaken for Hashimoto thyroiditis or lymphoma (if lymphoid population is monotonous or atypical)
- Papillary and follicular architectures can be seen
- Pleomorphic cells with characteristic PTC nuclear features may be subtle in some cases
- Stromal fibrosis and abundant psammoma bodies
- Squamous metaplasia is present and often extensive
- 3D clusters of follicular cells with abundant psammoma bodies and squamous metaplasia should alert one to this entity in appropriate clinical and US setting
- **Molecular**: *RET::PTCH1* in 46% and *RET::NCOA4* in 16%, *ALK* mutations in 13%
  - o *BRAF* V600E mutations in ~ 20% and *RAS* mutations absent
  - o High frequency of LOH of 3p24, 9p21, 17q21, 21q22, and 22q13

ONCOCYTIC SUBTYPE

General Features
- Behavior similar to conventional PTC

Papillary Thyroid Carcinoma Subtypes

Cytology

- Papillary or follicular architecture
- Polygonal cells with abundant granular eosinophilic cytoplasm
- Apically located nuclei with characteristic PTC nuclear features
- *BRAF* V600E mutation in in 40%, *NDUFA13* (GRIM19) (germline mutation), rarely, *RET* rearrangements
- **Differential diagnosis**: Oncocytic (Hürthle cell) tumors and medullary carcinoma
  - Round nuclei with prominent nucleoli in Hürthle cell tumors; powdery chromatin is rare
  - Medullary carcinomas are calcitonin and CEA (+), thyroglobulin (-)

WARTHIN-LIKE SUBTYPE

General Features

- Behavior similar to conventional PTC
- Often seen with lymphocytic/Hashimoto thyroiditis

Cytology

- Predominant lymphoid background
- Oval or polygonal cells with abundant eosinophilic/oncocytic cytoplasm
- Characteristic nuclear features of PTC are not easily identifiable
- **Molecular**: *BRAF* V600E detected in 75%

Differential Diagnosis

- Lymphocytic thyroiditis, TC variant of PTC

MACROFOLLICULAR SUBTYPE

General Features

- < 0.5% of PTC; female patients in their 20s and 30s, good prognosis
- Criteria: Histologically composed exclusively or predominantly (> 50%) of macrofollicles > 200 µm in > 50% of cross-sectional area
- *BRAF* and *RAS* mutations generally not seen

Cytology

- Difficult to diagnose cytologically and often mistaken for benign adenomatous/follicular nodule
- Abundant watery colloid with low to variable cellularity of follicular cells, which are often in sheets on low power
- Nuclear features of PTC are subtle and patchy
  - Large sheets with some nuclear crowding and powdery chromatin
  - Intranuclear inclusions and grooves are rare
  - Peripheral micronucleoli are seen but papillae or avascular papillary fronds are rare
  - Attention to nuclear detail in what looks like benign nodule on low power is key to correct diagnosis on histology and may be completely missed on cytology
  - Cytologically often classified as AUS or benign

Differential Diagnosis

- Adenomatous/hyperplastic nodule: Abundant watery colloid in background and subtle nuclear features may mimic benign nodule

SOLID SUBTYPE

General Features and Cytology

- Rare, < 3% of PTC, but common in children and radiation exposure survivors
- Solid sheets, 3D cohesive, or syncytial clusters with rounded outlines or papillary-like structures of tumor cells with characteristic PTC nuclear features
- Often diagnosed cytologically as positive or suspicious for malignancy Bethesda categories
- Microfollicular pattern of solid subtype may be difficult to separate from FVPTC or other follicular patterned neoplasms
- Molecular: *RET/NCOA4* or *ETV6/NTRK3* rearrangements in radiation-exposed cases
- *BRAF* V600 is rare
- **Differential diagnosis**: Poorly differentiated thyroid carcinoma, which has necrosis and mitosis
  - More recently, significant overlap with secretory carcinoma [mammary analogue secretory carcinoma (MASC)], in thyroid gland
  - Perhaps PTCs with *ETV6/NTRK3* rearrangements are actually secretory carcinomas

CLEAR CELL SUBTYPE

General Features and Cytology

- Abundant vacuolated clear cytoplasm

DIAGNOSTIC CHECKLIST

Pathologic Interpretation Pearls

- PTC subtypes are typically found in combination with each other
- Tumor should be dominated by certain features to be categorized as specific subtype
- Usually it is not possible or necessary to determine all subtypes by cytology

SELECTED REFERENCES

1. Baloch ZW et al: Overview of the 2022 WHO Classification of Thyroid Neoplasms. Endocr Pathol. 33(1):27-63, 2022
2. Haaga E et al: Non-invasive follicular thyroid neoplasm with papillary-like nuclear features is not a cytological diagnosis, but it influences cytological diagnosis outcomes: a systematic review and meta-analysis. Acta Cytol. 66(2):85-105, 2022
3. De Graef A et al: Papillary thyroid carcinoma with hobnail features showing rapid progression and therapy resistance. Acta Chir Belg. 121(2):77-85, 2021
4. Donaldson LB et al: Hobnail variant of papillary thyroid carcinoma: a systematic review and meta-analysis. Endocrine. 72(1):27-39, 2021
5. Roukain A et al: Papillary thyroid carcinoma with desmoid-type fibromatosis: review of published cases. Cancers (Basel). 13(17):4482, 2021
6. Coca-Pelaz A et al: Papillary thyroid cancer-aggressive variants and impact on management: a narrative review. Adv Ther. 37(7):3112-28, 2020
7. Ohashi R: Solid variant of papillary thyroid carcinoma: an under-recognized entity. Endocr J. 67(3):241-8, 2020
8. Bongiovanni M et al: Impact of non-invasive follicular thyroid neoplasms with papillary-like nuclear features (NIFTP) on risk of malignancy in patients undergoing lobectomy/thyroidectomy for suspected malignancy or malignant fine-needle aspiration cytology findings: a systematic review and meta-analysis. Eur J Endocrinol. 181(4):389-96, 2019
9. Lewiński A et al: Correlations between molecular landscape and sonographic image of different variants of papillary thyroid carcinoma. J Clin Med. 8(11):1916, 2019
10. Rossi ED et al: Cytologic features of aggressive variants of follicular-derived thyroid carcinoma. Cancer Cytopathol. 127(7):432-46, 2019
11. Pusztaszeri M et al: Update on the cytologic features of papillary thyroid carcinoma variants. Diagn Cytopathol. 45(8):714-30, 2017

Papillary Thyroid Carcinoma Subtypes

Follicular Variant of PTC
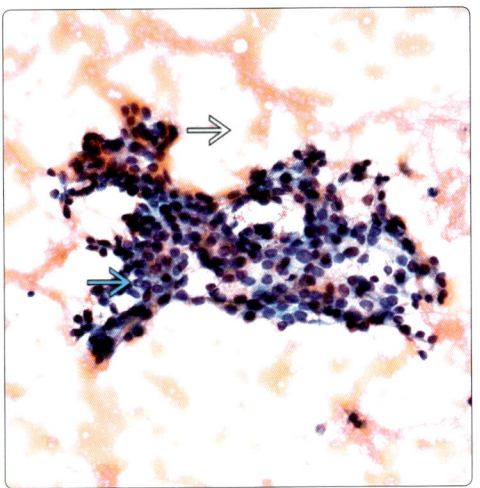

Follicular Variant of PTC Histology
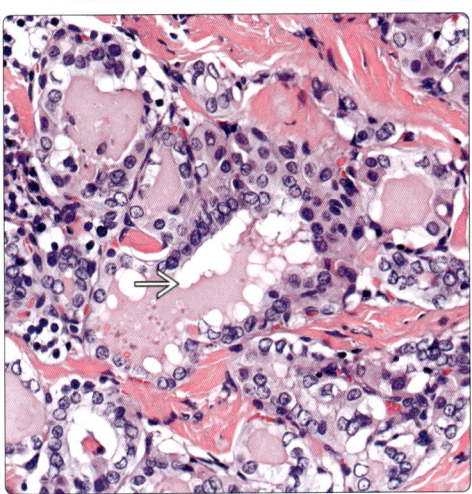

(Left) Pap stain of a thyroid nodule suspicious for FVPTC shows abundant watery colloid ➡ and branching staghorn-like sheets of cells with occasional nuclear grooves and a rare intranuclear cytoplasmic inclusion ➡. (Right) H&E section of the subsequent thyroidectomy shows FVPTC. Note the intrafollicular colloid with peripheral scalloping ➡, a common finding in FVPTC. The colloid tends to be hypereosinophilic. Capsular or vascular invasion distinguishes it from NIFTP.

Microfollicular Pattern
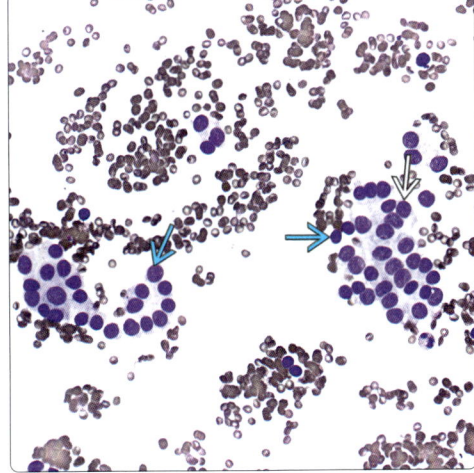

Low Magnification of FVPTC
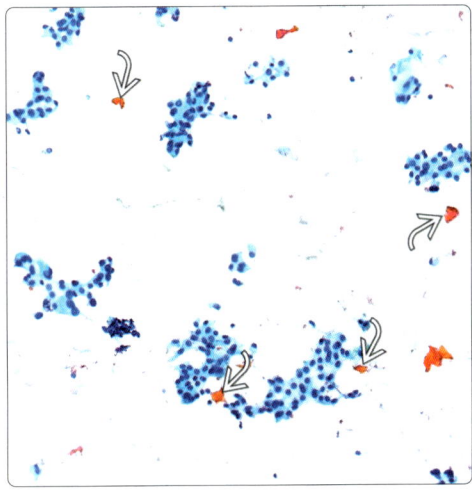

(Left) Diff-Quik stain shows a microfollicular pattern ➡ with an open nuclear chromatin and a rare small nucleolus ➡. Nuclear grooves, intranuclear cytoplasmic inclusions, or papillae are not seen. This was originally interpreted as a follicular neoplasm. Resection was diagnosed as FVPTC. (Right) Pap-stained smear on low magnification shows small sheets and microfollicular pattern. The colloid from the follicles trails the cellular groups ➡.

FVPTC, Diff-Quik Appearance
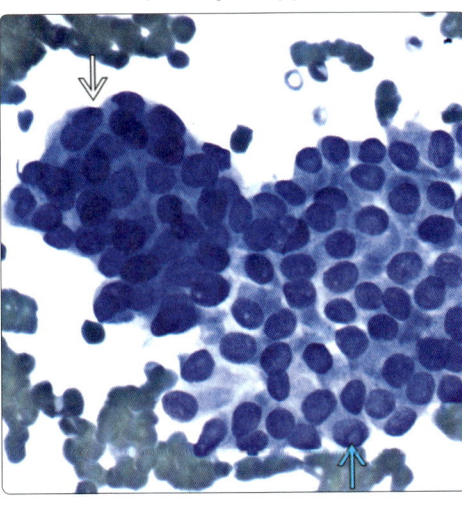

FVPTC/NIFTP
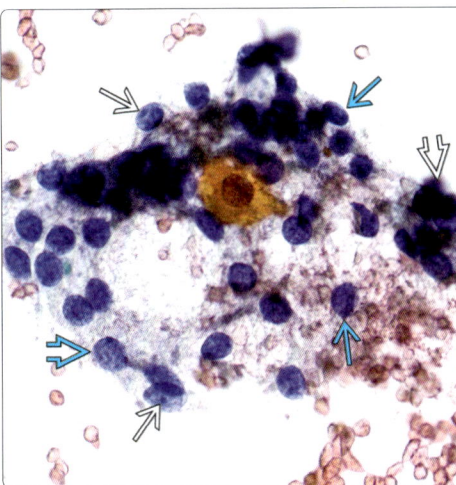

(Left) Diff-Quik stain shows a 3D cluster ➡ with tight microfollicles and a more flat, sheet-like area adjacent to it. The nuclei are larger with open chromatin and questionable nuclear inclusions ➡. (Right) Pap-stained smear shows a microfollicular pattern with nuclear overlap ➡. The chromatin is fine and powdery ➡ with small nucleoli ➡. Nuclear grooves ➡ are few and intranuclear cytoplasmic inclusions are absent. The resection showed an NIFTP.

Papillary Thyroid Carcinoma Subtypes

Cystic PTC Subtype
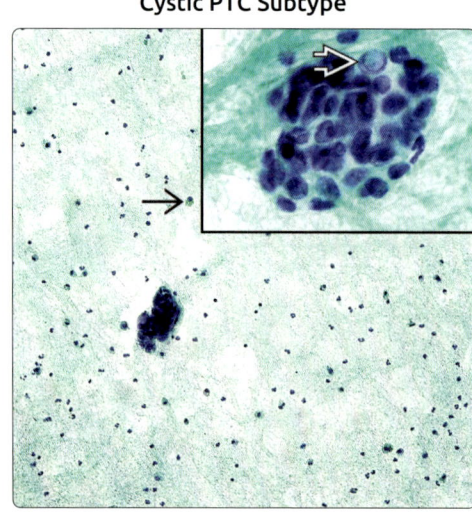

Cystic Subtype on ThinPrep
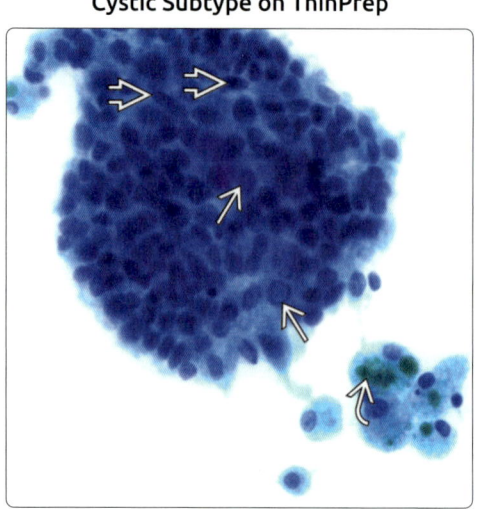

(Left) Pap stain shows a thyroid aspirate with numerous macrophages ➡ and only a few groups of follicular cells (inset), some with nuclear irregularities and intranuclear inclusions ➡. Quantitatively, the follicular cells were not sufficient for a definitive diagnosis of PTC. (Right) Pap-stained ThinPrep shows a cluster of cells in a clean background with hemosiderin-laden macrophages ➡. There are nuclear contour irregularities ➡, powdery chromatin, nucleoli, and well-defined nuclear holes ➡.

PTC, Cystic Subtype
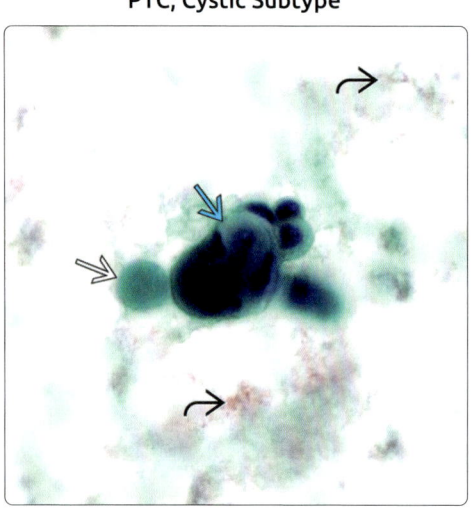

High-Power View of Cystic Subtype

(Left) Pap-stained smear of thyroid cyst contents showed a rare group of degenerated ➡ vacuolated ➡ cells in a bloody background ➡. This case was initially diagnosed as AUS. (Right) Pap-stained image of the rare groups seen in cystic PTC shows elongated nuclei with nuclear grooves ➡ and irregularity. Quantitatively, the follicular cells were not sufficient for a definitive diagnosis of PTC.

PTC, Cystic Subtype on Resection
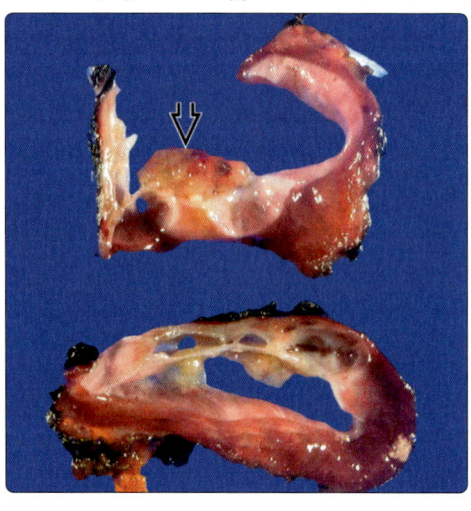

PTC, Macrofollicular Subtype
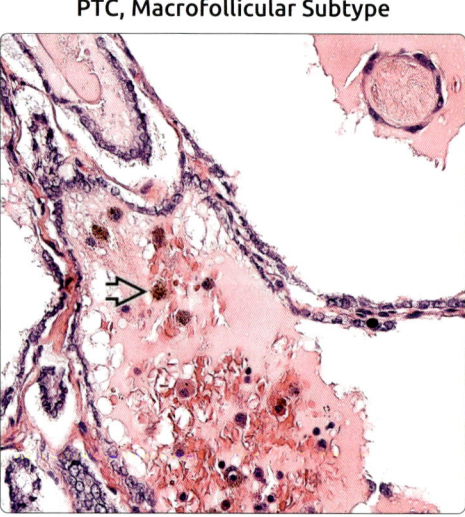

(Left) Gross photograph of cystic subtype of PTC shows a small solid area attached to the cyst wall ➡. (Right) H&E section of a macrofollicular variant of PTC shows large follicles with abundant colloid and a few hemosiderin-laden macrophages ➡. The nuclei lining the follicles have features of PTC, which can be focal and subtle and easily missed.

Papillary Thyroid Carcinoma Subtypes

Tall Cell Subtype of PTC

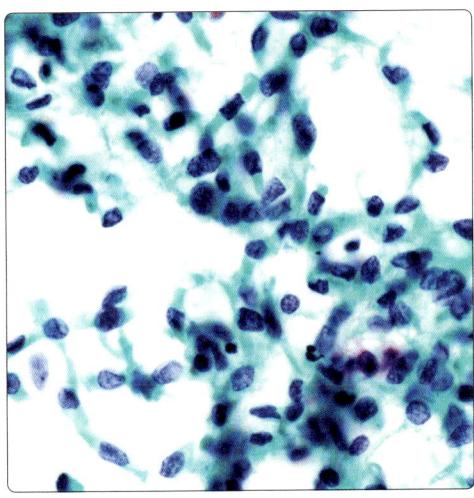

Tall Cell Subtype With Pleomorphism

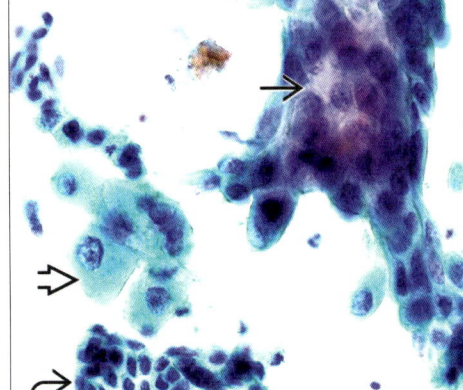

(Left) Pap stain of a tall cell subtype of PTC shows dyscohesive tall single cells with round to oval nuclei. Cell height is at least 2-3x the cell width. Most cells have cytoplasmic tails, a common finding in tall cell subtype of PTC. (Right) Pap stain shows a tall cell subtype of PTC with moderate to severe pleomorphism. Some cells are slightly elongated ➡. Other cells have clear ➡ to oncocytic ➡ cytoplasm and moderate nuclear atypia.

Tall Cell Subtype, Soap Bubble Nuclei on ThinPrep

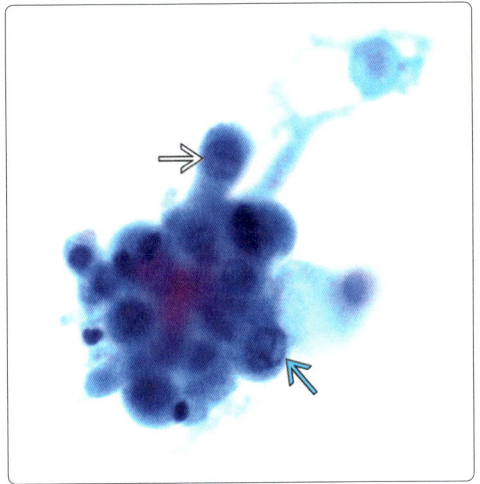

Tall Cell Subtype of PTC on Resection

(Left) Pap-stained ThinPrep shows an elongated cell ➡ with pale powdery chromatin and nucleoli. The soap bubble intranuclear inclusions are easily seen ➡, even on this liquid-based preparation, raising the possibility of tall cell subtype. (Right) H&E section shows tall cells with height 2-3x their width. Cells have elongated nuclei with characteristic nuclear features of PTC. There is abundant eosinophilic cytoplasm resulting in low nuclear:cytoplasmic ratio.

Columnar Cell Subtype of PTC

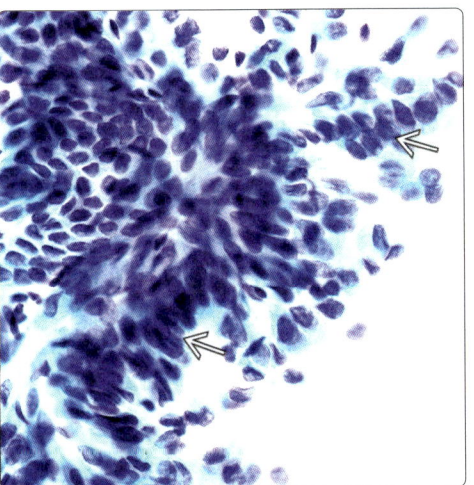

Columnar Cell Subtype of PTC on Resection

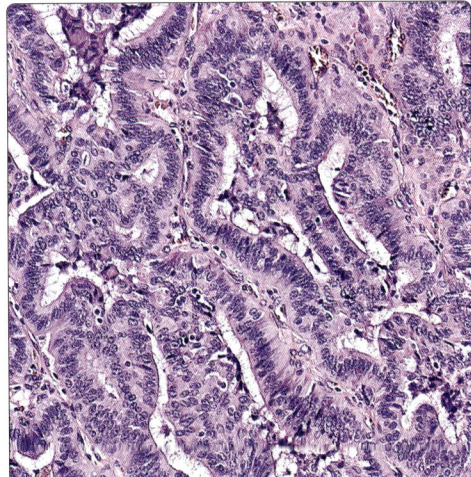

(Left) Pap stain of a columnar cell subtype shows complex papillae lined by elongated cells with pseudostratified nuclei ➡ and scant cytoplasm. In contrast to tall cell PTC, these cells have high nuclear:cytoplasmic ratios. Characteristic nuclear features of PTC are rare. (Right) H&E section of a columnar subtype of PTC shows elongated nuclei with pseudostratification. The tumor mimics metastatic colon or endometrial carcinoma. Columnar PTC can be CDX2 and BRAF (+), complicating the diagnosis.

Papillary Thyroid Carcinoma Subtypes

Sclerosing Subtype of PTC With Stroma

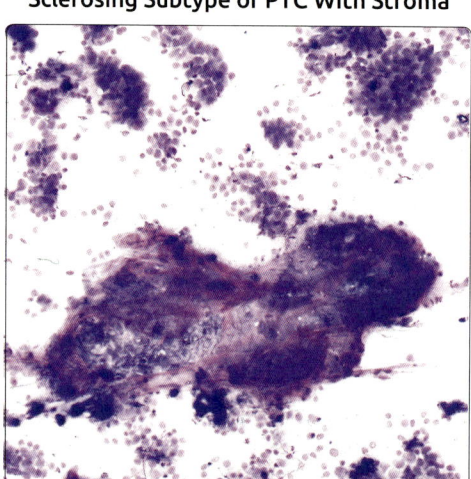

Sclerosing Subtype of PTC

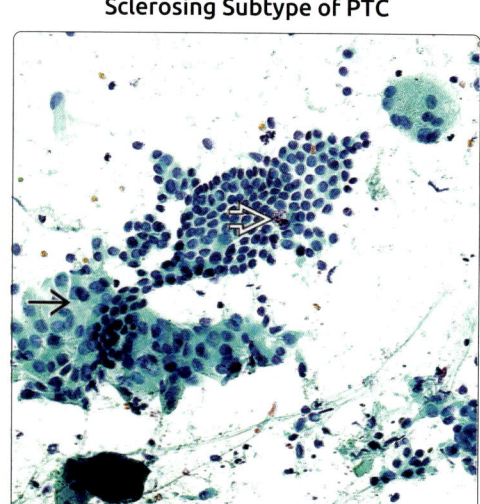

(Left) Diff-Quik stain of a sclerosing subtype of PTC illustrates syncytial clusters of atypical cells embedded in a magenta-colored stroma. (Right) Pap stain of a sclerosing subtype of PTC shows clusters of cells with characteristic nuclear features of PTC. Some cells have abundant hard squamoid cytoplasm ➡. There is a small psammoma body ➡ in the syncytial sheet.

Sclerosing Subtype of PTC on Resection

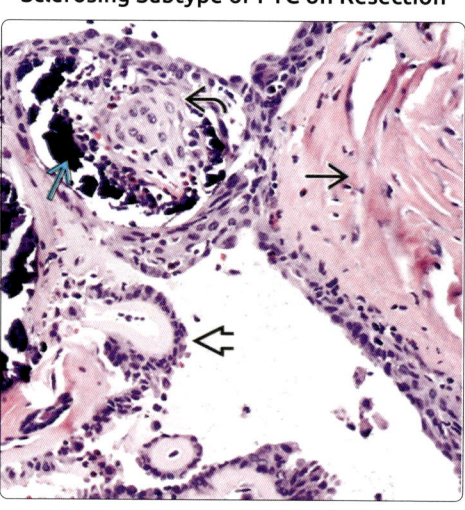

Oncocytic Subtype of PTC

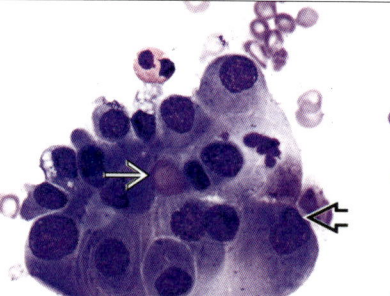

(Left) H&E section shows papillary structures with nuclear features of PTC ➡, focal squamous metaplasia ➡, and amorphous stroma with sclerosis ➡. Calcifications ➡ are abundant. (Right) Diff-Quik stain of an oncocytic subtype of PTC shows oncocytic (Hürthle) cells with irregular nuclear membranes ➡, abundant granular cytoplasm, and a possible intranuclear inclusion ➡. Nuclear features are essential for diagnosis of PTC and should be present in most cells.

PTC, Oncocytic Subtype on ThinPrep

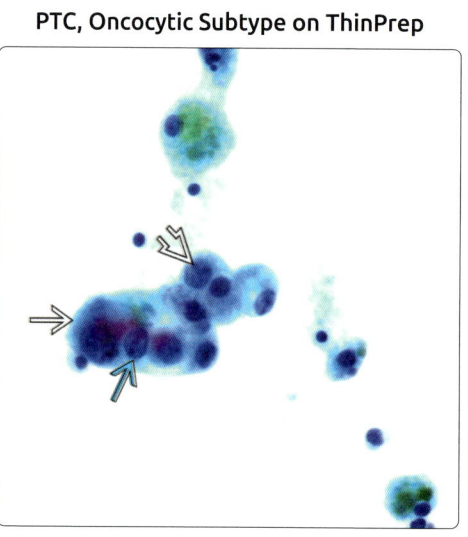

Histology of Oncocytic Subtype

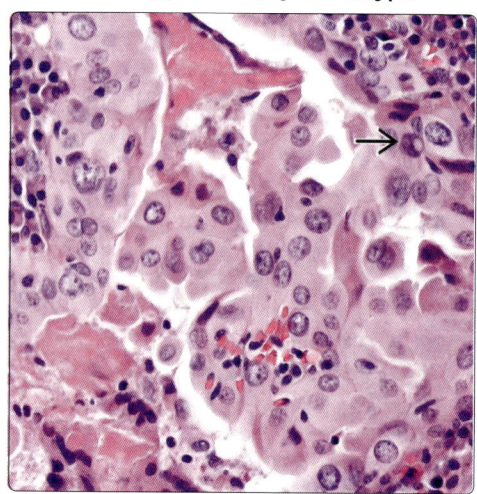

(Left) Pap-stained ThinPrep shows large cells with abundant granular cytoplasm ➡. The nuclei are large with fine, powdery chromatin, grooves ➡, and nucleoli ➡. No intranuclear inclusions are seen in this field, therefore, diagnosis of malignancy cannot be made on the basis of this field alone. (Right) H&E section of an oncocytic subtype of PTC shows cells with abundant eosinophilic cytoplasm. Nuclei have characteristic features of classic PTC, such as grooves, clearing, and intranuclear cytoplasmic inclusions ➡.

Papillary Thyroid Carcinoma Subtypes

Warthin-Like PTC
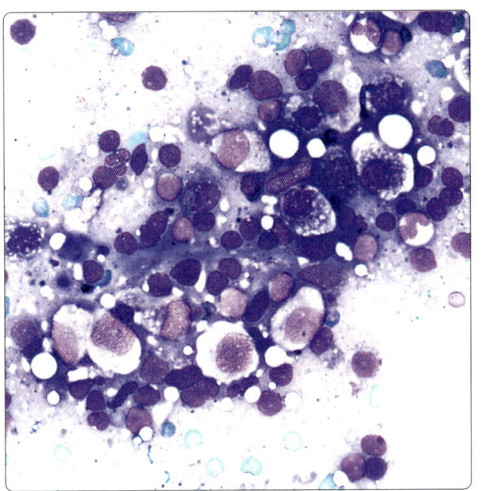

Trabecular Pattern in Warthin-Like PTC
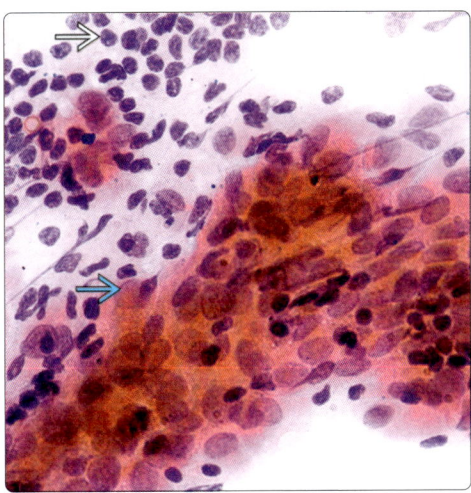

(Left) *Diff-Quik stain of a Warthin-like PTC shows oncocytic cells admixed with polymorphous lymphocytes. Characteristic nuclear features of PTC are rare. There is a possibility of false-negative diagnosis as lymphocytic thyroiditis.* (Right) *Pap stain of the same case shows oncocytic cells arranged in a trabecular pattern ➡ with occasional nuclear irregularities and grooves. There are lymphocytes in the background ➡.*

Warthin-Like PTC on Resection
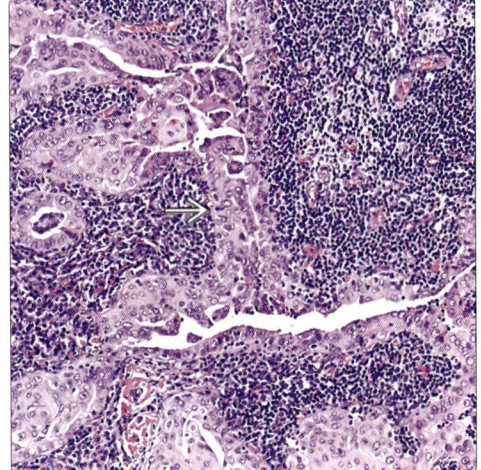

Tall Cell Subtype With Lymphocytes
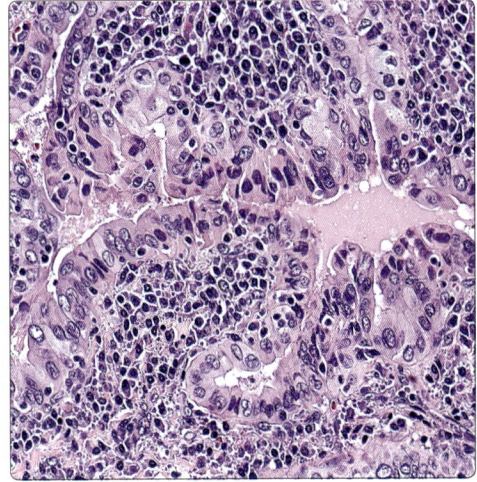

(Left) *H&E section of a Warthin-like PTC illustrates trabeculae of oncocytic cells with abundant eosinophilic cytoplasm ➡. Nuclei are round to oval and show nuclear clearing and grooves. Differential diagnosis includes the tall cell variant of PTC.* (Right) *H&E section of a tall cell subtype of PTC shows papillary structures with marked lymphocytic infiltration. Cells are elongated, and some have oncocytic cytoplasm. Compared with Warthin-like PTC, there is more nuclear atypia and pleomorphism.*

Hobnail Subtype of PTC
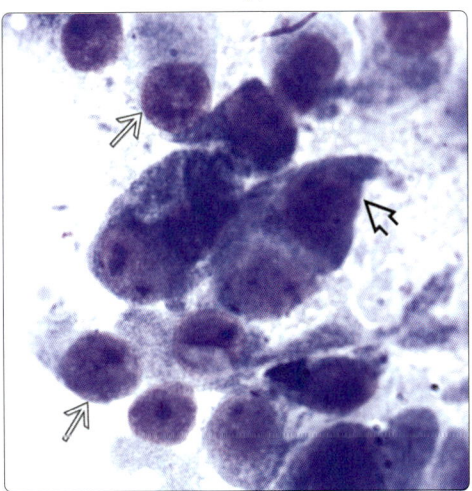

Hobnail Subtype on Histology
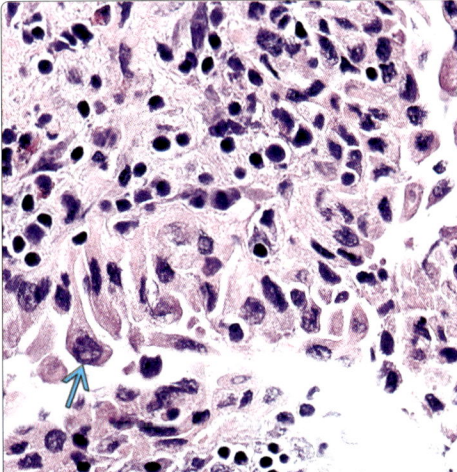

(Left) *Diff-Quik stain of a hobnail subtype of PTC illustrates oval or teardrop-shaped cells ➡ with marked atypia and abundant cytoplasm. Nuclei are apically placed ➡, producing a bulge that leads to a hobnail appearance.* (Right) *H&E section illustrates focal hobnail features ➡ in this example of papillary carcinoma.*

Medullary Thyroid Carcinoma

KEY FACTS

CLINICAL ISSUES
- Medullary thyroid carcinoma (MTC) arises from C cells
- 5-10% of all thyroid malignancies
  - 75-80% sporadic, 20-25% hereditary
- Increased serum calcitonin and CEA levels
- *RET* gene mutation analysis important for prognosis and management
- 5-year survival rate: 60-80%
- 10-year survival rate: 40-70%
- High grade: Mitosis ≥ 5/10 HPF (~ 2 mm²), Ki-67 ≥ 5% or necrosis

CYTOPATHOLOGY
- Spindle, polygonal, or bipolar cells often with eccentric nuclei and ill-defined cell borders
- Hyperchromatic nuclei with coarse chromatin and moderate pleomorphism
- Abundant eosinophilic or amphophilic cytoplasm with fibrillar quality
- Metachromic red (azurophilic) cytoplasmic granules in DQ
- Several variants present; subclassification of MTC has no management or prognostic value
- Grading in small sample not recommended

ANCILLARY TESTS
- Positive for calcitonin and CEA [poorly differentiated MTC may be calcitonin (-)]

TOP DIFFERENTIAL DIAGNOSES
- Papillary thyroid carcinoma (PTC), follicular neoplasm, oncocytic neoplasm, hyalinizing trabecular adenoma, melanoma, metastatic neuroendocrine tumor, lymphoma
- **PTC**
  - Intranuclear inclusions can be seen in MTC and PTC
  - Thyroglobulin (+), calcitonin (-)
- **Oncocytic (Hürthle cell) adenoma/carcinoma**
  - Oncocytic MTC may resemble oncocytic neoplasm
  - Thyroglobulin (+), calcitonin (-)

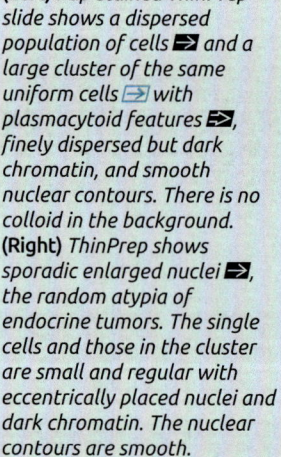

(Left) *Pap-stained ThinPrep slide shows a dispersed population of cells ➡ and a large cluster of the same uniform cells ➡ with plasmacytoid features ➡, finely dispersed but dark chromatin, and smooth nuclear contours. There is no colloid in the background.* (Right) *ThinPrep shows sporadic enlarged nuclei ➡, the random atypia of endocrine tumors. The single cells and those in the cluster are small and regular with eccentrically placed nuclei and dark chromatin. The nuclear contours are smooth.*

Medullary Thyroid Carcinoma, Liquid Based

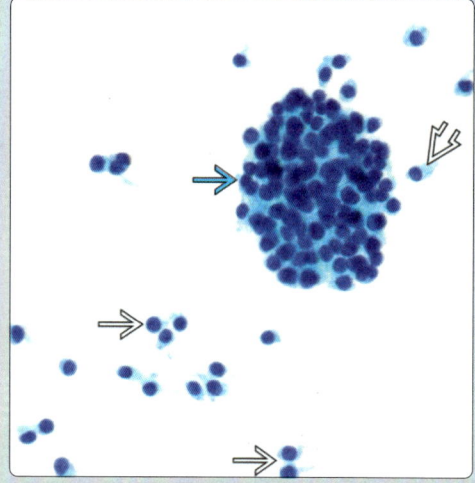

Endocrine Atypia, Medullary Carcinoma

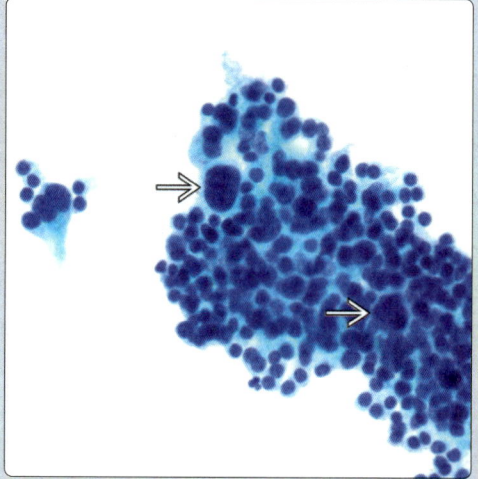

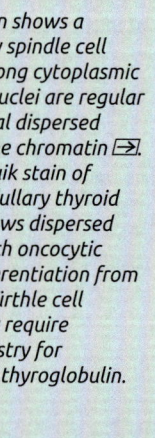

(Left) *Pap stain shows a predominantly spindle cell pattern with long cytoplasmic tails ➡. The nuclei are regular with the typical dispersed neuroendocrine chromatin ➡.* (Right) *Diff-Quik stain of oncocytic medullary thyroid carcinoma shows dispersed single cells with oncocytic features. Differentiation from a oncocytic/Hürthle cell neoplasm may require immunochemistry for calcitonin and thyroglobulin.*

Medullary Thyroid Carcinoma, Spindle Cell Pattern

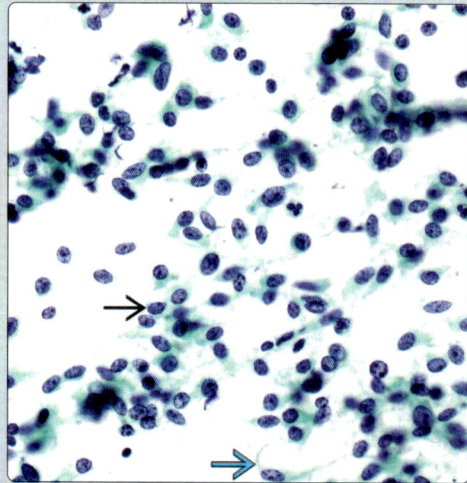

Medullary Carcinoma, Oncocytic Type

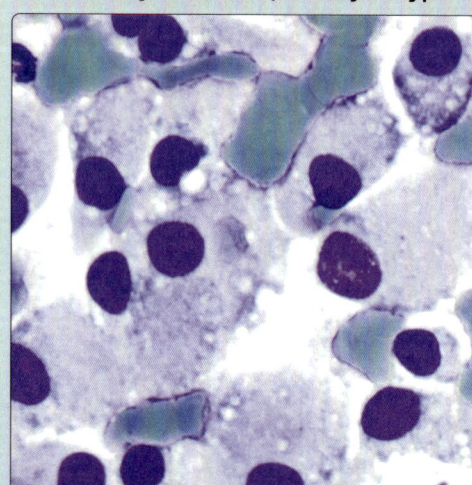

Medullary Thyroid Carcinoma

TERMINOLOGY

Abbreviations
- Medullary thyroid carcinoma (MTC)

Definitions
- Malignant neuroendocrine tumor derived from C cells (parafollicular cells) of thyroid

ETIOLOGY/PATHOGENESIS

Genetic Predisposition
- **Multiple endocrine neoplasias (MEN2 syndrome)**
  - Autosomal dominant, usually with high penetrance
  - Caused by activating point mutations in *RET* gene
  - Fusion genes with tyrosine kinase domain of *RET* also occur
  - **MEN2A**: MTC, parathyroid hyperplasia, pancreatic endocrine tumors, and pheochromocytoma
    - Most common mutation on exon 11 codon 634
  - **MEN2B**: MTC, pheochromocytoma, and mucosal soft tissue tumors (notably neuromas)
    - Most common mutations involve exon 16 codon 918T and less often exon 15 (A883F)
- **Familial MTC-only syndrome**: Not associated with other tumors

Sporadic
- May have **somatic** *RET* mutation at codon 918
- Somatic *HRAS*, *KRAS*, and *NRAS* mutations can occur

Precursor Lesions
- **Reactive C-cell hyperplasia (CCH)**
  - Physiologic increase in C-cells due to thyroid neoplasms, hyperparathyroidism, hypergastrinemia
  - Cell clusters < 50 cells
  - Lack pleomorphism, amyloid, fibrosis, or invasion
- **Neoplastic CCH (NCCH)**
  - > 50 C cells surrounding or invading follicles
  - Harbors germline *RET* mutations

CLINICAL ISSUES

Epidemiology
- Incidence
  - 5-10% of all thyroid malignancies
    - 75-80% sporadic
    - 20-25% familial/hereditary
  - Rising detection due to calcitonin screening protocols and *RET* genetic testing
- Age
  - 50-60 years in sporadic cases
  - Familial cases can present from early childhood
- Sex
  - Slight female predominance in sporadic cases

Presentation
- Often presents as painless "cold" nodule
- May present with lymph node or distant metastases
  - MTC tends to metastasize early: Liver, lungs, bone, soft tissue, brain, and bone marrow
- Paraneoplastic syndrome
  - Symptoms of carcinoid or Cushing syndromes
- Dysphagia and airway obstruction in large tumors
- Nonthyroid findings in hereditary cases
  - Mucosal neuromas
  - Parathyroid, adrenal, pituitary, and pancreatic tumors

Laboratory Tests
- Increased serum calcitonin &/or CEA levels
- Abnormal pentagastrin-stimulated calcitonin response
- *RET* gene mutation analysis
- Screening and monitoring tests for high-risk patients

Treatment
- Surgical approaches
  - Total thyroidectomy
  - Neck dissections considered for tumors > 1 cm
  - Prophylactic thyroidectomy for familial MTC
    - Evidence-based guidelines are developed for timing of thyroidectomy on basis of specific *RET* germline mutations and family history
    - Codons 611, 618, 620, or 634, MEN2A: By 5 years of age
    - Codons 883, 918, MEN2B: By 1 year of age
    - Most familial MTCs: Thyroidectomy by 5 years of age
    - More aggressive mutations: Thyroidectomy < 1 year of age
  - Genetic counseling recommended
- Adjuvant therapy
  - Targeted tyrosine kinase, hormone therapy, chemotherapy, and anti-CEA treatments
- Radiation
  - For residual disease and palliation

Prognosis
- Variable, overall 5- and 10-year survival rates of 60-80% and 40-70%, respectively
- Better prognostic factors: Low tumor stage, young age, women, and familial forms
- Poor prognostic factors: Necrosis, squamous metaplasia, < 50% calcitonin immunoreaction, and CEA reactivity in absence of calcitonin, increased mitosis
- Some genetic mutations associated with more aggressive behavior (e.g., M918T or A883F *RET* mutations)

IMAGING

Scintigraphic Scan
- "Cold" nodule on iodine scan

CYTOPATHOLOGY

Cellularity
- Hypercellular, loosely cohesive to noncohesive cells

Pattern
- Single cells or small clusters with papillary, trabecular, microfollicular, or syncytial pattern

Background
- Amyloid (on cytologic preparations resembles colloid)
- Colloid absent

Medullary Thyroid Carcinoma

Cells
- Cells can be any size and any shape: Spindle, polygonal, oncocytic, bipolar, or small cells
- Binucleated and multinucleated tumor cells common
- Occur in combination; 1 cell type may predominate
- Occasional bizarre cells, typical of neuroendocrine tumors

Nuclear Details
- Round to oval usually eccentric nuclei
- Stippled or coarse salt and pepper chromatin, typical of neuroendocrine tumors
- Inconspicuous nucleoli
- Intranuclear inclusions or nuclear molding may occur

Cytoplasmic Details
- Usually abundant eosinophilic or amphophilic cytoplasm with fibrillar quality and ill-defined borders
- Metachromic red cytoplasmic granules in Diff-Quik
- Cytoplasmic extension (dendritic processes) common
- Rarely may have melanin-like pigment, intracytoplasmic vacuoles, or mucin-like material

Cell Block Findings
- Can be used for Congo red and immunohistochemical studies

MACROSCOPIC

General Features
- Hereditary tumors usually multicentric and bilateral
- Usually not encapsulated but well circumscribed
- Firm, yellow-white, gritty cut surface
- Mostly in upper pole of thyroid in lateral aspect, where higher concentration of C cells
  - Usually does not arise in isthmus

Size
- Microscopic to large tumors replacing entire gland
- Medullary microcarcinomas: < 1 cm in diameter

MICROSCOPIC

Histologic Features
- Variants: Follicular, papillary, clear cell, oncocytic, small cell, giant cell, melanotic, paraganglioma-like, and squamous

ANCILLARY TESTS

Histochemistry
- Congo red shows apple green birefringence under polarized light

Immunohistochemistry
- Calcitonin, chromogranin, synaptophysin, keratin, TTF-1, and CEA (+)
- Calcitonin (-) tumor may be CEA(+)
- Thyroglobulin (-)
- S100(+) in 60% of familial MTC (negative in sporadic cases)

Genetic Testing
- RET gene analysis for prognosis and timing of prophylactic thyroidectomy

Electron Microscopy
- Membrane-bound neurosecretory granules

DIFFERENTIAL DIAGNOSIS

Malignant Neoplasms
- Papillary thyroid carcinoma (PTC)
  - MTC lacks characteristic nuclear features of PTC
  - Intranuclear inclusions can be seen in MTC and PTC
  - Calcitonin (-), thyroglobulin (+)
- Oncocytic neoplasm
  - Oncocytic MTC may resemble oncocytic adenoma/carcinoma
  - Neuroendocrine chromatin in MTC
  - Calcitonin (-), thyroglobulin (+)
- Insular carcinoma
  - Difficult to distinguish from small cell MTC
  - Calcitonin (-), thyroglobulin (+)
- Undifferentiated carcinoma
  - Pleomorphism, necrosis, and high mitotic activity
  - Calcitonin (-)
- Metastatic neuroendocrine tumors
  - Can be calcitonin (+), CEA (+) in rare cases
- Metastatic melanoma
  - S100, melan-A (+); cytokeratin (-)
- Mixed medullary and follicular (follicular/parafollicular) carcinomas
  - Extremely rare
  - Show endocrine-neuroendocrine differentiation
  - Express both calcitonin and thyroglobulin
- Lymphoma
  - Small cell MTC may mimic lymphoma
  - Flow cytometry and immunostains required

Benign Neoplasms
- Hyalinizing trabecular tumor
  - Spindled cells may mimic MTC
  - Hyalin material may mimic amyloid
  - Calcitonin (-), thyroglobulin (+)
- Intrathyroid parathyroid tumor
  - PTH(+); calcitonin, thyroglobulin (-)
  - Clear delicate cytoplasm, numerous naked nuclei
- Paraganglioma
  - Calcitonin, thyroglobulin, CEA (-)

DIAGNOSTIC CHECKLIST

Pathologic Interpretation Pearls
- Consider MTC and calcitonin staining in any suspicious thyroid tumor without colloid production
- Cytologic diagnosis of MTC must be confirmed by Congo red &/or immunostain
  - Can be done on cell block or unstained smears
  - Fluid rinse can be used for calcitonin and CEA testing
  - Tumors may be positive for CEA only

SELECTED REFERENCES
1. Liu CY et al: Constitutive cytomorphologic features of medullary thyroid carcinoma using different staining methods. Diagnostics (Basel). 11(8):1396, 2021

Medullary Thyroid Carcinoma

Metachromatic Neurosecretory Granules

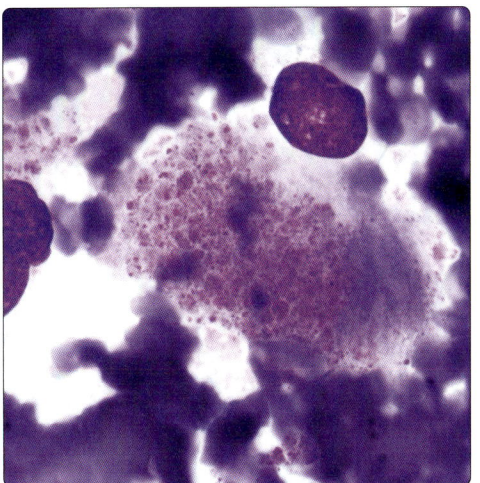

Uniform Cells of Medullary Carcinoma

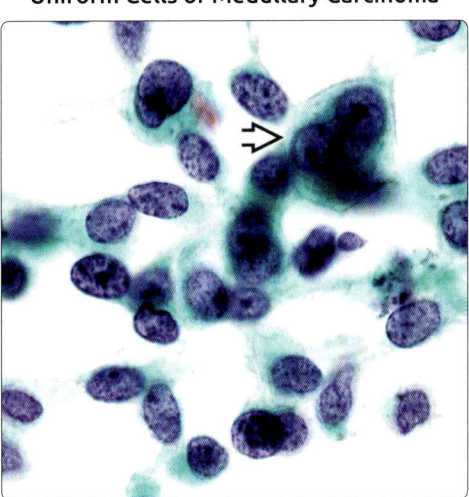

(Left) Diff-Quik stain of oncocytic medullary thyroid carcinoma highlights a bulging eccentric nucleus and metachromatic (azurophilic) neurosecretory granules. *(Right)* Pap stain of medullary thyroid carcinoma shows deceptively uniform cells with round to oval nuclei and coarse chromatin. There is a binucleated cell ⇨, which is a common finding in medullary thyroid carcinoma.

Amyloid on Diff-Quik

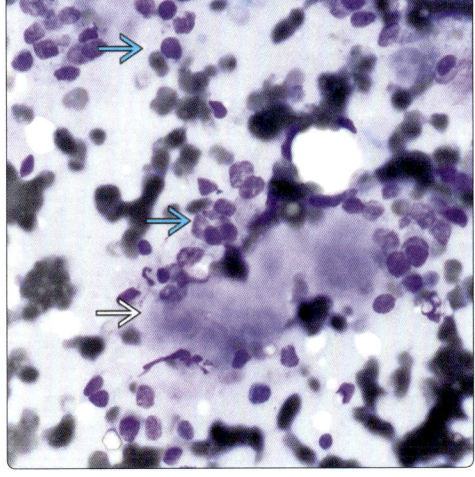

Amyloid on Congo Red With Polarization

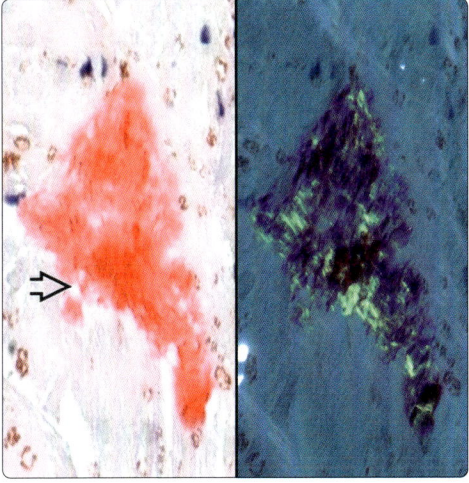

(Left) Diff-Quik stain of medullary thyroid carcinoma shows round and regular cells ⇨ surrounding amorphous material, which is amyloid ⇨. *(Right)* On the left, Congo red stain performed on a cell block of medullary thyroid carcinoma demonstrates a salmon pink color deposit ⇨, characteristic of amyloid. On the right, apple green birefringence under polarized light is diagnostic for amyloid.

Mixed Medullary-Follicular Carcinoma

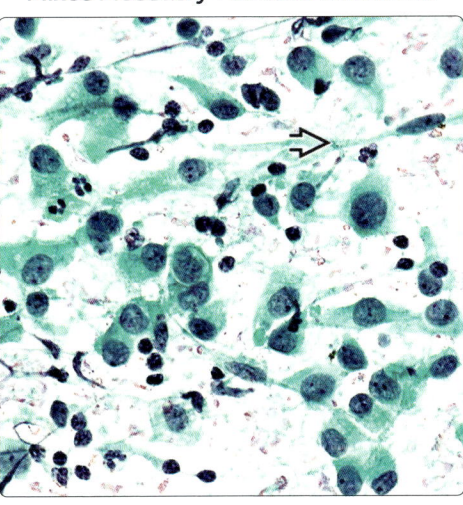

Mixed Medullary-Follicular Carcinoma Immunohistochemistry

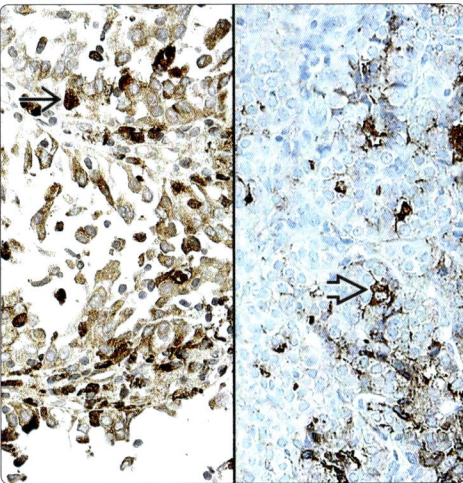

(Left) Pap stain of a mixed follicular-parafollicular carcinoma shows pleomorphic cells with cytoplasmic (dendritic) processes ⇨. The nuclei have coarse chromatin and rare prominent nucleoli. *(Right)* Subsequent thyroidectomy shows a poorly differentiated mixed follicular-parafollicular carcinoma with oncocytic features. The tumor cells are positive for CEA ⇨ and TTF-1, focally positive for thyroglobulin ⇨, and negative for calcitonin immunostains.

Poorly Differentiated Thyroid Carcinoma

KEY FACTS

CLINICAL ISSUES
- Patients often present with locally advanced disease and widespread metastases
- Prognosis is intermediate between well- and undifferentiated thyroid carcinomas
- Death from disease is common, often years later
- Not responsive to conventional therapy

CYTOPATHOLOGY
- Definitive diagnosis requires histologic examination
- Highly cellular smears with scant colloid
- Monotonous, small to intermediate-sized cells
- Bland nuclei with fine chromatin and small nucleoli
- Necrosis and mitoses are common

ANCILLARY TESTS
- Thyroglobulin and TTF-1 are usually positive
- Cytokeratin, cyclin-D1, and BCL2 are usually positive
- Neuroendocrine markers and calcitonin are negative

- TERT, TP53, CTNNB1 mutations are common

TOP DIFFERENTIAL DIAGNOSES
- Follicular or well-differentiated carcinoma
  - Uniform cells arranged in microfollicles, no mitosis, necrosis
- Papillary thyroid carcinoma
  - Diagnosis is based on conventional nuclear features
  - Presence of isolated cells suggests diagnosis of poorly differentiated thyroid carcinoma (PDTC)
- Medullary thyroid carcinoma
  - Often has increased mitotic activity and necrosis
  - Microfollicles and colloid support diagnosis of PDTC
  - Positive for calcitonin and neuroendocrine markers; negative for thyroglobulin
- Anaplastic thyroid carcinoma
  - Aggressive tumor with rapid disease course
  - Isolated cells with marked nuclear pleomorphism
  - Thyroglobulin and TTF-1 are usually negative

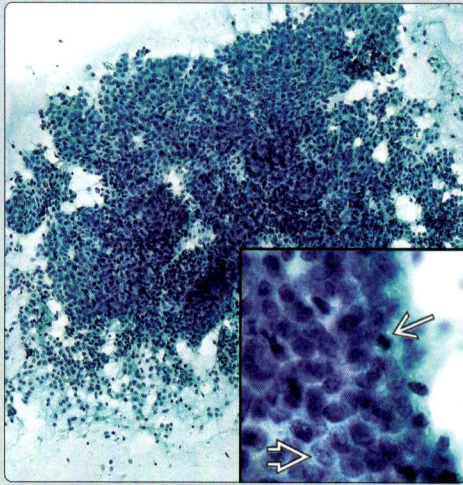

Trabecular Pattern of Poorly Differentiated Carcinoma

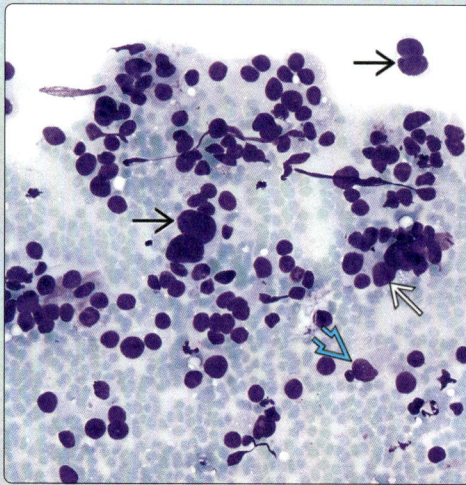

Cellular Patterns on Diff-Quik

(Left) Pap stain shows a cellular smear with trabecular architecture. The inset illustrates small uniform cells with high nuclear:cytoplasmic ratios and few cells with convoluted nuclei ➡. Mitosis is also present ➡. (Right) Diff-Quik stain shows single cells within a bloody background devoid of colloid. Some vague microfollicles ➡, random single atypical cells ➡, and rare oncocytic/Hürthle ➡ cells are seen.

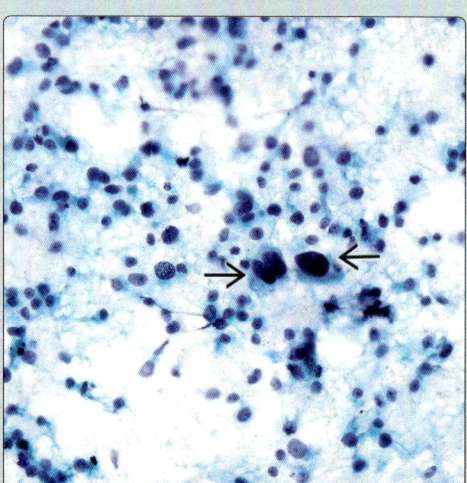

Single Cells With Occasional Large Cell Pattern

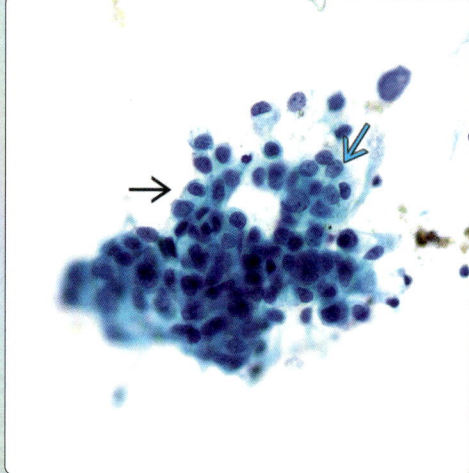

Trabeculae and Vague Microfollicular Pattern

(Left) On Pap stain, single cells predominate. Most are uniformly small and round to oval, but a few larger, more markedly atypical cells ➡ are present. (Right) On Pap stain, these cells are arranged in vague microfollicles ➡ and trabeculae ➡. Most are small and bland with a moderate amount of ill-defined cytoplasm.

Poorly Differentiated Thyroid Carcinoma

TERMINOLOGY

Abbreviations
- Poorly differentiated thyroid carcinoma (PDTC)

Synonyms
- Insular thyroid carcinoma

Definitions
- Malignant epithelial thyroid neoplasm showing features intermediate between differentiated and undifferentiated thyroid carcinomas

ETIOLOGY/PATHOGENESIS

Origin
- May arise from preexisting papillary or follicular carcinoma or as de novo neoplasm

CYTOPATHOLOGY

Overview
- Definitive diagnosis requires histologic examination
- Most FNA specimens are diagnosed as follicular neoplasms or metastatic carcinoma

Cellularity
- Cellular aspirates; bloody, scant colloid; variable necrosis

Pattern
- Variable: Microfollicular, insular, or trabecular patterns
- Single cells predominate, usually small, round, and monotonous, similar to follicular cells
- Also see clusters of overlapping cells forming microfollicles and rare papillae

Nuclear Details
- Bland nuclei with fine chromatin and small nucleoli
- Mild nuclear atypia and pleomorphism may be seen
- May have intranuclear inclusions and nuclear grooves
- Necrosis and mitoses are variably common

Cytoplasmic Details
- Moderate, poorly defined, and slightly vacuolated, eosinophilic

MICROSCOPIC

Histologic Features
- Definitive diagnosis made on histology (Turin criteria)
- Solid, trabecular, or insular growth pattern, plus
  - Presence of at least 1 of following: Convoluted nuclei, > 3 mitoses per 10 HPF, or tumor necrosis

ANCILLARY TESTS

Immunohistochemistry
- Cytokeratin, TTF-1, thyroglobulin, cyclin-D1 usually positive
- Neuroendocrine markers and calcitonin are negative
- Ki-67 proliferative index is high

Genetic Testing
- TP53, CTNNB1, and TERT mutations are common
- HRAS, KRAS, or NRAS mutations in 50% cases
- BRAF mutations are **not** detected

DIFFERENTIAL DIAGNOSIS

Follicular or Well-Differentiated Carcinoma
- Uniform cells arranged in microfollicles, no mitosis, necrosis

Papillary Thyroid Carcinoma
- Presence of isolated cells suggests diagnosis of PDTC

Medullary Thyroid Carcinoma
- Positive for calcitonin and neuroendocrine markers; negative for thyroglobulin

Anaplastic Thyroid Carcinoma
- Thyroglobulin and TTF-1 are usually negative

SELECTED REFERENCES
1. Kim NR et al: Contribution of cytologic examination to diagnosis of poorly differentiated thyroid carcinoma. J Pathol Transl Med. 54(2):171-8, 2020

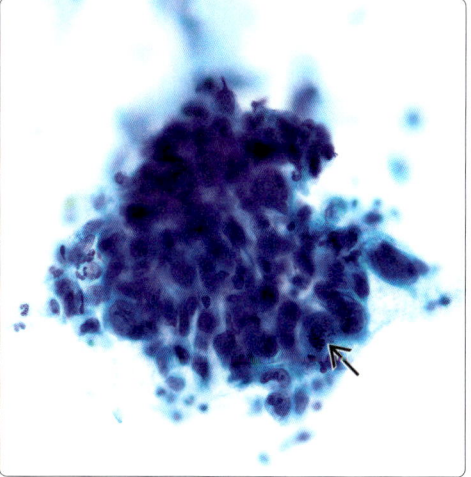

Nuclear Atypia and Mitosis

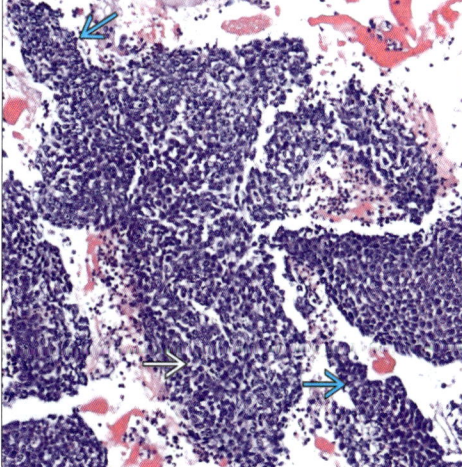

Poorly Differentiated Carcinoma, Core Needle Biopsy

(Left) On Pap stain, this cell cluster demonstrates nuclear atypia and a mitotic figure ➡. Mitoses and necrosis may be seen in poorly differentiated thyroid carcinoma. (Right) Core needle biopsy of large thyroid mass shows solid ➡ and trabecular pattern ➡ of poorly differentiated carcinoma. Appropriate immunohistochemical and molecular work-up can be performed on cell blocks and core needle biopsies.

Anaplastic Thyroid Carcinoma

KEY FACTS

CLINICAL ISSUES
- Most patients have history of nodular hyperplasia
- Rapidly progressive with poor prognosis
- Considered T4 and stage IV tumor by definition

CYTOPATHOLOGY
- Highly cellular neoplasm with absent colloid
- Background of necrotic debris and inflammatory cells
- Markedly pleomorphic nuclei with prominent nucleoli and ample eosinophilic cytoplasm
- Varying malignant cellular population consisting of osteoclastic and pleomorphic giant cells, squamoid, signet-ring, spindle, rhabdoid, stellate, and carcinosarcomatous patterns
- Paucicellular and angiomatoid variants also described
- Primary squamous cell carcinoma of thyroid is categorized as anaplastic thyroid carcinoma

ANCILLARY TESTS
- Vimentin, keratin, and PAX8 (nuclear) (+) in > 80%
- p53 and p63 usually diffusely (+); KI67 index > 80%
- TTF-1, thyroglobulin, desmin, HMB-45, CD31, and CD34 (-)
- Most consistent finding is *TP53* and *CTNNB1* gene mutation [IHC nuclear (+)]
- *BRAF* V600E testing important for management; *RAS* mutations also common
- Poor response on chemotherapy but targeted therapies show promise based on mutation: Protease inhibitors, multikinase inhibitors, vascular targeting agents, and gene therapies
- Primary squamous cells carcinoma express PAX8 and TTF-1 in 91% and 38% of cases, respectively

TOP DIFFERENTIAL DIAGNOSES
- Primary sarcoma, malignant melanoma, poorly differentiated thyroid carcinoma, medullary carcinoma, and Riedel thyroiditis

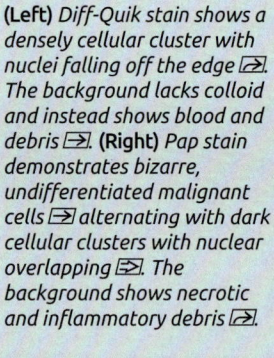

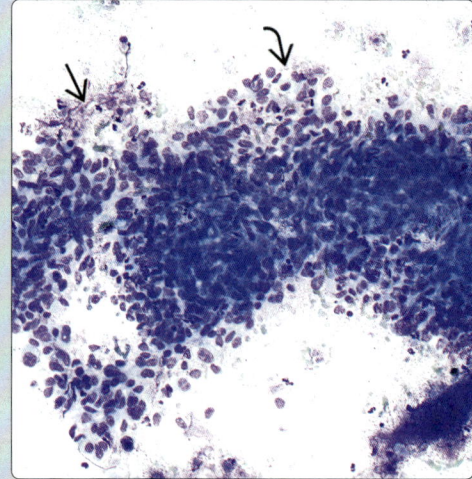

Anaplastic Thyroid Carcinoma, Cellular Clusters

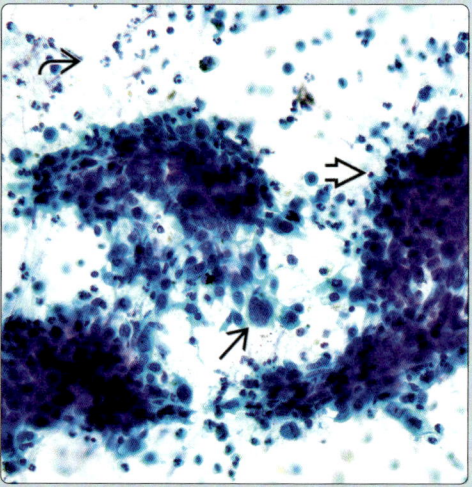

Cellular With Bizarre Malignant Cells

(Left) Diff-Quik stain shows a densely cellular cluster with nuclei falling off the edge ➔. The background lacks colloid and instead shows blood and debris ➔. (Right) Pap stain demonstrates bizarre, undifferentiated malignant cells ➔ alternating with dark cellular clusters with nuclear overlapping ➔. The background shows necrotic and inflammatory debris ➔.

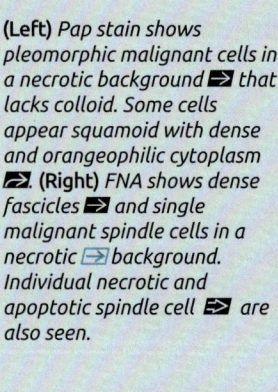

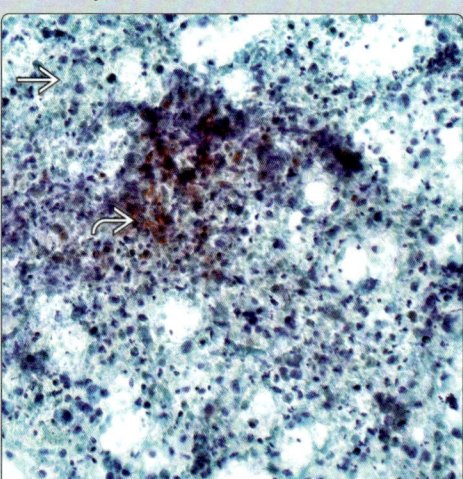

Squamoid Cells With Necrosis

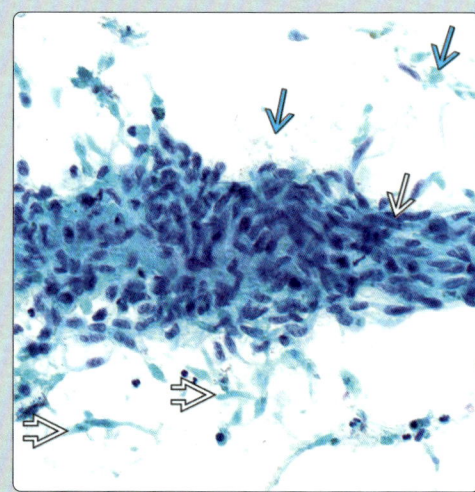

Spindle Cell Pattern of Anaplastic Thyroid Carcinoma

(Left) Pap stain shows pleomorphic malignant cells in a necrotic background ➔ that lacks colloid. Some cells appear squamoid with dense and orangeophilic cytoplasm ➔. (Right) FNA shows dense fascicles ➔ and single malignant spindle cells in a necrotic ➔ background. Individual necrotic and apoptotic spindle cell ➔ are also seen.

Anaplastic Thyroid Carcinoma

TERMINOLOGY

Definitions
- Highly malignant tumor of undifferentiated cells with ultrastructural or IHC features of epithelial differentiation
- Primary squamous cell carcinoma of thyroid now considered anaplastic thyroid carcinoma per 2022 WHO Classification of Thyroid Neoplasms
  - *BRAF* V600E mutations in 87% and outcome similar to anaplastic carcinoma

CLINICAL ISSUES

Presentation
- Most patients have long history of nodular hyperplasia, radiation exposure, or iodine deficiency
- Presents as rapidly expanding neck mass
- 75% of patients > 60 years old; F:M = 1.5:1
- Usually symptomatic and involves surrounding tissues

Prognosis
- Rapidly progressive with overall poor prognosis
- *BRAF* V600E mutation testing mandatory for management (*BRAF* and *MEK* inhibitor therapy)
- Lymph node and distant metastases common

CYTOPATHOLOGY

Cellularity and Pattern
- Highly cellular, except in cases of marked desmoplasia
- Cells arranged in clusters, sheets, or dispersed
- Follicles, papillae, and colloid absent
- May be accompanied by differentiated thyroid cancer component (e.g., papillary thyroid carcinoma)

Background
- Dirty background composed of necrotic debris, inflammatory cells, and diathesis
- Tumor cells may be difficult to identify within background debris; scant/absent colloid

Cells
- Variable appearance: May appear spindle-shaped, polygonal, pleomorphic, epithelioid, or giant cell-like
- Cells appear highly malignant and often bizarre
- Rarely myxoid change, cartilaginous or osseous metaplasia
- Primary squamous cell carcinoma of thyroid is also considered anaplastic carcinoma

Nuclear Details
- Markedly pleomorphic with irregular nuclear contours
- Chromatin abnormal, coarse, and dark
- Macronucleoli prominent
- Intranuclear cytoplasmic inclusions may be present
- Mitotic figures frequent, including abnormal forms
- Apoptotic bodies common

Cytoplasmic Details
- Cytoplasm abundant and variable in appearance
- May appear pale and vacuolated to granular (hürthleoid) or dense (squamoid)

ANCILLARY TESTS

Immunohistochemistry
- Vimentin, keratin (AE1/AE3), and PAX8 (nuclear) (+) in > 80%
- p53, p63 diffusely (+); Ki67 index > 80%: TTF-1, thyroglobulin mostly (-)
- Primary squamous cells carcinoma express PAX8 and TTF-1 in 91% and 38% of cases, respectively

Genetic Testing
- Most consistent finding: *TP53* mutation [IHC nuclear (+)]
- β-catenin (*CTNNB1*) mutations in 80%; *RAS* (50%); *BRAF* V600E mutation testing for management
- *PTEN* and *PIK3CA* mutations may also be seen

SELECTED REFERENCES

1. Xu B et al: Dissecting anaplastic thyroid carcinoma: a comprehensive clinical, histologic, immunophenotypic, and molecular study of 360 cases. Thyroid. 30(10):1505-17, 2020

Anaplastic Thyroid Carcinoma
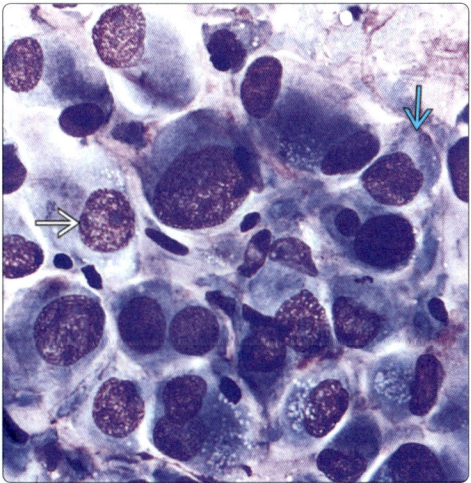

Cell Block With Highly Malignant Cells
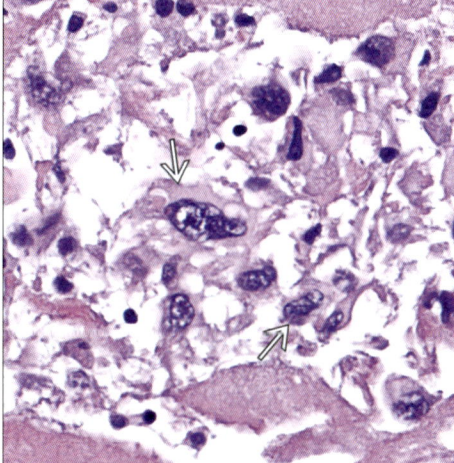

(Left) Diff-Quik-stained smear shows rhabdoid tumor cells with eccentrically placed nuclei ➡ and prominent nucleoli (single and multiple). The cytoplasm can be dense and rarely may show a hof-like structure ➡. *(Right)* H&E-stained cell block with large and small markedly pleomorphic malignant cells ➡ is shown.

Thyroid Lymphoma

KEY FACTS

CLINICAL ISSUES

- Generally associated with lymphocytic thyroiditis
  - **80x** increased risk
- < 5% of thyroid tumors; 3-7% of extranodal lymphomas
- Most are non-Hodgkin lymphomas of B-cell lineage
- 60-80% of thyroid lymphomas are EMZBCL or DLBCL
- Follicular, Hodgkin, and T-cell lymphomas are less common
- Can be associated with hypothyroidism
- Symptoms: Sudden enlargement of longstanding goiter, pain, dyspnea, dysphagia, hemoptysis, hoarseness, cough

CYTOPATHOLOGY

- Hypercellular aspirate of noncohesive lymphoid cells
- Lymphoglandular bodies are usually present; best seen on Diff-Quik
- May see lymphoepithelial lesions or germinal centers
- DLBCL: Large, round, immature lymphocytes
- EMZBCL: Mix of small, atypical lymphocytes

ANCILLARY TESTS

- CD20 and CD79a, PAX5 confirm B-cell immunophenotype
- Flow cytometry is helpful to characterize clonality
- Cytogenetic and molecular features are less useful than in other sites

TOP DIFFERENTIAL DIAGNOSES

- Lymphocytic thyroiditis
  - Crucial differential diagnosis
  - Tends to be confused with lymphoma
  - No germinal center colonization
  - No light chain restriction
- Undifferentiated thyroid carcinoma
  - Cytokeratin (+); CD45 and CD20 (-)
- Melanoma
  - S100, HMB-45, and Melan-A (+); CD45 and CD20 (-)
- Ectopic thymoma
- Sclerosing mucoepidermoid carcinoma with eosinophilia

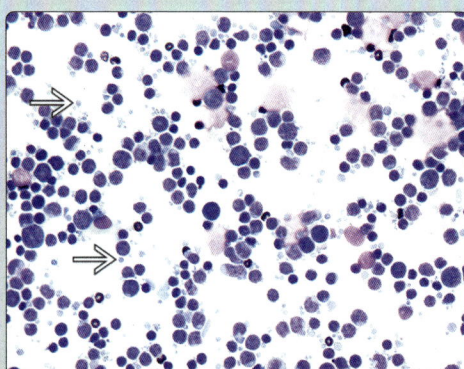

Monotonous Dyshesive Population of Cells

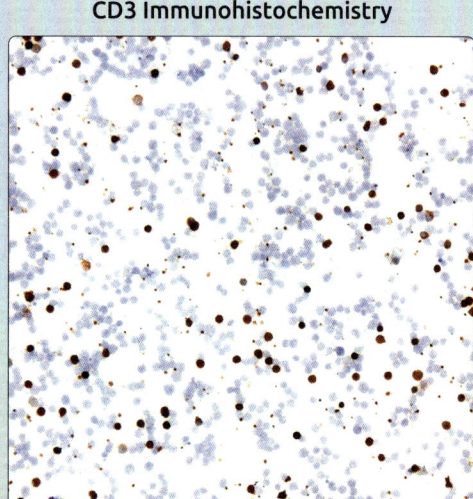

CD3 Immunohistochemistry

(Left) Diff-Quik is the ideal stain to assess hematopoietic lesions because of its similarity to the Wright stain. This smear shows a dyshesive population of round, monotonous cells with high nuclear:cytoplasmic ratios and background lymphoglandular bodies ➡. Colloid is lacking. (Right) Immunohistochemical stains can help characterize a lymphoma, particularly if flow cytometry is unavailable. This CD3 stain highlights only rare T lymphocytes in this B-cell lymphoma.

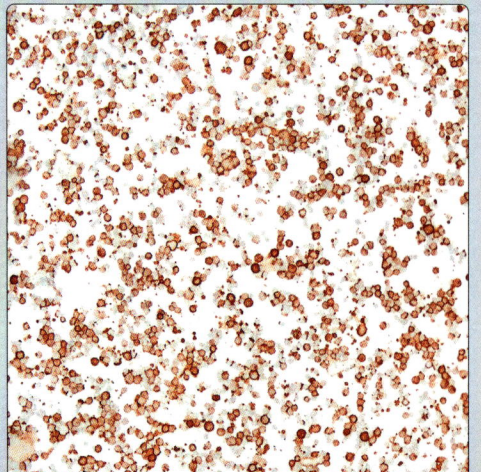

κ-Light Chain

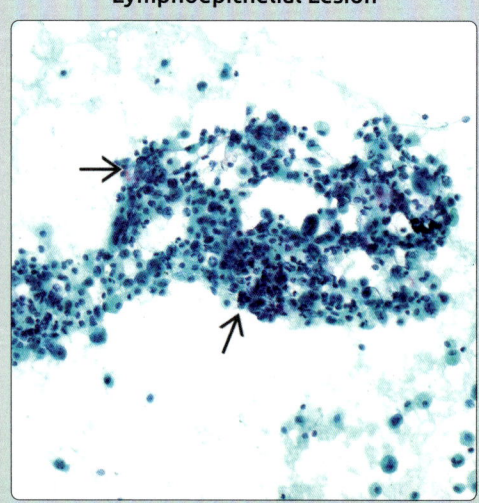

Lymphoepithelial Lesion

(Left) Clonality is confirmed by this κ stain, which demonstrates extensive κ-light chain restriction. (Right) Benign follicular cells are extensively infiltrated by lymphocytes ➡ in this Pap-stained image. This finding should raise concern for the possibility of extranodal marginal zone B-cell lymphoma.

Thyroid Lymphoma

TERMINOLOGY

Abbreviations
- Diffuse large B-cell lymphoma (DLBCL)
- Extranodal marginal zone B-cell lymphoma (EMZBCL)

Definitions
- Primary lymphoma arising in thyroid

CLINICAL ISSUES

Epidemiology
- Incidence
  - < 5% of thyroid tumors; 3-7% of extranodal lymphomas
  - Most are non-Hodgkin lymphomas of B-cell lineage
  - 95% of thyroid lymphomas are EMZBCL or DLBCL

Presentation
- Almost always associated with lymphocytic thyroiditis
- Can be associated with hypothyroidism
- Symptoms: Sudden enlargement of longstanding goiter, pain, dyspnea, dysphagia, hemoptysis, hoarseness, cough

CYTOPATHOLOGY

Cellularity
- Hypercellular aspirates composed predominantly of lymphoid cells

Pattern
- Noncohesive sheets of single cells
- Distinction from reactive process is often difficult, especially for EMZBCL
- Lymphoid cells may form prominent lymphoepithelial lesions

Background
- Lymphoglandular bodies are usually present
- Karyorrhexis may be extensive

Cells
- Morphology best appreciated with Diff-Quik stain
- **DLBCL**: Usually large, round, immature lymphocytes resembling centroblasts, immunoblasts, monocytoid B cells, and plasmacytoid cells
- **EMZBCL**: Mix of small atypical lymphocytes, centrocytes, monocytoid B cells, immunoblasts, and plasma cells

Nuclear Details
- Chromatin is relatively fine
- Nuclear membranes can be cleaved or noncleaved
- Nucleoli are usually prominent and marginated
- Cytoplasm can be scant or moderate

ANCILLARY TESTS

Immunohistochemistry
- B-cell immunophenotype can be confirmed with positivity for CD20 &/or CD79a
- BCL2 reactivity in neoplastic cells is present (not seen in reactive germinal centers)
- Immunoglobulin light chain restriction is often seen
- Cytokeratin highlights epithelial component in lymphoepithelial lesions
- DLBCL is subclassified as germinal center B-cell-like (GCB) or non-GCB using CD10, BCL6, and MUM1

Flow Cytometry
- Very helpful in characterizing lymphoid cells
- Needle rinse material from lesions with monotypic lymphocytes should be collected in RPMI medium

Genetic Testing
- Cytogenetic and molecular genetic features are not as useful as in other sites
- EMZBCL can be associated with loss of BCL2 expression and increased p53 inactivation
- May see *FAS* gene mutations and clonal rearrangement of heavy chain variable region

SELECTED REFERENCES

1. Huang CG et al: The diagnosis of primary thyroid lymphoma by fine-needle aspiration, cell block, and immunohistochemistry technique. Diagn Cytopathol. 48(11):1041-7, 2020

Large Atypical Lymphocytes

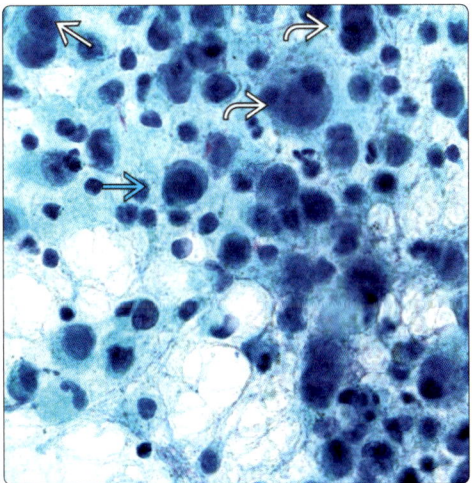

Cell Block for Lymphoma Work-Up

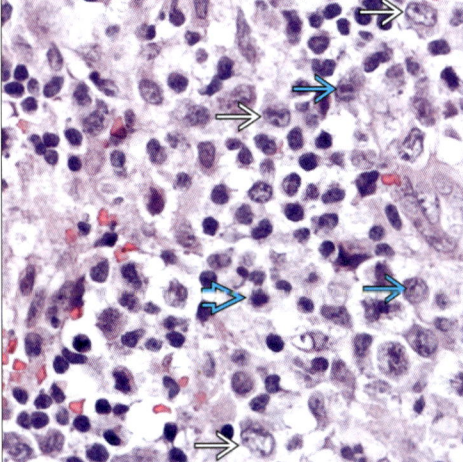

(Left) Dispersed large atypical cells on Pap-stained smear ➡, many with vesicular chromatin and nucleoli ➡, are shown. Further work-up on cell block was confirmatory for diffuse large B-cell lymphoma. These large cells ➡ often rupture on flow cytometry, resulting in a nondiagnostic flow due to low cellularity. *(Right)* Cell block shows large atypical lymphocytes ➡ with prominent nucleoli ➡ and mitotic activity ➡. Cell blocks can be effectively utilized for lymphoma work-up.

Metastatic Carcinoma to Thyroid

KEY FACTS

CLINICAL ISSUES
- Thyroid is vascular and predisposed to metastases
- Incidence depends on incidence of underlying tumor
- Carcinomas are most common metastases (~ 80%)
- Renal cell carcinoma is most common carcinoma; melanoma and leiomyosarcoma are most common noncarcinomas

CYTOPATHOLOGY
- Cytomorphology resembles primary tumor
- Smears are cellular with 2 distinct cell populations if background thyroid is sampled
- Thyroglobulin may diffuse into adjacent tissue or become "entrapped" within metastatic deposits

ANCILLARY TESTS
- Metastatic tumors share immunohistochemical profile with primary tumor, distinctly different from thyroid
  - Exceptions include lung adenocarcinoma and small cell carcinoma (TTF-1)
- Genetic testing: Helpful but with overlapping results
  - *BRAF*: Papillary thyroid carcinoma, melanoma, and colorectal, ovarian, and lung carcinomas
  - *KRAS*: Codon 12/13 mutations are more likely in lung, colon, and other sites than thyroid

TOP DIFFERENTIAL DIAGNOSES
- Thyroid follicular neoplasm (follicular neoplasm with clear cell features, Hürthle cell neoplasm)
  - Colloid usually present; lacks prominent vascularity and hemorrhage
  - TTF-1, thyroglobulin, PAX8 (+)
- Medullary thyroid carcinoma
  - Calcitonin, CEA, TTF-1, synaptophysin, chromogranin (+)
- Anaplastic (giant cell and spindle) carcinoma
  - TTF-1, thyroglobulin (-); PAX8(+)
- Direct extension of squamous cell carcinoma

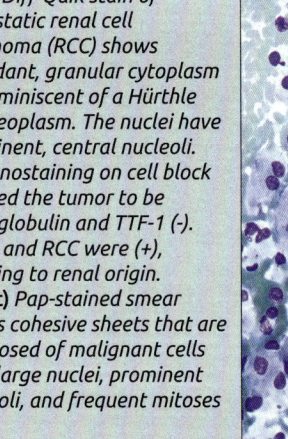

(Left) *Diff-Quik stain of metastatic renal cell carcinoma (RCC) shows abundant, granular cytoplasm ➡ reminiscent of a Hürthle cell neoplasm. The nuclei have prominent, central nucleoli. Immunostaining on cell block showed the tumor to be thyroglobulin and TTF-1 (-). PAX8 and RCC were (+), pointing to renal origin.* (Right) *Pap-stained smear shows cohesive sheets that are composed of malignant cells with large nuclei, prominent nucleoli, and frequent mitoses ➡.*

Oncocytic Cells of Metastatic Renal Cell Carcinoma

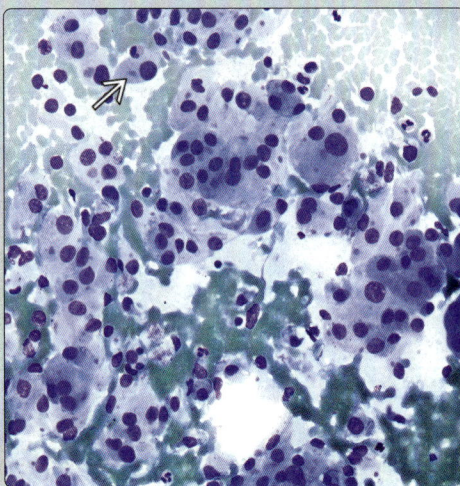

Metastatic Breast Carcinoma

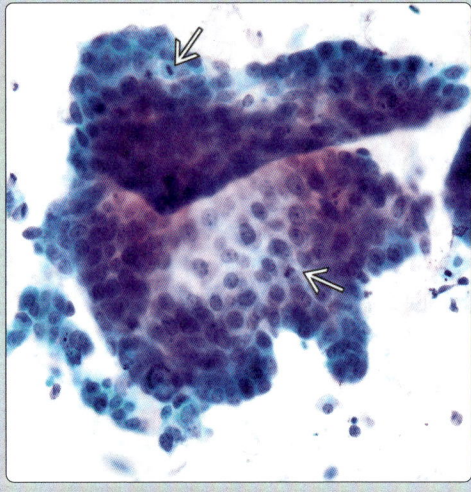

(Left) *Diff-Quik-stained smear shows glands and acini lined by columnar cells ➡ with a necrotic background ➡.* (Right) *Metastatic colon carcinoma can be confirmed by nuclear positivity for CDX2 on cell block material.*

Metastatic Colon Cancer

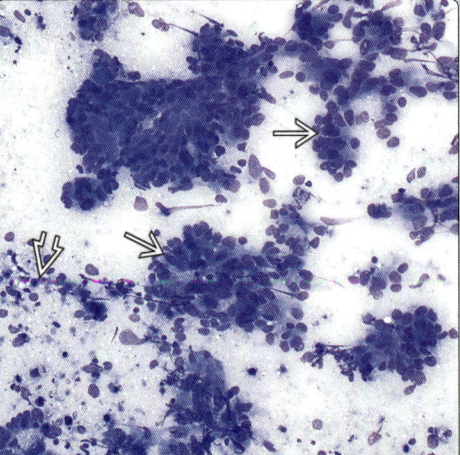

CDX2(+) Nuclei in Cell Block

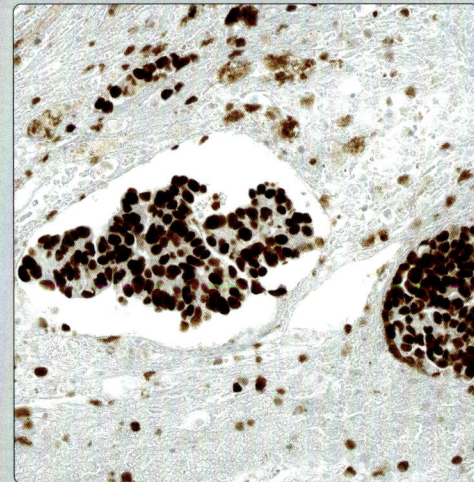

Metastatic Carcinoma to Thyroid

TERMINOLOGY

Definitions
- Tumor secondarily involving thyroid as result of primary malignancy spreading from another site

CLINICAL ISSUES

Epidemiology
- Incidence
  - Depends on incidence of underlying tumor
  - Detection increasing due to improved radiology and increased use of FNA
  - All ages can be affected; F:M = 1.2:1.0

Presentation
- Most patients present with known history of cancer
- Hyperthyroidism may result from thyroid parenchymal destruction and release of hormones

Natural History
- Clinical history is important in diagnosing metastases
- Renal cell carcinoma (RCC) is most common primary
- Other common sites are melanomas, lymphomas, colorectal, lung, and breast

Prognosis
- Usually poor clinical outcome, depending on primary
- If metastatic disease is limited to thyroid, prolonged survival is possible with surgical removal

CYTOPATHOLOGY

Pattern
- Cytologic appearance depends on primary tumor
- Smears are cellular with 2 distinct cell populations if background thyroid is sampled
- Background necrosis and mitoses are frequently seen

Cells
- RCC
  - Abundant, clear, vacuolated cytoplasm
  - Large, oval nuclei with large nucleoli
  - Bloody background with stripped nuclei, no colloid
- Adenocarcinoma
  - Gland formation with well-defined cell borders
  - Coarse nuclear chromatin and prominent nucleoli
- Squamous cell carcinoma
  - Coarse to pyknotic chromatin, irregular nuclear contours, and prominent nucleoli
  - Vacuolated to dense and orangeophilic cytoplasm
- Melanoma
  - Cellular aspirate of dyscohesive cells
  - Prominent nucleoli, intranuclear inclusions, multinucleation, and cytoplasmic melanin pigment

MICROSCOPIC

Histologic Features
- Distinctly different histology from thyroid
- Generally resembles primary tumor
- Carcinomas are most common metastases (~ 80%)
- Melanomas and leiomyosarcomas are most common noncarcinomas
- Differential include anaplastic and medullary carcinomas

ANCILLARY TESTS

Immunohistochemistry
- Metastatic tumors share immunohistochemical profile of primary site, distinctly different from thyroid

Genetic Testing
- Helpful but with overlapping results
- *BRAF*: Papillary thyroid carcinoma, melanoma, and colorectal, ovarian, and lung carcinomas
- *KRAS*: Codon 12/13 mutations are more likely in lung, colon, and other sites than thyroid

SELECTED REFERENCES

1. Ghossein CA et al: Metastasis to the thyroid gland: a single-institution 16-year experience. Histopathology. 78(4):508-19, 2021
2. Pastorello RG et al: Metastases to the thyroid: potential cytologic mimics of primary thyroid neoplasms. Arch Pathol Lab Med. 143(3):394-9, 2019

Metastatic Melanoma

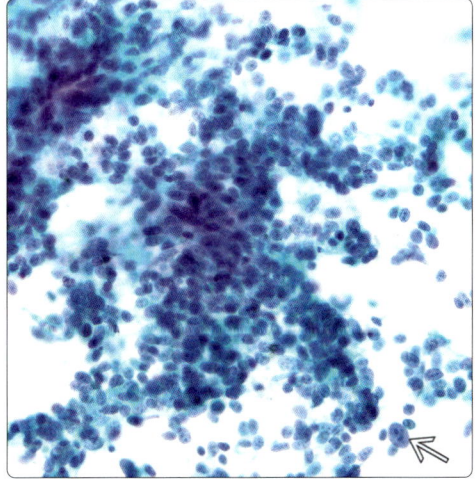

Keratinizing Squamous Cell Carcinoma

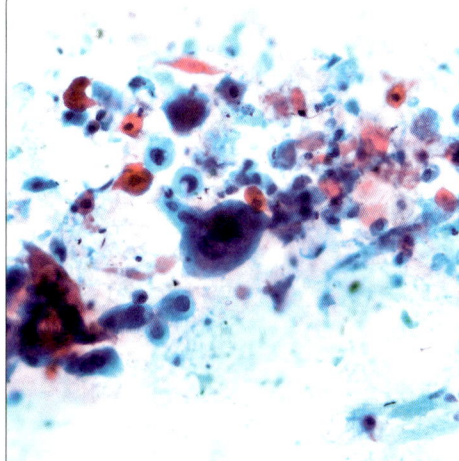

(Left) On Pap stain, this metastatic melanoma is cellular and composed of dispersed cells in a background devoid of colloid. Even at low magnification, prominent nucleoli can be seen ➡. *(Right)* Pap-stained slide highlights the orangeophilic cells, angulated nuclei, and keratin debris of metastatic keratinizing squamous cell carcinoma.

Other Nonneoplastic and Neoplastic Thyroid Lesions Encountered on Thyroid FNA

RARE PRIMARY MALIGNANT THYROID NEOPLASMS

Cribriform-Morular Carcinoma

- General features
  - Rare; young age (< 35 years), and female sex
  - Associated with familial adenomatous polyposis (FAP) in 40% of cases, 60% are sporadic
    - Autosomal dominant syndrome
    - Germline mutations of *APC* gene (5q21) and somatic *RET* (PTC) gene rearrangement
    - Genetic testing/counseling of patient and family members is recommended
    - In 25-30% of cases, this might be 1st presentation of FAP syndrome
  - Usually good prognosis but may be multifocal and more aggressive when associated with FAP
- Cytology
  - Cellular aspirates with complex tissue fragments
  - Absent colloid, typical nuclear features of PTC are rare or absent
  - Squamoid morulae, whorls of spindle cells, and fenestrated sheets of uniform hyperchromatic cells
  - Biotin accumulation in nuclei causes peculiar nuclear clearing resulting in ground-glass nuclei
    - Psammamoma bodies, colloid, multinucleated giant cells absent
  - Mostly round to oval tumor cells; rarely, papillary arrangement of tall columnar cells may be seen
  - Exact diagnosis on cytology is challenging
- Ancillary testing
  - β-catenin nuclear and cytoplasmic positivity is important for definitive diagnosis
  - PAX8 and thyroglobulin usually (-)
    - TTF-1(+) in cribriform elements only
    - CD5, CDX2, CK5 (+) in morules only
  - *CTNNB1* (encoding β-catenin) and *APC* mutations most common in FAP cases
  - *PIK3CA* mutation is seen in sporadic cases

Carcinoma Showing Thymus-Like Differentiation

- Resembles thymic lymphoepithelioma-like carcinoma
- Synonym: Intrathyroidal epithelial thymoma
- Average age: 50 years; more common in women
- Possibly arising from multipotential stem cell, thymic remnants, or solid cell nests
- Cytology: Large cell clusters without papillary or follicular architecture, round or spindle cells with prominent nucleoli, occasional keratinizing cells, lymphocytic background
- TTF-1, thyroglobulin (-); CD5, p63, high molecular weight cytokeratin (HMWCK), BCL2 (+), neuroendocrine markers focally (+); CEA(+/-); *TERT* promoter mutation has been reported
- Prognosis: Variable but usually good; may relapse
- Differential diagnosis: Squamous cell carcinoma (SCC), primary thymic carcinoma

Spindle Epithelial Tumor With Thymus-Like Differentiation (SETTLE)

- Usually young adults; average age: 15 years
- Probably arising from thymic remnants or branchial pouch
- Cytology: Highly cellular, uniform bland spindle cells, fine chromatin, naked oval nuclei
- HMWCK(+); TTF-1, thyroglobulin, calcitonin, CD5, neuroendocrine markers, desmin (-)
- Differential diagnosis: Invasive thymoma, medullary thyroid carcinoma (MTC), synovial sarcoma

Sclerosing Mucoepidermoid Carcinoma With Eosinophilia

- Age range: 40-70 years; female predilection
- WHO: Uncertain histogenesis tumor
- Usually low grade (high-grade cases may occur)
- Associated with lymphocytic/Hashimoto thyroiditis
- Squamous cells/pearls, epithelial nests, lymphoid population, eosinophils, and various amount of mucin
- May have PAS(+) hyalin bodies
- p63(+); TTF-1 usually (-), thyroglobulin usually (-), and calcitonin (-)

Cribriform-Morular Thyroid Carcinoma

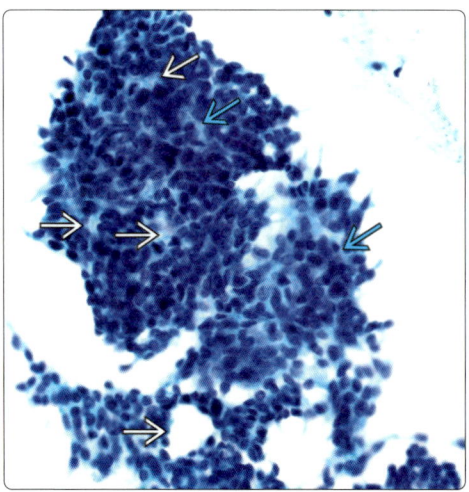

Morule and Cribriform Areas

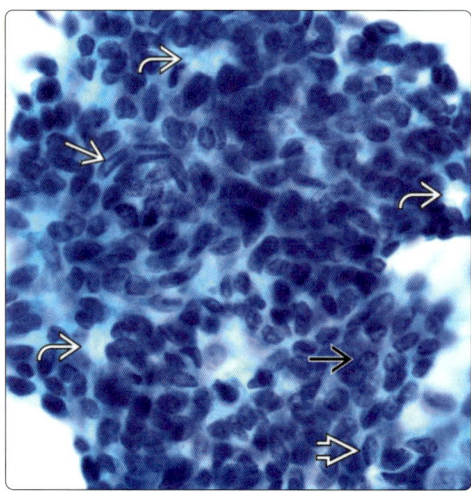

(Left) Pap-stained smear shows large, cohesive, complicated fragments in the absence of background colloid. Regular round ➔, punched-out, and slit-like spaces ➔ are seen. The nuclei are hyperchromatic. (Right) Pap-stained smear shows spindled cells in a circular pattern forming a morule ➔ along with punched-out circular and slit-like spaces corresponding to the cribriform component ➔. The nuclei are hyperchromatic with grooves ➔ and chromatin clearing ➔.

Other Nonneoplastic and Neoplastic Thyroid Lesions Encountered on Thyroid FNA

- Differential diagnosis: Primary or metastatic SCC, thymic carcinoma, papillary thyroid carcinoma (PTC)

Neuroendocrine/Small Cell Carcinoma
- Poorly differentiated carcinoma
- Morphologically similar to lung small cell carcinoma
- Neuroendocrine markers, thyroglobulin, TTF-1 (+); CEA, calcitonin (-)
- Differential diagnosis: MTC, insular carcinoma, metastatic small cell carcinoma

RARE PRIMARY THYROID LESIONS/NEOPLASMS

Hyalinizing Trabecular Tumor (HTT)
- Predilection for women; average age: 40 years
- Some features resemble PTC
  - PTC can have HTT-like areas
  - Prognosis: Low-risk neoplasm
- Cytologic findings
  - Spindle cells arranged in parallel/trabecular arrays
  - Pointed nuclei, intranuclear inclusions and grooves
  - Cytoplasms with ill-defined borders
  - Cytoplasmic "hyalin bodies" have been described: Yellow in H&E, blue-green in Pap, pink in Diff-Quik
  - Metachromatic fibrillar hyalin stroma with feathery edges between trabeculae is important diagnostic feature [PAS-D(+)]
- Histology: Encapsulated tumor with hyalinized stroma and eosinophilic spindle cells in trabecular pattern
- Thyroglobulin, TTF-1, PAX8, MIB-1 (membranous) (+); calcitonin (-)
- *GLIS* gene rearrangement; *PAX8::GLIS3* (more common) and *PAX8::GLIS1*
- Differential diagnosis: PTC, MTC, paraganglioma, granuloma

Amyloidosis
- Primary amyloid goiter: Rare
- Secondary amyloidosis: In systemic amyloidosis
- Irregular acellular deposits
  - Blue-green in Pap, metachromatic in Diff-Quik
  - Congo red stain: Characteristic salmon pink color with apple green birefringence under polarized light
- May have rare stromal cells embedded in deposits
- Differential diagnosis: Hard colloid, skeletal muscle

Dyshormonogenetic Goiter
- Genetic defect in thyroid hormone metabolism
  - Lack of responsiveness to TSH
- Usually hypothyroid
- No sex predilection; 75% present < 20 years of age
- Gross: Diffusely enlarged multinodular, dull brown (not glistening) thyroid
- Hypercellular, predominantly solid nodules
- Microfollicular architecture with marked atypia
- Minimal or absent colloid, fibrosis common

Riedel Thyroiditis
- Fibrosis with infiltrative borders, grossly suggests carcinoma
- Usually fibrosing disease of other organs present
- Cytology: Usually acellular or rare spindle cells

Therapy/Radiation Effects
- Radiation effect
  - Randomly scattered bizarre cells with coarse chromatin or smudged nuclei and vacuolated cytoplasm
- Antithyroid or antipsychotic medications
  - Hyperchromasia, pleomorphism, scant colloid, bizarre Hürthle cells, cytoplasmic black pigment (lipofuscin)

RARE EXTRATHYROIDAL LESIONS PRESENTING AS THYROID NODULES

Parathyroid Adenoma
- Delicate clear to eosinophilic cytoplasm, uniform nuclei with fine chromatin, numerous naked nuclei, absent colloid
- PTH(+); thyroglobulin, TTF-1 (-)

Epidermal Inclusion Cyst (EIC)
- EIC anterior to thyroid may present as thyroid nodule
- Rare primary thyroid EIC reported
- Abundant anucleated or superficial squamous cells
- Follicular cells, colloid, and cytologic atypia absent

Zenker (Esophageal) Diverticulum
- May mimic thyroid nodule on ultrasonography
- Squamous cells, numerous cocci and bacilli, undigested food matter and debris
- Usually requires barium swallow study for diagnosis

Thyroglossal Duct Cyst
- Due to incomplete closure of thyroglossal duct
- Rarely presents as solitary thyroid nodule
- Sinus tract or cyst lined by pseudostratified ciliated or squamous epithelium
- Mucous glands and thyroid follicles in stroma
- Cytologic findings
  - Ciliated columnar epithelium &/or squamous cells
  - Mucoid/myxoid material and macrophages ± inflammatory debris
- Diagnostic pitfall: Squamous metaplasia with reactive atypia may mimic SCC
- Differential diagnosis: Bronchogenic cyst, branchial cleft cyst, cystic PTC, SCC
- Any thyroid neoplasm can arise in thyroglossal duct cyst
  - Papillary carcinoma is most common carcinoma arising in wall

Paraganglioma
- Oval or spindle cells with ill-defined cytoplasm
- May have intranuclear inclusions: Mimics PTC
- Neuroendocrine markers (+); thyroglobulin (-): Mimics MTC

Other Neoplasms
- Desmoid tumor, mesenchymal tumor, thyroid teratomas, lymphomas may present as thyroid nodule

SELECTED REFERENCES
1. Boyraz B et al: Cribriform-morular thyroid carcinoma Is a distinct thyroid malignancy of uncertain cytogenesis. Endocr Pathol. 32(3):327-35, 2021

Other Nonneoplastic and Neoplastic Thyroid Lesions Encountered on Thyroid FNA

Cribriform-Morular Thyroid Carcinoma Nuclei

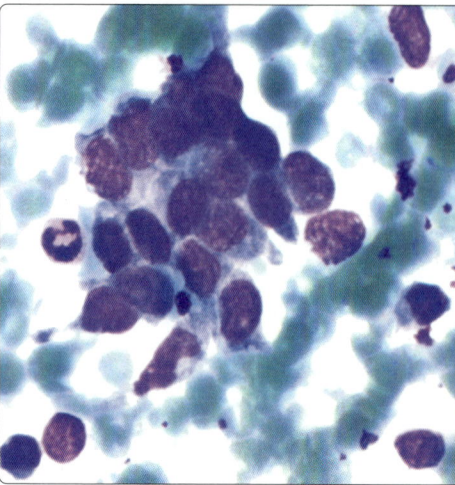

Cribriform-Morular Carcinoma, Nuclear Details

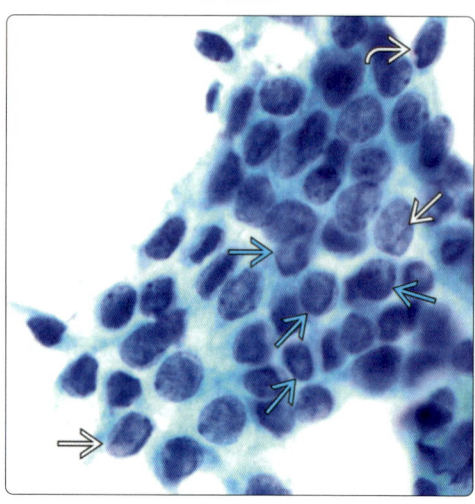

(Left) Diff-Quik-stained smear shows a cluster of malignant cells with irregular nuclear contours but lacking the fully developed features of papillary thyroid carcinoma. (Right) Pap-stained thyroid FNA shows abnormal cells with nuclear irregularities ⇨, hyperchromasia, dispersed chromatin, and occasional grooves ⇨ but lacking well-developed intranuclear cytoplasmic inclusions. Note the rim-like chromatinic condensation with open chromatin ⇨.

SETTLE

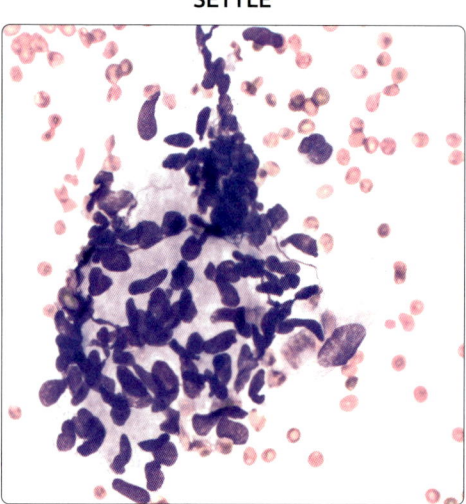

SETTLE With Uniform Spindle Cells

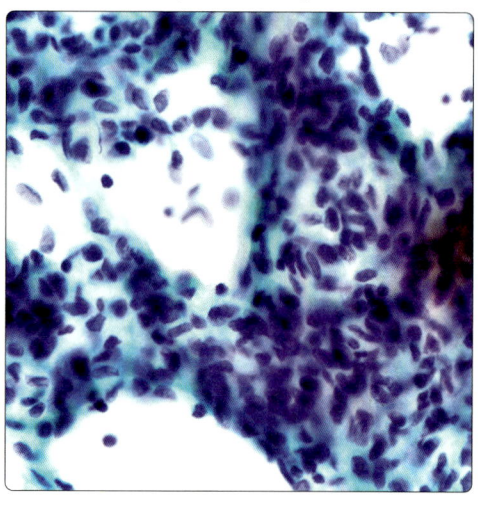

(Left) Diff-Quik-stained smear of spindle epithelial tumor with thymus-like differentiation (SETTLE) shows spindle cells in a bloody background. Note the lack of colloid and necrosis or mitosis. Granuloma and medullary thyroid carcinoma (MTC) enter into the differential. (Right) Pap stain of SETTLE shows uniform spindle cells with bland nuclei, suggesting MTC, synovial sarcoma, or paraganglioma. The tumor was HMWCK(+) and calcitonin, thyroglobulin, CEA, and neuroendocrine markers (-).

Mucoepidermoid Carcinoma, Low Power

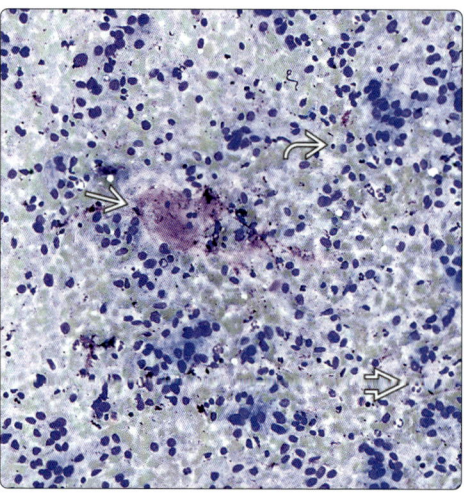

Squamous Pearls in Mucoepidermoid Carcinoma

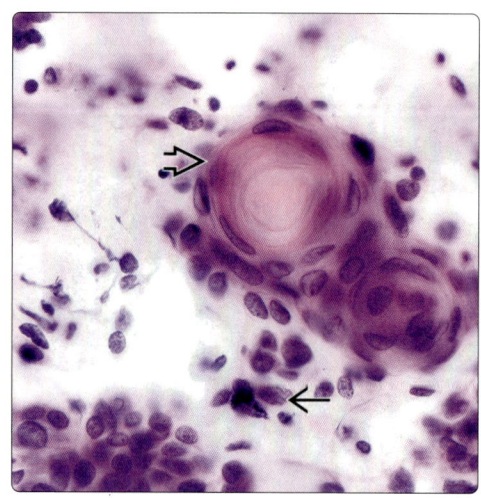

(Left) Low magnification of a Diff-Quik-stained smear with mucin ⇨ shows magenta-stained material. The cells are in loose groups with scattered lymphocytes ⇨ and other inflammatory cells ⇨ in the background. (Right) H&E stain of mucoepidermoid carcinoma (MEC) illustrates squamous cells forming pearls ⇨ and cells with nuclear grooves ⇨. Squamous cells are TTF-1 and thyroglobulin (-).

Other Nonneoplastic and Neoplastic Thyroid Lesions Encountered on Thyroid FNA

Hyalinizing Trabecular Tumor

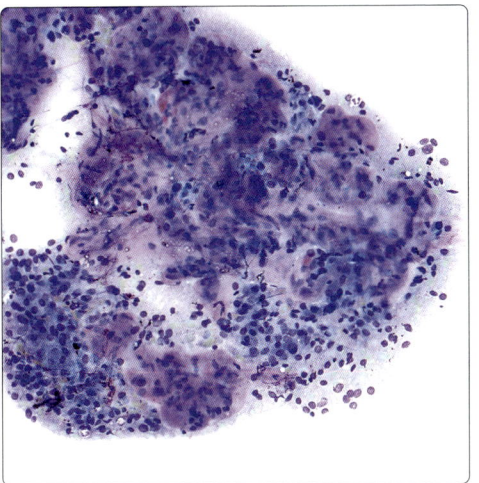

Hyalinizing Trabecular Tumor, Stroma

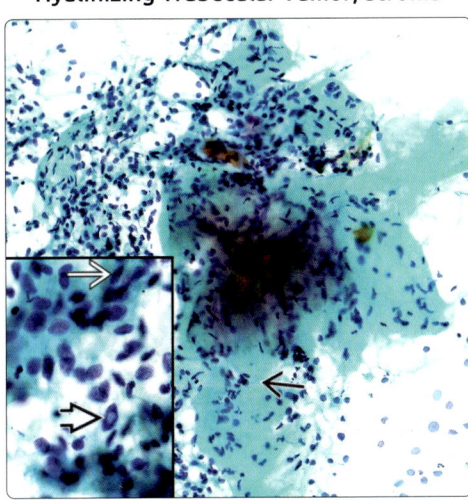

(Left) Diff-Quik stain of hyalinizing trabecular tumor (HTT) illustrates eosinophilic cells arranged in trabeculae. There is fibrillary metachromatic stroma with feathery edges between the cells. (Right) Pap stain shows oval to spindle cells arranged in a parallel array and embedded in abundant basement membrane-like stroma ⇒. High-power inset illustrates spindle cells with ill-defined borders, nuclear grooves, nuclei with pointed ends ⇒, and an intranuclear pseudoinclusion ⇒.

Histology of Hyalinizing Trabecular Tumor

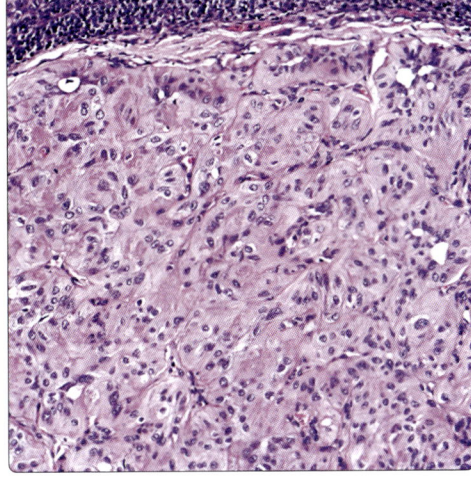

Riedel Thyroiditis

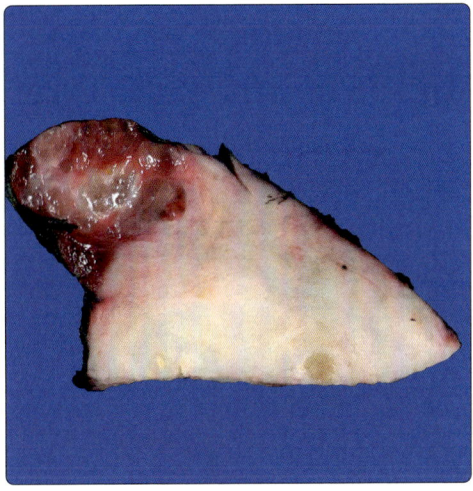

(Left) H&E section of the subsequent lobectomy shows HTT with characteristic trabecular pattern and extracellular basement membrane-like stroma. (Right) Gross photograph of Riedel thyroiditis illustrates a fibrotic, tan-white, firm nodule with an infiltrative border resembling carcinoma. Aspirates of these lesions are usually paucicellular to acellular with rare fibroplastic spindle cells.

Amyloid

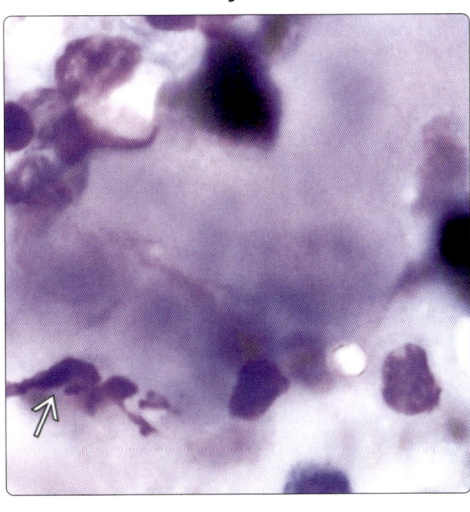

Amyloid Amorphous Deposit on Cell Block

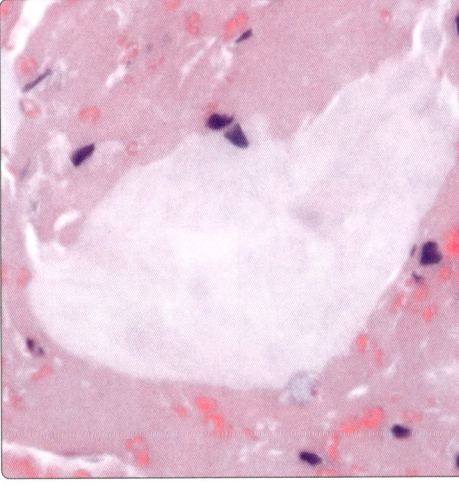

(Left) Diff-Quik stain of an amyloid goiter shows amyloid deposits and rare follicular cells. It is very difficult to distinguish amyloid from colloid on cytologic preparation. Entrapment of fibroblasts ⇒ favors amyloid. (Right) H&E stain of cell block of amyloid goiter illustrates amorphous pink material. Special stain for Congo red showed characteristic apple green birefringence consistent with amyloid.

Other Nonneoplastic and Neoplastic Thyroid Lesions Encountered on Thyroid FNA

Benign Bizarre Cells

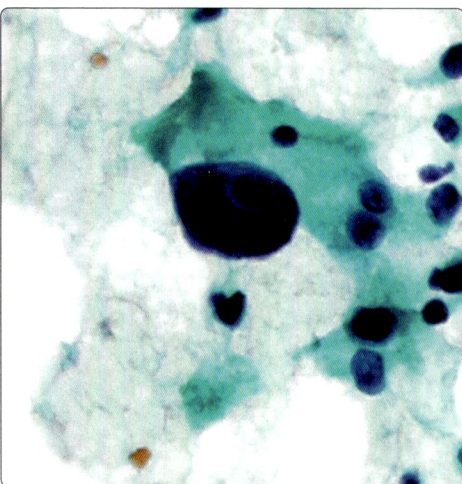

Benign Bizarre Cell With Pigment

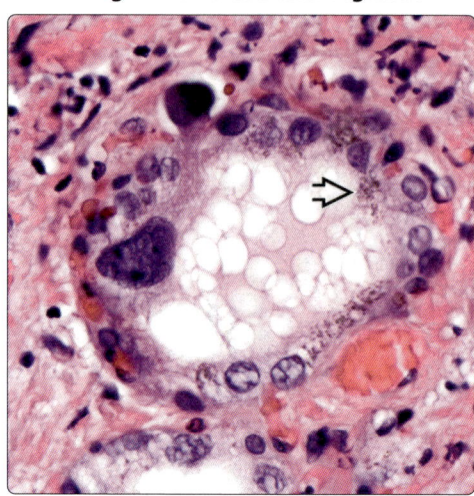

(Left) Pap stain illustrates therapy effect. There is a bizarre cell with a large nucleus, smudged chromatin, and abundant cytoplasm. This can be secondary to radiation, antithyroid therapy, or antipsychotic drugs. In the absence of previous treatment history, a possibility of dyshormonogenetic goiter should be considered. (Right) H&E section of Graves disease, status post antithyroid therapy, shows atypical follicular cells and intracytoplasmic brown pigment deposits ➡.

Parathyroid Adenoma in Thyroid

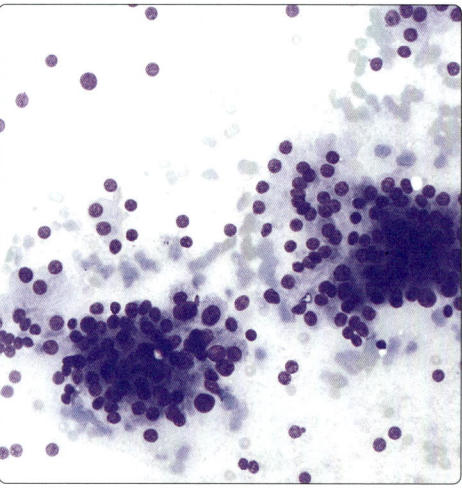

Parathyroid Adenoma

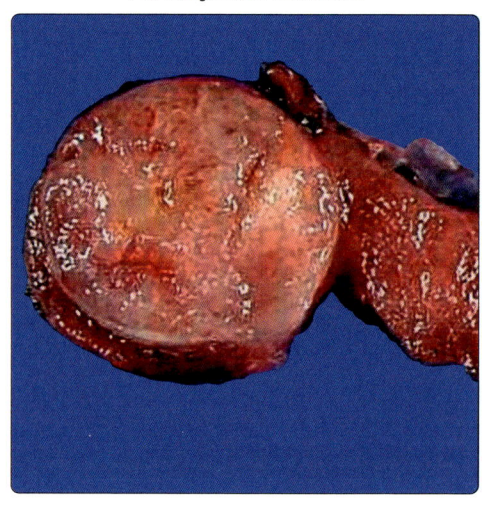

(Left) Diff-Quik stain of parathyroid adenoma presenting as thyroid nodule shows abundant uniform cells with fragile, delicate cytoplasm and round nuclei. Distinguishing parathyroid adenoma from follicular neoplasm can be difficult without clinical or laboratory findings. Numerous naked nuclei and absence of colloid are diagnostic clues and warrant additional immunostain on smears or cell block. (Right) Gross photograph shows parathyroid adenoma presenting as solitary thyroid nodule.

Anucleated Squamous Cells of Epidermal Inclusion Cyst

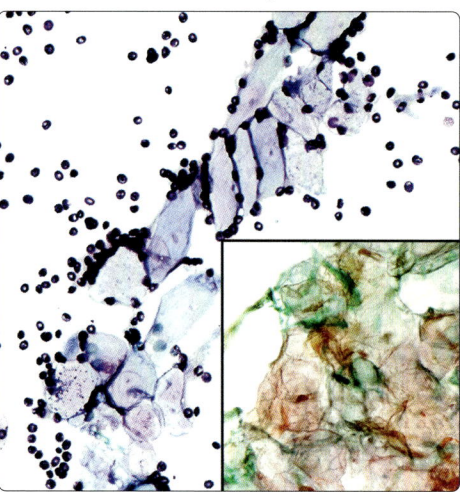

Low-Grade Chondrosarcoma

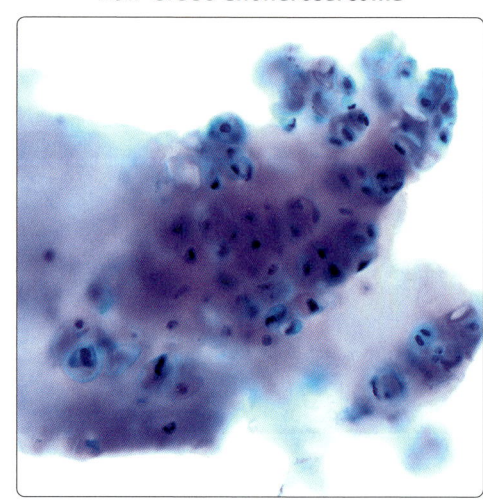

(Left) Diff-Quik and Pap (inset) stains of an epidermal inclusion cyst presenting as a palpable thyroid nodule show anucleated squamous cells and rare superficial squamous cells with no significant atypia. Subsequent ultrasonography showed that the lesion was immediately anterior to the thyroid gland. (Right) Pap stain of a hyalin cartilage tumor (low-grade chondrosarcoma) of thyroid cartilage presenting as a thyroid lesion shows mildly atypical chondrocytes embedded in chondroid stroma.

Other Nonneoplastic and Neoplastic Thyroid Lesions Encountered on Thyroid FNA

Debris in Zenker Diverticulum

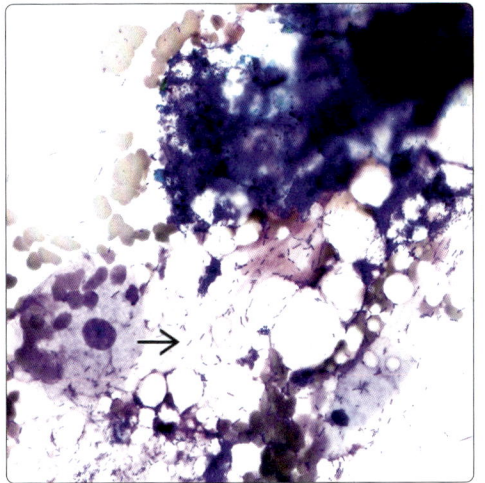

Skeletal Muscle in Zenker Diverticulum

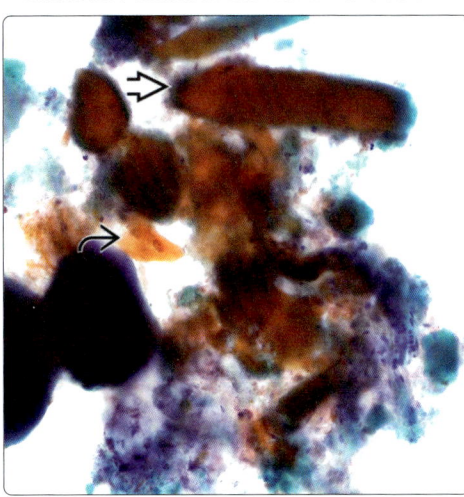

(Left) Diff-Quik stain shows squamous cells, bacilli ⇨, and debris consistent with Zenker (esophageal) diverticulum. The case was initially diagnosed as a thyroid nodule on ultrasonography. (Right) Pap stain shows bland squamous cells ⇨, undigested food matter ⇨, bacteria, and debris. Subsequent barium swallow confirmed the diagnosis of esophageal diverticulum.

Paraganglioma

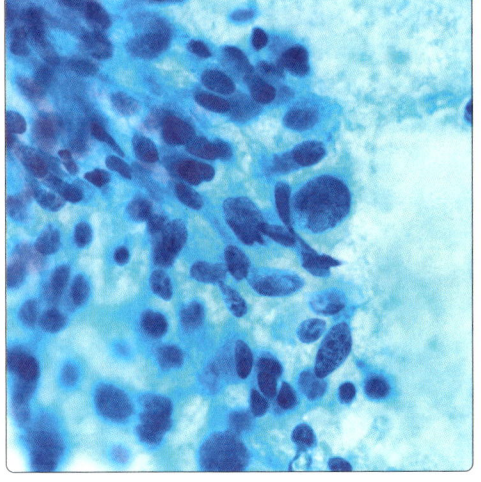

Cyst Contents and Wall

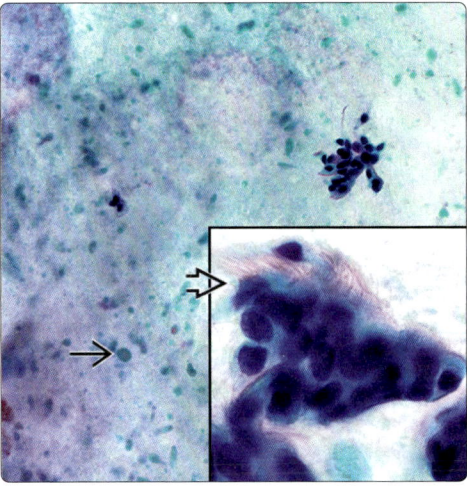

(Left) Pap stain of paraganglioma presenting as a thyroid nodule shows spindle cells with coarse chromatin resembling MTC. The tumor was neuroendocrine markers (+) and calcitonin and CEA (-). (Right) Pap stain of a cyst in the thyroid shows macrophages ⇨ and clusters of ciliated epithelium ⇨ in a background of mucoid/myxoid material. Differential diagnosis includes thyroglossal duct cyst, bronchogenic cyst, and branchial cleft cyst.

Thyroglossal Duct Cyst With Atypia

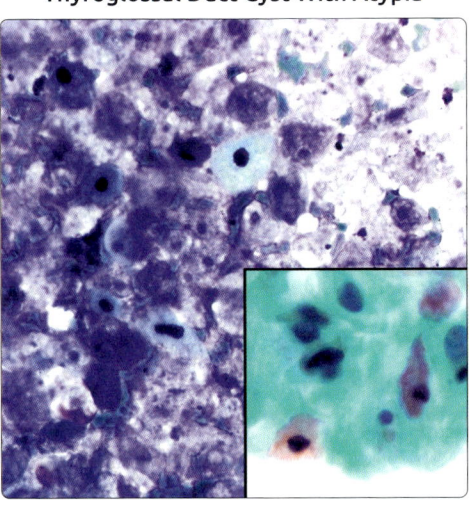

Squamous Metaplasia With Reactive Atypia

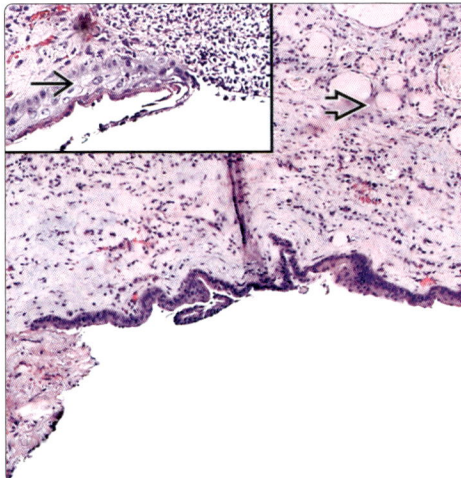

(Left) Diff-Quik and Pap (inset) stains of an inflamed thyroglossal duct cyst show atypical squamous metaplasia and necrotic debris mimicking squamous cell carcinoma. (Right) H&E of a subsequent resection shows a thyroglossal duct cyst containing thyroid tissue in the stroma ⇨ and lined by ciliated epithelium. There is squamous metaplasia with reactive atypia ⇨ associated with marked inflammation.

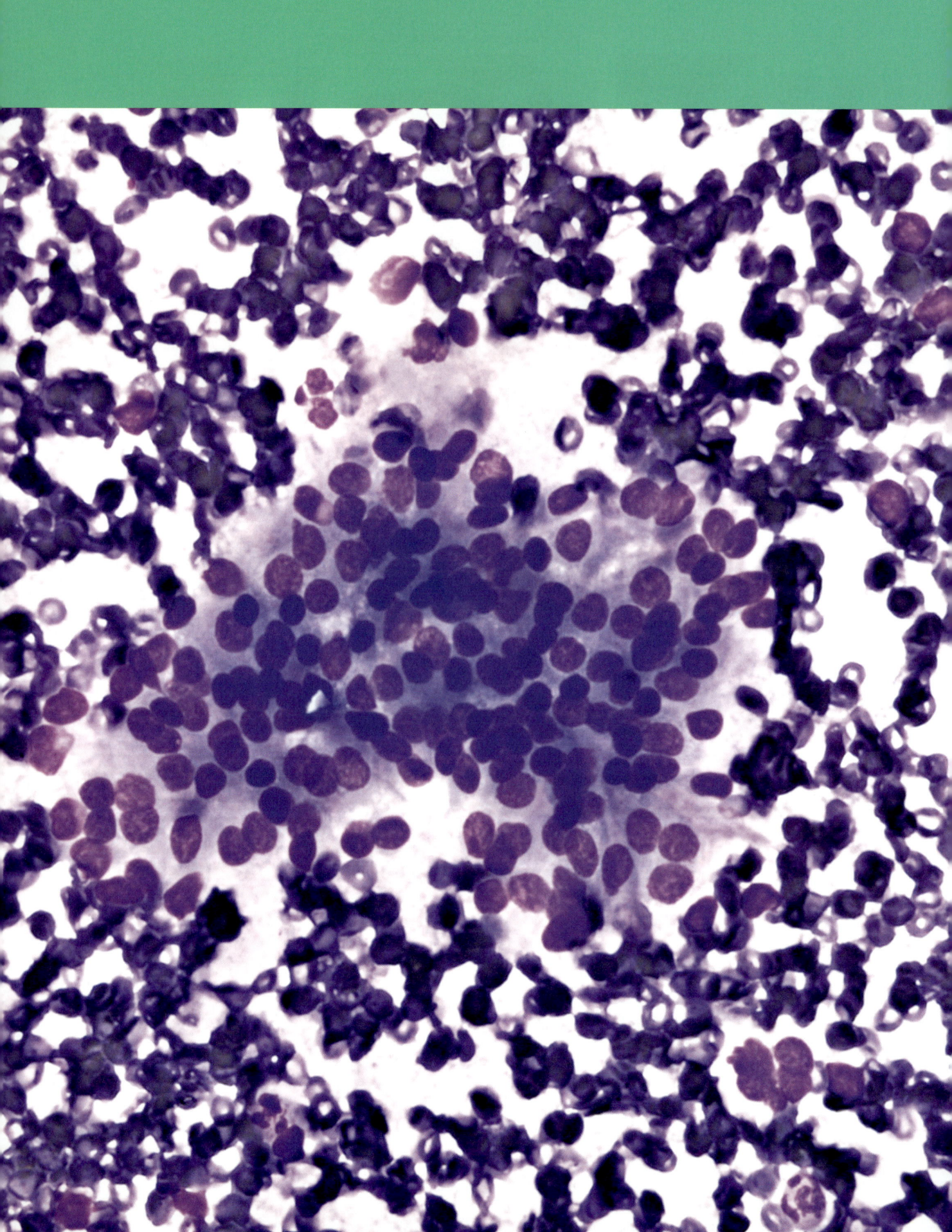

PART III
SECTION 3
Parathyroid Gland

Parathyroid Cyst, Adenoma, and Carcinoma 318

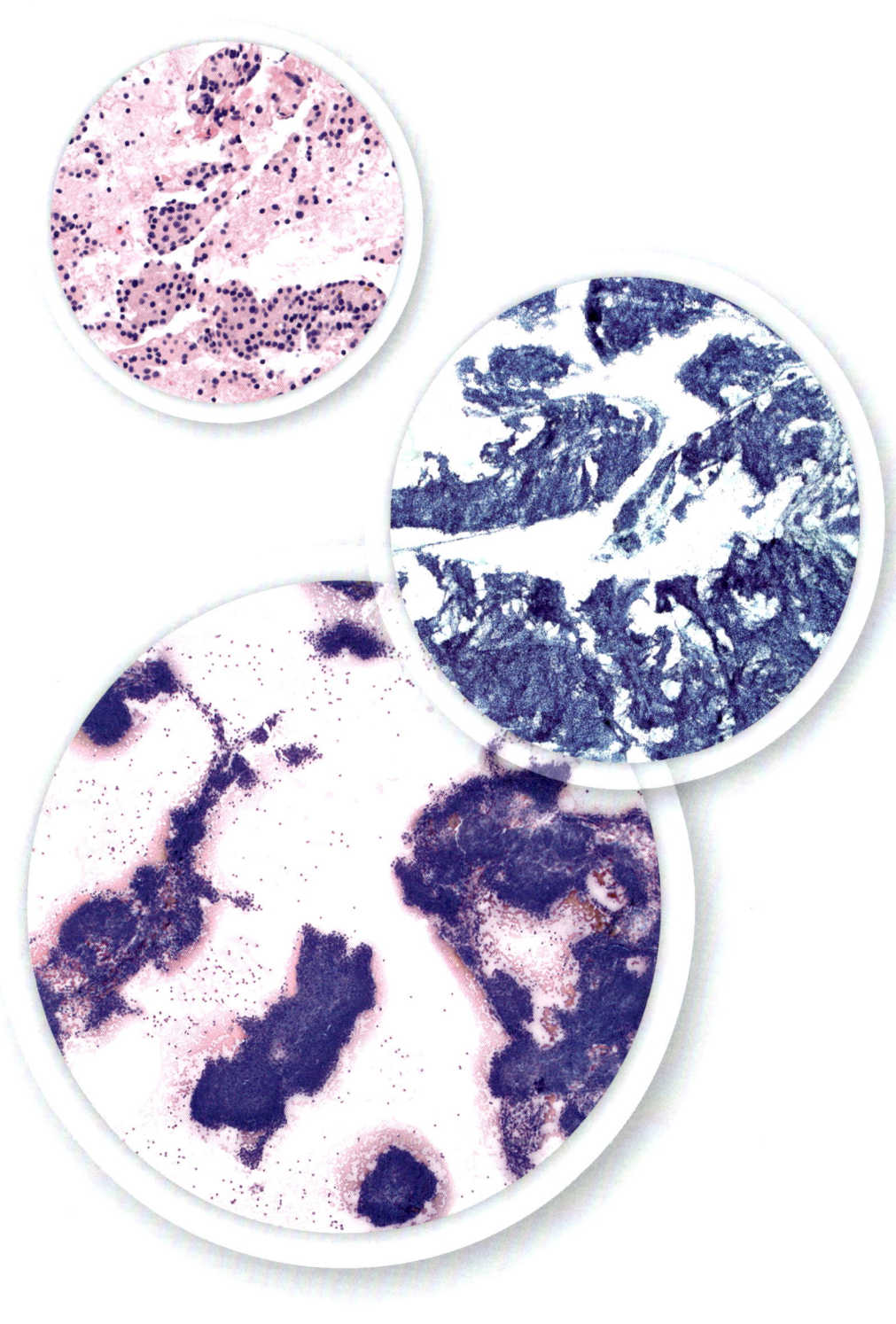

Parathyroid Cyst, Adenoma, and Carcinoma

KEY FACTS

CLINICAL ISSUES
- Enlarged parathyroid glands are often aspirated as clinically suspected solitary thyroid nodules
- Arise in parathyroid tissues and in ectopic sites
- Imaging studies can identify lesion but cannot separate adenoma (PA) from carcinoma (PC)
- Laboratory tests
  - Elevated serum calcium and PTH levels
  - Hypophosphatemia, hyperphosphaturia
  - Derangements more severe with PC than with PA

CYTOPATHOLOGY
- Cyst, adenoma, and carcinoma share similar cytology
- Cyst: Hypocellular aspirate of thin, water-clear fluid
- Adenoma and carcinoma
  - Naked nuclei; cells arranged in acini and follicles
  - Small, round nuclei with coarse chromatin and inconspicuous nucleoli
  - Neuroendocrine atypia is common
  - Atypical mitoses, anaplasia, and necrosis favor PC

ANCILLARY TESTS
- Immunohistochemistry is often necessary to distinguish parathyroid cells from thyroid cells
- Positive: Chromogranin, synaptophysin, keratin (particularly CAM5.2), and PTH
- Negative: TTF-1, thyroglobulin, and calcitonin
- Decreased expression of Rb and p27 in PC (vs. PA)
- **PA**: Positive Rb, p27, Bcl-2, MDM2; low Ki-67 index
- **PC**: Low/absent Rb, p27, and MDM2; high Ki-67 index
- Parafibromin: Protein product of *HRPT2* gene
  - Uniform nuclear staining is seen in PA, lost in PC

TOP DIFFERENTIAL DIAGNOSES
- Thyroid follicular lesion/neoplasm
- Hürthle cell lesion/neoplasm
- Medullary carcinoma
- Metastasis

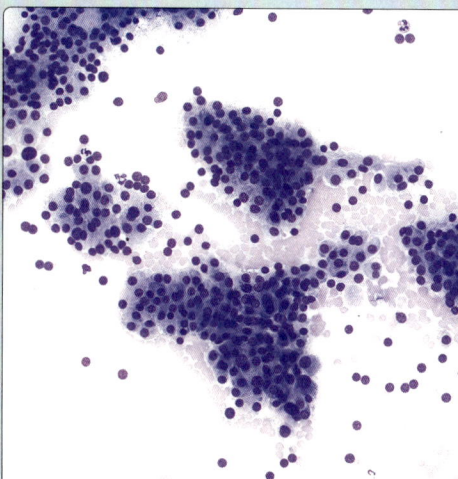

Cellular Aspirate of Parathyroid Adenoma

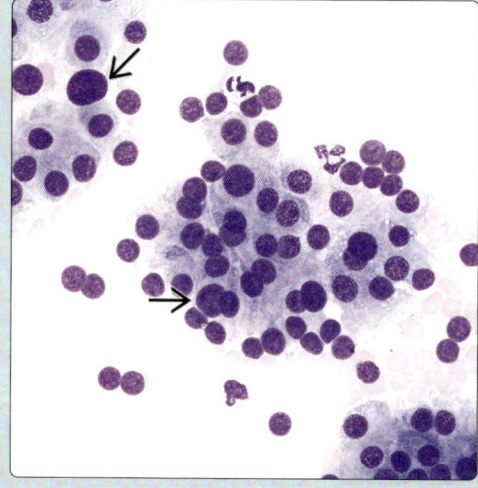

Bland Nuclear Features

(Left) Diff-Quik-stained cellular aspirate shows a microfollicular pattern that lacks follicular or background colloid. *(Right)* Nuclear features are seen on this Diff-Quik stain. The nuclei are round and central with smooth contours, coarsely stippled chromatin, and absent nucleoli. No nuclear grooves or pseudoinclusions are noted. The abundant granular cytoplasm resembles that of Hürthle cells. A few larger nuclei ➡ are also present, so-called "endocrine atypia."

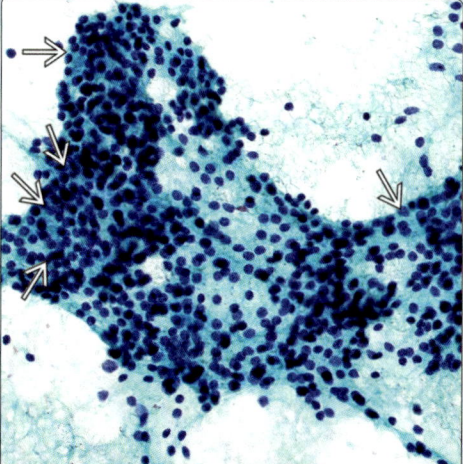

Microfollicles in Parathyroid Aspirate

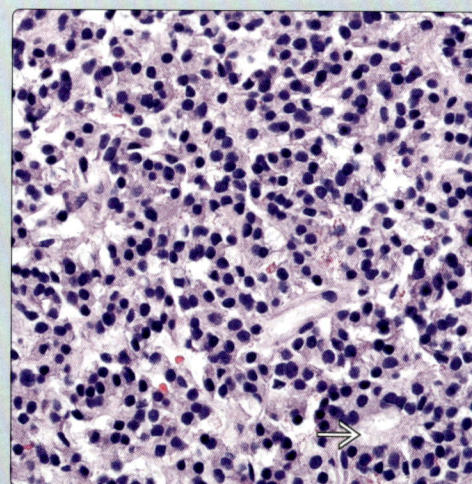

Core Needle Biopsy of Neck Mass

(Left) Pap-stained thyroid FNA shows a tightly packed conglomeration of microfollicles ➡ but without the dense colloid in the center of the follicles or the background colloid. The clean background should raise the suspicion of an intrathyroidal parathyroid adenoma. *(Right)* H&E-stained core needle biopsy shows a tightly packed microfollicular pattern ➡ of uniform cells with low-grade endocrine-type cells. Colloid is absent. Immunohistochemistry was TTF-1 and thyroglobulin negative. PTH was positive.

Parathyroid Cyst, Adenoma, and Carcinoma

TERMINOLOGY

Definitions
- Parathyroid cyst
  - Rare, benign, cystic lesion of parathyroid tissue
- Parathyroid adenoma (PA)
  - Benign neoplasm of parathyroid
- Parathyroid carcinoma (PC)
  - Malignant neoplasm of parathyroid

CLINICAL ISSUES

Presentation
- Cyst and PA: Asymptomatic or with mild symptoms
- PC: Most are functional and produce symptoms

Treatment
- Cyst: FNA may be curative; surgery if functional
- PA: Excision of adenomatous gland
- PC: Surgical resection en bloc with adjacent tissues

CYTOPATHOLOGY

Overview
- Enlarged parathyroid glands are often aspirated as clinically suspected solitary thyroid nodules
- Parathyroid cysts, adenomas, and carcinomas share similar basic cytomorphology
- Parathyroid tissue typically contains
  - Numerous naked nuclei and small sheets of cells
  - Cells arranged in acinar and follicular structures
  - Few small aggregates of dense, colloid-like material
  - Small cells with round to oval nuclei
    - Chromatin is coarse and neuroendocrine
    - Anisonucleosis is common
- May closely resemble thyroid follicular epithelium
  - Parathyroid cells are usually smaller and have more finely stippled chromatin
  - Colloid and macrophages favor thyroid
  - Immunohistochemistry often needed for diagnosis

Parathyroid Cyst
- Characteristically has thin, colorless, water-clear fluid
- Some are filled with golden-brown fluid, grossly resembling thyroid cysts
- Usually poorly cellular
- Diagnosis can be confirmed by analyzing fluid for parathormone (high) and thyroglobulin (low)

Parathyroid Adenoma and Carcinoma
- Cellular aspirates
  - Cells are arranged as naked nuclei, small cords, thick groups, and cohesive sheets
  - May form microfollicular or papillary structures
- Palisading may be present around capillaries
- Cells are usually small and uniform but can be markedly pleomorphic
  - Nuclei are round to oval and smaller than red cells
  - Chromatin is variable but often has typical salt and pepper appearance
  - Nucleoli are **usually** inconspicuous
  - Occasional larger, atypical nuclei are common
  - May contain cytoplasmic fat
- Features that favor carcinoma
  - Extreme cellularity, crowding, and dyshesion
  - Diffuse, marked anaplasia
  - Necrosis, atypical mitoses, and metastasis

MACROSCOPIC

General Features
- Cyst: Large, unilocular cyst filled with clear fluid
- PA: Rounded borders and delicate capsule
- PC: Adherent or invasive into adjacent structures (microscopic invasion is required for diagnosis)

ANCILLARY TESTS

Immunohistochemistry
- Positive for chromogranin, synaptophysin, keratin (CAM5.2 most helpful), and parathyroid hormone
- Negative for TTF-1, thyroglobulin, and calcitonin
- Decreased expression of Rb and p27 in PC (vs. PA)
- **PA**: Positive Rb, p27, Bcl-2, MDM2; low Ki-67 index
- **PC**: Low/absent Rb, p27, and MDM2; high Ki-67 index

Genetic Testing
- *HRPT2* mutation (tumor suppressor gene that encodes parafibromin, 1q21-q31)
- Cyclin-D1/*CCND1* (11q13)
- *RET* mutation (protooncogene, 10q11.2)
- *MEN1* mutation (tumor suppressor gene, 11q13, results in truncated Menin protein)
- Adenoma: Loss of 11q (*MEN1* gene location)
- Carcinoma: Loss of 1p and 13q; gain of 11
  - Loss of heterozygosity on 13q (*RB* and *BRCA2* gene locations)

DIFFERENTIAL DIAGNOSIS

Thyroid Follicular or Hürthle Cell Neoplasm
- Follicular growth pattern; background colloid
- Lacks well-defined cytoplasmic membranes
- Positive for TTF-1 and thyroglobulin
- Negative for PTH and chromogranin

Medullary Thyroid Carcinoma
- Lacks colloid and is positive for neuroendocrine markers and keratins (like PC)
- Positive for calcitonin and CEA; negative for PTH

Metastasis
- Metastatic tumors to parathyroid/thyroid have immunoprofile of primary site

SELECTED REFERENCES

1. Obołończyk Ł et al: The current role of parathyroid fine-needle biopsy (P-FNAB) with iPTH-washout concentration (iPTH-WC) in primary hyperparathyroidism: a single center experience and literature review. Biomedicines. 10(1), 2022
2. Suzuki A et al: Fine-needle aspiration of parathyroid adenomas: Indications as a diagnostic approach. Diagn Cytopathol. 49(1):70-6, 2021
3. Ha HJ et al: Major clues and pitfalls in the differential diagnosis of parathyroid and thyroid lesions using fine needle aspiration cytology. Medicina (Kaunas). 56(11), 2020

Parathyroid Cyst, Adenoma, and Carcinoma

Hypocellular Cyst Aspirate With Watery Fluid

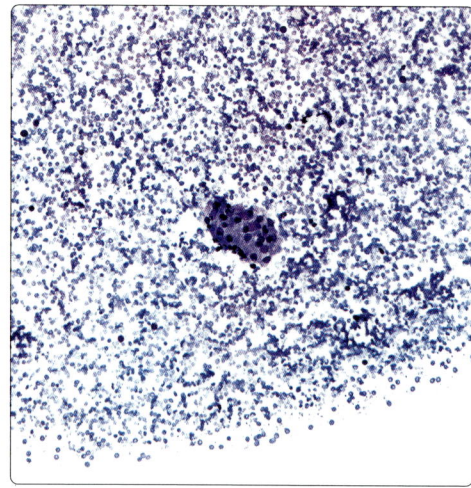

Cyst Fluid With Rare Cells

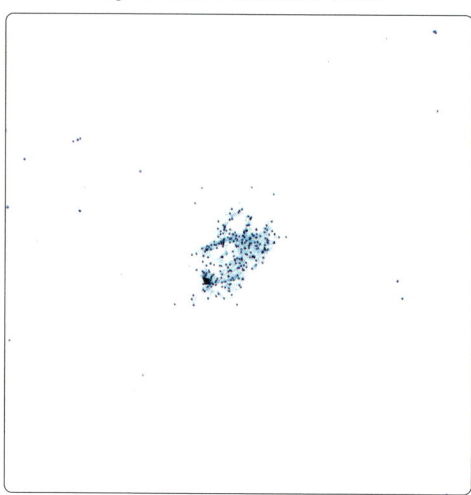

(Left) *Parathyroid cysts classically yield a water-clear fluid that is poorly cellular. At low magnification on Diff-Quik, this parathyroid cyst has very low cellularity with only rare, small clusters of epithelial cells.* **(Right)** *Low cellularity and a clean background of a typical parathyroid cyst are also seen on this Pap-stained slide.*

Details of Cells With Clean Background

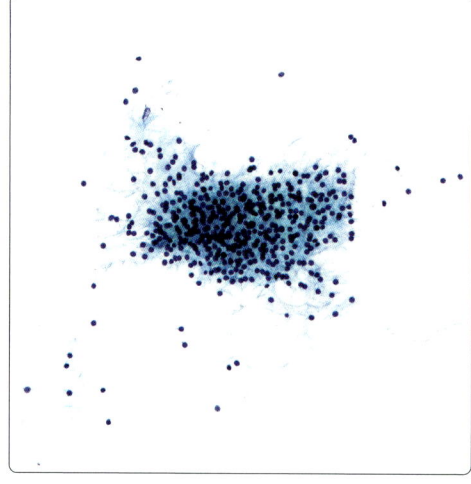

Regular Cells With Microfollicular Pattern

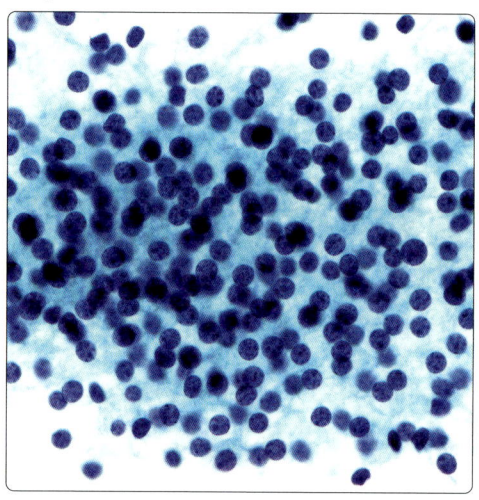

(Left) *At intermediate magnification, there is a group of epithelial cells with no associated colloid.* **(Right)** *At higher magnification, the group is composed of uniform cells with small, bland nuclei and a moderate amount of granular, pale cytoplasm. The cells are arranged in vague follicles, mimicking thyroid tissue. The lack of colloid and the fine cytoplasm should make one consider a parathyroid origin.*

Hypercellular With Trabecular Pattern in Parathyroid Neoplasms

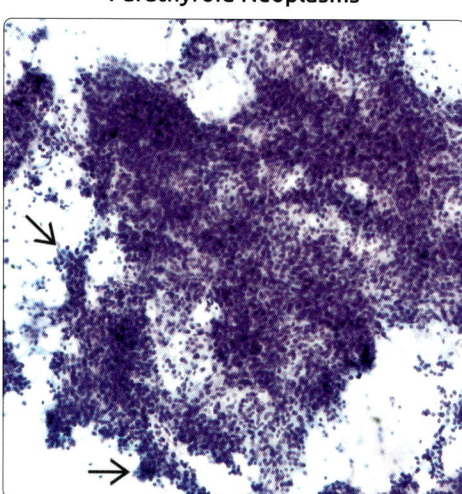

Cell Block of Parathyroid Adenoma

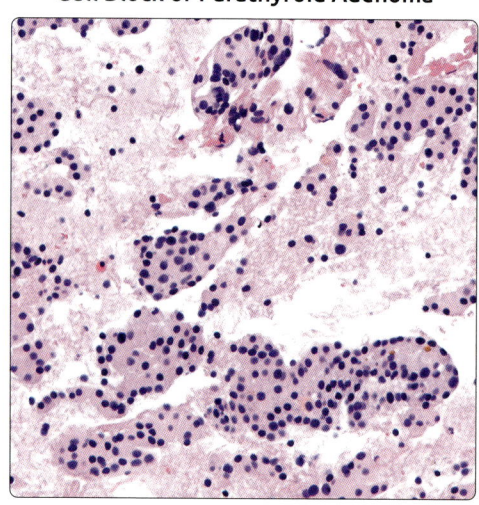

(Left) *Hypercellularity is also seen on this Pap-stained slide. The cells are arranged in thick sheets, trabeculae, and vague papillae ➔ but without follicle formation.* **(Right)** *H&E-stained cell block section nicely demonstrates the cellularity of this parathyroid adenoma. The follicular architecture is even more prominent on this preparation.*

Parathyroid Cyst, Adenoma, and Carcinoma

Oxyphil Cells

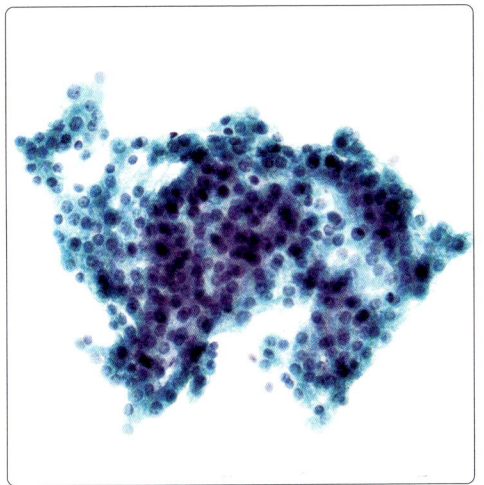

Parathyroid Carcinoma

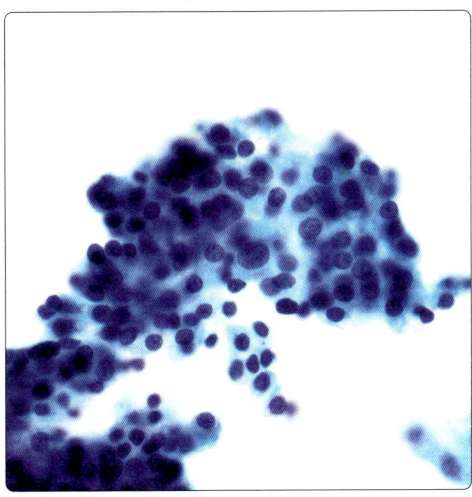

(Left) The abundant granular cytoplasm of parathyroid oxyphil cells is well-visualized on this Pap-stained smear. The nuclei are round and uniform with inconspicuous nucleoli. (Right) Pap-stained slide of a parathyroid carcinoma shows a 3D cluster of follicular cells that have finely stippled chromatin, inconspicuous nucleoli, and abundant chromatin. Occasional larger nuclei are present, a feature commonly seen in neuroendocrine tissues that is not specific for malignancy.

Microacinar Pattern

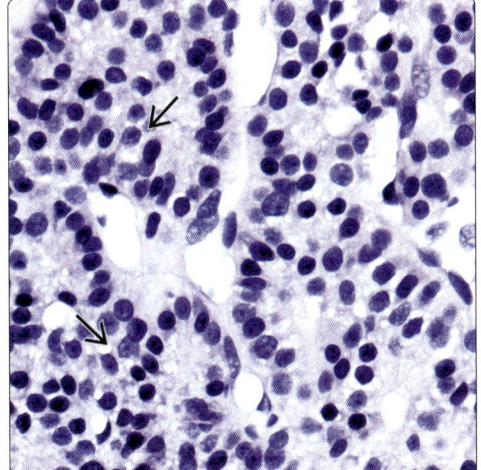

Negative TTF-1 Stain

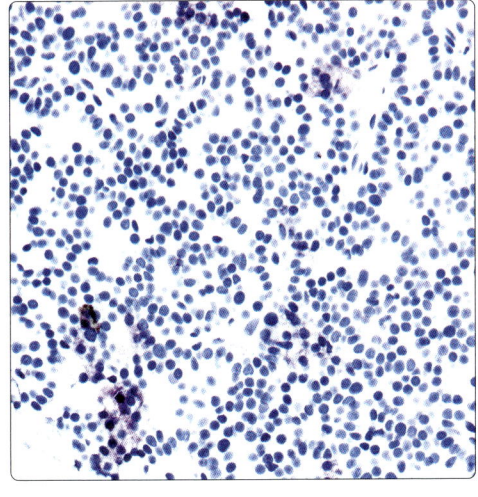

(Left) H&E-stained cell block section shows parathyroid cells arranged in small acini, cords, and follicles. Most of the nuclei are bland and oval, although there are a few larger nuclei and scattered small nucleoli ➡. (Right) Immunohistochemistry can be very helpful in distinguishing parathyroid from thyroid tissue. TTF-1 characteristically shows strong nuclear positivity in thyroid tissue. The negative staining seen here supports a diagnosis of parathyroid cells.

Positive Parathormone on IHC

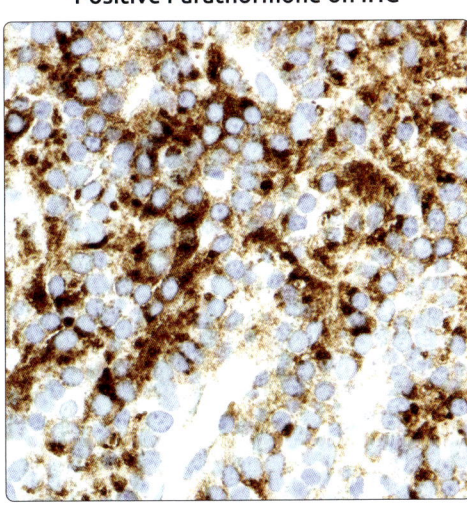

Strong Positive Rb on IHC

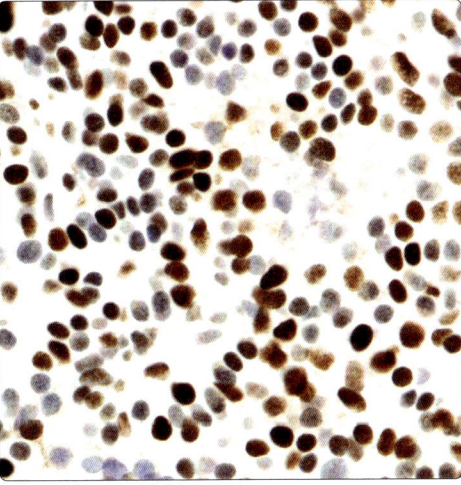

(Left) Immunoperoxidase stain for parathormone (PTH) shows diffuse, strong cytoplasmic positivity, consistent with parathyroid cells. (Right) Immunoperoxidase staining may also help differentiate parathyroid adenomas from carcinomas. The retinoblastoma gene (RB1) encodes a tumor suppressor protein that is frequently inactivated in parathyroid carcinomas. The strong nuclear staining seen here supports a diagnosis of adenoma; most carcinomas are negative.

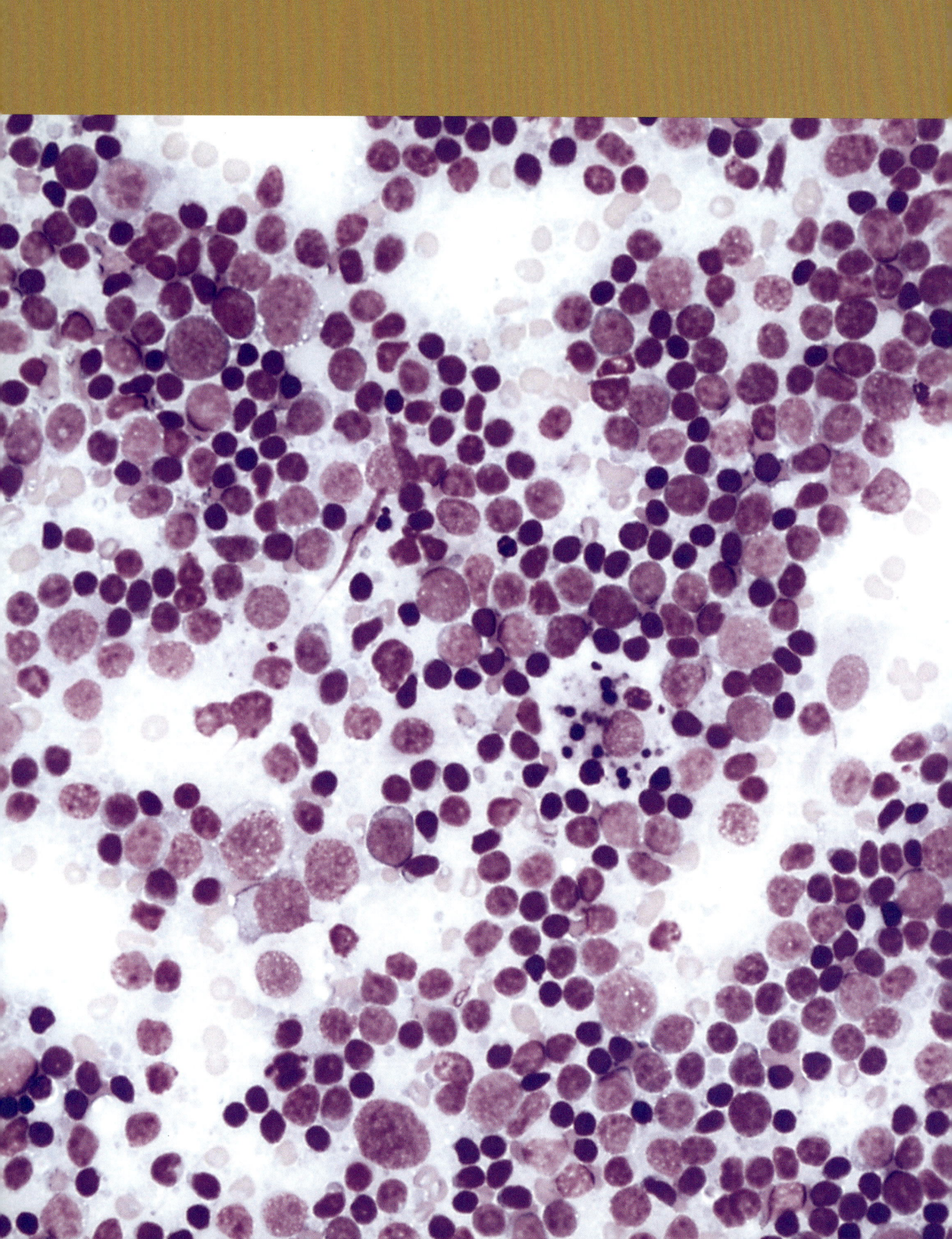

PART III
SECTION 4
Lymph Nodes

Overview

Lymph Node Aspiration: Indications, Techniques, and Reporting	324
FNA Sample Prep and Triage in Evaluating Suspected Lymphoma	326

Benign, Infectious, and Reactive Hyperplasia

Inflammatory and Reactive Lymphoid Hyperplasia	328
Granulomatous Lymphadenitis, Infectious and Sarcoid	330
Rosai-Dorfman Disease	334

Metastatic Malignancies

Metastatic Malignancies (Carcinoma, Melanoma)	336
HPV-Positive Head and Neck Squamous Cell Carcinoma	338

Nodal B-Cell Lymphoma

Small Lymphocytic Lymphoma	342
Lymphoplasmacytic Lymphoma	344
Mantle Cell Lymphoma	346
Nodal Marginal Zone Lymphoma	348
Follicular Lymphoma	350
Burkitt Lymphoma	352
Large B-Cell Lymphoma	354

Extranodal B-Cell Lymphoma

Plasmacytoma	356
Mediastinal Large B-Cell Lymphoma	358
Plasmablastic Lymphoma	360

T-Cell Lymphoma

Peripheral T-Cell Lymphoma	362
Mycosis Fungoides	364
Angioimmunoblastic Lymphoma	366
ALK(+) Anaplastic Large Cell Lymphoma	368
T-Cell Lymphoblastic Lymphoma	370

Hodgkin Lymphoma

Nodular Lymphocyte-Predominant Hodgkin Lymphoma	372
Classic Hodgkin Lymphoma	374

Lymph Node Aspiration: Indications, Techniques, and Reporting

TYPES OF PROCEDURES

Superficial Lymph Nodes (Not Image Guided)
- Often performed in outpatient clinics or physician offices on large, easily palpable nodes

Deep Lymph Nodes (Image Guided)
- CT-guided, endobronchial ultrasound (EBUS)-guided, or endoscopic ultrasound (EUS)-guided

GENERAL POINTS

Indications
- **To evaluate lymphadenopathy**
  - To evaluate presence or absence of malignancy
  - In cases of known malignancy, to quickly confirm metastatic disease to initiate treatment modalities, hospice care
- **To quickly obtain material for ancillary studies**
  - If infectious etiology suspected, can obtain material for cultures
  - Molecular tests, genetic studies, flow cytometry, etc.
- Faster, safer, more cost-effective than core biopsy
  - Main disadvantages are sampling errors and lack of intact architecture for evaluation

TECHNIQUE

Image Guided
- Techniques may vary based on location, size, patient

CYTOLOGIC FEATURES

Lymphocytes
- Small lymphocytes
  - Most frequent component of benign lymph node aspirate
  - Small, round nuclei; hyperchromatic, inconspicuous nucleoli; scant cytoplasm
- Centrocyte
  - Large or small, cleaved cells; hyperchromatic, inconspicuous nucleoli; scant cytoplasm
- Centroblast

Reactive Lymph Node
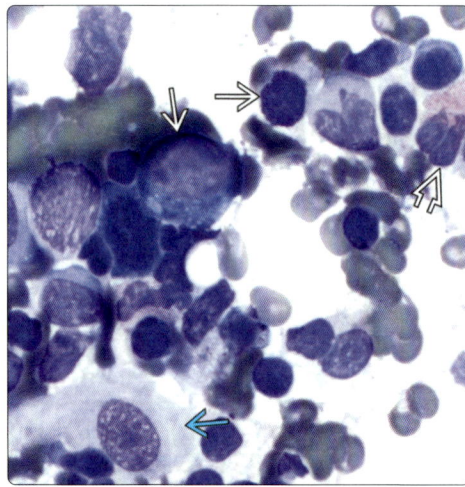

Polymorphous Lymphocytes and Tingible Body Macrophage
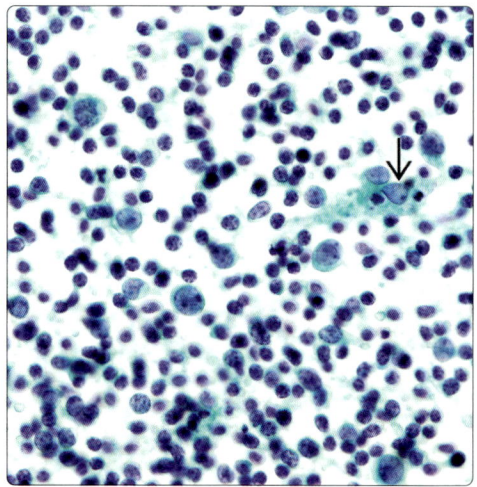

(Left) Diff-Quik stain shows a polymorphous population of lymphocytes ➡, histiocytes ➡, and eosinophils ➡ in this lymph node that was confirmed as being reactive. **(Right)** Lymphocytes of varying sizes are demonstrated in this Pap-stained aspirate of a reactive lymph node. A tingible body macrophage ➡ is included.

Monotonous Population of Cells
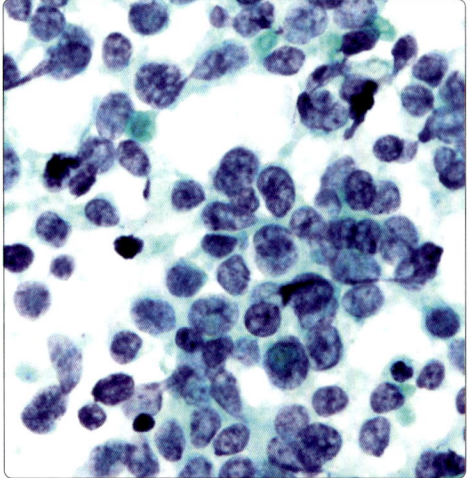

Monotonous Cells and Lymphoglandular Bodies
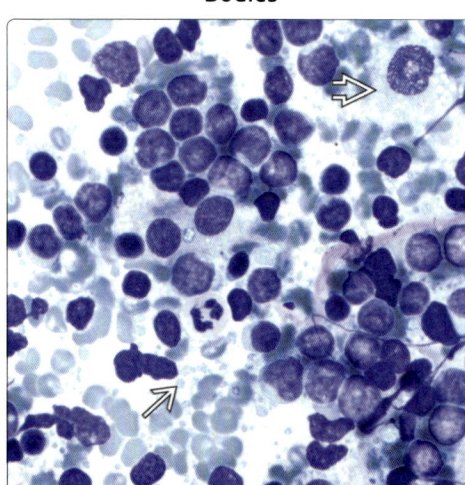

(Left) In contrast to the previous image, this group of monotonous cells on Pap stain is worrisome for lymphoma or carcinoma. **(Right)** Diff-Quik stain at the time of rapid on-site evaluation shows a somewhat monotonous population of cells with lymphoglandular bodies ➡ as well as an occasional histiocyte ➡. Appropriate triage (flow cytometry and molecular testing) was confirmatory for a follicular lymphoma (grade 3A), along with a core needle biopsy for architecture.

Lymph Node Aspiration: Indications, Techniques, and Reporting

Proposed 2-Tiered System for Reporting Lymph Node FNAB and Recommendations (Sydney System)

Diagnostic Level	Reporting Terminology	Management Recommendations
1st Diagnostic Level		
	Inadequate/Nondiagnostic (scant cellularity, necrosis, technical)	Repeat FNAB or CNB or excision
	Benign (inflammation, granulomas, specific infections, heterogenous lymphoid population with flow or serologies)	Clinical follow-up/specific treatment (based on results)
	AUS/ALUS (heterogenous lymphoid population but discrepancy on flow or clinically)	Repeat FNA with acquisition of material for ancillary studies (flow, cell block, microbiology) &/or CNB or excision
	Suspicious for lymphoma or carcinoma but falls short of definitive diagnosis of malignancy	Repeat FNA and acquire material for appropriate ancillary studies or CNB or excision
	Malignant (specify type; carcinoma, lymphoma, etc., if possible)	Request biopsy or excision if needed for further work-up and clinically indicated
2nd Diagnostic Level		
	Provide specific etiology in reactive process (if possible based on ancillary studies)	Clinical follow-up or specific treatment based on ancillary studies (serologies, cultures, etc.)
	Subtyping NHL and specific diagnosis if possible (based on flow/molecular); HL with subtyping or primary site of metastasis if possible	

CNB = core needle biopsy; FNAB = fine-needle aspiration biopsy; NHL = Non-Hodgkin lymphoma; HL = Hodgkin lymphoma; AUS/ALUS = atypical undetermined significance, atypical lymphoid undetermined significance.

Al-Abbadi MA et al: A Proposal for the performance, classification, and reporting of lymph node fine-needle aspiration cytopathology: the Sydney system. Acta Cytol. 64(4):306-22, 2020.

- Large cells, noncleaved with 1 or multiple nucleoli and scant cytoplasm
- Immunoblast
  - Large nuclei with prominent nucleoli and fair amount of associated cytoplasm

Histiocytes
- Large cells with oval, elongated, or round nuclei with abundant cytoplasm
- If degenerated cellular debris is visible in cytoplasm, type of cell is referred to as tingible body macrophage

Plasma Cells
- Eccentric nuclei, often with clockface chromatin pattern
- Paranuclear clear zone (Golgi)

Others, rare
- Eosinophils
- Neutrophils
- Basophils
- Mast cells
- Endothelial cells

DIAGNOSTIC CHECKLIST
Pathologic Interpretation Pearls
- Lymphoglandular bodies represent cytoplasmic fragments of disrupted lymphocytes, indicate lymphocytes (benign or malignant) are component of lesion
- Tingible body macrophages are reassuring sign that node is reactive but are frequently seen in high-grade malignancies as well
- Presence of polymorphous lymphocytic population is often indicative of reactive process but is not pathognomonic of benignity
  - Must be correlated with flow cytometric studies

Laboratory Work-up of Lymphoma in Adults
- Evidence-based recommendations for work-up of lymphomas in adults
- ASCP, CAP, and ASH convened expert panel of pathologists and hematologists
- 13 guideline statements published in 2021

SELECTED REFERENCES
1. Rabe K et al: Effects of COVID-19 pandemic on cytology: specimen adequacy in fine-needle aspiration of palpable head and neck masses. J Am Soc Cytopathol. 11(4):234-40, 2022
2. Zadeh SL et al: Global cytopathology-hematopathology practice trends. Am J Clin Pathol. 157(2):196-201, 2022
3. Davey DD: Impact of laboratory work-up of lymphoma guidelines on cytopathology practices. J Am Soc Cytopathol. 10(3):338-40, 2021
4. Kroft SH et al: Laboratory workup of lymphoma in adults: guideline from the American Society for Clinical Pathology and the College of American Pathologists. Arch Pathol Lab Med. 145(3):269-90, 2021
5. Seviar D et al: Image-guided core needle biopsy as the first-line diagnostic approach in lymphoproliferative disorders-a review of the current literature. Eur J Haematol. 106(2):139-47, 2021
6. Shah A et al: An approach to small lymph node biopsies: pearls and pitfalls of reporting in the real world. J Am Soc Cytopathol. 10(3):328-37, 2021
7. Shyu S et al: Image guided lymph node fine-needle aspiration: the Johns Hopkins Hospital experience. J Am Soc Cytopathol. 10(6):543-57, 2021
8. Al-Abbadi MA et al: A Proposal for the performance, classification, and reporting of lymph node fine-needle aspiration cytopathology: the Sydney system. Acta Cytol. 64(4):306-22, 2020
9. Chi PD et al: Rinsing sampling of core needle biopsy for flow cytometric analysis: a favorable method for lymphoma diagnosis. Cancer Med. 9(24):9336-45, 2020

FNA Sample Prep and Triage in Evaluating Suspected Lymphoma

SUSPICION FOR LYMPHOMA

Unexplained Adenopathy
- With predisposing factors (e.g., immunodeficiency)
- With clinical symptoms (e.g., B symptoms)
- With worrisome imaging findings
- In older patients

Adenopathy With History of Lymphoma
- Staging or ruling out relapsed disease

UTILITY AND LIMITATIONS OF FNA

Utility of FNA
- Good screening test for B-cell lymphoma (BCL) and classic Hodgkin lymphoma (HL)
- Detects recurrent or relapsed lymphoma
- Detects large cells of diffuse large B-cell lymphoma (DLBCL) and transformed low-grade BCL
- Accurately classifies most cases of Burkitt lymphoma (BL), follicular lymphoma (FL), mantle cell lymphoma (MCL), and small lymphocytic lymphoma (SLL)

Limitations of FNA
- Loss of histologic features (e.g., follicular vs. diffuse in FL, or nodular vs. diffuse in MCL)
- Accurate grading is problematic (e.g., HL and FL)
- Poor detection of lymphocyte-predominant HL, T-cell/histiocyte-rich large BCL (TCRLBCL), some T-cell lymphoma (TCL)
- Distinguishing HL, anaplastic large cell lymphoma (ALCL), and TCRLBCL is not always possible
- Subclassification of TCL, ALCL, HL, DLBCL, and low-grade BCL with atypical phenotype can be unreliable
- Potential misclassification of gray zone lymphomas

Comments
- Nodal fibrosis/necrosis, sample preparation, laboratory capabilities, and skill of operator procuring aspirate can be limiting factors

Immunophenotypes of Common Lymphoid Neoplasms

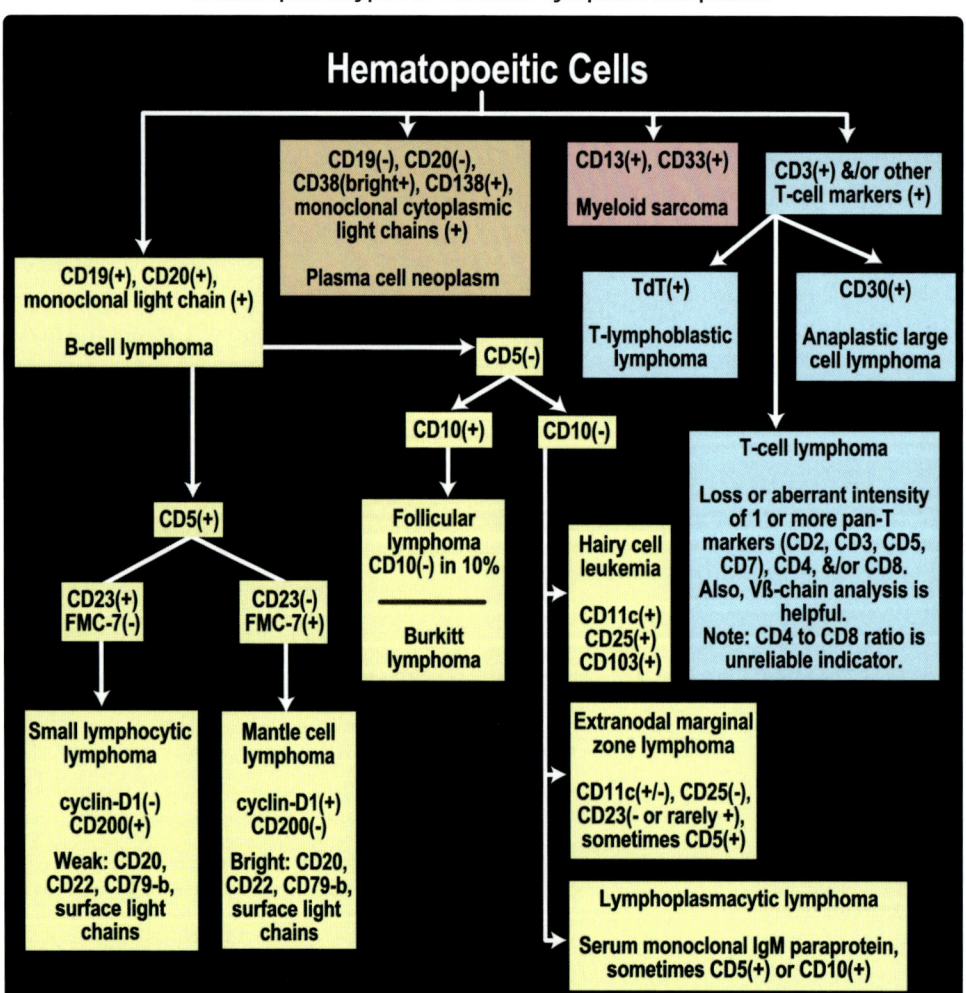

Flow cytometric immunophenotype analysis is essential for accurate classification of most lymphomas evaluated by FNA. This dendrogram shows the typical immunophenotypes of the common lymphoid neoplasms. The immunophenotype must be correlated with the cytomorphology and available clinical findings, immunostains, and molecular results. Exceptions occur. Some lymphomas with classic morphology have an abnormal immunophenotype, whereas others with a classic immunophenotype exhibit an atypical morphology. Note also that negative flow cytometry results do not exclude lymphoma.

FNA Sample Prep and Triage in Evaluating Suspected Lymphoma

- FNA is useful adjunct to core biopsy
- Many limitations of FNA are shared by higher gauge (i.e., 18/20) core needle biopsies
- Negative FNA result does not exclude lymphoma
- Excisional biopsy (not needle core biopsy) is gold standard and is recommended if feasible for confirmation, subclassification, and grading in most cases of newly diagnosed lymphoma

FNA PROCESSING AND TRIAGE

Morphology
- Direct smears or liquid-based preparations for Diff-Quik and Pap stains

Immunophenotype
- Collect needle passes in RPMI media (or Hank solution) for flow cytometry
  - Adequacy can be assessed by visual inspection of turbidity, concurrently prepared smears, or preferably by Coulter counter
  - Negative flow cytometry results do not exclude lymphoma, and correlation with morphology is always needed
    - Aspirated material composed of mainly peripheral blood
    - Large cells of DLBCL may not survive processing
    - Partial nodal involvement may be missed
    - TCRLBCL may not be detected
    - TCL may have normal immunophenotype
    - HL is typically undetected
- Process portion of aspirate in RPMI through density gradient (e.g., LymphoPrep); use buffy coat to prepare cytospin slides for ancillary testing
  - Stain with Diff-Quik &/or Pap
  - Use for immunoperoxidase stains
  - Use for FISH or molecular studies, as needed
  - Air-dried/methanol-fixed unstained slides can be stored in freezer for future use
- Prepare cell block from clot/sediment from RPMI rinse following centrifugation

Mutational Analysis
- FISH assays: Use cytospin slides or cell block
- Next-generation sequencing/PCR-based assays: Use cell suspension, cell block, or cytospins
- Karyotyping: Use cell suspension

DIAGNOSING LYMPHOMA IN CYTOPATHOLOGY LABORATORY

Establish Differential Diagnosis Based on Cell Size
- Small cell predominant
  - SLL
  - Lymphoplasmacytic lymphoma
  - FL, grade 1
  - MCL
  - Marginal zone lymphoma (MZL)
  - TCL
- Mixed small and large cells
  - FL, grades 2 and 3
  - TCL (most)
- Intermediate cell predominant
  - Lymphoblastic lymphoma (LBL)
  - BL
  - MCL, blastoid variant
- Large cell predominant
  - DLBCL
  - Follicular lymphoma, grade 3 (some)
  - MCL, pleomorphic variant
  - TCL
- Atypical large cells in small/mixed cell background
  - Classic HL
  - ALCL
  - TCRLBCL

Refine Differential Diagnosis Based on Immunophenotype
- Flow cytometry &/or immunostains

Molecular Testing
- Translocation *ALK* 2p23
  - ALCL: Usually t(2;5) but variants in 25%
- Translocation *BCL2* 18q21
  - FL: t(14;18) in 80-90%
  - DLBCL (subset)
- Translocation *BCL6* 3q27
  - FL, DLBCL (subsets)
- Translocation *MYC* 8q24
  - BL: t(8;14) in 80%; t(8;22) or t(2;8) in 20%
  - FL, DLBCL (subsets)
- Translocation *CCND1* 11q13
  - MCL: t(11;14)

Utility of CD3 and Ki-67 Stains in BCL
- CD3 accounts for T cells (nodal or blood) to normalize Ki-67 expression to B cells in BCL
- Ki-67 can help assess biologic grade
  - Ki-67 > 30% for SLL, MZL, and FL suggests accelerated phase, more aggressive course, or large cell transformation
  - Ki-67 for MCL is usually < 25%; > 40% suggests aggressive variant (i.e., blastoid or pleomorphic)
  - Ki-67 > 95% is seen in BL and LBL

SELECTED REFERENCES

1. Caputo A et al: Nodal and extra-nodal diagnosis of lymphoma by fine-needle cytology: different diagnostic levels and clinical relevance. Diagn Cytopathol. 49(8):968-9, 2021
2. Kroft SH et al: Laboratory workup of lymphoma in adults: guideline from the American Society for Clinical Pathology and the College of American Pathologists. Arch Pathol Lab Med. 145(3):269-90, 2021
3. Wang H et al: Diagnostic accuracy of fine-needle aspiration cytology for lymphoma: a systematic review and meta-analysis. Diagn Cytopathol. 49(9):975-86, 2021
4. Al-Abbadi MA et al: A proposal for the performance, classification, and reporting of lymph node fine-needle aspiration cytopathology: the Sydney system. Acta Cytol. 64(4):306-22, 2020
5. Barroca H et al: A basic approach to lymph node and flow cytometry fine-needle cytology. Acta Cytol. 60(1):284-301, 2016
6. Frederiksen JK et al: Systematic review of the effectiveness of fine-needle aspiration and/or core needle biopsy for subclassifying lymphoma. Arch Pathol Lab Med. 139(2):245-51, 2015
7. Ochs RC et al: Molecular genetic characterization of lymphoma: application to cytology diagnosis. Diagn Cytopathol. 40(6):542-55, 2012
8. Shetuni B et al: Optimal specimen processing of fine needle aspirates of non-Hodgkin lymphoma. Diagn Cytopathol. 40(11):984-6, 2012

Inflammatory and Reactive Lymphoid Hyperplasia

KEY FACTS

ETIOLOGY/PATHOGENESIS

- Environmental exposure
  - Pollutants, chemicals, therapeutic drugs
  - Vaccine administration (1-3 weeks post vaccination)
- Infectious agents
  - Viral infection: Epstein-Barr virus (EBV), cytomegalovirus, herpes simplex virus (type 1 or 2)
  - Bacterial infection
  - Fungal infection

CLINICAL ISSUES

- Patients typically present with enlarged lymph nodes, either localized or widespread
- Systemic symptoms can be present
- Size, location, and consistency of lymph nodes as well as duration and patient age are important factors in identifying etiology

CYTOPATHOLOGY

- Lymphocytes in varying stages of maturation
- Lymphohistiocytic aggregates (lymphocytes admixed with histiocytes)
- Tingible body macrophages (macrophages with cellular debris in vacuoles)
- Numerous neutrophils suggest bacterial or fungal infection

TOP DIFFERENTIAL DIAGNOSES

- Hodgkin lymphoma
  - Infectious mononucleosis may have Reed-Sternberg-like cells and mixed inflammatory cells in background
  - Ancillary immunostaining useful: CD15(+), CD30(+), PAX5 [(dim (+)], CD45/LCA(-)
- Non-Hodgkin lymphoma: Rule out with flow cytometry
  - Usually more monotonous lymphocytic population
  - Demonstrates monoclonal population of lymphoid cells

Polymorphous Lymphocytes

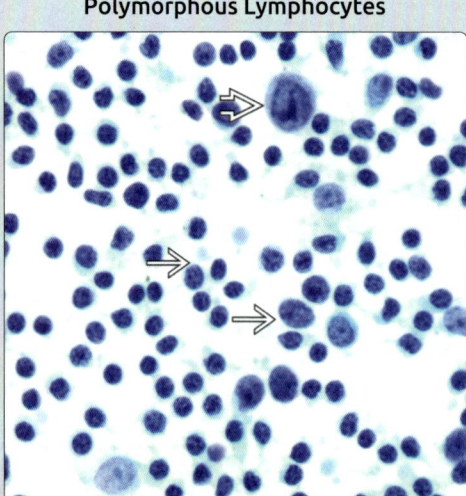

Tingible Body Macrophage

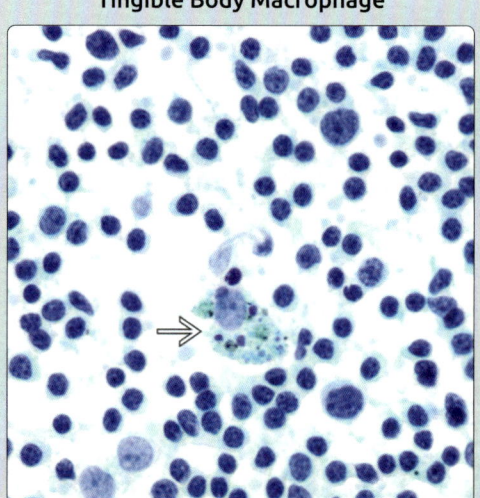

(Left) Pap-stained FNA smear of a reactive lymph node shows a polymorphous population of lymphoid cells, including small- and intermediate-sized lymphoid cells ➡ and an immunoblast ➡. (Right) Pap-stained FNA smear of a reactive lymph node shows a polymorphous population of lymphoid cells, including a tingible body macrophage ➡ with cellular debris in the cytoplasm.

Lymphoglandular Bodies

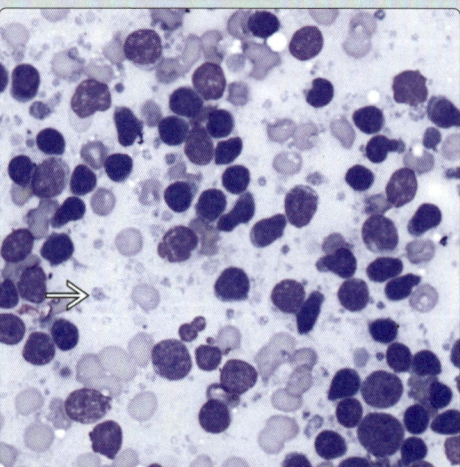

Lymphohistiocytic Aggregate

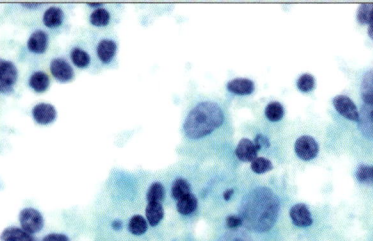

(Left) Diff-Quik-stained FNA smear shows a polymorphous population of lymphoid cells with many lymphoglandular bodies ➡ in the background. (Right) Pap-stained FNA smear of a reactive lymph node shows a lymphohistiocytic aggregate, including small lymphoid cells ➡ and histiocytes ➡.

Inflammatory and Reactive Lymphoid Hyperplasia

ETIOLOGY/PATHOGENESIS

Environmental Exposure
- Pollutants, chemicals, therapeutic drugs
- Vaccine administration (1-3 weeks post vaccination)

Infectious Agents
- Viral infection
  - Epstein-Barr virus (EBV), cytomegalovirus, herpes simplex virus (type 1 or 2)
- Bacterial infection
- Fungal infection

CLINICAL ISSUES

Presentation
- Patients present with enlarged lymph nodes that are either localized or widespread
- Systemic symptoms can be present
  - Fever, fatigue, and weight loss
- Laboratory abnormalities may be present
- Clues to etiology derived from
  - Age, duration of symptoms, and site
  - Size and consistency of lymph node(s)

Treatment
- Localized lymph node enlargement in absence of other symptoms can be followed
  - If no resolution after 3-4 weeks, investigation needed

CYTOPATHOLOGY

Pattern
- Dyshesive

Cells
- Lymphocytes in varying stages of maturation
- Lymphohistiocytic aggregates (lymphocytes admixed with histiocytes)
- Tingible body macrophages (macrophages with cellular debris in vacuoles)
- Numerous neutrophils suggest bacterial or fungal infection

MICROSCOPIC

Histologic Features
- Overall lymph node architecture distorted but preserved

ANCILLARY TESTS

Immunohistochemistry
- Evidence of virus in EBV-associated cases: EBV-LMP(+)

In Situ Hybridization
- Evidence of virus in virally induced cases

DIFFERENTIAL DIAGNOSIS

Hodgkin Lymphoma
- Classic Reed-Sternberg cells present
  - CD15(+), CD30(+), PAX5 [dim (+)], CD45/LCA(-)

Non-Hodgkin Lymphoma
- Usually more monotonous lymphocytic population
- Flow cytometry helpful

DIAGNOSTIC CHECKLIST

Pathologic Interpretation Pearls
- At time of aspiration, obtain material for cultures and flow cytometry (rule out clonal population)
- Lymphoglandular bodies indicate that aspirate contains lymphocytes; not helpful in determining malignancy
- Infectious mononucleosis may have false-negative serologic studies and lead to aspiration
  - Presence of Reed-Sternberg-like cells and mixed inflammatory background simulates Hodgkin lymphoma
  - Flow cytometry not helpful
  - May require repeat serology &/or excision for in situ hybridization and immunohistochemistry for EBV

SELECTED REFERENCES

1. Hagen C et al: Fine needle aspiration in COVID-19 vaccine-associated lymphadenopathy. Swiss Med Wkly. 151:w20557, 2021

Infectious Mononucleosis, Many Large Lymphocytes

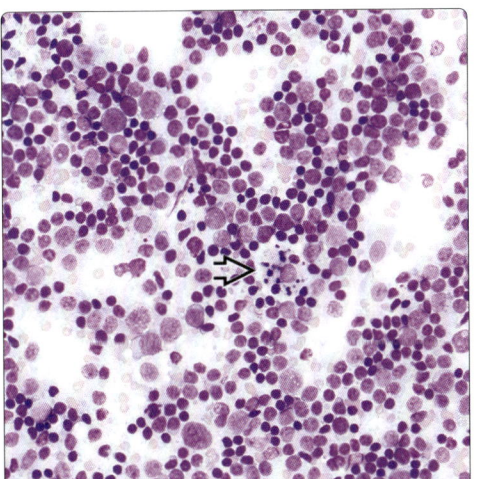

Infectious Mononucleosis, Reed-Sternberg-Like Cell

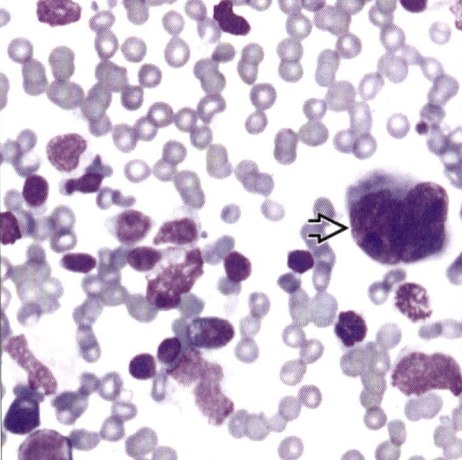

(Left) Diff-Quik-stained FNA smear of lymph node aspiration from a patient with infectious mononucleosis shows a polymorphous population of lymphoid cells, including a tingible body macrophage ➡. (Right) Diff-Quik-stained FNA smear of a lymph node aspirate shows Reed-Sternberg-like cells ➡ in a patient with infectious mononucleosis.

Granulomatous Lymphadenitis, Infectious and Sarcoid

KEY FACTS

CLINICAL ISSUES
- Cervical lymph nodes most commonly involved

CYTOPATHOLOGY
- Epithelioid histiocytes and inflammatory cells can be identified in FNA smears
- Histiocytes have elongated nuclei, may show grooves, and are often boomerang- or kidney-shaped or resemble "footprints in sand"
- Necrosis may be present in background
- Special stains can be performed on smears or cell block

ANCILLARY TESTS
- Special stains
  - Acid-fast bacilli can be demonstrated by Ziehl-Neelsen, Kinyoun, or Fite-Faraco stain
  - Fungal-like organisms can be highlighted with PAS or GMS stain
  - Warthin-Starry stain for *Bartonella henselae* (cat-scratch disease) or *Treponema pallidum* (syphilis)
- Immunohistochemistry: Useful for identification of selected infectious agents
- PCR allows identification of infectious agents in cases where special stains &/or immunostaining fails to demonstrate infectious agent

TOP DIFFERENTIAL DIAGNOSES
- *Mycobacterium tuberculosis* lymphadenitis
- Atypical mycobacterial lymphadenitis
- Fungal lymphadenitis
  - *Histoplasma, Coccidioides, Cryptococcus* (most common)
- Bacterial lymphadenitis
  - *B. henselae* (most common)
- Malignancy
- Sarcoidosis
- Foreign body

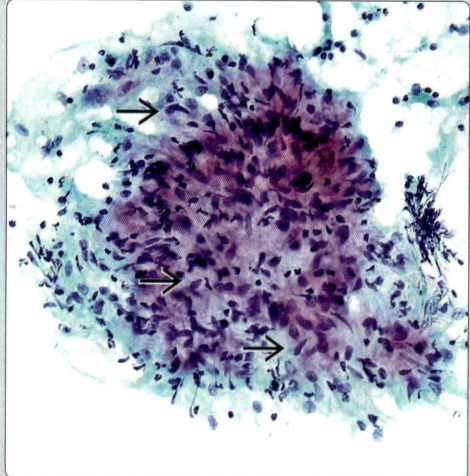

Epithelioid Granuloma, Pap Stain

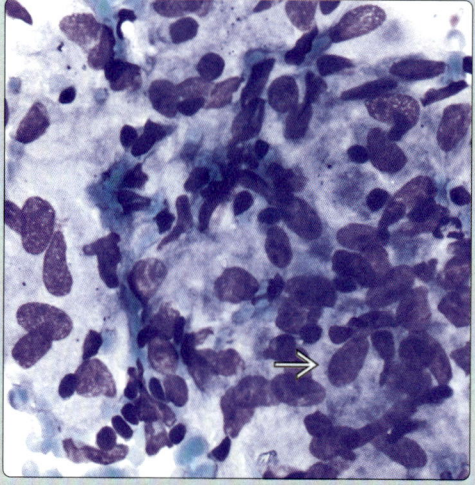

Epithelioid Granuloma, Diff-Quik Stain

(Left) Pap-stained FNA smear shows an intact granuloma composed of epithelioid histiocytes ➡ with oval to elongated nuclei. (Right) Diff-Quik-stained FNA smear shows a nonnecrotizing granuloma with epithelioid histiocytes ➡.

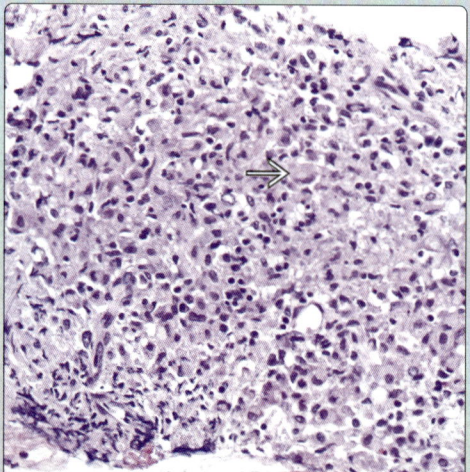

Epithelioid Granuloma, Cell Block

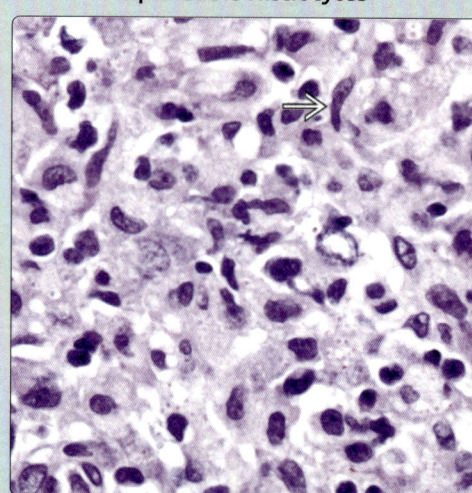

Epithelioid Histiocytes

(Left) H&E-stained cell block section shows a nonnecrotizing granuloma composed of epithelioid histiocytes ➡. (Right) Pap-stained FNA smear shows many epithelioid histiocytes ➡ with elongated nucleus and a moderate amount of delicate and vacuolated cytoplasm.

Granulomatous Lymphadenitis, Infectious and Sarcoid

TERMINOLOGY

Definitions
- Granulomatous inflammation is specific type of inflammatory response
  - Characterized by accumulation of modified macrophages (epithelioid cells)
  - Initiated by infectious or noninfectious agents

ETIOLOGY/PATHOGENESIS

Infectious Agents
- Usually caused by one of wide variety of infectious agents, including mycobacteria, bacteria, viruses, fungi, and parasites
- Infectious granulomas can be classified into 3 subgroups based on etiology
  - Infections caused by well-recognized organisms
    - *Mycobacterium tuberculosis* is most common
  - Infections caused by organisms identified by molecular methods but not readily isolated by conventional microbiologic methods
  - Infectious etiology is strongly suspected, but causal organisms have not yet been identified

Other Causes
- Foreign body reaction
- Autoimmune diseases (e.g., sarcoidosis)
- Malignancies (carcinomas, sarcomas, lymphomas)

CLINICAL ISSUES

Site
- Lymph node group involved depends in part on
  - Initiating agent
  - Route of entry into body
- Cervical lymph nodes are most common
- Any lymph node or lymph node group can be affected

Presentation
- Lymphadenopathy, localized or general
- May be accompanied by systemic symptoms

Laboratory Tests
- Microbiologic culture and identification by biochemical methods
- Serologic tests are helpful in
  - Identifying infectious agents
  - Determining timing of exposure to organism
- PCR methods detect infectious agents with high sensitivity
  - Infectious agents have been identified in diseases that were previously of unknown etiology

Prognosis
- Depends on specific etiology and therapy administered
- Benign clinical course with good prognosis

CYTOPATHOLOGY

Cellularity
- Often cellular smears

Pattern
- Epithelioid histiocytes can occur singly or in groups

Background
- Scattered lymphocytes and plasma cells, neutrophils (bacteria, fungus), eosinophils (parasite)
- Necrosis may be present (not seen in sarcoidosis)

Cells
- Histiocytes, multinucleated giant cells, lymphocytes, plasma cells, neutrophils, eosinophils

Nuclear Details
- Histiocytes have elongated nuclei, may show grooves, and are often boomerang- or kidney-shaped or resemble "footprints in sand"

Cytoplasmic Details
- Histiocytes often have abundant pale cytoplasm and indistinct cell boundaries

MACROSCOPIC

General Features
- Yellow areas can be seen corresponding to necrotic foci

MICROSCOPIC

Histologic Features
- Immune type
  - Caused by insoluble particles (e.g., bacteria) that elicit cell-mediated immune response
  - Can further divide these into caseating and noncaseating granulomas
  - Caseating granulomas
    - Composed of central areas of coagulative necrosis
    - Peripheral concentric layers of epithelioid cells, Langhans giant cells, lymphocytes, and fibroblasts
    - Organisms may be identified by using special stains
    - *M. tuberculosis* is most common cause of caseating granulomas
  - Noncaseating granulomas
    - Composed of collection of epithelioid cells, Langhans giant cells, lymphocytes, and histiocytes
- Foreign body type
  - Caused by inert substances, such as talc, suture, lipid
    - Usually no necrosis
  - Can often detect foreign body by using polarized light

ANCILLARY TESTS

Immunohistochemistry
- Mycobacterial antigens can be detected and typed with monoclonal antibodies conjugated to peroxidase

PCR
- Highly sensitive and has identified infectious agents in diseases that previously had no known etiology

Special Stains
- Acid-fast bacilli can be demonstrated by Ziehl-Neelsen, Kinyoun, or Fite-Faraco stain
- Fungal-like organisms can be highlighted with PAS or GMS stain

Granulomatous Lymphadenitis, Infectious and Sarcoid

- Gram-positive and gram-negative organisms can be seen with Gram stain
- Parasites can be highlighted by Giemsa stain
- Warthin-Starry stain for *Bartonella henselae* (cat-scratch disease) or *Treponema pallidum* (syphilis)

DIFFERENTIAL DIAGNOSIS

M. tuberculosis Lymphadenitis

- Decreasing incidence in resource-rich nations
  - Except resurgence has occurred in HIV(+) patients
- Common in resource-limited countries and immigrants to resource-rich countries
- Common lymph node groups: Cervical, supraclavicular
- Abnormal chest radiograph common
- Positive tuberculin test
- Cultures for *M. tuberculosis* are reliable but slow
  - Organism grows slowly over weeks
- PCR is rapid and reliable alternative method for diagnosis

Atypical Mycobacterial Lymphadenitis

- There are number of nontuberculous or atypical mycobacteria
  - Most common include
    - *Mycobacterium marinum, Mycobacterium fortuitum, Mycobacterium kansasii*
    - *Mycobacterium scrofulaceum, Mycobacterium avium-intracellulare*
- *M. marinum* has been associated with swimming pool use
- *M. kansasii* causes infection of cervical lymph nodes in children
  - Also displays increased prevalence in patients with hairy cell leukemia
- *M. scrofulaceum* is known for causing cervical lymphadenitis, a.k.a. scrofula in children
- *M. avium-intracellulare* is common in HIV(+) patients

Fungal Lymphadenitis

- Number of fungi can infect lymph nodes and cause granulomatous lymphadenitis
  - Common organisms include
    - *Histoplasma capsulatum, Blastomyces dermatitidis, Paracoccidioides brasiliensis*
    - *Coccidioides immitis, Sporothrix schenckii, Cryptococcus neoformans*
    - *Aspergillus, Mucor,* and *Candida* in immunodeficient patients
  - Histoplasmosis is most common in North America
    - Endemic in central United States
    - Dimorphic fungus with narrow-based budding yeasts at body temperature
  - Cytologic findings
    - Granulomas are often associated with acute inflammation
    - Yeast forms are intracellular within histiocytes on GMS stain
    - Caseation is often not prominent

Sarcoidosis

- More common in Black than White or Asian patients
- Multisystemic disease of unknown etiology
- Hypercalcemia, hypergammaglobulinemia, and elevated angiotensin-converting enzyme common
- Kveim test positive
- Commonly involves lymph nodes and lungs, but any site can be affected
- Cytologic findings
  - Nonnecrotizing/noncaseating granulomas

Nonmycobacterial Infections of Lymph Nodes

- Number of bacterial infections can cause granulomatous lymphadenitis
- Examples of organisms include
  - *B. henselae*, gram-negative bacillus that causes cat-scratch disease
    - Granulomas occur late, often with suppuration
  - *Chlamydia* serotypes L1, L2, and L3 cause lymphogranuloma venereum
    - Typically involve inguinal lymph nodes
    - Granulomas occur late, often with suppuration
  - *Brucella abortus, Brucella melitensis,* or *Brucella suis*
    - Related to consumption of unpasteurized milk or cheese
    - Lymph nodes show granulomatous inflammation often associated with suppuration
  - *Francisella tularensis*
    - History of handling rabbits
    - Lymphadenopathy can be prominent
    - Lymph nodes show granulomatous inflammation often associated with suppuration
  - *T. pallidum* (syphilis)
    - Chronic granulomatous inflammation is uncommon but can occur
    - Granulomas are typically noncaseating
    - Spirochetes on Warthin-Starry stain
    - Antitreponemal antibodies detected by serology tests

Foreign Body Granulomas

- Number of foreign bodies can cause chronic granulomatous lymphadenitis
  - Lipid: Causes lipogranulomas
  - Talc: Presents as result of previous surgical procedure

DIAGNOSTIC CHECKLIST

Clinically Relevant Pathologic Features

- Chronic granulomatous lymphadenitis has large number of causes
- Microbiologic cultures/special stains are essential component of aspiration

SELECTED REFERENCES

1. Faraz M et al: Reactive lymphadenopathies. Clin Lab Med. 41(3):433-51, 2021
2. Gosavi AV et al: FNAC of lymph nodes in HIV positive patients-a diagnostic boon. J Am Soc Cytopathol. 6(2):59-65, 2017
3. Madan K et al: Conventional transbronchial needle aspiration versus endobronchial ultrasound-guided transbronchial needle aspiration, with or without rapid on-site evaluation, for the diagnosis of sarcoidosis: a randomized controlled trial. J Bronchology Interv Pulmonol. 24(1):48-58, 2017

Granulomatous Lymphadenitis, Infectious and Sarcoid

Sarcoidosis, Boomerang-Shaped Nuclei

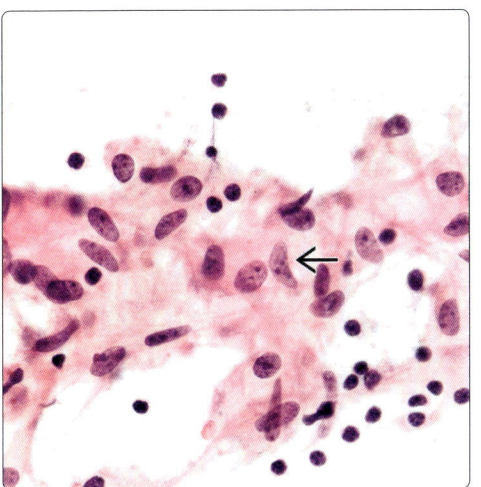

Cryptococcus neoformans

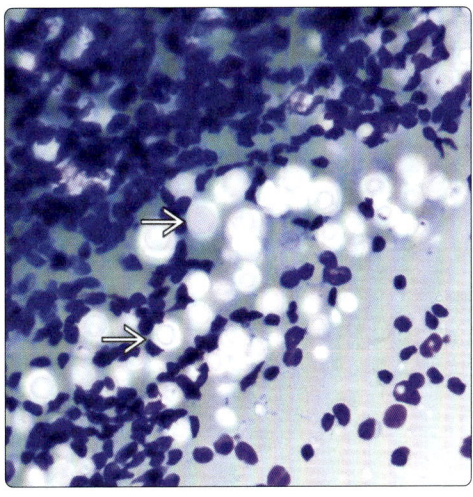

(Left) Pap-stained FNA smear of a lymph node aspiration from a patient with sarcoidosis shows epithelioid histiocytes with a characteristic boomerang shape ➡. (Right) Diff-Quik-stained FNA smear shows many yeast forms ➡ of variable sizes surrounded by a clear halo, consistent with Cryptococcus neoformans.

Mycobacterium tuberculosis, Ziehl-Neelsen Stain

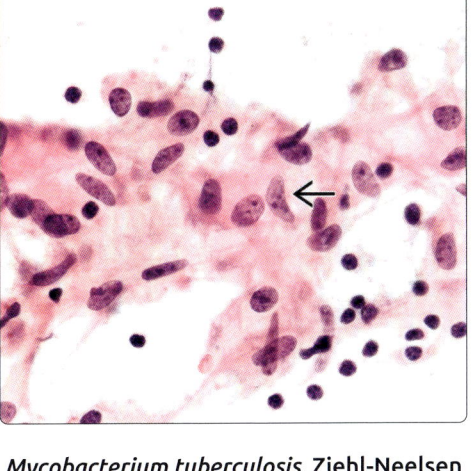

Mycobacterium tuberculosis, Negative Image on Diff-Quik

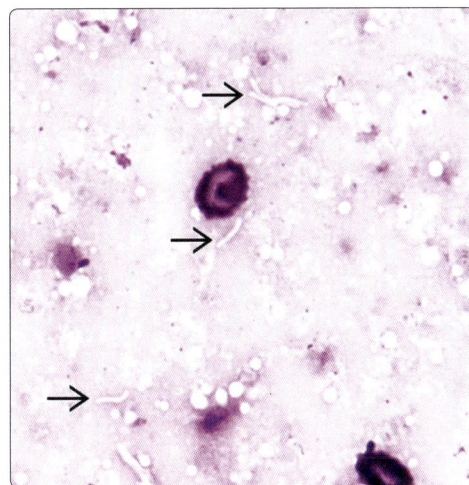

(Left) Ziehl-Neelsen stain of a cell block section shows many acid-fast bacilli with prominent beading of the red stain ➡. (Right) Under oil immersion, negative images of Mycobacterium tuberculosis ➡ can be seen on a Diff-Quik stain. Nocardia also produces negative images but they are more elongate.

Histoplasma capsulatum

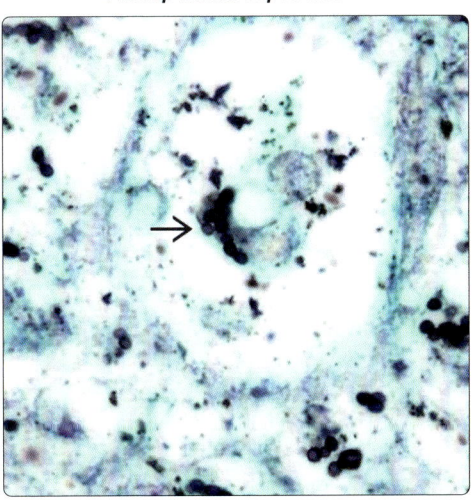

Coccidioides immitis

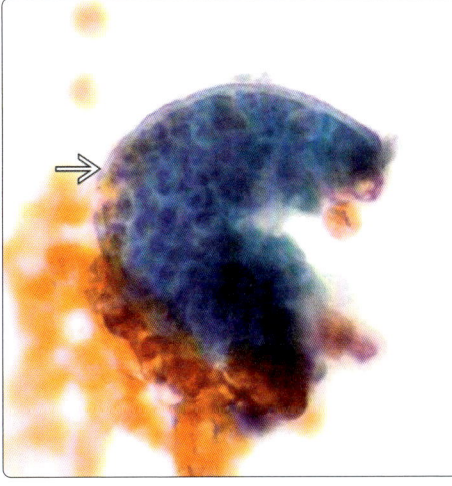

(Left) GMS stain of a cell block section shows numerous intracellular organisms of histoplasmosis ➡. (Right) Rarely, intact Coccidioides immitis spherules containing endospores ➡ may be seen on Pap-stained aspirate smears. (Courtesy M. Amrikachi, MD.)

Rosai-Dorfman Disease

KEY FACTS

TERMINOLOGY
- Benign proliferation of histiocytes with characteristic cytologic features

CLINICAL ISSUES
- Usually asymptomatic adenopathy in young patients
- Extranodal sites involved in ~ 40% of patients
- Spontaneous regression occurs in most patients
- No specific therapy is required except rare aggressive subset

CYTOPATHOLOGY
- Rosai-Dorfman disease (RDD) histiocytes
  - Large size with abundant eosinophilic cytoplasm
  - Defined cell border
  - Emperipolesis is usual
- Round, vesicular nucleus
  - Distinct central nucleolus

ANCILLARY TESTS
- Immunohistochemistry
  - S100, CD1a, langerin (-)
- Histiocyte markers: CD4(+/-); CD14, CD68, CD163 (+)
- B-cell antigens, T-cell antigens (-)

TOP DIFFERENTIAL DIAGNOSES
- Langerhans cell histiocytosis
  - Cells have twisted nuclei with nuclear grooves
  - No emperipolesis
  - S100, CD1a, langerin/CD207 (+)
- Chronic granulomatous inflammation
  - Epithelioid histiocytes and multinucleated cells
  - Histiocytes do not resemble RDD histiocytes
  - S100 (focal -/+)
- Kikuchi lymphadenitis
  - No emperipolesis
  - Necrosis without neutrophils

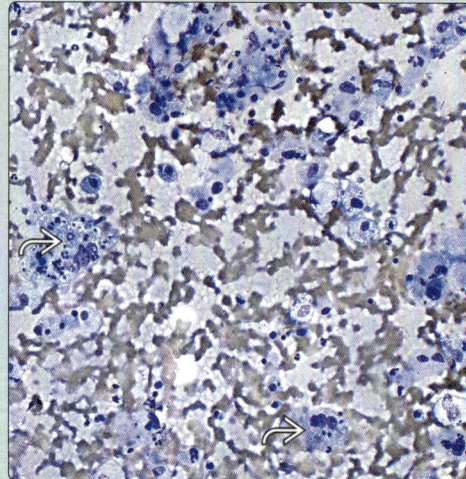
Rosai-Dorfman Disease Histiocytes

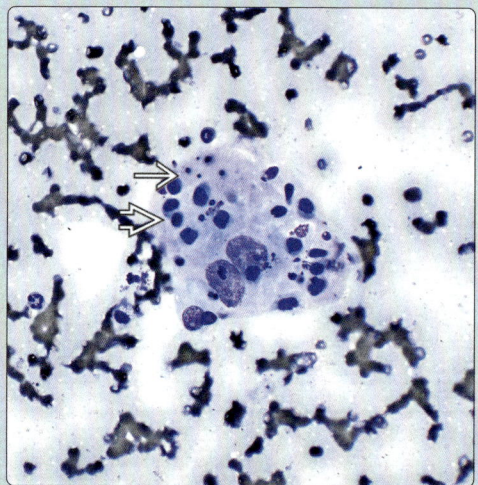
Intracytoplasmic Lymphocytes and Tingible Debris

(Left) Diff-Quik-stained FNA smear shows histiocytes, including some that demonstrate varying degrees of emperipolesis ➡ with lymphocytes and tingible debris in the cytoplasm. (Right) Diff-Quik-stained FNA smear shows a Rosai-Dorfman disease histiocyte containing lymphocytes ➡ and sparse tingible debris ➡.

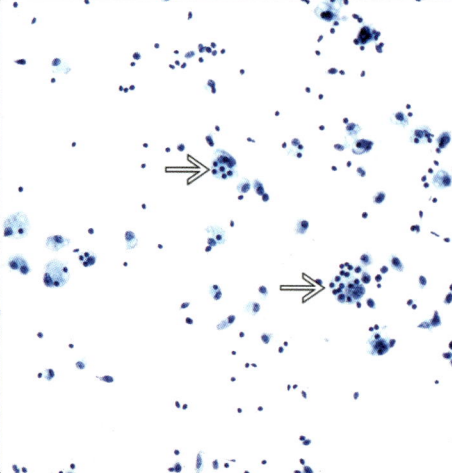
Emperipolesis

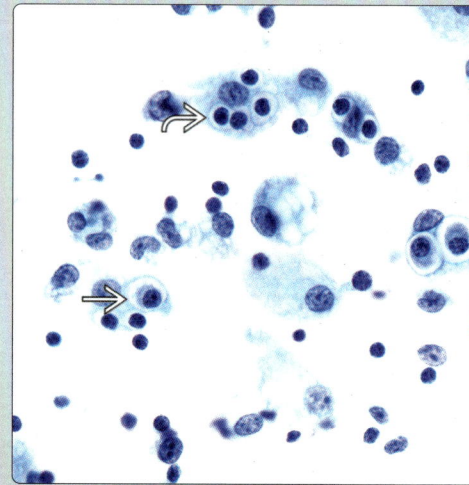
Viable Lymphocytes and Plasma Cells Within Cytoplasm

(Left) Pap-stained FNA smear shows Rosai-Dorfman disease histiocytes with variable numbers of lymphocytes in the background. Note that some of the histiocytes demonstrate significant emperipolesis ➡. (Right) Pap-stained FNA smear shows histiocytes exhibiting emperipolesis. Note that the lymphocytes ➡ and plasma cells ➡ appear viable and enclosed in a defined space within the cytoplasm of the Rosai-Dorfman disease histiocyte.

Rosai-Dorfman Disease

TERMINOLOGY

Abbreviations
- Rosai-Dorfman disease (RDD)

Synonyms
- Sinus histiocytosis with massive lymphadenopathy

Definitions
- Benign proliferation of histiocytes with characteristic cytologic features

CLINICAL ISSUES

Site
- Lymph nodes; extranodal sites in ~ 40% of patients
  - Head and neck region are commonly involved
  - Almost any site can be involved

Presentation
- Lymphadenopathy, often without symptoms
- Can be associated with Hodgkin or non-Hodgkin lymphomas

Prognosis
- Excellent for most affected patients
- Rare cases can be clinically aggressive

CYTOPATHOLOGY

Cells
- RDD histiocytes are characterized by large size with abundant cytoplasm and well-defined cell borders

Nuclear Details
- Round, vesicular nucleus with small central nucleolus

Cytoplasmic Details
- Emperipolesis is typical but can be absent in extranodal sites

ANCILLARY TESTS

Immunohistochemistry
- RDD histiocytes
  - S100(+); CD1a, langerin/CD207
  - Histiocyte markers: CD4(+/-); CD14, CD68, CD163 (+)
  - Adhesion molecules: CD11b, CD11c, CD18, CD31 (+)
  - B-cell antigens, T-cell antigens (-)
- Intracytoplasmic T and B cells
- Plasma cells are polytypic

Flow Cytometry
- Polytypic B cells
- T cells with normal immunophenotype

DIFFERENTIAL DIAGNOSIS

Langerhans Cell Histiocytosis
- Eosinophils and necrosis are common
- Cells have twisted nuclei with nuclear grooves
  - Less cytoplasm than RDD histiocytes
  - No emperipolesis
- Birbeck granules demonstrated by electron microscopy
- S100, CD1a, langerin/CD207 (+)

Chronic Granulomatous Inflammation
- Associated necrosis and acute/chronic inflammation
- Epithelioid histiocytes and multinucleated cells
  - Histiocytes do not resemble RDD histiocytes
  - S100 (focal -/+)

Kikuchi Lymphadenitis
- No emperipolesis
- Necrosis without neutrophils

SELECTED REFERENCES
1. Doglioni C: Rosai-Dorfman disease. A legacy of Professor Rosai that is still not exploited completely. Pathologica. 113(5):388-95, 2021
2. Bruce-Brand C et al: Rosai-Dorfman disease: an overview. J Clin Pathol. 73(11):697-705, 2020

Large Histiocyte Containing Many Lymphocytes

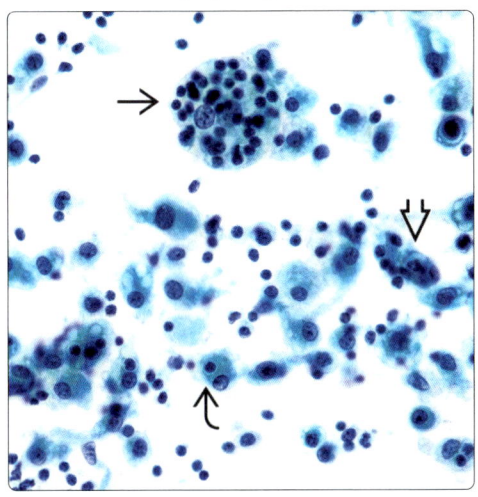

Ill-Defined Clusters of Histiocytes

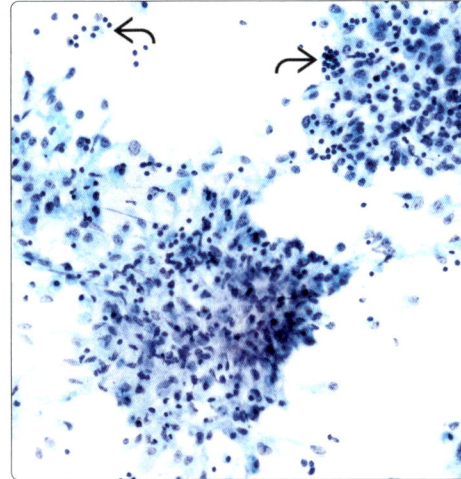

(Left) Pap-stained FNA smear shows a large histiocytoid cell containing > 30 lymphocytes ➡. Smaller cells contain 1 or 2 lymphocytes ➡ or (rarely) neutrophils ➡. (Right) Pap-stained FNA smear shows ill-defined clusters of histiocytes, including some that demonstrate emperipolesis ➡.

Metastatic Malignancies (Carcinoma, Melanoma)

KEY FACTS

CLINICAL ISSUES
- Usually history of prior malignancy
- May be initial presentation
- Cervical lymphadenopathy: Head and neck, skin, thyroid, lung, and oral cavity most likely
- Axillary: Breast and lung most likely
- Supraclavicular: Lung, breast, and genitourinary most likely
- Inguinal: Genitourinary, gynecologic, gastrointestinal, and skin most likely

CYTOPATHOLOGY
- Hyperchromatic nuclei with sharp angulations, dense, glassy cytoplasm in squamous cell carcinoma
- Vesicular chromatin and prominent nucleoli in adenocarcinomas in general
- Elongated, cigar-shaped hyperchromatic nuclei in large bowel primary
- Nuclear molding, increased cellular dyshesion, high N:C ratio, and coarse chromatin in high-grade neuroendocrine carcinomas
- Melanoma may have any nuclear pattern but often shows prominent nucleoli or intranuclear cytoplasmic inclusions and binucleation and may have cytoplasmic pigment

ANCILLARY TESTS
- Squamous cell carcinoma: p63, p40
- Lung: TTF-1, CK7, napsin A
- Thyroid: TTF-1, thyroglobulin, CK7
- Breast: Mammaglobin, ER, PR, GATA3
- Kidney: RCC, CD10, PAX8
- Liver: HepPar1, glypican-3, arginase-1
- Ovary: WT1, PAX8
- Large intestine: CK20, CDX2, villin
- Prostate: PSA, PAP, NKX3.1
- Melanoma: S100, Melan-A, HMB-45, SOX10

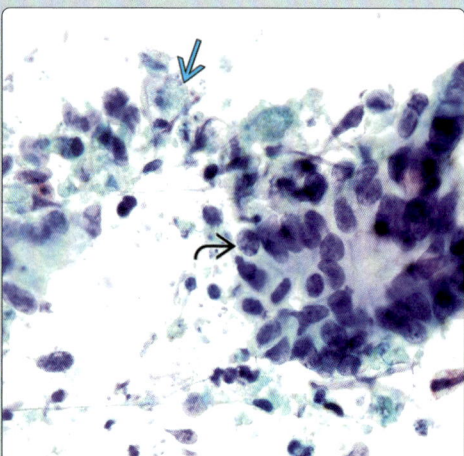

Cigar-Shaped Hyperchromatic Nuclei

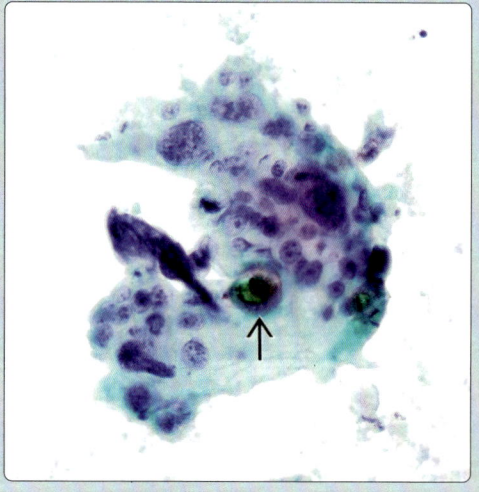

Psammoma Bodies and Pleomorphic Cells

(Left) On Pap stain, a smear of a metastatic colorectal adenocarcinoma often consists of elongated (cigar-shaped) hyperchromatic nuclei ⇨ in a "dirty", necrotic background ⇨. (Right) Malignant cells that are highly pleomorphic, often with associated psammoma bodies ⇨ and cytoplasm that may contain large vacuoles, favors a papillary serous carcinoma, usually from the ovary, as seen in this Pap stain.

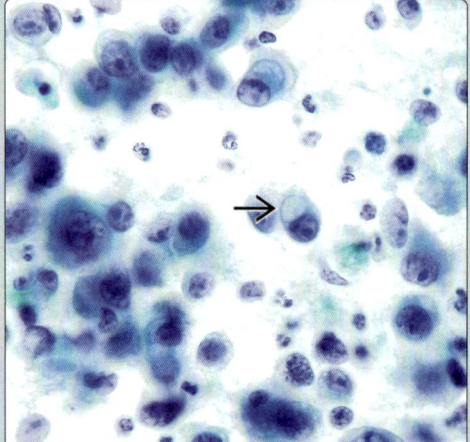

Intracytoplasmic Mucin

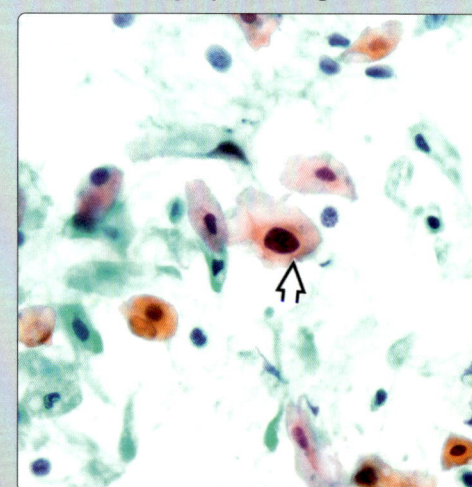

Keratinized Cytoplasm, Angulated Nuclei

(Left) An adenocarcinoma that consists of relatively small cells and shows intracytoplasmic mucin ⇨ suggests stomach or breast origin. (Right) This Pap stain shows angulated, hyperchromatic nuclei ⇨ of a keratinizing squamous cell carcinoma.

Metastatic Malignancies (Carcinoma, Melanoma)

CLINICAL ISSUES

Presentation
- ± history of prior malignancy
  - May be initial presentation
- Cervical lymphadenopathy: Head and neck, skin, thyroid, lung, and oral cavity most likely
- Axillary: Breast and lung most likely
- Supraclavicular: Lung, breast, and genitourinary most likely
- Inguinal: Genitourinary, gynecologic, gastrointestinal, and skin most likely

CYTOPATHOLOGY

Pattern
- Generally cellular smears
- Carcinomas generally show some degree of cohesion
- Melanomas may be cohesive or dyshesive
- High-grade neuroendocrine carcinomas (NECs) and melanomas may be dyshesive and raise possibility of lymphoma
  - Material for flow cytometry may be requested at adequacy check to help with differential
- Features of adenocarcinoma and squamous carcinoma in lung, pancreas, and urothelial carcinoma
  - Cercariform cells may be seen in urothelial carcinoma
- If bland cells in small acinar pattern, then think prostate

Background
- Any malignancy (especially high grade) may show associated necrosis, but large bowel primaries ("dirty" necrosis) and small cell carcinomas are classically described as having necrosis in background
- Associated endothelial cells in renal cell carcinoma and NECs
- Psammoma bodies in papillary adenocarcinomas
- Mucin may be seen in background of adenocarcinomas
- Tigroid background is classically associated with seminomas

Nuclear Details
- May vary from small and bland (think breast, stomach) to overtly malignant
- Hyperchromatic nuclei with sharp angulations in squamous cell carcinoma
- Elongated, cigar-shaped hyperchromatic nuclei in large bowel primary
- Vesicular chromatin and prominent nucleoli in adenocarcinomas in general
- Melanoma may exhibit any nuclear pattern but often has eccentrically placed (plasmacytoid) nuclei, binucleation, prominent nucleoli, or intranuclear cytoplasmic inclusions
  - May show epithelioid, small cell, or spindle pattern
    - Spindle shape may suggest sarcoma, but sarcomas rarely metastasize to lymph nodes
- Nuclear molding, increased cellular dyshesion, high N:C ratio, and coarse chromatin in high-grade NECs

Cytoplasmic Details
- Dense/glassy cytoplasm in squamous cell carcinoma
- Intracytoplasmic mucin dot in adenocarcinomas (often breast or stomach)
- Larger vacuoles/clear cytoplasm in ovary, thyroid, lung, and renal cell carcinoma
- Melanoma may or may not display cytoplasmic pigment

ANCILLARY TESTS

Immunohistochemistry
- Lung: TTF-1, CK7, napsin A
- Breast: Mammaglobin, ER, PR, GATA3
- Kidney: RCC, CD10, PAX8
- Ovary: WT1, PAX8, arginase-1
- NEC: CD56, synaptophysin, chromogranin, TTF-1, INSM1
- Melanoma: S100, Melan-A, HMB-45, SOX10

SELECTED REFERENCES
1. Bellizzi AM: An algorithmic immunohistochemical approach to define tumor type and assign site of origin. Adv Anat Pathol. 27(3):114-63, 2020

Cohesive Epithelioid Cells
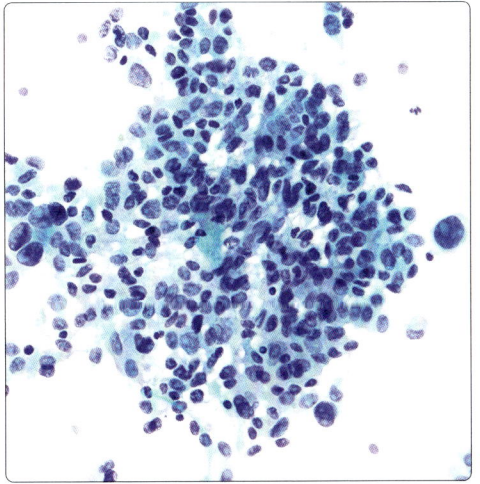

Amelanotic Melanoma
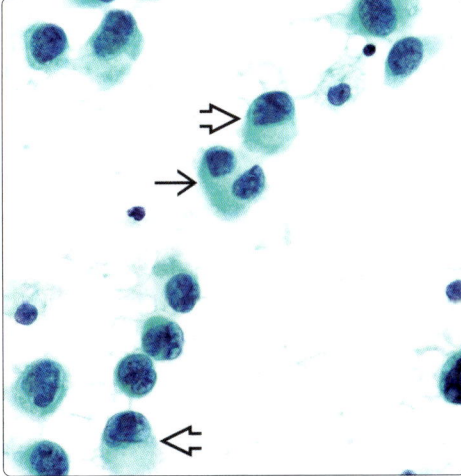

(Left) Pap stain shows a cohesive group of epithelioid cells with marked pleomorphism. Although the features are suggestive of a carcinoma, this is actually an example of nonpigmented melanoma. (Right) This is another example of a melanoma that lacks pigment on Pap stain. The presence of plasmacytoid cells ⇨ and binucleation ⇨ suggests melanoma.

HPV-Positive Head and Neck Squamous Cell Carcinoma

KEY FACTS

ETIOLOGY/PATHOGENESIS
- 90-95% associated with HPV-16
- Differs from conventional squamous cell carcinoma, major risk factors of which are cigarette smoking, other tobacco use, and heavy alcohol use

CLINICAL ISSUES
- There has been dramatic increase in incidence of oropharyngeal HPV-positive squamous carcinoma
- Different demographics and molecular biology; better prognosis than conventional head and neck squamous carcinoma
- Cervical lymphadenopathy is most common presentation
- Cervical nodes are often large and cystic (clue for HPV-positive squamous carcinoma)

CYTOPATHOLOGY
- Cohesive fragments of basaloid cells, generally nonkeratinizing
- Intermediate-sized hyperchromatic nuclei
- More single cells and smaller groups in FNA of cystic nodal component

ANCILLARY TESTS
- IHC for p16
- High-risk HPV DNA by in situ hybridization
- PCR for high-risk HPV DNA
- HPV E6/E7 mRNA in situ hybridization
- Liquid-based assays (as used for cervicovaginal cytology)
- **Please also see College of American Pathologists (CAP) consensus guidelines (2018) for details**

TOP DIFFERENTIAL DIAGNOSES
- Conventional squamous cell carcinoma
- Small cell carcinoma
- Nasopharyngeal carcinoma
- Merkel cell carcinoma

Cystic Squamous Cell Carcinoma Lymph Node Aspirate

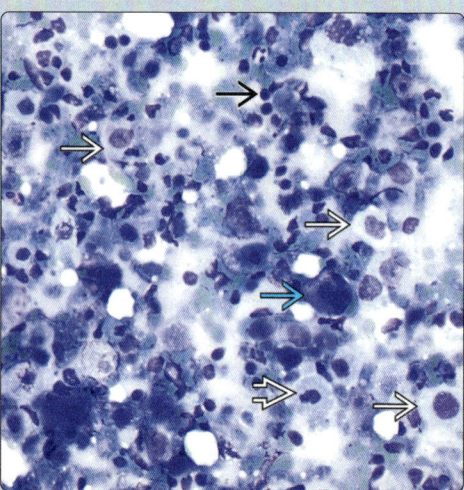

Abrupt Keratinization

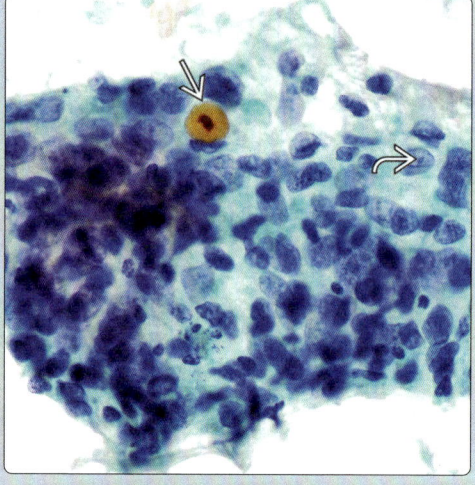

(Left) Diff-Quik-stained smear from a cystic neck node aspirate shows large malignant cells ➡ with dense/hard ➡ cytoplasm. Cells in varying stages of degeneration ➡ are also seen. See background lymphocytes ➡ for size comparison. *(Right)* Pap stain shows focal abrupt keratinization ➡, more vesicular chromatin, and small nucleoli ➡, which may occasionally be seen in this type of carcinoma.

Metastatic HPV-Positive Squamous Cell Carcinoma

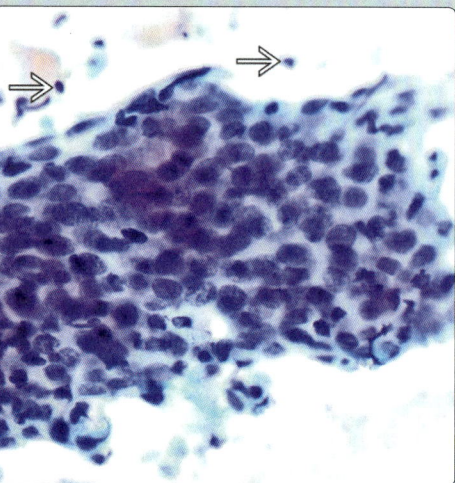

p16 IHC and High-Risk HPV In Situ Hybridization

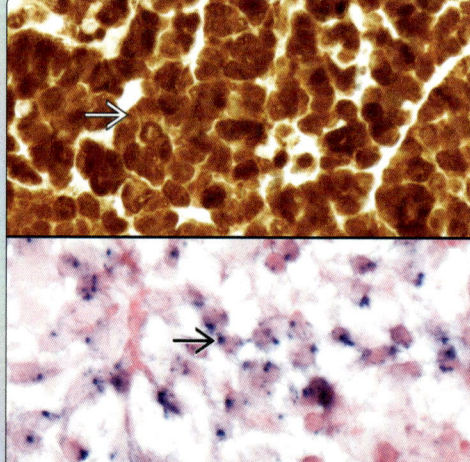

(Left) Pap-stained smear of a cervical lymph node aspirate shows a fragment of metastatic nonkeratinizing squamous cell carcinoma. Note background lymphocytes ➡ for size comparison. *(Right)* IHC stain for p16 shows diffuse strong nuclear and cytoplasmic immunoreactivity ➡. In situ hybridization for high-risk HPV RNA shows positive nuclear and cytoplasmic signal ➡ in this HPV-positive head and neck squamous cell carcinoma.

HPV-Positive Head and Neck Squamous Cell Carcinoma

TERMINOLOGY

Definitions
- HPV-positive head and neck squamous cell carcinoma (HNSqCa)
  - Terms "basaloid" or "poorly differentiated" not recommended, as can be confused with basaloid variant, which is clinically more aggressive
  - Tumor grading not recommended, as classic grading does not correlate with biologic behavior, prognosis, or clinical outcome in HPV-positive SqCa
  - Most are nonkeratinizing SqCas
  - Less common variants of oropharyngeal SqCa (OPSqCa) include those with papillary, basaloid, adenosquamous, sarcomatoid, and lymphoepithelioma-like features

ETIOLOGY/PATHOGENESIS

Infectious Agents
- 90-95% associated with HPV-16
- Integration of host DNA into host genome leads to increased transcription of HPV oncoproteins E6 and E7; E6 overexpression leads to proteolytic degradation of p53, which results in accumulation of DNA aberrations
- Major risk factor: Increased number of sexual partners
- Greater risk for oral-genital and oral-anal sex
- Cigarette smoking and immunosuppression may be additional corisk factors
- Differs from conventional SqCa, major risk factors of which are cigarette smoking, other tobacco use, and heavy alcohol use
- HPV-positive HNSqCa (oropharyngeal) has better prognosis than conventional smoking-related HNSqCa
- HPV-positive small cell carcinoma has poor prognosis

CLINICAL ISSUES

Epidemiology
- Dramatic increase over past 5 decades compared to marked decreased incidence of smoking-related HNSqCa (viral "epidemic")
- OPSqCa now accounts for > 30% of all HNSqCas in USA
- Currently, > 80% of OPSqCa in USA are HPV positive
- Age and sex: Mostly men 40-60 years of age and higher socioeconomic status; average age has been drifting up in recent years
- Conventional smoking-related SqCa: Mostly men > 60 years

Site
- Mostly oropharyngeal, especially tonsil and base of tongue
- HPV detected in 8-30% of sinonasal SqCa
- HPV DNA is detected in variable percentage of HNSqCa at nonoropharyngeal sites, but HPV status not associated with better prognosis or better therapeutic response at these sites
- Therefore, no current indication to test for HPV status outside of oropharynx or nodal metastasis

Presentation
- Most present with low T stage (T1-2) with small or occult primaries
- Often present with advanced N stage (N2-3)
- Cervical lymphadenopathy is most common presentation
- Cervical nodes are often large and cystic, clue for HPV-positive OPSqCa
- It is usually nodal metastases, which are aspirated, as primaries are difficult to access
- Determination of HPV status in level 2 or level 3 cervical lymph node of unknown primary (CUP) may be helpful in identifying occult oropharyngeal primary

Treatment
- Radiotherapy ± chemotherapy, surgery, immunotherapy with more aggressive therapy for higher stage disease
- Clinical trials of transoral robotic surgery (TORS) as part of multimodality therapy
- Clinical trials assessing whether therapy can be deescalated (deintensified) to reduce significant treatment-associated morbidity

CYTOPATHOLOGY

Cellularity
- Generally cellular or cystic
  - Aspirates of cystic component are less cellular or paucicellular unless wall of cystic area is sampled
- Patients generally present with cervical lymphadenopathy
  - Primary tumors are generally small and hard to access
  - Hence, usual cytologic assessment is FNA of enlarged node

Pattern
- Mostly cohesive fragments of variable size, some looser
- Single cells and small groups if cystic

Background
- Lymph node metastasis with cystic component may have predominantly macrophages, inflammatory cells, anucleate squamous cells, and degenerated nucleated cells
- Variable number of lymphocytes, depending on how much of node is replaced by tumor

Cells
- Most have basaloid appearance
- Uncommonly, have small cell carcinoma or undifferentiated carcinoma morphology

Nuclear Details
- Most commonly, intermediate-sized hyperchromatic nuclei without enlarged nucleoli
- Undifferentiated pattern has larger nucleus with vesicular chromatin and prominent nucleolus
- May see nuclear molding, increased mitosis, apoptosis

Cytoplasmic Details
- Generally nonkeratinizing with scant cytoplasm
  - Occasionally may see abruptly keratinized cells
  - Less commonly may be keratinizing

Cell Block Findings
- Helpful for IHC staining for p16, in situ hybridization, or other tests for HPV status

ANCILLARY TESTS

Immunohistochemistry
- p16 is surrogate marker for transcriptionally active HPV

- Can be performed on tissue biopsies or cell block of FNA; some perform on smears but harder to control variables and less data on cut-off values
- No consensus on what cut-off for positive p16 should be in cell blocks; reported cut-offs range from any staining to nuclear and cytoplasmic staining of ≥ 70% of tumor cells

In Situ Hybridization
- DNA in situ hybridization for HPV: More specific but less sensitive than PCR
- E6/E7 mRNA in situ hybridization: More sensitive than DNA in situ hybridization; detection of mRNA E6/E7 transcripts generally regarded as gold standard for HPV detection
- Can be performed using automated IHC equipment

PCR and Other
- PCR for HPV DNA may be too sensitive; may not be able to distinguish between passenger virus or viral contamination and clinically relevant HPV integrated into host genome
- Commercial methods for high-risk (HR) HPV detection: Hybrid Capture II, Cervista, Roche cobas, Aptima
  - Support that carcinoma is HPV positive
  - Help to identify most likely primary site (most HPV-positive HNSqCas are oropharyngeal)
  - Guide treatment and selection for clinical trials
  - Help distinguish new 2nd primary SqCa from metastasis in patient with HPV-positive HNSqCa

Highlights of College of American Pathologists (CAP) Consensus Guidelines (2018)
- CAP consensus evidence-based guidelines recommend assessing HPV status on primary or nodal metastasis of all newly diagnosed OPSqCa; for tissue biopsies, recommend IHC for p16 or nodal metastasis
- For tissue biopsies of oropharyngeal primary or of level 2 or 3 cervical nodal metastases, > 70% nuclear and cytoplasmic staining considered supportive of diagnosis of HPV-positive (p16-positive) SqCa
- HPV-specific testing recommended for patients with positive IHC staining for p16 who have multisite tumor involving oropharynx, level of cervical node sampled not known, or nonclassic morphology of nodal metastasis
- Because of limited published data, no recommendation was made for or against any specific testing methodology for HPV testing of FNAs

DIFFERENTIAL DIAGNOSIS

Conventional Squamous Cell Carcinoma
- More keratinized cells; IHC for p16 and HPV is negative

Basaloid Variant of Squamous Cell Carcinoma
- Clinical history; IHC for p16/HPV testing is negative

Small Cell Carcinoma
- Less cellular cohesion, more single cells, fragile nuclei with chromatin streaking
- Both small cell carcinoma and HPV-positive HNSqCa have absent or small nucleoli, scant cytoplasm, and nuclear molding

Nasopharyngeal Carcinoma
- Vesicular chromatin and prominent nucleoli vs. hyperchromasia and absence of prominent nucleoli in typical HPV-positive HNSqCa
- Associated with EBV; lymph nodes often in posterior triangle

Merkel Cell Carcinoma
- Clinical history of skin nodule in sun-exposed skin, usually in older individual
- Loosely cohesive and dyshesive and finer chromatin vs. cohesive fragments in HPV-positive HNSqCa
- Synaptophysin, chromogranin, and CK20 positive by IHC

Medullary Carcinoma
- Clinical history of thyroid nodule
- Polymorphous population of cells, which may have intranuclear inclusions
- May see fine neuroendocrine granules on Diff-Quik
- Calcitonin, CEA, TTF-1, synaptophysin, chromogranin are positive by IHC

Adenoid Cystic Carcinoma
- Less nuclear pleomorphism; more uniform acinar structures with more abundant intraluminal basement membrane material

Malignant Lymphoma
- Noncohesive cells, immunophenotyping by flow cytometry or IHC

Branchial Cleft Cyst
- Carefully search for atypical squamous cells to rule out HPV-positive HNSqCa
- p16 IHC is often positive (diagnostic pitfall)
- Have high suspicion for cystic neck masses in adults
  - Consider HR-HPV testing

DIAGNOSTIC CHECKLIST

Pathologic Interpretation Pearls
- Metastatic nonkeratinizing carcinoma in cystic level 2 or 3 cervical lymph nodes is most often metastasis from HPV-positive OPSqCa
- Strong diffuse nuclear and cytoplasmic IHC staining for p16 supportive with classic morphology and site
- No current consensus on threshold for defining p16 positivity in FNAs
- When nonclassic cytomorphology in level 2 or 3 cervical nodal metastasis or exact site of cervical nodal metastasis not known, recommend additional HPV-specific testing to assess HR-HPV status

HPV-Related Multiphenotypic Sinonasal Carcinoma
- Formerly known as HPV-related carcinoma with adenoid cystic-like features
- Arises in nasal cavity and paranasal cavity; typically surgical biopsy/resection, but touch preps for ROSE may be encountered in cytology
- ~ 1/3 of patients have local recurrence and few have distant metastasis; in contrast to HPV-positive OPSqCa, it does not metastasize to lymph nodes

HPV-Positive Head and Neck Squamous Cell Carcinoma

HPV-Positive Squamous Cell Carcinoma and Mimics

	HPV-Positive Squamous Carcinoma	Non-HPV Squamous Carcinoma	Small Cell Carcinoma	Nasopharyngeal Carcinoma	Merkel Cell Carcinoma
Primary site	Oropharynx	Head and neck, lung, skin, other	Lung, head and neck, other	Nasopharynx	Skin
Cell type	Nonkeratinizing, may have focal abrupt keratinization; rarely undifferentiated or keratinizing	Variable (keratinizing and nonkeratinizing)	Small blue cells	Dyshesive epithelioid undifferentiated cells with high N:C ratio; rarely keratinizing and nonkeratinizing variants	Small blue cells (small cell carcinoma of skin)
IHC	p16(+), p40(+)	p16(-), p40(+)	Chromogranin, CD56, synaptophysin all (+), TTF-1(+) (lung)	p40(+) p16 may be (+)	CK20 [dot-like (+)], chromogranin (+), synaptophysin (+), CM2B4 (anti-MCPyV) (+)
Molecular	HR-HPV(+) (usually HPV-16)	HR-HPV(-)	HR-HPV(-), unless rare oropharyngeal primary small cell carcinoma	HR-HPV(-) EBV by ISH (EBER) (+)	Polyomavirus (by ISH or PCR)

HR-HPV = high-risk HPV; ISH = in situ hybridization.

- Less aggressive behavior than sinonasal SqCa, sinonasal undifferentiated carcinoma, and *SMARCB1*-deficient sinonasal carcinoma
- Epithelial and myoepithelial differentiation with solid nests of basaloid cells having focal cribriform and occasional tubule formation
- May have squamous, chondroid, and other sarcomatoid differentiation
- HPV positive, mainly HPV-33; p16 positive

CAP Consensus Guidelines (2018)

- Multidisciplinary expert panel convened by CAP recently published evidenced-based guidelines for testing for HPV in head and neck cancer; these guidelines were vetted by multiple cancer and other subspecialty societies
- Guidelines are currently being updated based on review of recent published literature
- Key recommendations of 2018 guidelines include
  o All patients with newly diagnosed OPSqCa, including all histologic subtypes, should have HR-HPV testing on primary tumor or regional lymph node metastasis
  o Routine HR-HPV testing should **not** be performed on nonsquamous OPSqCa or on nonoropharyngeal primary head and neck cancers, as HPV status in these subtypes and at these sites is not associated with statistically significant better outcome
  o If HPV status is known, HPV testing should **not** be repeated on locoregional recurrences or persistent tumor
  o Routine HR-HPV testing should not be performed on distant metastases if HPV status of primary is known; however, HR-HPV testing may be performed if there is uncertainty about whether tumor is metastasis or new primary (e.g., SqCa in lung)
  o Routine HR-HPV testing should be performed on all metastatic SqCa of unknown primary in cervical level 2 of 3 lymph node or cervical lymph node where exact site not known
  o For tissue, IHC for p16, surrogate marker for transcriptionally active HPV, should be performed on oropharyngeal biopsies and on cervical nodal metastases; algorithm is provided for when additional HPV-specific testing (PCR, in situ hybridization) is needed
  o HR-HPV testing should be performed on head and neck FNAs of SqCa from all patients with known OPSqCa not previously tested for HR-HPV, with suspected OPSqCa, or with metastatic SqCa of unknown primary in cervical lymph node; if FNA is HR-HPV-negative, testing should be repeated if tissue becomes available
  o There is currently insufficient data to recommend specific testing modality for HR-HPV testing in FNAs
  o If IHC for p16 is used on FNAs, pathologists need to validate cut-off for defining positive result
  o There is **no** role for routine testing for low-risk HPV in HNSqCa; low-risk HPV does not drive HPV-positive OPSqCa
  o Smoking history should not modify approach to HR-HPV testing since smoking does not directly alter results of p16 IHC or HPV-specific testing; however, multiple studies have shown that tobacco use is associated with decreased survival and lower locoregional therapeutic response among those with HPV-positive OPSqCa

SELECTED REFERENCES

1. Ribeiro EA et al: p16 immunostaining in cytology specimens: its application, expression, interpretation, and challenges. J Am Soc Cytopathol. 10(4):414-22, 2021
2. Lewis JS Jr et al: Human papillomavirus testing in head and neck carcinomas: guideline from the College of American Pathologists. Arch Pathol Lab Med. 142(5):559-97, 2018

Small Lymphocytic Lymphoma

KEY FACTS

CLINICAL ISSUES
- Presents as generalized lymphadenopathy in people > 50 years old

CYTOPATHOLOGY
- Primarily small lymphocytes with clumped chromatin and scattered prolymphocytes and paraimmunoblasts

ANCILLARY TESTS
- Immunohistochemistry
  - Positive for B-cell antigens (CD20 expression can be very weak/dim), CD5, CD23, LEF1
- Flow cytometry
  - Expression of CD19, CD20 (dim +), CD79a, CD5, CD23, CD200, CD43, LEF1; κ- or λ-light chain restriction
  - CD11c(+/-), CD10(-), FMC7(-)
  - Expression of ZAP70, CD38 on > 30% of cells associated with worse prognosis

TOP DIFFERENTIAL DIAGNOSES
- Follicular lymphoma
  - Neoplastic lymphocytes: Centrocytes and centroblasts
  - CD10(+), CD19(+), CD20(+), CD22(+), CD5(-), CD11c(-), CD43(-)
- Mantle cell lymphoma
  - Lymphocytes: Intermediate in size with irregular nuclei
  - CD5(+), CD19(+), CD20(+), CD22(+), CD43(+), CD10(-), CD23(-/+)
  - Cyclin-D1 (+), SOX11(+); t(11;14)(q13;q32)
- Marginal zone lymphoma
  - Typically bright CD19, CD20, CD22; CD5(-), CD23(-)
- Lymphoplasmacytoid lymphoma
  - Variants can closely mimic small lymphocytic lymphoma; some are CD5(+)
  - CD23 usually negative or dim; elevated serum IgM
- Reactive process
  - Polyclonal B-cell population

Predominantly Small Lymphocytes

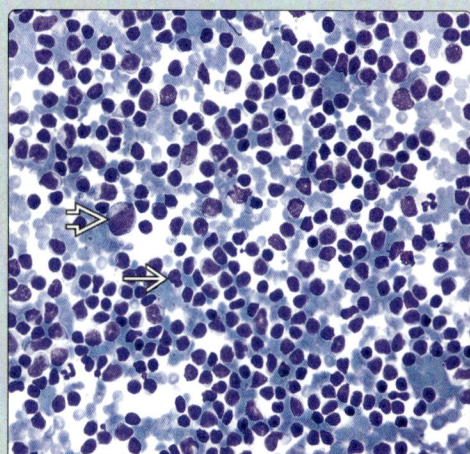

Rare Prolymphocytes

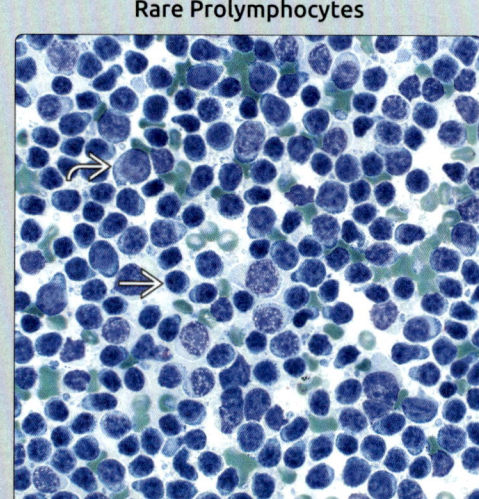

(Left) Diff-Quik-stained FNA smear of small lymphocytic lymphoma shows predominantly small lymphoid cells ➡ with a rare prolymphocyte ➡. **(Right)** Diff-Quik-stained FNA smear of small lymphocytic lymphoma shows admixed prolymphocytes ➡ with larger nuclei, more open chromatin, and nucleoli. Most of the neoplastic cells are small lymphocytes ➡.

Nuclear Features of Small Lymphocytes

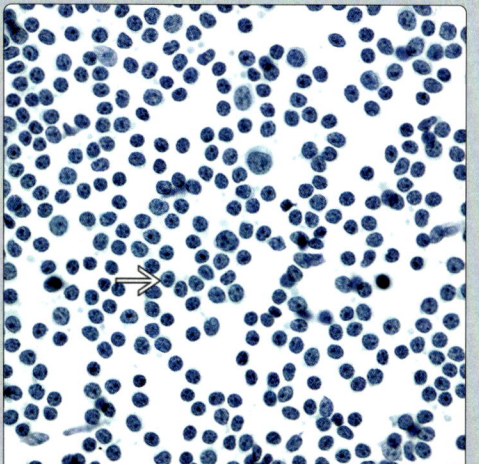

Small Lymphocytic Lymphoma Biopsy

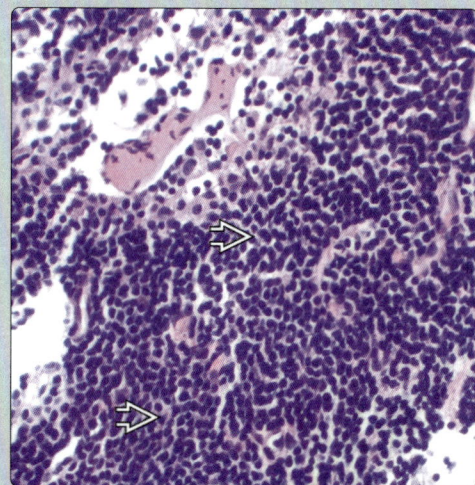

(Left) Pap-stained FNA smear shows predominantly small lymphoid cells ➡ with round nuclei, clumped chromatin, and scant cytoplasm. **(Right)** Core biopsy of small lymphocytic lymphoma stained with H&E shows a population of uniform, small lymphoid cells ➡ with condensed nuclear chromatin and scant cytoplasm.

Small Lymphocytic Lymphoma

TERMINOLOGY

Definitions
- Neoplasm composed of monomorphic, small, round B cells in peripheral blood, bone marrow, lymph nodes, or spleen
- Small lymphocytic lymphoma (SLL) is terminology for nonleukemic cases with morphology and immunophenotype of chronic lymphocytic leukemia (CLL)

CLINICAL ISSUES

Presentation
- Generalized lymphadenopathy

Prognosis
- Not curable with available therapy
- 2-8% of patients develop Richter (large-cell) transformation
- ~ 0.5% develop classic Hodgkin lymphoma

CYTOPATHOLOGY

Cells
- Predominantly small lymphocytes with scattered prolymphocytes and paraimmunoblasts

Nuclear Details
- Small lymphocytes: Small, round nuclei and clumped chromatin; rarely, irregular nuclear membranes
- Prolymphocytes: Medium-sized cells with dispersed chromatin and distinct nucleoli
- Paraimmunoblasts: Medium to large cells with round to oval nuclei, dispersed chromatin, and central nucleoli

ANCILLARY TESTS

Immunohistochemistry
- Positive for B-cell antigens (CD20 expression can be very weak/dim), CD5, CD23, LEF1

Flow Cytometry
- Expression of CD19, CD20 (dim +), CD79a, CD5, CD23, CD200, CD43, LEF1; κ- or λ-light chain restriction
- CD11c(+/-), CD10(-), FMC7(-)
- Expression of CD38 on > 30% of cells is seen in ~ 1/2 of cases and reported to be associated with worse prognosis
- Cases with ZAP70 on > 30% of cells by flow cytometry have worse prognosis than ZAP70(-) cases

DIFFERENTIAL DIAGNOSIS

Follicular Lymphoma
- Neoplastic lymphocytes: Centrocytes and centroblasts
- CD10(+), CD19(+), CD20(+), CD22(+), CD5(-), CD11c(-), CD43(-)

Mantle Cell Lymphoma
- Lymphocytes: Intermediate in size with irregular nuclear contours
- CD5(+), CD19(+), CD20(+), CD22(+), CD43(+), CD10(-), CD23(-/+)
- Cyclin-D1 (+), SOX11(+); t(11;14)(q13;q32)

Nodal Marginal Zone Lymphoma
- Typically bright CD19, CD20, CD22; CD5(-), CD23(-)

Lymphoplasmacytic Lymphoma
- Variants can closely mimic SLL; some are CD5(+)
- CD23 usually negative or dim
- Elevated serum IgM

Reactive Process
- Polyclonal B-cell population

SELECTED REFERENCES

1. Yoshino T et al: Differential diagnosis of chronic lymphocytic leukemia/small lymphocytic lymphoma and other indolent lymphomas, including mantle cell lymphoma. J Clin Exp Hematop. 60(4):124-9, 2020
2. Menter T et al: Diagnostic utility of lymphoid enhancer binding factor 1 immunohistochemistry in small B-cell lymphomas. Am J Clin Pathol. 147(3):292-300, 2017
3. Scarfò L et al: Chronic lymphocytic leukaemia. Crit Rev Oncol Hematol. 104:169-82, 2016

Accelerated Phase
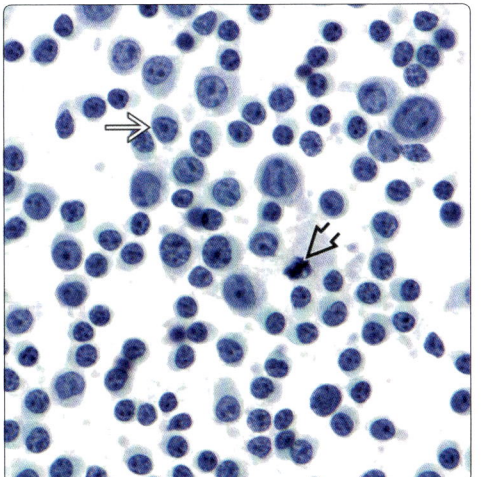

Large-Cell (Richter) Transformation
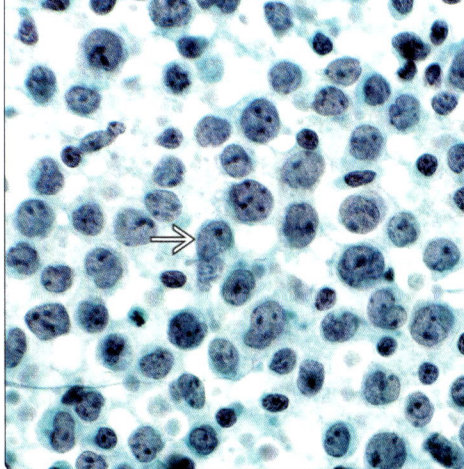

(Left) Pap-stained FNA smear of small lymphocytic lymphoma/chronic lymphocytic leukemia, accelerated phase, shows increased numbers of paraimmunoblasts and prolymphocytes ➡. A mitotic figure ➡ is present. (Right) Pap-stained FNA smear of large cell transformation of small lymphocytic lymphoma (Richter syndrome) shows the typical centroblastic morphology ➡ of the large lymphoid cells.

Lymphoplasmacytic Lymphoma

KEY FACTS

CLINICAL ISSUES

- Neoplasm of small B lymphocytes, plasmacytoid lymphocytes, and plasma cells
  - Usually associated with serum monoclonal paraprotein; usually IgM; rarely IgG or IgA; not required
- Waldenström macroglobulinemia involves bone marrow with associated IgM paraprotein

CYTOPATHOLOGY

- Lymphoplasmacytoid subtype: Monotonous small cells with varying degrees of plasmacytoid features
- Lymphoplasmacytic subtype: Lymphocytes and plasmacytic cells ± Dutcher &/or Russell bodies
- Polymorphous subtype: Small lymphocytes, plasmacytoid cells, and immunoblasts (> 10% of cells)

ANCILLARY TESTS

- 2 immunophenotypic components: B cells and plasmacytoid/plasma cells

TOP DIFFERENTIAL DIAGNOSES

- Marginal zone lymphoma
  - Cytomorphologic and immunophenotypic features overlap with those of lymphoplasmacytic lymphoma
  - Centrocyte-like cells with scattered large forms can be encountered
- Chronic lymphocytic leukemia/small lymphocytic lymphoma with plasmacytic differentiation
  - Morphologically resembles lymphoplasmacytoid variant of lymphoplasmablastic lymphoma
  - Neoplastic cells are sIg(dim +), CD5(+), CD23(+), CD200(+)
  - Serum IgM levels are rarely > 3 g/dL
- Plasma cell myeloma, small cell variant
  - ± clinical features of myeloma, such as lytic bone lesions and renal insufficiency
  - Myeloma plasma cells may be CD20(+)/CD138(+) but usually CD19(-)/CD45(dim +/-)
  - *IGH* translocation present in 40-60% of cases

Mature Lymphocytes

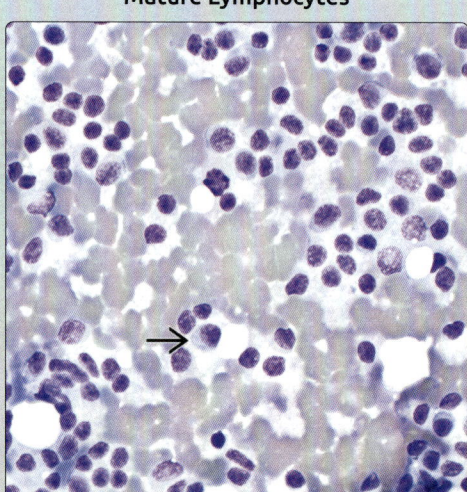

Clumped Chromatin

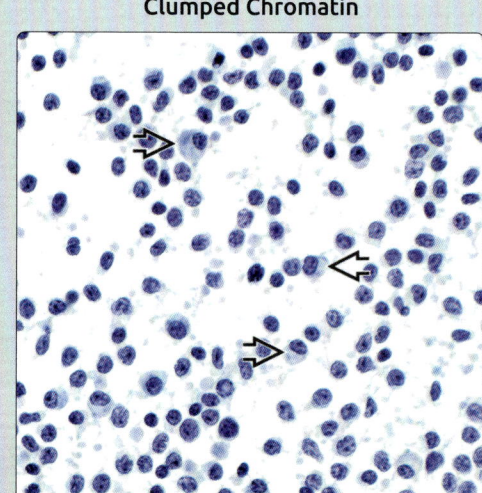

(Left) *Diff-Quik-stained FNA smear of lymphoplasmacytic lymphoma shows small to medium-sized mature lymphocytes, some with slight plasmacytoid features ➡.* (Right) *Pap-stained FNA smear demonstrates small lymphoid cells with clumped chromatin and varying degrees of plasmacytic differentiation ➡.*

Small Lymphocytes and Plasmacytoid Cells

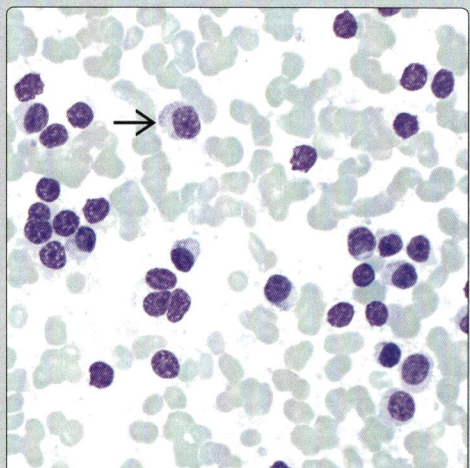

Lymphoplasmacytic Lymphoma Biopsy

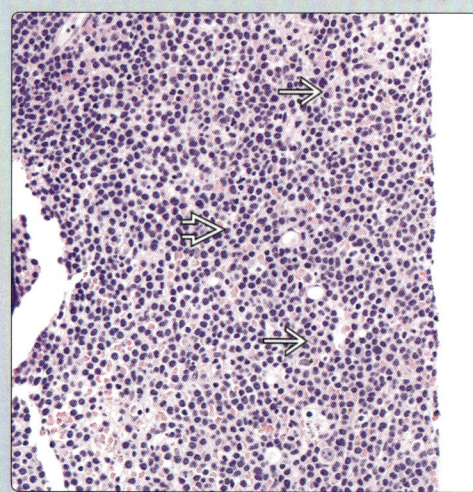

(Left) *Diff-Quik-stained FNA smear of lymphoplasmacytic lymphoma shows small lymphocytes, some with plasmacytoid features ➡.* (Right) *Core biopsy of lymphoplasmacytic lymphoma shows proliferation of small lymphoid cells ➡, including scattered plasma cells ➡.*

Lymphoplasmacytic Lymphoma

TERMINOLOGY

Abbreviations
- Lymphoplasmacytic lymphoma (LPL)

Definitions
- LPL: Neoplasm of small B lymphocytes, plasmacytoid lymphocytes, and plasma cells that does not meet criteria for any other type of small B-cell lymphoma showing plasmacytic differentiation
  - Usually associated with serum monoclonal paraprotein
- Waldenström macroglobulinemia (WM): LPL involving bone marrow and associated with IgM paraprotein
  - WM represents great majority of LPL cases

CYTOPATHOLOGY

Cells
- Lymphoplasmacytoid subtype: Monotonous small cells with varying degrees of plasmacytoid features
- Lymphoplasmacytic subtype: Lymphocytes and plasmacytic cells ± Dutcher &/or Russell bodies
- Polymorphous subtype: Small lymphocytes, plasmacytoid cells, and immunoblasts (> 10% of cells)

Nuclear Details
- Plasmacytoid: Round, eccentrically located nucleus with clumped chromatin
- Dutcher bodies: Nuclear pseudoinclusions

Cytoplasmic Details
- Russell bodies: Cytoplasmic inclusions of Ig

ANCILLARY TESTS

Immunohistochemistry
- LPL and WM have 2 components: B cells and plasmacytoid/plasma cells
- B cells
  - CD19(+), CD20(+), CD22(+), PAX5(+)
  - CD45/LCA(+), BCL2(+), cytoplasmic Ig(-)
- Plasmacytoid/plasma cells
  - CD38(+), CD138(+), CD20(-), PAX5(-/+)
  - Monotypic cytoplasmic Ig light chain(+), IgM(+)
- Ki-67 typically low

Flow Cytometry
- B cells
  - Surface IgM(+), Ig light chain(+), CD19(+), CD20(+)
  - Usually CD5(-), CD10(-), CD23(-)
  - Subset of cases may express CD5, CD10, or CD23
  - CD11c(+/-), CD22(dim +/-), FMC7(+/-), CD43(+/-)
- Plasma cells
  - Cytoplasmic IgM(+), Ig light chain(+)
  - CD19(+), CD38(+), CD138(+)

Genetic Testing
- t(9;14)(p13;q32) and rearrangement of *PAX5* in up to 50%

DIFFERENTIAL DIAGNOSIS

Nodal Marginal Zone Lymphoma
- Cytomorphologic and immunophenotypic features overlap with those of LPL
  - Unlike WM/LPL, centrocyte-like cells with scattered large forms can be encountered

Chronic Lymphocytic Leukemia/Small Lymphocytic Lymphoma With Plasmacytic Differentiation
- Neoplastic cells are sIg(dim +), CD5(+), CD23(+), CD200(+)

Plasma Cell Myeloma, Small Cell Variant
- ± clinical features of myeloma, such as lytic bone lesions and renal insufficiency
- Myeloma plasma cells may be CD20(+)/CD138(+) but usually CD19(-)/CD45(dim +/-)

SELECTED REFERENCES

1. Gertz MA: Waldenström macroglobulinemia: 2021 update on diagnosis, risk stratification, and management. Am J Hematol. 96(2):258-69, 2021
2. Wang W et al: Lymphoplasmacytic lymphoma and Waldenström macroglobulinaemia: clinicopathological features and differential diagnosis. Pathology. 52(1):6-14, 2020

PAS Stain for Dutcher Bodies

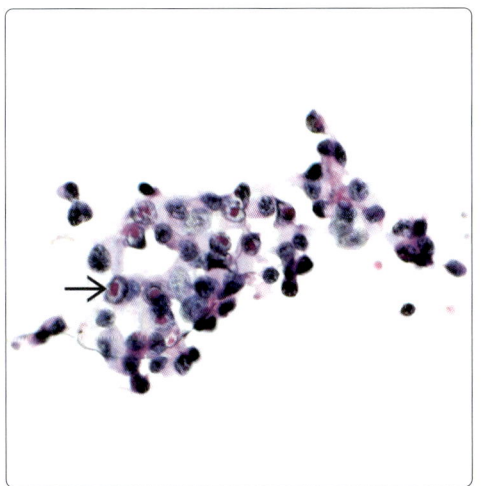

Plasmacytic Differentiation

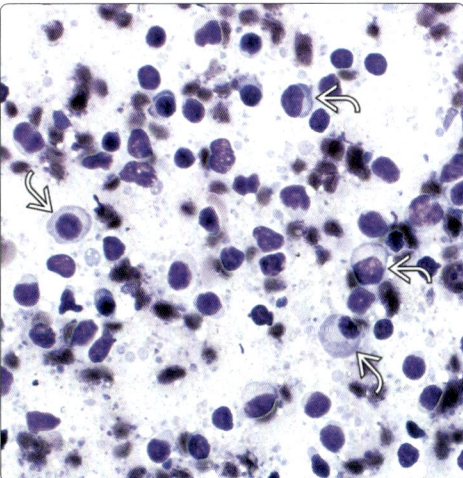

(Left) *PAS-stained FNA smear (performed using a destained Pap slide) shows intranuclear inclusions (Dutcher bodies), an interesting but nonspecific finding sometimes seen in lymphoplasmacytic lymphoma* ➡. (Right) *Diff-Quik-stained FNA smear shows small lymphocytes with varying degrees of plasmacytic differentiation* ➡.

Mantle Cell Lymphoma

KEY FACTS

CLINICAL ISSUES
- Clinically aggressive B-cell lymphoma composed of monomorphic small to medium-sized cells
- Associated with t(11;14) resulting in cyclin-D1 overexpression
- Median age: 6th-7th decades; male predominance
- Most patients present with clinical stage III/IV disease
- Presents with B symptoms, lymphadenopathy, extranodal involvement
- Currently considered incurable
  - Median survival: 2-5 years

CYTOPATHOLOGY
- Classic type: Monotonous population of small to medium-sized lymphoid cells
  - Slightly irregular nuclear contours, condensed chromatin, indistinct to small nucleolus
- Blastoid variant: Monotonous population of medium to large cells
  - Immature nuclear chromatin, enlarged nucleolus, and high mitotic index
- Pleomorphic variant: Heterogeneous population of large cells
  - Prominent nucleoli and high mitotic index

ANCILLARY TESTS
- Immunohistochemistry: Cyclin-D1 (+)
- Flow cytometry: CD5(+), CD19(+), CD20(+), CD43(+/-), FMC7(+), CD10(-), CD23(-), CD200(-)
- Cytogenetics: t(11;14)(q13;q32)

TOP DIFFERENTIAL DIAGNOSES
- For classic type
  - Chronic lymphocytic leukemia/small lymphocytic lymphoma, follicular lymphoma, nodal marginal zone B-cell lymphoma
- For blastoid/pleomorphic variant
  - Lymphoblastic lymphoma, diffuse large B-cell lymphoma

Classic Variant, Pap Stain
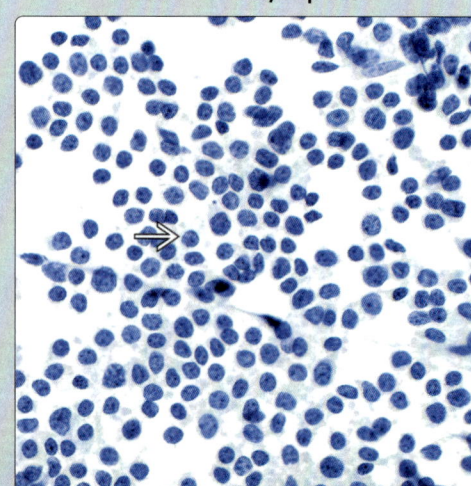

Classic Variant, Diff-Quik
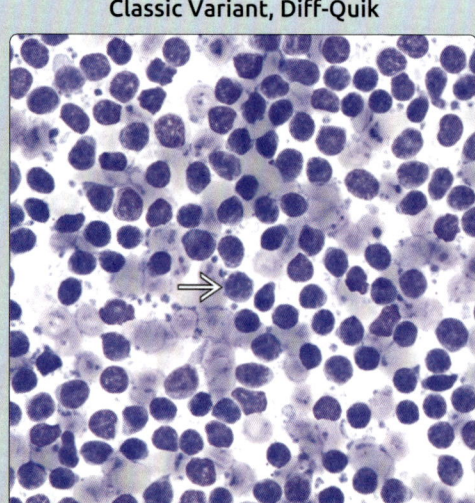

(Left) Pap-stained FNA smear of classic mantle cell lymphoma shows a monomorphous population of small lymphoid cells ➡. (Right) Diff-Quik-stained FNA smear of mantle cell lymphoma shows atypical small lymphoid cells ➡ with nuclear contour irregularities and condensed chromatin.

Mantle Cell Lymphoma Biopsy
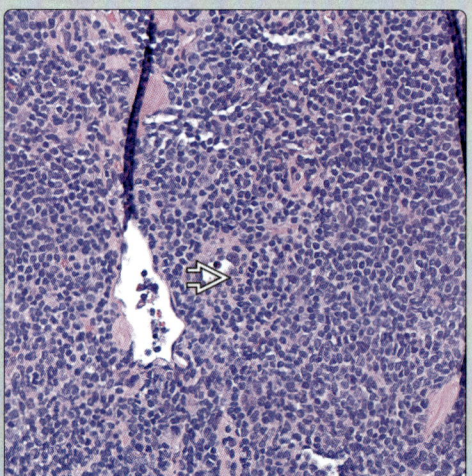

Cyclin-D1 (+)
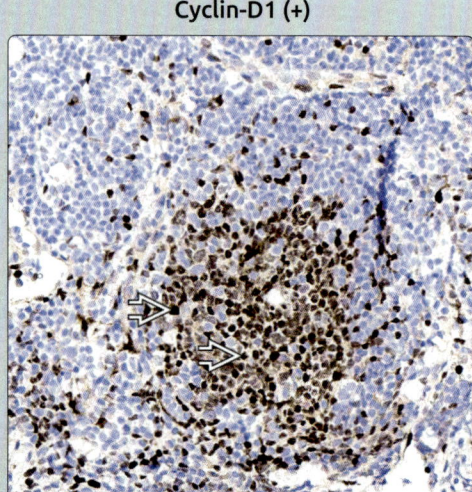

(Left) Core biopsy of mantle cell lymphoma stained with H&E shows a monomorphous population of small lymphoid cells ➡. (Right) Immunostaining of core biopsy for cyclin-D1 shows positive nuclear staining on many of the atypical small lymphoid cells ➡, which supports the diagnosis of mantle cell lymphoma.

Mantle Cell Lymphoma

TERMINOLOGY

Definitions
- Clinically aggressive B-cell lymphoma, usually composed of monomorphic small to medium-sized cells and associated with t(11;14)

ETIOLOGY/PATHOGENESIS

t(11;14)(q13;q32)
- Juxtaposes *CCND1* at 11q13 with *IGH* at 14q32 and results in cyclin-D1 overexpression

CLINICAL ISSUES

Presentation
- Median age: 6th-7th decades; male predominance
- Generalized lymphadenopathy
- Extranodal sites commonly involved
  - Particularly GI tract, bone marrow, spleen, peripheral blood

CYTOPATHOLOGY

Cells
- Classic: Monotonous population of small to medium-sized lymphoid cells with irregular nuclear contours, condensed chromatin, indistinct to small nucleoli
- Blastoid variant: Monotonous population of medium to large cells with immature chromatin, enlarged nucleolus, and high mitotic index
- Pleomorphic variant: Heterogeneous population of large cells often with prominent nucleoli and high mitotic index

ANCILLARY TESTS

Immunohistochemistry
- Cyclin-D1 overexpression (+), SOX11(+)

Flow Cytometry
- CD5(+), CD19(+), CD20(+), CD22(+), CD79b(+), FMC7(+), and monotypic Ig
- CD3(-), CD10(-), CD23(-), CD43(+/-), CD200(-)

Genetic Testing
- PCR detects 1 major breakpoint (MTC) in 30-50% of cases
- Numerous methods can be used for demonstrating t(11;14)(q13;q32)
  - FISH convenient because it can be performed on fixed tissue sections
  - Conventional cytogenetics if fresh material available

DIFFERENTIAL DIAGNOSIS

Follicular Lymphoma
- Centrocytes and centroblasts express CD10 but not CD5, CD43, or cyclin-D1

Small Lymphocytic Lymphoma/Chronic Lymphocytic Lymphoma
- Mixture of small lymphocytes, prolymphocytes, and paraimmunoblasts
- Expresses CD5, CD23, and CD200 but not cyclin-D1

Nodal Marginal Zone B-Cell Lymphoma
- Neoplastic B cells ± monocytoid cytoplasm
- Reactive germinal centers are common
- CD5(-) and cyclin-D1 (-)

Lymphoblastic Lymphoma
- Mimics blastoid variant of mantle cell lymphoma (MCL)
- Younger patients; TdT(+) and cyclin-D1 (-)

Diffuse Large B-Cell Lymphoma
- Mimics pleomorphic variant of MCL
- CD5(-) and cyclin-D1 (-)

Reactive Follicular Hyperplasia
- No evidence of monoclonality

SELECTED REFERENCES
1. Cortelazzo S et al: Mantle cell lymphoma. Crit Rev Oncol Hematol. 153:103038, 2020

Blastoid Variant, Pap Stain

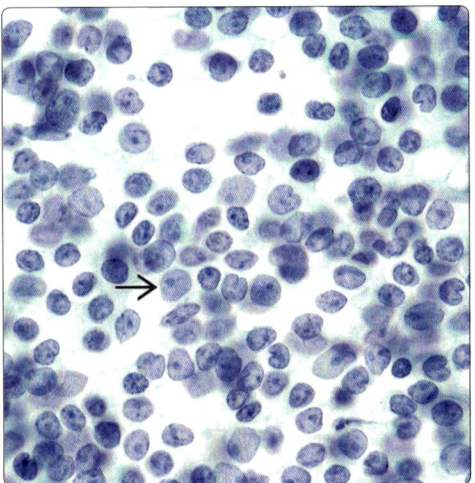

Pleomorphic Variant

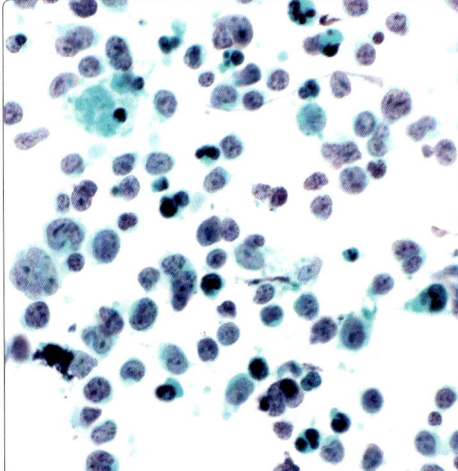

(Left) Pap-stained FNA smear of blastoid variant of mantle cell lymphoma shows neoplastic cells ➡ with fine nuclear chromatin, nucleoli, and scant cytoplasm. *(Right)* Lymph node aspirate of mantle cell lymphoma, pleomorphic variant, shows large neoplastic cells with convoluted nuclei and prominent nucleoli on Pap-stained smear.

Nodal Marginal Zone Lymphoma

KEY FACTS

CLINICAL ISSUES
- Age: 5th-6th decades
- No evidence of extranodal or splenic lymphoma
- Clinically indolent
  - \> 60% of patients have overall survival > 5 years
- Can transform to diffuse large B-cell lymphoma

CYTOPATHOLOGY
- Polymorphous, closely resembling reactive process
- Typically increased monocytoid cells, plasmacytoid cells, and plasma cells, which can be subtle
  - Monocytoid cells are best seen on Diff-Quik; have excess pale to light blue cytoplasm

ANCILLARY TESTS
- Positive for monotypic Ig (bright) and B-cell markers
- Aberrantly express CD43 in ~ 50% of cases
- Usually negative for CD5, CD10, and CD23

TOP DIFFERENTIAL DIAGNOSES
- Lymphoplasmacytic lymphoma (LPL)
  - Almost all patients with LPL also have Waldenström macroglobulinemia (WM)
  - Immunophenotypes of both entities overlap
- Mantle cell lymphoma
  - Clinically more aggressive disease
  - CD5(+), cyclin-D1 (+), t(11;14)(q13;q32)
- Chronic lymphocytic leukemia/small lymphocytic lymphoma (CLL/SLL)
  - Plasmacytoid differentiation can occur but is unusual
  - Dim monotypic surface Ig; CD5(+), CD23(+), dim CD20(+)
- Follicular lymphoma
  - Composed of centrocytes and centroblasts
  - CD10(+), BCL6(+), t(14;18)(q32;q21)
- Reactive lymphoid hyperplasia
  - B cells express polytypic Ig light chains

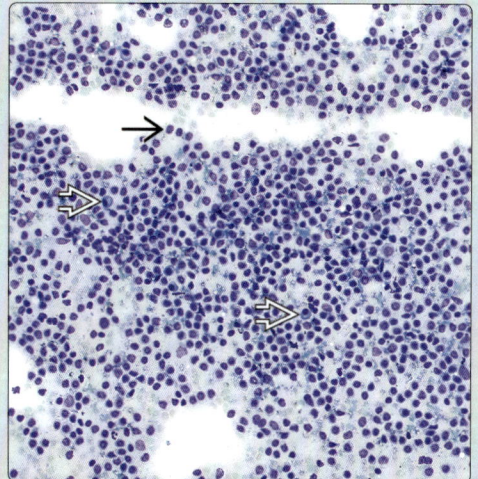

Occasional Plasma Cells Among Lymphocytes

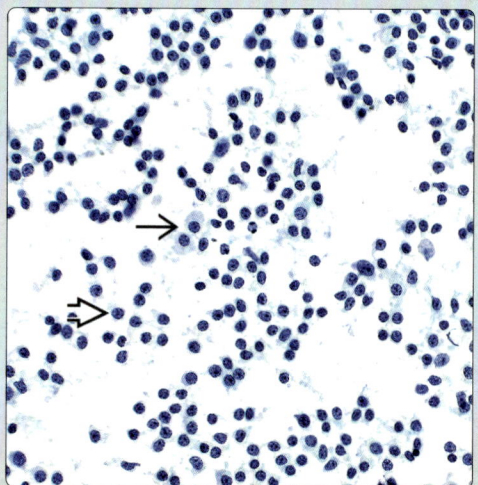

Slight Nuclear Irregularity in Lymphocytes

(Left) Diff-Quik-stained FNA smear of nodal marginal zone lymphoma shows small to medium-sized lymphocytes ➡ and scattered plasma cells ➡. (Right) Pap-stained FNA smear shows small and medium-sized lymphocytes ➡ with slight nuclear irregularity and occasional plasma cells ➡.

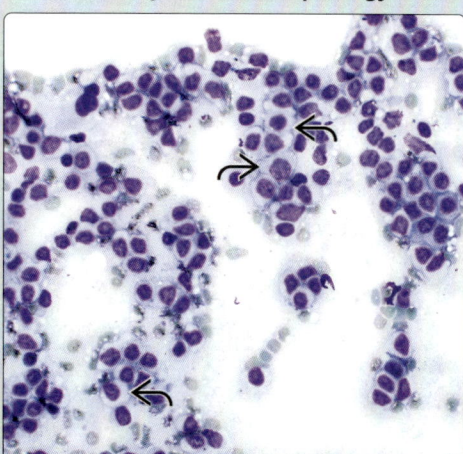

Monocytoid Cell Morphology

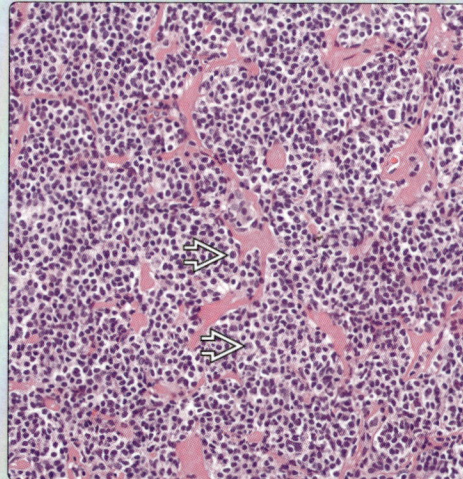

Nodal Marginal Zone Lymphoma Biopsy

(Left) Diff-Quik-stained FNA smear of nodal marginal zone lymphoma shows cells with abundant pale cytoplasm and bland nuclei, typical of monocytoid cells ➡. (Right) Core biopsy of nodal marginal zone lymphoma shows small lymphoid cells ➡ with monocytoid features, including slight nuclear irregularity and moderate amount of pale cytoplasm.

Nodal Marginal Zone Lymphoma

TERMINOLOGY

Abbreviations
- Nodal marginal zone B-cell lymphoma (NMZL)

Definitions
- NMZL cytologically resembles lymph nodes involved by marginal zone lymphoma of extranodal or splenic types
  - There can be no evidence of extranodal or splenic disease

CLINICAL ISSUES

Presentation
- Lymphadenopathy (localized or widespread)

Prognosis
- Clinically indolent
  - > 60% of patients have overall survival > 5 years
- Patients can undergo transformation to diffuse large B-cell lymphoma

CYTOPATHOLOGY

Pattern
- Polymorphous, difficult or impossible to distinguish from reactive lymph node

Cells
- Increased centrocytic or monocytoid cells with plasmacytoid cells and plasma cells

Nuclear Details
- Minor nuclear membrane irregularity typical

Cytoplasmic Details
- Monocytoid cells, usually subtle and best seen on Diff-Quik; have excess pale to light blue cytoplasm

ANCILLARY TESTS

Flow Cytometry
- Usually express monotypic surface Ig
- Brightly positive for pan-B-cell antigens (CD19, CD20, CD22) and negative for CD10

PCR
- Ig gene rearrangements present

Genetic Testing
- No consistent translocations identified

DIFFERENTIAL DIAGNOSIS

Lymphoplasmacytic Lymphoma
- Almost all patients with lymphoplasmacytic lymphoma (LPL) also have Waldenström macroglobulinemia (WM)
- Immunophenotypes of NMZL and LPL/WM overlap

Mantle Cell Lymphoma
- Clinically more aggressive disease
- CD5(+), cyclin-D1 (+), t(11;14)(q13;q32)

Chronic Lymphocytic Leukemia/Small Lymphocytic Lymphoma
- Cytomorphologic features:
  - Small cells tend to be round with little cytoplasm
  - Plasmacytoid differentiation can occur but is unusual
- Dim monotypic surface Ig; CD5(+), CD23(+), CD20 [dim (+)]

Follicular Lymphoma
- CD10(+), BCL6(+), t(14;18)(q32;q21)

Peripheral T-Cell Lymphoma
- Neoplastic cells express T-cell markers

Reactive Follicular and Interfollicular Hyperplasia
- B cells express polytypic Ig light chains

SELECTED REFERENCES

1. Nakamura S et al: Marginal zone B-cell lymphoma: lessons from Western and Eastern diagnostic approaches. Pathology. 52(1):15-29, 2020
2. Juárez-Salcedo LM et al: Lymphoplasmacytic lymphoma and marginal zone lymphoma. Hematol Oncol Clin North Am. 33(4):639-56, 2019
3. Tadmor T et al: Nodal marginal zone lymphoma: clinical features, diagnosis, management and treatment. Best Pract Res Clin Haematol. 30(1-2):92-8, 2017

Subtle Pale Cytoplasm on Pap Stain
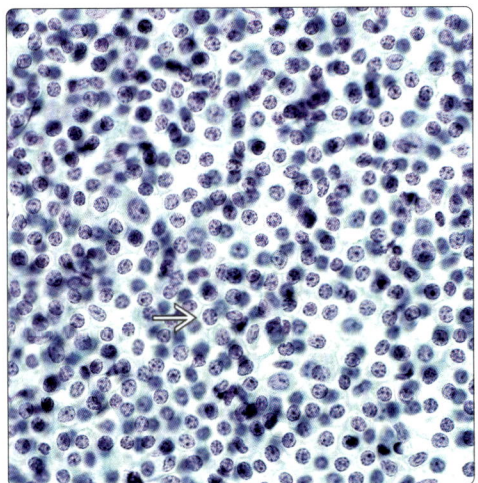

Cytoplasm Better Seen on Diff-Quik
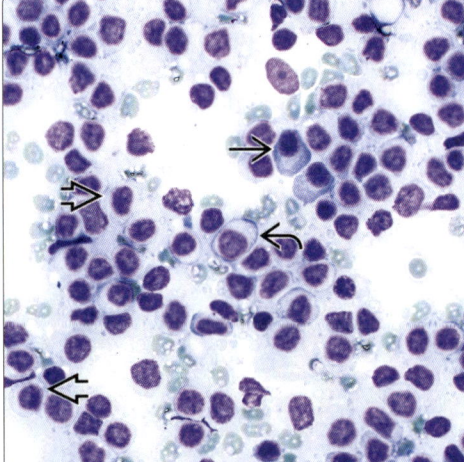

(Left) Pap-stained FNA smear of nodal marginal zone lymphoma shows monocytoid cells ➡ with slight nuclear membrane irregularity and pale cytoplasm, which can be subtle on Pap-stained smears. (Right) Diff-Quik-stained FNA smear demonstrates plasma cells ➡, plasmacytoid lymphocytes ➡, and monocytoid cells ➡ with a moderate amount of cytoplasm.

Follicular Lymphoma

KEY FACTS

CLINICAL ISSUES
- 2nd most common non-Hodgkin lymphoma
- Usually asymptomatic, although disseminated at presentation

CYTOPATHOLOGY
- Variable mixture of centrocytes and centroblasts
  - Centrocytes: Small to large cells with cleaved or angulated nuclei with condensed chromatin
  - Centroblasts: Large cells with oval or multilobulated nuclei, vesicular chromatin, and 1-3 nucleoli
- Germinal aggregates are often present
- Grading: Controversial, especially distinguishing grade 2 from grade 3; grades 1 and 2 combined as low grade

ANCILLARY TESTS
- Monotypic B cells, CD10(+), CD5(-)
- t(14;18)(q32;q21) results in overexpression of BCL2
- Ki-67 can help in estimation of biologic grade

TOP DIFFERENTIAL DIAGNOSES
- Reactive process
  - Affects children and young adults; patients with autoimmune disease; polytypic B cells
- Mantle cell lymphoma
  - Monotypic B cells with irregular nuclear contours, CD5(+), CD10(-); no centroblasts; detection of t(11;14)(q13;q32)
- Nodal marginal zone lymphoma
  - Neoplastic lymphocytes include small lymphocytes, lymphocytes with monocytoid nuclei, and large cells; frequent plasmacytic differentiation; monotypic B cells, CD5, CD10 (-)
- Nodular lymphocyte-predominant Hodgkin lymphoma
  - Most cells in nodules are small, round lymphocytes admixed with few lymphocyte-predominant cells; lymphocyte-predominant cells are CD20, CD45 (+); CD10, BCL2 (-)

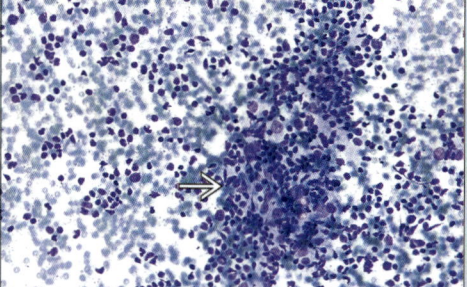
Low-Grade Follicular Lymphoma, Diff-Quik

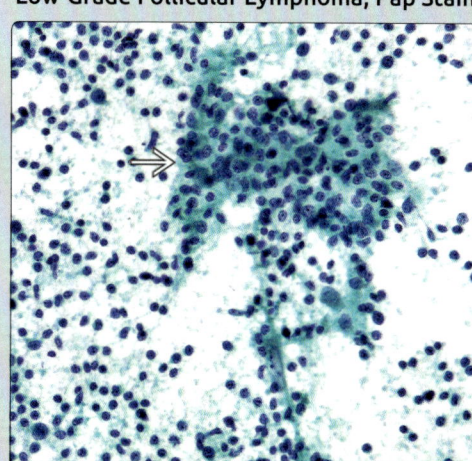
Low-Grade Follicular Lymphoma, Pap Stain

(Left) Diff-Quik-stained FNA smear of low-grade follicular lymphoma (FL) shows a follicular aggregate ➡ of small lymphoid cells and follicular dendritic cells. (Right) Pap-stained FNA smear of low-grade FL shows a follicular aggregate ➡ composed primarily of small lymphocytes.

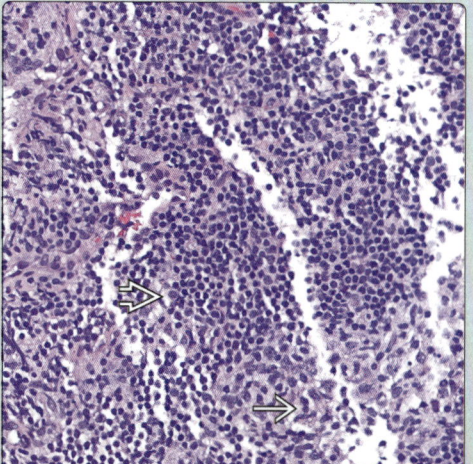
Low-Grade Follicular Lymphoma

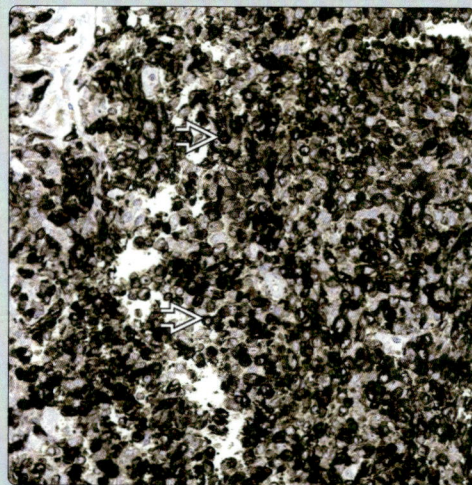
BCL2(+)

(Left) Core biopsy of FL shows a follicular aggregate of small lymphoid cells ➡ with dendritic reticulum cells ➡ in the immediate vicinity. (Right) Core biopsy immunostained for BCL2 shows cytoplasmic positivity in the lymphoid cells ➡, which is useful for distinguishing neoplastic from reactive lymphoid follicles.

Follicular Lymphoma

TERMINOLOGY

Abbreviations
- Follicular lymphoma (FL)

Definitions
- B-cell neoplasm composed of germinal center B cells (centrocytes and centroblasts)
  - Follicular, follicular and diffuse, and diffuse growth patterns
    - Growth patterns cannot be accurately accessed on cytology specimens

ETIOLOGY/PATHOGENESIS

Genetics
- BCL2 is antiapoptotic and confers survival advantage
- t(14;18) is considered to be initiating molecular event of FL

CYTOPATHOLOGY

Cells
- Variable mixtures of centrocytes and centroblasts
  - May form germinal aggregates

Nuclear Details
- Centrocytes: Small to large cells with cleaved or angulated nuclei with condensed chromatin
- Centroblasts: Large cells with oval or multilobulated nuclei, vesicular chromatin, and 1-3 nucleoli

Cytoplasmic Details
- Scant to moderate

Cytology-Histology Correlation
- Smears are unreliable for histologic pattern

Grading
- WHO classification recommends combining grades 1 and 2 as low grade
- Grading based on smears is controversial, especially distinguishing grade 2 from grade 3
- Ki-67 expression normalized to B cells can help estimate biologic grade

ANCILLARY TESTS

Immunohistochemistry
- Monotypic surface Ig, pan-B-cell markers (+)
- CD10(+), CD23(+/-)
- Usually CD5, CD43 (-)
- Proliferation rate assessed by Ki-67
  - Percentage of Ki-67(+) cells correlates with grade

In Situ Hybridization
- Fluorescent in situ hybridization (FISH) can detect t(14;18) in up to 90% of cases

Genetic Testing
- Rare cases have t(2;18)(p12;q21)
  - Juxtaposes *BCL2* with light chain gene on chromosome 2
- Additional breaks, most commonly involving chromosomes 1, 2, 4, 5, 13, and 17 or additions of X, 7, 12, or 18
- Abnormalities at 6q25-27 can be found in 10-40% and are most common 2nd abnormality in cases with t(14;18)

DIFFERENTIAL DIAGNOSIS

Reactive Process
- Polytypic B cells

Mantle Cell Lymphoma
- Monotypic B cells, CD5(+), CD10(-)

Nodal Marginal Zone Lymphoma
- Monotypic B cells, CD5, CD10 (-)

Nodular Lymphocyte-Predominant Hodgkin Lymphoma
- Lymphocyte-predominant cells are CD20, CD45 (+); CD10, BCL2 (-)

SELECTED REFERENCES
1. Freedman A et al: Follicular lymphoma: 2020 update on diagnosis and management. Am J Hematol. 95(3):316-27, 2020

Follicular Lymphoma, Grade 1

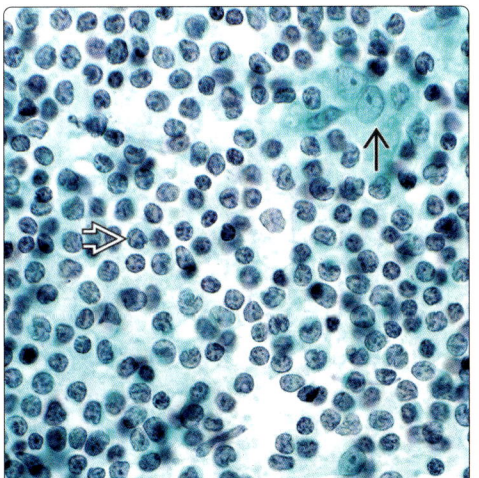

Follicular Lymphoma, Grade 1-2

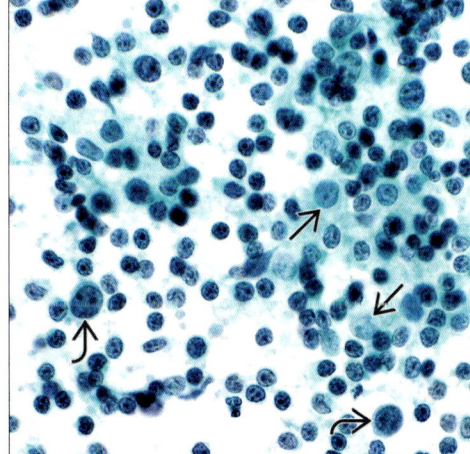

(Left) Pap-stained smear of FL shows follicular dendritic cells ⇨ and centrocytes ⇨, corresponding to grade 1 histology. (Right) Pap-stained smear of FL shows follicular dendritic cells ⇨, centrocytes, and a few centroblasts ⇨, corresponding to low-grade (FL grades 1-2) histology.

Burkitt Lymphoma

KEY FACTS

CLINICAL ISSUES
- Highly aggressive B-cell lymphoma with very short doubling time
- Has 3 clinical variants
  - Endemic Burkitt lymphoma (BL) occurs in equatorial Africa and is associated with EBV in almost all cases
  - Sporadic BL occurs in immunocompetent patients
  - AIDS-associated BL in patients infected with HIV

CYTOPATHOLOGY
- Monotonous population of cells with round to oval nuclei, coarse chromatin, and several nucleoli
- Cytoplasm is moderate in amount and highly basophilic, often containing vacuoles on Romanowsky-stained slides
- Background of necrosis, apoptosis, and tingible body macrophages

ANCILLARY TESTS
- Immunohistochemistry
  - Pan-B-cell markers (+), CD10(+), EBER(+/-)
  - Ki-67 strongly positive in > 90% of cells
- Flow cytometry
  - Pan-B-cell markers (+), CD10(+), CD38(+), FMC7(+), monotypic surface IgM(+); κ > λ
- In situ hybridization
  - EBER(+) in > 95% of endemic cases, ~ 30-40% of immunodeficiency-associated cases, and ~ 10-20% of sporadic cases of BL
  - Fluorescence in situ hybridization is useful for detecting *MYC* translocations

TOP DIFFERENTIAL DIAGNOSES
- Diffuse large B-cell lymphoma (DLBCL)
- High-grade B-cell lymphoma with *MYC* and *BCL2* &/or *BCL6* rearrangements
- Lymphoblastic leukemia/lymphoma
- Mantle cell lymphoma, blastoid variant
- Burkitt-like lymphoma with 11q aberrations

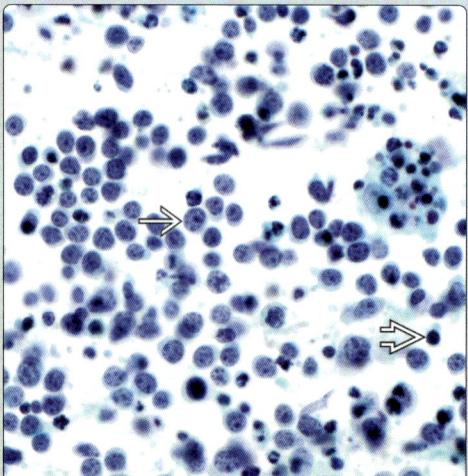

Burkitt Lymphoma, Pap Stain

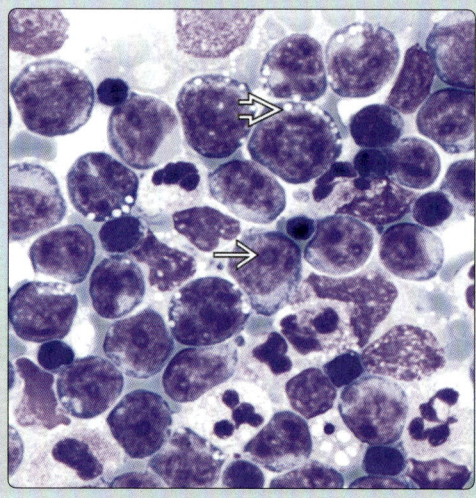

Burkitt Lymphoma, Diff-Quik

(Left) Pap-stained FNA smear of Burkitt lymphoma shows medium-sized lymphocytes ➡ with coarsely clumped chromatin, multiple nucleoli, and scant cytoplasm with many apoptotic cells in the background ➡. (Right) Diff-Quik-stained FNA smear of Burkitt lymphoma shows medium-sized lymphoid cells with multiple nucleoli ➡ and a moderate amount of deeply basophilic cytoplasm with vacuoles ➡ in some of the tumor cells.

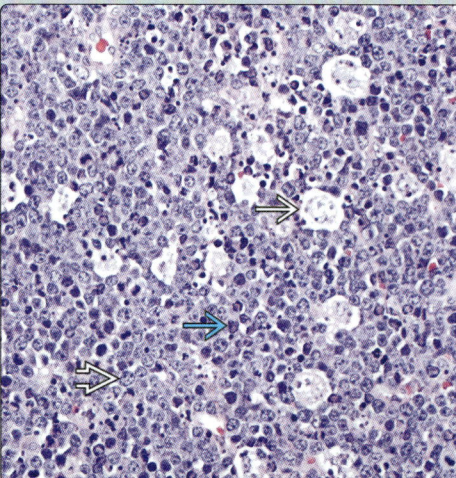

Burkitt Lymphoma Biopsy

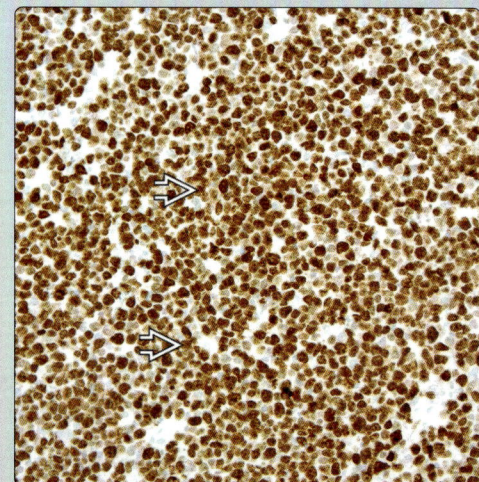

Burkitt Lymphoma, Very High Ki-67

(Left) Core biopsy of Burkitt lymphoma shows medium-sized uniform lymphoid cells with round nucleus, multiple nucleoli ➡, and scant cytoplasm, associated with apoptotic cells ➡ and tingible body macrophages ➡, giving a starry-sky appearance in the background. (Right) Core biopsy of Burkitt lymphoma immunostained for Ki-67 shows labeling in nearly all neoplastic cells ➡.

Burkitt Lymphoma

TERMINOLOGY

Definitions
- Highly aggressive B-cell lymphoma with very short doubling time
- 3 clinicopathologic variants
  - Endemic Burkitt lymphoma (BL) occurs in equatorial Africa and is associated with Epstein-Barr virus (EBV)
  - Sporadic BL occurs outside endemic areas (where it is ~ 1% of lymphomas) in immunocompetent patients
  - Immunodeficiency-associated BL is typically seen in patients infected with HIV

ETIOLOGY/PATHOGENESIS

Infectious Agents
- Association with EBV infection

MYC Protooncogene
- Translocations juxtapose intact MYC with enhancer elements of IGH genes, resulting in MYC upregulation

CYTOPATHOLOGY

Background
- Apoptosis, necrosis, tingible body macrophages

Cells
- Monomorphic population of medium-sized lymphoid cells

Nuclear Details
- Typically round to oval nuclei with coarse chromatin and 2-5 nucleoli

Cytoplasmic Details
- Cytoplasm is moderate in amount and highly basophilic, often containing vacuoles on Romanowsky-stained slides

ANCILLARY TESTS

Immunohistochemistry
- Pan-B-cell antigens (+), CD10(+), CD45/LCA (+)
- Ki-67, strong staining in most (> 90%) nuclei

Flow Cytometry
- Pan-B-cell markers (+), CD10(+), CD38(+), FMC7(+), monotypic surface IgM(+); κ > λ

In Situ Hybridization
- EBER(+) in > 95% of endemic cases, ~ 30-40% of immunodeficiency-associated cases, and ~ 10-20% of sporadic cases of BL
- Fluorescence in situ hybridization is useful for detecting MYC translocations

Genetic Testing
- MYC translocations are characteristic: t(8;14)(q24;q32) in 80%; others t(8;22)(q24;q11) or t(2;8)(p11;q24)
- ~ 5-10% of reported cases do not carry MYC translocation

DIFFERENTIAL DIAGNOSIS

Diffuse Large B-Cell Lymphoma
- Subset of diffuse large B-cell lymphoma (DLBCL) cases has immunophenotype identical to BL but EBER(-) and Ki-67 usually < 90%

High-Grade B-Cell Lymphoma With MYC and BCL2 &/or BCL6 Rearrangements
- Mimics BL morphologically but has atypical immunophenotype

Lymphoblastic Leukemia/Lymphoma
- TdT(+), CD34(+), surface Ig (-)

Mantle Cell Lymphoma, Blastoid Variant
- CD5(+), cyclin-D1(+), t(11;14)(q13;q32)(+)

Burkitt-Like Lymphoma With 11q Aberrations
- Lacks MYC rearrangements and has 11q alterations

SELECTED REFERENCES
1. Chen MT et al: A novel prognostic index for sporadic Burkitt lymphoma in adult patients: a real-word multicenter study. BMC Cancer. 22(1):45, 2022
2. Evens AM et al: Burkitt lymphoma in the modern era: real-world outcomes and prognostication across 30 US cancer centers. Blood. 137(3):374-86, 2021

Burkitt Lymphoma, EBER(+)
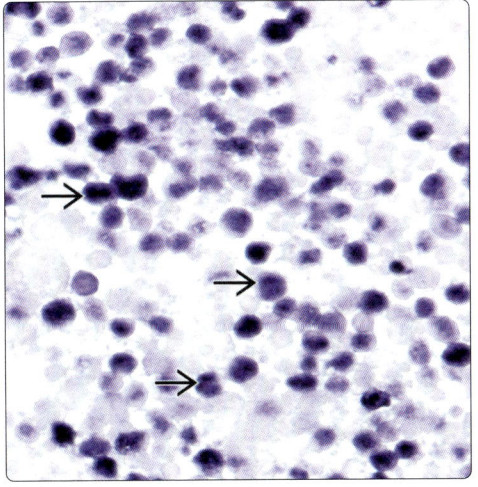

Burkitt Lymphoma, Apoptotic Bodies
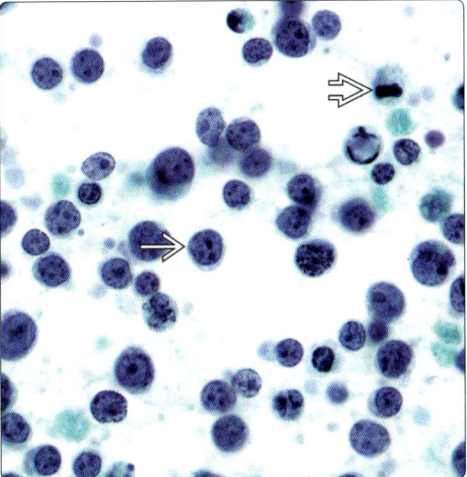

(Left) In situ hybridization performed on a cell block preparation of Burkitt lymphoma shows cells reactive for EBER ➡. (Right) Pap-stained FNA smear of Burkitt lymphoma shows medium-sized lymphoid cells with multiple nucleoli and scant cytoplasm ➡. Note apoptotic cells in the background ➡.

Large B-Cell Lymphoma

KEY FACTS

CLINICAL ISSUES
- 20-30% of non-Hodgkin lymphoma (NHL) in adults
- De novo or secondary to underlying low-grade NHL
- Enlarging mass in nodal or extranodal sites
- Primarily disease of older adults, rarely children
- 5-year survival rate: 25-75%

CYTOPATHOLOGY
- Typically composed primarily of centroblasts; less common variants: Immunoblastic and anaplastic
- Centroblastic variant: Medium to large cells
  - Typically noncleaved nuclei with 2-4 small, peripheral nucleoli and scant, basophilic cytoplasm
  - Less commonly multilobated nuclei (> 3 lobes)
- Immunoblastic variant: Large cells
  - Vesicular chromatin; single large, central nucleolus
  - More abundant cytoplasm, sometimes plasmacytoid
- Anaplastic variant: Large to very large cells with bizarre and anaplastic morphology

ANCILLARY TESTS
- Variable but at least 1 (+) pan-B-cell antigen (CD19, CD20, CD22, CD79-a) and (-) for T-cell, myeloid antigens
- Germinal center type (GCB): CD10(+) or CD10(-)/BCL6(+)/MUM1(-)
- Activated B-cell type (ABC): CD10(-) with BCL6(-) or BCL6(+)/MUM1(+)
- Anaplastic: frequently CD30(+)
- CD5(+) in 10%, often de novo, may be aggressive
- Flow cytometry has false-negative results in up to 25% of cases due to disruption of large cells in acquisition/processing

TOP DIFFERENTIAL DIAGNOSES
- Other high-grade B-cell lymphoma, Burkitt lymphoma, high-grade follicular lymphoma, pleomorphic mantle cell lymphoma, nonhematological malignancies

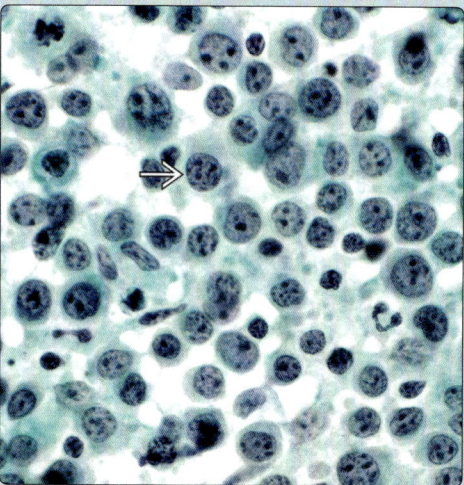

Centroblastic Variant, Multiple Nucleoli

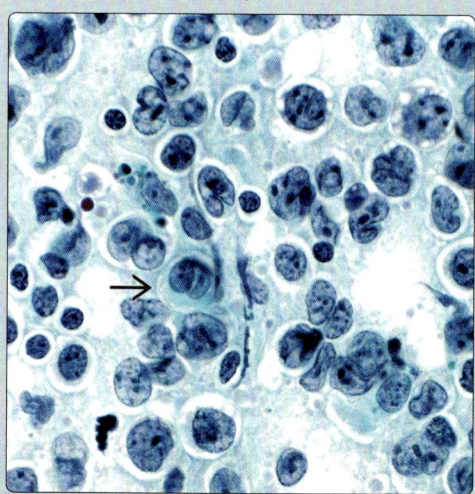

Centroblastic Variant, Multilobated Nuclei

(Left) Pap-stained FNA smear of diffuse large B-cell lymphoma, centroblastic variant, shows large cells ➡ with rounded nuclei and multiple nucleoli. (Right) Pap-stained FNA smear of diffuse large B-cell lymphoma, centroblastic variant, demonstrates neoplastic cells ➡ with multilobated nuclei and multiple nucleoli.

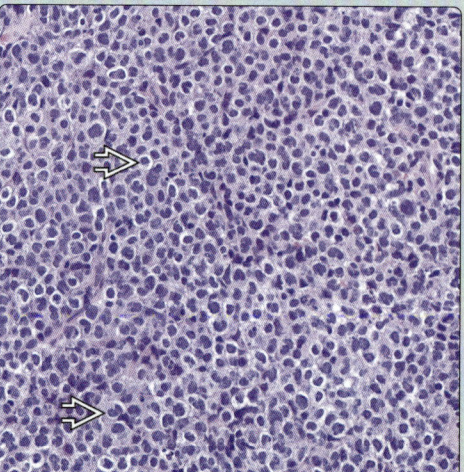

Centroblastic Type

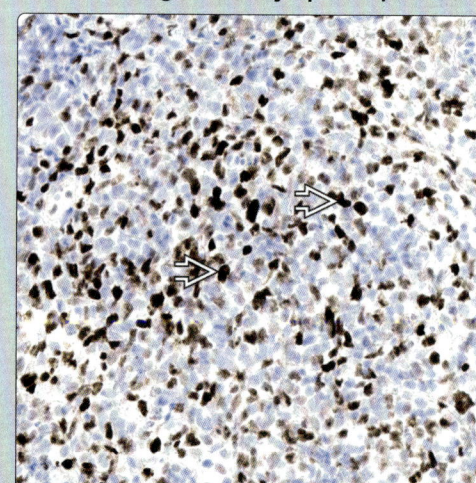

Diffuse Large B-Cell Lymphoma, c-MYC

(Left) Core biopsy of diffuse large B-cell lymphoma shows large, atypical lymphoid cells ➡ with a polymorphic and polylobated appearance, consistent with the centroblastic type. (Right) Core biopsy of diffuse large B-cell lymphoma immunostained for c-MYC shows positive staining in many tumor cells ➡.

Large B-Cell Lymphoma

TERMINOLOGY

Abbreviations
- Large B-cell lymphoma (LBCL)

CLINICAL ISSUES

Presentation
- De novo or secondary to underlying low-grade non-Hodgkin lymphoma (NHL)
- Enlarging mass in nodal or extranodal sites

CYTOPATHOLOGY

Cells
- Centroblastic variant: Medium to large cells
  - Typically noncleaved nuclei with 2-4 small, peripheral nucleoli and scant, basophilic cytoplasm
  - Less commonly, multilobated nuclei (> 3 lobes)
- Immunoblastic variant: Large cells
  - By definition, > 90% immunoblasts
  - Vesicular chromatin; single large, central nucleolus
  - More abundant cytoplasm, sometimes plasmacytoid
- Anaplastic variant: Large to very large cells with bizarre and anaplastic morphology
- T-cell/histiocyte rich: Majority of cells are nonneoplastic T cells ± histiocytes, < 10% are large, neoplastic B-cells

ANCILLARY TESTS

Immunohistochemistry
- Variable but at least 1 (+) pan-B-cell antigen (CD19, CD20, CD22, CD79a) and (-) for T-cell, myeloid antigens
- Germinal center type (GCB): CD10(+) or CD10(-)/BCL6(+)/MUM1(-)
- Activated B-cell type (ABC): CD10(-) with BCL6(-) or BCL6(+)/MUM1(+)
- Anaplastic: Frequently CD30(+)
- CD5(+) in 10%, often de novo, may be aggressive; CD5(+) diffuse LBCL are (-) for cyclin-D1 expression
- Double expressor lymphoma (a.k.a. double-positive lymphoma); MYC(+), BCL2(+) but lacks dual translocation
- BCL2(+) in 30-50%

Flow Cytometry
- False-negative results in up to 25% of cases due to disruption of large cells in acquisition/processing
- Up to 40% of cases lack surface light chain expression

DIFFERENTIAL DIAGNOSIS

High-Grade B-Cell Lymphoma
- Morphology: High grade with Burkitt-like features
- MYC, BCL2, &/or BCL6 rearrangements
  - EBV + LBCL; ALK + LBCL; HHV8 + diffuse LBCL; T-cell/histiocyte-rich LBCL; LBCL with IRF4; primary mediastinal LBCL

Burkitt Lymphoma
- Ki-67 strongly positive in virtually 100% of cells
- MYC gene translocations (8q24) are characteristic

Follicular Lymphoma (Grade 3)
- Distinction cannot be made by FNA in some cases

Mantle Cell Lymphoma, Pleomorphic Variant
- Cyclin-D1 (+); t(11;14)

Nonhematologic Malignancies
- Small cell carcinoma: TTF-1(+), neuroendocrine (+)
- Melanoma: HMB-45(+), S100(+), Melan-A (+)
- Seminoma: OCT4(+)
- Pediatric-type small round cell tumors
  - Immunohistochemistry variable according to type

SELECTED REFERENCES

1. Plaça JR et al: Reproducibility of gene expression signatures in diffuse large B-cell lymphoma. Cancers (Basel). 14(5):1346, 2022
2. Rohilla M et al: Application of Hans algorithm for subcategorization of diffuse large B-cell lymphoma in fine-needle aspiration biopsy cytology. Acta Cytol. 66(1):14-22, 2022
3. Swerdlow SH et al: The 2016 revision of the World Health Organization (WHO) classification of lymphoid neoplasms. Blood. 127(20):2375-90, 2016

Anaplastic Variant
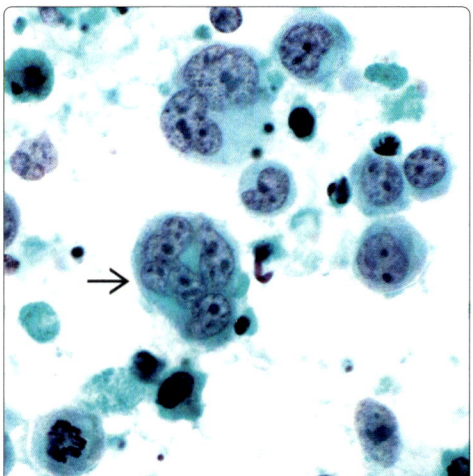

Diffuse Large B-Cell Lymphoma, Diff-Quik
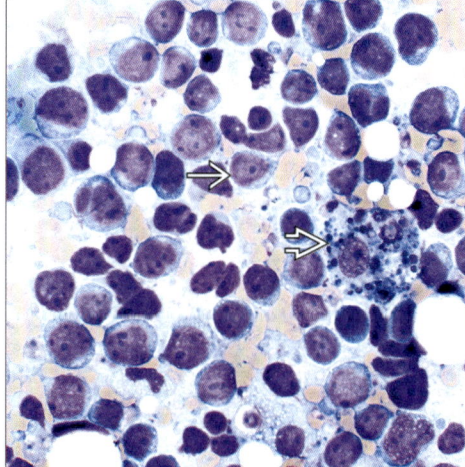

(Left) Pap-stained FNA smear of diffuse large B-cell lymphoma, anaplastic variant, reveals pleomorphic cells ➡. (Right) Diff-Quik-stained FNA smear of diffuse large B-cell lymphoma shows large tumor cells ➡ with prominent nucleolus and scant basophilic cytoplasm. Note the presence of a tingible body macrophage ➡.

Plasmacytoma

KEY FACTS

TERMINOLOGY
- Neoplasm composed of monoclonal plasma cells
  - Features diagnostic of plasma cell myeloma not present
- Extramedullary plasmacytoma (EP): Arises outside bone
  - Head and neck (90%), also GI tract
- Solitary plasmacytoma of bone (SPB)
  - Vertebrae are commonly involved

CYTOPATHOLOGY
- Plasma cells show spectrum of maturation
- Mature: Clumped peripheral chromatin, inconspicuous to absent nucleoli, and cytoplasmic perinuclear hof
- Immature: Pleomorphic nuclei, fine or immature chromatin, and prominent nucleoli
- Plasmablastic or anaplastic: Large nuclei, less cytoplasm, often prominent nucleoli

ANCILLARY TESTS
- CD138(+), CD38(+), CD19(-), CD20(-), light chain restriction

TOP DIFFERENTIAL DIAGNOSES
- Low-grade lymphoma with marked plasmacytic differentiation
  - Presence of monoclonal B-cell population (usually MALT lymphoma)
- Castleman disease, plasma cell variant
  - Plasma cells are polytypic
- Plasma cell granuloma
  - Polytypic and lacks cytologic atypia
- Plasmablastic lymphoma
  - EBER usually positive (negative in plasmacytoma)
- ALK(+) diffuse large B-cell lymphoma
  - Typically CD138(+), ALK(+), CD30(-), CD20(-), CD45 (weak)
- Poorly differentiated carcinoma
  - CD138(+), cytokeratin (+), Ig(-)
- Metastatic melanoma
  - CD38(-), S100(+), HMB-45(+)

(Left) *Pap-stained FNA smear of plasmacytoma shows plasma cells with a clumped clockface chromatin pattern ⇨, inconspicuous nucleoli, and perinuclear hof ⇨.* (Right) *Diff-Quik-stained FNA smear of plasmacytoma shows a mixture of less differentiated plasma cells ⇨, as demonstrated by higher N:C ratio, and more prominent nucleoli. Well-differentiated plasma cells ⇨ are also present.*

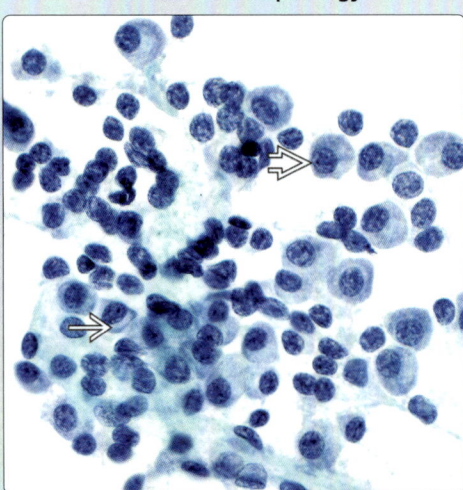
Plasma Cell Morphology

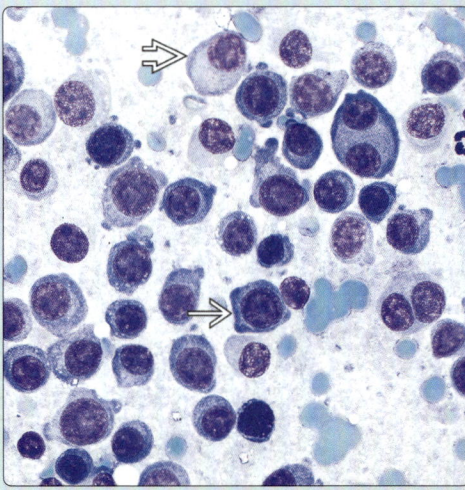
Mixed Mature and Immature Plasma Cells

(Left) *Core biopsy of plasmacytoma stained with H&E shows sheets of plasma cells ⇨ with eccentrically placed nucleus, including rare binucleated forms ⇨.* (Right) *Core biopsy of plasmacytoma immunostained for CD138 shows diffuse and strong positivity in the tumor cells ⇨.*

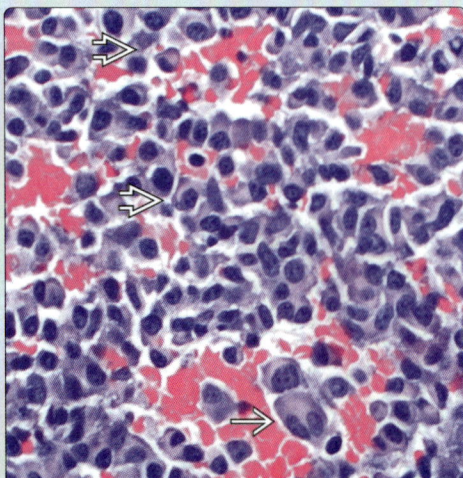
Plasmacytoma

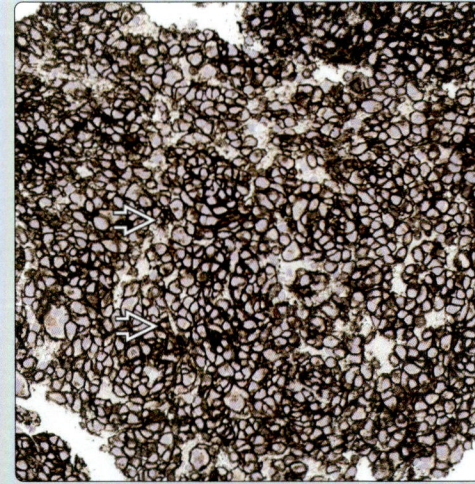
Plasmacytoma

Plasmacytoma

TERMINOLOGY

Definitions
- Neoplasm composed of monoclonal plasma cells
  - No evidence of bone marrow involvement
  - No clinical features of plasma cell myeloma
  - Small or absent monoclonal component in urine or serum

CLINICAL ISSUES

Epidemiology
- Incidence
  - Rare; < 5% of all plasma cell malignancies

Presentation
- Extramedullary plasmacytoma (EP)
  - Head and neck (90%), also GI tract
- Solitary plasmacytoma of bone (SPB)
  - Bone pain, pathologic fracture
  - Vertebrae are commonly involved (thoracic > lumbar/cervical)

CYTOPATHOLOGY

Cells
- Plasma cells may show spectrum of maturation from well to poorly differentiated
  - Mature: Clumped peripheral chromatin, inconspicuous to absent nucleoli, and cytoplasmic perinuclear hof
  - Immature: Pleomorphic nuclei, fine or immature chromatin, and prominent nucleoli
  - Plasmablastic or anaplastic: Large nuclei, less cytoplasm, often prominent nucleoli

ANCILLARY TESTS

Immunohistochemistry
- CD138(+), CD38(+), CD79a(+), MUM1/IRF4(+), usually IgG(+)/IgA(+)
- IHC &/or ISH show light chain restriction
- CD19(-), usually PAX5(-), CD20(-), CD45(-)
- CD56(+) in 50% in bone and 10% of others

Flow Cytometry
- Immunophenotype similar to IHC

DIFFERENTIAL DIAGNOSIS

Low-Grade Lymphoma With Marked Plasmacytic Differentiation
- Presence of monoclonal B-cell population (usually MALT lymphoma)

Castleman Disease, Plasma Cell Variant
- Plasma cells are polytypic

Plasma Cell Granuloma
- Polytypic and lacks cytologic atypia

Plasmablastic Lymphoma
- Antigen profile similar to that of plasmacytoma
- EBER usually positive (negative in plasmacytoma)

ALK(+) Diffuse Large B-Cell Lymphoma
- Usually occurs in children and young adults
- Typically CD138(+), ALK(+), CD30(-), CD20(-), CD45 (weak)

Poorly Differentiated Carcinoma
- CD138(+), cytokeratin (+), Ig(-)

Metastatic Melanoma
- CD38(-), S100(+), HMB-45(+)

SELECTED REFERENCES

1. Shi L et al: Extramedullary plasmacytoma of the pancreas diagnosed by EUS-guided fine-needle biopsy (with videos). Endosc Ultrasound. 10(2):143-4, 2021
2. Pham A et al: Solitary plasmacytoma: a review of diagnosis and management. Curr Hematol Malig Rep. 14(2):63-9, 2019
3. Caers J et al: Diagnosis, treatment, and response assessment in solitary plasmacytoma: updated recommendations from a European Expert Panel. J Hematol Oncol. 11(1):10, 2018
4. de Waal EG et al: Progression of a solitary plasmacytoma to multiple myeloma. A population-based registry of the northern Netherlands. Br J Haematol. 175(4):661-7, 2016

Variation in Cell Size

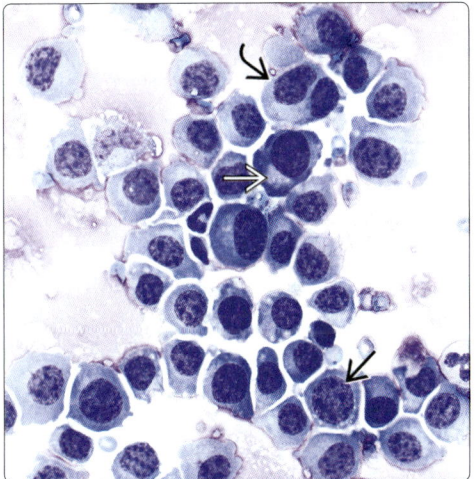

Eccentric Nuclei and Perinuclear Hof

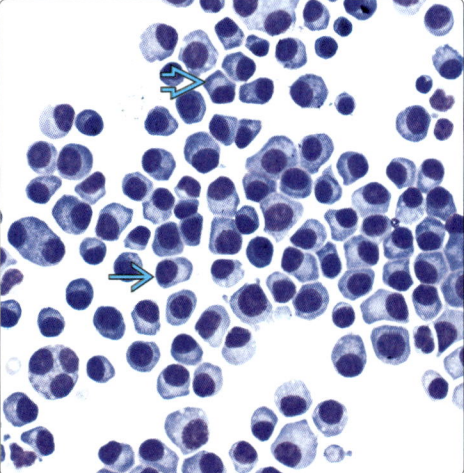

(Left) Diff-Quik-stained cytospin of plasmacytoma shows plasma cells with a clockface chromatin pattern ➡, perinuclear hof ➡, and binucleation ➡. Note the variation in cell size, which is typical of a plasma cell neoplasm. (Right) Diff-Quik-stained FNA smear of plasmacytoma shows plasma cells with eccentrically placed nuclei ➡ and perinuclear hof ➡.

Mediastinal Large B-Cell Lymphoma

KEY FACTS

CLINICAL ISSUES
- Enlarging mass in anterior-superior mediastinum
- Most patients 20-35 years of age; M:F = 1:2
- Prognosis is similar to patients with other types of diffuse large B-cell lymphoma (DLBCL)

CYTOPATHOLOGY
- Large lymphoma cells; not readily distinguished from other types of large B-cell lymphoma
  o Extensive sclerosis can reduce yield of neoplastic cells
- Nuclei round to convoluted, often containing nucleoli
- Crush artifact, lymphoglandular bodies, necrosis variable

ANCILLARY TESTS
- CD45/LCA(+), CD20(+), CD30(+/-), usually weak or focal, CD10(-), CD15(-)
- Monoclonal Ig gene rearrangements
- Discordance in B-cell receptor expression is common; surface Ig(-) and CD79a(+)

TOP DIFFERENTIAL DIAGNOSES
- Nodular sclerosis Hodgkin lymphoma
  o Mediastinal involvement in ~ 80%
  o CD45/LCA(-), CD30(+), CD15(+/-), PAX5 (dim +), EMA(-)
- DLBCL
  o Older adults but also occurs at younger ages
  o Pan B-cell markers, PAX5(+), CD45/LCA(+), CD10 (+/-); typically surface Ig(+)
- T-lymphoblastic lymphoma
  o Small to medium lymphoblasts with fine nuclear chromatin
  o Typically immature T-cell lineage; TdT(+) in almost all cases
- Metastatic carcinoma
  o Cohesive groups of tumor cells
  o Keratin (+), CD45/LCA(-)
- Seminoma
  o SALL4(+), PLAP(+), OCT3/4(+), CD45/LCA(-)

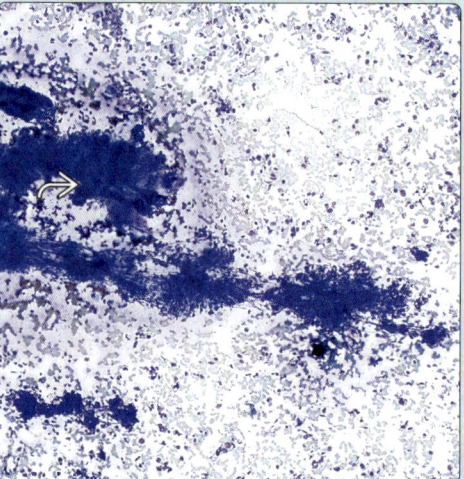

Large Fragments Due to Sclerosis

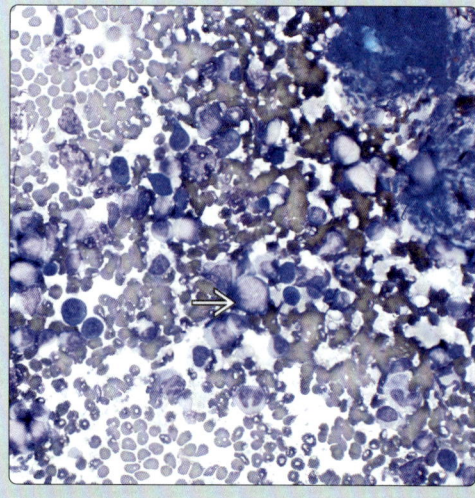

Large Lymphocytes

(Left) Diff-Quik-stained smear of primary mediastinal large B-cell lymphoma (PMLBCL) shows large fragments with cell crush artifact due to sclerosis ➡ and variable numbers of intact lymphocytes. (Right) Diff-Quik-stained FNA smear of mediastinal large B-cell lymphoma shows increased numbers of large lymphoid cells ➡.

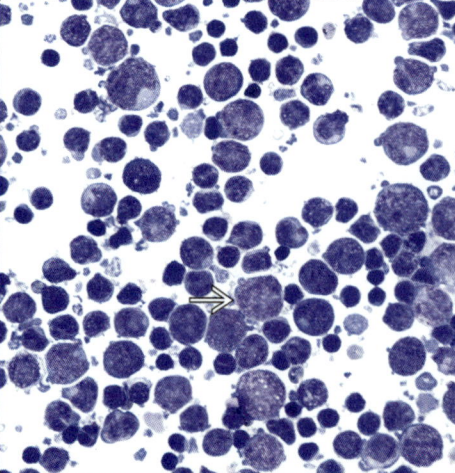

Polymorphous Lymphocytes

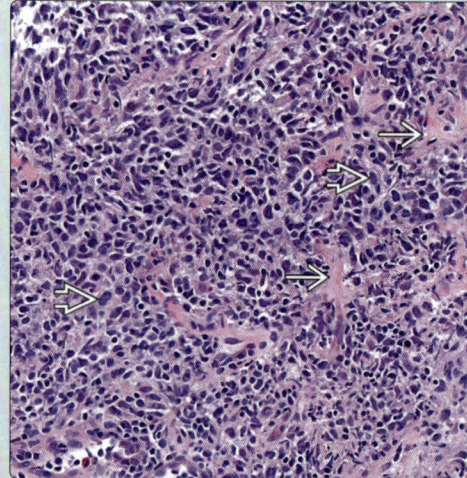

Mediastinal Large B-Cell Lymphoma Biopsy

(Left) Diff-Quik-stained cytospin preparation of mediastinal large B-cell lymphoma demonstrates medium and large-sized lymphoid cells ➡ with scant basophilic cytoplasm. (Right) Core biopsy of mediastinal large B-cell lymphoma shows distorted, predominantly large lymphoid cells ➡ with associated delicate interstitial fibrosis ➡.

Mediastinal Large B-Cell Lymphoma

TERMINOLOGY

Definitions
- Diffuse large B-cell lymphoma (DLBCL) arising in mediastinum of putative thymic B-cell origin

CLINICAL ISSUES

Epidemiology
- Incidence
  - 2% of all non-Hodgkin lymphomas
- Age and sex
  - Most frequent: 20-35 years; M:F = 1:2

Presentation
- Enlarging mass in anterior-superior mediastinum
- Patients have distinctive serum chemistry profile
  - Low serum β-2 microglobulin and high lactate dehydrogenase levels

CYTOPATHOLOGY

Cellularity
- Variable due to sclerosis

Background
- Crush artifact, lymphoglandular bodies, necrosis variable

Cells
- Large lymphoid cells not readily distinguishable from other types of large B-cell lymphoma

Nuclear Details
- Round to convoluted, often containing nucleoli

Cell Block Findings
- Typically limited by sclerosis and cell crush artifact

ANCILLARY TESTS

Immunohistochemistry
- Positive for common pan-B-cell markers
- CD45/LCA(+), p63(+) in ~ 95%
- CD30(+/-); weak/focal in ~ 75%
- CD10(-), CD15(-)

Flow Cytometry
- B-cell immunophenotype
- Discordance in B-cell receptor expression is common; surface Ig(-) and CD79a(+)

In Situ Hybridization
- EBER(-)

DIFFERENTIAL DIAGNOSIS

Nodular Sclerosis Classic Hodgkin Lymphoma
- CD45/LCA(-), CD30(+), CD15(+/-), PAX5(dim +), EMA(-)

Diffuse Large B-Cell Lymphoma
- Pan B-cell markers, PAX5(+), CD45/LCA(+), CD10 (+/-), typically surface Ig(+)

T-Lymphoblastic Leukemia/Lymphoma
- Small to medium-sized lymphoblasts with fine nuclear chromatin
- Typically immature T-cell lineage
- TdT(+) in almost all cases

Metastatic Carcinoma
- Cohesive groups of tumor cells
- Keratin(+), CD45/LCA(-)

Germ Cell Tumor
- Seminoma: OCT3/4(+), CD45/LCA(-)

SELECTED REFERENCES

1. Ahmed Z et al: Primary mediastinal B-Cell lymphoma: a 2021 update on genetics, diagnosis, and novel therapeutics. Clin Lymphoma Myeloma Leuk. 21(11):e865-75, 2021
2. Savage KJ: Primary mediastinal large B-cell lymphoma. Blood. ePub, 2021
3. Yu Y et al: Primary mediastinal large B cell lymphoma. Thorac Cancer. 12(21):2831-7, 2021
4. Vitagliano G et al: Large-cell lymphoma with features intermediate between Hodgkin's, primary mediastinal B-cell and grey-zone lymphoma: a conundrum on fine needle aspiration cytology. Cytopathology. 31(4):325-8, 2020

Cytospin Appearance
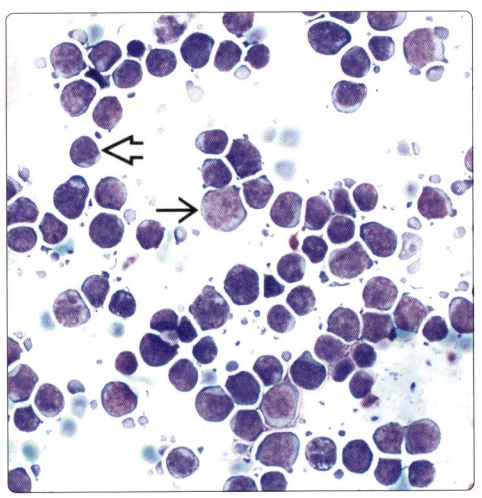

Necrosis and Debris in Background
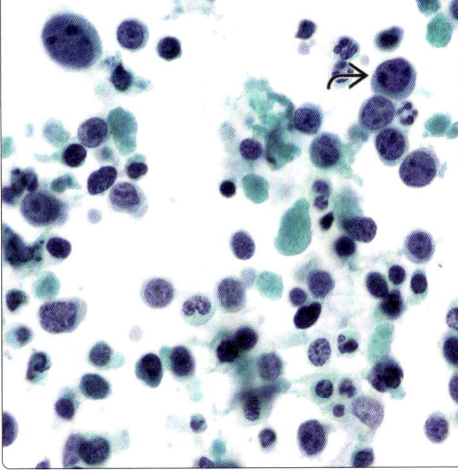

(Left) Diff-Quik-stained cytospin preparation of mediastinal large B-cell lymphoma shows medium-sized ⇨ and large ⇨ lymphoid cells. (Right) Pap-stained aspirate is hypocellular, containing few well-preserved large cells ⇨, in a background of necrotic cells and cellular debris.

Plasmablastic Lymphoma

KEY FACTS

CLINICAL ISSUES
- Frequently originates in mucosa of oral cavity
- EBV(+); strongly associated with HIV infection

CYTOPATHOLOGY
- Cytologic spectrum ranging from plasmablastic (abundant cytoplasm and eccentric nuclei) to immunoblastic (less cytoplasm and prominent central nucleoli)
- Cytoplasm of plasmablastic lymphoma (PBL) cells is usually deeply basophilic
- Binucleation or multinucleation is common in PBL

ANCILLARY TESTS
- Plasma cell markers (+)
- Weak or absent pan-B-cell antigens
- EBER(+); HHV8(-)
- Monoclonal *IGH* gene rearrangements
- High proliferation index (Ki-67)

TOP DIFFERENTIAL DIAGNOSES
- Large B-cell lymphoma, immunoblastic variant
  - CD20(+), CD19(+), CD45(+), CD10(+/-)
- Plasmablastic plasma cell myeloma
  - Can have virtually identical immunophenotypic profile to that of PBL
  - Favored by serum monoclonal protein (paraprotein), lytic bone lesions, and EBER(-)
- Multicentric Castleman disease, HHV8(+)
  - Patients have clinical and histologic features of multicentric Castleman disease
  - CD20(+/-), CD138(-), EBER(-), HIV(+)
- ALK(+) large B-cell lymphoma
  - ALK(+) in all cases; commonly CD4(+) and CD45/LCA(+)
  - Usually pan-B- and pan-T-cell markers (-), CD30(-)
- Melanoma
  - S100(+), HMB-45(+), Melan-A (+)

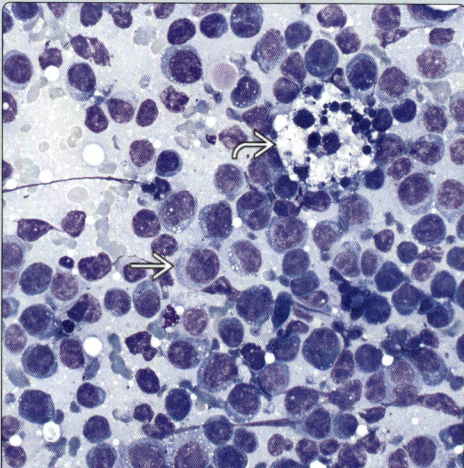

Plasmablastic Cells

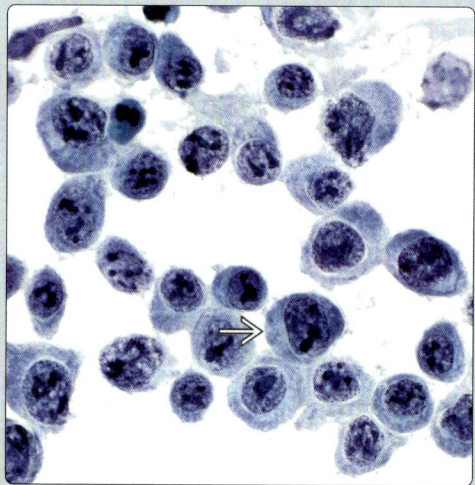

Basophilic Cytoplasm

(Left) Diff-Quik-stained FNA smear of plasmablastic lymphoma shows large cells with eccentric round nuclei and variably abundant basophilic cytoplasm as well as a tingible body macrophage. (Right) Pap-stained FNA smear of plasmablastic lymphoma shows plasmacytoid tumor cells of varying sizes with eccentrically placed nuclei and moderate amounts of basophilic cytoplasm.

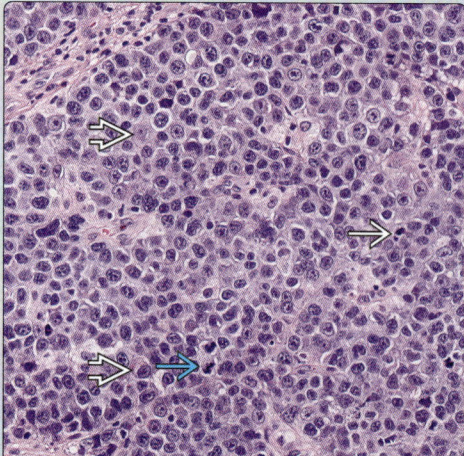

Plasmablastic Lymphoma Biopsy

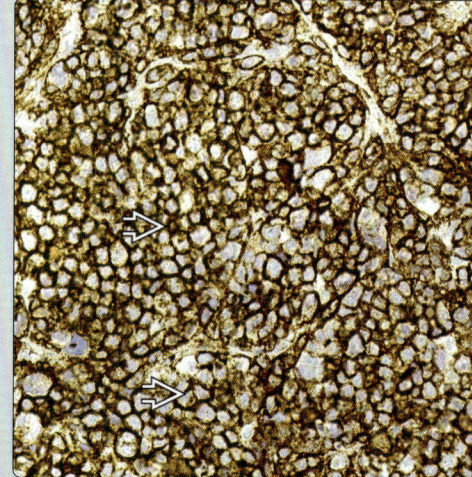

Plasmablastic Lymphoma, CD138 Stain

(Left) Core biopsy of plasmablastic lymphoma shows plasmacytoid cells with eccentrically placed large nuclei containing prominent central nucleoli. Apoptotic bodies and mitotic figures are seen among the tumor cells. (Right) Core biopsy of plasmablastic lymphoma immunostained for CD138 shows diffuse positive staining in all the tumor cells.

Plasmablastic Lymphoma

TERMINOLOGY

Definitions
- Diffuse proliferation of large neoplastic cells
  - Immunoblastic or plasmablastic cytologic features
  - Plasma cell immunophenotype: CD38(+), CD138(+), CD20(-)

ETIOLOGY/PATHOGENESIS

Infectious Agents
- EBV(+)
- Strongly associated with HIV infection

CLINICAL ISSUES

Presentation
- Most often originates in mucosal extranodal sites
- Oral cavity is most common site in HIV(+) patients

CYTOPATHOLOGY

Cells
- Plasmablastic
  - Cells have more abundant cytoplasm and eccentrically located nuclei
- Immunoblastic
  - Cells have prominent central nucleoli

Nuclear Details
- Binucleation or multinucleation is common in plasmablastic lymphoma (PBL)

Cytoplasmic Details
- Cytoplasm of PBL cells is usually deeply basophilic

ANCILLARY TESTS

Immunohistochemistry
- Common pan-B-cell markers are usually absent
- Strong positivity for plasma cell-associated markers
- High Ki-67 (> 70% in most cases)
- EMA is often positive; CD30(+) in subset
- Aberrant expression of T-cell markers in some cases
- HHV8(-); EBV-LMP1 and EBV-LMP2 are not expressed

In Situ Hybridization
- EBER(+) in ~ 75%

PCR
- Monoclonal *IGH* gene rearrangements

DIFFERENTIAL DIAGNOSIS

Large B-Cell Lymphoma, Immunoblastic Variant
- CD20(+), CD19(+), CD45(+), CD10(+/-)

Plasmablastic Plasma Cell Myeloma
- Greatly overlaps with PBL cytomorphologically and immunophenotypically
  - Favored by serum monoclonal protein (paraprotein), lytic bone lesions, and EBER(-)

Multicentric Castleman Disease, HHV8(+)
- CD20(+/-), CD138(-), EBER(-), HIV(+)

ALK(+) Diffuse Large B-Cell Lymphoma
- Immunophenotype is distinctive
  - ALK(+) in all cases
  - Usually pan-B- and pan-T-cell markers (-), CD30(-)

Myeloid Sarcoma
- Immunophenotype is helpful
  - MPO(+), lysozyme (+), CD68(+), CD117(+)

Melanoma
- S100(+), HMB-45(+), Melan-A (+)

SELECTED REFERENCES

1. Mori H et al: Heterogeneity in the diagnosis of plasmablastic lymphoma, plasmablastic myeloma, and plasmablastic neoplasm: a scoping review. Int J Hematol. 114(6):639-52, 2021
2. Pileri SA et al: Plasmablastic lymphoma: one or more tumors? Haematologica. 106(10):2542-3, 2021

Multinucleated Cells

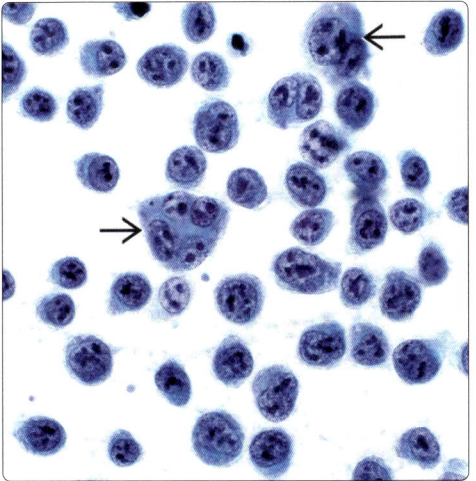

Eccentric Nuclei

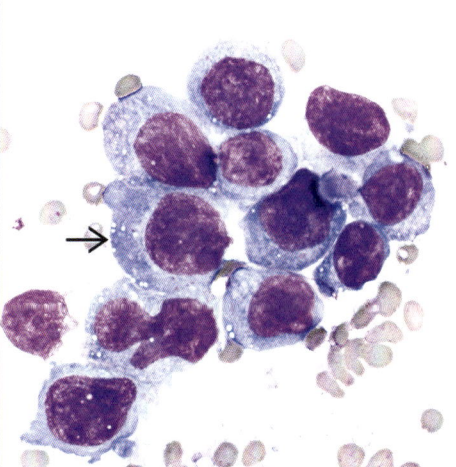

(Left) Pap-stained FNA smear shows plasmablastic tumor cells of various sizes, including scattered multinucleated tumor cells ➡. (Right) Diff-Quik-stained FNA smear of plasmablastic lymphoma highlights large tumor cells ➡ with eccentrically placed nuclei and moderate amounts of basophilic cytoplasm.

Peripheral T-Cell Lymphoma

KEY FACTS

CLINICAL ISSUES
- Represents ~ 6.0% of all non-Hodgkin lymphomas
- Mainly arises in middle-aged adults; rare in children
- Advanced stage disease with B symptoms
- Poor prognosis with frequent relapses
- Lymphadenopathy; extranodal sites are often involved

CYTOPATHOLOGY
- Wide spectrum of neoplastic T cells of small, intermediate, or large size
  - Most common: Numerous intermediate-sized &/or large cells
- Variable nuclear features: Round, cleaved/highly irregular
  - Multinucleated or Reed-Sternberg-like nuclei can occur
- Variable cytoplasmic features: Sparse to moderately abundant
  - Clear, eosinophilic, or basophilic
- Variable numbers of inflammatory cells (eosinophils, plasma cells, and epithelioid histiocytes) in background

ANCILLARY TESTS
- Immunophenotype best assessed by flow cytometry
- Pan-T-cell antigens (+)
- CD4(+)/CD8(-) or CD4(-)/CD8(+)
- Aberrant T-cell immunophenotypes in ~ 80% of cases
- Can be CD30(+); rarely CD15(+)
- Monoclonal TCR gene rearrangements

TOP DIFFERENTIAL DIAGNOSES
- Other T-cell lymphomas
  - Subclassification is based on histology; peripheral T-cell lymphoma (PTCL) is diagnosis of exclusion
- Classic Hodgkin lymphoma
  - Malignant cells: CD15(+), CD30(+), PAX5 (dim +)
- Granulomatous lymphadenitis
  - PTCL can present with associated chronic granulomatous inflammation
- B-cell lymphomas
  - Cytomorphologic overlap with many B-cell lymphomas

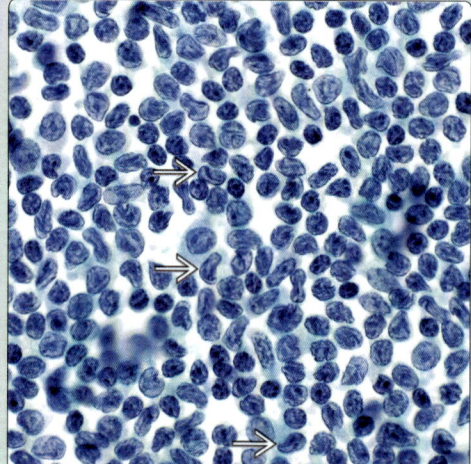

Nuclear Membrane Irregularities

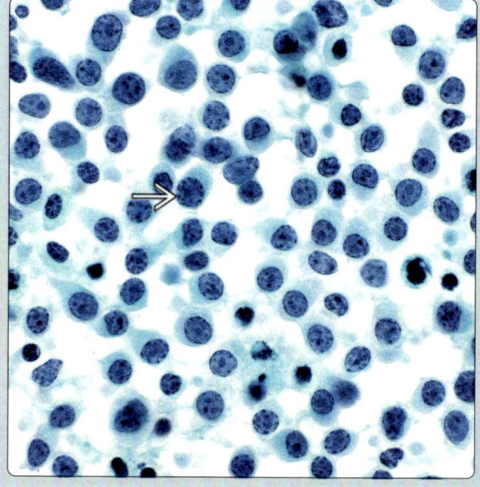

Eccentric Nuclei

(Left) Pap-stained FNA smear of peripheral T-cell lymphoma shows small- to medium-sized lymphoid cells with prominent nuclear membrane irregularities ➡. (Right) Pap-stained FNA smear of peripheral T-cell lymphoma shows predominantly medium-sized lymphoid cells ➡ with eccentric rounded nuclei and moderately abundant cytoplasm.

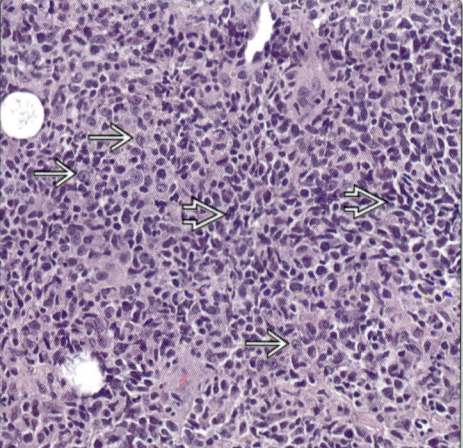

T-Cell Lymphoma Biopsy

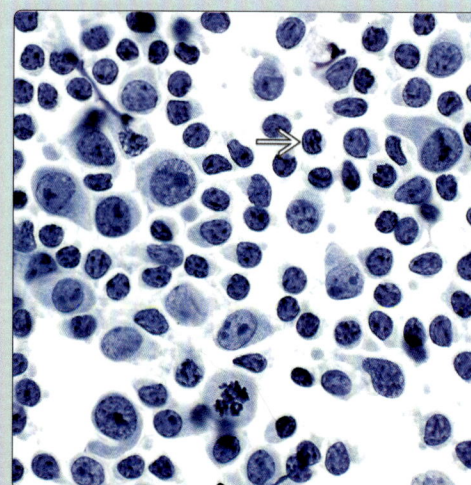

Mixed Small, Medium, and Large Cells

(Left) Core biopsy of peripheral T-cell lymphoma shows small lymphoid cells ➡ with irregular nuclear outlines associated with intermediate and large atypical lymphoid cells ➡. (Right) Pap-stained FNA smear of peripheral T-cell lymphoma shows a mixture of small, medium, and large lymphoid cells. Note that many of the smaller cells have irregular nuclei ➡.

Peripheral T-Cell Lymphoma

TERMINOLOGY

Definitions
- Mature T-cell lymphoma that cannot be classified into specific T-cell categories
  - Heterogeneous group in current WHO classification
  - In part, diagnosis of exclusion

CLINICAL ISSUES

Site
- Lymph nodes are usually involved
- Involvement of extranodal sites is common
  - Bone marrow, spleen, liver, lung, and skin

CYTOPATHOLOGY

Background
- Variable numbers of inflammatory cells (eosinophils, plasma cells, and epithelioid histiocytes)

Cells
- Wide spectrum of neoplastic T cells of small, intermediate, or large size
  - Numerous intermediate-sized &/or large cells are most common

Nuclear Details
- Wide spectrum: Vesicular, hyperchromatic, or pleomorphic
- Multinucleated or Reed-Sternberg-like nuclei can occur

Cytoplasmic Details
- Variable, from sparse to moderately abundant
- Clear, eosinophilic, or basophilic

ANCILLARY TESTS

Immunohistochemistry
- Mature T-cell immunophenotype
  - CD4(+)/CD8(-) or CD4(-)/CD8(+)
  - TdT(-), CD1a(-), CD99(-), pan-B-cells antigens (-)
- Aberrant T-cell immunophenotype in ~ 80% of cases
  - Loss or deletion of ≥ 1 pan-T-cell antigen
    - Frequent absence of CD2, CD3, CD5, CD7, or TCR
    - Decreased (dim) intensity of antigen expression compared with normal T cells
- Can be CD30(+), rarely CD15(+)
- Proliferation rate (Ki-67) is highly variable

Flow Cytometry
- More reliably assesses aberrant immunophenotype

Genetic Testing
- Monoclonal TCR gene rearrangements

DIFFERENTIAL DIAGNOSIS

Other T-Cell Lymphomas
- Subclassification is based on histology; peripheral T-cell lymphoma (PTCL) is diagnosis of exclusion

Classic Hodgkin Lymphoma
- Hodgkin-Reed-Sternberg (HRS)-like cells can occur in PTCL and mimic classic Hodgkin lymphoma
- HRS cells: CD15(+), CD30(+), PAX5 (dim +)

Granulomatous Lymphadenitis
- PTCL can present with associated chronic granulomatous inflammation
- Aberrant T-cell immunophenotype or monoclonal TCR gene rearrangements support PTCL

B-Cell Lymphoma
- Cytomorphologic overlap, particularly with follicular lymphoma, marginal zone lymphoma, diffuse large B-cell lymphoma, and T-cell/histiocyte-rich large B-cell lymphoma

SELECTED REFERENCES

1. Luminari S et al: What's new in peripheral T-cell lymphomas. Hematol Oncol. 39 Suppl 1:52-60, 2021
2. Fiore D et al: Peripheral T cell lymphomas: from the bench to the clinic. Nat Rev Cancer. 20(6):323-42, 2020
3. Basha BM et al: Application of a 5 marker panel to the routine diagnosis of peripheral T-cell lymphoma with T-follicular helper phenotype. Am J Surg Pathol. 43(9):1282-90, 2019

Reed-Sternberg-Like Cell

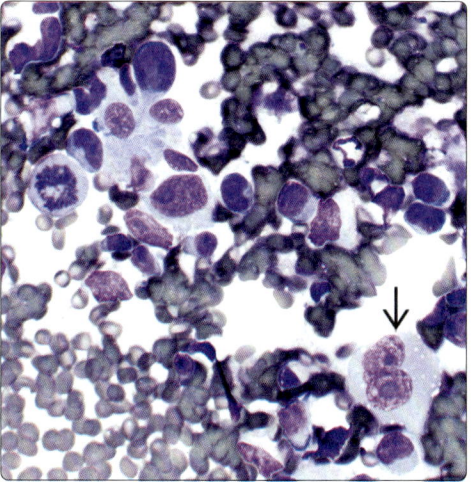

Atypical Mitosis

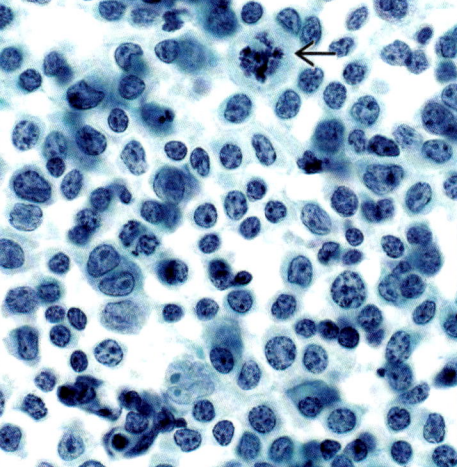

(Left) Diff-Quik-stained FNA smear of peripheral T-cell lymphoma shows many large lymphoid cells, including 1 that demonstrates Reed-Sternberg-like morphology ➡. *(Right)* Pap-stained FNA smear of peripheral T-cell lymphoma shows a polymorphous population of lymphoid cells, including small, medium, as well as large lymphoid, cells. Note the presence of an atypical mitotic figure ➡ in one of the neoplastic cells.

Mycosis Fungoides

KEY FACTS

CLINICAL ISSUES
- Primary cutaneous T-cell lymphoma characterized by epidermotropism and stepwise evolution of patches, plaques, and tumors
- 50% of all cases of primary cutaneous lymphoma
- Adults (5th-6th decades); M:F = 2:1
- Overall indolent clinical course
- Clinical stage is most important predictor of prognosis
- Nodal involvement changes therapy and indicates poor prognosis

CYTOPATHOLOGY
- Small to medium-sized lymphocytes
- Some cells are elongated with trailing cytoplasm
- Irregular (cerebriform) nuclear contours with hyperchromasia
- May undergo large cell transformation

ANCILLARY TESTS
- Immunophenotype
  - CD3(+), CD5(+), TCR-αβ(+)
  - Typically CD4(+), CD8(-), CD7(-), CD26(-)
  - CD30(+/-), usually expressed by large cells
- Flow cytometry
  - Typical immunophenotype: CD3(+), CD4(+), CD8(-), CD5(+), TCR-αβ(+)
    - CD4:CD8 ratio is often increased
    - Frequent immunophenotypic aberrancies
      - CD26(-), loss of/decreased CD7; dim expression of CD2, CD3, CD4, or CD5
- Genetic testing
  - Monoclonal TCR gene rearrangements

TOP DIFFERENTIAL DIAGNOSES
- Reactive process
- Peripheral T-cell lymphoma
- Anaplastic large cell lymphoma

Elongated Cells With Trailing Cytoplasm
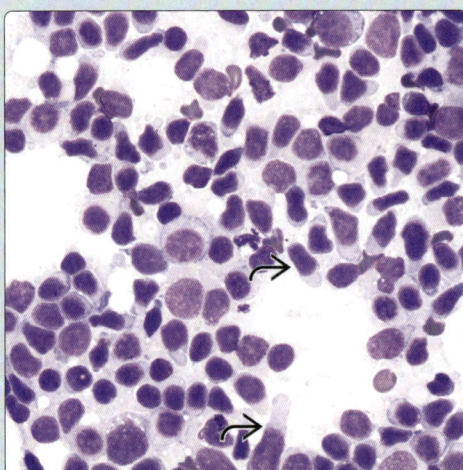

Cerebriform Nuclei
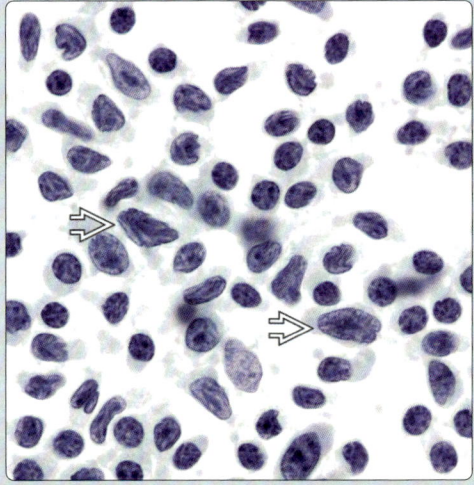

(Left) Diff-Quik-stained FNA smear of a lymph node involved by mycosis fungoides shows a polymorphous population of lymphocytes with elongated cells, some with trailing cytoplasm ➤. (Right) Pap-stained FNA smear of a lymph node involved by mycosis fungoides shows large lymphoid cells with highly irregular, cerebriform nuclei ➤.

Mycosis Fungoides Biopsy
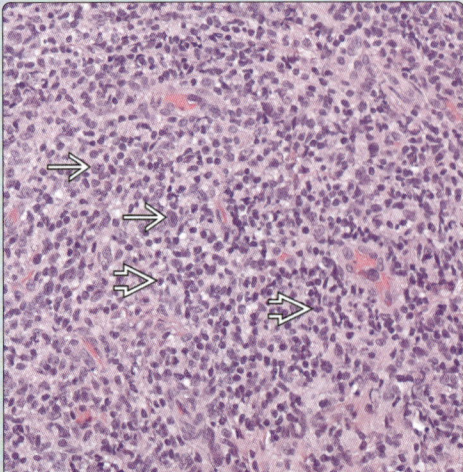

Mycosis Fungoides, CD4(+)
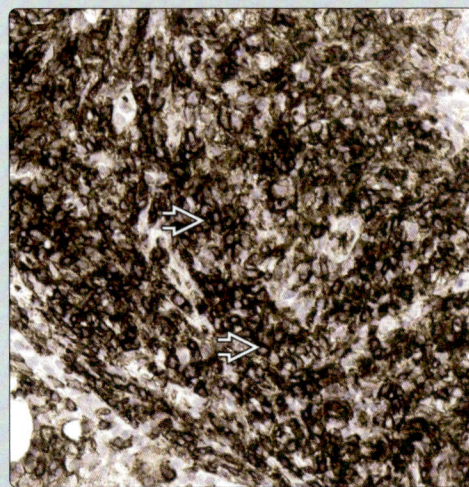

(Left) Core biopsy of mycosis fungoides stained with H&E shows small lymphoid cells ➤ with irregular nuclear contours associated with few intermediate and large lymphoid cells ➤. (Right) Core biopsy of mycosis fungoides immunostained for CD4 shows all the neoplastic lymphoid cells to be positive ➤.

Mycosis Fungoides

TERMINOLOGY

Definitions
- Primary cutaneous T-cell lymphoma characterized by
  - Epidermotropism
  - Clinical course showing stepwise evolution of patches, plaques, and tumors

CLINICAL ISSUES

Epidemiology
- Incidence
  - 50% of all cases of primary cutaneous lymphoma
- Age
  - Adults (5th-6th decades)
- Sex
  - M:F = 2:1
- Ethnicity
  - Incidence is 1.7x higher in Black than in White populations

CYTOPATHOLOGY

Cells
- Small to medium-sized
- Some appear elongated or twisted

Nuclear Details
- Cerebriform nuclear contours and hyperchromatic nuclei

Cytoplasmic Details
- Some cells have trailing cytoplasm

Cytology-Histology Correlation
- FNA is useful in setting of extensive involvement by mycosis fungoides (MF) (N3 disease)

ANCILLARY TESTS

Immunohistochemistry
- CD2(+), CD3(+), CD5(+)
- Often shows CD7 loss (all disease stages)
- CD4(+), CD8(-); rare cases can be CD4(-), CD8(+)
- CD45/LCA(+), CD52(+), CD25(-/+)
- CD30(+/-), usually expressed by large cells

Flow Cytometry
- CD4:CD8 ratio is often increased
- Typical immunophenotype: CD3(+), CD4(+), CD8(-), CD5(+), TCR-αβ(+)
- Frequent immunophenotypic aberrancies
  - CD26(-), loss of/decreased CD7
  - Dim expression of CD2, CD3, CD4, or CD5

Genetic Testing
- Monoclonal TCR gene rearrangements
- Complex karyotypes occur in subset of patients
  - Most common in patients with advanced-stage disease

DIFFERENTIAL DIAGNOSIS

Reactive Hyperplasia
- No atypical T cells
- Polyclonal B cells

Peripheral T-Cell Lymphoma
- Clinical history or histologic evidence of MF elsewhere is helpful

Anaplastic Large Cell Lymphoma
- Cases of MF with large cell transformation can be uniformly CD30(+), mimicking anaplastic large cell lymphoma
- Clinical history or histologic evidence of MF elsewhere is helpful

SELECTED REFERENCES

1. Sidiropoulou P et al: The different faces of mycosis fungoides: results of a single-center study. Int J Dermatol. 59(3):314-20, 2020
2. Hodak E et al: Mycosis fungoides: a great imitator. Clin Dermatol. 37(3):255-67, 2019
3. Kamijo H et al: Two distinct variants of mycosis fungoides (MF): folliculotropic MF and erythrodermic MF. J Dermatol. 46(12):1136-40, 2019
4. Cerroni L: Mycosis fungoides-clinical and histopathologic features, differential diagnosis, and treatment. Semin Cutan Med Surg. 37(1):2-10, 2018

Mitotically Active Large Cells

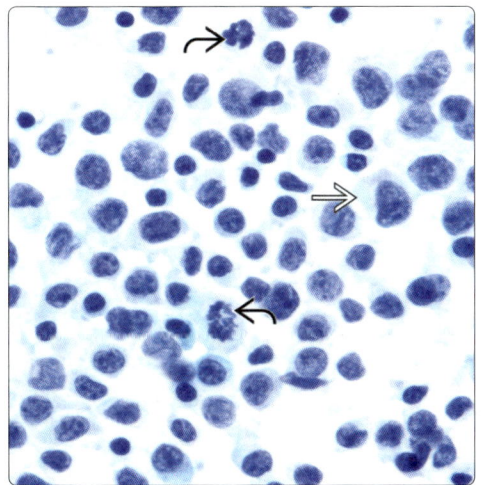

Nuclear Membrane Irregularities

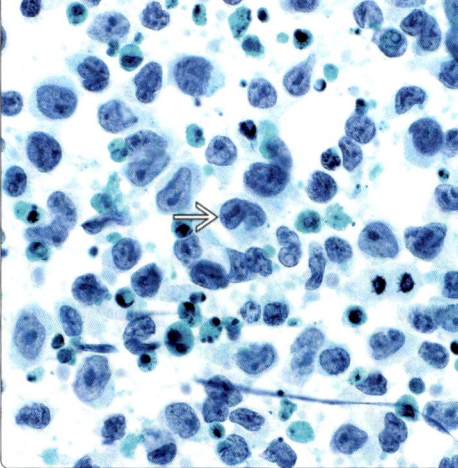

(Left) Pap-stained FNA smear of a lymph node aspiration from a patient with mycosis fungoides shows increased numbers of large lymphoid cells ➡ and scattered mitotic figures ➡. (Right) Pap-stained FNA smear of a lymph node involved by mycosis fungoides shows large lymphoid cells ➡ with striking nuclear membrane irregularities and prominent nucleoli. Apoptosis is also prominent.

Angioimmunoblastic Lymphoma

KEY FACTS

CLINICAL ISSUES
- ~ 20% of all peripheral T-cell lymphomas (PTCL); age range: 59-65 years
- Subacute or acute systemic illness
- Advanced stage with generalized lymphadenopathy, hepatomegaly, &/or splenomegaly
- Aggressive; median survival of < 3 years

CYTOPATHOLOGY
- Arborizing vasculature; increased follicular dendritic cells, eosinophils, and plasma cells; polymorphous lymphocytes with infrequent immunoblasts
- With advanced disease, fraction of large cells increases, and inflammatory background decreases

ANCILLARY TESTS
- Aberrant T-cell markers, CD7 (dim -), CD10(+/-), CXCL13(+/-), PD-1(+/-), TCR-αβ(+)
- B-immunoblasts in variable numbers
- Monoclonal TCR rearrangements
- EBER(+) in ~ 80-90% of cases
- Neoplastic cells have gene expression profile of follicular T-helper cells

TOP DIFFERENTIAL DIAGNOSES
- Reactive processes
  - Absence of atypical T-cells that are positive for CD10 or follicular T-helper cell markers
  - Usually no evidence of monoclonal TCR rearrangements
- Hodgkin lymphoma
  - No evidence of aberrant T-cell immunophenotype or monoclonal TCR rearrangements
- PTCL, not otherwise specified (NOS)
  - Lacks features that allow diagnosis of angioimmunoblastic T-cell lymphoma (AITL)
  - Markedly reduced B-cells; most cases are EBV(-)
  - Overlap in features between AITL and subset of PTCL, NOS

Polymorphous Population of Cells / Follicular Dendritic Reticulum

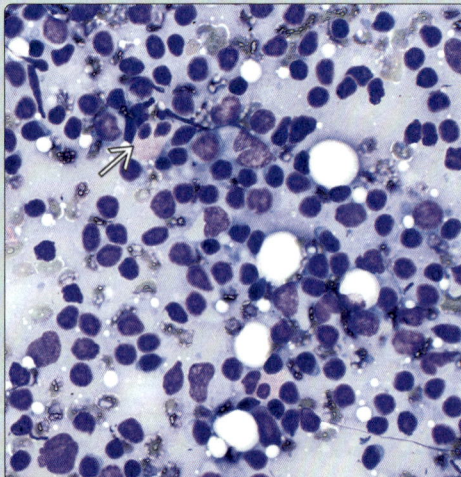 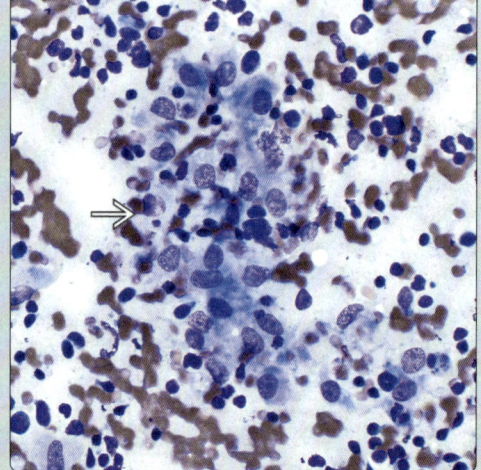

(Left) Diff-Quik-stained FNA smear of angioimmunoblastic T-cell lymphoma (AITL) shows a polymorphous population of lymphocytes as well as a few eosinophils ⇒. (Right) Diff-Quik-stained FNA smear of AITL shows an aggregate of follicular dendritic reticulum cells ⇒, which is a common finding in this entity though not specific.

Angioimmunoblastic Lymphoma Biopsy / Angioimmunoblastic Lymphoma, CD3 Stain

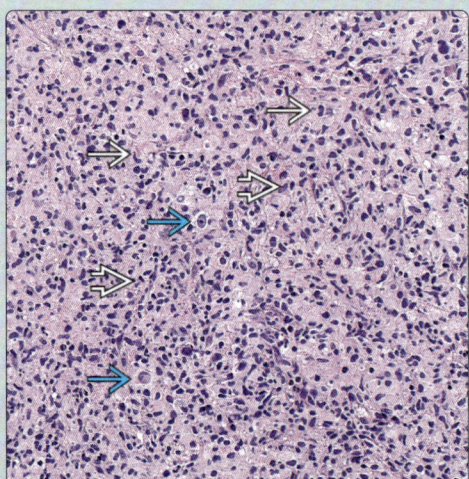 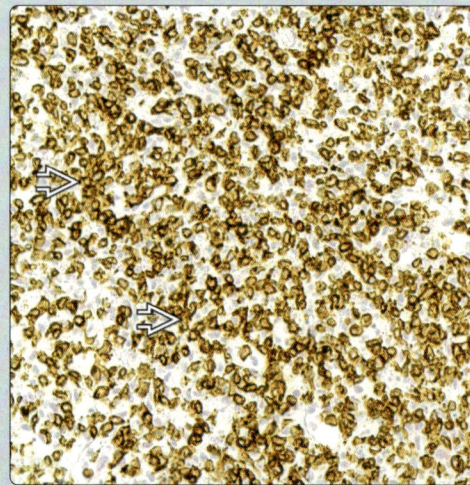

(Left) Core biopsy of angioimmunoblastic lymphoma stained with H&E shows numerous small, slightly irregular lymphocytes ⇒, histiocytes ⇒, and occasional large atypical cells resembling Hodgkin cells ⇒. (Right) Core biopsy of angioimmunoblastic lymphoma immunostained for CD3 shows that almost all of the small lymphoid cells in the tumor are CD3(+) ⇒.

Angioimmunoblastic Lymphoma

TERMINOLOGY

Abbreviations
- Angioimmunoblastic T-cell lymphoma (AITL)

Definitions
- Peripheral T-cell lymphoma (PTCL) derived from CD4(+) follicular T-helper cells characterized by lymphadenopathy, systemic disease, and (usually) immunodysregulation and immunodeficiency

ETIOLOGY/PATHOGENESIS

Viral Infection
- EBV(+) B-cells are detected in most cases of AITL

CYTOPATHOLOGY

Pattern
- Lymphoid fragments with arborizing vasculature and cell crush artifact, smaller fragments composed of follicular dendritic cells and lymphocytes, and dispersed single cells

Background
- Increased eosinophils, plasma cells, and dendritic cells
- Infrequent immunoblasts

Cells
- Polymorphous, mostly small- to medium-sized lymphocytes

Nuclear Details
- Irregular nuclei, often with minimal atypia

Cytoplasmic Details
- Clear to pale cytoplasm

ANCILLARY TESTS

Immunohistochemistry
- CD2(+), CD3(+), CD5(+), TCR-αβ(+)
- CD7(+/-), usually CD4(+) and CD8(-)
- CD10(+), BCL6(+), CXCL13(+), PD-1(+/-)
- Follicular dendritic cell-associated marker expression: CD21, CD23, CD35, clusterin
- B-immunoblasts are present in variable number
  - Commonly EBER(+); subset EBV-LMP1(+/-)

Flow Cytometry
- Normal CD4:CD8 ratio is common
  - Reactive T-cells often outnumber neoplastic T-cells
- Decreased expression or loss of CD7 &/or CD26
- Coexpression of CD10 in subset of T-cells
- Monotypic B-cells can be detected in ~ 15% of cases

In Situ Hybridization
- EBER(+) in ~ 80-90% of cases, but T-cells are EBER(-)

Genetic Testing
- TCR rearrangements in 75-90% of cases

DIFFERENTIAL DIAGNOSIS

Reactive Hyperplasia
- Absence of atypical T-cells that are positive for CD10 or follicular T-helper cell markers
- EBV(-) with exception of EBV(+) infectious mononucleosis
- Usually no evidence of monoclonal TCR rearrangements

Classic Hodgkin Lymphoma
- No evidence of aberrant T-cell immunophenotype or monoclonal TCR rearrangements

Peripheral T-Cell Lymphoma, Not Otherwise Specified (NOS)
- Gene expression profiling has shown that subset of PTCL, NOS has follicular T-helper cell profile
  - This suggests that some cases of early AITL are included within current PTCL, NOS category

SELECTED REFERENCES

1. Fei M et al: Cytopathological characteristics of angioimmunoblastic T-cell lymphoma diagnosed by fine needle aspiration. Cytopathology. ePub, 2022
2. Chiba S et al: Advances in understanding of angioimmunoblastic T-cell lymphoma. Leukemia. 34(10):2592-606, 2020

Cell Block Findings

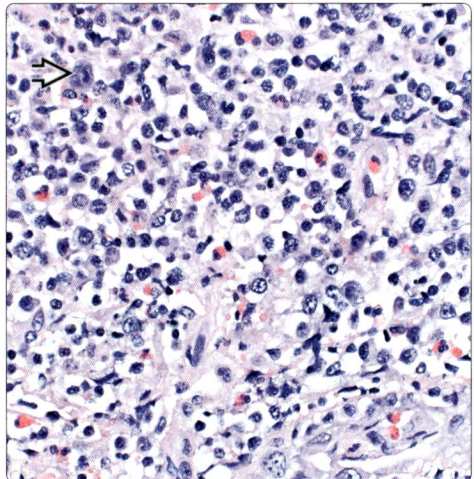

Dendritic Cells and Small Lymphocytes

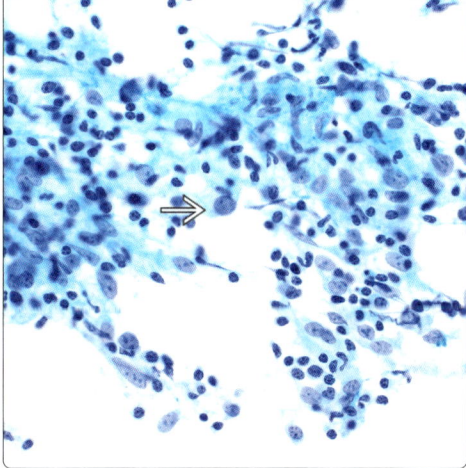

(Left) H&E-stained cell block preparation of a case of AITL shows prominent eosinophils, occasional plasma cells, and rare immunoblasts ➡. (Right) Pap-stained FNA smear of AITL shows many follicular dendritic reticulum cells ➡ associated with small lymphocytes.

ALK(+) Anaplastic Large Cell Lymphoma

KEY FACTS

CLINICAL ISSUES
- Usually presents in children and young adults
- Most patients present with clinical stage III/IV
- Extranodal involvement is common (60%)
- 5-year survival: 80-90%

CYTOPATHOLOGY
- Cytologic spectrum of neoplastic cells from small to large
- Characteristic hallmark cells: Large cells with eccentric horseshoe- or kidney-shaped nuclei and prominent paranuclear Golgi region
- Variants include lymphohistiocytic, small cell, and sarcomatoid

ANCILLARY TESTS
- Strongly and uniformly positive for CD30 and ALK
  - T- or null-cell lineage
- Characterized by translocations involving *ALK* gene at 2(p23); most commonly t(2;5)

TOP DIFFERENTIAL DIAGNOSES
- Classic Hodgkin lymphoma
  - Hodgkin Reed-Sternberg cells are positive for PAX5 (nuclear and weak) and ALK(-)
  - ALK(+) ALCL tumor cells are PAX5(-) and ALK(+)
- ALK(-) anaplastic large cell lymphoma (ALCL)
  - Morphologically similar to ALK(+) ALCL
  - Strong, uniform expression of CD30 but lacking ALK protein expression
- Peripheral T-cell lymphoma
  - Cytologic features not anaplastic
  - CD3(+), CD5(+), TCR(+)
  - CD30(-) or variably positive
- Diffuse large B-cell lymphoma expressing CD30
  - Some positive for CD30, but PAX5(+) and ALK(-)
  - Rarely expresses ALK; rarely carries either t(2;5) or t(2;17)

Hallmark Cell in Pleomorphic Population
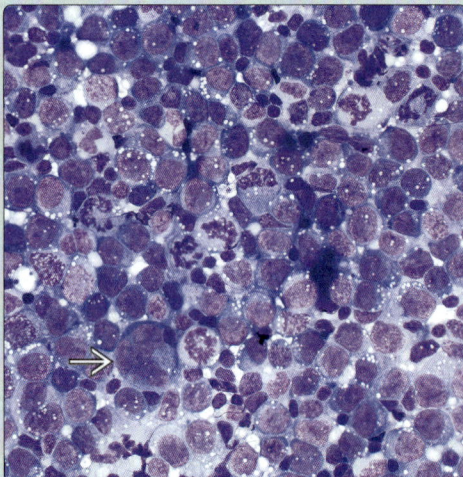

Horseshoe-Shaped Nucleus
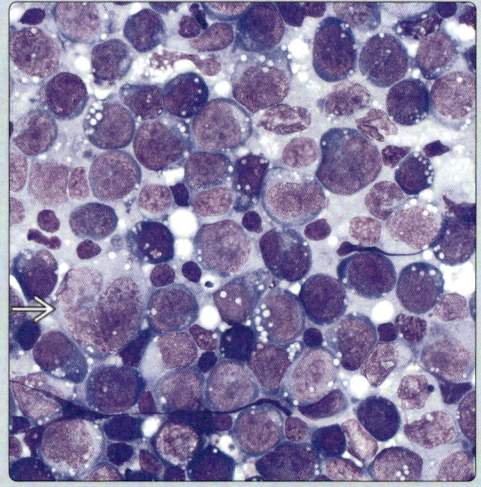

(Left) Diff-Quik-stained smear of ALK(+) anaplastic large cell lymphoma [ALK(+) ALCL] contains a hallmark cell ➡. The other lymphocytes are pleomorphic. (Right) Diff-Quik-stained FNA smear highlights the horseshoe-shaped nucleus of a hallmark cell ➡.

Anaplastic Large Cell Lymphoma
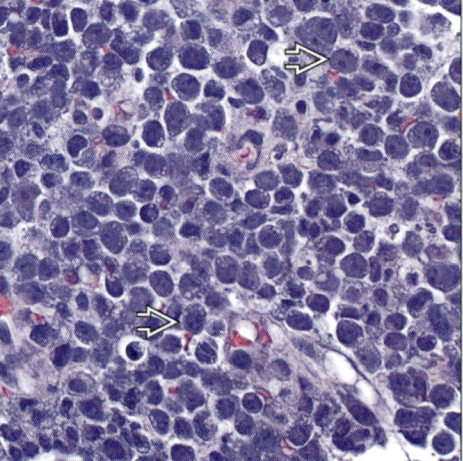

ALK(+)
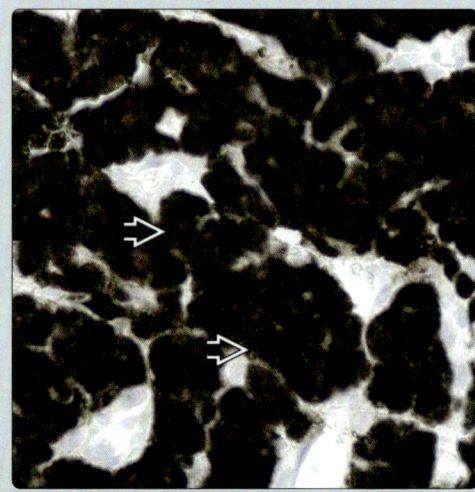

(Left) Core biopsy of ALCL stained with H&E shows monomorphic large lymphoid cells ➡ with round nuclei and prominent nucleoli in many tumor cells. (Right) Core biopsy of ALCL immunostained with ALK shows diffuse and strong nuclear and cytoplasmic positivity ➡ in the tumor cells.

ALK(+) Anaplastic Large Cell Lymphoma

TERMINOLOGY

Abbreviations
- Anaplastic large cell lymphoma (ALCL)

Definitions
- CD30(+) systemic lymphoma of T- or null-cell lineage with chromosomal abnormalities involving 2p23 and *ALK*

CLINICAL ISSUES

Presentation
- Children and young adults
- Most patients present with clinical stage III/IV disease and B symptoms
- Extranodal involvement is common (60%)
  - Particularly skin, soft tissue, and lungs

CYTOPATHOLOGY

Background
- Often necrotic; small lymphocytes

Cells
- Cytologic spectrum of neoplastic cells from small to large
- Hallmark cells: Large cells with eccentric horseshoe- or kidney-shaped nuclei and prominent paranuclear Golgi region
- Variants include lymphohistiocytic, small cell, and sarcomatoid

Nuclear Details
- Large, irregular, and pleomorphic; often polylobated

Cytoplasmic Details
- Variable (from scant to moderate)

ANCILLARY TESTS

Immunohistochemistry
- Strongly and uniformly positive for CD30 (membranous/Golgi) and for ALK in 60-85%
  - ALK(+) in 60-85%; ALK staining can be nuclear and cytoplasmic or restricted to nucleus or cytoplasm
- Can be of T- or null-cell lineage
  - In cases of T-cell lineage, aberrant T-cell immunophenotype is common
- EMA(+/-), CD45/LCA(+/-), EBV(-), B-cell antigens (-)

Genetic Testing
- ALK(+) ALCL characterized by chromosomal translocations involving *ALK* gene at 2p23
- Chromosomal translocations
  - 75-80% of cases t(2;5)(p23;q35)
    - t(2;5) juxtaposes nucleophosmin (*NPM1*) gene at 5q35 with *ALK* gene at 2p23, resulting in fusion protein NPM::ALK

DIFFERENTIAL DIAGNOSIS

Classic Hodgkin Lymphoma
- Hodgkin Reed-Sternberg cells are positive for PAX5 (nuclear and weak)
- Negative for EMA, CD45/LCA, and ALK

ALK(-) Anaplastic Large Cell Lymphoma
- Morphologically similar to ALK(+) ALCL
  - Strong, uniform expression of CD30 but lacking ALK protein expression

Peripheral T-Cell Lymphoma
- Cytologic features not anaplastic
- CD3(+), CD5(+), TCR(+)
- CD30(-) or variably positive

Diffuse Large B-Cell Lymphoma
- Some positive for CD30, but PAX5(+) and ALK(-)
- Rarely expresses ALK; rarely carries either t(2;5) or t(2;17)

SELECTED REFERENCES

1. Leventaki V et al: Pathology and genetics of anaplastic large cell lymphoma. Semin Diagn Pathol. 37(1):57-71, 2020

CD30(+) Tumor Cells

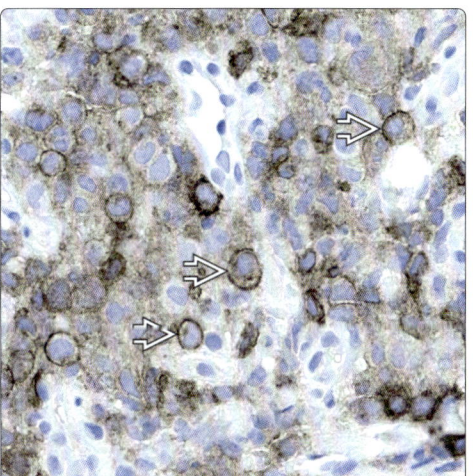

Resemblance to Carcinoma

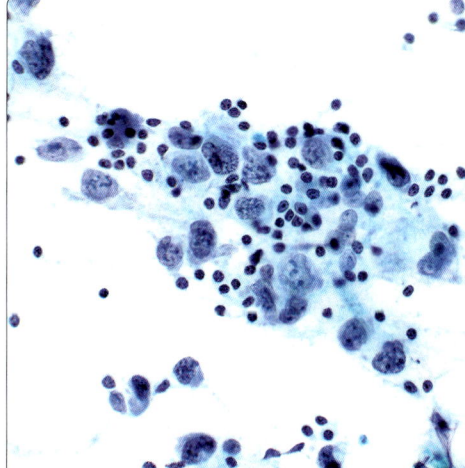

(Left) Core biopsy of ALCL immunostained for CD30 shows positive staining in the tumor cells ➡. **(Right)** Pap-stained FNA smear of ALK(+) ALCL shows a loosely cohesive group of tumor cells cytomorphologically mimicking a poorly differentiated carcinoma.

T-Cell Lymphoblastic Lymphoma

KEY FACTS

CLINICAL ISSUES
- Primarily affects adolescents and young adults
- Male predominance
- Rapidly growing anterior mediastinal mass (~ 75% of patients)
- Lymphadenopathy is typically supradiaphragmatic

CYTOPATHOLOGY
- Monomorphic population of lymphoblasts
- Small to intermediate nuclei with immature chromatin, variably present nucleoli, and scant cytoplasm
  - Convoluted or round nuclear contours
- High mitotic activity

ANCILLARY TESTS
- Immunophenotype
  - T-cell antigens (+), TdT(+)
  - CD1a(+) and CD10(+) in pre-T and cortical T stages
- TCR gene rearrangements

TOP DIFFERENTIAL DIAGNOSES
- B-lymphoblastic leukemia/lymphoma (B-LBL)
  - Morphologically similar; immunophenotype is needed
  - Pan-B-cell antigens (+) in B-LBL; TdT(+) and CD10(+/-) [similar to T-cell lymphoblastic lymphoma (T-LBL)]
- Large B-cell lymphoma
  - Pan-B-cell antigens (+); TdT(-) and CD10(+/-)
- Burkitt lymphoma
  - Monotonous, medium-sized cells with 2-5 distinct nucleoli; deeply basophilic cytoplasm with many vacuoles
  - Pan-B-cell markers (+), CD10(+); T-cell antigens (-), TdT(-), BCL2(-); Ki-67 > 90%
- Thymoma
  - Thymic epithelial cells can be appreciated in lymphocyte-rich thymoma using keratin immunostain
  - Mitotic activity in thymoma is low to moderate and not high as in T-LBL
  - No evidence of monoclonal TCR gene rearrangements

Homogenous, Medium-Sized Cells
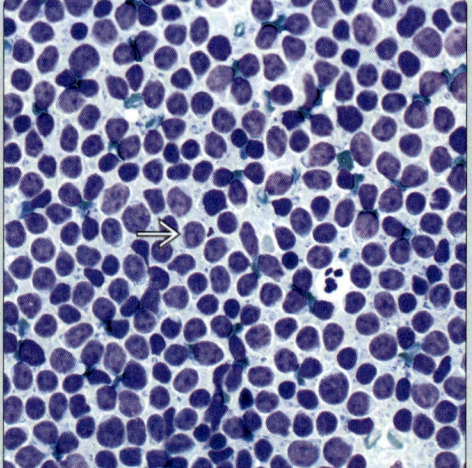

Fine Nuclear Chromatin
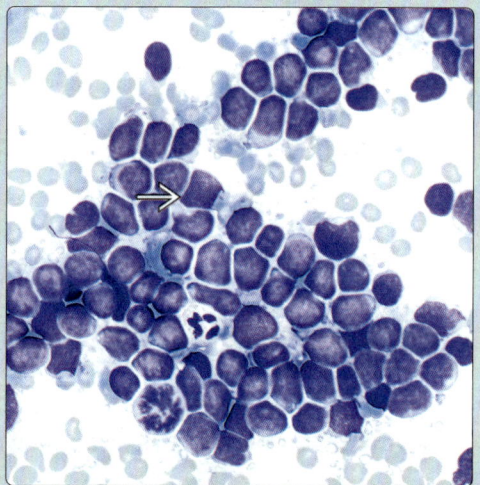

(Left) Diff-Quik-stained FNA smear of T-cell lymphoblastic lymphoma shows a relatively homogeneous population of medium-sized lymphoid cells with fine nuclear chromatin ➡. **(Right)** Diff-Quik-stained FNA smear of T-cell lymphoblastic lymphoma shows neoplastic cells ➡ with fine nuclear chromatin and scant cytoplasm.

Variable Nuclear Contour Irregularities
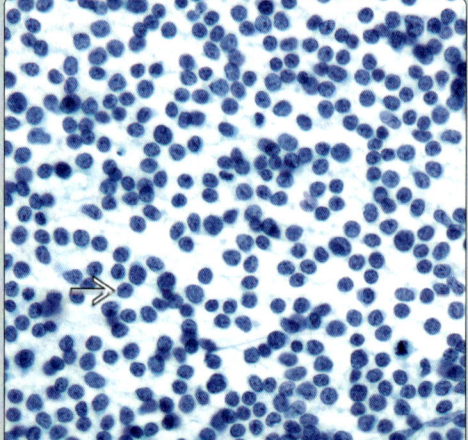

T-Cell Lymphoblastic Lymphoma Biopsy
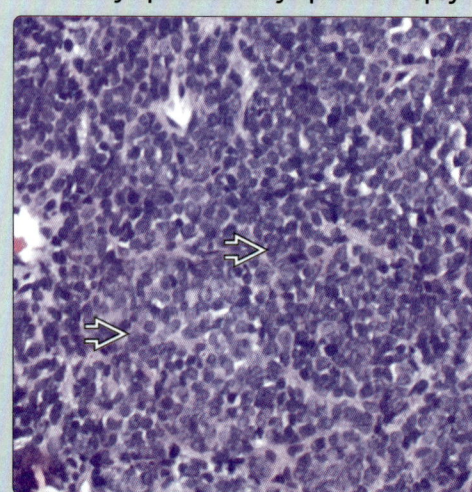

(Left) Pap-stained FNA smear of T-cell lymphoblastic lymphoma shows medium-sized lymphoid cells with round nuclei and nuclear membrane irregularities ➡ of varying degrees. **(Right)** Core biopsy of T-cell lymphoblastic lymphoma stained with H&E shows a uniform population of medium-sized lymphoid cells ➡ with fine nuclear chromatin and scant cytoplasm.

T-Cell Lymphoblastic Lymphoma

TERMINOLOGY

Abbreviations
- T-cell lymphoblastic lymphoma (T-LBL)

Definitions
- Neoplasm composed of lymphoblasts committed to T-cell lineage
- T-lymphoblastic lymphoma
  - Presentation with involvement of thymus, lymph nodes, &/or extranodal sites
  - No or minimal involvement of peripheral blood (PB) or bone marrow (BM)
- T-lymphoblastic leukemia (T-ALL)
  - Presentation with involvement of PB and BM

CLINICAL ISSUES

Presentation
- T-ALL
  - Rapidly growing anterior mediastinal mass (~ 75% of patients)
  - ~ 75% of patients present with stage III or IV disease

CYTOPATHOLOGY

Cells
- Monomorphic population of lymphoblasts
- High mitotic activity

Nuclear Details
- Small to intermediate nuclei with immature chromatin and variably present nucleoli

Cytoplasmic Details
- Scant cytoplasm

ANCILLARY TESTS

Immunohistochemistry
- T-cell antigens (+), TdT(+), CD1a(+), CD45(-/+), CD20(-)
- CD34(+/-), CD99(+/-), CD117/C-kit(-/+)
- Proliferation rate usually high but variable: Ki-67 ~ 50-90%

Flow Cytometry
- T-cell antigens are expressed in sequence as precursor T cells mature
  - T-LBL and T-ALL arise from precursor cell "frozen" in differentiation
  - T-ALL cases are more immature than T-LBL cases
- CD13(-/+) or CD33(-/+) in 20-30% of cases

Genetic Testing
- Gene rearrangements
  - Monoclonal TCR gene rearrangements in almost all cases

DIFFERENTIAL DIAGNOSIS

B-Lymphoblastic Leukemia/Lymphoma (B-LBL)
- Immunophenotype is needed to distinguish B- from T-LBL

Large B-Cell Lymphoma
- Pan-B-cell antigens (+)

Burkitt Lymphoma
- Morphologic features differ from those of T-LBL
- Pan-B-cell markers (+), CD10(+); Ki-67 > 90%

Thymoma
- Immunophenotype
  - Keratin (+) interlocking pattern of thymic epithelial cells in thymoma
  - Flow cytometry shows T cells in various stages of maturation

SELECTED REFERENCES

1. Luca DC: Update on lymphoblastic leukemia/lymphoma. Clin Lab Med. 41(3):405-16, 2021
2. Xu X et al: Genomic and clinical characterization of early T-cell precursor lymphoblastic lymphoma. Blood Adv. 5(14):2890-900, 2021
3. Kroeze E et al: T-cell lymphoblastic lymphoma and leukemia: different diseases from a common premalignant progenitor? Blood Adv. 4(14):3466-73, 2020
4. Cortelazzo S et al: Lymphoblastic lymphoma. Crit Rev Oncol Hematol. 113:304-17, 2017

Round to Oval Nuclei

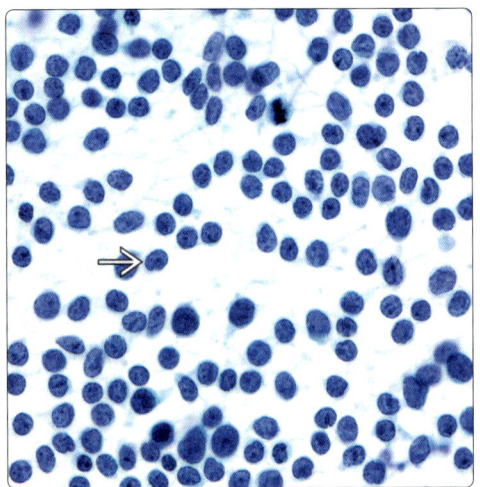

TdT(+)

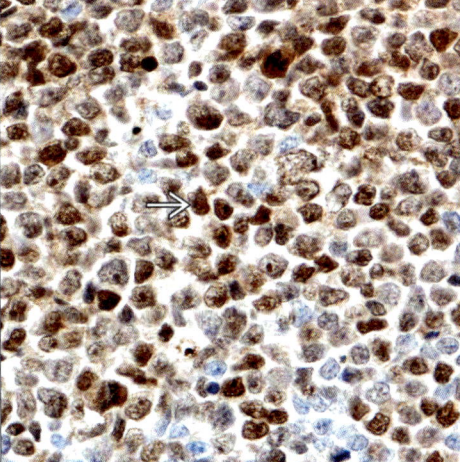

(Left) Pap-stained FNA smear of T-cell lymphoblastic lymphoma shows medium-sized lymphoid cells exhibiting round to oval nuclei with nuclear membrane irregularities ➡. (Right) TdT immunohistochemical stain performed on the cell block preparation of T-cell lymphoblastic lymphoma shows that the neoplastic cells are positive for TdT ➡.

Nodular Lymphocyte-Predominant Hodgkin Lymphoma

KEY FACTS

CLINICAL ISSUES
- 5-6% of all Hodgkin lymphomas
- All age groups are affected; peak incidence in 4th decade
- Presentation: Peripheral lymphadenopathy
  - Most commonly affected groups include cervical, axillary, or inguinal lymph nodes
- Good prognosis with 10-year survival rate > 80%
- Survival rate is higher than in classic Hodgkin lymphoma

CYTOPATHOLOGY
- Scattered large, neoplastic B cells called lymphocyte-predominant (LP) cells associated with small lymphocytes and epithelioid histiocytes
  - Eosinophils, neutrophils, and plasma cells are unusual
  - Classic Hodgkin and Reed-Sternberg cells are absent or rare
- LP cells have variety of appearances
  - Multilobated "popcorn" cells with vesicular chromatin and multiple small nucleoli
  - Multinucleated or mummified cells
  - Can be round without multilobation
- Diagnosis is difficult to establish in FNA specimens

ANCILLARY TESTS
- Immunophenotype of LP cells
  - CD20(+), CD22(+), CD45/LCA(+), CD79a(+), PAX5(+)
  - EMA(+) and MUM1(+) in ~ 50% of cases
  - CD15(-), CD30(-), EBV(-), BCL2(-)
- Background inflammatory infiltrate
  - Small lymphocytes are mixture of B and T cells

TOP DIFFERENTIAL DIAGNOSES
- Classic Hodgkin lymphoma
- T-cell/histiocyte-rich large B-cell lymphoma
- Follicular lymphoma
- Reactive lymphoid hyperplasia
- Viral lymphadenopathies

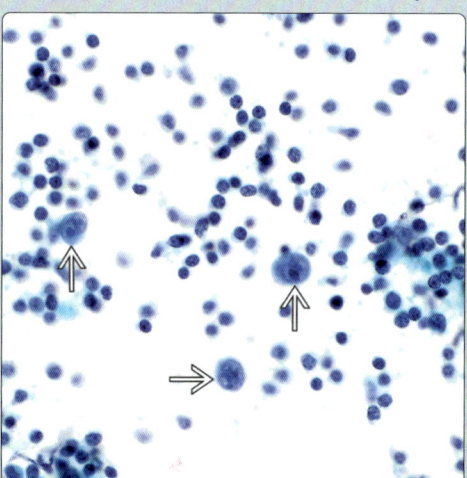

Lymphocyte-Predominant Cells: Pap

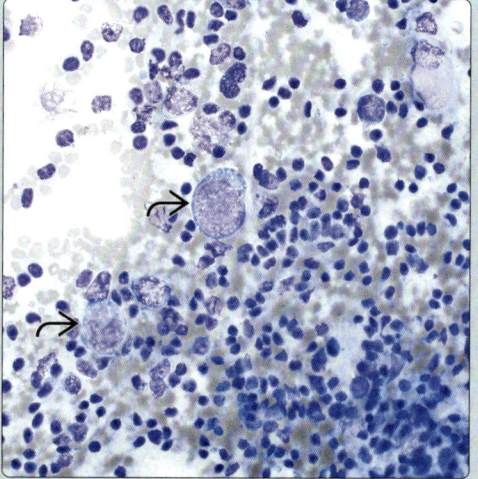

Lymphocyte-Predominant Cells: Diff-Quik

(Left) Pap-stained FNA smear of nodular lymphocyte-predominant (LP) Hodgkin lymphoma shows 3 LP cells ➡ with large, irregular nuclei and multiple nucleoli. (Right) Diff-Quik-stained FNA smear of LP Hodgkin lymphoma shows 2 LP cells ➡ in a background of small lymphocytes.

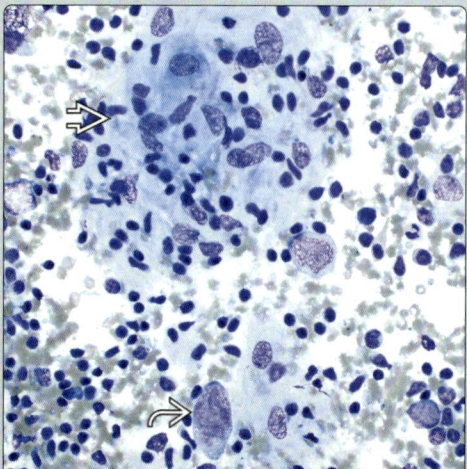

Background Histiocytes

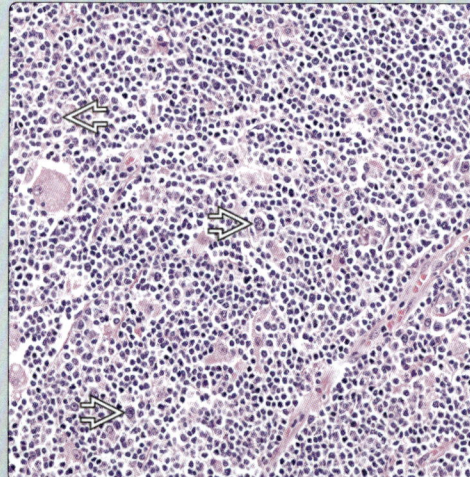

Nodular Lymphocyte-Predominant Hodgkin Lymphoma Biopsy

(Left) Diff-Quik-stained FNA smear of LP Hodgkin lymphoma shows an aggregate of epithelioid histiocytes ➡ and an LP cell ➡. (Right) Core biopsy of nodular LP Hodgkin lymphoma stained with H&E shows scattered neoplastic cells referred to as LP cells, a.k.a. "popcorn" cells ➡, in a background of small lymphocytes and histiocytes.

Nodular Lymphocyte-Predominant Hodgkin Lymphoma

TERMINOLOGY

Definitions

- Nodular proliferation of scattered large neoplastic B-cells associated with numerous chronic inflammatory cells
  - Neoplastic cells are designated as lymphocyte-predominant (LP) cells
    - a.k.a. "popcorn" cells because of their hyperlobated nuclei with vesicular chromatin
  - Background infiltrate of nonneoplastic small lymphocytes and histiocytes

CYTOPATHOLOGY

Background

- Diagnosis is difficult to establish in FNA specimens
  - Small, polymorphous lymphocytes and epithelioid histiocytes
  - Eosinophils, neutrophils, and plasma cells are unusual

Cells

- LP cells are large, rare, and scattered amongst abundant small lymphocytes and histiocytes
- Classic Hodgkin and Reed-Sternberg cells are absent or rare

Nuclear Details

- LP cells have variety of appearances
  - Multilobated "popcorn" cells with vesicular chromatin and multiple small nucleoli
  - Multinucleated or mummified cells
  - Can be round without multilobation

Cytoplasmic Details

- Pale, often disrupted on smears

ANCILLARY TESTS

Immunohistochemistry

- LP cells
  - CD20(+), CD22(+), CD79a(+)
  - CD45/LCA(+), PAX5(+), high Ki-67 (increased proliferation)
  - EMA(+) and MUM1(+) in ~ 50% of cases
  - Pan-T-cell antigens (-), BCL2(-)
  - CD15(-) and CD30(-)
  - EBV-LMP1(-)
- Background inflammatory infiltrate
  - Small lymphocytes are mixture of B and T cells

DIFFERENTIAL DIAGNOSIS

Classic Hodgkin Lymphoma

- Reed-Sternberg and Hodgkin cells are CD15(+), CD30(+), CD45/LCA(-)

T-Cell/Histiocyte-Rich Large B-Cell Lymphoma

- Immunophenotype
  - Large cells are of B-cell lineage
    - Pan-B-cell antigens (+), CD45/LCA(+), CD30(+/-)

Follicular Lymphoma

- Immunophenotype
  - CD10(+), BCL6(+), BCL2(+)
  - Flow cytometry immunophenotype shows monotypic B lymphocytes, CD10(+)

Reactive Lymphoid Hyperplasia

- Small and large centrocytes and centroblasts without atypia; tingible body macrophages

Viral Lymphadenopathies

- Acute clinical symptoms, usually in young patients
- Large cells stain with T- and B-cell markers

SELECTED REFERENCES

1. Connors JM et al: Hodgkin lymphoma. Nat Rev Dis Primers. 6(1):61, 2020
2. Gupta S et al: Role of FNA with core biopsy or cell block in patients with nodular lymphocyte-predominant Hodgkin lymphoma. Cancer Cytopathol. 128(8):570-9, 2020
3. Hartmann S et al: Nodular lymphocyte predominant Hodgkin lymphoma: pathology, clinical course and relation to T-cell/histiocyte rich large B-cell lymphoma. Pathology. 52(1):142-53, 2020
4. Fan Z et al: Characterization of variant patterns of nodular lymphocyte predominant Hodgkin lymphoma with immunohistologic and clinical correlation. Am J Surg Pathol. 27(10):1346-56, 2003

"Popcorn" Lymphocyte-Predominant Cell

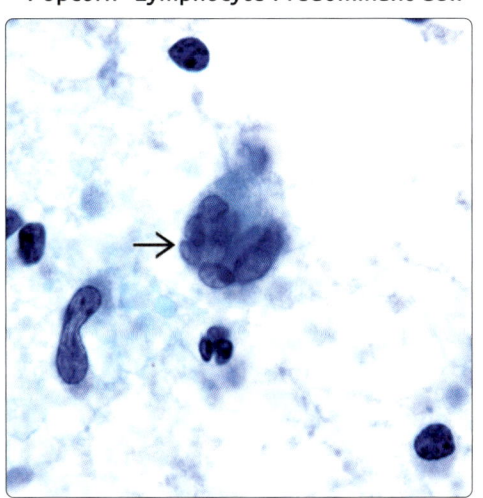

CD20(+) Lymphocyte-Predominant Cell

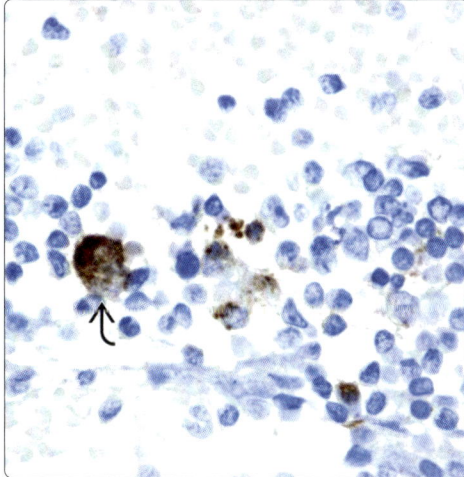

(Left) Pap-stained FNA smear of LP Hodgkin lymphoma shows a "popcorn" LP cell ➡. **(Right)** Cell block section of LP Hodgkin lymphoma shows an LP cell positive for CD20 ➡.

Classic Hodgkin Lymphoma

KEY FACTS

CLINICAL ISSUES
- Lymphoid neoplasm composed of Hodgkin and Reed-Sternberg (HRS) cells in variable inflammatory background
- 4 subtypes: Nodular sclerosis, lymphocyte rich, mixed cellularity, and lymphocyte depleted
- Epstein-Barr virus (EBV) present in HRS cells in ~ 20% of cases and has probable pathogenetic role
- Typical presentation: Age 15-34 years; mediastinal or cervical lymph nodes
- > 90% survival at 5 years in patients with early-stage disease

CYTOPATHOLOGY
- Variable numbers of HRS cells in background of spectrum of small lymphocytes, eosinophils, &/or histiocytes
- Reed-Sternberg (RS) cells: Large with binucleated nuclei and very prominent nucleoli
- Hodgkin cells: Large with single nuclei and prominent nucleoli
- Lacunar cells: Large with lobated nuclei and less prominent nucleoli than other HRS cells; often associated with nodular sclerosis subtype

ANCILLARY TESTS
- CD30(+) in > 95%; CD15(+) in ~ 70-80%, PAX5 (dim +) in ~ 90%, CD79a(+) in ~ 10-20%, GATA3(+)
  - CD30 has characteristic membranous pattern with accentuation in Golgi area
- CD20 (variably +) in ~ 20%
- EBV(+) in ~ 20%, CD45/LCA(-), EMA(-)
- Flow cytometry: polytypic B-cells and T-cells with normal immunophenotype, often elevated CD4:CD8 ratio

TOP DIFFERENTIAL DIAGNOSES
- Primary mediastinal and other large B-cell lymphomas
- Anaplastic large cell lymphoma
- Peripheral T-cell lymphoma
- Metastatic carcinoma

Reed-Sternberg Cells
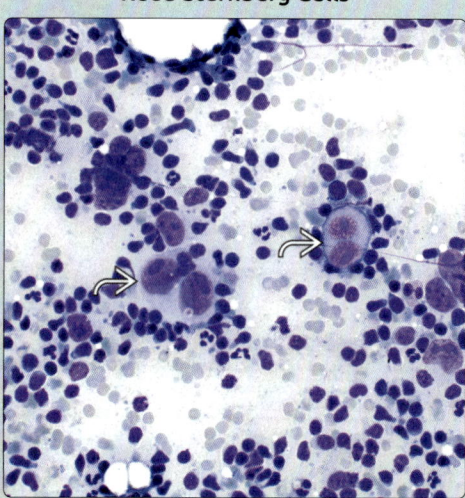

Hodgkin Cells
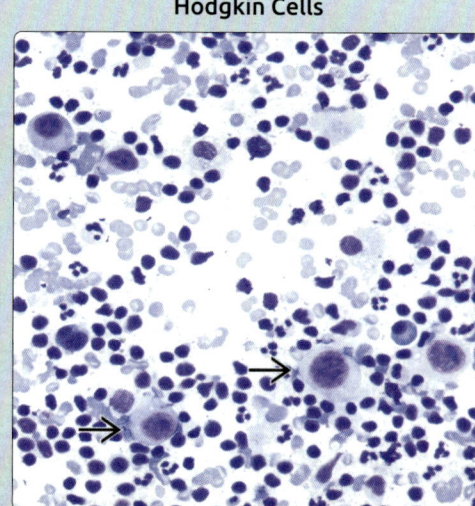

(Left) Diff-Quik-stained FNA smear of classic Hodgkin lymphoma shows 2 Reed-Sternberg cells ⇨, which are large with binucleated nuclei and very prominent nucleoli. (Right) Diff-Quik-stained FNA smear shows Hodgkin cells ⇨, which are large and mononucleated with prominent nucleoli, in a background of lymphocytes, histiocytes, neutrophils, and eosinophils.

Classic Hodgkin Lymphoma Biopsy
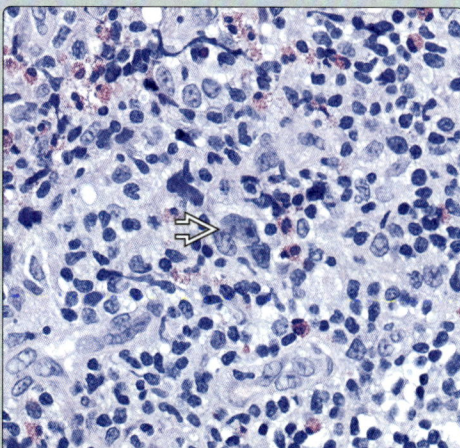

Reed-Sternberg Cell, Pap Stain
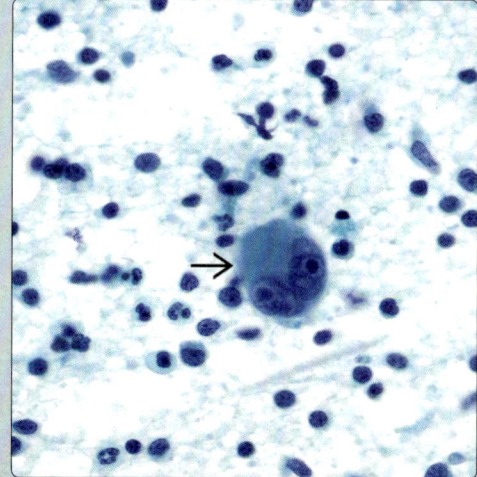

(Left) Core biopsy of classic Hodgkin lymphoma shows a Hodgkin cell with prominent nucleolus ⇨ in a background of small lymphocytes, histiocytes, and eosinophils. (Right) Pap-stained FNA smear of classic Hodgkin lymphoma shows a classic Reed-Sternberg cell ⇨. Note the prominent nucleoli giving an appearance sometimes referred to as owl's eyes.

Classic Hodgkin Lymphoma

TERMINOLOGY

Definitions
- Lymphoid neoplasm composed of Hodgkin and Reed-Sternberg (HRS) cells in variable inflammatory background
- 4 subtypes: Nodular sclerosis, lymphocyte rich, mixed cellularity, and lymphocyte depleted

ETIOLOGY/PATHOGENESIS

Infectious Agents
- Epstein-Barr virus (EBV) present in HRS cells in ~ 20% of cases and has probable pathogenetic role

CLINICAL ISSUES

Presentation
- B symptoms in ~ 40% of cases
- Peak age range: 15-34 years
- Typically seen in mediastinal or cervical nodes

CYTOPATHOLOGY

Cellularity
- Variable depending on associated sclerosis

Background
- Variable numbers of small lymphocytes, eosinophils, &/or histiocytes

Cells
- Reed-Sternberg (RS): Large with binucleated nuclei and very prominent nucleoli
- Hodgkin: Large with single nuclei and prominent nucleoli
- Lacunar: Large with lobated nuclei and less prominent nucleoli than other HRS cells; often associated with nodular sclerosis subtype

Cytology-Histology Correlation
- Difficult to subtype and grade on FNA specimens

ANCILLARY TESTS

Immunohistochemistry
- CD30(+) in > 95%; CD15(+) in ~ 70-80%; CD45/LCA(-), EMA(-), and GATA3(+)
- PAX5 (dim +) in ~ 90%: CD20 (variably +) in ~ 20%; CD79a(+) in ~ 10-20%
- EBV(+) with latency type II pattern in ~ 20% of cases

Flow Cytometry
- Polytypic B-cells and T-cells with normal immunophenotype, often elevated CD4:CD8 ratio

DIFFERENTIAL DIAGNOSIS

Primary Mediastinal Large B-Cell Lymphoma
- Immunophenotype of neoplastic monoclonal B cells, surface Ig(-)
  - CD45/LCA(+), CD10(-), CD15(-), CD30 (often dim, +/-)

Large B-Cell Lymphoma
- CD20(+), CD45/LCA(+), CD30(+/-), CD15(-); light chain restriction establishes clonality

Anaplastic Large Cell Lymphoma
- CD30(+), CD15(-), PAX5(-); aberrant T-cell immunophenotype by flow cytometry; T-cell clonality by molecular studies

Peripheral T-Cell Lymphoma, Not Otherwise Specified
- T-cell markers (+), CD15(-), CD30(-/+), PAX5(-); aberrant T-cell immunophenotype by flow cytometry; T-cell clonality by molecular studies

Metastatic Carcinoma
- Cytokeratin (+), CD15(-), CD45/LCA(-), PAX5(-), EBV(-)

SELECTED REFERENCES
1. Cozzolino I et al: CD15, CD30, and PAX5 evaluation in Hodgkin's lymphoma on fine-needle aspiration cytology samples. Diagn Cytopathol. 48(3):211-16, 2020

Cell Block Findings

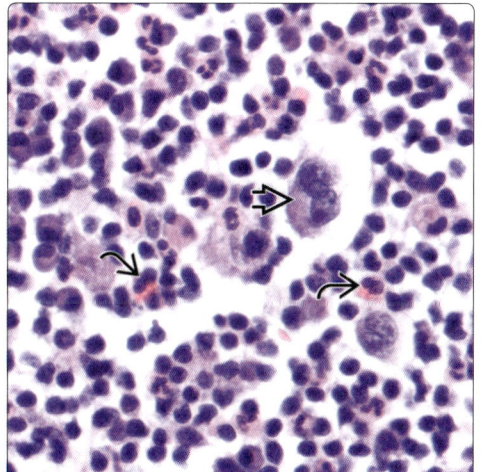

CD30(+)

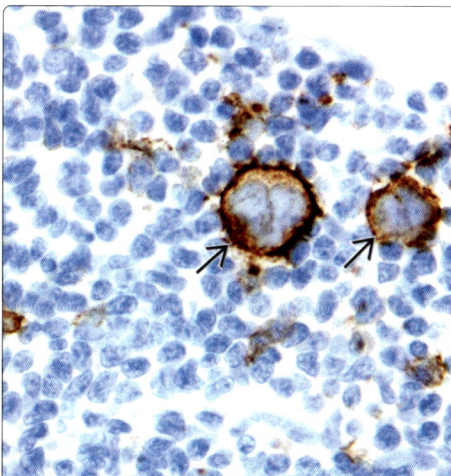

(Left) H&E-stained cell block section of classic Hodgkin lymphoma shows a Reed-Sternberg cell ➡ in a background of lymphocytes, plasma cells, and eosinophils ➡. (Right) Immunostained cell block section of classic Hodgkin lymphoma shows that the large, atypical cells are positive for CD30 ➡.

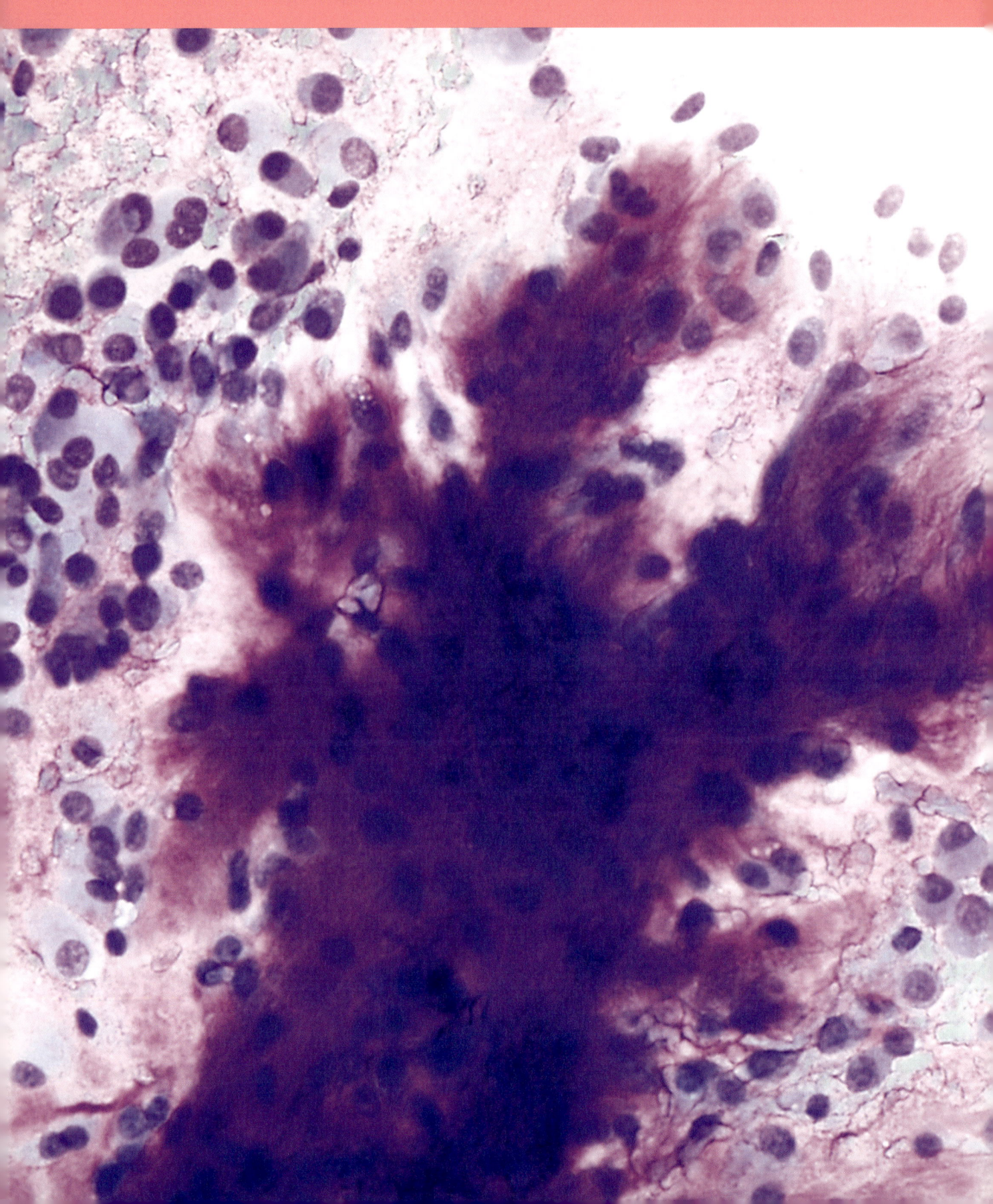

PART III
SECTION 5

Salivary Gland

Overview

Approach to Interpretation of Salivary Gland Aspiration Biopsies and Reporting Terminology (Milan System)	378

Benign Lesions

Normal Salivary Gland and Sialadenitis on Aspiration	382
Cysts	384
Pleomorphic Adenoma	386
Warthin Tumor	388
Myoepithelioma	390
Oncocytoma, Salivary Gland	391

Malignant Neoplasms

Adenoid Cystic Carcinoma	392
Acinic Cell Carcinoma	394
Mucoepidermoid Carcinoma	396
Basaloid Neoplasms, Benign and Malignant	398
Carcinoma Ex Pleomorphic Adenoma	400
Adenocarcinoma, NOS	402
Polymorphous Adenocarcinoma	404
Salivary Duct Carcinoma	406
Secretory Carcinoma	408
Myoepithelial Carcinoma	410
Cribriform Adenocarcinoma	411
Metastatic Carcinoma	412
Primary and Metastatic Nonepithelial Tumors	414

Approach to Interpretation of Salivary Gland Aspiration Biopsies and Reporting Terminology (Milan System)

PATTERNS OF SALIVARY GLAND ASPIRATES

Cystic Lesions
- Acellular clear fluid
  - Normal gland
  - Sialocele
  - Lymphoepithelial cyst (LEC)
- Cloudy/mucoid fluid ± cells
  - Duct obstruction
  - Abscess
  - Mucocele
  - LEC
  - Warthin tumor
  - Low-grade mucoepidermoid carcinoma (MEC)
  - Acinic cell carcinoma (ACC) (rarely)
  - Cystic degeneration in any neoplasm, benign or malignant

Inflammatory Cells
- Abscess
- Chronic sialadenitis
- Lymphoepithelial sialadenitis
- LEC
- Warthin tumor
- Lymph node
- Lymphoma (monotonous)

Granulomas
- Sarcoid
- Tuberculous, fungal, or other infection

Oncocytic Cell Pattern
- Nodular oncocytic hyperplasia
- Warthin tumor
- Oncocytoma/oncocytic carcinoma
- MEC, oncocytic variant
- ACC
- Mammary analog secretory carcinoma (MASC)
- Metastatic carcinoma (e.g., renal cell)
- Salivary duct carcinoma (SDCA)

Lymphocytic Cell Pattern
- Chronic sialadenitis
- Lymphoepithelial sialadenitis
- LEC
- Lymph node
- Lymphoma (monotonous cells)
- Warthin tumor
- ACC

Basaloid Cell Pattern
- Basal cell (monomorphic) adenoma or carcinoma
- Cellular pleomorphic adenoma (PA)
- Adenoid cystic carcinoma (AdCC)
- Myoepithelial carcinoma
- Polymorphous (low-grade) adenocarcinoma
- Small cell carcinoma, primary or metastatic
- Secondary involvement by cutaneous basal cell carcinoma
- Sialoblastoma

Stroma Patterns in Neoplasms
- PA: Fibrillary stroma
- AdCC: Discrete, round globules
- Basal cell adenoma/carcinoma: Dense, ropy, membranous
- Nodular fasciitis: Loose myxoid stroma
- Spindle cell myoepithelioma: Fibrillary
- Polymorphous (low-grade) adenocarcinoma: Fibrillary
- Myoepithelial carcinoma: Fibrillary

Clear Cells and Clear Cell Neoplasms
- Normal salivary gland
- Lipoma
- ACC
- MEC
- Clear cell myoepithelioma or myoepithelial carcinoma
- Epithelial myoepithelial carcinoma
- Sebaceous lymphadenoma or carcinoma
- Metastatic clear cell carcinoma (e.g., renal or squamous)

High-Grade Malignant Neoplasms
- High-grade MEC

(Left) Diff-Quik stain highlights the magenta fibrillary stroma ➡, which blends into the plasmacytoid cells ➡ of a myoepithelial cell-rich pleomorphic adenoma. (Right) Diff-Quik stain highlights distinct, well-defined globular stroma ➡, consisting of basement membrane-like material surrounded by a wreath of basaloid cells ➡ in an adenoid cystic carcinoma.

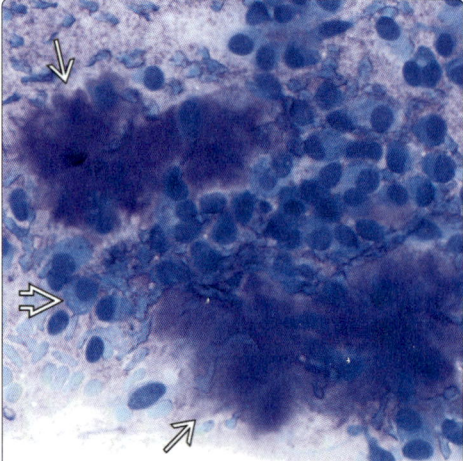
Fibrillary Stroma of Pleomorphic Adenoma

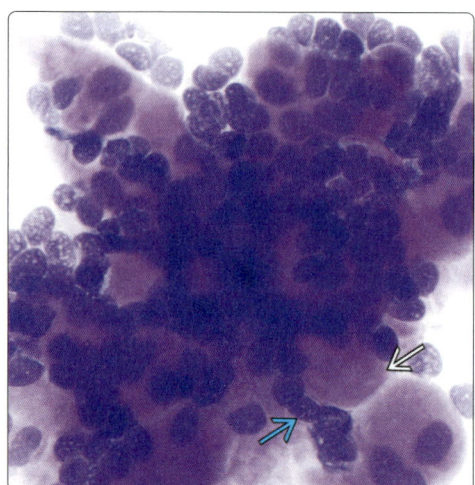
Well-Defined Stroma of Adenoid Cystic Carcinoma

Approach to Interpretation of Salivary Gland Aspiration Biopsies and Reporting Terminology (Milan System)

- Adenocarcinoma, not otherwise specified (NOS)
- SDCA
- Carcinoma ex PA
- Secretory carcinoma
- Squamous cell carcinoma
- Merkel cell carcinoma
- Metastatic malignancy
- Melanoma
- Angiosarcoma

Mucinous Pattern
- Normal submandibular or sublingual glands
- Florid adenomatoid hyperplasia
- Mucocele
- Low-grade MEC

Spindle Cells in Aspirate
- Schwannoma/neurofibroma
- Nodular fascitis
- Myoepithelioma
- Myoepithelial-predominant PA
- Angiosarcoma
- Metastatic spindle cell malignancy

Normal Salivary Gland Tissue Aspirated
- Sampling variance, lesion not aspirated
- Lipoma
- Hamartoma
- Sialadenosis
- Sialadenitis
- Idiopathic enlargement
- Accessory lobe of parotid

Crystals in Salivary Glands
- Tyrosine crystals: Daisy petal appearance, seen in PA
- Amylase: Elongated hexagons, seen in chronic sialadenitis and various cysts
- Cholesterol crystals: Clear and colorless, seen in cysts and Warthin tumors
- Asteroid bodies and calcium oxalate: Seen in sarcoidosis
- Calcium crystals: Purplish on Pap stain, colorless on Diff-Quik; retained products of saliva
- Psammoma bodies: In normal or inflamed salivary gland; in benign or malignant neoplasms

MILAN REPORTING SYSTEM

Milan System for Reporting Salivary Gland Cytopathology, 2nd Edition

- **Nondiagnostic**: Insufficient material, qualitative or quantitative, for diagnosis (after everything is processed and examined and correlated clinically and radiologically)
  - No validated criteria yet; exceptions include acellular matrix or mucinous cyst contents
  - Reported range for risk of malignancy (ROM) in literature post 1st edition of MSRSGC is 0-50%; mean: ~ 15%
  - Targeted reporting rate: < 10%
- **Nonneoplastic**: Chronic and granulomatous sialadenitis, sialolithiasis, reactive lymph nodes within or adjacent to salivary gland (flow cytometry if clinically or cytologically worrisome or older age), benign cysts
  - ROM post 1st edition of MSRSGC ranges from 0-100%; mean: ~ 11%
- **Atypia of undetermined significance (AUS)**: Heterogeneous category in which neoplasm cannot be entirely excluded
  - Usually compromised specimen due to sampling or preparation; usually reactive process or poorly sampled neoplasm
  - Typical examples would be oncocytic metaplasia vs. oncocytoma/carcinoma, mucinous cyst contents vs. low-grade MEC
  - Targeted reporting rate: < 10%
  - ROM post 1st edition of MSRSGC ranges from 10-100%; mean: ~ 30%
- **Neoplasm, benign**: Easily diagnosable benign neoplasms if all criteria met, i.e., PA, Warthin tumor, oncocytoma, lipoma, schwannoma, hemangioma, lymphangioma
  - ROM reported range is 0-50%; mean: < 3%
- **Salivary gland neoplasm of uncertain malignant potential (SUMP)**: Cytologic features of neoplasm, but malignancy cannot be excluded
  - These are usually cellular benign neoplasms or with atypia, e.g., cellular basaloid, or clear cell, or oncocytic neoplasms; e.g., PA, Warthin with atypia, basaloid tumors (adenoma vs. carcinoma), myoepitheliomas, cystadenomas
  - Post 1st edition of MSRSGC literature review shows ROM from 0-100%; mean: 26%
- **Suspicious for malignancy**: Aspirate is highly suggestive of carcinoma/malignancy but qualitatively or quantitatively falls short of definitive diagnosis
  - Indicate suspicion of primary low- or high-grade malignancy, or lymphoma or metastasis
  - Literature review shows ROM from 50-100%; mean: 83%
- **Malignant**: Aspirate diagnostic of malignancy; make every attempt to classify low grade vs. high grade or specific diagnosis or type of metastasis
  - ROM ranges from 80-100%; mean: 98%

Causes of False-Negative Aspirates
- Sampling and interpretive variances
- Underdiagnosis of ACC, low-grade MEC, AdCC, lymphoma
- Cutaneous angiosarcoma with extension into parotid/submandibular gland (bloody, poor sampling)

Salivary Gland FNA Statistics
- From post 1st edition of MSRSGC
  - Overall accuracy: 94% (93-95%)
  - Sensitivity: 93% (91-94%); specificity: 96% (95-97%)
  - PPV: 97% (97-98%); NPV: 89% (87-91%)

SELECTED REFERENCES

1. Faquin W and Rossi ED et al: The Milan System for Reporting Salivary Gland Cytopathology. 2nd Ed. Springer International, 2022
2. Cormier CM et al: Utility of the Milan System for Reporting Salivary Gland Cytology, with focus on the incidence and histologic correlates of atypia of undetermined significance (AUS) and salivary gland neoplasm of uncertain malignant potential (SUMP): a 3-year institutional experience. Cancer Cytopathol. 130(4):303-12, 2022
3. Manucha V et al: Impact of the Milan System for Reporting Salivary Gland Cytology on risk assessment when used in routine practice in a real-time setting. J Am Soc Cytopathol. 10(2):208-15, 2021
4. Kurtycz DFI et al: Milan Interobserver Reproducibility Study (MIRST): Milan System 2018. J Am Soc Cytopathol. 9(3):116-25, 2020

Approach to Interpretation of Salivary Gland Aspiration Biopsies and Reporting Terminology (Milan System)

Patterns of Salivary Gland Aspirates/Small Biopsies

Basaloid	Clear Cell	Cystic	Inflammatory	Mucinous	Oncocytic	Stromal	Spindle	Normal Gland	HGMT
AdCC	Normal	Abscess	Abscess	Mucocele	ACC	AdCC	Angiosarcoma	Sampling variance	Adeno-CA NOS
BCA/CA	ACC	ACC, rarely	ACC	Low-grade MEC	MASC	BCA/CA	MYE	Accessory lobe	Angiosarcoma
Skin basal cell CA	Clear cell MYE	Low-grade MEC	Chronic sialadenitis	Normal gland	MEC	MYE/CA	Nodular fasciitis	Idiopathic enlargement	SC
Cellular PA	Epithelial/myoep CA	LEC	LEC/sialadenitis		Oncocytic hyperplasia	Nodular fasciitis	Pleomorphic adenoma	Hamartoma	MEC (high grade)
MYE	MEC	Mucocele	LN/lymphoma		OCY/CA	Pleomorphic adenoma	Schwannoma	Lipoma	Merkel cell CA
PLGA	Lipoma	Warthin tumor	MEC			SDCA	PLGA	Other mets	Sialadenosis	SDCA
Small cell CA	Renal and other mets	Cystic tumor degen	Warthin tumor		Warthin tumor				Other mets

ACC = acinic cell carcinoma; AdCC = adenoid cystic carcinoma; BCA = basal cell adenoma; CA = carcinoma; degen = degeneration; HGMT = high-grade malignant tumor; LEC = lymphoepithelial carcinoma; LN = lymph node; MASC = mammary analogue secretory carcinoma; MEC = mucoepidermoid carcinoma; mets = metastases; MYE = myoepithelioma; myoep = myoepithelial; NOS = not otherwise specified; OCY = oncocytoma; PA = pleomorphic adenoma, PLGA = polymorphous (low-grade) adenocarcinoma; SDCA = salivary duct carcinoma; SC = secretory carcinoma.

Milan System for Reporting Salivary Gland Cytopathology and ROM Percentage

Milan System Category (ROM %)	Suggested/Possible Management Options
Nondiagnostic (15%)	Clinical/radiologic correlation, repeat FNA
Nonneoplastic (11%)	Clinical/radiologic correlation, follow-up
Atypia of undetermined significance (AUS) (30%)	Repeat FNA or surgery
Neoplasm: Benign (< 3%)	Conservative surgery or close clinical follow-up
Salivary gland neoplasm of uncertain malignant potential (SUMP) (26%)	Surgery with intraoperative consultation if necessary
Suspicious for malignancy (83%)	Surgical management depending on suspected tumor grade and intraoperative consultation
Malignant (low vs. high grade) (98%)	Surgical management depending on type and tumor grade

ROM = risk of malignancy.

Ancillary Testing for Major Salivary Gland Tumors

Tumor	Immunohistochemistry (Useful Positive Markers)	Molecular Testing, Genes Involved (Prevalence in %)
Acinic cell carcinoma	DOG1, SOX10, NR4A3	NR4A3 FISH
Adenoid cystic carcinoma	Myb, DOG1, CD117, SOX10, S100, calponin, CK5/6, p63, p40, CK7, CEA	MYB-NFIB translocation (25-64%), diagnostic and therapeutic
Basal cell adenoma/carcinoma	β-catenin overexpression, CK7, myoepithelial markers, GATA3*, PLAG-1*	CTNNB1 mutations (60-70%); CYLD1 loss (75-80%)
Hyalinizing clear cell carcinoma	Pan CK, low/high molecular weight keratins, p63*	EWSR1::ATF gene fusion (85%)
Mammary analogue secretory carcinoma	GATA-3, S100, keratins, mammaglobin	ETV6::NTRK3 gene fusion (90-100%)
Mucoepidermoid carcinoma	p63, p40, GATA3*, CD117*	CRTC1::MAML2 gene fusion (40-80%); CTRC3::MAML2 gene fusion (~ 5%)
Pleomorphic adenoma	PLAG1, SMA, calponin, p63, p40, SOX10, GFAP, CK7, S100, GATA3*	PLAG1::CTNNB1 or LIFR gene fusion (50-60%); HMGA2 amplification or fusion
Salivary duct carcinoma	GATA3, AR, HER2*	ERBB2 amplification (~ 40%); PIK3CA mutation (~ 20%)

*Variable positivity.

Approach to Interpretation of Salivary Gland Aspiration Biopsies and Reporting Terminology (Milan System)

Basaloid Pattern With Dense Ribbon-Like Stroma

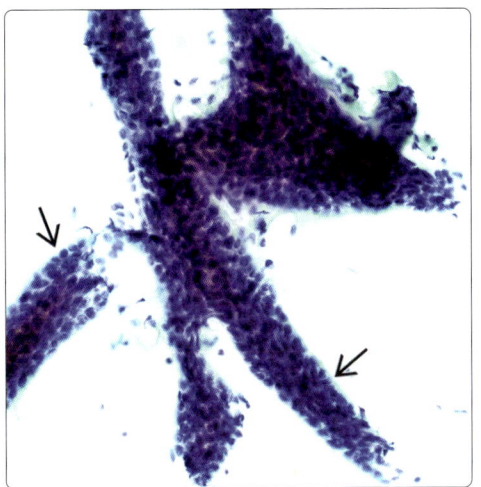

Mucinous Pattern

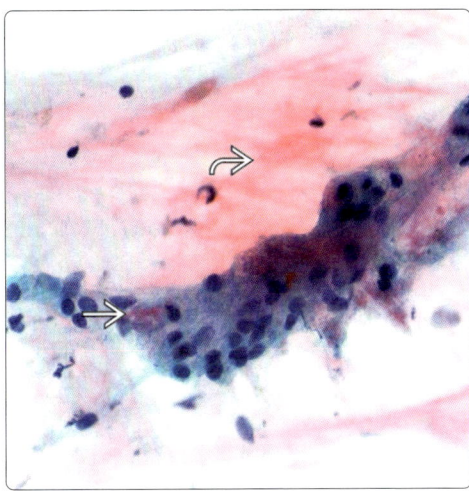

(Left) Pap stain shows a basaloid neoplasm characterized by branching tubules of small basaloid cells with a dense peripheral matrix ribbon ➡. (Right) Pap-stained smear of a low-grade mucoepidermoid carcinoma shows neoplastic cells with cytoplasmic mucin ➡ floating in a sea of mucin ➡.

Clear Cell Pattern

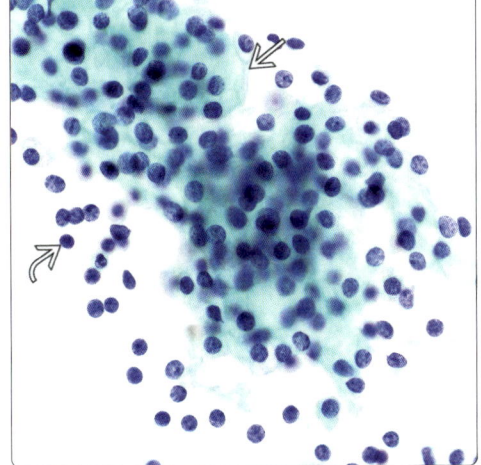

Oncocytic Pattern

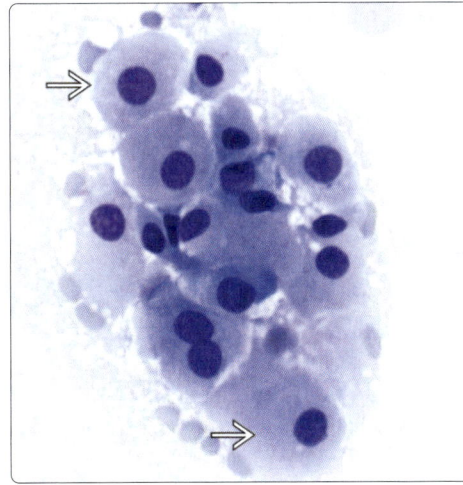

(Left) Pap stain shows clear acinar cells ➡ and bare nuclei ➡ of acinar cells in a clear cell pattern. (Right) Diff-Quik-stained smear shows oncocytic cells with abundant finely granular cytoplasm ➡ in this case of oncocytic mucoepidermoid carcinoma.

Spindle Cell Pattern

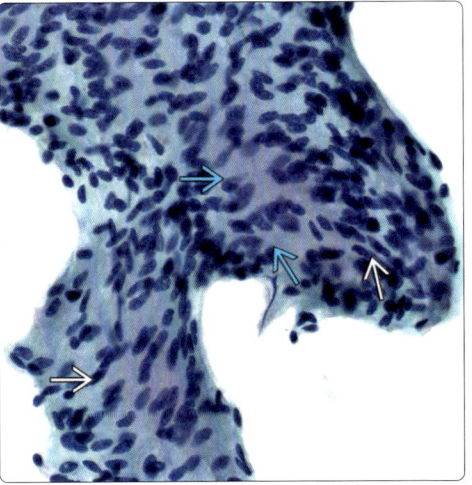

Inflammatory Pattern With Granulomas

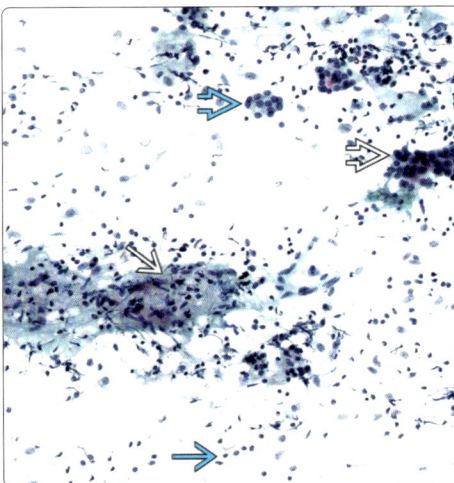

(Left) Pap-stained salivary gland FNA shows a spindle cell pattern ➡ with a hint of Verocay bodies ➡ in this case of schwannoma. (Right) Pap-stained aspirate from a granulomatous sialadenitis shows noncaseating granulomas ➡ in a background of lymphocytes ➡ and salivary ductal ➡ and acinar ➡ tissue.

Normal Salivary Gland and Sialadenitis on Aspiration

CLINICAL IMPLICATIONS

Clinical Presentation

- Acute sialadenitis
  - Red, firm gland with associated pain
  - Etiology: Bacterial (usually *Streptococcus*, *Staphylococcus*, or gram negative) or viral
  - Risk factors: Stone, immunodeficiency, malnutrition, or poor oral hygiene
- Chronic sialadenitis
  - Firm gland
  - More common than acute sialadenitis
  - Risk factors: Autoimmune disorders or stone
- Granulomatous sialadenitis
  - Sarcoidosis, infection, or duct obstruction by stone with resulting rupture and reactive granulomatous response

CYTOLOGIC FEATURES

Normal Salivary Tissue

- Aspirates are usually paucicellular
- Composed of
  - Acini typically arranged in small, cohesive groups resembling clusters of grapes
  - Acini composed of tightly cohesive cells with small, dark nuclei peripherally located in abundant granular or vacuolated cytoplasm
  - Cytoplasm is fragile; hence, smears often show stripped, naked nuclei in granular background
  - May show squamous, mucous, or oncocytic metaplasia
  - Ductal (cuboidal or low columnar) cells arranged in cohesive sheets with nonoverlapping, honeycomb arrangement and little pleomorphism
  - Adipose tissue is minor component
  - Myoepithelial cells have small, dark, oval nuclei and scant cytoplasm and are rarely seen

Acute Sialadenitis

- Numerous polymorphonuclear leukocytes, macrophages
- Rare, often degenerating acini
- Multinucleated giant cells in background
- Stone fragments or crystals may be seen

Normal Salivary Acini and Ducts

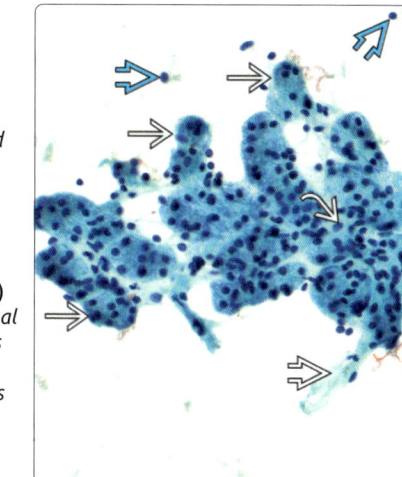

Higher Magnification of Normal

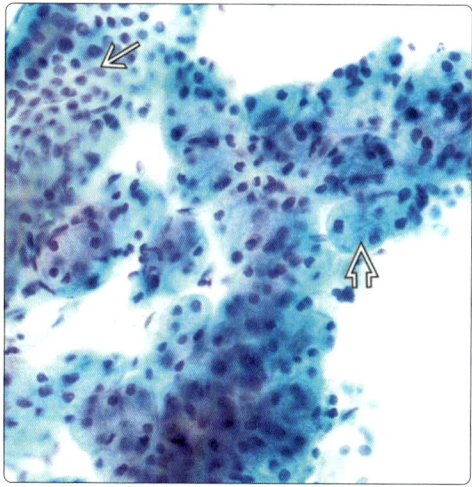

(Left) Pap-stained normal salivary acinar and ductal tissue show a grape-like cluster of acini ➡ with low nuclear:cytoplasmic ratios, finely granular to vacuolated cytoplasm, and small, peripherally arranged nuclei ➡. A central duct ➡ is seen as well as vessels ➡. Bare nuclei from ruptured acinar cells are also seen ➡. (Right) Pap-stained smear of a normal salivary gland shows clusters of acini ➡ with an adjacent sheet of bland columnar cells of ductal origin ➡.

Chronic Sclerosing Sialadenitis

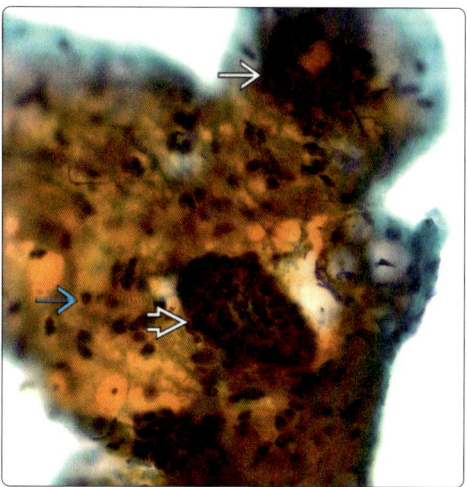

Granuloma

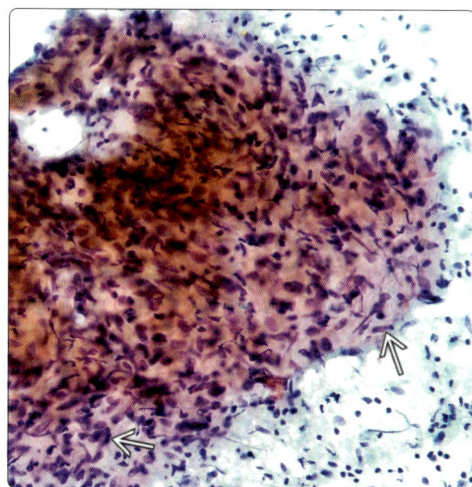

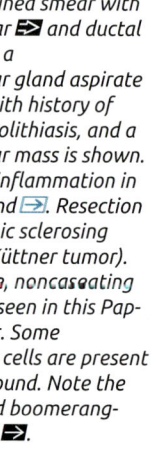

(Left) Pap-stained smear with atrophic acinar ➡ and ductal units ➡ from a submandibular gland aspirate in a patient with history of radiation, sialolithiasis, and a submandibular mass is shown. Note chronic inflammation in the background ➡. Resection showed chronic sclerosing sialadenitis (Küttner tumor). (Right) A large, noncaseating granuloma is seen in this Pap-stained smear. Some inflammatory cells are present in the background. Note the elongated and boomerang-shaped nuclei ➡.

Normal Salivary Gland and Sialadenitis on Aspiration

Chronic Sialadenitis
- Paucicellular, rare acini, mostly lymphocytes
- Fragments of fibrous tissue with ductal structures

Chronic Sclerosing Sialadenitis (Küttner Tumor)
- Most are considered IgG4-related systemic autoimmune disease
- Few due to chronic inflammation, stones, radiation
- Usually submandibular gland with pain and swelling
- Lymphoplasmacytic infiltration of lobules with sclerosis, acinar atrophy, and squamous metaplasia of ducts
- FNAs painful with scant cellularity due to fibrosis and atrophy
- Atrophic ducts and acini with plasma cells and lymphocytes
- Serum IgG4 elevated in autoimmune variant

Granulomatous Sialadenitis
- Cellular with tightly cohesive epithelioid histiocytes
  - Oval to elongated, kidney-shaped nuclei and ample cytoplasm
- Necrosis is present in infections (tuberculosis and fungal)
- No necrosis in sarcoidosis
- Lymphocytes and multinucleated giant cells

Intraglandular Lymph Nodes
- May be enlarged benign/reactive intraglandular lymph nodes, especially in young
- Older individuals (> 50 yr), usually due to lymphoma or mets
- Flow cytometry helpful in cases of reactive and nonmetastatic nodes
- Interpreted as nonneoplastic under Milan System for reporting, if benign

DIFFERENTIAL DIAGNOSIS

Warthin Tumor
- Sialadenitis may show oncocytic metaplasia, lymphocytes, and cellular debris similar to cystic material of Warthin tumor
- Larger clusters of oncocytes in papillary arrangement favor Warthin tumor

Squamous Cell Carcinoma
- Smears show abundant neutrophils if central cystic portion is aspirated
  - Complicated by fact that normal salivary glands may undergo squamous metaplasia as reactive change to inflammation
  - Careful search of background cells to identify intact, well-preserved cells with overt features of malignancy should be performed

Low-Grade Mucoepidermoid Carcinoma
- Benign salivary tissue may show mucous metaplasia
- Because these tumors often show bland cytologic features, diagnosis should always be considered whenever mucous cells are seen on aspirates
- Mucoepidermoid carcinomas are usually more cellular and have mucin in background and admixed intermediate cells

Lymphoma
- Presence of lymphocytes raises possibility of lymphoma, especially in older adults
  - Obtain material for flow cytometry at time of adequacy

DIAGNOSTIC CHECKLIST

Pathologic Interpretation Pearls
- Salivary glands (especially parotid) may contain intraglandular lymph nodes
  - Aspirates that contain lymphocytes should broaden differential to include following
    - Normal lymph node, sialadenitis, autoimmune disorders, cysts (lymphoepithelial and branchial cleft)
    - Neoplasms (Warthin tumor and lymphoma)
- Cases of acute sialadenitis should prompt additional passes at time of adequacy check for cultures

SELECTED REFERENCES
1. Liu Y et al: Needle biopsy compared with surgical biopsy: pitfalls of small biopsy in histologial diagnosis of IgG4-related disease. Arthritis Res Ther. 23(1):54, 2021
2. Salehi S et al: Diagnostic challenges and problem cases in salivary gland cytology: a 20-year experience. Cancer Cytopathol. 126(2):101-11, 2018

Chronic Sclerosing Sialadenitis
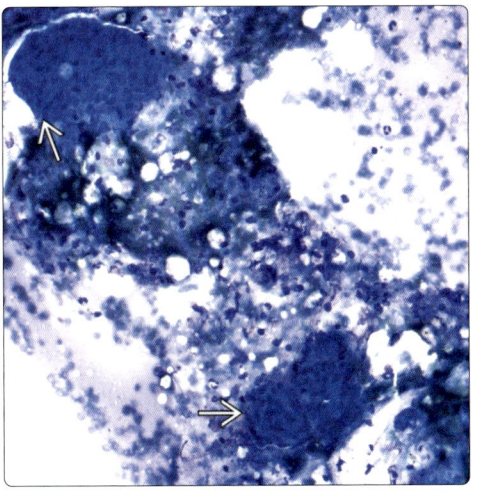

Lymph Node in Salivary Gland
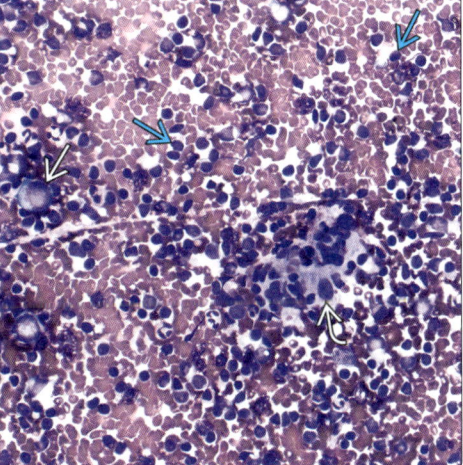

(Left) Diff-Quik-stained smear shows atrophic salivary ductal and lobular units ➡ in a background of chronic inflammation. These aspirates are hypocellular and bloody with scattered fibrous fragments and inflammation. (Right) Diff-Quik-stained smear of a parotid aspirate in a young individual shows a polymorphous population of large ➡ and small ⇨ lymphocytes and macrophages ➡. Monospot test for Epstein-Barr virus was positive.

Cysts

KEY FACTS

ETIOLOGY/PATHOGENESIS

- Cysts can be intrinsic or extrinsic, mucinous or nonmucinous, single or multiple
- Parotid gland is most frequent site
- Lymphoepithelial cysts are associated with history of HIV or Sjögren syndrome
- Retention cysts are secondary to obstruction from stone (sialolithiasis)
- Cysts may derive from inclusions in salivary glands or intraglandular lymph nodes

CLINICAL ISSUES

- Primary locations: Parotid gland and minor salivary glands of lips, buccal mucosa, and palate
- In Milan System for salivary gland cytology reporting, cysts, depending upon their contents and findings, will be reported in categories from nondiagnostic (acellular) to malignant (as in cystic malignancies)
  - Clinical and radiologic correlation and examination of material is important for accurate diagnosis so as not to miss cystic neoplasm or malignancy
  - Risk of malignancy or neoplasm varies depending upon reporting category

CYTOPATHOLOGY

- Lymphoepithelial cyst: Lymphocytes; epithelial cells may be present in background
- Branchial cleft cyst: Lymphocytes and squamous cells
- Epidermal inclusion cyst: Squamous cells; inflammation may be present in background
- Retention cyst: Mucin and macrophages; rare epithelial cells

TOP DIFFERENTIAL DIAGNOSES

- Mucoepidermoid carcinoma
- Squamous cell carcinoma
- Lymphoma
- Warthin tumor

Cyst Contents, Macrophages Only

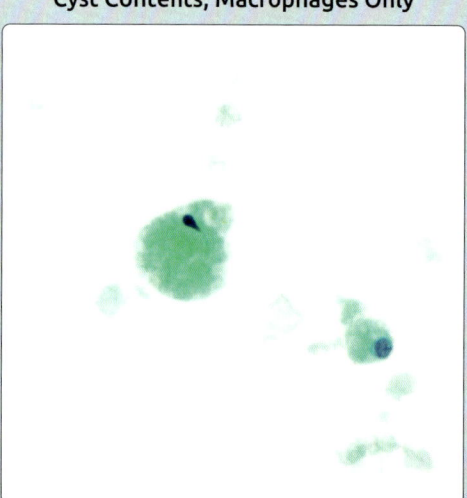

Amylase Crystals

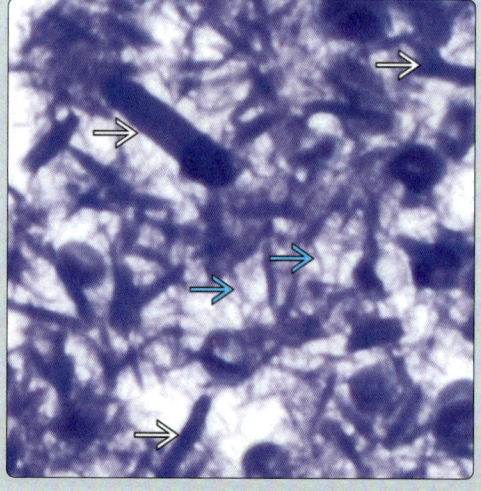

(Left) Smears of benign cysts, as seen in this Pap stain, are often paucicellular and consist of only rare, usually degenerated, macrophages. (Right) Diff-Quik stain of an aspirated salivary cyst shows large, rectangular ⇒, as well as small and fragmented, needle-shaped ⇒ amylase crystals.

Mucous Retention Cyst

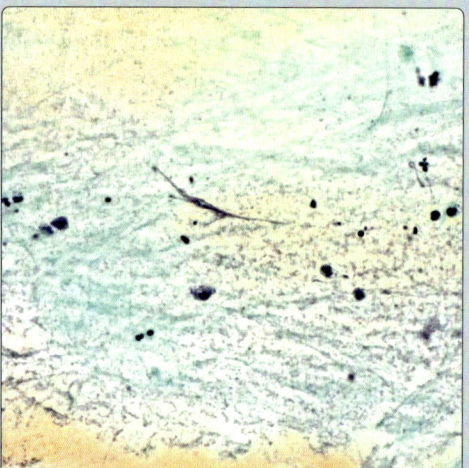

Lymphoepithelial Cyst

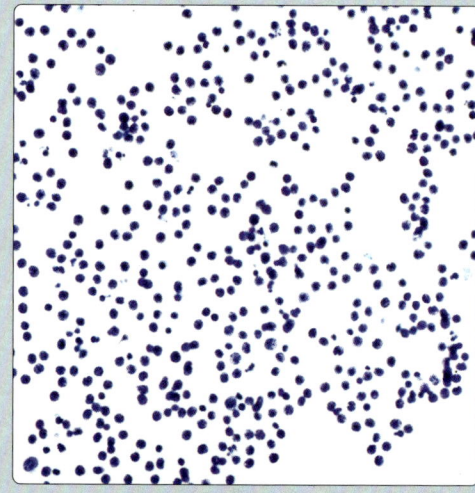

(Left) A mucous or retention cyst, depicted in this Pap smear, consists of mucus and rare macrophages. It may be difficult to rule out low-grade mucoepidermoid carcinoma in such cases. Additional sampling after draining the cyst can provide reassurance of a benign process. (Right) Lymphoepithelial cyst on Pap stain shows a polymorphous lymphocytic population. Correlation with radiology is needed to confirm a cystic lesion.

Cysts

ETIOLOGY/PATHOGENESIS

Congenital or Acquired
- Cysts can be intrinsic or extrinsic, mucinous or nonmucinous
- Mucinous cysts can be nonneoplastic (e.g. mucocele) or neoplastic (low-grade mucoepidermoid carcinoma)
- Nonmucinous cysts can be lymphocytic (lymphoepithelial cysts or neoplastic like Warthin's
- Nonlymphocytic cysts can be nonneoplastic (inflammatory) or neoplastic/malignant
- Parotid gland is most frequent site
- Lymphoepithelial cysts are associated with HIV and Sjögren syndrome
- Retention cysts are secondary to obstruction from stone (sialolithiasis)
- Cysts may derive from inclusions in salivary glands or intraglandular lymph nodes

CYTOPATHOLOGY

Cells
- Lymphoepithelial cyst
  - Lymphocytes
  - Background may contain macrophages and epithelial cells (squamous &/or glandular)
  - Often bilateral and recurs following aspiration
- Branchial cleft cyst
  - Lymphocytes
  - Squamous cells or, less commonly, ciliated columnar cells
- Epidermal inclusion cyst (keratinous cyst)
  - Abundant squamous cells, usually keratinizing
  - Multinucleated giant cells and acute inflammation may be present in background
  - Scant lymphocytic component
- Retention cyst
  - Paucicellular, usually only mucin with few macrophages and inflammatory cells if infected
  - Rare squamous, goblet, or cuboidal epithelial cells; rule out cystic neoplasm/malignancy

DIFFERENTIAL DIAGNOSIS

Mucoepidermoid Carcinoma
- May contain significant cystic component
- Often has greater cellularity
- Mixture of epidermoid, intermediate, mucous, &/or clear cells

Warthin Tumor (Papillary Cystadenoma Lymphomatosum)
- Cloudy, hemorrhagic fluid on aspiration
- Numerous oncocytes, often in papillary arrangement
- Associated lymphocytic component

Squamous Cell Carcinoma
- Malignant squamous cells, often keratinizing
- Well-differentiated carcinomas may show minimal cytologic atypia

Lymphoma
- Many benign cysts contain lymphocytic component
- Numerous lymphocytes should raise suspicion of lymphoma, especially in older population
- Obtain material for flow cytometric studies

Pilomatrixoma
- Dermal-based tumor, often affects younger population
- Mixture of inflammatory cells, mature squamous cells, basaloid cells, multinucleated giant cells, and ghost cells

DIAGNOSTIC CHECKLIST

Pathologic Interpretation Pearls
- If cyst collapses after aspiration, subsequent passes of residual mass should be performed to exclude cystic neoplasm; see Milan System for reporting guidance

SELECTED REFERENCES
1. Maleki Z et al: Application of the Milan system for reporting salivary gland cytopathology to cystic salivary gland lesions. Cancer Cytopathol. 129(3):214-25, 2021

Branchial Cleft Cyst

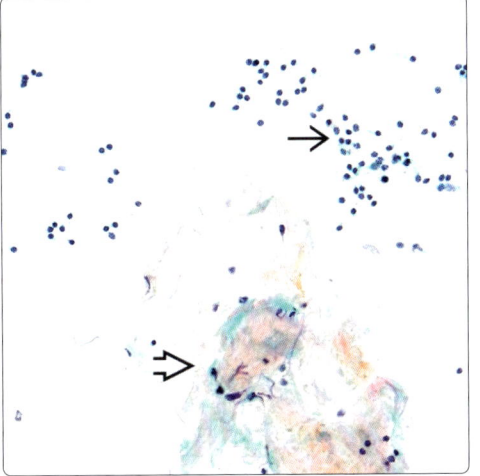

Cystic Keratinizing Squamous Cell Carcinoma

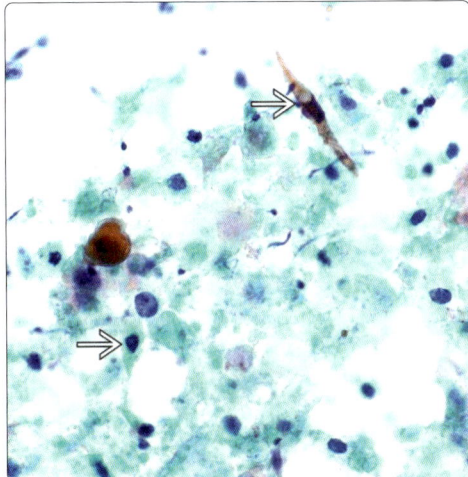

(Left) Branchial cleft cyst on Pap stain consists of a polymorphous lymphocytic population ➡ and squamous cells ➡. These findings are nonspecific; definitive diagnosis requires clinical and radiologic correlation. *(Right)* Pap-stained smear of amber-colored to clear cyst contents in an area of the parotid shows mostly dead cells and only rare, viable nucleated squamous cells ➡ in this patient with history of resected squamous carcinoma of the face.

Pleomorphic Adenoma

KEY FACTS

CLINICAL ISSUES
- Most common neoplasm of salivary gland origin
- Parotid gland is most common site

CYTOPATHOLOGY
- Fibrillary chondromyxoid stroma (may be scant)
  - Metachromatic on Diff-Quik stain
  - Grayish-blue on Pap stain
- Myoepithelial cells: Shapes include spindle, polygonal, plasmacytoid, round, clear
- Ductal cells: Clusters of small cuboidal to polygonal cells in ducts or small sheets
  - Bland but can show focal atypia
- Squamous, mucinous, sebaceous metaplasia as well as tyrosine and oxalate crystals can be seen

ANCILLARY TESTS
- Cytokeratin, p63, GFAP, S100, calponin, SOX10, and SMA are variably positive
- ~ 70% show *PLAG1* or *HMGA2* rearrangements (nuclear stain on IHC)

TOP DIFFERENTIAL DIAGNOSES
- Myoepithelioma
  - No fibrillary chondromyxoid stroma or ductal cells
- Basal cell adenoma
  - Uniform proliferation of basaloid cells
  - No myoepithelial cells or fibrillary chondromyxoid stroma
  - Dense basal stroma encircles cell nests
- Adenoid cystic carcinoma
  - Cells are predominantly uniform in size with oval to angulated shape; MYB and C-kit (+)
  - Basement membrane-like material is dense and homogeneous (not fibrillary) on Diff-Quik stain
- Carcinoma ex pleomorphic adenoma
  - Marked pleomorphism, mitotic figures, necrosis

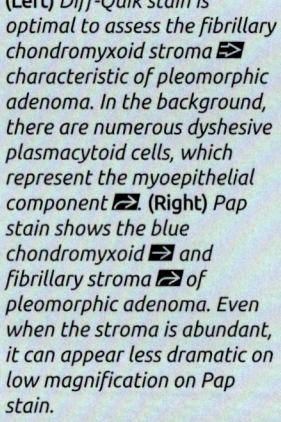

(Left) Diff-Quik stain is optimal to assess the fibrillary chondromyxoid stroma ⇒ characteristic of pleomorphic adenoma. In the background, there are numerous dyshesive plasmacytoid cells, which represent the myoepithelial component ⇒. (Right) Pap stain shows the blue chondromyxoid ⇒ and fibrillary stroma ⇒ of pleomorphic adenoma. Even when the stroma is abundant, it can appear less dramatic on low magnification on Pap stain.

Fibrillary Stroma and Myoepithelial Cells

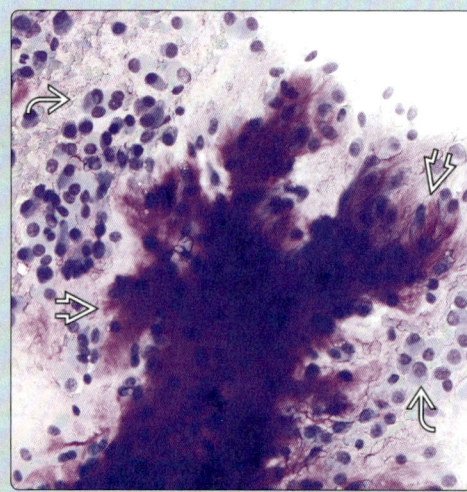

Fibrillary and Chondromyxoid Stroma on Pap Stain

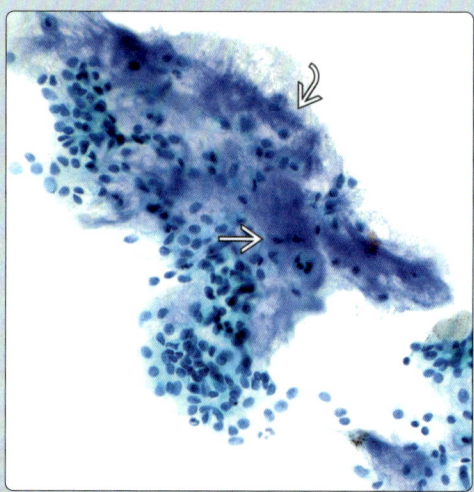

(Left) Thrombin cell block with an embedded microtissue fragment shows ductal ⇒, myoepithelial ⇒, and myxoid stromal ⇒ components of a pleomorphic adenoma. (Right) Pap stain of a cellular pleomorphic adenoma with a predominance of myoepithelial cells ⇒ in which the stroma appears well-defined and ropy ⇒ rather than fibrillary is shown. This finding brings up the differential of adenoid cystic carcinoma.

Pleomorphic Adenoma Cell Block

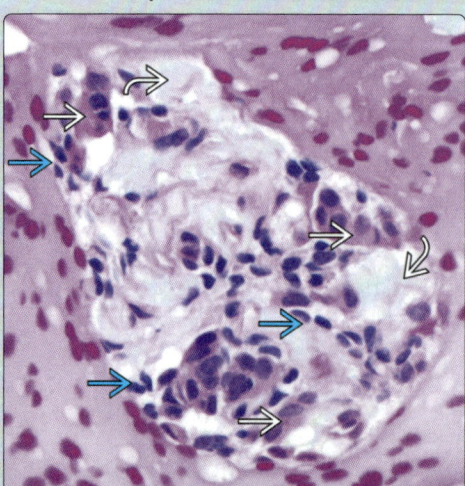

Ropy Stroma

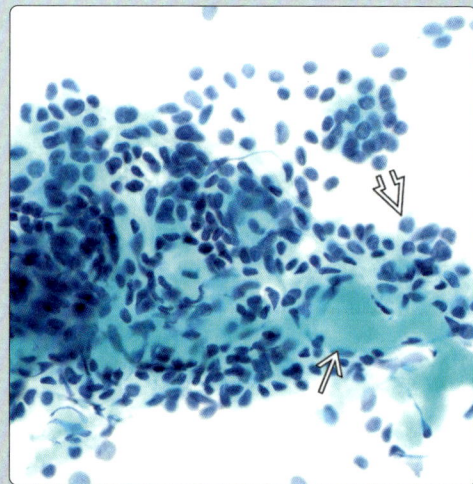

Pleomorphic Adenoma

TERMINOLOGY

Synonyms
- Benign mixed tumor

Definitions
- Benign tumor that shows epithelial, myoepithelial, and mesenchymal (myxoid, mucoid, or chondroid) elements

CLINICAL ISSUES

Epidemiology
- Most common salivary gland tumor
- Peak in 4th-6th decades
- ~ 75% occur in superficial lobe of parotid

Presentation
- Usually painless, slow-growing mass
- Single smooth, mobile, firm nodule

Prognosis
- Malignant transformation in up to 7% of cases

CYTOPATHOLOGY

Background
- Fibrillary chondromyxoid stroma (may be scant)
  - Metachromatic on Diff-Quik stain
  - Grayish-blue on Pap stain
- Tyrosine crystals may be seen

Cells
- Ductal cells
  - Clusters of small cuboidal to polygonal cells
  - Squamous, oncocytic, or sebaceous metaplasia may occur
- Myoepithelial cells
  - Small, dyshesive, variety of shapes (polygonal, plasmacytoid, spindle, round, clear)

Nuclear Details
- Bland, even chromatin; focal atypia occasionally

ANCILLARY TESTS

Immunohistochemistry
- Cytokeratin, p63, GFAP, S100, calponin, SOX10, and SMA are variably positive
- Nuclear staining for *PLAG1* or *HMGA2*

Genetic Testing
- ~ 70% show *PLAG1* or *HMGA2* rearrangements

DIFFERENTIAL DIAGNOSIS

Myoepithelioma
- No fibrillary chondromyxoid stroma or ductal cells

Basal Cell Adenoma
- Uniform proliferation of basaloid cells
- No myoepithelial cells or fibrillary chondromyxoid stroma
- Dense basal stroma encircles cell nests

Adenoid Cystic Carcinoma
- Cells are predominately uniform in size with oval to angulated shape; MYB and C-kit (+)
- Basement membrane-like material is dense and homogeneous (not fibrillary) on Diff-Quik stain

Carcinoma Ex Pleomorphic Adenoma
- Marked pleomorphism, mitotic figures, necrosis

DIAGNOSTIC CHECKLIST

Pathologic Interpretation Pearls
- Recognition of fibrillary chondromyxoid stroma is key
- Classic cases reported under Neoplasm in Milan System; more cellular cases or cases lacking stroma may end up under SUMP

SELECTED REFERENCES

1. Nix JS et al: Navigating small biopsies of salivary gland tumors: a pattern-based approach. J Am Soc Cytopathol. 9(5):369-82, 2020
2. Faquin WC et al: The Milan System for Reporting Salivary Gland Cytopathology. Springer, 2018

Dense Nonfibrillary Stroma Occasionally Seen in Pleomorphic Adenoma

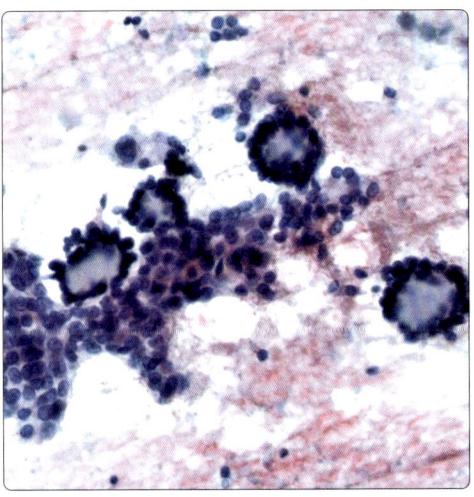

Sebaceous Metaplasia

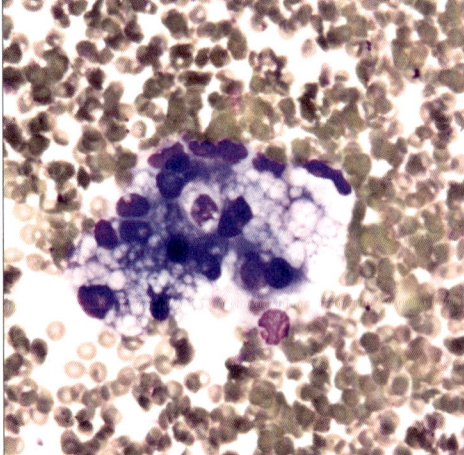

(Left) Smear of parotid FNA shows a field of nonfibrillary dense stroma surrounded by cells. Such foci can be seen in pleomorphic adenomas, which raises the differential of adenoid cystic carcinoma. IHC &/or molecular testing helps to resolve the issue. *(Right)* Ductal cells in this Diff-Quik stain demonstrate sebaceous metaplasia with numerous small vacuoles within the cytoplasm.

Warthin Tumor

KEY FACTS

CLINICAL ISSUES
- 2nd most common benign salivary gland tumor (following pleomorphic adenoma)
- Almost exclusively involves parotid gland, especially tail
- Soft and doughy feel on palpation is characteristic
- Usually 1-8 cm in diameter

CYTOPATHOLOGY
- Aspiration may yield thick, tan-brown fluid
  - Dirty, granular, proteinaceous background on smears
- Combination of oncocytic-appearing epithelial cells and mature lymphocytes
  - Oncocytic cells usually in cohesive, flat, 2D sheets
  - Nuclei are round and regular with nucleoli
  - Abundant granular cytoplasm (due to mitochondria)
  - Mixed small and larger lymphocytes, plasma cells, and lymphohistiocytic aggregates
  - Small lymphocytes predominate

- Squamous and mucinous (metaplastic) cells may be identified in up to 30% of cases
  - Metaplasias lack significant pleomorphism or mitotic activity
  - Metaplastic cells are usually degenerated

TOP DIFFERENTIAL DIAGNOSES
- Oncocytoma
  - Lacks lymphocytic component of Warthin tumor
- Low-grade mucoepidermoid carcinoma with oncocytic cells
  - Look for mucus-producing cells
  - Cells are usually in 3D clusters rather than flat sheets
- Squamous cell carcinoma
  - Warthin can show squamous metaplasia with marked atypia, but squamous carcinomas are usually more cytologically atypical with well-preserved cells
  - Metaplastic cells show degenerative changes with smudged nuclear chromatin

Warthin Tumor on Diff-Quik Stain
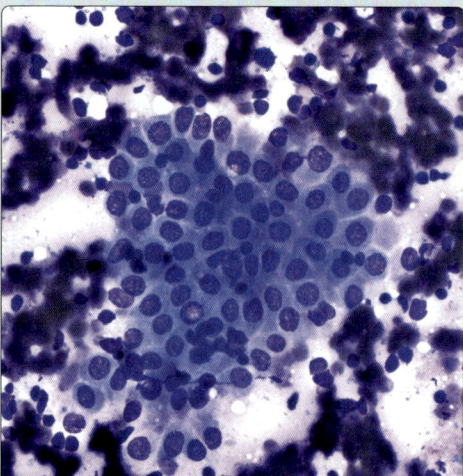

Warthin Tumor on Pap Stain
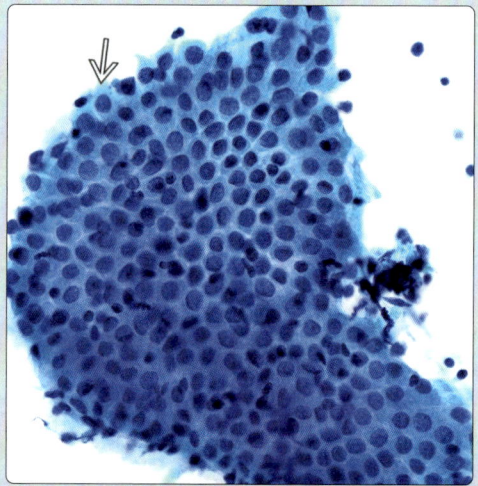

(Left) FNA specimen contains a flat sheet of oncocytic cells with distinct cell borders in a mixed lymphocytic background. (Right) A flat sheet of oncocytes with distinct cell borders and abundant granular cytoplasm ➡ is present in this Pap-stained FNA. Scattered small lymphocytes are seen in the background.

Warthin Tumor Cells and Background
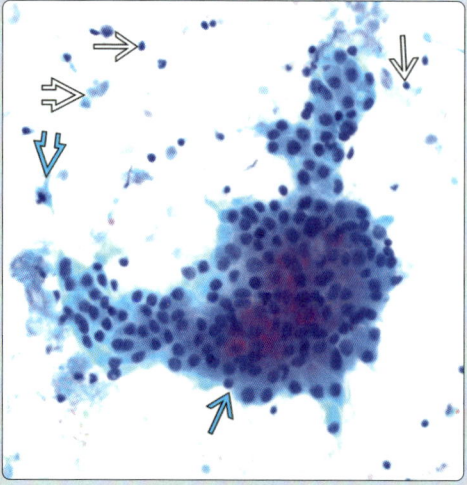

Core Needle Biopsy of Warthin Tumor
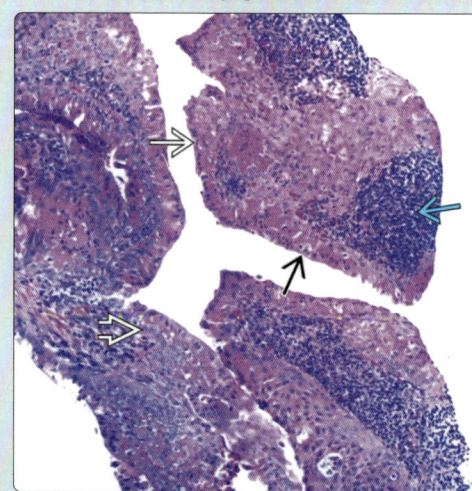

(Left) FNA of a PET-avid mass at the angle of the jaw shows flat sheets of cells with dense, granular/oncocytic cytoplasm, low nuclear:cytoplasmic ratios, and lack of atypia ➡. The background shows small lymphocytes ➡ and necrotic debris ➡ along with a rare squamous cell ➡. (Right) H&E-stained core needle biopsy shows an oncocytic population of dual-layered columnar ➡ and cuboidal cells ➡ with underlying mature lymphoid population ➡. The nuclei of the columnar cells are polarized to the luminal surface ➡.

Warthin Tumor

TERMINOLOGY

Synonyms
- Adenolymphoma, papillary cystadenoma lymphomatosum

ETIOLOGY/PATHOGENESIS

Environmental Exposure
- Associated with cigarette smoking

CLINICAL ISSUES

Epidemiology
- Incidence
  o 2nd most common benign salivary gland tumor
  o Most common in 5th-7th decades of life
  o Historically M > F but increasing in women

Site
- Almost exclusively involves parotid gland, superficial lobe along inferior pole
- Bilateral in up to 10%; can be multifocal
- Presents as painless mass (1-8 cm) in tail of parotid with soft, doughy feel

CYTOPATHOLOGY

Pattern
- Oncocytes in cohesive sheets or papillary clusters as well as individual cells, often in honeycomb arrangement with distinct cell borders

Background
- Background of aspirate may appear dirty with cellular debris
- Lymphocytes may be abundant (usually) or scant

Cells
- Combination of oncocytic-appearing epithelial cells and mature lymphocytes
- Squamous and mucinous (metaplastic) cells may be identified

Nuclear Details
- Oncocytes with uniform round nuclei, granular chromatin, and prominent nucleoli

Cytoplasmic Details
- Oncocytes show abundant granular cytoplasm

MICROSCOPIC

Histologic Features
- Papillary projections of double layer of eosinophilic cells with underlying lymphocytes
- May undergo degenerative change (spontaneously or following FNA biopsy) with necrosis, squamous metaplasia, and cytologic atypia

DIFFERENTIAL DIAGNOSIS

Oncocytoma
- May be considered in lymphocyte-poor Warthin cases
  o Both are benign and treated same

Salivary Gland Carcinomas With Oncocytic Cells
- Oncocytic cells may be seen in wide variety of tumors (e.g., mucoepidermoid carcinoma, acinic cell carcinoma, salivary duct carcinoma)
  o Look for more cytologic atypia in malignancies
  o Low-grade mucoepidermoid carcinoma can be bland; look for mucus-producing cells

Squamous Cell Carcinoma
- May be primary, direct extension from overlying skin, or metastasis
  o Squamous metaplastic cells in Warthin can show marked atypia secondary to infarct/degenerative change
  o Patient examination and history are key

SELECTED REFERENCES

1. Allison DB et al: Assessing the diagnostic accuracy for pleomorphic adenoma and Warthin tumor by employing the Milan System for Reporting Salivary Gland Cytopathology: an international, multi-institutional study. Cancer Cytopathol. 129(1):43-52, 2021

Luminal Nuclear Polarization of Oncocytic Columnar Cells

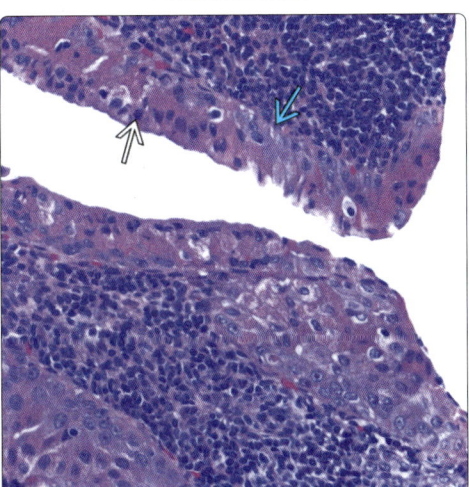

Low-Grade Mucoepidermoid Carcinoma

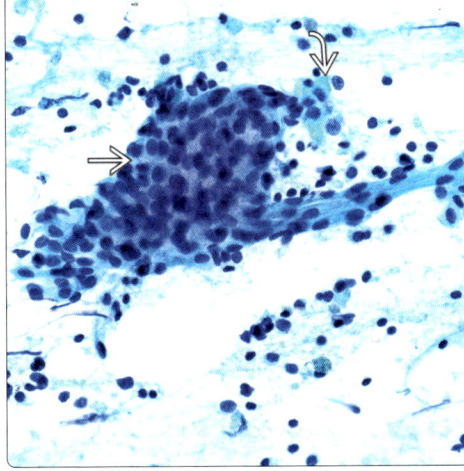

(Left) H&E-stained core needle biopsy shows an epithelial component consisting of tall columnar cells with luminal polarization of the nuclei ➡ and basal cuboidal cells ➡. Mature lymphocytes underlie the epithelial component. (Right) Pap-stained smear shows a 3D cluster of cells without distinct cell borders in most cells. The cells contain a subtle vacuolated cytoplasm ➡ as well as extracellular mucin ➡. A lymphocytic background can be seen in these tumors.

Myoepithelioma

KEY FACTS

TERMINOLOGY
- Neoplasm of myoepithelial cells, which can have varied appearance (spindled, clear, plasmacytoid, epithelioid)
- Average age at presentation: 44 years
- 1.5% of all salivary gland and ~ 6% of minor salivary gland neoplasms
- 50% occur in parotid, followed by hard and soft palate
- No ductal component and absence of chondroid areas

CYTOPATHOLOGY
- Usually cellular smears with absence of obvious fibrillary or chondroid stroma
- Cells may be spindle-shaped to plasmacytoid and even epithelioid with bland, even chromatin
- Usually 1 cellular component dominates but can be mixed
- Absence of ductal component seen in pleomorphic adenoma
- Stroma is typically scant and collagenous or fibrillary; cartilaginous stroma is not seen
- Absence of necrosis, mitosis or significant atypia, unless myoepithelial carcinoma

ANCILLARY TESTS
- **Positive**: AE1/AE3, CK7, CK14, p63, GFAP, S100 protein, actins, calponin
- Unlike pleomorphic adenomas, *PLAG1* rarely detected

TOP DIFFERENTIAL DIAGNOSES
- Pleomorphic adenoma
  - Also has component of ductal cells and distinct chondromyxoid fibrillary stroma
- Adenoid cystic carcinoma
  - Small basaloid cells may resemble myoepithelial cells but have less cytoplasm
- Schwannoma
  - Spindle cells with nuclear palisading; cytokeratins (-)
- Plasmacytoma
  - Spoke-wheel chromatin and cytoplasmic hof

Spindled Myoepithelial Cells and Stroma

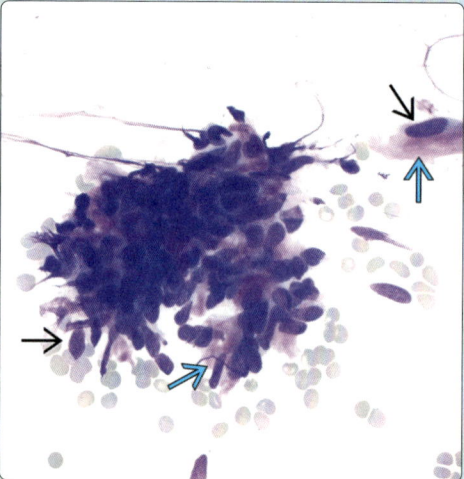

Spindle Cell Pattern of Myoepithelioma

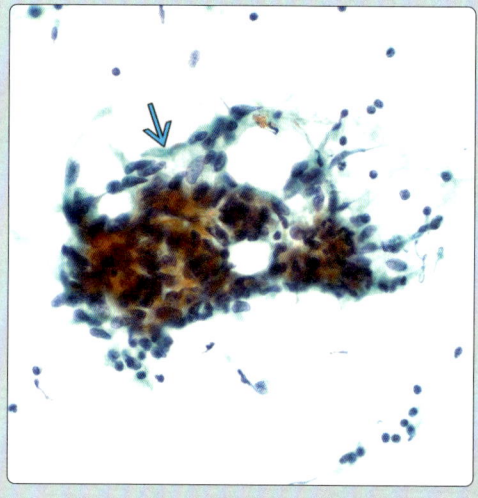

(Left) Diff-Quik-stained smear shows spindle cells ➡ admixed with magenta-colored scant fibrillary and collagenous stroma ➡. (Right) Pap-stained smear shows a spindle cell pattern of a myoepithelioma. Note lack of ductal cells and minimal ➡ to absent stroma.

Myoepithelioma and Normal Salivary Acini

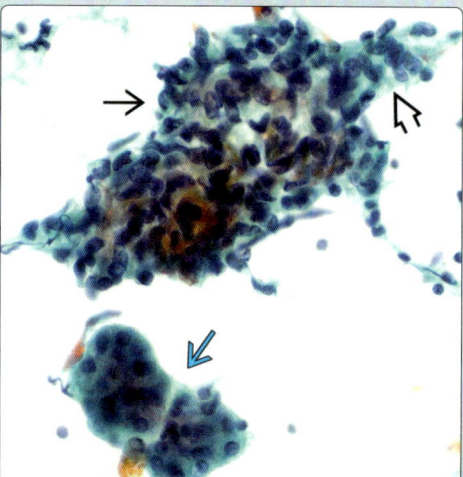

Plasmacytoid Myoepithelioma

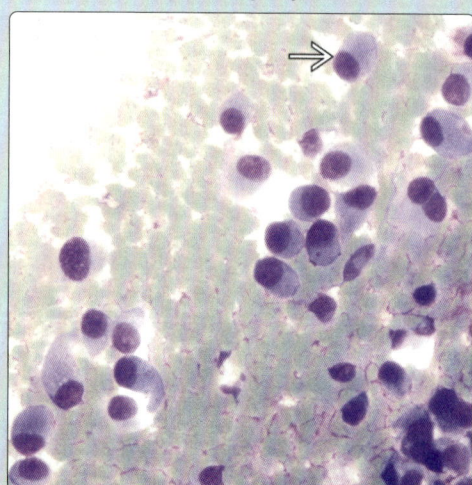

(Left) Pap-stained smear shows a tight cluster of spindled myoepithelial cells ➡ with scant stroma ➡ and no ductal cells. Two normal salivary acini ➡ are also seen. (Right) Diff-Quik stain depicts the plasmacytoid ➡ myoepithelial cells without stroma. Note that the cells are dyscohesive. The chromatin does not show the spoke-wheel or clockface pattern of true plasma cells, aiding in recognition of the true nature of the cells.

Oncocytoma, Salivary Gland

KEY FACTS

TERMINOLOGY
- Neoplasm of oncocytes; usually in parotid; occurs in 6th-8th decades; 2% of salivary neoplasms
  - History of ionizing radiation in younger individuals

CYTOPATHOLOGY
- Increased cellularity compared with nonneoplastic salivary gland or oncocytosis in gland
- Cells can rupture on aggressive smearing, resulting in granular background
- Lack of lymphocytes or mucus in background
- Oncocytes demonstrate round, regular nuclei that have centrally placed prominent nucleoli
  - Cytoplasm is abundant, well defined, and granular
  - Cytoplasmic granularity due to numerous mitochondria
  - Cells may acquire glycogen and have clear cytoplasm

ANCILLARY TESTS
- Immunohistochemistry
  - Positive: EMA, CK8/18, CK7, CK19, α-1 antitrypsin, SDHB, antimitochondrial Ab, p63, and CK5/6 (basal cells only)
  - Negative: S100, PAX8, calponin, GFAP, actins, DOG1, SOX10
  - Limited initial panel of p63, SOX10, and DOG1 helpful

TOP DIFFERENTIAL DIAGNOSES
- **Warthin tumor**
  - Epithelial cells cytologically similar but has lymphocytic component and cyst contents
- **Oncocytic metaplasia**
  - Many benign and malignant tumors can have oncocytes
- **Pleomorphic adenoma**
  - Oncocytic metaplasia is usually focal; has characteristic stromal, ductal, and myoepithelial components
- **Mucoepidermoid carcinoma**
  - Look for glandular differentiation and mucin production
- **Nodular oncocytic hyperplasia**
  - Low cellularity, not distinct/circumscribed mass

Cohesive Clusters of Oncocytic Cells / Abundant Granular Cytoplasm

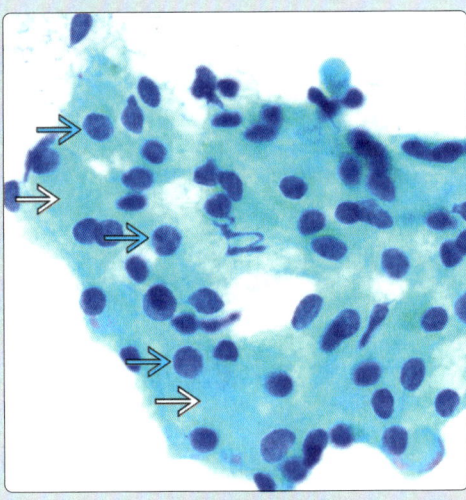

(Left) Diff-Quik stain shows acinar-like structures ➡ of cells with abundant cytoplasm, low nuclear:cytoplasmic ratios, and round regular nuclei with nucleoli (which may be difficult to see on low magnification). (Right) Pap-stained smear from an oncocytic neoplasm shows cords of cells with abundant granular cytoplasm ➡, low nuclear:cytoplasmic ratios with round regular nuclei ➡, and occasional nucleoli.

Oncocytoma Cells in Large Cluster / Oncocytoma, Histology

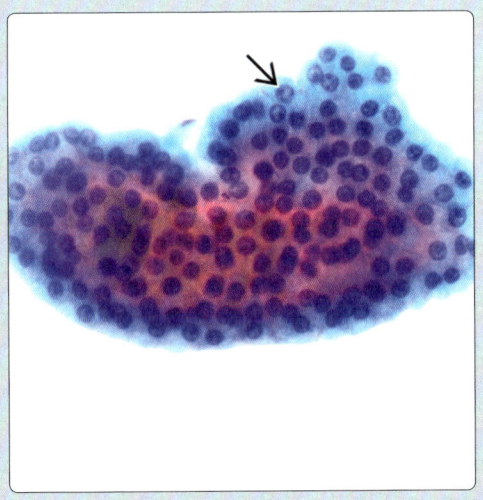
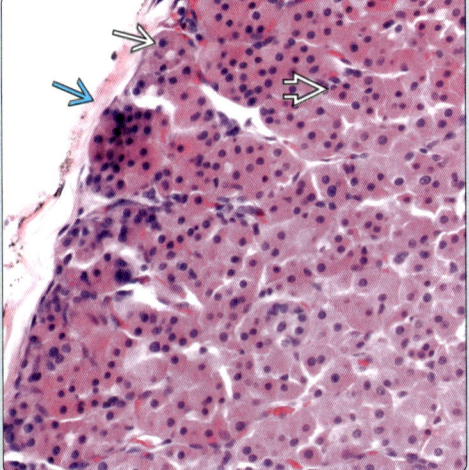

(Left) Oncocytoma resembles a Warthin tumor but with absence of the lymphocytic component on a Pap stain. The tumor cells have round, regular nuclei with prominent nucleoli ➡ and ample granular cytoplasm. (Right) H&E-stained resected tumor shows a thin capsule ➡. The cells are arranged in cords ➡ and acini ➡. The cytoplasm is abundant, pink, and granular. The nuclei are small and round with nucleoli visible on higher magnification.

Adenoid Cystic Carcinoma

KEY FACTS

CLINICAL ISSUES
- Presentation
  - Mass with pain/facial paralysis
- Adults (peak in 6th decade, rare in children); M:F = 3:2

CYTOPATHOLOGY
- Cohesive cellular clusters surrounding balls of mucopolysaccharide material
- Small to medium cells with eosinophilic to clear cytoplasm
- Nuclei oval to sharply angulated
- Characteristic round, scattered fragments of mucopolysaccharide material surrounded by cells
  - Diff-Quik: Purple-pink to magenta, bubblegum-like
  - Papanicolaou: Light green
  - Cells at periphery, not embedded within material
- High nuclear:cytoplasmic ratio
- Coarse nuclear chromatin

TOP DIFFERENTIAL DIAGNOSES
- Pleomorphic adenoma, basaloid tumors

DIAGNOSTIC CHECKLIST
- Recognition of dense, nonfibrillary basement membrane-like material is key
- Difficulty arises with solid variant of adenoid cystic carcinoma (ACCa), which has little to no acellular material
- Differential includes some benign lesions (pleomorphic adenoma, basal cell adenoma)
- Immunohistochemistry: CK7(+), CEA(+), SMA(+), S100(+), CK5/6(+), p63(+), SOX10(+), calponin (+); c-kit (+) in 90%
- Molecular: Chromosomal 6:9 translocation results in *MYB*::*NFIB* fusion with resulting overexpression of MYB oncoprotein
- Nuclear MYB stain on IHC, FISH probe supports diagnosis
- *MYB* RNA in situ hybridization more sensitive and specific

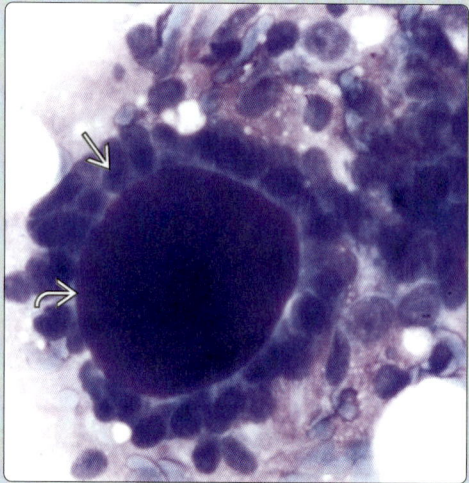

Adenoid Cystic Carcinoma Cells and Stromal Interface

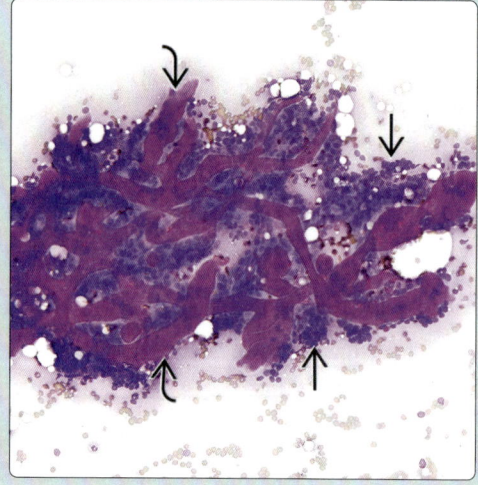

Ropey Stroma of Adenoid Cystic Carcinoma

(Left) The presence of dense, acellular material ➡ surrounded by small dark epithelial cells ➡ is a helpful feature on Diff-Quik stain in this adenoid cystic carcinoma (ACCa). **(Right)** The basement membrane material may also be arranged in long strands or tubules ➡ and stains dark purple on Diff-Quik. Islands of malignant epithelial cells ➡ are loosely attached at the periphery.

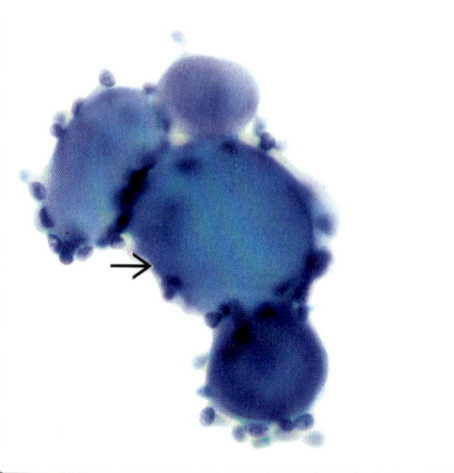

Stroma and Cells of Adenoid Cystic Carcinoma

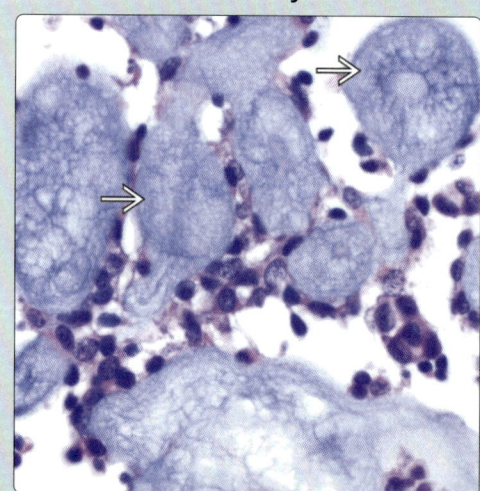

Cell Block of Adenoid Cystic Carcinoma

(Left) On Pap stain, the acellular material stains a pale blue-green ➡ but still has a dense appearance. The separation between the cells and stroma is distinct, unlike the fibrillary or chondromyxoid stroma of pleomorphic adenoma, which merges with the cells. **(Right)** H&E stained section shows well-defined globular myxohyaline spherules ➡ in punched-out spaces. The surrounding epithelium is distinct from the stroma, unlike pleomorphic adenomas.

Adenoid Cystic Carcinoma

TERMINOLOGY

Abbreviations
- Adenoid cystic carcinoma (ACCa)

CLINICAL ISSUES

Presentation
- Mass often with associated pain/facial paralysis due to extensive perineural invasion

Prognosis
- High incidence of recurrence, late metastasis
- Patients with solid pattern tumors have worse prognosis

CYTOPATHOLOGY

Pattern
- Cohesive cellular clusters surrounding balls of mucopolysaccharide material if classic cribriform type
- Solid pattern type lacks stroma and shows small basaloid cells, difficult to diagnose cytologically

Cells
- Small with scant cytoplasm
- Nuclei are oval to sharply angulated
  - Occasional small nucleoli
  - Mitotic figures are rare
- Characteristic round, scattered fragments of mucopolysaccharide material surrounded by cells
  - Diff-Quik: Purple-pink to magenta, bubblegum-like
  - Papanicolaou: Light green
  - Cells at periphery, not embedded within material

Nuclear Details
- High nuclear:cytoplasmic ratio
- Coarse nuclear chromatin

DIFFERENTIAL DIAGNOSIS

Polymorphous Adenocarcinoma
- Most difficult to distinguish from ACCa
- Only identified in minor salivary glands

Pleomorphic Adenoma
- Chondromyxoid matrix material different (fibrillary, not dense as seen in ACCa)

Basal Cell Adenocarcinoma
- Shows well-developed peripheral palisading
- Lacks glycosaminoglycan material

Basal Cell Adenoma
- Solid ACCa variant will show similar features
- No history of pain/facial paralysis

Epithelial-Myoepithelial Carcinoma
- Clear cell component

Basaloid Squamous Cell Carcinoma
- Usually found in base of tongue or hypopharynx

DIAGNOSTIC CHECKLIST

Pathologic Interpretation Pearls
- Recognition of dense, nonfibrillary basement membrane-like material is key
- Difficulty arises with solid variant of ACCa, which has little to no acellular material
  - Differential includes some benign lesions (pleomorphic adenoma, basal cell adenoma)
  - Hence, may be interpreted as SUMP or "suspicious for malignancy" under Milan System for Reporting
- Immunohistochemistry: CK7(+), CEA(+), SMA(+), S100(+), CK5/6(+), p63(+), SOX10(+), calponin (+), c-kit (+) in 90%
- Chromosomal 6:9 translocation results in *MYB*::*FIB* fusion with resulting overexpression of MYB oncoprotein
- Nuclear MYB stain on IHC, FISH probe supports diagnosis
- *MYB* RNA in situ hybridization more sensitive and specific

SELECTED REFERENCES
1. The Milan System for Reporting Salivary Gland Cytopathology Faquin and Rossi, Springer 2018

Variable Stroma in Adenoid Cystic Carcinoma

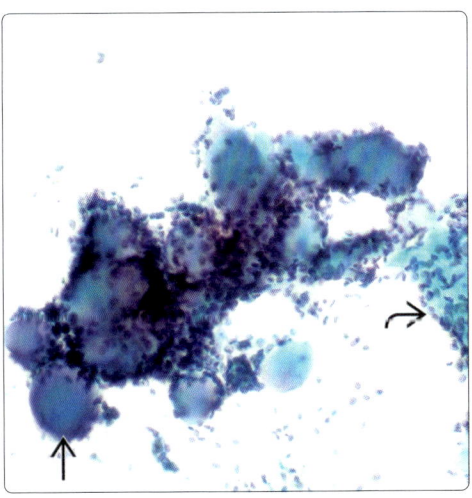

Hyperchromatic Nuclei in Adenoid Cystic Carcinoma

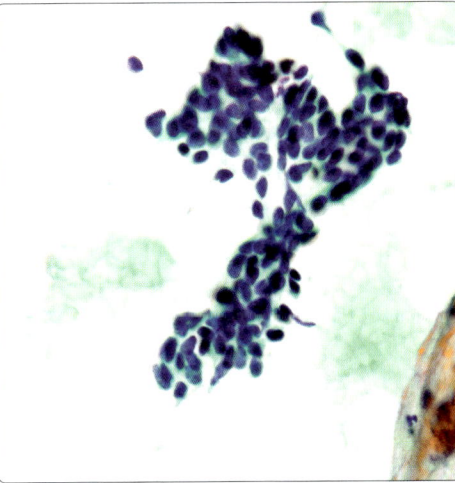

(Left) Pap stain shows obvious acellular material ➡ amid the basaloid cells. In other areas ➡, it is not so apparent. *(Right)* The tumor cells on this Pap stain are small and hyperchromatic and contain scant cytoplasm. Without the acellular material, a wide variety of basaloid tumors (benign and malignant) enter the differential.

Acinic Cell Carcinoma

KEY FACTS

CLINICAL ISSUES
- Parotid gland is most commonly affected (80%)
- 6% of salivary gland tumors, 10-12% of malignant salivary gland tumors

CYTOPATHOLOGY
- Usually high cellularity
- Cohesive, small and large, loose and tight acinar clusters and sheets, which, unlike normal parotid, lack ducts and adipocytes
  - Rarely papillary and microfollicular clusters
- Many stripped, bare tumor nuclei may be present in background
  - Background may consist of lymphocytes ± bare nuclei from ruptured tumor cells
- Large, uniform cells with small, round, and regular nuclei with coarse chromatin and nucleoli may be prominent
- Ample, granular to vacuolated cytoplasm, lacking coarse granules
- Cytoplasmic zymogen granules are PAS positive and diastase resistant
- Rarely, high-grade transformation, which may be difficult to distinguish from other high-grade tumors
- Acinar cell carcinomas show strong and diffuse as well as canalicular pattern of DOG1 positivity
  - NR4A3(NOR-1) nuclear positive
  - Mammaglobin and S-100 negative

TOP DIFFERENTIAL DIAGNOSES
- Normal salivary gland
  - Most common cause of false-negative
  - Tight acinar clusters, ducts, adipocytes
- Secretory carcinoma
  - Mammaglobin (+), *ETV6* translocation (+)
- Mucoepidermoid carcinoma
  - Mucicarmine (+), *CRTC1-MAML2*; t(11;19)(q21;p13)
- Papillary cystadenocarcinoma
  - Lacks zymogen granules, mucicarmine (+)

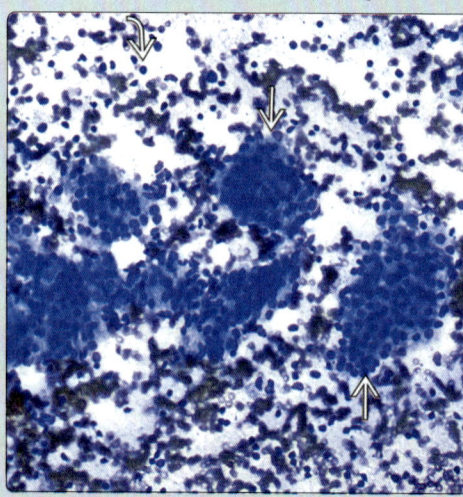

Acinic Cell Carcinoma Diff-Quik

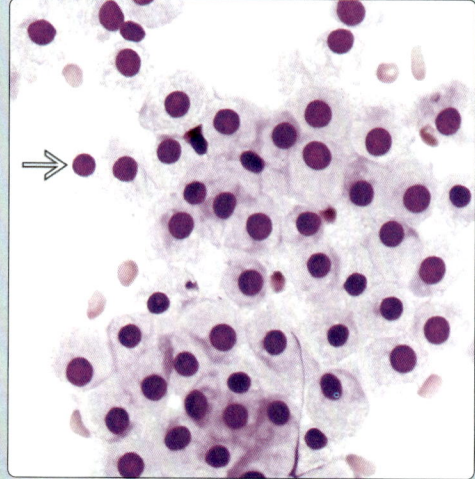

Acinic Cell Carcinoma Cytoplasmic and Nuclear Features

(Left) Intermediate-power view demonstrates a cellular smear consisting of many large acinar ➡ structures without ducts or adipose tissue. The background contains many lymphocytes as well as bare nuclei ➡, which are identical to the nuclei of the intact cells in the clusters. *(Right)* The finely vacuolated cells with distinct cell boundaries are clearly seen on this Diff-Quik stain. The nuclei are round with smooth nuclear contours ➡. The delicate cells can rupture, leaving only bare nuclei, which may resemble lymphocytes.

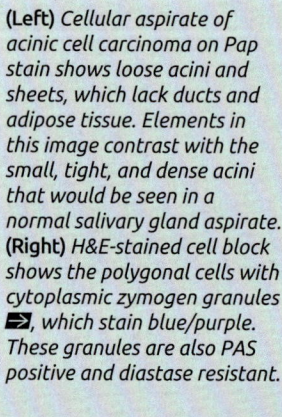

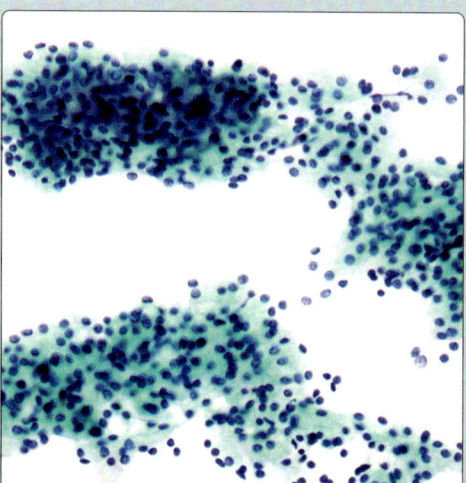

Acinic Cell Carcinoma Without Ducts

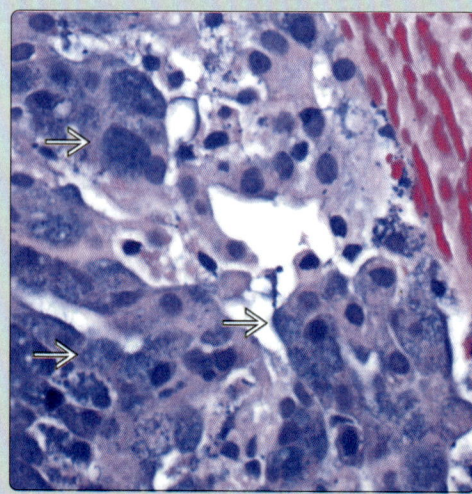

Zymogen Granules in Acinic Cell Carcinoma

(Left) Cellular aspirate of acinic cell carcinoma on Pap stain shows loose acini and sheets, which lack ducts and adipose tissue. Elements in this image contrast with the small, tight, and dense acini that would be seen in a normal salivary gland aspirate. *(Right)* H&E-stained cell block shows the polygonal cells with cytoplasmic zymogen granules ➡, which stain blue/purple. These granules are also PAS positive and diastase resistant.

Acinic Cell Carcinoma

TERMINOLOGY

Abbreviations
- Acinic cell carcinoma (AcCC)

CLINICAL ISSUES

Epidemiology
- Incidence
  - Accounts for ~ 6% of salivary gland tumors, with 80% occurring in parotid gland
  - Wide age range with mean in mid 40s
  - 10-12% of malignant salivary gland tumors; 2nd most common malignant salivary gland tumor in children
  - Most common bilateral salivary gland malignancy
  - F:M = 3:2

Presentation
- Slowly enlarging solitary mass; may be mobile or fixed
- History of pain is present in up to 1/2 of patients
- Facial nerve paralysis is present in 5-10% of cases

CYTOPATHOLOGY

Cellularity
- Usually high cellularity

Pattern
- Cohesive, small, tight clusters resembling normal acini
  - Fibrovascular core may be noted
- May be dyshesive and lack acinar formation

Background
- Many stripped, bare tumor nuclei may be present
  - Cytoplasm is fragile and easily disrupted with pressure during smear preparation

Cells
- Large, uniform cells with small, round, and regular nuclei with coarse chromatin and nucleoli may be prominent
  - Carcinoma cells are slightly larger than nonneoplastic acinar cells
- Ducts and adipocytes are absent

Cytoplasmic Details
- Ample, granular to vacuolated, lacking coarse granules
  - Stripped cytoplasm creates naked nuclei

ANCILLARY TESTS

Immunohistochemistry
- DOG1 strong and diffuse positivity as well as intercanalicular positivity, helpful in distinguishing from secretory carcinoma and salivary duct carcinomas
- NR4A3(NOR-1) nuclear stain is highly sensitive and specific for AcCC; SOX10 nuclear positive in AcCC

DIFFERENTIAL DIAGNOSIS

Normal Salivary Gland, Sialadenitis
- Scant cellularity on smears with admixed ducts and adipocytes
- Very well-differentiated tumors may be incorrectly interpreted as normal (high false-negative rate)

Secretory Carcinoma
- Mammaglobin, S100 positive by IHC; *ETV6* gene rearrangement by molecular testing

Warthin Tumor
- Look for background of lymphocytes, oncocytes, and cyst contents

Mucoepidermoid Carcinoma
- Look for glandular differentiation/mucicarmine positivity

Metastatic Renal Cell Carcinoma
- Clear cell variant of AcCC is rare, and clear cells are usually limited and focal
- Renal cell shows more pleomorphism and larger nucleoli

SELECTED REFERENCES

1. Owosho A et al: NR4A3 (NOR-1) immunostaining shows better performance than DOG1 immunostaining in acinic cell carcinoma of salivary gland: a preliminary study. J Oral Maxillofac Res. 12(1):e4, 2021

Nuclear SOX-10 Positive

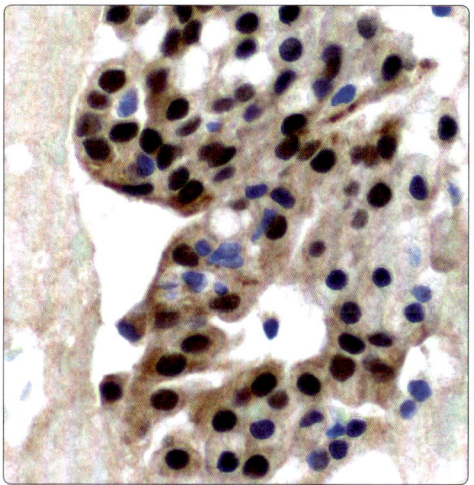

DOG1 Positive

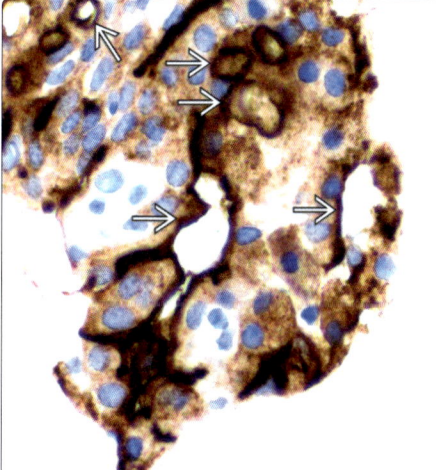

(Left) Acinic cell carcinoma shows nuclear SOX-10 positivity, as seen in this cell block example. **(Right)** Cell block containing fragments of acinic cell carcinoma, which, on DOG1 immunohistochemical stain, shows a distinct canalicular staining pattern ➡. The combination of SOX-10 and DOG1 on cell block or core biopsies is helpful in small biopsy diagnosis of acinic cell carcinoma.

Mucoepidermoid Carcinoma

KEY FACTS

CLINICAL ISSUES
- Mucoepidermoid carcinoma (MEC): Most common malignant salivary gland tumor

CYTOPATHOLOGY
- May be hypocellular or acellular if cystic areas sampled
- Variable amounts of mucin in background
- Lymphocytes may be seen in background
- Low grade: Clusters of bland intermediate or epithelial cells and mucocytes
- High grade: Simulates poorly differentiated squamous cell carcinoma; mucous cells rarely seen

ANCILLARY TESTS
- t(11;19)(q21-22;p13) identified in 60%
  - Testing by FISH or next-gen sequencing
- Fuses MEC translocation 1 (*MECT1*) (exon 1 of gene at 19p13) with mastermind-like gene family (*MAML2*) (exons 2-5 of gene at 11q21)
  - Identified in low- to intermediate-grade tumors only
- Mucicarmine (+) mucocytes identified in cell block
- IHC not helpful due to lack of distinctive markers

TOP DIFFERENTIAL DIAGNOSES
- Sialometaplasia
- Mucus extravasation reaction
- Warthin tumor (especially Warthin's-like variant)
- Squamous cell carcinoma

DIAGNOSTIC CHECKLIST
- Aspirates of low-grade tumors may be paucicellular and result in false-negative diagnosis
- Think of MEC whenever mucin seen
- Mucous cells may be difficult to identify
- Cell block and mucin stain helpful
- Poorly differentiated MECs resembles any other poorly differentiated carcinomas (primary or metastatic) and cannot reliably be differentiated from them

Mucin, Epithelioid, and Transitional Cells

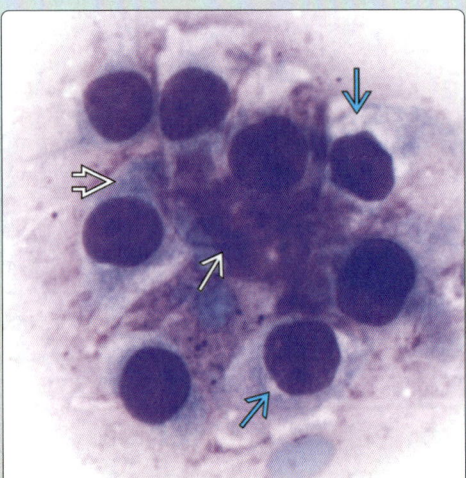

Mucin and Mucous Cells

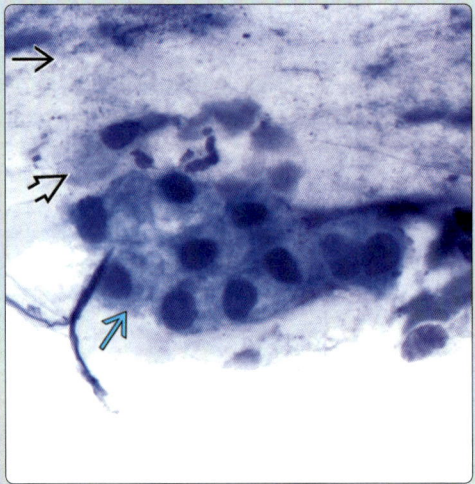

(Left) Touch preparation of core needle biopsy shows a ring of cells surrounding mucin ➡. The cells have cytoplasm that ranges from vacuolated ➡ to finely granular ➡ in this case of mucoepidermoid carcinoma (MEC). (Right) Diff-Quik stain shows abundant background mucin ➡ in which a few free-floating mucous cells are seen. These can be uni- ➡ or multivacuolated ➡. Low-grade MECs typically have abundant mucin and few cells, and may be underdiagnosed as mucocele or atypical in the Milan System.

Abundant Intracellular Mucin

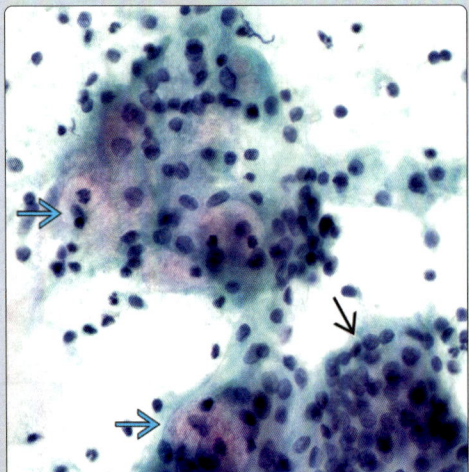

Oncocytic Mucoepidermoid Carcinoma

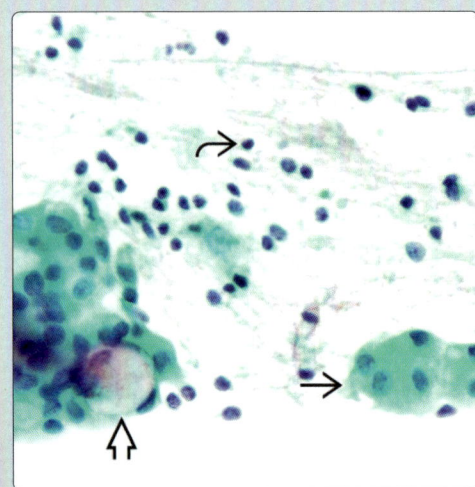

(Left) Pap-stained smear shows intermediate cells ➡ with relatively scant cytoplasm as well as mucous cells with abundant pink mucin ➡ in cytoplasmic vacuoles. (Right) Pap-stained smear shows an oncocytic MEC. Numerous epithelial cells show abundant granular cytoplasm ➡ with scattered mucous cells ➡. Lymphocytes ➡ are present in the background.

Mucoepidermoid Carcinoma

TERMINOLOGY

Abbreviations
- Mucoepidermoid carcinoma (MEC)

Definitions
- Malignant salivary gland tumor composed of mucous, squamous, and intermediate cells

CLINICAL ISSUES

Site
- Major and minor salivary glands
  - Parotid gland most common location

Prognosis
- Low grade: Rarely metastasizes
- High grade: 55-80% metastasize or result in death

CYTOPATHOLOGY

Cellularity
- May be hypocellular or acellular if cystic areas sampled in low-grade carcinoma

Background
- Variable amounts of mucin in background
- Scattered lymphocytes my be present

Cells
- Low grade: Sheets or clusters of bland epithelial cells and intermediate cells with scattered mucous cells
  - Mucous cells may be columnar, cuboidal, or histiocytoid
- High grade: Simulates poorly differentiated squamous cell carcinoma; mucous cells rarely seen
- Mucin-secreting cells may be identified by mucicarmine stain

ANCILLARY TESTS

Genetic Testing
- t(11;19)(q21-22;p13) identified in 60%
  - Fuses MEC translocation 1 (*MECT1*) (exon 1 of gene at 19p13) with mastermind-like gene family (*MAML2*) (exons 2-5 of gene at 11q21)
  - Testing by FISH for *MAML2* rearrangement or next-gen sequencing

DIFFERENTIAL DIAGNOSIS

Chronic Sialadenitis/Sialometaplasia
- Paucicellular smears, lacks cystic growth, intermediate or mucous cells

Mucus Extravasation Reaction
- Lacks intermediate cells and epithelial cells
- Mucus found primarily in macrophages

Warthin Tumor
- Aspirate consists of bloody cyst fluid
- Like MEC, may show mucous cells
- Usually more pronounced lymphocytic infiltrate
- Less cytologic atypia

Squamous Cell Carcinoma
- Morphologically indistinguishable from high-grade MEC

DIAGNOSTIC CHECKLIST

Pathologic Interpretation Pearls
- Aspirates of low-grade tumors may be paucicellular and result in false-negative diagnosis
  - Think of MEC whenever mucin seen
- Mucous cells may be difficult to identify
  - Cell block and mucin stain helpful
- Poorly differentiated MECs resembles any other poorly differentiated carcinomas (primary or metastatic) and cannot reliably be differentiated from them

SELECTED REFERENCES

1. Fehr A et al: Mucoepidermoid carcinoma of the salivary glands revisited with special reference to histologic grading and CRTC1/3-MAML2 genotyping. Virchows Arch. 479(5):975-85, 2021

Oncocytic Mucoepidermoid Carcinoma

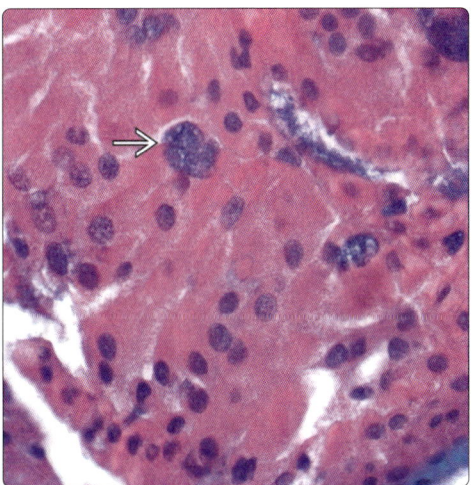

Cell Block of High-Grade Mucoepidermoid Carcinoma

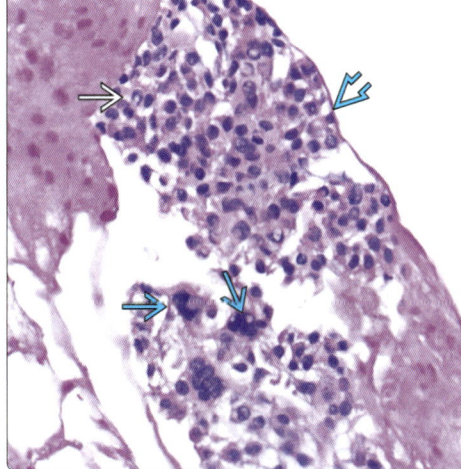

(Left) H&E-stained section of a core needle biopsy with an oncocytic neoplasm of the salivary glands is shown. The bluish mucin ➡ raised the possibility of MEC, which was confirmed on FISH for MAML2. *(Right)* Thrombin cell block with trapped fragments of intermediate/transitional ➡ and high pleomorphic epithelial cells ➡ from high-grade MEC is shown. Rare cells with cytoplasmic vacuoles ➡ are also seen.

Basaloid Neoplasms, Benign and Malignant

KEY FACTS

CLINICAL ISSUES
- Most basal cell adenomas (BCA) and adenocarcinomas (BCAC) arise in parotid gland

CYTOPATHOLOGY
- FNA is highly sensitive at detecting basaloid neoplasm in salivary gland
    - Richly cellular cohesive groups, cords, or irregular clusters of uniform basaloid cells
    - Branching tubules or cohesive trabecular or insular groups surrounded by thin peripheral ribbon of basement membrane material may be present
    - Peripheral palisading may be seen
    - Squamous differentiation (e.g., squamous morules), if present, is characteristic of BCA/BCAC
    - Intracellular globules of matrix material can be seen
    - Extracellular metachromatic hyaline material, ranging from minimal to abundant, easily distinguishable from chondrofibrillary material seen in pleomorphic adenoma

- Distinction between BCA and BCAC cannot be reliably performed on basis of cytologic features
- In Milan System for Reporting, most will end up under salivary neoplasm of uncertain malignant potential
- Immunohistochemistry: Positive for CK-PAN, CK7, CD117
- Myoepithelial cells positive for S100, actin-sm, p63, CK5/6, and calponin; nuclear β-catenin (+) in 75%
- *CTNNB1* activating mutation on molecular testing

TOP DIFFERENTIAL DIAGNOSES
- Adenoid cystic carcinoma (especially solid type)
    - Presence of intracellular matrix globules, squamous morules, or peripheral palisading favors BCA/BCAC
- Cellular pleomorphic adenoma
    - Well-sampled specimen is required for identification of characteristic fibrillary matrix material by Diff-Quik stain
- Distinguishing among these differentials is usually not crucial: All are treated with surgical resection

Cohesive Cellular Sheets of Basaloid Cells
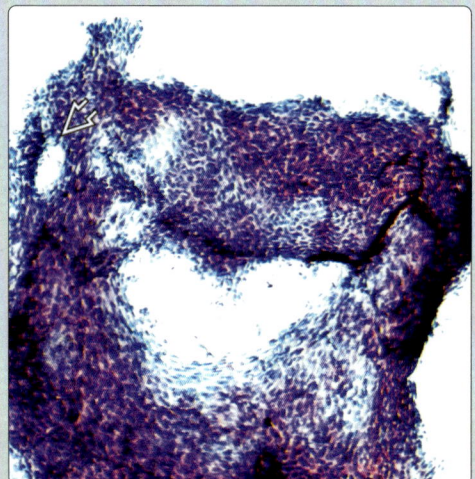

Peripheral Palisading
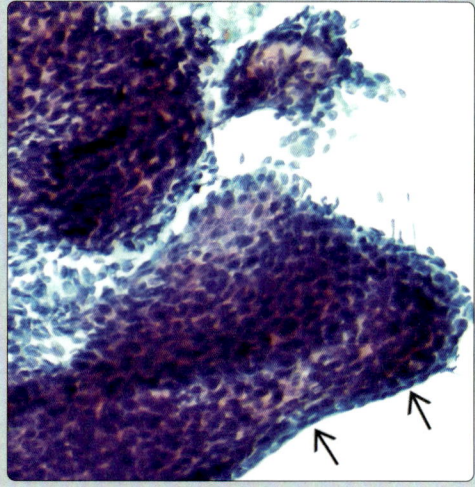

(Left) Pap-stained FNA of basal cell adenoma (BCA) shows cohesive cellular sheets of basaloid cells with focal tubule formation ⮕. (Right) Pap-stained FNA of BCA shows cellular clusters of basaloid cells with peripheral palisading ⮕.

Peripheral Basement Membrane
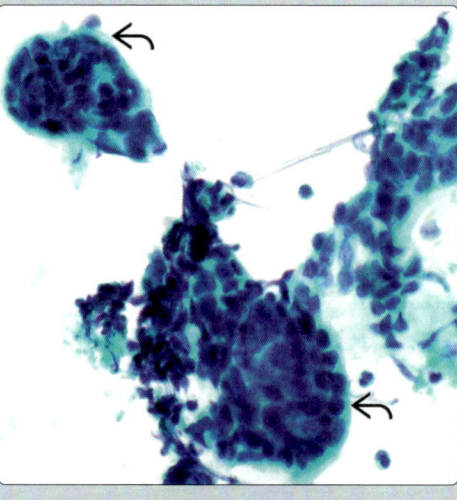

Basal Cell Adenoma vs. Carcinoma Histology
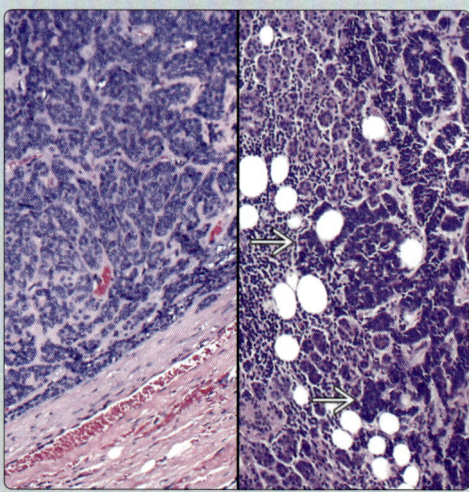

(Left) Pap-stained FNA of BCA shows 2 tight cohesive groups of basaloid tumor cells that are surrounded by a thin peripheral ribbon of basement membrane material ⮕. (Right) H&E section of BCA (left) shows a well-circumscribed border. H&E section of basal cell adenocarcinoma (right) shows an infiltrating border ⮕.

Basaloid Neoplasms, Benign and Malignant

TERMINOLOGY

Abbreviations
- Basal cell adenoma (BCA)
- Basal cell adenocarcinoma (BCAC)

Synonyms
- BCA is formerly known as monomorphic adenoma
- BCAC is synonymous with basaloid salivary carcinoma, basal cell carcinoma, and malignant BCA

Definitions
- BCA and BCAC
  - Uncommon salivary gland tumors composed of basaloid cell proliferation forming nests, cords, and glandular structures
- BCAC is distinguished from BCA by infiltrative growth pattern and perineural and angiolymphatic invasions

CLINICAL ISSUES

Epidemiology
- Age
  - Both BCA and BCAC occur in older individuals

Site
- Majority of BCAs and BCACs arise in parotid gland

Prognosis
- BCAC is locally destructive and often recurs with only occasional metastasis (low-grade malignancy)
- BCA is usually nonrecurrent tumor after resection

Brooke-Spiegler Syndrome
- Disease of autosomal dominant inheritance pattern (tumor suppressor gene CYLD mutations), characterized by multiple cutaneous adnexal tumors
- Basal cell neoplasms in salivary gland are known to occur, although they are not frequent

CYTOPATHOLOGY

Cellularity
- Richly cellular

Pattern
- Cohesive (fragmented) groups, cords, or irregular clusters, with variable numbers of single cells
- Branching tubules or cohesive trabecular or insular groups surrounded by thin peripheral ribbon of basement membrane material may be present
- Peripheral palisading may be seen
- Squamous differentiation (e.g., squamous morules), if present, is characteristic of BCA/BCAC
  - Adenoid cystic carcinoma can be excluded from differential diagnosis if squamous cells are present
- Extracellular metachromatic hyaline material is present, ranging from minimal to abundant
  - This is easily distinguishable from chondrofibrillary material seen in pleomorphic adenoma

Background
- Clean background; usually no necrosis

- Fibromyxoid stroma seen in pleomorphic adenoma is **not** seen

Cells
- Small, uniform basaloid cells with small amount of cytoplasm (i.e., high nuclear:cytoplasmic ratio)
- Mild nuclear atypia &/or pleomorphism may be seen in BCAC
- Significant cellular atypia, increased mitotic activity, &/or necrosis, if present, exclude BCA

Nuclear Details
- Round to oval, uniform, dark nuclei with granular chromatin and small, indistinct nucleoli

Cytoplasmic Details
- Intracellular globules of matrix material can be seen

Cytology-Histology Correlation
- Cytologically, BCAC and BCA cannot be reliably distinguished; infiltrative growth pattern needs to be identified histologically for diagnosis of BCAC

MICROSCOPIC

Histologic Features
- 4 subtypes are known: Solid, tubular, trabecular, and membranous
  - Tumors may present with > 1 of these patterns
- Cystic change, squamous differentiation in form of whorls or "eddies," or (rarely) cribriform patterns can be seen
- Immunohistochemistry: Positive for CK-PAN, CK7, CD117
- Myoepithelial cells positive for S100, actin-sm, p63, CK5/6, and calponin; nuclear β-catenin (+) in 75%
- CTNNB1 activating mutation on molecular testing

DIFFERENTIAL DIAGNOSIS

Salivary Gland Basaloid Lesions
- Adenoid cystic carcinoma (ACC)
  - Peripheral ribbon of matrix surrounding tumor cells (BCA/BCAC) vs. branching of globular matrix surrounded by tumor cells (ACC)
    - Solid type of ACC particularly difficult to differentiate given characteristically scant or absent matrix
  - Intracellular matrix globules, squamous morules, peripheral palisading, &/or absence of cellular atypia favor BCA/BCAC
- Cellular pleomorphic adenoma
  - Characteristically sparse fibrillar matrix material
  - Adequate sampling with careful search for characteristic fibrillary matrix material by Diff-Quik stain is crucial

SELECTED REFERENCES

1. Cantley RL: Fine-needle aspiration cytology of cellular basaloid neoplasms of the salivary gland. Arch Pathol Lab Med. 143(11):1338-45, 2019
2. Pal S et al: Fine needle aspiration cytology of basal cell adenoma of parotid simulating adenoid cystic carcinoma. J Cytol. 35(1):55-7, 2018
3. Jurczyk M et al: Pitfalls of fine-needle aspiration cytology of parotid membranous basal cell adenoma-a review of pitfalls in FNA cytology of salivary gland neoplasms with basaloid cell features. Diagn Cytopathol. 43(5):432-7, 2015

Carcinoma Ex Pleomorphic Adenoma

KEY FACTS

TERMINOLOGY
- Carcinoma arising from pleomorphic adenoma (PA)
- Requires concurrent PA histologically or history of PA at same site
- Carcinoma can be any number of neoplasms
  - Salivary duct carcinoma (most common), myoepithelial carcinoma, epithelial myoepithelial carcinoma, and others

CLINICAL ISSUES
- Parotid > > minor salivary glands
- Parotid (80%) > submandibular (18%) > > sublingual gland (< 2%)
- Long clinical history of painless mass with recent rapid enlargement and nerve palsy
- Accounts for ~ 4% of all salivary tumors
- Usually in 6th and 7th decades
- Patients ~ 10-12 years older than age at presentation of PA

CYTOPATHOLOGY
- Cellular smears with population of predominantly epithelial cells
- Background may be necrotic
- May show 2 distinct patterns
  - Unequivocal groups and single malignant cells admixed with benign epithelial and stromal components of PA
  - Variably pleomorphic cells without clear-cut malignant criteria and with mixture of epithelial and stromal components of PA
- Adequate sampling is critical to exclude malignancy

ANCILLARY TESTS
- Fluorescence in situ hybridization for *PLAG1* or *HMGA2* can be used to distinguish between PA and carcinoma ex-PA and their morphologic mimics and de novo counterparts

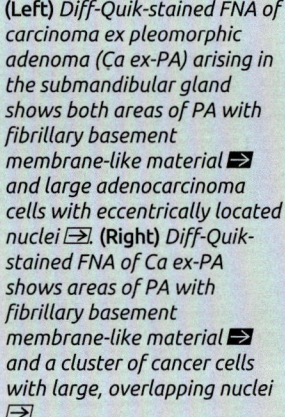

(Left) Diff-Quik-stained FNA of carcinoma ex pleomorphic adenoma (Ca ex-PA) arising in the submandibular gland shows both areas of PA with fibrillary basement membrane-like material ⇨ and large adenocarcinoma cells with eccentrically located nuclei ⇨. (Right) Diff-Quik-stained FNA of Ca ex-PA shows areas of PA with fibrillary basement membrane-like material ⇨ and a cluster of cancer cells with large, overlapping nuclei ⇨.

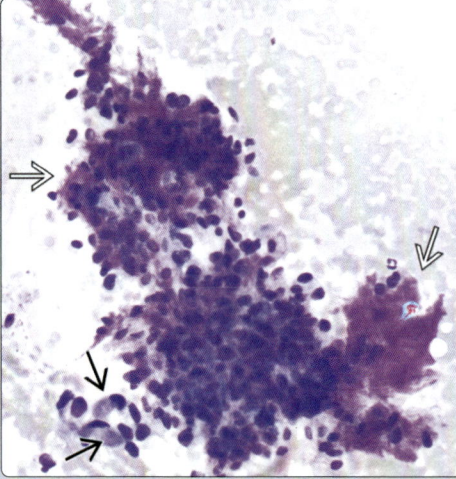

Carcinoma Ex Pleomorphic Adenoma Aspirate (Diff-Quik)

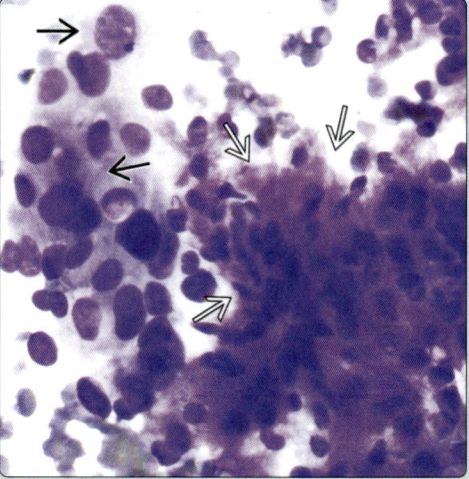

Carcinoma Ex Pleomorphic Adenoma Aspirate (Diff-Quik)

(Left) Pap-stained FNA of Ca ex-PA in the same case shows a loosely cohesive cluster of cancer cells ⇨ and a PA component with bland nuclei and hyalinized/fibrillary stroma ⇨. Note the differences in nuclear size and atypia between these 2 areas. (Right) Pap-stained FNA of Ca ex-PA in the same case shows a bland PA area with a fibrillary background ⇨ and a loose aggregate of adenocarcinoma cells with vesicular chromatin and prominent nucleoli ⇨.

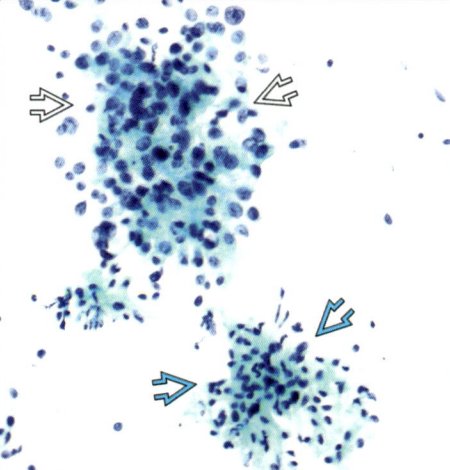

Carcinoma Ex Pleomorphic Adenoma Aspirate (Pap)

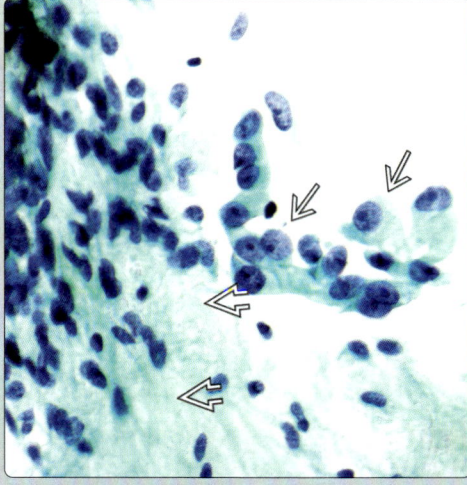

Carcinoma Ex Pleomorphic Adenoma Aspirate (Pap)

Carcinoma Ex Pleomorphic Adenoma

TERMINOLOGY

Abbreviations
- Carcinoma ex pleomorphic adenoma (Ca ex-PA)

Definitions
- Carcinoma arising from PA
  - Requires concurrent PA histologically or history of PA at same site
  - Carcinomatous components can be any number of neoplasms, mostly high grade
    - Salivary duct carcinoma (most common), myoepithelial carcinoma, epithelial myoepithelial carcinoma, and others

CLINICAL ISSUES

Site
- Major salivary glands most often (80%)
  - Parotid (80%) > submandibular (18%) > > sublingual (< 2%) glands

Presentation
- Long clinical history of PA
  - Greater length of time with tumor = higher risk of malignant transformation
- Usually, recent rapid enlargement

CYTOPATHOLOGY

Cellularity
- Cellular smears with population of predominantly epithelial cells, necrotic background

Pattern
- May show 2 distinct patterns
  - Unequivocal groups and single malignant cells admixed with benign epithelial and stromal components of PA
    - Groups, sheets, papillary structures, cribriform pattern
    - Large cells, pleomorphic nuclei, prominent nucleoli, increased mitotic figures, necrosis
  - Variably pleomorphic cells, without clear-cut malignant criteria, with mixture of epithelial and stromal components of PA

Cells
- Variation in type and grade of carcinoma, coupled with unknown benign and malignant proportions, makes FNA interpretation difficult

MICROSCOPIC

Histologic Features
- Carcinomatous component may be specific tumor type
  - Adenocarcinoma, not otherwise specified
  - Salivary duct carcinoma
  - Adenoid cystic carcinoma
  - Mucoepidermoid carcinoma
  - Myoepithelial carcinoma
  - Polymorphous low-grade adenocarcinoma
  - Epithelial-myoepithelial carcinoma
- Separated into low and high grade
  - Based on degree of pleomorphism, necrosis, increased mitoses
- Concurrent PA is very frequently extensively hyalinized (fibrotic, scarred)
- Separation based on invasion: Noninvasive, minimally invasive (≤ 1.5 mm), and invasive

ANCILLARY TESTS

Genetic Testing
- Fluorescence in situ hybridization for *PLAG1* or *HMGA2* can be used to distinguish between PA and CA ex-PA and their morphologic mimics and do novo counterparts

SELECTED REFERENCES
1. Okano K et al: Cytological features of carcinoma ex pleomorphic adenoma of the salivary glands: a diagnostic challenge. Diagn Cytopathol. 48(2):149-53, 2020
2. Covinsky M et al: Low grade carcinoma ex-pleomorphic adenoma: Diagnosis and diagnostic challenges caused by fine needle aspiration: report of three cases and review of literature. Head Neck Pathol. 12(1):82-8, 2018

Complex Epithelial Groups of Salivary Duct Carcinoma Ex Pleomorphic Adenoma

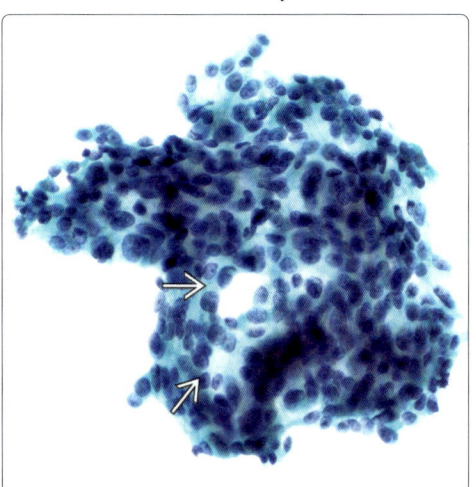

Microacini and Micropapillae in Carcinoma Ex Pleomorphic Adenoma

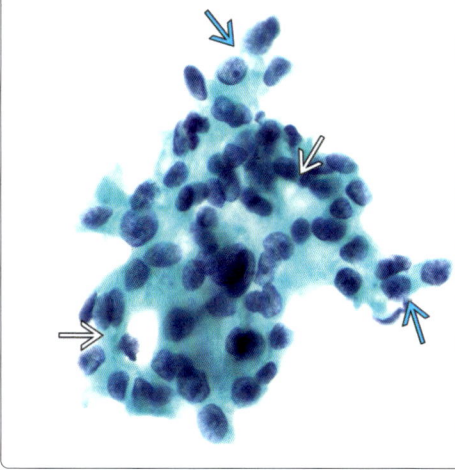

(Left) Pap stain shows a cohesive group of malignant epithelial cells arranged in a complex architectural pattern with microacinar formation ➡ corresponding to cribriform glands seen on histology. *(Right)* Pap stain shows malignant epithelial cells in microacinar ➡ and micropapillary formations ➡ of a salivary duct carcinoma.

Adenocarcinoma, NOS

KEY FACTS

TERMINOLOGY
- Adenocarcinoma, not otherwise specified (ANOS)
  - Malignant salivary gland neoplasm with ductal differentiation that lacks any histologic features characteristic of other defined types of salivary gland carcinomas

CLINICAL ISSUES
- Parotid gland most common site, 40% in minor salivary glands
- Usually asymptomatic

CYTOPATHOLOGY
- Diverse cytological and architectural features
  - Cells display variable pleomorphism, mitotic figures, and nucleoli
  - Background may be necrotic, myxoid, or hemorrhagic
  - Clear, oncocytoid, melanoma-like, mucinous, sebaceous, and plasmacytoid cells can be seen
- Lacks features characteristic of specific tumor

ANCILLARY TESTS
- Limited practical use except to exclude other defined salivary malignancies or metastasis
- However, molecular alterations unique to recently described entities should be ruled out

TOP DIFFERENTIAL DIAGNOSES
- Other primary salivary gland tumors or metastasis: Diagnosis of exclusion
- Metastatic adenocarcinomas: History crucial; immunohistochemistry helpful to identify primary site
- Cutaneous angiosarcoma infiltrating underlying salivary gland
  - Acinar &/or rosette formation in low-grade angiosarcomas can be easily mistaken for ANOS
  - CD31 immunohistochemistry for confirmation

Adenocarcinoma, Not Otherwise Specified
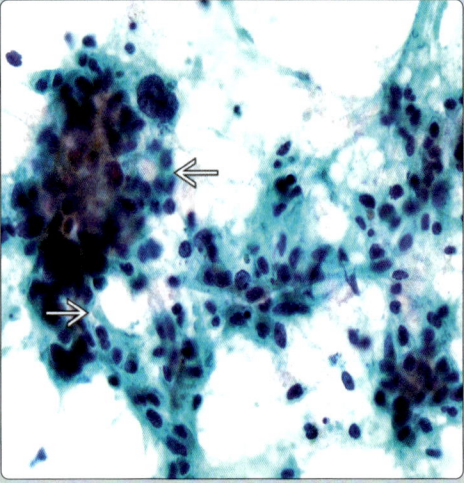
(Left) Pap-stained FNA of high-grade adenocarcinoma, not otherwise specified (ANOS) reveals multiple clusters of pleomorphic cancer cells with scattered, gland-like structures ➡. The background is somewhat dirty due to necrosis. (Right) Pap-stained higher-power view of the same lesion shows markedly pleomorphic and hyperchromatic cells.

High Magnification of High-Grade Adenocarcinoma, Not Otherwise Specified
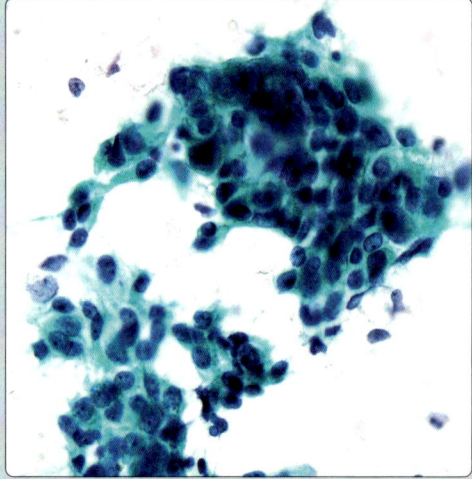

Low-Grade Adenocarcinoma, Not Otherwise Specified
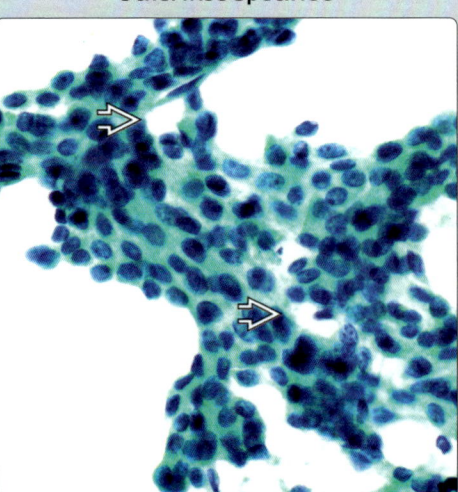
(Left) Pap-stained FNA of low-grade ANOS shows a sheet of mildly pleomorphic tumor cells forming occasional gland-like structures ➡ in a clean background. (Right) Pap-stained FNA of low-grade ANOS of parotid reveals monomorphic tumor cells with vesicular chromatin around blood vessels ➡. A somewhat papillary architecture is noted. Mitotic figures are not conspicuous.

Low-Grade Adenocarcinoma, Not Otherwise Specified
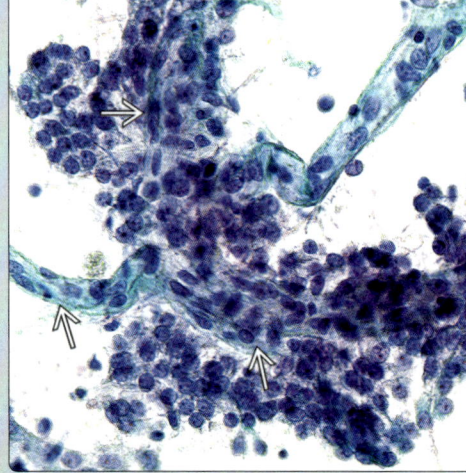

Adenocarcinoma, NOS

TERMINOLOGY

Abbreviations
- Adenocarcinoma, not otherwise specified (ANOS)

Definitions
- Malignant salivary gland neoplasm with ductal differentiation that lacks any histologic features characteristic of other defined types of salivary gland carcinomas

CLINICAL ISSUES

Epidemiology
- Incidence
  - Depends on workup to rule out metastasis and other salivary gland primaries

Site
- Majority in major glands (parotid specifically)
- Minor glands account for ~ 40% of cases

CYTOPATHOLOGY

Cellularity
- Richly cellular, lacks features characteristic of specific salivary malignancies
  - Background may be necrotic, myxoid, or hemorrhagic

Cells
- Display variable pleomorphism, mitotic figures, and nucleoli
- Distinct cell borders
- Clear, oncocytoid, melanoma-like, mucinous, sebaceous, and plasmacytoid cells can be seen

MICROSCOPIC

Histologic Features
- Glandular or duct-like structures that vary within individual tumors invariably present
- Variety of growth patterns, with infiltration into surrounding tissue
  - Glandular, papillary, cystic, cribriform, solid, lobular, nest-like, and strand-like differentiation
  - Perivascular or intravascular, perineural invasion
- No features characteristic of other defined salivary adenocarcinomas
- Stroma can be collagenized or myxoid

DIFFERENTIAL DIAGNOSIS

Other Primary Salivary Gland Tumors
- ANOS is diagnosis of exclusion

Metastatic Diseases
- History of other malignancy crucial
- Immunohistochemistry helps to confirm specific sites of origin

Cutaneous Angiosarcoma Infiltrating Salivary Gland
- Occurs in older population
- Acinar &/or rosette formation in low-grade angiosarcomas can be easily mistaken for ANOS
- Intracytoplasmic lumina with lymphocytes and many single or spindle cells should be clue
- CD31 immunohistochemistry for confirmation
  - CK-PAN could be positive in both

GRADING

Reflected by Cytologic Atypia (3 Grades)
- Grade 1: Well-formed ductal/tubular structures; mild pleomorphism, small nucleoli, few mitoses
- Grade 2: Less ductal/tubular structures; moderate pleomorphism, increased mitoses
- Grade 3: Limited ductal/tubular structures; moderate to severe pleomorphism; hyperchromasia; increased mitoses, including atypical forms; necrosis and hemorrhage

SELECTED REFERENCES
1. Speight PM et al: Salivary gland tumours: diagnostic challenges and an update on the latest WHO classification. Diagn Histopathol. 26(4):147-58, 2020

Histology of Adenocarcinoma, Not Otherwise Specified

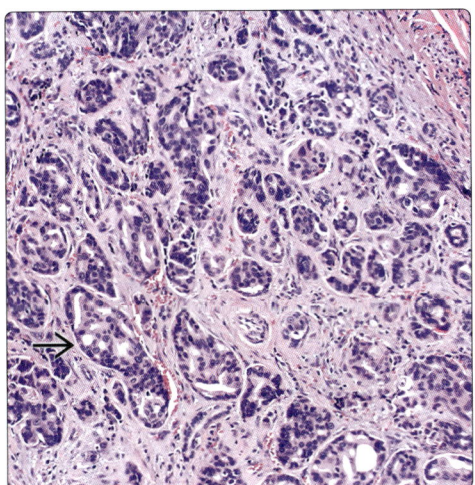

Angiosarcoma Mimicking Adenocarcinoma

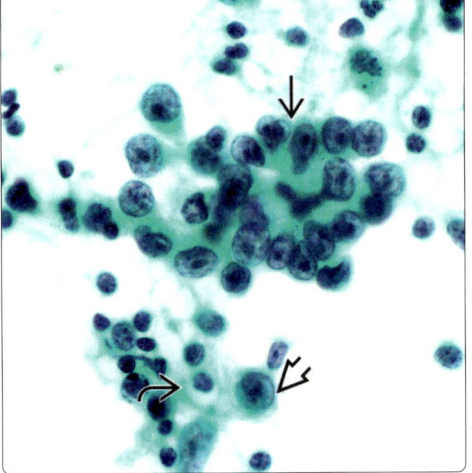

(Left) H&E stain shows infiltrating cancer cells forming nests in a desmoplastic stroma. Cribriform pattern ➡ is focally noted. (Right) Cutaneous angiosarcoma is shown with rosette and acinar ➡ structures as well as single cells ➡ with cytoplasmic lumina ➡ mimicking ANOS.

Polymorphous Adenocarcinoma

KEY FACTS

TERMINOLOGY
- Polymorphous adenocarcinoma (PAC): Malignant epithelial tumor characterized by infiltrative growth of cytologically uniform cells arranged in architecturally diverse patterns

CLINICAL ISSUES
- 2nd most common intraoral minor salivary gland malignant tumor (~ 25%)
- **Almost always** in minor glands (palate: 60%)
- Slow-growing nontender mass with excellent long-term prognosis

CYTOPATHOLOGY
- Hypercellular smear with sheets showing branching papillae, globular and tubular structures of tumor cells
- Uniformly bland (isomorphic) tumor cells with dispersed chromatin, no/inconspicuous nucleoli, some grooves, and rare nuclear holes
- Myxoid/hyaline stromal fragments and hyaline globules similar to pleomorphic adenoma and adenoid cystic carcinoma
- Bare nuclei are frequently seen in background

ANCILLARY TESTS
- Immunoreactive for cytokeratin 7, CAM5.2, S100 protein, Variable p63 positivity
  - *PRKD1* (E710D) mutation in 73-89% of PAC

TOP DIFFERENTIAL DIAGNOSES
- Pleomorphic adenoma
  - Biphasic (ductal and myoepithelial) pattern: Use immunohistochemistry to support.
- Adenoid cystic carcinoma
  - Dark, basaloid cells with peg-shaped, carrot-shaped, or angular nuclei

Polymorphous Adenocarcinoma Cells and Background
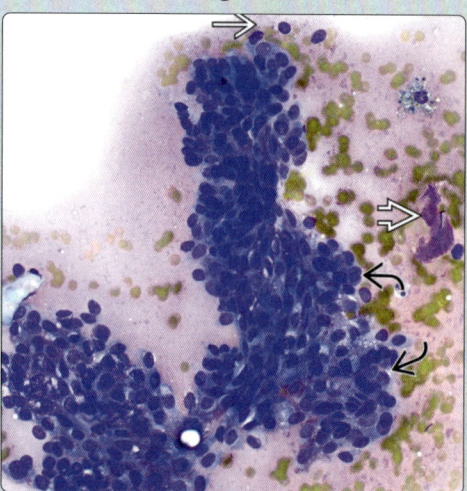

Polymorphous Adenocarcinoma Variable Architecture
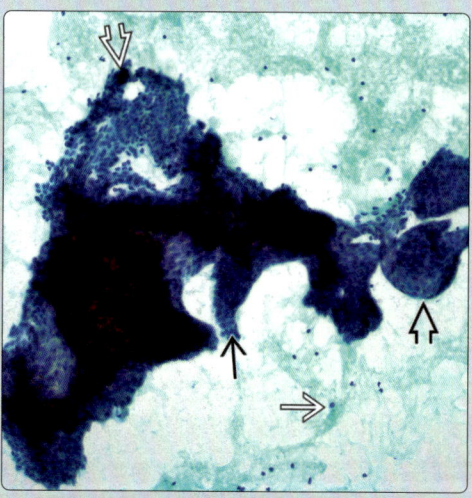

(Left) Sheets of Diff-Quik-stained cells show a streaming pattern, microcaini ⇒ with bare nuclei ⇒ in background, and a magenta-colored stromal fragment ⇒. **(Right)** Pap stain shows a large sheet of cells with complex and branching tubular ⇒, globular ⇒, and pseudopapillary ⇒ structures with bare nuclei ⇒ in the background, corresponding to the various architectural patterns characteristic of polymorphous adenocarcinoma (PAC).

Nuclear and Architectural Details of Polymorphous Adenocarcinoma
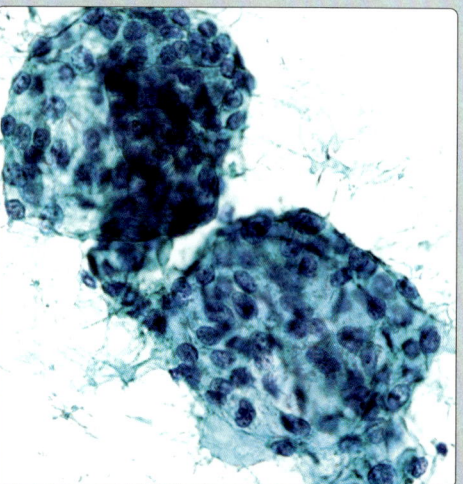

Cytologic Details of Polymorphous Adenocarcinoma
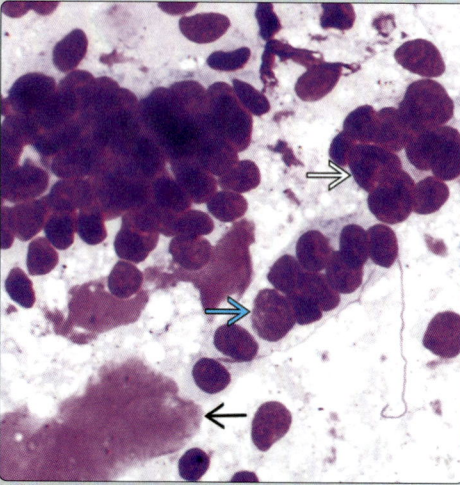

(Left) Pap-stained FNA smear shows ball-like globular clusters of tumor cells with slightly irregular, small- to medium-sized nuclei and fine chromatin. (Courtesy A. Kawahara, CT, CMIAC.) **(Right)** Diff-Quik-stained smear shows monomorphic tumor cells with bland nuclei. Focal small duct ⇒ and linear nest ⇒ formations are seen. Basement membrane-like material ⇒ is also noted.

Polymorphous Adenocarcinoma

TERMINOLOGY

Abbreviations
- Polymorphous adenocarcinoma (PAC)

Synonyms
- Formerly known as polymorphous low-grade adenocarcinoma
- Terminal duct carcinoma

Definitions
- Malignant epithelial tumor characterized by infiltrative growth of cytologically uniform cells arranged in architecturally diverse patterns

CLINICAL ISSUES

Epidemiology
- Incidence
  - 2nd most common intraoral minor salivary gland malignant tumor (~ 25%)

Site
- **Almost always** in minor glands (60% palate)

Prognosis
- Overall excellent long-term prognosis

CYTOPATHOLOGY

Cellularity
- Richly cellular with various patterns and bare nuclei in background

Pattern
- Various possibilities, including branching papillae, sheets, and clusters (± duct formation)

Background
- Myxoid/hyaline stromal fragments and metachromatic globules similar to pleomorphic adenoma and adenoid cystic carcinoma

Cells
- Bland uniform cells

Nuclear Details
- Bland, round or oval nuclei with dispersed fine chromatin and absent or inconspicuous nucleoli
- Minimal to no nuclear pleomorphism

Cytoplasmic Details
- Scant to moderate amount of eosinophilic cytoplasm

ANCILLARY TESTS

Immunohistochemistry
- Positive: Low molecular cytokeratin (e.g., cytokeratin 7 and CAM5.2), SOX10, and S100 protein
  - Focal expression of myoepithelial markers (smooth muscle actin, muscle specific actin, and GFAP) can be seen
  - Variable p63 positivity (typically diffuse or random, not biphasic pattern seen in pleomorphic adenoma)
  - *PRKD1* (E710D) mutation in 73-89% of PAC

DIFFERENTIAL DIAGNOSIS

Pleomorphic Adenoma
- Cytomorphological distinction may be very difficult
- Fibrillary chondromyxoid stroma (highlighted with Diff-Quik stain)
- Hyaline myoepithelial cells (plasmacytoid cells)

Adenoid Cystic Carcinoma
- Dark, basaloid cells with hyperchromatic, peg-shaped, carrot-shaped, or angular nuclei
- Prominent metachromatic hyaline globules and cylinders (highlighted with Diff-Quik stain)

SELECTED REFERENCES

1. Jiménez-Heffernan JA et al: Fine needle aspiration cytology of polymorphous adenocarcinoma of the salivary glands: a report of 11 patients and review of the literature. Diagn Cytopathol. 48(11):1013-20, 2020

Cytologic Details on Pap Stain of Polymorphous Adenocarcinoma

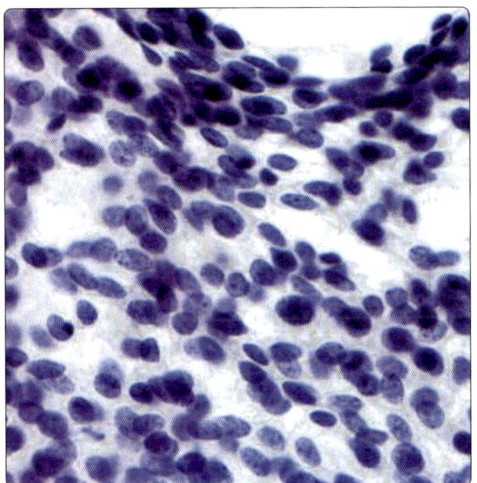

Cell Block of Polymorphous Adenocarcinoma

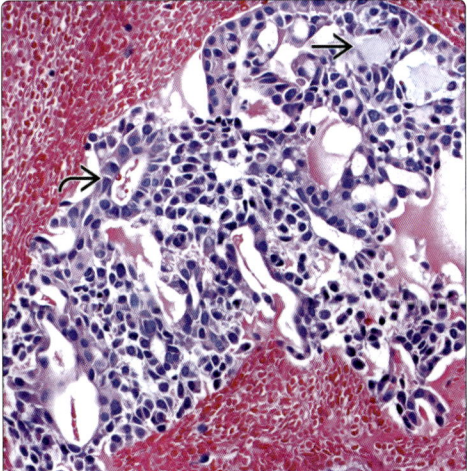

(Left) Pap-stained FNA shows a cellular smear composed of relatively uniform, basaloid tumor cells. Mitoses are not evident. (Courtesy F-M. Deng, MD.) **(Right)** Cell block shows various tubular, acinar ➔, and cribriform patterns. Some mucin/basement membrane-like material ➔ is seen in the cribriform areas, which may be mistaken for adenoid cystic carcinoma

Salivary Duct Carcinoma

KEY FACTS

CLINICAL ISSUES
- Parotid gland most commonly involved
- Poor prognosis overall (5-year survival rate: < 35%)

CYTOPATHOLOGY
- Features of high-grade adenocarcinoma
- Cellular smear with background necrotic debris
- Cohesive 3D clusters and broad flat sheets with cribriform/papillary pattern
- Polygonal or low columnar epithelial cells
- Mitotic figures usually present

ANCILLARY TESTS
- Immunoreactive for androgen receptor, HER2/neu protein, and GCDFP-15
- HER2 gene amplification detected by FISH in 10-30% of cases

TOP DIFFERENTIAL DIAGNOSES
- High-grade mucoepidermoid carcinoma
  - Lacks prominent papillary and cribriform patterns
  - Goblet, epidermoid, and intermediate cells
  - Salivary duct carcinoma (SDC) cells with large cytoplasmic vacuoles may simulate mucocytes of mucoepidermoid carcinoma
- Oncocytic carcinoma
  - Lacks papillary and cribriform patterns, no necrosis in background
  - Cytoplasmic granularity is more prominent
- Other types of salivary carcinomas with high-grade transformation
  - Search for cells from better differentiated areas
- Squamous cell carcinomas metastatic to parotid area
  - Obvious keratinization is not a feature of SDC
  - Clinical history is crucial

Large Papillary Forms
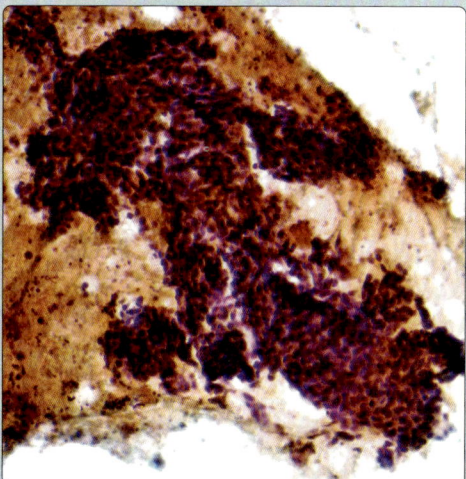

Cribriform-Like Pattern
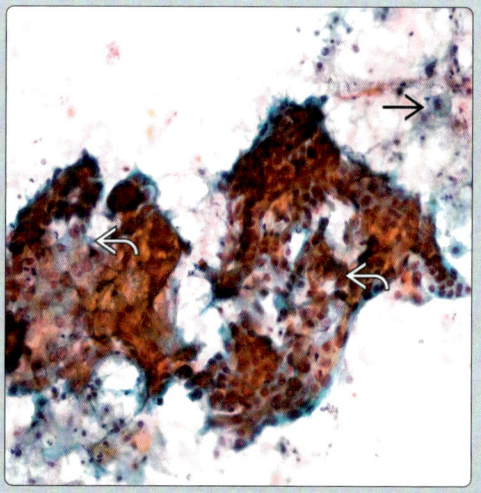

(Left) Pap-stained FNA of salivary duct carcinoma shows a hypercellular smear characterized by multiple 3D cellular sheets and papillary structures of tumor cells in a hemorrhagic and necrotic background. (Right) Pap-stained FNA shows cellular sheets of polygonal to low columnar tumor cells with a cribriform-like pattern ➔. Necrotic debris with foamy macrophages ➔ is noted in the background.

High-Grade Nuclei and Mitosis (Diff-Quik)
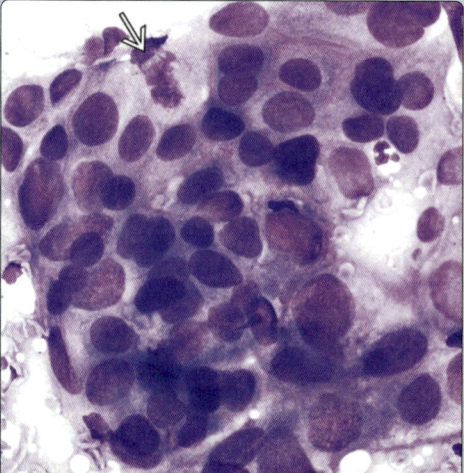

High-Grade Nuclear Features (Pap)
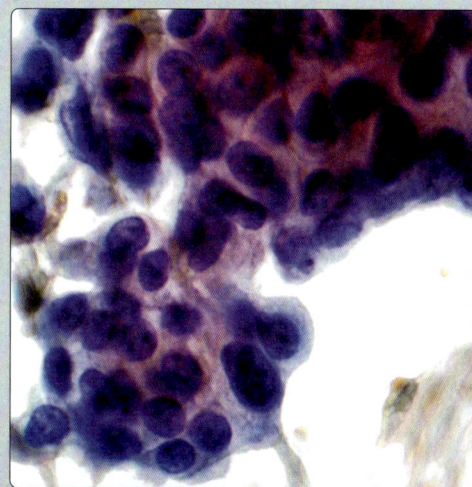

(Left) Diff-Quik-stained FNA smear shows a cohesive cluster of pleomorphic polygonal tumor cells with relatively abundant, well-defined cytoplasm, high-grade nuclei, and mitosis ➔. (Right) Pap-stained FNA smear shows a sheet of tumor cells with finely vacuolated cytoplasm and overlapping nuclei with vesicular chromatin. Some nuclei have irregular contour.

Salivary Duct Carcinoma

TERMINOLOGY

Abbreviations
- Salivary duct carcinoma (SDC)

Definitions
- High-grade adenocarcinoma resembling high-grade breast ductal carcinoma and thought to be derived from intralobular and interlobular excretory ducts
  - Important to recognize as specific category/entity with clinical implications

CLINICAL ISSUES

Epidemiology
- Incidence
  - Uncommon salivary gland malignancy
    - De novo &/or part of carcinoma ex pleomorphic adenoma (50%)
  - Up to 9% of malignant salivary gland neoplasms
- Sex
  - M:F = 2-4:1

Site
- Parotid gland is most commonly involved
  - ~ 70-95% of cases
- Submandibular gland, minor salivary glands (palate specifically), and (rarely) sublingual gland
- Maxillary sinus and larynx (very uncommon)

Prognosis
- Poor prognosis overall (5-year survival rate < 35%)
  - One of most aggressive salivary gland malignancies

CYTOPATHOLOGY

Cellularity
- Richly cellular

Pattern
- Features of high-grade adenocarcinoma
- Cohesive 3D clusters and broad flat sheets with cribriform/papillary architecture
- Isolated, individual atypical epithelial cells scattered at periphery of clusters

Background
- Necrotic debris common, often abundant

Cells
- Medium to large, polygonal or low columnar epithelial cells
- Mitotic figures are usually present

Nuclear Details
- Round to oval, hyperchromatic nuclei
- Prominent nucleoli can be seen
- Intranuclear inclusions may be observed

Cytoplasmic Details
- Finely granular or vacuolated cytoplasm
- Oncocytic feature can be noted

Cell Block Findings
- Androgen receptor, HER2/neu, and GCDFP-15 immunostains on cell block section can confirm diagnosis

DIFFERENTIAL DIAGNOSIS

Other Types of Salivary Carcinomas With High-Grade Transformation
- Search for cells from better-differentiated areas

Squamous Cell Carcinomas, Metastatic to Parotid Area
- Positive for p63/p40, but negative for AR
- Clinical history is crucial

SELECTED REFERENCES

1. Goswami A et al: Oncocytic features in salivary duct carcinoma, a potential pitfall for misdiagnosis as Warthin tumor in fine needle aspiration specimens: a cytomorphologic analysis of 14 cases. Diagn Cytopathol. 48(7):604-9, 2020
2. Nakaguro M et al: Salivary duct carcinoma: updates in histology, cytology, molecular biology, and treatment. Cancer Cytopathol. 128(10):693-703, 2020

Cell Block Section (H&E Stain)

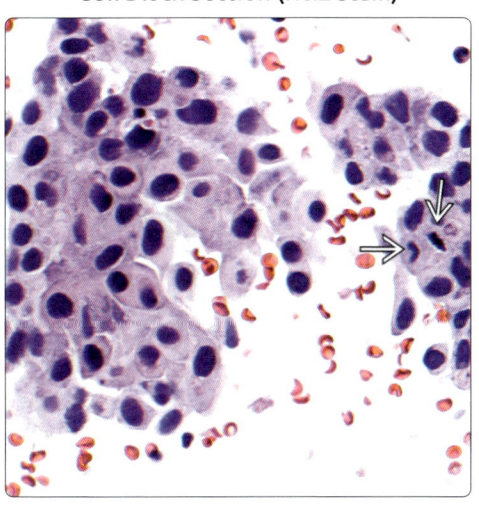

Liquid-Based Cytology

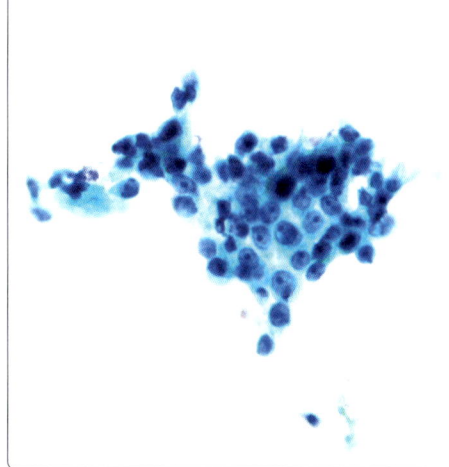

(Left) H&E-stained cell block section of salivary duct carcinoma shows loosely cohesive clusters of cancer cells with hyperchromatic nuclei, well-defined cytoplasm, and mitotic figures ➡. *(Right)* Pap-stained FNA (liquid-based preparation) shows cancer cells with prominent nucleoli, vesicular chromatin, and thick nuclear membranes.

Secretory Carcinoma

KEY FACTS

TERMINOLOGY
- Previously known as mammary analogue secretory carcinoma and zymogen-poor acinic cell carcinoma

CLINICAL ISSUES
- Usually slow-growing, painless mass
  - Uncommon high-grade variants may present with faster growth and nerve injury
- Most (70%) are in parotid
  - Can also arise in other major and minor salivary glands and in thyroid

CYTOPATHOLOGY
- Diverse architecture
  - Papillary configurations with transgressing vessels
  - Acinar-like cell clusters
  - Sheets of cells
- Cystic tumors may have abundant secretory material
- Histiocyte-like cells are characteristic
- Abundant cytoplasm with vacuoles, mostly small, but may be large with signet-ring appearance
- Nuclei are typically uniform and bland

MOLECULAR
- *ETV6* translocations are characteristic, usually detected by FISH break-apart probes
- t(12;15)(p13;q25) *ETV6-NTRK3* translocation is typical
  - Specific to secretory carcinoma (in salivary gland)
- *ETV6* can also rarely have other translocation partners

ANCILLARY TESTS
- Mammaglobin and S100 positive
- Pan-TRK immunostain is more specific
- Mucin vacuoles stain with mucicarmine, Alcian blue, and PAS without diastase

TOP DIFFERENTIAL DIAGNOSES
- Acinic cell carcinoma
- Low-grade intraductal carcinoma

Secretory Carcinoma With High Cellularity
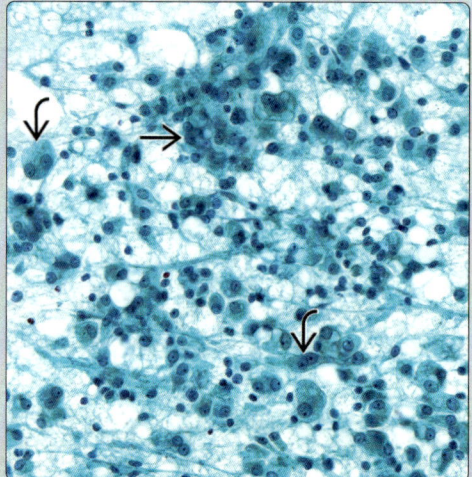

Small and Large Cytoplasmic Vacuoles
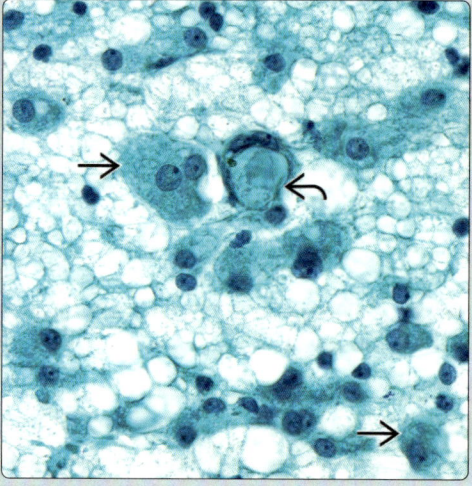

(Left) Pap-stained smear contains numerous tumor cells with focal cohesive sheets ⇨ but predominantly dispersed individual cells. Note the occasional binucleated cells ⇨ present in this example. *(Courtesy S. Ali, MD.)* **(Right)** Higher-power smear shows that many of the cells have obvious cytoplasmic vacuoles visible by Pap stain. Most cells have multiple small vacuoles ⇨, but occasional cells have a single large vacuole ⇨ creating a configuration similar to a signet-ring with nuclear displacement. *(Courtesy S. Ali, MD.)*

Uniform Cell Population
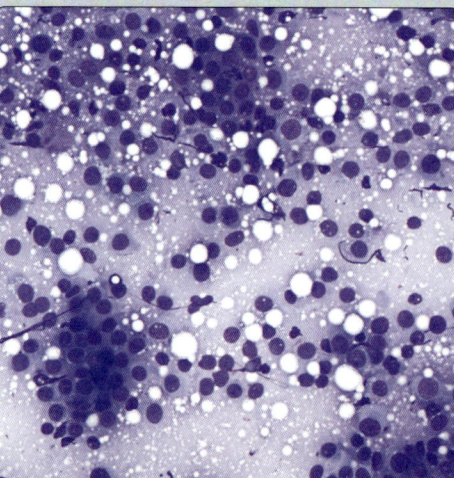

Histiocyte-Like Appearance of Tumor Cells
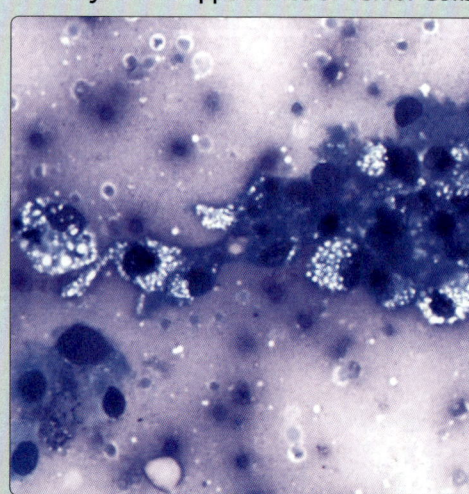

(Left) Diff-Quik-stained smear demonstrates a fairly uniform population of cells with round nuclei that have smooth contours. Abundant secretory material is seen in the background. *(Courtesy S. Krishnamurthy, MD.)* **(Right)** This cluster of mammary analogue secretory carcinoma cells stained with Diff-Quik shows numerous small clear vacuoles present in many of the cells. These cells could easily be mistaken for histiocytes in a specimen with low cellularity. *(Courtesy S. Kane, MD.)*

Secretory Carcinoma

TERMINOLOGY

Synonyms
- Mammary analogue secretory carcinoma

Definitions
- Salivary gland tumor characterized by *ETV6* translocations, identical to secretory carcinoma of breast

CLINICAL ISSUES

Presentation
- Slow-growing, painless mass
  - Uncommon high-grade variants may present with faster growth and nerve injury
- Most (70%) are in parotid
  - Can also arise in other major and minor salivary glands and in thyroid

CYTOPATHOLOGY

Cellularity
- Moderate to high cellularity

Pattern
- Papillary configurations with transgressing vessels
- Acinar-like cell clusters
- Sheets of cells

Background
- Cystic tumors may have abundant secretory material

Cells
- Bland, histiocyte-like cells are characteristic

Nuclear Details
- Typically uniform and bland with prominent nucleoli

Cytoplasmic Details
- Abundant cytoplasm containing vacuoles, mostly small, but maybe be large with signet-ring appearance
- Diff-Quik may highlight metachromatic hyaline globules &/or granules in some cases

MICROSCOPIC

Histologic Features
- Solid, microcystic, tubular, papillocystic, and cribriform patterns can be seen in varying proportions
- Cystic areas often contain colloid-like or frothy secretions

ANCILLARY TESTS

Histochemistry
- Secretory material is stained by mucicarmine, Alcian blue, and PAS without diastase

Immunohistochemistry
- Mammaglobin and S100 positive
- Pan-TRK is new marker more specific for secretory carcinoma

In Situ Hybridization
- *ETV6* translocations are usually detected with FISH break-apart probes
- t(12,15)(p13;q25) *ETV6::NTRK3* is characteristic

DIFFERENTIAL DIAGNOSIS

Acinic Cell Carcinoma
- Usually more cytologic diversity than secretory carcinoma
- Distinct zymogen granules are PAS(+)
- DOG1 (+); Pan-TRK, mammaglobin, and S100 (-)

Low-Grade Intraductal Carcinoma
- Cytoplasm is not vacuolated, may contain yellow lipofuscin-like pigment
- Overlapping immunohistochemistry: Both mammaglobin and S100 (+)

SELECTED REFERENCES
1. Egusa Y et al: Cytopathological findings of secretory carcinoma of the salivary gland and the diagnostic utility of Giemsa staining. Diagnostics (Basel). 11(12):2284, 2021
2. Bell D et al: Pan-Trk immunohistochemistry reliably identifies ETV6-NTRK3 fusion in secretory carcinoma of the salivary gland. Virchows Arch. 476(2):295-305, 2020

Prominent Nucleoli

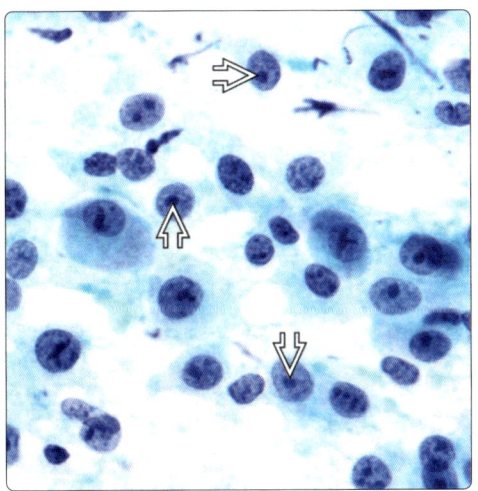

Transgressing Vessels

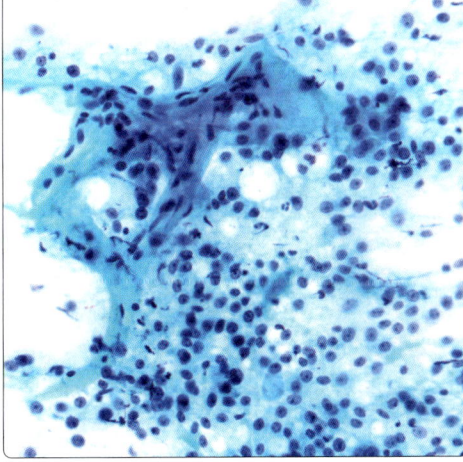

(Left) On Pap stain, prominent nucleoli ➡ can readily be seen in the malignant cells. The nuclear features are otherwise bland, however, with minimal nuclear membrane irregularity and pale chromatin. (Courtesy S. Krishnamurthy, MD.) (Right) Pap-stained cluster of cells is poorly cohesive but surrounds a cluster of vessels, likely corresponding to a papillary structure that has lost its integrity during the smearing process. (Courtesy S. Krishnamurthy, MD.)

Myoepithelial Carcinoma

KEY FACTS

TERMINOLOGY
- Malignant myoepithelial tumor (infiltrative or metastatic)

CLINICAL ISSUES
- Uncommon tumor of major or minor salivary glands
- Often underdiagnosed as pleomorphic adenoma

CYTOPATHOLOGY
- Crowded sheets and clusters, cord-like patterns, nests with cribriforming, and papillary-like clusters; no ductal cells
    - Dissociated cells are always seen in background
- Though cells are of same lineage, can have varied morphology in same smear
    - Epithelioid: Polygonal cells with central nuclei and moderate cytoplasm; most common morphology
    - Plasmacytoid: Round to oval cells with round hyperchromatic eccentric nuclei and moderate dense cytoplasm; binucleate cells can be seen
    - Basaloid, clear cell, and spindle cell morphology also seen
- Rounded nuclei with coarse chromatin; intranuclear cytoplasmic pseudoinclusions and nucleoli may be seen
- Stroma is variable and can be either myxoid or hyaline
    - Dense metachromatic stroma on Diff-Quik stain
- Necrosis and mitosis favor malignancy; in absence, tumors can be labeled as "myoepithelial neoplasm"

ANCILLARY TESTS
- Positive for AE1/AE3, CK7, p63, SMA, calponin, S100
- t(19;22)(q13; q12) translocation; *EWSR1::ZNF444* gene

TOP DIFFERENTIAL DIAGNOSES
- Myoepithelioma; no necrosis or mitosis, often not distinguishable by cytomorphology
- Myoepithelial-rich pleomorphic adenoma; ductal component, more fibrillary and chondroid stroma
- Adenoid cystic carcinoma; basaloid cells, matrix globules
- Plasmacytoma; true plasma cells with spoke-wheel or clockface nuclei and perinuclear hof, minimal stroma

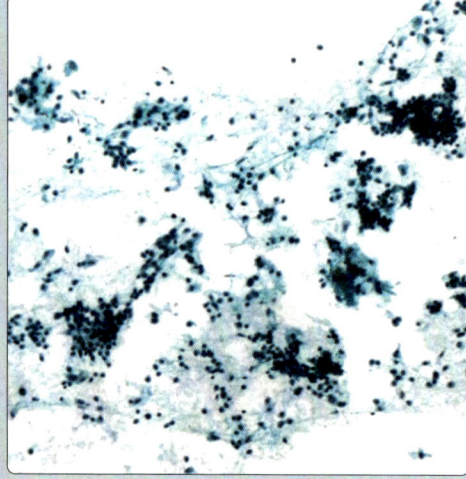

Irregular Clusters and Dissociated Cells in Background

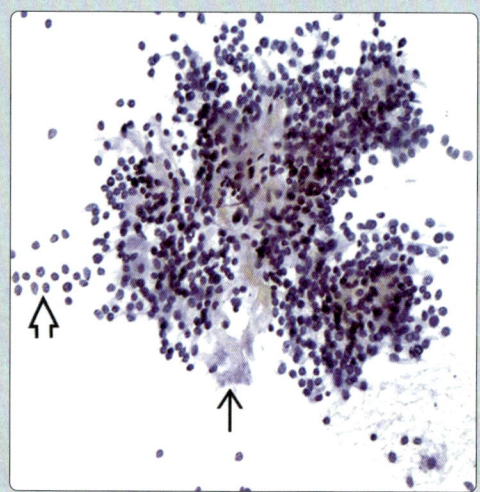

Large Cluster With Uniform Cells and Dense Stroma

(Left) Pap-stained smear at low power demonstrates the presence of many irregular clusters as well as numerous individual myoepithelial cells in the background. *(Right)* This large, irregular cluster of tumor cells has uniform nuclei. There is associated dense stroma ➡ easily appreciated even on Pap stain. Scattered individual cells are seen in the background ➡.

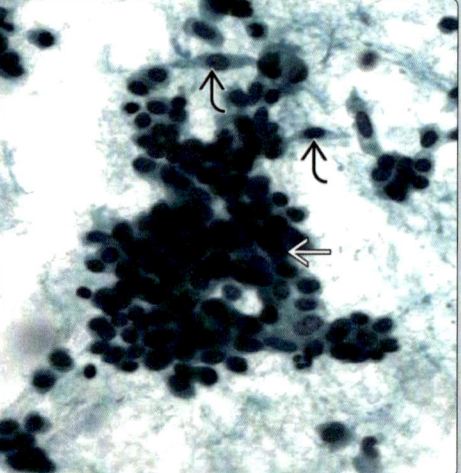

Epithelioid and Spindled Morphology

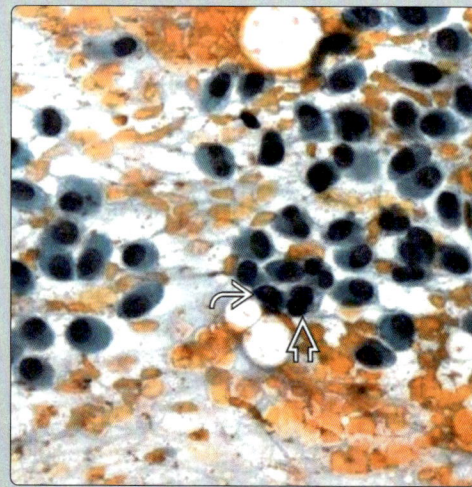

Plasmacytoid Morphology

(Left) Pap-stained cluster of cells shows predominantly epithelioid morphology with moderate cytoplasm and overlapping nuclei ➡, though occasional spindled cells ➡ are also seen. *(Right)* Pap-stained example of plasmacytoid myoepithelial cells demonstrates dyscohesion and eccentric nuclei with coarse chromatin. Note the presence of a binucleated cell ➡ and an intranuclear pseudoinclusion ➡.

Cribriform Adenocarcinoma

KEY FACTS

TERMINOLOGY
- Known as cribriform adenocarcinoma of minor salivary gland (CAMSG) or tongue (CAT)
- May be subtype of polymorphous adenocarcinoma but has different clinicopathologic features

CLINICAL ISSUES
- Very rare with no sex predilection
- Arises in minor salivary gland sites, primarily base of tongue
- Indolent despite nodal metastasis at presentation in 3/4

CYTOPATHOLOGY
- Sheets and clusters of cells with irregular outline; focal papillary patterns may be seen
  - Cribriform pattern in sheets is characteristic
- Very few dissociated cells imparting clean background
- Nuclei resemble papillary carcinoma of thyroid
  - Overlapping, ground-glass appearance with grooves and pseudoinclusions
- Cytoplasm is pale eosinophilic with focal vacuolization
- Metachromatic stroma is variable, reminiscent of colloid, seen in background or within spaces

ANCILLARY TESTS
- Positive immunohistochemistry: S100, vimentin, CK7
- Variable expression of myoepithelial markers: p63(+/-) and calponin (+/-)
- Negative: C-Kit, thyroglobulin, TTF-1
- Rearrangement of PRKD genes

TOP DIFFERENTIAL DIAGNOSES
- Papillary thyroid carcinoma metastatic to lymph nodes
  - Primary tumor in thyroid seen by ultrasound
  - Thyroglobulin and TTF-1 (+)
- Polymorphous adenocarcinoma
  - Nuclei not as reminiscent of papillary thyroid carcinoma
  - Nodal involvement at presentation is rare
  - Palate is most common site with female predilection

Irregular Branching Sheets
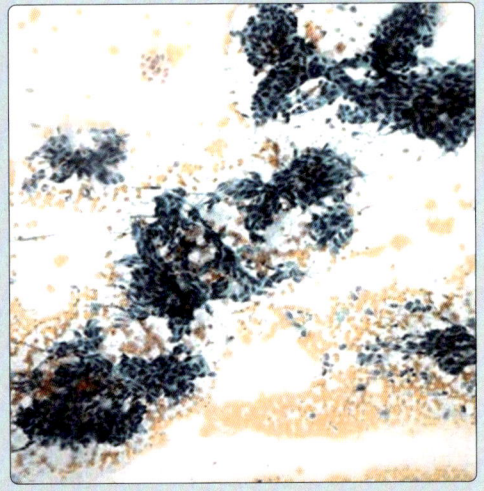

Monomorphic Tumor Cells
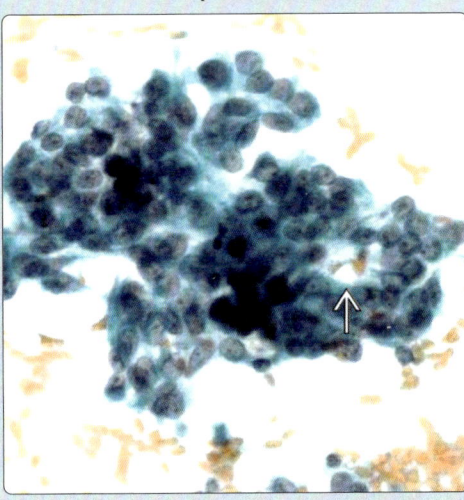

(Left) Low-power view of this Pap-stained FNA shows several large clusters of tumor cells forming sheets of cells with irregular branching projections. *(Right)* On higher power of the same Pap-stained sample, the uniformity of the tumor cells is apparent. A cribriform structure ➔ can be seen within the sheet of cells. Very few dissociated cells are seen in the background.

Nuclear Grooves and Pseudoinclusions
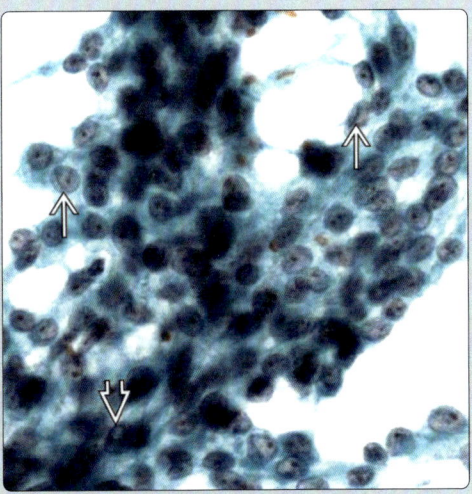

Metachromatic Stroma
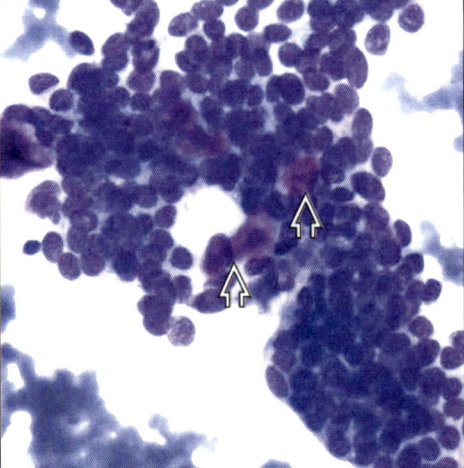

(Left) This sheet of Pap-stained tumor cells demonstrates the resemblance of the nuclei to papillary thyroid carcinoma, including grooves ➔ and pseudoinclusions ➔. Lymph node metastases may therefore be mistaken for the much more common thyroid carcinoma. *(Right)* Diff-Quik stain highlights scanty metachromatic stroma ➔ in this example, though this feature is not always evident. The stroma can be mistaken for colloid in samples from cervical lymph nodes, leading to misdiagnosis.

Metastatic Carcinoma

KEY FACTS

CLINICAL ISSUES

- Metastasis to major salivary gland "regions" is not rare
  - 2-16% of all salivary gland tumors are metastatic tumors
- Older age, M > F
- Most common "recipient" is parotid
- Most common "donors" are squamous cell carcinoma and melanoma in ipsilateral head and neck region
- For staging purposes/therapeutic management, differential diagnosis between primary and metastasis is important
- Metastases from infraclavicular sites account for only 20%
  - Lung, kidney, breast, liver (hepatocellular carcinoma), or gastrointestinal or genitourinary sites
  - Significant numbers of cases of metastatic renal cell carcinoma have been reported
  - Can be initial presenting sign of primary renal tumor
- Sublingual gland metastasis is unusual

CYTOPATHOLOGY

- Usually high-grade cytomorphological features with mitoses

ANCILLARY TESTS

- Immunocytochemistry on cell block sections for identification of primary site

TOP DIFFERENTIAL DIAGNOSES

- Primary high-grade mucoepidermoid carcinoma
  - Consider mutation testing for mucoepidermoid carcinoma
- Acinic cell carcinoma vs. metastatic renal cell carcinoma
  - Renal cell carcinoma is PAX8 and RCC (+)
- Primary oncocytoma vs. hepatocellular carcinoma
  - Hepatocellular carcinoma is Hep-Par1(+)
- Primary salivary gland adenocarcinomas vs. metastasis from other sites

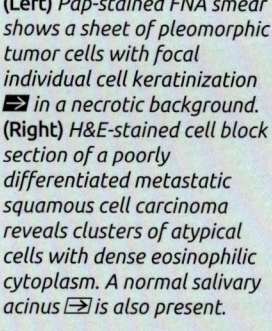

(Left) Pap-stained FNA smear shows a sheet of pleomorphic tumor cells with focal individual cell keratinization ➡ in a necrotic background. (Right) H&E-stained cell block section of a poorly differentiated metastatic squamous cell carcinoma reveals clusters of atypical cells with dense eosinophilic cytoplasm. A normal salivary acinus ➡ is also present.

Metastatic Squamous Cell Carcinoma, Moderately Differentiated

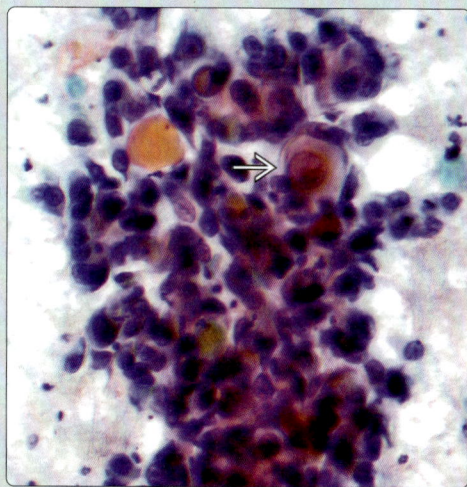

Cell Block of Squamous Cell Carcinoma

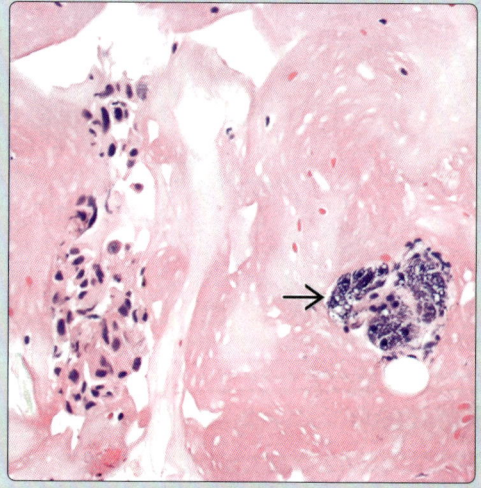

(Left) Pap-stained smear from a parotid aspirate in a patient with known melanoma of the scalp show dyscohesive and pleomorphic malignant cells with large nucleoli ➡. (Right) Pap-stained FNA of metastatic Merkel cell carcinoma (from a primary tumor of the face) to the parotid reveals loosely cohesive tumor cells with oval- to spindle-shaped nuclei and salt and pepper chromatin. Note necrosis in the background ➡.

Metastatic Melanoma

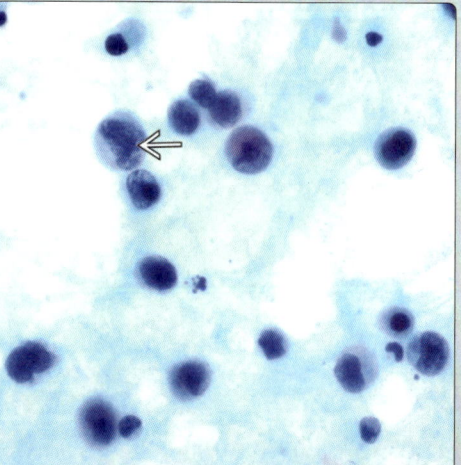

Metastatic Merkel Cell Carcinoma

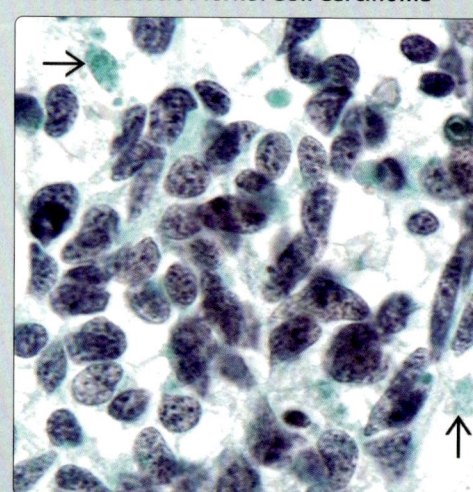

Metastatic Carcinoma

CLINICAL ISSUES

Epidemiology
- Metastasis to major salivary gland "regions" is not rare
- Mucosal or cutaneous malignancies (squamous cell carcinoma and melanoma) in ipsilateral head and neck areas are most common "donors"
- Metastases from infraclavicular sites (only 20%)
  - Lung, kidney, breast, liver (hepatocellular carcinoma), or gastrointestinal or genitourinary sites
  - Significant numbers of metastatic renal cell carcinoma cases have been reported
    - Can be initial presenting sign of primary renal tumor
- Of all major salivary glands, parotid gland is most common "recipient"
- Sublingual gland metastasis is unusual

Site
- Parotid gland metastasis
  - Usually metastasis to intraglandular lymph nodes
    - Multiple intraglandular lymph nodes are usually present in parotid
  - Sometimes difficult to differentiate metastasis to upper cervical lymph nodes from metastasis to lower pole of parotid
- Submandibular gland metastasis
  - Clinically indistinguishable from metastasis to retroglandular lymph nodes
    - No intraglandular lymph nodes are present in submandibular gland in contrast to parotid
  - Metastasis from site distant to head and neck is more frequent in submandibular gland than in parotid

Diagnostic Method
- FNA is extremely sensitive, rapid, and simple method to detect malignant cells

CYTOPATHOLOGY

Cellularity
- Usually high

Pattern
- Cohesive sheets and nests of tumor cells with scattered single cells

Background
- Necrosis can be seen

Cells
- Usually high-grade cytological features with mitoses

Cytoplasmic Details
- Keratinizing squamous tumor cells are highlighted with Pap stain
- Intracytoplasmic mucin is usually not seen

Cell Block Findings
- To identify site of origin, immunocytochemistry on cell block sections is very useful

MICROSCOPIC

Histologic Features
- Metastasis to parotid intraglandular lymph node: Residual lymph node structure may be seen in resected specimens
- Sharp border may be seen between retroglandular lymph node metastasis and submandibular gland in resected specimens

ANCILLARY TESTS

Immunohistochemistry
- Cell block section is useful for immunohistochemistry to identify primary site

DIFFERENTIAL DIAGNOSIS

Metastatic Squamous Cell Carcinoma
- Primary high-grade mucoepidermoid carcinoma (MEC)
  - Presence of mucin-containing cells and intermediate cells
  - Prominent keratinization is usually not seen
  - Mucinous background (although not common in high-grade MEC)
- Primary squamous cell carcinoma (rare)
  - Cytomorphologically indistinguishable
  - Clinicoradiologic correlation is crucial
- Warthin tumor with extensive squamous differentiation
  - Dirty background (from cyst content) mimics necrotic debris seen in squamous cell carcinoma
  - Single atypical squamous cells may be abundant, but atypia is not sufficient enough for malignancy
  - Clusters of oncocytic cells
  - Usually soft in consistency
- Infarcted pleomorphic adenoma with squamous differentiation
  - Ductal, myoepithelial, and fibromyxoid stromal components are present
    - Diff-Quik stain is helpful to highlight magenta myxofibrillary stroma
  - Atypia of reactive squamous cells is not sufficient for malignancy

Metastatic Renal Cell Carcinoma
- Primary salivary tumors with clear cell features (e.g., MEC, acinic cell carcinoma)
- Immunocytochemistry on cell block sections is very helpful (PAX8, RCC marker, CD10)

DIAGNOSTIC CHECKLIST

Clinically Relevant Pathologic Features
- Checking clinical history of malignancy is crucial

SELECTED REFERENCES
1. Lajara S et al: Metastatic malignant melanoma mimicking a salivary gland basaloid neoplasm after treatment with nivolumab. Diagn Cytopathol. 49(9):E370-3, 2021
2. Thomas S et al: Cytodiagnosis of unusual metastases in parotid gland. J Oral Maxillofac Pathol. 25(1):171-6, 2021

Primary and Metastatic Nonepithelial Tumors

KEY FACTS

CLINICAL ISSUES
- Metastatic malignant melanoma is 2nd most common metastatic salivary gland tumor, most often originating from head and neck region
- Extranodal marginal zone B-cell lymphoma (EMZBCL) of mucosa-associated lymphoid tissue is most common type of lymphoma of salivary gland origin
- Primary mesenchymal tumors: Benign > > malignant
  - Vascular tumors, neurogenic tumors, lipoma, and nodular fasciitis are most common

CYTOPATHOLOGY
- **Hemangioma**: Cohesive groups of elongated bland spindle cells in bloody background
  - Cell block section shows small open spaces (reminiscent of capillary spaces) lined by uniform plump to flattened cells in some areas
  - Immunohistochemical staining for endothelial markers (e.g., CD34, CD31) is helpful for diagnostic confirmation
- **EMZBCL**: Polymorphous lymphoid population
  - Flow cytometry is helpful for identifying immunoglobulin light chain restriction
  - Neoplastic B cells are negative for CD5, CD10, CD23, and cyclin-D1
- **Schwannoma**: Spindle tumor cells with wavy nuclei
  - No mitotic activity, random nuclear pleomorphism, positive for S100
- **Lipoma**: All types can occur in salivary glands
  - Spindle cell and pleomorphic lipomas can be cellular and result in misdiagnosis
  - Immunohistochemical staining for endothelial markers (e.g., CD34, CD31) is helpful for diagnostic confirmation
- **Nodular fasciitis**: Similar to that seen in head and neck, usually young individuals
  - Spindle and stellate cells with myxoid background and scattered lymphocytes and macrophages
  - Cellularity depends on age of lesion (recent more cellular)

Lipoma
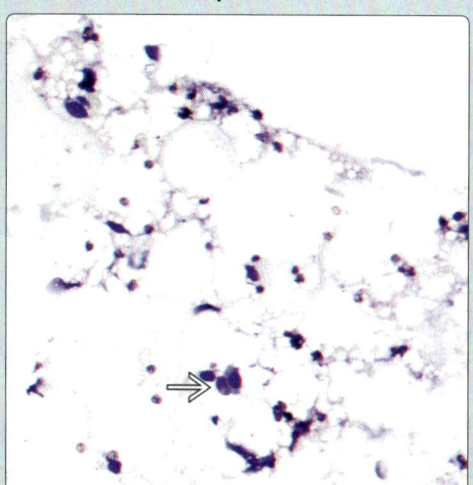

Schwannoma
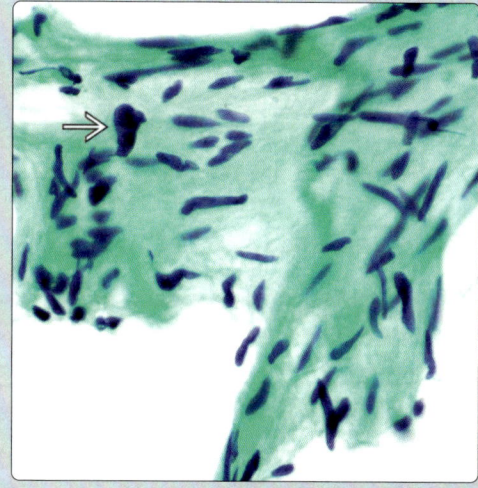

(Left) Diff-Quik-stained smear shows mature adipocytes, some with multivesicular cytoplasm. Few salivary ductal cells ➡ are also identified. (Right) Pap-stained FNA smear of a parotid schwannoma shows spindle tumor cells with wavy nuclei and random nuclear pleomorphism ➡.

Angiosarcoma With Acinar-Like Configuration
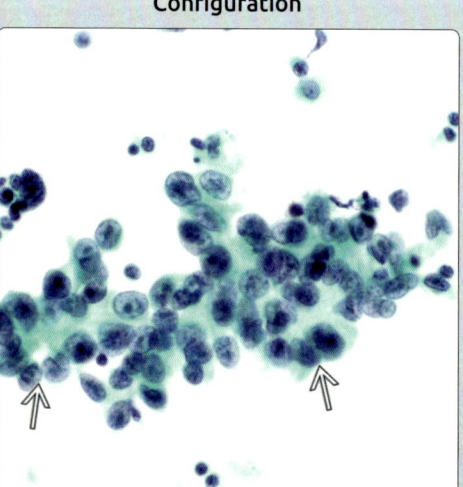

Desmoid-type Fibromatosis of Parotid
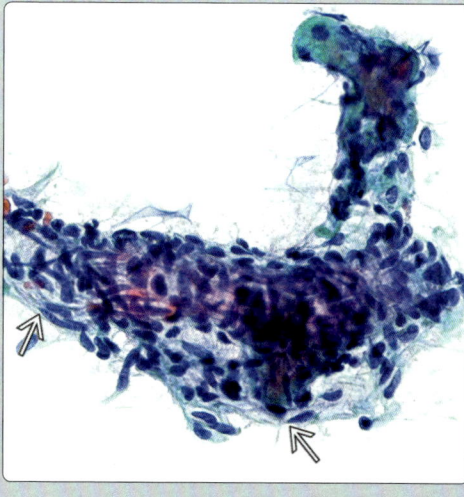

(Left) Pap-stained smear of a cutaneous angiosarcoma that infiltrated into the parotid, forming a mass, is shown. The cells form acinar/glandular-like structures ➡ that can easily be misinterpreted as an epithelial neoplasm. (Right) Pap-stained FNA smear of desmoid-type fibromatosis involving the parotid shows a cellular aggregate of spindled tumor cells with pointed nuclei ➡. No mitosis is seen.

Primary and Metastatic Nonepithelial Tumors

CLINICAL ISSUES

Epidemiology
- Metastatic melanoma
  - 2nd most common metastatic tumor to salivary gland
  - Most parotid metastases are from melanomas in head and neck region
- Lymphomas
  - Mostly non-Hodgkin B-cell lymphomas
- Mesenchymal tumors
  - Benign > > malignant
    - Benign: Vascular (hemangioma, lymphangioma) > neurogenic tumors (neurofibroma, schwannoma); others (lipoma, nodular fasciitis, giant cell tumor, solitary fibrous tumor)
    - Malignant: Hemangiopericytoma, malignant peripheral nerve sheath tumor, fibrosarcoma, rhabdomyosarcoma, angiosarcoma, undifferentiated pleomorphic sarcoma
  - Parotid > > submandibular gland

CYTOPATHOLOGY

Metastatic Melanoma
- Metastasis retains to some extent cytological characteristics of respective primary tumor

Extranodal Marginal Zone B-Cell Lymphoma
- Polymorphous lymphoid proliferation, including
  - Predominant population of intermediate-sized lymphoid cells with centrocyte-like or monocytoid features
  - Transformed lymphocytes
  - Variable numbers of plasma cells
- Often difficult to differentiate from reactive lymphoid process
- Neoplastic B cells are negative for CD5, CD10, CD23, and cyclin-D1
- Lymphoepithelial lesions may be present
- Flow cytometry is helpful for identifying immunoglobulin light chain restriction

Hemangioma (Juvenile Variant)
- Cohesive groups of elongated bland spindle cells with oval bland nuclei in bloody background
- Cell block section shows small open spaces (reminiscent of capillary spaces) lined by uniform plump to flattened cells in some areas
  - Immunohistochemical staining for endothelial markers (e.g., CD34, CD31) is helpful for diagnostic confirmation

Neurogenic Tumor (Schwannoma, Neurofibroma)
- Spindle tumor cells with wavy nuclei
  - No mitotic activity
- Random nuclear pleomorphism is commonly seen in schwannoma
- Hemosiderin is commonly seen in schwannoma
- Diffuse strong S100 protein immunoreactivity is seen

Lipomas
- All types can occur in salivary glands
- Spindle cell and pleomorphic lipomas can be cellular and result in misdiagnosis

Nodular Fasciitis
- Occurs in head and neck region, usually young individuals
- Cytology varies depending on age of lesion
- Spindle cells in loose myxoid stroma, rare macrophages, lymphocytes

Angiosarcomas
- Cutaneous angiosarcomas in older individuals can infiltrate underlying salivary gland
- Vary from low (usually) to high grade
- Epithelioid or spindle proliferation with malignant features
- Intracytoplasmic lumen with hematopoietic cells helpful
- Cells are CD31(+)

SELECTED REFERENCES
1. Torres JMV et al: Mesenchymal neoplasms of salivary glands: a clinicopathologic study of 68 cases. Head Neck Pathol. 16(2):353-6, 2022
2. Chandra SR et al: Parotid neurogenic tumors: MPNST sarcoma to schwannoma-review of literature and guidelines in management. J Maxillofac Oral Surg. 20(3):356-63, 2021

Metastatic Melanoma

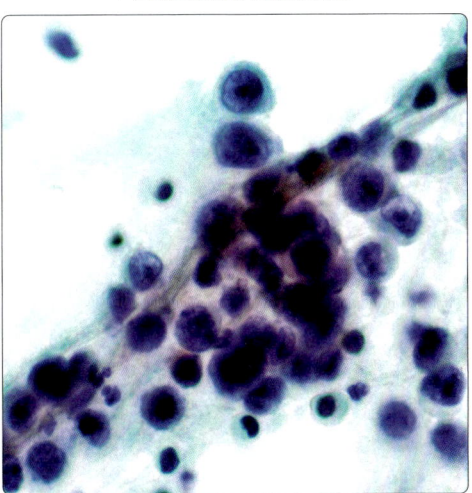

Giant Cell Tumor

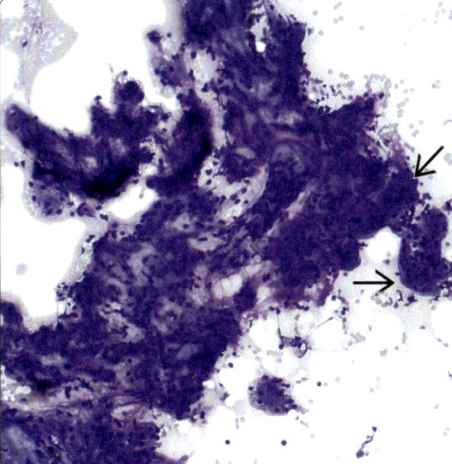

(Left) Pap-stained FNA smear of metastatic melanoma shows loosely cohesive, markedly atypical tumor cells with hyperchromasia and prominent nucleoli. Melanin pigments are not evident in this example. (Right) Giant cell tumor occurring in the parotid area on Diff-Quik stain shows numerous osteoclastic giant cells ➡. This tumor may arise from a temporomandibular joint.

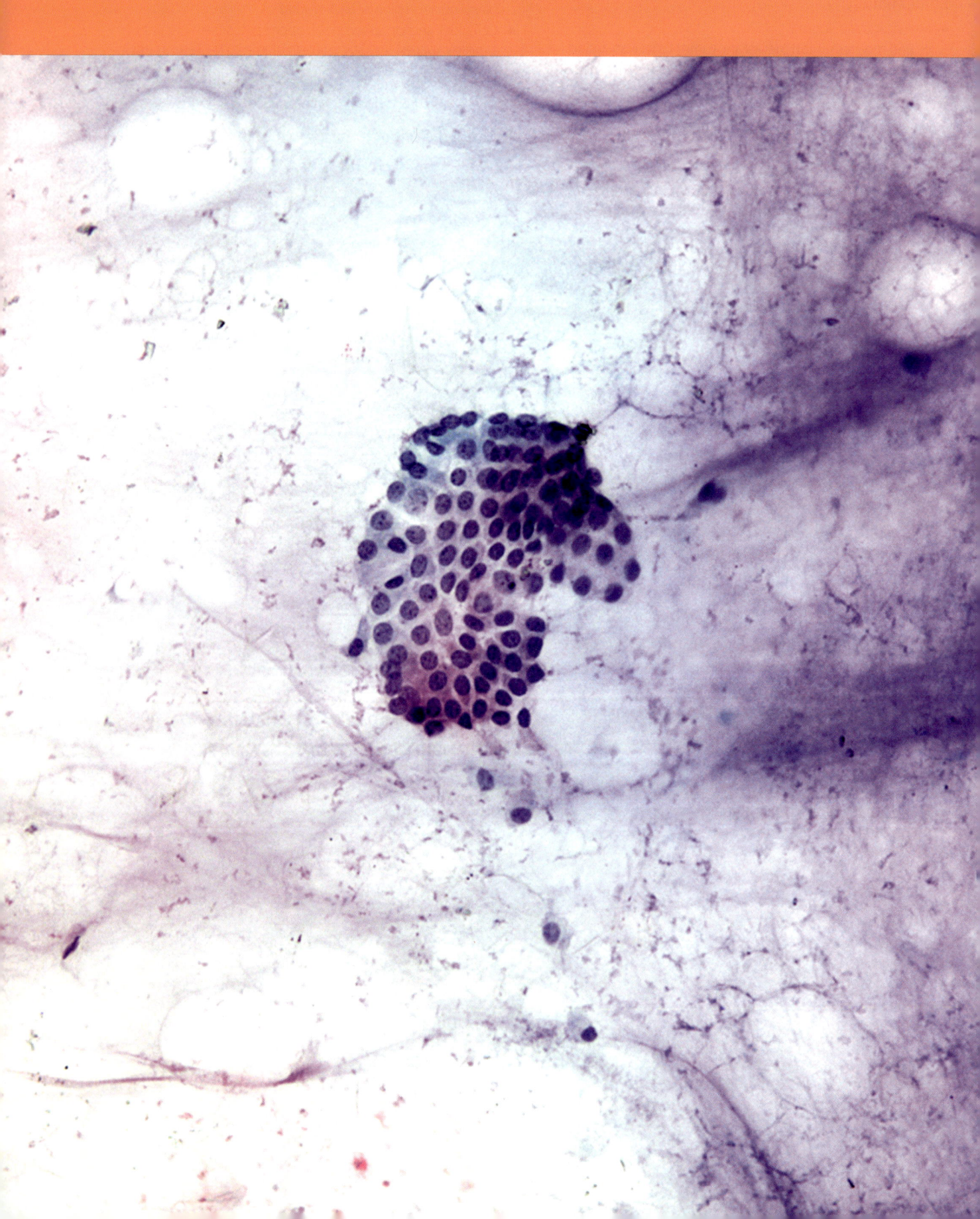

PART III
SECTION 6
Breast

Overview
Role of Fine-Needle Aspiration of Breast, Techniques and Triple Test	418

Benign Breast Lesions
Inflammatory and Granulomatous Conditions	420
Fat Necrosis	422
Nonproliferative and Proliferative Changes in Breast	424
Radial Scar/Complex Sclerosing Lesion	428
Gynecomastia	430
Mucocele-Like Lesion	432

Benign Neoplasms
Fibroadenoma	434
Granular Cell Tumor of Breast	438
Papillary Neoplasms	440
Myofibroblastoma, Mammary	446

Malignant Neoplasms
Ductal Carcinoma and Variants of Invasive Mammary Carcinoma	448
Lobular Carcinoma	456
Phyllodes Tumor	458
Angiosarcoma and Other Sarcomas	460
Lymphomas and Metastatic Tumors	464

Nipple Discharge
Cytology Specimens for Risk Assessment of Breast Cancer	466

Role of Fine-Needle Aspiration of Breast, Techniques and Triple Test

TERMINOLOGY

Definitions

- Fine-needle aspiration biopsy (FNAB)
  - Aspiration of palpable and nonpalpable breast lesions using 23- to 25-gauge needle ± image guidance and ± local anesthesia

BREAST FNAB

Advantages

- Minimally invasive technique
- Tolerated better by patient in comparison with core needle biopsy of breast
- Simple and easy to perform
- Cost effective
- Immediate evaluation of lesion
- Allows operator to maintain tactile sensitivity, which enhances accurate localization of lesion
- Allows investigation of different areas of lesion
- Safer for lesions located close to chest wall
- Safer for investigation of lesions in breast with implants

Disadvantages

- Success depends on skill of operator in procuring diagnostic material from targeted lesion
- Lesions associated with significant fibrosis may not yield diagnostic material
- Lack of tissue architecture may lower specificity of diagnosis
- Interpretation requires skilled cytopathologists
- Availability of immediate assessment is needed for success of technique
- Not very reliable for distinction of carcinoma in situ from invasive carcinoma
- Not recommended for evaluation of prognostic and predictive markers of index lesions of breast carcinoma

Complications

- Minor bleeding/hematoma, minimal local pain, rarely pneumothorax

REPORTING CRITERIA

International Academy of Cytology Yokohama System for Standardized Reporting of Breast FNAB

- 5 categories
  - Category 1: Insufficient/inadequate
    - Risk of malignancy: 2.6-4.8%
    - Management with availability of imaging and CNB: Review clinical and imaging; if imaging is indeterminate or suspicious, repeat FNAB or proceed to CNB; if imaging is benign, consider repeat FNAB
  - Category 2: Benign
    - Risk of malignancy: 1.4-2.3%
    - Management with availability of imaging and CNB: Review clinical and imaging; if triple test benign, no further biopsy; if clinical &/or imaging is suspicious, repeat FNAB or proceed to CNB
  - Category 3: Atypical
    - Risk of malignancy: 1.3-15.7%
    - Management with availability of imaging and CNB: Review clinical and imaging findings; repeat FNAB if atypia due to technical issues; if atypical with good material, repeat FNAB or preferably proceed to CNB
  - Category 4: Suspicious for malignancy
    - Risk of malignancy: 84.6-97.1%
    - Management with availability of imaging and CNB: Review clinical and imaging finding; CNB is mandatory
  - Category 5: Malignant
    - Risk of malignancy: 99.0-100%
    - Management with availability of imaging and CNB: Review clinical and imaging findings; CNB if any discrepant findings; if triple test is concordant malignant, proceed to definitive management
- Recommendations for breast FNAB structured reporting
  - Heading to include 1 of 5 categories
  - Brief cytologic description noting where possible presence or absence of key diagnostic features
  - Conclusion or summary: Specific diagnosis of lesion if possible or provide lost likely differential diagnoses

FNA of Breast Lesion

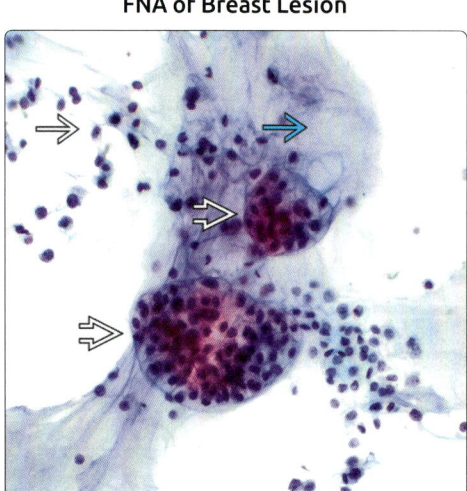

ER on Cell Block

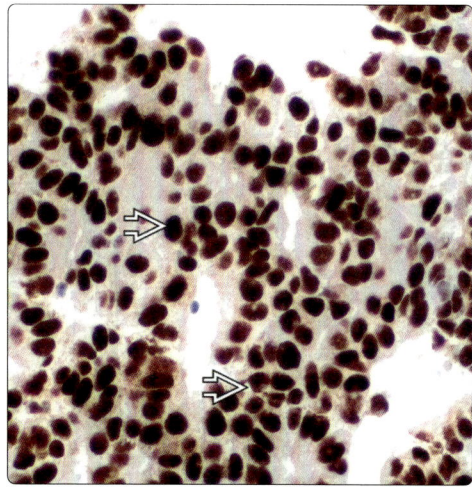

(Left) Pap-stained FNA smear of a satellite breast lesion away from the index tumor shows mucinous carcinoma with loose clusters ⇨ and single tumor cells ⇨ distributed in a background of extracellular mucin ⇨. (Right) Cell block of FNA of metastatic breast carcinoma in an axillary lymph node immunostained for ER shows strong and diffuse positivity ⇨ in the tumor cells.

Role of Fine-Needle Aspiration of Breast, Techniques and Triple Test

- Correlation of cytology, clinical, and imaging findings to indicate concordant or discordant triple test
  o Category number 1, 2, 3, 4, or 5 for insufficient, benign, atypical, suspicious, and malignant to be stated in body of report

Specimen Adequacy Criteria
- Determined based on
  o Size and nature of lesion
  o Accuracy of targeting lesion for sampling
  o Skill of operator performing procedure
- Mandatory to investigate further if not satisfactory
- Recommendations for adequacy of mass lesions that do not decrease in size or drain by FNAB by International Academy of Cytology Yokohama System for Reporting Breast FNAB Cytopathology
  o 7 tissue fragments with 20 or more epithelial cells

INTERPRETATION OF BREAST FNAB

Triple Test
- Interpretation of breast FNAB should always be performed in conjunction with clinical and imaging findings
- Correlation of cytologic findings with clinical and imaging findings is mandatory
- Triple testing of breast lesions includes evaluation of clinical, imaging, and pathologic findings of lesion
- Golden rule of breast FNAB practice is to always follow triple test
- Discordance in findings of breast FNAB with clinical &/or imaging findings should always be investigated further by CNB or surgical excision of lesion

Performance
- Widely variable in different reports
- Sensitivity: 35-95%
- Specificity: 48-100%
- False-positive diagnosis: 1-10%
- False-negative diagnosis: 5-29%

CURRENT APPLICATIONS

1st-Line Investigation of Breast Lesions
- Breast lesions suspected to be nonneoplastic by clinical &/or imaging studies
  o Breast FNAB is very useful for evaluation of lesions, such as abscess, hematoma, fat necrosis, nonproliferative and proliferative breast changes, and cysts
- Breast lesions suspected to be neoplastic
  o Benign: Breast FNAB can be used for initial investigation of lesions suspected to be fibroadenoma or papilloma by imaging studies
  o Malignant: Breast FNAB can be used for initial investigation of lesions that are very highly suspicious for malignancy
    - Diagnosis of malignancy can be made with high level of sensitivity and specificity in such cases
    - However, reliable diagnosis of carcinoma in situ or invasive carcinoma cannot be always made
    - Diagnostic yield of breast FNAB may be low in malignant breast lesions associated with sclerosis/fibrosis that can lead to false-negative diagnosis of malignancy
    - CNB is currently more popular than FNAB for initial investigation of breast lesions that are very suspicious for breast carcinoma
    - FNAB is very useful to collect material for ancillary immunophenotyping by flow cytometry in lesions suspected to be hematopoietic malignancies
- Investigation of satellite lesions around lesions proven to be malignant
  o Breast FNAB is useful for inclusion or exclusion of lesions in area of tissue to be included in breast conservation surgery for breast cancer
  o FNAB of satellite breast lesions to confirm malignancy can be useful for marking area with marker clips
    - Satellite area with marker clip can be monitored for response during course of neoadjuvant chemotherapy
    - Satellite area with marker clip can be appropriately sampled following resection ± neoadjuvant chemotherapy

Investigation of Lesions Suspected to Be Metastasis
- Breast FNAB is very often used for establishing diagnosis of metastatic tumors

Prognostic and Predictive Markers
- Breast FNAB can be used for evaluating currently recommended prognostic and predictive markers, e.g., estrogen receptor (ER), progesterone receptor (PR), and HER2 of recurrent and metastatic breast carcinomas
  o Useful when core needle biopsy is not available or has insufficient diagnostic material to perform testing
- Breast FNAB specimen preparations for evaluation of prognostic and predictive markers
  o Cell blocks: Optimal specimen for testing; fixation of cell blocks for ≥ 6 hours in formalin to be in compliance with American Society of Clinical Oncology (ASCO)/College of American Pathologists (CAP) guidelines for evaluation of prognostic and predictive markers
    - Cell blocks for immunostaining ER, PR, and HER2 should be validated with tissue specimens before routine usage
    - Cell blocks for performing FISH for HER2 should be validated with tissue specimens before routine usage if preparation differs in any way from surgical pathology specimens
  o FNA smears: Pap-stained smears and Diff-Quik-stained smears can be used provided testing is validated with tissue specimens before routine usage
  o Cell-transferred smears and cytospin smears can be used if validated with tissue specimens before routine usage

SELECTED REFERENCES

1. Sarangi S et al: Risk stratification of breast fine-needle aspiration biopsy specimens performed without radiologic guidance by application of the International Academy of Cytology Yokohama System for Reporting Breast Fine-Needle Aspiration Cytopathology. Acta Cytol. 65(6):483-93, 2021
2. Field AS et al: Breast fine needle aspiration biopsy cytology: the potential impact of the International Academy of Cytology Yokohama System for Reporting Breast Fine Needle Aspiration Biopsy Cytopathology and the use of rapid on-site evaluation. J Am Soc Cytopathol. 9(2):103-11, 2020
3. Krishnamurthy S: Relevance and impact of the International Academy of Cytology Yokohama System for standardized reporting of breast fine-needle aspiration biopsy cytology. J Am Soc Cytopathol. 9(2):63-6, 2020

Inflammatory and Granulomatous Conditions

TERMINOLOGY

Definitions
- Lesions of breast characterized by acute, chronic, or granulomatous inflammation

Conditions
- Acute mastitis/breast abscess, subareolar abscess, duct ectasia, lymphocytic mastitis, granulomatous mastitis

ACUTE MASTITIS

Etiology/Pathogenesis
- Usually occurs in lactating women due to abrasion or crack in nipple resulting from nursing
  o Leads to entry of bacteria followed by acute inflammation and eventually abscess formation
  o Nonlactational causes of acute mastitis are rare and often associated with smoking

Clinical Presentation
- Breast swelling, redness, and warmth with fever
  o Lymphadenopathy may also be present

Treatment
- Managed medically or with incision and drainage

Cytopathology
- Aspirate of breast abscesses can be thick, yellowish green, and purulent
- In acute phase, marked acute inflammation ± necrotic cellular debris in background
- In chronic phase, granulation tissue and histiocytic and chronic inflammatory infiltration, including multinucleated foreign body giant cells, can be present
- Few clusters and single ductal and mesenchymal cells ± reactive atypia with enlarged and prominent nucleus and mitotic figures

SUBAREOLAR ABSCESS

Etiology/Pathogenesis
- Squamous metaplasia of lactiferous ducts leads to keratin plugging

Acute Mastitis
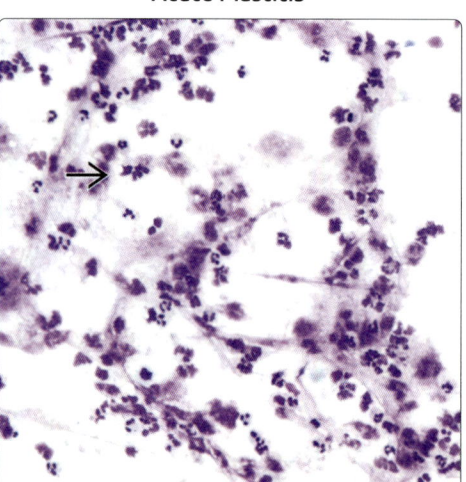

Subareolar Abscess
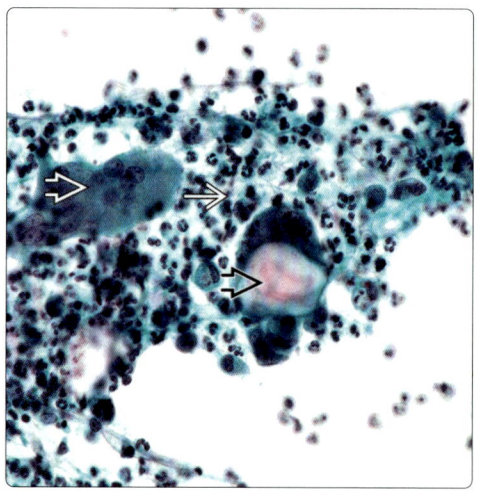

(Left) Diff-Quik-stained FNA smear from a case of acute mastitis shows acute inflammatory cells ➡ and proteinaceous debris in the background. (Right) Pap-stained smear of a subareolar abscess of the breast shows multinucleated giant cells ➡, one of which has keratinous material in the cytoplasm ➡ associated with acute inflammatory cells ➡ in the background.

Granulomatous Mastitis
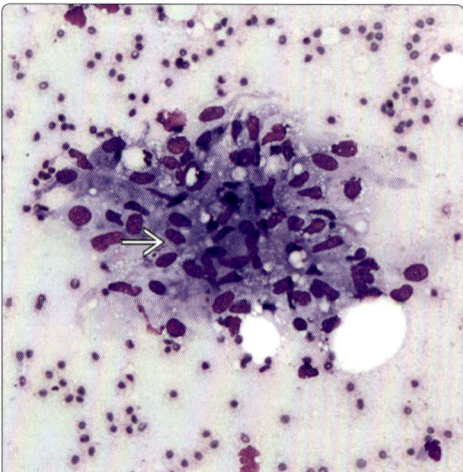

Acute Inflammatory Granulation Tissue
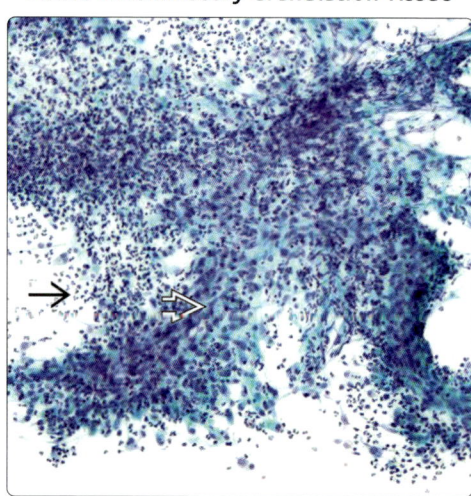

(Left) Diff-Quik-stained FNA smear of a case of idiopathic granulomatous mastitis of the breast shows a nonnecrotizing granuloma composed of epithelioid cells ➡. (Right) Pap-stained FNA smear shows acute inflammatory granulation tissue composed of acute inflammatory cells ➡ that are associated with vascular proliferation ➡.

Inflammatory and Granulomatous Conditions

Clinical Presentation
- Painful erythematous subareolar mass

Treatment
- Can recur with incision and drainage; surgical removal of keratin-producing epithelium may be necessary

Cytopathology
- Thick, yellow aspirate
- Marked acute inflammation associated with many squamous cells, including anucleate or nucleated squamous cells
- Multinucleated giant cells with engulfed keratinous material and squamous cells in cytoplasm are characteristic
- Granulation tissue, chronic inflammation, epithelioid, and foamy histiocytes can be present in longstanding lesions
- Reactive changes in few clusters of ductal and squamous cells with enlarged nucleus and prominent nucleolus can mimic malignant cells

DUCT ECTASIA

Etiology/Pathogenesis
- Age-related weakness of walls of large ducts, resulting in ectasia of ducts

Clinical Presentation
- Palpable, ill-defined subareolar mass that may be attached to skin and nipple; thick nipple discharge

Treatment
- No treatment is necessary if carcinoma is excluded

Cytopathology
- Thick, "cheesy" material showing amorphous granular debris, often with cholesterol clefts and calcifications
- Few clusters of ductal epithelial cells ± reactive changes associated with lymphocytes, plasma cells, lipofuscin-containing histiocytes referred to as ochrocytes, and multinucleated giant cells

LYMPHOCYTIC MASTITIS

Etiology/Pathogenesis
- Can be sporadic or associated with autoimmune diseases, such as type 1 diabetes mellitus, Hashimoto thyroiditis, or rheumatoid arthritis

Clinical Presentation
- Can present as mass

Cytopathology
- Few clusters of benign ductal epithelial cells associated with many lymphocytes

GRANULOMATOUS MASTITIS

Etiology/Pathogenesis
- Granulomatous inflammation
  - Idiopathic granulomatous mastitis occurs only in parous women

Clinical Presentation
- Can present as mass; may or may not be tender

Treatment
- Treatment of pertinent infection
- Idiopathic granulomatous mastitis: Excisional biopsy is curative; if inflammation persists, corticosteroids may be used

Cytopathology
- Granulomas composed of epithelioid histiocytes and multinucleated giant cells ± central necrosis or microabscesses
- Silicone mastitis: Silicone may be dissolved in preparations leaving empty spaces
  - If not dissolved, appears as homogeneous, faintly yellow or blue, refractile nonbirefringent material in smears
  - Abundant histiocytes with vacuoles, multinucleated giant cells often with asteroid bodies may be seen

DIFFERENTIAL DIAGNOSIS

Carcinoma
- Clinical presentation of subareolar mass in subareolar abscess or duct ectasia can mimic malignant lesion
- Abundant clusters and single atypical cells in carcinoma unlike few clusters of ductal cells ± reactive atypia; highly atypical cells are sparse in inflammatory lesions
- Breast cancers are generally not associated with marked acute inflammation

Lymphoma
- Entities, such as duct ectasia or lymphocytic mastitis, are generally associated with mild to moderate infiltration of small lymphocytes, including histiocytes and plasma cells, unlike lymphoma, which shows abundant lymphoid cells proven to be clonal

Inflammatory Breast Carcinoma
- Obstruction of dermal lymphatics by tumor cells causes erythema and edema of breast, which can mimic acute mastitis/breast abscess
- Usually not noted in lactational period, unlike acute mastitis or breast abscess; tissue biopsy and skin punch biopsy may be needed for distinction

SELECTED REFERENCES

1. Mohapatra S et al: Primary tuberculous mastitis. J Glob Infect Dis. 13(4):196-7, 2021
2. Scott DM: Inflammatory diseases of the breast. Best Pract Res Clin Obstet Gynaecol. ePub, 2021
3. Barreto DS et al: Granulomatous mastitis: etiology, imaging, pathology, treatment, and clinical findings. Breast Cancer Res Treat. 171(3):527-34, 2018
4. Ail DA et al: Clinical and cytological spectrum of granulomatous mastitis and utility of FNAC in picking up tubercular mastitis: an eight-year study. J Clin Diagn Res. 11(3):EC45-9, 2017
5. Helal TE et al: Idiopathic granulomatous mastitis: cytologic and histologic study of 65 Egyptian patients. Acta Cytol. 60(5):438-44, 2016
6. Troxell ML et al: Cystic neutrophilic granulomatous mastitis: association With Gram-positive bacilli and Corynebacterium. Am J Clin Pathol. 145(5):635-45, 2016
7. Cheng L et al: Mastitis, a radiographic, clinical, and histopathologic review. Breast J. 21(4):403-9, 2015
8. D'Alfonso TM et al: Cystic neutrophilic granulomatous mastitis: further characterization of a distinctive histopathologic entity not always demonstrably attributable to Corynebacterium infection. Am J Surg Pathol. 39(10):1440-7, 2015

Fat Necrosis

KEY FACTS

CLINICAL ISSUES
- Common benign inflammatory reaction secondary to injury of breast adipose tissue, including wide spectrum of clinical and radiologic appearances
- Should regress or resolve over time

CYTOPATHOLOGY
- Fragments of degenerated adipose tissue, infiltration by foamy histiocytes and multinucleated giant cells, presence of myospherulosis, hemosiderin pigment deposition, and calcifications
- Histiocytes and myofibroblasts in lesion generally exhibit vesicular nuclear chromatin without significant atypia
- Histiocytes and multinucleated giant cells demonstrate abundant foamy cytoplasm due to ingested lipid
- Foamy histiocytes with ingested lipid are also referred to as lipophages

TOP DIFFERENTIAL DIAGNOSES
- Spindle cell tumor of breast
  - Spindle-shaped histiocytes or myofibroblasts in fat necrosis (FN) do not exhibit cytologic atypia and are associated with chronic inflammatory cells and giant cells
- Granular cell tumor
  - Histiocytes in FN should be strongly (+) for CD68 and may be (+) for S100, whereas granular cells in granular cell tumors are strongly (+) for S100 and may be (+) for CD68
- Lupus mastitis
  - Features of FN associated with abundant lymphocytic infiltration and plasma cells are present
- Erdheim-Chester disease
  - Very rare non-Langerhans cell histiocytosis (polyostotic sclerosing histiocytosis) with mild lymphocytic infiltrate that may involve breast

(Left) Pap-stained FNA smear shows a fragment of degenerated adipose tissue ➡. (Right) Pap-stained FNA smear of intermediate-stage of fat necrosis (FN) shows abundant foamy macrophages ➡.

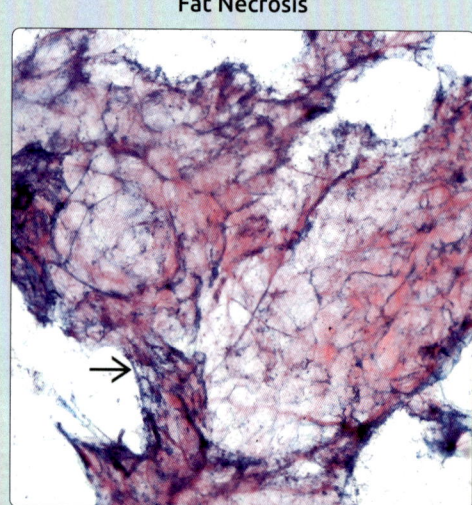
Fat Necrosis

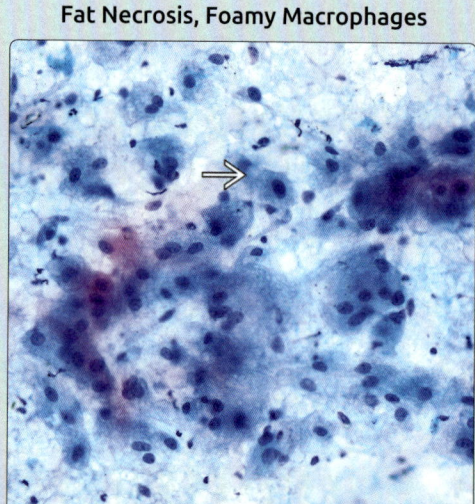
Fat Necrosis, Foamy Macrophages

(Left) Core biopsy of FN in the breast shows necrotic adipose tissue ➡ associated with chronic inflammation ➡, fibrosis, and calcifications ➡. (Right) Pap-stained FNA smear shows the details of a spherule of myospherulosis. The sac-like structure shows conglomerated and degenerated RBCs ➡.

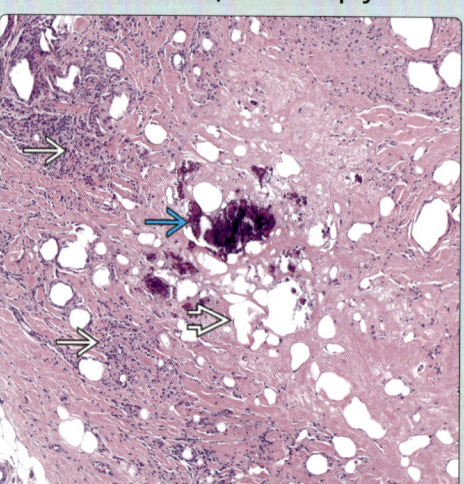
Fat Necrosis, Breast Biopsy

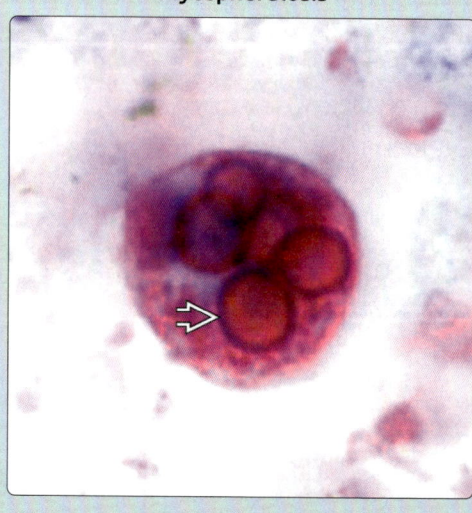
Myospherulosis

Fat Necrosis

TERMINOLOGY

Abbreviations
- Fat necrosis (FN)

Definitions
- Common benign inflammatory reaction secondary to injury of breast connective tissue and adipose tissue

CLINICAL ISSUES

Prognosis
- Should regress or resolve over time

IMAGING

Mammographic Findings
- Most common findings include dystrophic calcifications and radiolucent oil cysts

CYTOPATHOLOGY

Cellularity
- Early stage is characterized by fragments of degenerated fat with loss of nuclear details accompanied by hemorrhage and acute inflammation
- In intermediate stage, there is infiltration by foamy histiocytes and multinucleated giant cells
  - Degenerated RBCs conglomerate in setting of fat released by necrotic adipocytes and form sac-like structures containing degenerated RBCs known as myospherulosis
- In late stage, hemosiderin pigment deposition, calcification, and fibrosis are seen
  - Histiocytes and myofibroblasts can exhibit reactive atypia that may mimic malignancy
  - Rarely, there may be exuberant proliferation of spindle-shaped histiocytes and myofibroblasts with formation of pseudotumor that may mimic spindle cell sarcoma

Background and Cells
- Amorphous material, lipid, calcifications, and hemosiderin pigment
- Foamy histiocytes, acute and chronic inflammatory cells, and multinucleated giant cells

DIFFERENTIAL DIAGNOSIS

Spindle Cell Tumor of Breast
- Spindle-shaped histiocytes or myofibroblasts in FN do not exhibit cytologic atypia and are associated with chronic inflammatory cells and giant cells

Granular Cell Tumor
- Lipid-laden histiocytes in FN and cells of granular cell tumor can be similar in appearance
  - Histiocytes in FN should be strongly (+) for CD68 and may be (+) for S100, whereas granular cells are strongly (+) for S100 and may be (+) for CD68
    - Granular cell tumor lacks inflammatory infiltration and evidence of necrotic fat characteristic of FN

Lupus Mastitis
- Rare manifestation of lupus with single or multiple masses; features of FN associated with abundant lymphocytic infiltration and plasma cells are present

Erdheim-Chester Disease
- Very rare non-Langerhans cell histiocytosis (polyostotic sclerosing histiocytosis) with mild lymphocytic infiltrate that may involve breast
- Histiocytes are CD68(+), CD1a(-), and S100(-)

SELECTED REFERENCES

1. Lee J et al: Natural course of fat necrosis after breast reconstruction: a 10-year follow-up study. BMC Cancer. 21(1):166, 2021
2. Sciallis AP et al: Cellular spindled histiocytic pseudotumor complicating mammary fat necrosis: a potential diagnostic pitfall. Am J Surg Pathol. 36(10):1571-8, 2012
3. Hata S et al: Cytologic appearance of myospherulosis of the breast diagnosed by fine-needle aspirates: a clinical, cytological and immunocytochemical study of 23 cases. Diagn Cytopathol. 39(3):177-80, 2011

Fat Necrosis, Early Stage
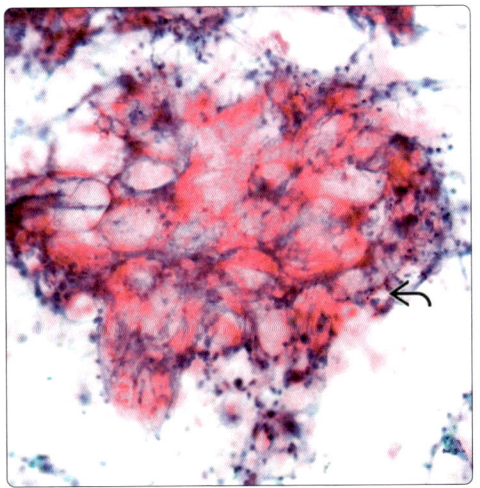

Calcifications in Fat Necrosis
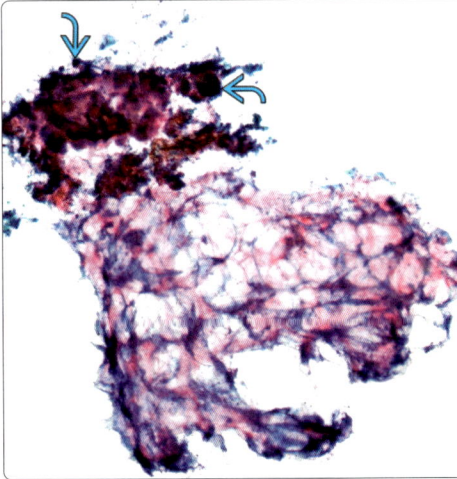

(Left) Pap-stained FNA smear shows changes of early-stage FN with degenerated adipose tissue associated with infiltration of acute inflammatory cells ➡. (Right) Pap-stained FNA smear shows a fragment of degenerated adipose tissue associated with calcification ➡.

Nonproliferative and Proliferative Changes in Breast

TERMINOLOGY

Synonyms
- Nonproliferative breast changes are also referred to as fibrocystic changes (FCCs)

Definitions
- Nonproliferative breast changes
  o Commonly encountered constellation of benign breast changes, including
    – Cysts
    – Apocrine metaplasia
    – Stromal fibrosis
    – Adenosis
- Proliferative breast changes
  o Usual ductal hyperplasia (UDH)
    – Represents benign intraductal proliferation without atypia
  o Atypical ductal hyperplasia (ADH)
    – Clonal intraductal proliferation with architectural and cytologic features approaching those seen in low-grade ductal carcinoma in situ

EPIDEMIOLOGY

Incidence
- Nonproliferative changes found in 40-70% of breast biopsies
- Proliferative breast disease without atypia: 30-60%
- UDH found in 25% of benign breast biopsies
- ADH can be found in 15-20% of breast biopsies performed to evaluate mammographic calcifications

Age Range
- Most commonly noted in women 30-50 years of age

ETIOLOGY/PATHOGENESIS

Hormonal Effects
- Responsiveness of breast tissue to monthly changes in estrogen and progesterone levels
- May be related to excess hormonal stimulation or hypersensitivity of breast tissue to hormonal stimulus
- Clinical factors associated with increased risk of benign breast disease
  o Late age at menopause
  o Estrogen replacement therapy
  o Nulliparity
  o Low body mass index
  o Family history of breast cancer
- Clinical factors associated with decreased risk of benign breast disease
  o High parity
  o Oral contraceptives
  o Physical activity
- Tamoxifen is associated with 28% reduction in prevalence of benign breast changes

CLINICAL IMPLICATIONS

Clinical Presentation
- Symptoms related to menstrual cycle
  o Premenstrual pain
  o Usually cease after menopause
  o May continue in women receiving hormone replacement therapy
- Lumpiness with multiple nodules
- Palpable nodularity in bilateral breasts but no symmetrical findings
- Tenderness and breast pain

Prognosis
- Nonproliferative changes
  o 4% lifetime risk of invasive carcinoma
- Proliferative disease without atypia
  o Associated with 1.5-2x increased risk for developing cancer
  o 5-7% increased lifetime risk of invasive cancer
- ADH is marker of increased risk for developing invasive carcinoma and nonobligate precursor of carcinoma
  o Associated with 4-5x increased relative risk or with 13-17% lifetime risk of invasive carcinoma

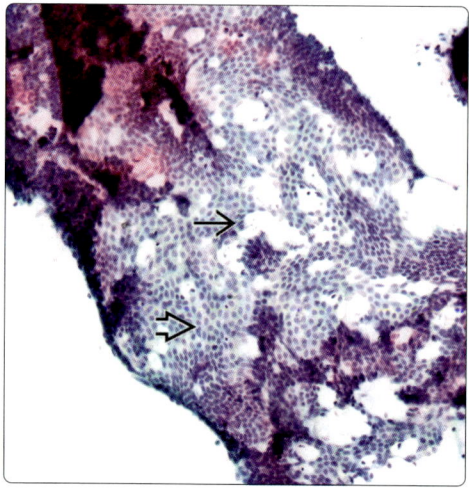

Ductal Epithelium With Slit-Like Spaces

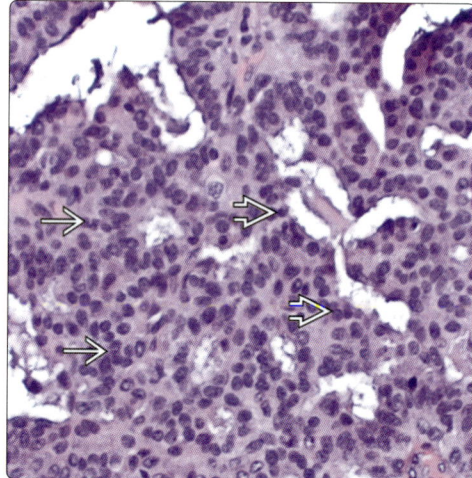

Florid Ductal Epithelial Hyperplasia Without Atypia

(Left) Pap-stained FNA smear of proliferative breast changes without atypia shows a large fragment of benign ductal epithelial cells ⇨ with slit-like spaces ⇨ amidst the hyperplastic ductal cells. *(Right)* Core biopsy stained with H&E shows florid ductal epithelial hyperplasia without atypia with the formation of slit-like spaces ⇨. The ductal epithelial cells are of varying shapes and sizes ⇨ and do not show the monotonous proliferation of uniform ductal epithelial cells as noted in atypical ductal hyperplasia.

Nonproliferative and Proliferative Changes in Breast

- o Cancer risk is ~ equal in both breasts
- Usually increased risk in women with positive family history of cancer

Imaging Findings
- Mammographic findings
  - o May present as ill-defined densities or clustered, indeterminate calcifications
  - o Cysts can present as rounded densities mimicking other benign tumors, such as fibroadenoma and papilloma

CYTOPATHOLOGY

Nonproliferative Changes
- Low cellularity
- Few clusters of benign ductal epithelial cells with associated myoepithelial cells and apocrine cells
- Few naked nuclei, foamy histiocytes, and small fragments of fibrocollagenous tissue in background
- Nuclei are regular with smooth nuclear membranes, fine nuclear chromatin, and inconspicuous nucleolus

Cysts
- Aspiration of fluid, which can be yellow, brown, or milky in appearance; lesion collapses following aspiration
  - o Few clusters of ductal cells, apocrine cells, and foamy histiocytes distributed in background of proteinaceous material
  - o Aggregated proteinaceous material can be present as extracellular globules of varying sizes
    - Liesegang rings, including slightly faceted concretions of proteinaceous material with laminations
  - o Fragments of calcifications, including birefringent calcium oxalate crystals, can be present
  - o Ductal epithelial cells and apocrine cells can demonstrate reactive/degenerative atypia with large, round or elongated nuclei with prominent nucleolus and abundant cytoplasm

Proliferative Breast Changes Without Atypia
- Cellularity is variable (usually moderate)
- Moderate- or large-sized fragments of cohesive ductal epithelial cells associated with other findings similar to nonproliferative breast changes
- Ductal epithelial cells in fragments show overlapping, have indistinct cell borders, and are often streaming, forming slit-like spaces
- Myoepithelial cells present in fragments
- Nuclei can be mildly pleomorphic with smooth nuclear membrane and inconspicuous nucleolus
- Small nucleoli and rare mitotic figures can be seen

Sclerosing Adenosis
- Low to moderate cellularity with few clusters of cohesive ductal epithelial cells with rounded, angulated, or tubular contours
- Few dyscohesive clusters of ductal epithelial cells, intact single cells, and fragments of fibroconnective tissue can be present
- Ductal epithelial cells in clusters and individually present in background can demonstrate focal mild to moderate atypia
- Myoepithelial cells are usually present in clusters but can be scant or even absent in some clusters

Proliferative Breast Changes With Atypia
- Cellularity is variable (usually moderate)
- Few fragments of cohesive ductal epithelial cells with abnormal architectural patterns associated with changes similar to proliferative changes without atypia
  - o Abnormal architectural patterns include cribriform, micropapillary, or solid forms
  - o Myoepithelial cells usually present in fragments
  - o Few naked nuclei, apocrine cells, and foamy histiocytes may be present in background of smear
  - o Ductal epithelial cells in abnormal fragments can be monotonous with distinct cell boundaries
  - o Nuclei are slightly enlarged, round or oval, and hyperchromatic
  - o Nuclear chromatin can be fine or clumped
  - o Nuclear membrane can be smooth or irregular
  - o Nucleoli may be present; rare mitotic figures may be noted in atypical ductal epithelial cells

DIFFERENTIAL DIAGNOSIS

Fibroadenoma
- Few clusters of benign ductal epithelial cells associated with some naked nuclei in background in hyalinized fibroadenoma can mimic nonproliferative breast changes
- Correlation with imaging findings may be useful for distinction

Carcinoma
- Clusters of low-grade ductal carcinoma can mimic nonproliferative FCCs
- Clusters in carcinoma show cytologic atypia and lack myoepithelial cells, unlike FCCs
- Imaging findings are generally different between these entities

Papilloma
- Smears of papilloma that do not contain fragments showing fibrovascular cores and are not very cellular may be similar to nonproliferative FCCs
- Papillomas often show columnar cells in clusters or as single cells with proteinaceous material and hemosiderin-laden macrophages in background
- Correlation of cytologic findings with imaging is also useful

SELECTED REFERENCES

1. Toktaş O et al: Relationship between proliferative breast lesions and breast cancer risk factors. Eur J Breast Health. 17(1):15-20, 2021
2. Agarwal C et al: Masood's and modified Masood's Scoring Index: an evaluation of fine needle aspiration cytology of breast lesions with histopathological correlation. Acta Cytol. 63(3):233-9, 2019
3. Kaur A et al: Feasibility of Masood's cytological index for screening breast lesions in low resource setting. Breast J. 25(3):434-8, 2019
4. Tanaka S et al: Usefulness of immunocytochemistry using a breast marker antibody cocktail targeting P63/cytokeratin7/18/cytokeratin5/14 for fine needle aspiration of the breast: a retrospective cohort study of 139 cases. Cytopathology. 27(6):465-71, 2016
5. Kundu UR et al: Fine needle aspiration cytology of sclerosing adenosis of the breast: a retrospective review of cytologic features in conjunction with corresponding histologic features and radiologic findings. Am J Clin Pathol. 138(1):96-102, 2012
6. Jensen KC et al: Cytologic diagnosis of columnar-cell lesions of the breast. Diagn Cytopathol. 35(2):73-9, 2007
7. Masood S: Cytomorphology of fibrocystic change, high-risk proliferative breast disease, and premalignant breast lesions. Clin Lab Med. 25(4):713-31, vi, 2005

Nonproliferative and Proliferative Changes in Breast

Breast Cyst, Concretions of Proteinaceous Material

Breast Cyst, Concretions Mimicking Necrosis

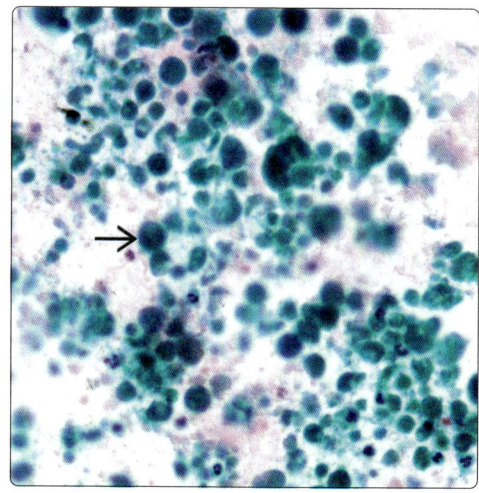

(Left) Pap-stained FNA smear of a breast cyst shows concretions of proteinaceous material ⇨ without any associated cells. (Right) Pap-stained FNA smear of a breast cyst shows many rounded concretions ⇨ of proteinaceous material, which can be mistaken for necrotic material.

Mildly Atypical Ductal Epithelial Cells

Breast Cyst, Spindling of Ductal Epithelial Cells

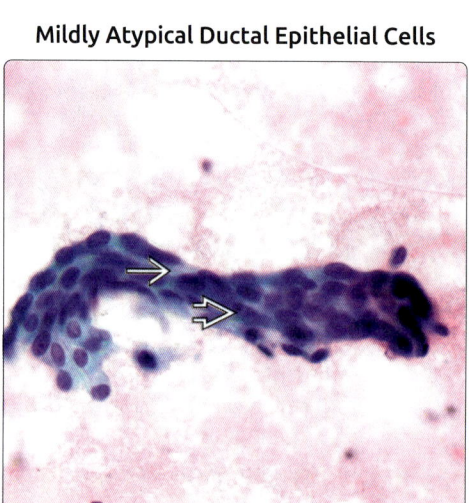
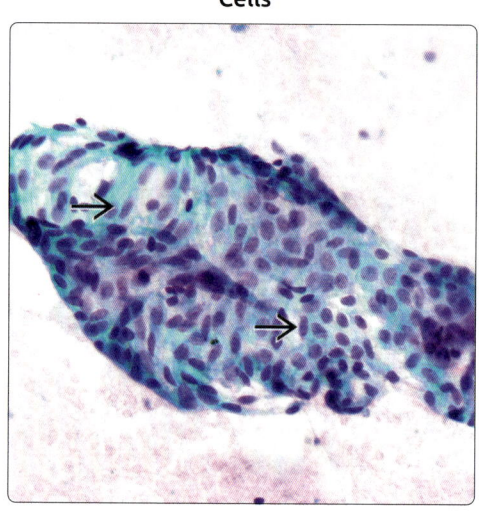

(Left) Pap-stained FNA smear of a breast cyst shows a fragment of mildly atypical ductal epithelial cells ⇨ with mildly enlarged and elongated nuclei ⇨ associated with proteinaceous material in the background. (Right) Pap-stained FNA smear of a breast cyst shows a fragment of ductal epithelial cells and myoepithelial cells with spindling of the nuclei ⇨.

Proliferative Ductal Epithelium Without Atypia

Breast Cyst Apocrine Cells

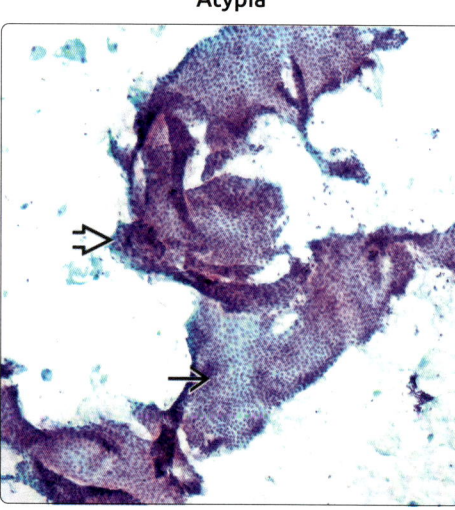
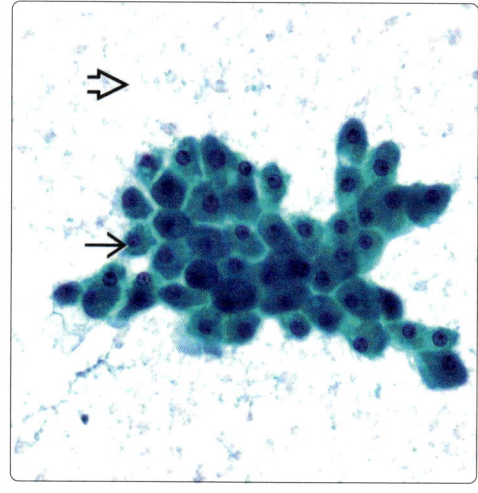

(Left) Pap-stained FNA smear of proliferative breast changes without atypia shows a large fragment ⇨ of uniform benign ductal epithelial cells, without any evidence of cytologic atypia, arranged in a honeycombed pattern ⇨. (Right) Pap-stained FNA smear of breast cyst contents shows a fragment of apocrine cells ⇨ with abundant granular cytoplasm and prominent nucleoli associated with proteinaceous material in the background ⇨.

Nonproliferative and Proliferative Changes in Breast

Benign Ductal Epithelium

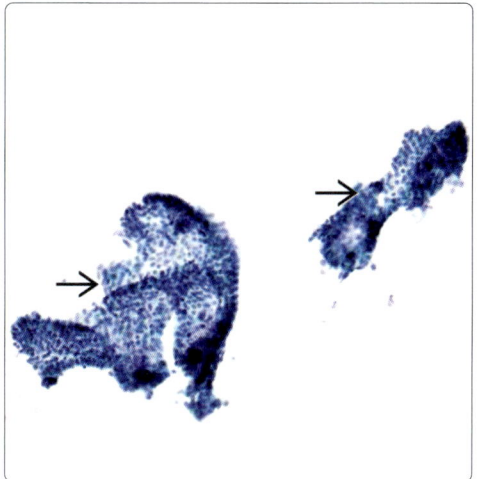

Hyperplastic Ductal Epithelium Without Atypia

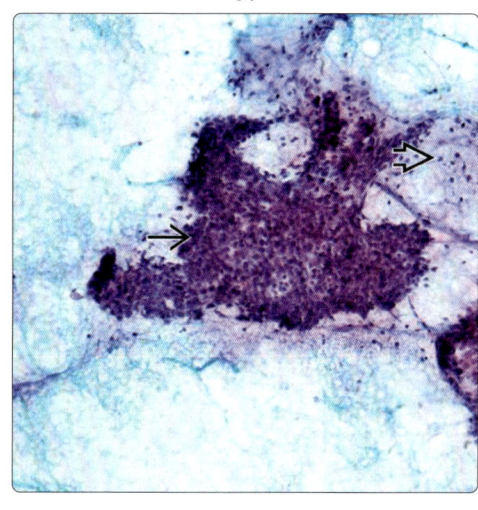

(Left) Pap-stained FNA smear of nonproliferative changes in the breast shows small fragments of benign ductal epithelial cells ➡ without any evidence of cytologic atypia. (Right) Pap-stained FNA smear shows a fragment of hyperplastic ductal epithelial cells ➡ with nuclear crowding and overlapping associated with few naked nuclei ➡ in the vicinity of the fragment.

Proliferative Ductal Epithelium With Spindling

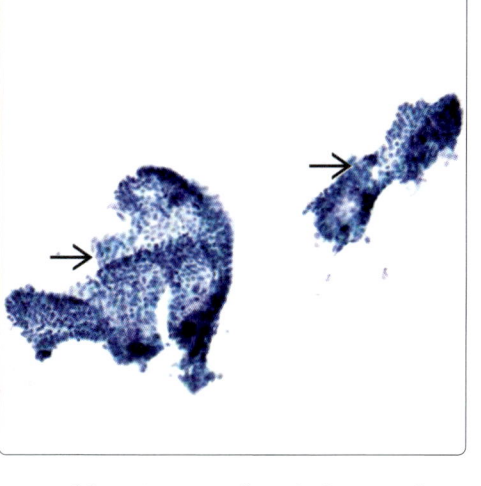

Atypical Ductal Hyperplasia Papillary Clusters

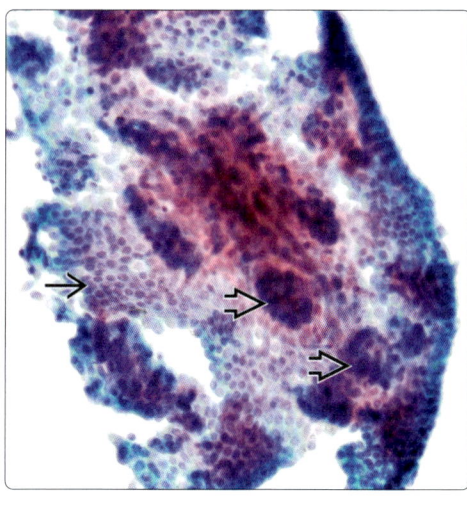

(Left) Pap-stained FNA smear of proliferative breast changes without atypia shows a fragment of benign ductal epithelial cells with spindling of the epithelial cells ➡. (Right) Pap-stained FNA smear of proliferative breast changes with atypia shows a fragment of monotonous ductal epithelial cells ➡ with several ball-like rounded papillary clusters of cells ➡.

Atypical Ductal Hyperplasia Cribriform Architecture

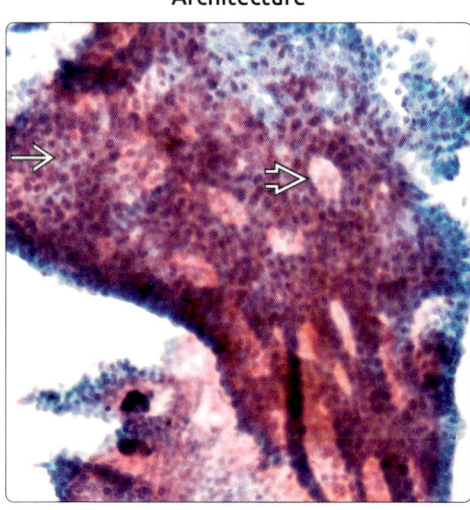

Atypical Ductal Hyperplasia

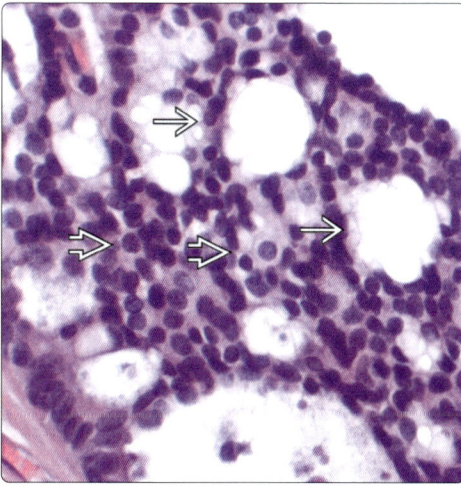

(Left) Pap-stained FNA smear of proliferative breast changes with atypia shows a large fragment of atypical monotonous ductal epithelial cells ➡ with abnormal cribriform architectural pattern with the formation of punched-out spaces ➡. (Right) Core biopsy stained with H&E shows atypical monotonous epithelial proliferation ➡ with the formation of punched-out spaces ➡, resulting in a cribriform architectural pattern.

Radial Scar/Complex Sclerosing Lesion

KEY FACTS

CLINICAL ISSUES
- Most radial sclerosing lesions (RSLs) are microscopic findings that are detected following investigation of mammographically found stellate lesions
- Risk factor for subsequent development of breast carcinoma; after adjusting for proliferative disease and atypical hyperplasia, risk is small
- Epithelial atypia, ↑ size, and multiple lesions are associated with ↑ risk for development of malignancy
- Both in situ and invasive carcinomas can occur in association with RSL

CYTOPATHOLOGY
- Variable cellularity with clusters of benign ductal epithelial cells of varying sizes ± hyperplasia, associated with few naked bipolar nuclei
- Fragments of elastoid and fibrocollagenous tissue in background
- Tubular and angular clusters with elongated contours may mimic neoplastic glands of tubular carcinoma (TC)
- Presence of myoepithelial cells in clusters and absence of rigid configuration are useful features for distinction of RSL from TC
- Cytologic findings are very similar to fibrocystic changes
- Correlation with imaging findings and further investigation with core needle biopsy are recommended for specific preoperative diagnosis

TOP DIFFERENTIAL DIAGNOSES
- TC
  - Significant overlap in imaging and cytologic features between RSL and TC
    - Proliferating neoplastic glands of TC show abnormal, sharply angulated tubular contours composed of ductal cells with mild cytologic atypia that, unlike RSL clusters, are not surrounded by myoepithelial cells

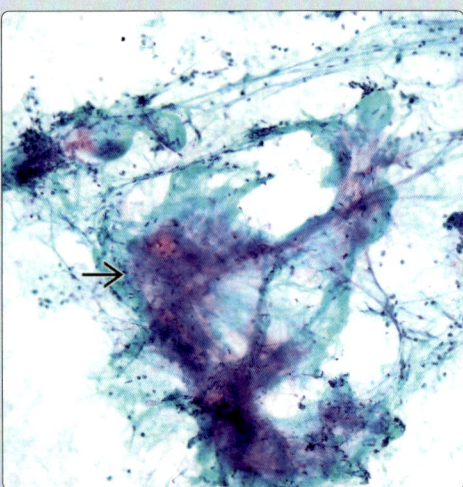

Radial Sclerosing Lesion: Elastoid Stromal Fragment

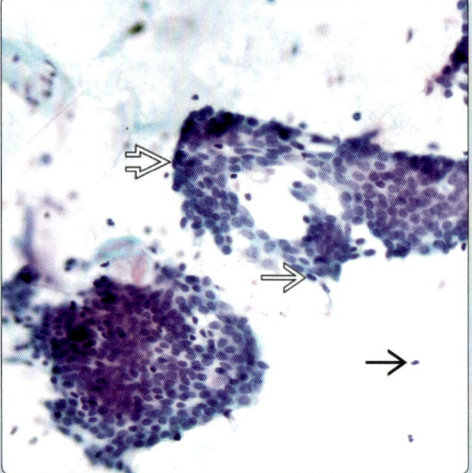

Radial Sclerosing Lesion: Ductal Hyperplasia

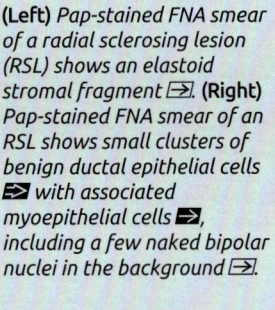

(Left) Pap-stained FNA smear of a radial sclerosing lesion (RSL) shows an elastoid stromal fragment ⇨. (Right) Pap-stained FNA smear of an RSL shows small clusters of benign ductal epithelial cells ⇨ with associated myoepithelial cells ⇨, including a few naked bipolar nuclei in the background ⇨.

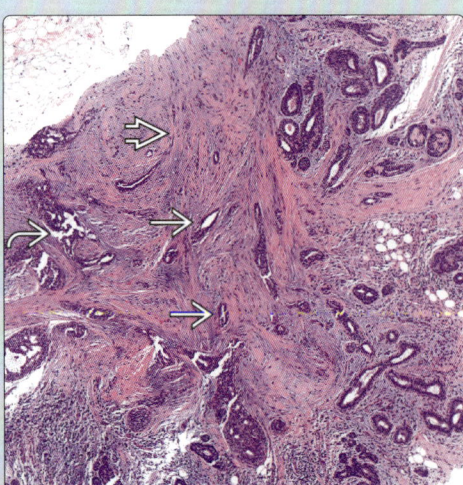

Radial Scar

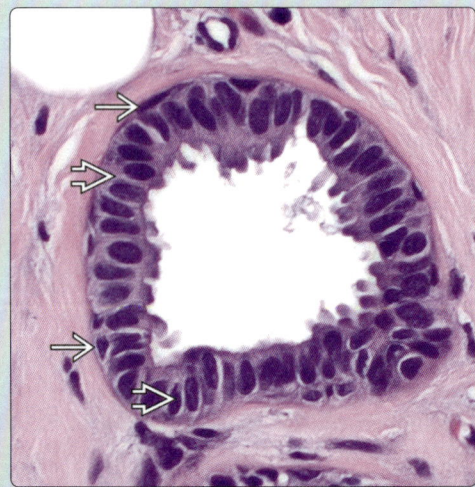

Radial Scar

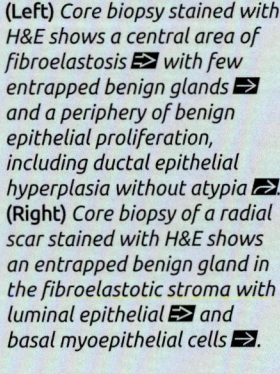

(Left) Core biopsy stained with H&E shows a central area of fibroelastosis ⇨ with few entrapped benign glands ⇨ and a periphery of benign epithelial proliferation, including ductal epithelial hyperplasia without atypia ⇨. (Right) Core biopsy of a radial scar stained with H&E shows an entrapped benign gland in the fibroelastotic stroma with luminal epithelial ⇨ and basal myoepithelial cells ⇨.

Radial Scar/Complex Sclerosing Lesion

TERMINOLOGY

Definitions
- Radial sclerosing lesion (RSL): Variable combinations of epithelial proliferation and stromal elastofibrosis, including dense sclerosis, resulting in irregular contours of lesion

CLINICAL ISSUES

Presentation
- Most are microscopic findings detected following investigation of mammographically identified abnormal stellate areas of density

Prognosis
- Histologic risk factor for subsequent development of breast carcinoma; after adjusting for proliferative disease and atypical hyperplasia, risk is small
- Epithelial atypia, ↑ size, and multiple lesions are associated with ↑ risk for development of malignancy
- Carcinoma in situ (ductal and lobular types) and invasive carcinoma can be associated with RSL

IMAGING

Mammographic Findings
- Presents as stellate lesion with lucent center usually < 2 cm with length of radiating arms being longer than size of mass ± associated calcifications

CYTOPATHOLOGY

Cells
- Variable cellularity with clusters of ductal epithelial cells of varying sizes associated with few scattered bipolar naked nuclei in background
- Elastoid and fibrotic stromal fragments may be present
- Epithelial cell clusters are associated with myoepithelial cells and may demonstrate ductal epithelial hyperplasia; ductal epithelial cells may exhibit mild cytologic atypia
- Tubular and angular clusters with elongated contours may mimic neoplastic glands of tubular carcinoma (TC)
- Presence of myoepithelial cells in clusters and absence of rigid configuration are useful features for distinction
- Apocrine cells and foamy macrophages may be present
- Overall findings are nonspecific and similar to fibrocystic changes
- Correlation with imaging findings and further investigation with core needle biopsy are recommended for specific preoperative diagnosis

DIFFERENTIAL DIAGNOSIS

Tubular Carcinoma
- Significant overlap in imaging and cytologic features between RSL and TC
  - Proliferating neoplastic glands of TC show abnormal, sharply angulated tubular contours composed of ductal cells with mild cytologic atypia that, unlike RSL clusters, are not surrounded by myoepithelial cells

SELECTED REFERENCES

1. Liu RQ et al: Upstage rate of radial scar/complex sclerosing lesion identified on core needle biopsy. Am J Surg. 221(6):1177-81, 2021
2. Gašljević G et al: Reducing indications for radial scar surgical excision in Slovenian breast cancer screening program. Ann Diagn Pathol. 45:151438, 2020
3. Woodward SG et al: Is radial scar on core needle biopsy a risk factor for malignancy? A single-center retrospective review and implications for management. Breast J. 26(10):2011-4, 2020
4. Chou WYY et al: Radial scar on image-guided breast biopsy: is surgical excision necessary? Breast Cancer Res Treat. 170(2):313-20, 2018
5. Donaldson AR et al: Radial scars diagnosed on breast core biopsy: frequency of atypia and carcinoma on excision and implications for management. Breast. 30:201-7, 2016
6. Li Z et al: Pathologic findings of follow-up surgical excision for radial scar on breast core needle biopsy. Hum Pathol. 48:76-80, 2016
7. Berg JC et al: Breast cancer risk in women with radial scars in benign breast biopsies. Breast Cancer Res Treat. 108(2):167-74, 2008
8. Manfrin E et al: Risk of neoplastic transformation in asymptomatic radial scar: analysis of 117 cases. Breast Cancer Res Treat. 107(3):371-7, 2008
9. Douglas-Jones AG et al: Radial scar lesions of the breast diagnosed by needle core biopsy: analysis of cases containing occult malignancy. J Clin Pathol. 60(3):295-8, 2007
10. Doyle EM et al: Radial scars/complex sclerosing lesions and malignancy in a screening programme: incidence and histological features revisited. Histopathology. 50(5):607-14, 2007

Radial Sclerosing Lesion: Ductal Hyperplasia

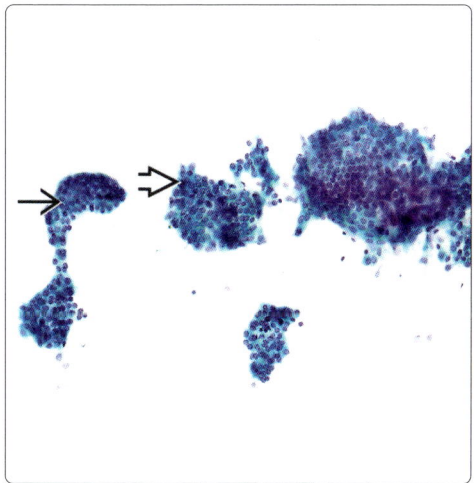

Radial Sclerosing Lesion: Calcifications

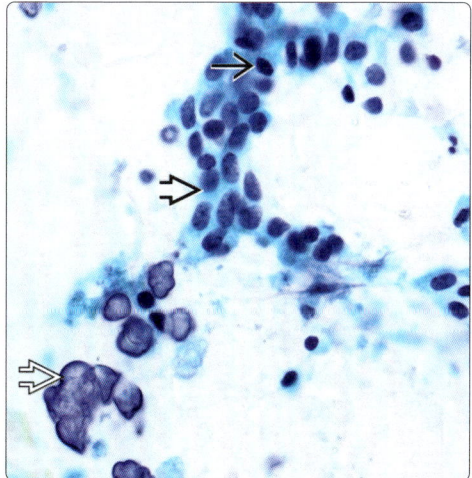

(Left) Pap-stained FNA smear of an RSL shows fragments of benign ductal epithelial cells of varying sizes ⇨, including a fragment with an angular configuration ⇨. *(Right)* Pap-stained FNA smear of RSL shows a small tubular fragment composed of benign ductal epithelial cells and myoepithelial cells ⇨ with associated calcifications ⇨. The ductal epithelial cells demonstrate mild cytologic atypia ⇨.

Gynecomastia

KEY FACTS

CLINICAL ISSUES
- Benign enlargement of male breast due to hyperplasia of epithelium and stroma
  - Occurs in 3 peaks (infancy, puberty, and old age)
- Benign condition; self-limited
- Develops because of alterations in ratio of free androgen:estrogen and in serum levels of sex hormone-binding globulin
- Obesity, liver or renal disease, or hormone deficiency due to primary or secondary gonadal failure and hormone-producing tumors can cause gynecomastia
- Consideration of surgical options or antiestrogen therapy in lesions associated with pain &/or cosmetic appearance

CYTOPATHOLOGY
- Clusters and sheets of benign ductal epithelial cells associated with myoepithelial cells ± proliferative changes and fragments of vascularized or sclerotic stroma in background
- Single intact epithelial cells generally absent in background
- Changes can be similar to fibrocystic changes in female breast, including epithelial hyperplasia and cytologic and architectural atypia
- Squamous metaplasia, apocrine metaplasia, and cystic change can be noted

TOP DIFFERENTIAL DIAGNOSES
- Pseudogynecomastia
  - Usually noted in obese older men as diffuse breast enlargement with fragments of adipose tissue alone on aspiration
  - Unlike subareolar palpable nodule in gynecomastia yielding benign ductal epithelium
- Male breast cancer
  - Firm, palpable, painless mass yielding cellular smears with clusters and single atypical epithelial cells
  - Unlike few clusters of cohesive benign ductal epithelial cells in gynecomastia

Gynecomastia
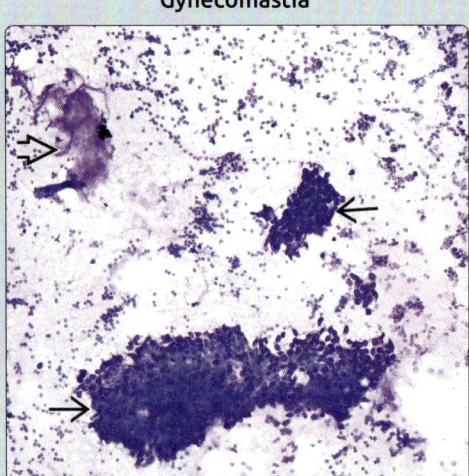

Gynecomastia, Ductal Hyperplasia
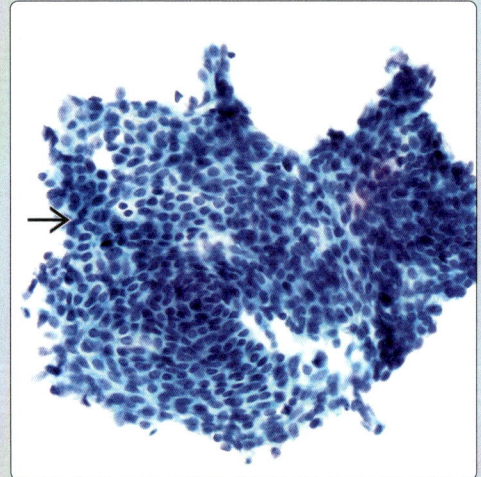

(Left) Diff-Quik-stained FNA smear of gynecomastia shows fragments of ductal epithelial cells of varying sizes ➡ and a stromal fragment ➡. (Right) Pap-stained FNA smear demonstrates tightly packed ductal epithelial cells in a fragment with interspersed myoepithelial cells ➡.

Gynecomastia
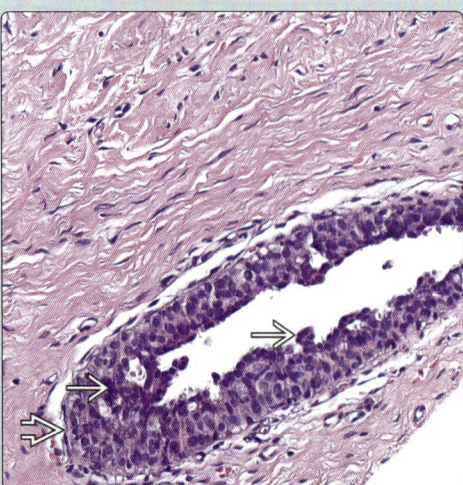

Gynecomastia, Ductal Hyperplasia
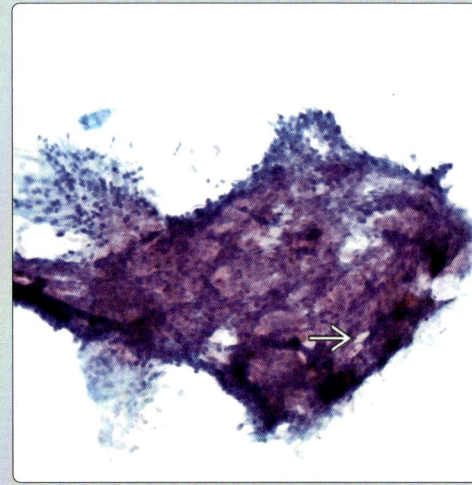

(Left) Core biopsy of gynecomastia stained with H&E shows a mammary duct ➡ with ductal epithelial hyperplasia without atypia ➡. (Right) Pap-stained FNA smear shows ductal epithelial hyperplasia without atypia in a case of gynecomastia. Note the slit-like spaces ➡ created by the hyperplastic ductal epithelial cells.

Gynecomastia

TERMINOLOGY

Definitions
- Nonneoplastic enlargement of male breast due to hyperplasia of both epithelium and stroma

ETIOLOGY/PATHOGENESIS

Several Causes
- Obesity, liver or renal disease, or hormone deficiency due to primary or secondary gonadal failure and hormone-producing tumors

CLINICAL ISSUES

Epidemiology
- Incidence
  - Common finding with 3 distinct peaks of occurrence: Infancy, puberty, and old age

Presentation
- Unilateral or bilateral; localized or diffuse; palpable, tender, firm, mobile, disc-shaped mound of tissue in subareolar region
- Aspiration of these lesions can be painful

Prognosis
- Benign condition; self-limited

IMAGING

Mammographic Findings
- Discrete, subareolar mass or flame-shaped central mass with linear projections; diffuse enlargement with dense, nodular parenchyma

CYTOPATHOLOGY

General Features
- Variable with clusters and sheets of cohesive, tightly packed, benign ductal epithelial cells associated with myoepithelial cells; overall findings can be similar to fibrocystic changes in female breast
- Fragments of vascularized or fibrotic stroma commonly noted in background of smears; single intact epithelial cells generally absent in background
- Proliferative changes, including ductal epithelial hyperplasia without atypia, commonly encountered
- Clusters of hyperplastic ductal epithelial cells can exhibit cytologic and architectural atypia
- Squamous metaplasia, apocrine metaplasia, and cystic change can be noted

DIFFERENTIAL DIAGNOSIS

Pseudogynecomastia
- Usually noted in obese older men as diffuse breast enlargement yielding fragments of adipose tissue alone on aspiration
  - Unlike subareolar palpable nodule in gynecomastia yielding benign ductal epithelium

Male Breast Cancer
- Firm, palpable, painless mass yielding cellular smears with clusters and single atypical epithelial cells
  - Unlike few clusters of cohesive benign ductal epithelial cells in gynecomastia

SELECTED REFERENCES

1. Laimon W et al: Prepubertal gynecomastia is not always idiopathic: case series and review of the literature. Eur J Pediatr. 180(3):977-82, 2021
2. Coopey SB et al: Atypical ductal hyperplasia in men with gynecomastia: what is their breast cancer risk? Breast Cancer Res Treat. 175(1):1-4, 2019
3. Hoda RS et al: Diagnostic value of fine-needle aspiration in male breast lesions. Acta Cytol. 63(4):319-27, 2019
4. Lapid O et al: Pathological findings in gynecomastia: analysis of 5113 breasts. Ann Plast Surg. 74(2):163-6, 2015
5. Narula HS et al: Gynaecomastia--pathophysiology, diagnosis and treatment. Nat Rev Endocrinol. 10(11):684-98, 2014
6. Kapila K et al: Cytomorphological spectrum in gynaecomastia: a study of 389 cases. Cytopathology. 13(5):300-8, 2002
7. Siddiqui MT et al: Breast masses in males: multi-institutional experience on fine-needle aspiration. Diagn Cytopathol. 26(2):87-91, 2002
8. Westenend PJ et al: Evaluation of fine-needle aspiration cytology of breast masses in males. Cancer. 96(2):101-4, 2002
9. Amrikachi M et al: Gynecomastia: cytologic features and diagnostic pitfalls in fine needle aspirates. Acta Cytol. 45(6):948-52, 2001

Gynecomastia, Apocrine Cells
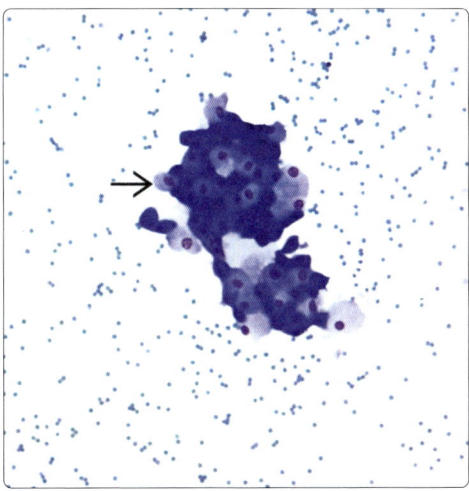

Gynecomastia, Cytologic Atypia
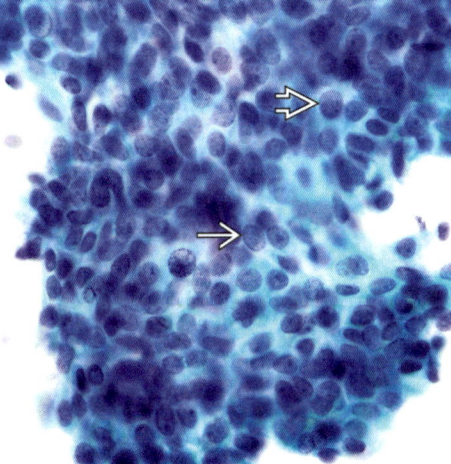

(Left) Diff-Quik-stained FNA smear of gynecomastia shows a small cluster of apocrine cells ➡. Apocrine cells can be encountered in gynecomastia. (Right) Pap-stained FNA smear of gynecomastia shows a fragment of mildly atypical hyperplastic ductal epithelial cells demonstrating nuclear enlargement ➡ and mild pleomorphism ➡.

Mucocele-Like Lesion

KEY FACTS

CLINICAL ISSUES
- Usually detected on screening mammograms as mass lesion or due to abnormal calcifications
- Uncommon breast lesion composed of mucin-containing cysts with extravasation of mucin in stroma
- Represents spectrum of lesions ranging from benign, atypical to malignant etiology

CYTOPATHOLOGY
- Benign mucocele-like lesion (MLL): Low cellularity with few clusters of benign ductal epithelial cells with associated myoepithelial cells in background of extracellular mucin
- Atypical MLL: Low cellularity with few clusters of atypical ductal epithelial cells with associated myoepithelial cells in background of extracellular mucin
- Malignant MLL: ↑ cellularity with 3D clusters without associated myoepithelial cells and individually distributed atypical epithelial cells in background of extracellular mucin

TOP DIFFERENTIAL DIAGNOSES
- Fibrocystic changes composed of dilated ducts filled with mucin
  - Cytologic features can be indistinguishable from benign MLL
- Myxoid fibroadenoma
  - Cellularity is generally higher and includes many fragments of benign epithelial and myoepithelial cells associated with numerous individual nuclei in background
    - Myxoid material can mimic mucin and is negative for mucicarmine, unlike mucin in MLL
- Mucinous carcinoma
  - ↑ cellularity with clusters of atypical epithelial cells without associated myoepithelial cells and single atypical cells, in contrast to absence of cells or few clusters of benign ductal cells in a background of abundant mucin
    - Features can be indistinguishable from those of malignant MLL

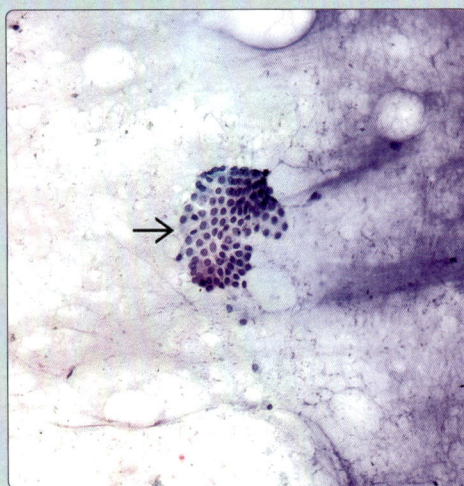
Benign Mucocele-Like Lesion

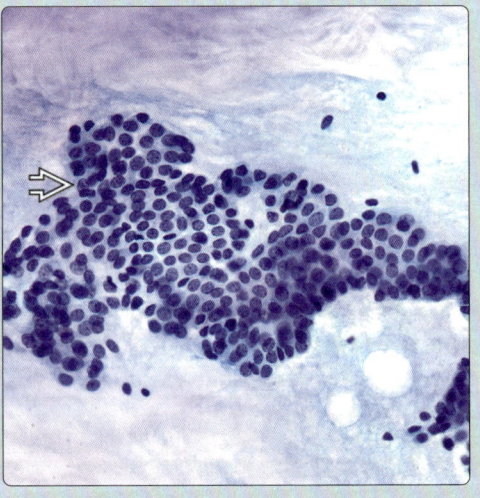
Benign Mucocele-Like Lesion

(Left) Pap-stained FNA smear of a benign mucocele-like lesion (MLL) shows a single small cluster of benign ductal epithelial and myoepithelial cells ➡ in a background of mucin. *(Right)* Pap-stained FNA smear of benign MLL shows a fragment of hyperplastic benign ductal epithelial and myoepithelial cells ➡ in a background of mucin.

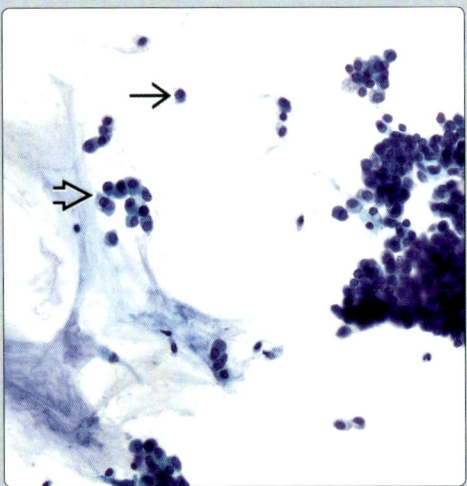
Malignant Mucocele-Like Lesion

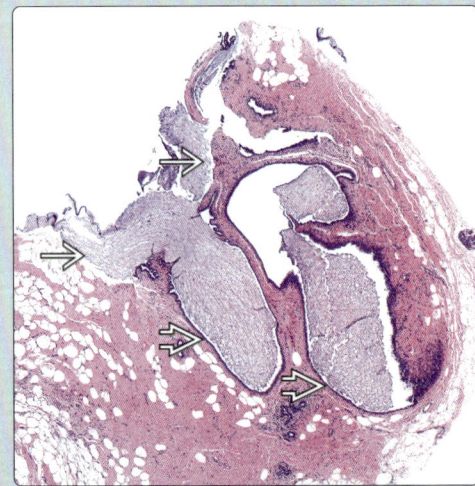
Benign Mucocele-Like Lesion Biopsy

(Left) Pap-stained FNA smear of malignant MLL shows few clusters ➡ and individually distributed atypical cells ➡ in a background of mucin. *(Right)* Core biopsy of benign MLL stained with H&E shows benign dilated ducts filled with mucin ➡ with extravasation of mucin into stroma ➡.

Mucocele-Like Lesion

TERMINOLOGY

Abbreviations
- Mucocele-like lesion (MLL)

Definitions
- Uncommon breast lesion composed of mucin-containing cysts that may rupture
- Represents spectrum of lesions ranging from benign to atypical to malignant etiology

CLINICAL ISSUES

Presentation
- Asymptomatic and detected on screening mammograms as mass or area of abnormal calcifications in women with wide age range at presentation: 27-79 years (mean: 48 years)
- MLL without atypical or malignant cells is entirely benign lesion

IMAGING

Mammographic Findings
- Pleomorphic and amorphous coarse calcifications are most commonly encountered; less commonly, lobulated and circumscribed mass may be present

Ultrasonographic Findings
- Multiple cysts with calcified or noncalcified solid components may suggest diagnosis; hypoechoic round or oval lobulated masses may be present

CYTOPATHOLOGY

Cellularity
- Varies from acellular to moderate cellularity; cell types can be benign, atypical, or malignant

Background
- Abundant extracellular mucin (+) for mucicarmine, PAS, and Alcian blue
- Intact epithelial cells are seldom noted, unlike macrophages, which are commonly present

- Benign MLL generally demonstrates few cohesive clusters of monolayered &/or hyperplastic ductal epithelial cells with associated myoepithelial cells that do not exhibit cytologic atypia
- Atypical MLL shows features similar to benign MLL but also includes several fragments of ductal epithelial cells with cytologic &/or architectural atypia
- Malignant MLL shows ↑ cellularity with many clusters of atypical epithelial cells that are not associated with myoepithelial cells and single dyscohesive atypical epithelial cells

DIFFERENTIAL DIAGNOSIS

Fibrocystic Changes With Dilated Ducts Containing Mucin
- Cytologic features can be indistinguishable from benign MLL with acellular mucin or mucin associated with small clusters of flattened and cuboidal epithelial cells without cytologic atypia

Myxoid Fibroadenoma
- Cellularity is generally higher and includes many fragments of benign epithelial and myoepithelial cells associated with numerous individual nuclei in background
- Myxoid material can mimic mucin and is negative for mucicarmine, unlike mucin in MLL

Mucinous Carcinoma
- ↑ cellularity with clusters of atypical epithelial cells without associated myoepithelial cells and single atypical cells, in contrast to absence of cells or few clusters of benign ductal cells in background of abundant mucin
- Features can be indistinguishable from those of malignant MLL

SELECTED REFERENCES
1. Towne WS et al: Mucocele-like lesion of the breast diagnosed on core biopsy. Arch Pathol Lab Med. 146(2):213-9, 2022
2. Ginter PS et al: A review of mucinous lesions of the breast. Breast J. 26(6):1168-78, 2020
3. Harrison BT et al: An update of mucinous lesions of the breast. Surg Pathol Clin. 11(1):61-90, 2018

Atypical Cells in Malignant Mucocele-Like Lesion

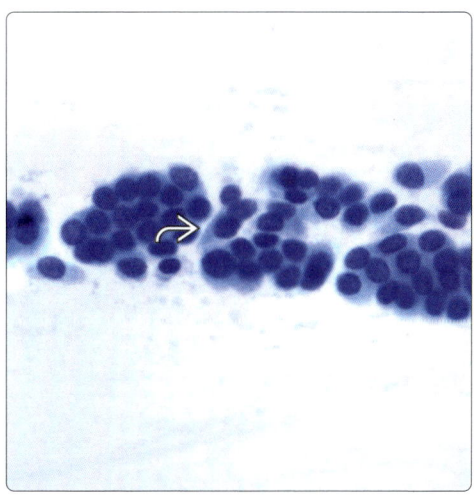

Benign Mucocele-Like Lesion

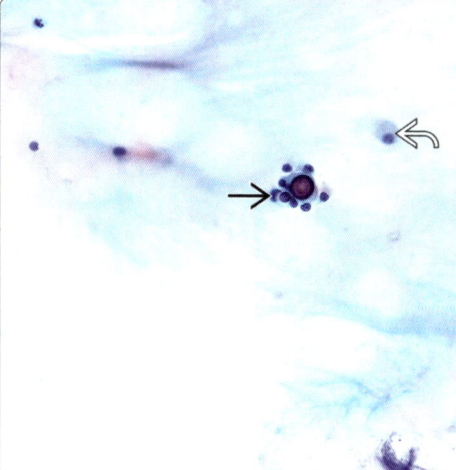

(Left) Pap-stained FNA smear of malignant MLL shows atypical ductal epithelial cells ➡ without associated myoepithelial cells in a background of extracellular mucin. *(Right)* Pap-stained FNA smear of benign MLL shows calcification ➡ surrounded by a few benign epithelial cells. Note the abundant mucin in the background of the smear with rare macrophages ➡.

Fibroadenoma

KEY FACTS

CLINICAL ISSUES
- Typically occurs in women 20-35 years of age
- Painless, slowly growing, mobile, well-defined mass
- Most common solid benign breast tumor
- Stroma typically undergoes hyalinization, which can serve as substrate for calcification
- Can grow rapidly during pregnancy; if rapid growth occurs, they can undergo infarction

CYTOPATHOLOGY
- Triad of changes: Epithelial cells, stromal fragments, and abundant naked nuclei in background
- Epithelial cells arranged as honeycomb sheets, papillary fronds, tubule-like or tight clusters with associated myoepithelial cells
- Cytologic atypia can be noted in epithelial cells
- Naked nuclei in background, round/oval or elongated with condensed chromatin
- Few intact stromal cells with elongated vesicular nucleus and scant cytoplasm
- Stromal fragments are well-defined and fibrotic, fibromyxoid, or myxoid
- Myxoid fibroadenoma has myxoid stromal fragments and myxoid material in background of smears

TOP DIFFERENTIAL DIAGNOSES
- Fibrocystic changes
- Phyllodes tumor
- Ductal carcinoma
- Papilloma
- Mucinous carcinoma
- Hamartoma (fibroadenolipoma)
- Pseudoangiomatous stromal hyperplasia
- Tubular adenoma
- Nodular adenosis/adenosis tumor
- Adenomyoepithelioma

Papillary Fronds
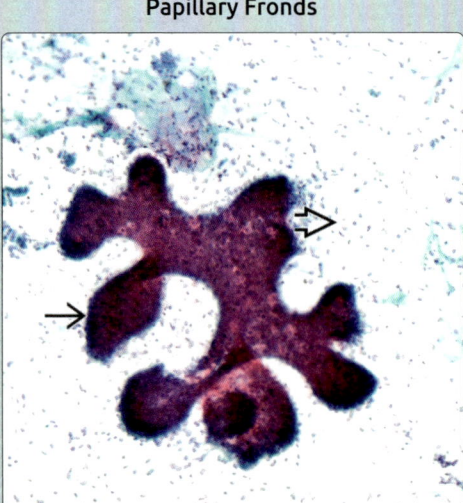

Epithelial and Myoepithelial Cells
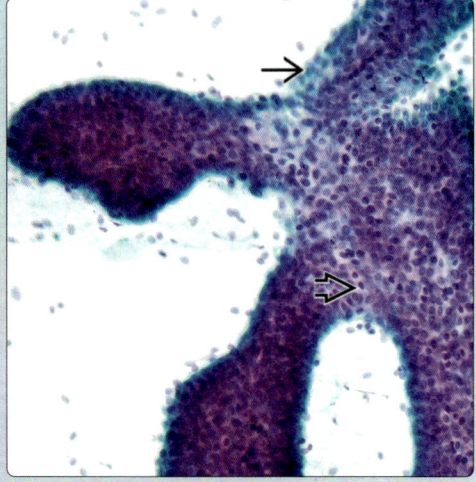

(Left) Pap-stained FNA smear in a case of fibroadenoma (FA) shows complex papillary fronds of benign epithelial cells ➡ associated with abundant naked nuclei ➡ in the background. (Right) Pap-stained FNA smear shows papillary epithelial fronds in FA, which are composed of benign ductal epithelial cells ➡ and myoepithelial cells ➡. The presence of numerous myoepithelial cells is a clue to the benign nature of the lesion.

Fibroadenoma
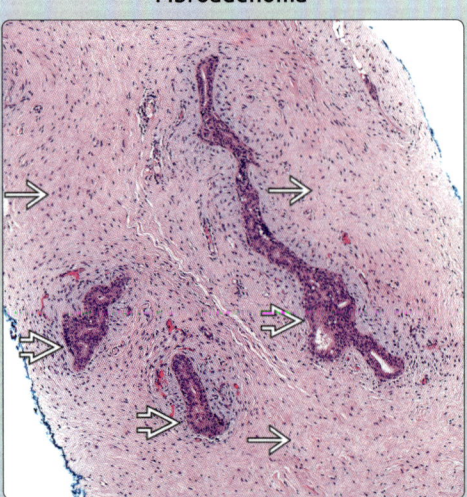

Naked Nuclei and Stromal Cell
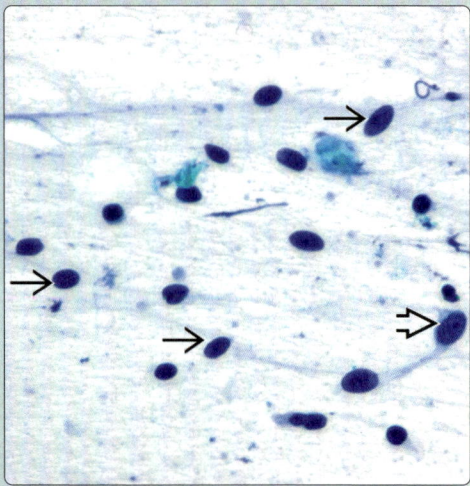

(Left) Core biopsy stained with H&E shows benign epithelial elements ➡ associated with stroma composed of spindle cells without significant nuclear pleomorphism, mitotic activity, or stromal overgrowth ➡. The overall findings of the fibroepithelial tumor is consistent with FA. (Right) Pap-stained FNA smear in a case of FA shows naked nuclei ➡ that are oval/elongated with condensed nuclear chromatin and an intact stromal cell with elongated nucleus and scant cytoplasm ➡.

Fibroadenoma

TERMINOLOGY

Abbreviations
- Fibroadenoma (FA)

Definitions
- Biphasic, benign fibroepithelial tumor consisting of intralobular stromal cells associated with epithelial cells

ETIOLOGY/PATHOGENESIS

Abnormal Growth of Intralobular Stromal Cells
- **Hormonal stimulation**
  o Most FAs are polyclonal hyperplasias of lobular stroma
    – Some stromal cells have estrogen receptor β &/or progesterone receptors
  o FAs occur most commonly in young, premenopausal women
    – Can change slightly in size with menstrual cycle
    – Can grow rapidly during pregnancy; if rapid growth occurs, they can undergo infarction
- **Iatrogenic**
  o Cyclosporine in kidney transplant recipients is associated with increase in FAs
- **Genetic/hereditary**
  o More common in Black women
  o Myxoid FAs occur in Carney complex
- **Neoplastic**
  o Some FAs are monoclonal stromal tumors with clonal genetic changes in stromal cells
    – Associated epithelial cells are usually polyclonal
  o FAs have few genetic changes
    – Some have gain of 1q similar to phyllodes tumor
  o As stromal proliferation becomes more pronounced and autonomous, changes seen in FAs can overlap with low-grade phyllodes tumors
    – Some phyllodes tumors likely arise from FAs

CLINICAL ISSUES

Epidemiology
- Incidence
  o Most common solid benign breast tumor
- Age
  o Typically occurs in younger women (20-35 years)
    – In older women, associated with continued elevated hormone levels due to either hormone replacement therapy or obesity

Presentation
- Most commonly presents as painless, slowly growing, mobile, well-defined, palpable nodule in young woman
- In older women, may be detected as mammographic circumscribed density or calcifications

Natural History
- May regress in size with age
  o Stroma typically undergoes hyalinization, which can serve as substrate for calcification

Treatment
- Surgical approaches
  o Surgery to remove FA may be indicated for large lesions, if patient requests removal, or for rare lesions that continue to grow in size

IMAGING

Mammographic Findings
- Circumscribed or lobulated mass, usually < 3 cm
- Calcifications may be present, particularly in older women, and will appear as cluster
- Calcifications may be coarse (large popcorn calcifications) or numerous and small
- Clustered calcifications may mimic those seen in ductal carcinoma in situ

Ultrasonographic Findings
- Circumscribed or lobulated mass

MR Findings
- Smooth-bordered mass
- May have nonenhancing internal septations
- Enhancement is generally slower than that seen with carcinomas

CYTOPATHOLOGY

Pattern
- Fragments of benign ductal cells and stroma associated with abundant naked nuclei in background form triad of findings in FA
- FAs can be cellular with stromal fragments of mildly increased cellularity and mildly increased numbers of individual stromal cells without cytologic atypia
- Stromal fragments are sharply demarcated fibrotic, myxoid, or fibromyxoid; usually of low cellularity composed of few spindle cells that do not exhibit atypia
  o Stromal fragments are metachromatic on Diff-Quik
- Cytologic features of cellular FA overlap with low-grade phyllodes tumor

Background
- Naked nuclei in background of smear are derived from myoepithelial cells or stromal cells
  o Naked nuclei are small, oval, bipolar, or elongated with condensed chromatin
  o Few individual stromal cells with elongated vesicular nucleus, small nucleolus, and scant cytoplasm are present
- Myxoid degeneration of stroma in myxoid FA results in presence of myxoid stromal fragments and thin myxoid material in background of smear
  o Fragments of benign epithelial cells and naked nuclei are distributed in myxoid background in myxoid FA

Cells
- Epithelial cells arranged as honeycomb sheets, papillary fronds, tubule like or tight clusters with associated myoepithelial cells
- Single epithelial cells can be present in background
- Apocrine metaplasia can be noted
- FA can undergo infarction, particularly during pregnancy; reactive/degenerative changes in epithelial cells can mimic malignancy

Fibroadenoma

Nuclear Details
- Epithelial cells usually demonstrate round/oval nuclei with smooth nuclear membrane and fine, evenly distributed chromatin
- Epithelial cells in fragments and single cells in background can show cytologic atypia, including nuclear enlargement, pleomorphism, presence of nucleolus, and mitotic figures

MACROSCOPIC
Gross Appearance
- FNA of FA yields shiny, gelatinous, sticky mucoid material

DIFFERENTIAL DIAGNOSIS
Fibrocystic Changes
- Usually low cellularity with few clusters of benign ductal epithelial cells, rare fragments of dense stroma, few naked nuclei, and scattered, foamy macrophages in background
- Clinical and imaging findings are different; fibrocystic changes are associated with ill-defined areas of thickening, whereas FAs present as well-defined nodules

Phyllodes Tumor
- Uncommon fibroepithelial neoplasm accounting for < 1% of primary mammary tumors
- Typically occurs in older patients than FA does (median age at diagnosis: 45 years)
- Cytologic features of low-grade phyllodes tumor overlap with cellular FA and cannot be distinguished on FNA
- Malignant phyllodes tumor can be easily distinguished from FA based on presence of very cellular stromal fragments with cytologically and mitotically active spindle cells, unlike FA

Ductal Carcinoma
- FA is most common cause of false-positive and false-negative diagnoses of malignancy
- Cytologic atypia in epithelial cells in fragments and in background can be mistaken for ductal carcinoma
  - Clusters of low-grade ductal carcinoma with few intact tumor cells in background can mimic FA
- Well-defined mobile mass in FA, unlike ductal carcinoma
- Recognition of fragments of benign ductal cells with associated myoepithelial cells, fibromyxoid fragments, and abundant naked bipolar nuclei in background supports FA over ductal carcinoma

Papilloma
- Very often shows dilated duct adjacent to vascular mass by imaging
- Papillary fronds of epithelial cells in FA can be mistaken for papillomas; papillary fronds in FAs lack fibrovascular cores, unlike papillomas
- Cytologic findings can overlap with those of FA when fibrovascular cores are absent in aspirated material
- Does not show fibromyxoid stromal fragments noted in FA
  - Generally shows proportionately more intact epithelial cells, including columnar cells, than FA does

Mucinous Carcinoma
- Myxoid FA with abundant myxoid material in background can mimic mucinous carcinoma
- Shows clusters of atypical cells without myoepithelial cells, unlike myxoid FA
- Atypical cells distributed in mucin, unlike benign epithelial fragments, and many naked nuclei in background mucin in myxoid FA

Hamartoma (Fibroadenolipoma)
- Well-circumscribed lesion composed of overgrowth of epithelial and stromal cells
- Considerable overlap in cytologic findings between FA and hamartoma
- Fragments of mature adipose tissue are usually encountered in hamartoma and not in FA

Pseudoangiomatous Stromal Hyperplasia
- Proliferation of interlobular myofibroblasts that surround rather than distort epithelial elements
  - Characteristic clefting of stroma; can form circumscribed or ill-defined mass or involve FAs
  - Findings can be similar with FAs except for increase in number of elongated, intact spindle cells in background of smear in pseudoangiomatous stromal hyperplasia

Tubular Adenoma
- Circumscribed lesion usually occurring in young women, similar to FA
- Clusters of benign ductal epithelial cells with rounded contours without stromal fragments
- Usually demonstrate much lower numbers of naked nuclei in background
- These lesions are most likely hyperplasias with predominance of epithelial elements, unlike both epithelial and stromal elements in FAs

Nodular Adenosis/Adenosis Tumor
- Conglomeration of lobules with sclerosing adenosis can form well-defined mass similar to FA
- Clusters of benign ductal epithelial cells, associated with naked nuclei and fragments of fibrotic stroma in background, can mimic FA

Adenomyoepithelioma
- Well-defined breast mass similar to FA
- Fragments of benign ductal cells with associated myoepithelial cells similar to FA
  - Naked bipolar nuclei, small clusters or single myoepithelial cells with epithelioid morphology can be noted
- Significant overlap in cytologic findings between FA and adenomyoepithelioma

SELECTED REFERENCES
1. Cheng CL et al: Artificial intelligence modelling in differentiating core biopsies of fibroadenoma from phyllodes tumor. Lab Invest. 102(3):245-52, 2022
2. Li JJX et al: Core needle biopsy diagnosis of fibroepithelial lesions of the breast: a diagnostic challenge. Pathology. 52(6):627-34, 2020
3. Sim Y et al: A novel genomic panel as an adjunctive diagnostic tool for the characterization and profiling of breast fibroepithelial lesions. BMC Med Genomics. 12(1):142, 2019
4. Dessauvagie BF et al: Interobserver variation in the diagnosis of fibroepithelial lesions of the breast: a multicentre audit by digital pathology. J Clin Pathol. 71(8):672-9, 2018
5. Krings G et al: Fibroepithelial lesions; the WHO spectrum. Semin Diagn Pathol. 34(5):438-52, 2017

Fibroadenoma

Stromal Fragment

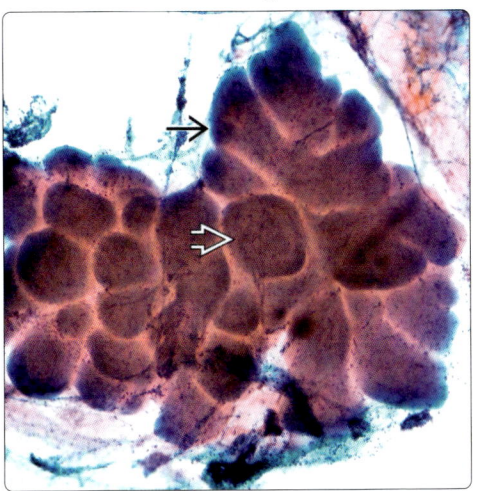

Metachromatic Stroma

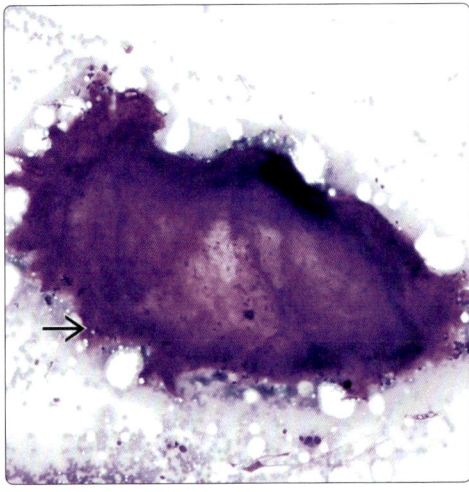

(Left) Pap-stained FNA smear of FA with a well-defined fibrotic stromal fragment ➡ shows many bulbous projections ➡. Note the large size and complexity of the fragment. (Right) Diff-Quik-stained FNA smear shows a metachromatic, well-defined fibromyxoid stromal fragment ➡ in a case of FA.

Myxoid Stromal Fragment

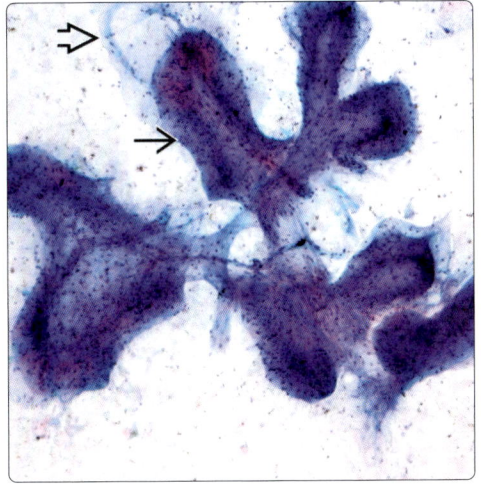

Spindle Cells in Myxoid Stroma

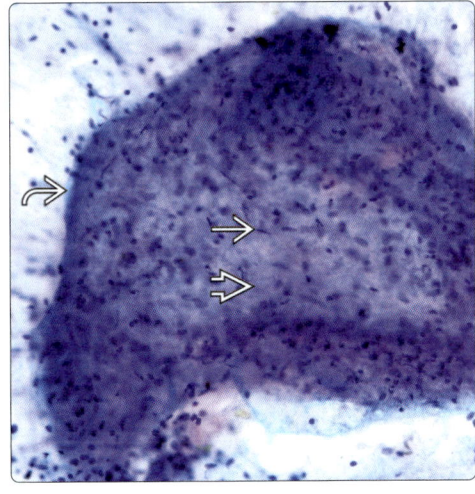

(Left) Pap-stained FNA smear of a myxoid FA shows a well-defined myxoid stromal fragment ➡. Wisps of myxoid material can also be seen in the background ➡. (Right) Pap-stained FNA smear shows a myxoid stromal fragment ➡ with spindle cells ➡ embedded within the myxoid stroma ➡.

Benign Epithelial Cells and Naked Nuclei

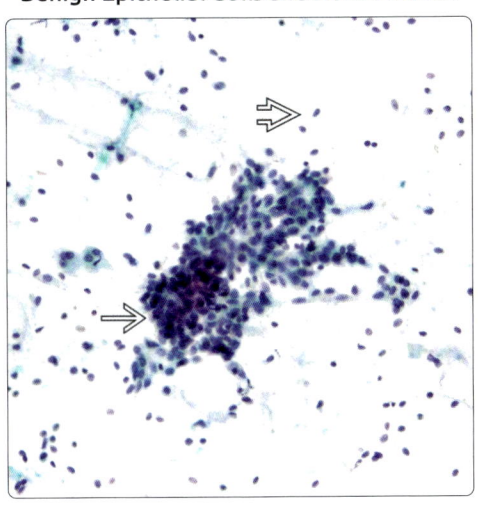

Honeycomb Sheet of Epithelial Cells

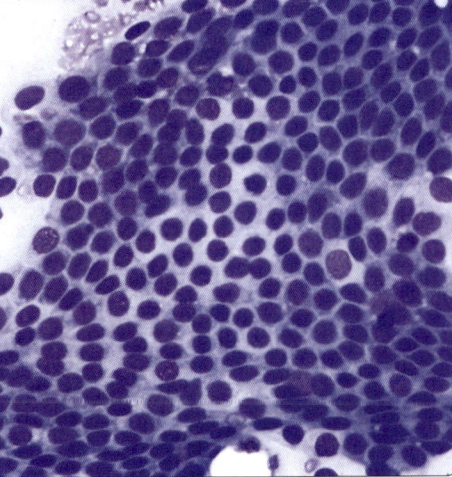

(Left) Pap-stained FNA smear shows a cohesive fragment of epithelial cells with associated myoepithelial cells ➡. Note the increased numbers of naked nuclei in the background of the smear ➡. (Right) Diff-Quik-stained FNA smear shows a honeycombed sheet of benign epithelial cells in FA. Despite the high cellularity, the uniform nuclei and architectural regularity indicate a benign process.

Granular Cell Tumor of Breast

KEY FACTS

CLINICAL ISSUES
- Rare breast tumor derived from Schwann cells
- Occurs most commonly in women of childbearing age

CYTOPATHOLOGY
- Moderately to highly cellular smears with polygonal or elongated cells, well-defined cell borders, and eccentric or centrally placed uniform round or oval nuclei
- Inconspicuous nucleolus with coarsely granular eosinophilic cytoplasm
- Mitotic activity insignificant; cells fragile and prone to disruption, resulting in naked nuclei and background filled with coarse granules
- Rarely, malignant granular cell tumor with large size, cellular pleomorphism, prominent nucleoli, significant mitotic activity, and necrosis can occur

ANCILLARY TESTS
- Granular cells: S100, NSE, vimentin, and CD68 (+); cytokeratin, myoglobin, desmin, ER, and PR (-)
- Granules seen on light microscopy correspond to numerous lysosomes seen on electron microscopy
- Granules PAS(+) and diastase resistant, better appreciated on Pap than on Diff-Quik stains

TOP DIFFERENTIAL DIAGNOSES
- Benign lesions containing histiocytes or apocrine cells
- Invasive carcinoma with apocrine, histiocytoid, or secretory features
- Metastatic tumors such as renal cell carcinoma or melanoma
- Alveolar soft part sarcoma

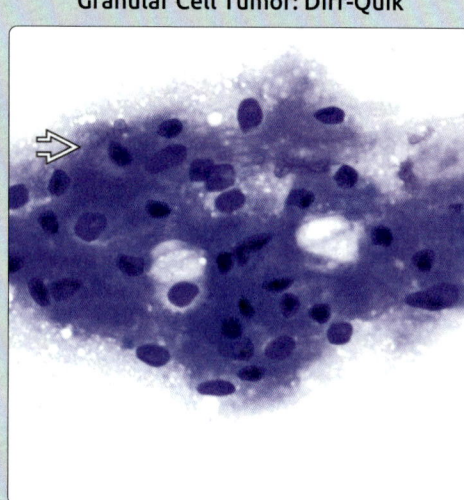

Granular Cell Tumor: Diff-Quik

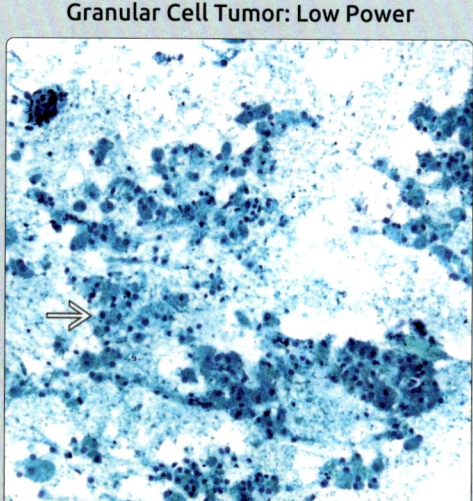

Granular Cell Tumor: Low Power

(Left) Diff-Quik-stained FNA smear shows a fragment of tumor cells with a low nuclear:cytoplasmic ratio ⇨; however, the granules in the cytoplasm are not apparent in comparison with Pap-stained smears. (Right) Pap-stained FNA shows a moderately cellular smear with loose clusters of tumor cells ⇨.

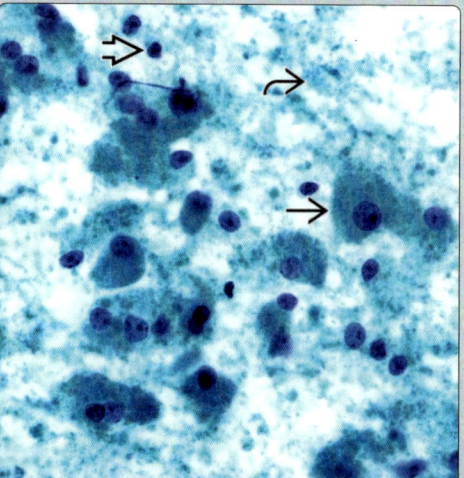

Granular Cell Tumor: Details

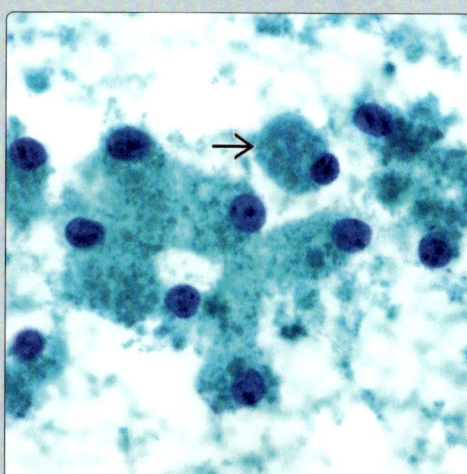

Granular Cell Tumor: Details

(Left) Pap-stained FNA smear shows tumor cells with granular cytoplasm ⇨ with few naked nuclei ⇨ and granular material in the background ⇨. (Right) Pap-stained FNA smear shows tumor cells with eccentric nucleus and abundant coarsely granular cytoplasm ⇨.

Granular Cell Tumor of Breast

TERMINOLOGY

Abbreviations
- Granular cell tumor (GCT)

Definitions
- Tumor of breast derived from Schwann cells, consisting of tumor cells with abundant eosinophilic, coarsely granular cytoplasm that ultrastructurally corresponds to lysosomes

CLINICAL ISSUES

Epidemiology
- Rare tumor; only 1 GCT per 100-200 cases of carcinoma
  - More common in women, with only 10% of tumors occurring in men
    - More common in Black than in White women

IMAGING

Mammographic Findings
- Mass with irregular, circumscribed, or lobulated borders; usually single but can be multiple in 5-10% of cases; calcifications generally absent

CYTOPATHOLOGY

Cells
- Moderately to highly cellular smears with polygonal or elongated cells, well-defined cell borders, and eccentric or centrally placed uniform round or oval nuclei
- Inconspicuous nucleolus with coarsely granular eosinophilic cytoplasm
- Mitotic activity insignificant; cells fragile and prone to disruption resulting in naked nuclei and background filled with coarse granules
- Rarely, malignant GCT with large size, cellular pleomorphism, prominent nucleoli, significant mitotic activity, and necrosis can occur

ANCILLARY TESTS

Histochemistry
- Granules PAS(+) and diastase resistant, better appreciated on Pap than on Diff-Quik stains

Immunohistochemistry
- Positive for S100, CD68, NSE, and vimentin
- Negative for cytokeratin, myoglobin, neurofilament, GFAP, ER, and PR

DIFFERENTIAL DIAGNOSIS

Benign Lesions
- With histiocytes/apocrine cells
  - Cause of inflammatory lesions, including histiocytes, usually apparent; inflammatory cells generally present
  - Apocrine cells have finely granular cytoplasm, CK(+)

Invasive Carcinoma
- Carcinomas with apocrine or histiocytoid features can resemble GCT
- Carcinomas exhibit cytologic atypia and CK(+)

Metastatic Tumors
- Tumor cells of metastatic melanoma and renal cell carcinoma may exhibit granular cytoplasm, have different immunoprofile (unlike GCT), and invariably show cytologic atypia

Alveolar Soft Part Sarcoma
- Tumor cells S100(-) and have translocation
  - der(17)t(X;17)(p11;q25), immunoreactive for TFE3

SELECTED REFERENCES

1. Mobarki M et al: Granular cell tumor a study of 42 cases and systemic review of the literature. Pathol Res Pract. 216(4):152865, 2020
2. Corso G et al: Granular cell tumor of the breast: molecular pathology and clinical management. Breast J. 24(5):778-82, 2018

Granular Cell Tumor: Cell Block
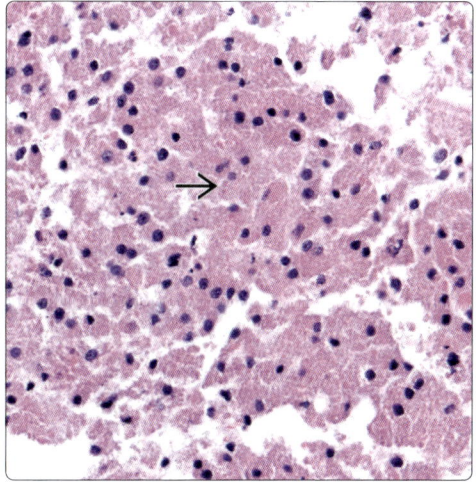

Granular Cell Tumor: S100 Positive
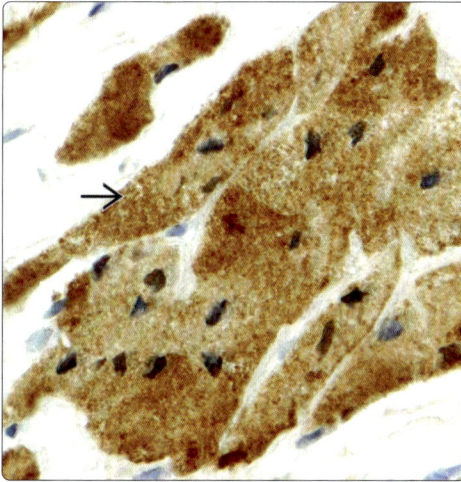

(Left) H&E-stained section of cell block prepared from FNA of granular cell tumor of the breast shows sheets of loosely cohesive tumor cells with abundant coarsely granular, eosinophilic cytoplasm ➡. (Right) Granular cell tumor shows cells diffusely and strongly positive for S100 ➡.

Papillary Neoplasms

KEY FACTS

CLASSIFICATION
- Lesions characterized by presence of fibrovascular stalks surrounded by benign or malignant epithelial proliferation
- Benign: Large duct papilloma, small duct papilloma
- Atypical: Partial involvement by malignancy (< 1/3)
- Malignant: Ductal carcinoma in situ, encapsulated papillary carcinoma, invasive papillary carcinoma

CYTOPATHOLOGY
- Characteristic feature of papillary neoplasms is presence of fibrovascular cores with associated epithelial proliferation
- Papillomas show variety of cells: Ductal cells, myoepithelial cells, apocrine metaplasia
  - Papillary clusters of benign ductal cells, often columnar in type, with associated myoepithelial cells
  - Naked bipolar nuclei and single epithelial cells in background
- Papillary carcinoma shows single type of atypical cells with wide range in degree of atypia without associated myoepithelial cells
  - Papillary carcinomas often show hyperchromatic stratified columnar nuclei ± mitotic activity
  - Tend to have more slender papillae than papillomas
  - Individual atypical cells in background without naked bipolar nuclei
- Proteinaceous material with hemosiderin-laden and foamy macrophages may be seen in background of benign and malignant papillary neoplasms
- Infarction can occur in benign and malignant papillary neoplasms, resulting in hemorrhage and necrosis

TOP DIFFERENTIAL DIAGNOSES
- Fibroadenoma
- Fibrocystic changes
- Ductal carcinoma
- Invasive micropapillary carcinoma

Papilloma, Branching Fibrovascular Stalk

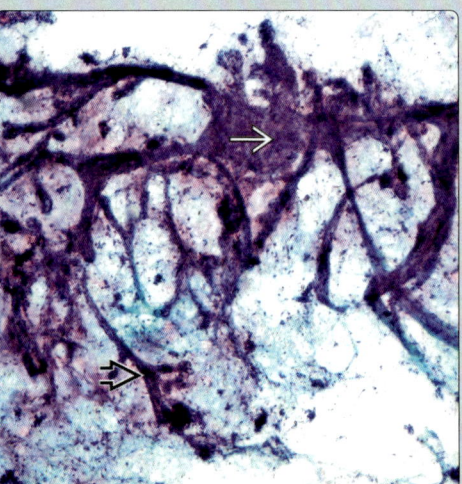

Papilloma With Complex Architecture

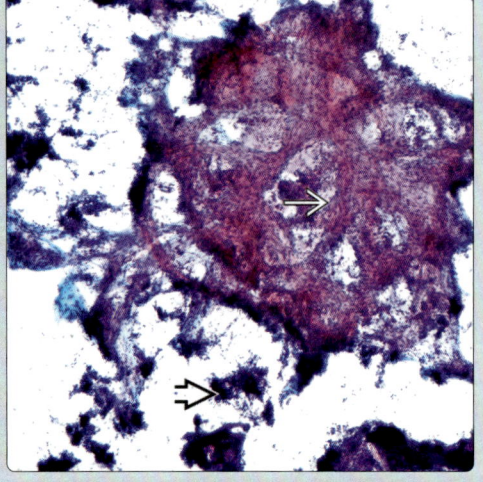

(Left) Pap-stained FNA smear of a papilloma shows the intricate branching ⮕ of the fibrovascular stalk ⮕ of a papilloma. (Right) Pap-stained FNA smear of a papilloma shows a fibrovascular core ⮕ with attached fragments of epithelial cells ⮕ of varying sizes.

Papilloma on Cell Block

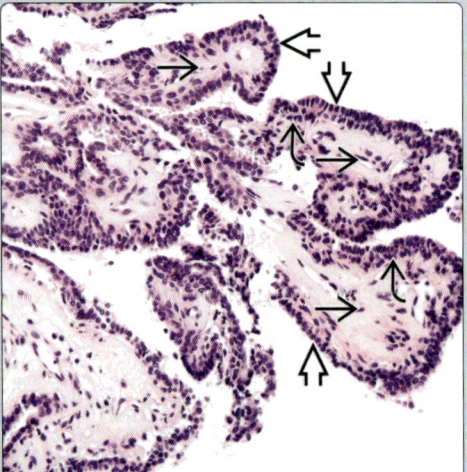

Papilloma, p63(+) Myoepithelial Cells

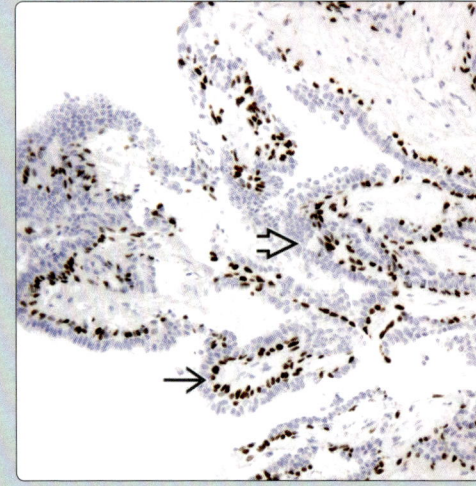

(Left) H&E-stained cell block section of a papilloma shows fibrovascular cores ⮕ surrounded by a luminal layer of benign ductal epithelial cells ⮕ and a basal layer of myoepithelial cells ⮕. (Right) Cell block section of a papilloma immunostained for the myoepithelial marker p63 highlights the presence of myoepithelial cells ⮕ beneath the luminal epithelial cells ⮕. The overall findings support the diagnosis of papilloma.

Papillary Neoplasms

TERMINOLOGY

Definitions
- Lesions characterized by fibrovascular cores surrounded by benign or malignant epithelial proliferation
  - **Benign**
    - Large duct papilloma (LDP)
    - Small duct papilloma (SDP)
  - **Atypical**
    - Partial involvement of papilloma by neoplastic cells
    - < 1/3 of lesion
  - **Malignant**
    - Ductal carcinoma in situ (DCIS): Papillary and nonpapillary types
    - Encapsulated papillary carcinoma (EPC): Intracystic papillary carcinoma, solid papillary carcinoma (SPC)
    - Invasive papillary carcinoma (IPC)

CLINICAL ISSUES

Epidemiology
- Age
  - LDP: Most common in women 35-50 years
  - SDP: Seen in younger women
  - DCIS: Seen in pre- and postmenopausal women
  - EPC: Most common in older women (70 years)
  - IPC: More common in postmenopausal women (65-70 years)

Presentation
- **LDP**
  - Palpable subareolar mass
    - Lobulated mass in imaging studies
  - Nipple discharge, unilateral, spontaneous
    - Sanguineous/serosanguineous in 80%
    - Can be bloody with malignancy or with infarction due to twisting on stalk of papillary lesion
- **SDP**
  - Usually does not cause mass or nipple discharge
  - Incidental finding on imaging or tissue biopsy
  - DCIS papillary and nonpapillary types, if present
  - Mammographic calcifications (85%); palpable mass or radiologic density (10%); nipple discharge (5%)
- **EPC**
  - Often presents as single palpable mass or circumscribed mammographic density
    - Mass can be multinodular with SPC
  - Location is usually central below nipple and deeper in breast than LDPs
    - May present with nipple discharge

Treatment
- Surgical excision for symptomatic or large papillomas and all papillary carcinomas
- Radiation therapy and hormonal therapy [ER(+) tumors] for papillary carcinoma

Prognosis
- Papillomas are benign
- Mild increased risk of subsequent carcinoma: 1.5-2.0x relative risk or 5-7% lifetime risk
  - Classified as proliferative disease without atypia
- Breast cancer risk is slightly higher for women with multiple peripheral SDPs (papillomatosis)
- EPC: Survival > 95% at 10 years; rarely metastasizes to lymph nodes or recurs
- DCIS: Recurrence rate is < 10% if treated by breast conservation surgery, radiation therapy, and hormonal therapy, and < 5% following mastectomy
- IPC: Prognosis is generally better than for invasive carcinoma of no special type

IMAGING

Mammographic Findings
- LDP: May not be visible on mammogram
- SDP: Can present as lobulated mass or cluster of calcifications
- EPC: Lobulated, well-circumscribed mass or multinodular in SPC
- DCIS papillary and nonpapillary types: Calcifications or density
- IPC: Ill-defined mass

Ultrasonographic Findings
- LDP: Intraductal, well-defined hypoechoic mass near nipple; may have solid and cystic components with dilatation of adjacent ducts
- SDP: Small, circumscribed or lobulated masses
- EPC: Lobulated hypoechoic mass
- IPC: Ill-defined hypoechoic mass

CYTOPATHOLOGY

General Features
- Cellularity usually high, often with proteinaceous material in background containing hemosiderin-laden and foamy macrophages
- Cellularity can be low if cystic content around papillary growth alone is aspirated or due to sclerosis of papillary lesion
- Characteristic feature of papillary neoplasms is presence of fibrovascular cores with associated epithelial proliferation
- Papillary carcinomas tend to have more slender papillae than papillomas
- Proliferative epithelial component of papillary neoplasm alone may be sampled, resulting in absence of fibrovascular cores in aspirated material in some cases
- Papillary clusters of epithelial cells, including balls of cells, are commonly present
- Infarction can occur in benign and malignant papillary neoplasms, resulting in hemorrhage and necrosis
- Psammoma bodies can be seen in benign and malignant papillary neoplasms

Papilloma
- Shows variety of cells, including epithelial cells, myoepithelial cells, and apocrine cells
- Shows fragments of ductal epithelial cells with associated myoepithelial cells; hyperplasia of ductal epithelial cells without atypia can be noted
- Naked bipolar nuclei are commonly present in background of smears in papillomas
- Can show many single or loose clusters of epithelial cells without atypia in background

Papillary Neoplasms

- Palisades of benign columnar cells composed of fragments and individually distributed columnar cells are commonly noted in papillomas
- Fragments of epithelial cells with dense eosinophilic cytoplasm ± vacuolation can often be noted in papillomas
- Apocrine metaplasia can be present in papillomas
- Cytologic atypia, including nuclear enlargement, pleomorphism, prominent nucleoli, and mitotic figures, can be present in epithelial cells in papillomas
- Squamous metaplasia and cytologic atypia can be noted in papillomas following infarction, which can mimic malignancy
- Collagenous spherulosis composed of rounded balls of collagen cores can be noted in papillomas but are not specific findings

Atypical Papillary Neoplasms
- Show fragments of atypical monotonous epithelial cells with abnormal architectural patterns, including solid or cribriform areas
- Other features similar to papillomas

Papillary Carcinoma
- Shows fragments of atypical epithelial cells without associated myoepithelial cells
- Naked bipolar nuclei are absent from background
- Individually distributed atypical epithelial cells can be noted in papillary carcinomas
- Often shows hyperchromatic stratified columnar nuclei ± mitotic activity and without associated myoepithelial cells
- Fragments of atypical monotonous epithelial cells with varying grades of atypia without columnar morphology can be present in association with fibrovascular cores in some papillary carcinomas
- Shows single population of malignant cells, unlike papillomas

Cell Block Findings
- Aspirates of papillary neoplasms are very cellular, which allows preparation of cell blocks directly from aspiration or scraped from cellular smears
- Fibrovascular cores surrounded by epithelial and myoepithelial cells in papillomas and atypical epithelial cells alone without associated myoepithelial cells in papillary carcinomas can be easily appreciated in cell blocks

ANCILLARY TESTS

Immunohistochemistry
- Cell blocks of papillary neoplasms can be used for immunostaining to demonstrate presence or absence of myoepithelial cells
- Myoepithelial markers, such as p63, calponin, SMMHC, and SMA, can be used
- CK5/6 may be useful to distinguish atypical hyperplasia/DCIS involving papillomas from florid hyperplasia without atypia
  - Atypical hyperplasia/DCIS involving papillomas will be negative, whereas florid hyperplasia will have some positive cells
- Tumor cells of SPC can be positive for neuroendocrine markers
- Papillary carcinomas are usually positive for ER and PR

DIFFERENTIAL DIAGNOSIS

Fibroadenoma
- Papillomas that lack fibrovascular cores in aspirated material can mimic fibroadenomas (FAs) due to high cellularity and complex architecture
- Papillomas commonly show clusters and single columnar cells
- Papillomas very often show proteinaceous material in background with hemosiderin-laden and foamy macrophages, unlike FAs
- FAs usually show well-defined fibromyxoid stromal fragments

Fibrocystic Changes
- Papillomas of low cellularity that do not contain fibrovascular cores in aspirated material can mimic fibrocystic change (FCC)
- FCC can also be associated with proteinaceous material with foamy macrophages in background similar to papillomas
- Imaging findings are different between 2 entities
- Areas of ill-defined thickening of breast parenchyma in FCC
  - Relatively well-circumscribed intraductal mass ± adjacent dilated duct in papillomas
- Papillomas commonly show clusters and single columnar cells more often than FCC

Ductal Carcinoma
- Fragments of atypical ductal epithelium without associated myoepithelial cells in papillary carcinoma may mimic ductal carcinomas
- Presence of fibrovascular cores in papillary carcinomas, unlike ductal carcinomas
- Papillary carcinoma may demonstrate fragments and single hyperchromatic columnar cells, unlike ductal carcinomas

Invasive Micropapillary Carcinoma
- Unusual type of invasive carcinoma with clusters of tumor cells in clear spaces, which is represented in smears by clusters of tumor cells with inside-out/inverted pattern
- Fibrovascular cores are absent, unlike papillary carcinoma
- Tumor cells are not columnar and stratified, unlike many papillary carcinomas

SELECTED REFERENCES

1. Kulka J et al: Papillary lesions of the breast. Virchows Arch. 480(1):65-84, 2022
2. Ross DS et al: Papillary neoplasms of the breast: diagnostic features and molecular insights. Surg Pathol Clin. 15(1):133-46, 2022
3. Brogi E et al: Papillary neoplasms of the breast including upgrade rates and management of intraductal papilloma without atypia diagnosed at core needle biopsy. Mod Pathol. 34(Suppl 1):78-93, 2021
4. Jamidi SK et al: Papillary lesions of the breast: a systematic evaluation of cytologic parameters. Cancer Cytopathol. 129(8):649-61, 2021
5. Salemis NS et al: Encapsulated papillary carcinoma of the breast. Breast J. 27(3):280-3, 2021
6. Vielh P: Deep learning of breast papillary lesions. Cancer Cytopathol. 129(8):577-8, 2021
7. Rakha EA et al: Diagnostic challenges in papillary lesions of the breast. Pathology. 50(1):100-10, 2018
8. Rageth CJ et al: First International Consensus Conference on lesions of uncertain malignant potential in the breast (B3 lesions). Breast Cancer Res Treat. 159(2):203-13, 2016

Papillary Neoplasms

Papilloma, Ductal Epithelial Hyperplasia

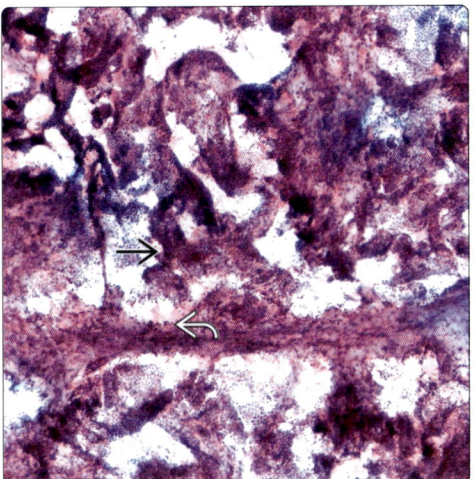

Papilloma Mimicking Fibroadenoma

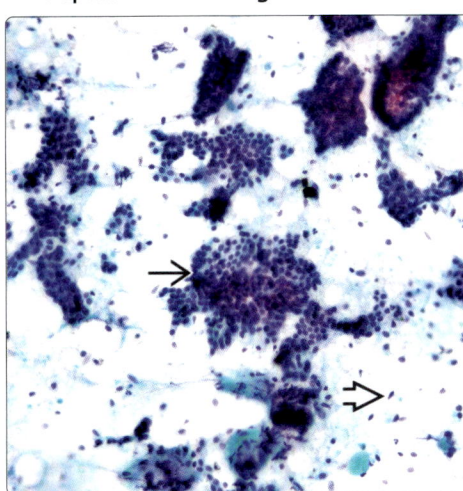

(Left) Pap-stained FNA smear of a papilloma shows the fibrovascular core ➡ associated with large sheets of benign ductal epithelial cells with features consistent with florid ductal epithelial hyperplasia ➡. (Right) Pap-stained FNA smear of a papilloma shows fragments of cohesive benign ductal epithelial cells ➡ with many naked bipolar nuclei ➡ in the background. This pattern is reminiscent of fibroadenoma.

Papilloma With Proteinaceous Material

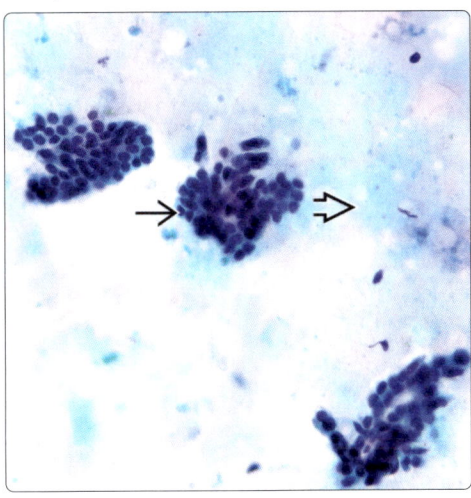

Papilloma Mimicking Ductal Carcinoma

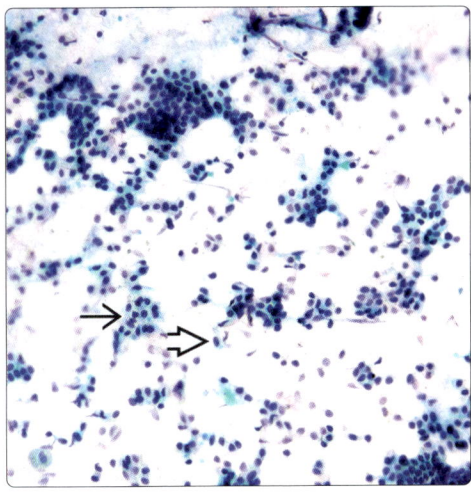

(Left) Pap-stained FNA smear of a papilloma shows fragments of tightly cohesive benign ductal epithelial cells ➡ associated with proteinaceous material ➡ in the background. This is a commonly encountered cytologic finding in papillomas. (Right) Pap-stained FNA smear of a papilloma shows high cellularity composed of many loose clusters ➡ and single benign ductal epithelial cells ➡. These features can mimic ductal carcinoma and lead to a false-positive diagnosis.

Papilloma, Columnar Cells

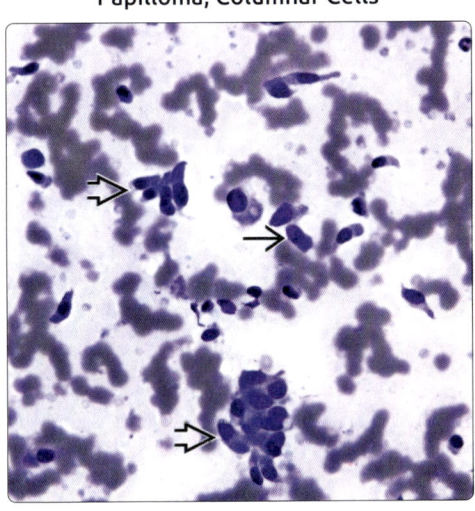

Papilloma, Collagenous Spherulosis

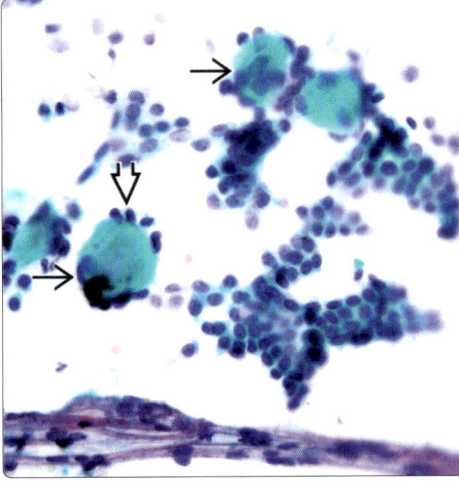

(Left) Diff-Quik-stained FNA smear of a papilloma shows a few clusters ➡ as well as single benign columnar cells ➡. Papillomas commonly demonstrate benign ductal epithelial cells with columnar features. (Right) Pap-stained FNA smear of a papilloma shows collagenous spherulosis ➡. Note the rounded balls of collagen bordered by naked nuclei ➡ derived from myoepithelial cells.

Papillary Neoplasms

(Left) *Pap-stained FNA smear of a papilloma shows strips of epithelial cells ➡ with moderate amounts of dense cytoplasm. The presence of such benign epithelial cells can be noted in focal areas of the smear in papillomas.* **(Right)** *Pap-stained FNA smear of a papilloma shows higher magnification of ductal epithelial cells. Note that the fragment of ductal epithelial cells demonstrates moderate amounts of dense, well-defined cytoplasm ➡ with a vesicular, centrally or eccentrically placed nucleus.*

Papilloma, Benign Epithelial Strips
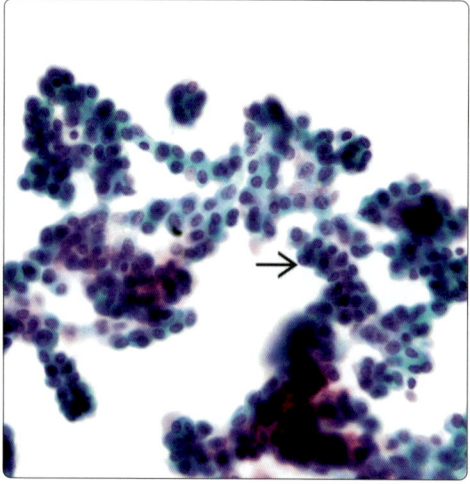

Papilloma, Ductal Epithelial Cells
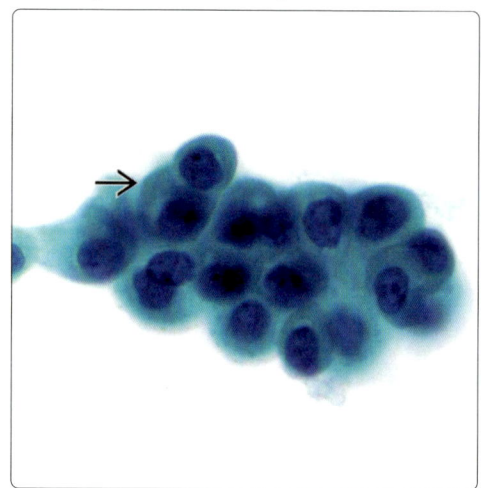

(Left) *Pap-stained FNA smear of a papilloma shows the intricate branching ➡ of the fibrovascular core.* **(Right)** *Cell block section of papilloma immunostained for SMA highlights the myoepithelial cells ➡ beneath the luminal epithelial cells.*

Papilloma, Fibrovascular Core
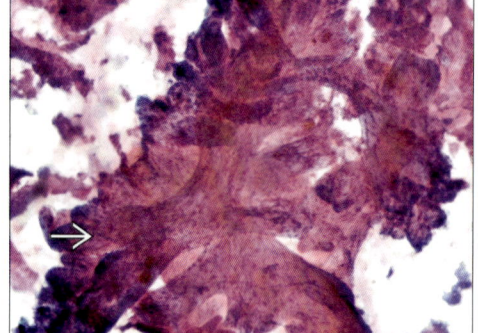

Papilloma, SMA(+) Myoepithelial Cells
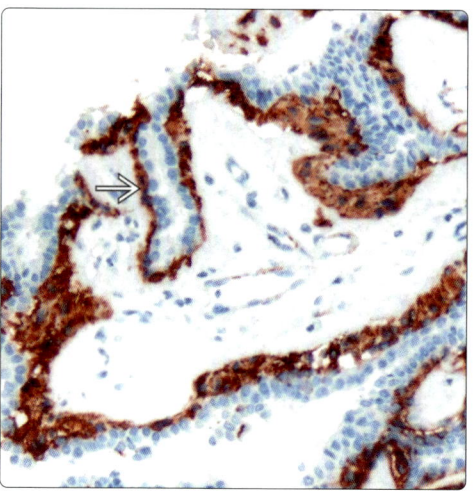

(Left) *Pap-stained FNA smear of papillary carcinoma shows fragments of hyperchromatic tumor cells ➡. Note that, unlike papillomas, there are no naked bipolar nuclei in the background of the smear.* **(Right)** *Pap-stained FNA smear of papillary carcinoma shows higher magnification of the tumor cells. Note the strip of columnar hyperchromatic tumor cells ➡ and end-on view of the same cells ➡ in an adjacent fragment of tumor cells. Myoepithelial cells are absent from the clusters.*

Papillary Carcinoma, Hyperchromasia
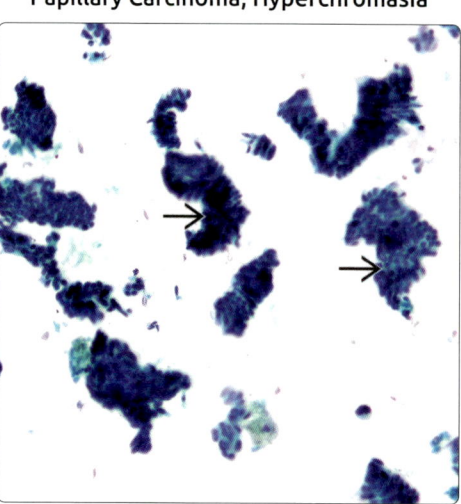

Papillary Carcinoma on High Power
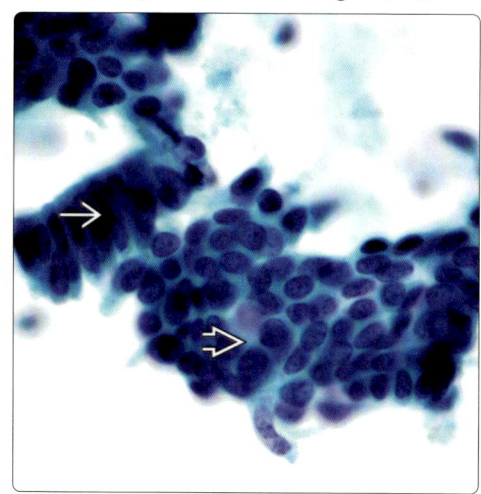

Papillary Neoplasms

Papillary Carcinoma, Columnar Cells

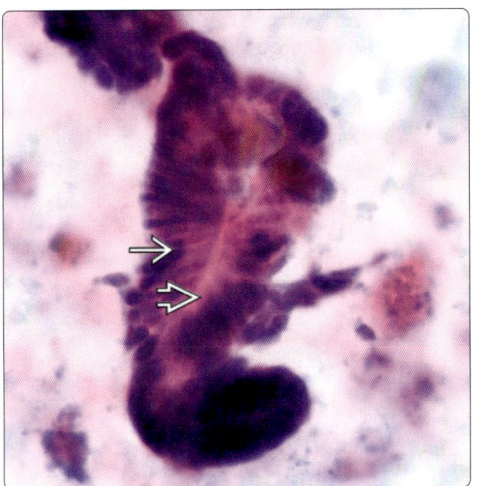

Papillary Carcinoma on Cell Block

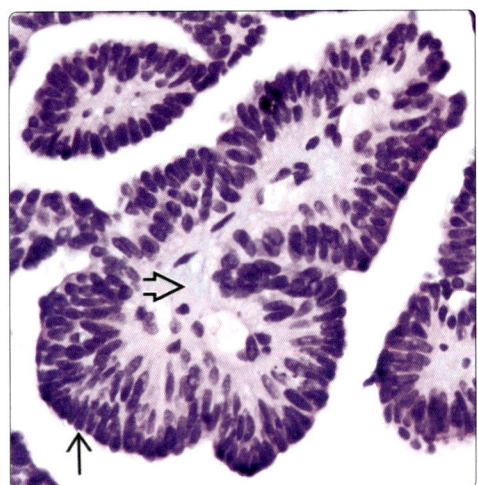

(Left) Pap-stained FNA smear in a case of intracystic papillary carcinoma shows a fragment of stratified columnar tumor cells ⇨. The tumor cells are arranged around a thin fibrovascular core ⇨. (Right) H&E-stained cell block section in a case of intracystic papillary carcinoma shows stratified columnar tumor cells ⇨ associated with a fibrovascular core ⇨. Note the absence of a basal layer of myoepithelial cells beneath the luminal layer of columnar cells.

Papillary Lesion With Infarction

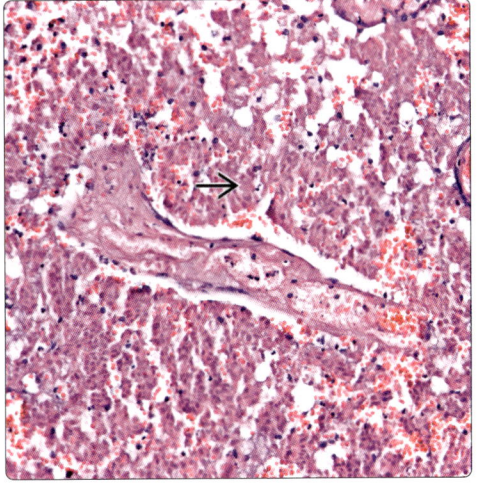

Papillary Carcinoma, Necrosis

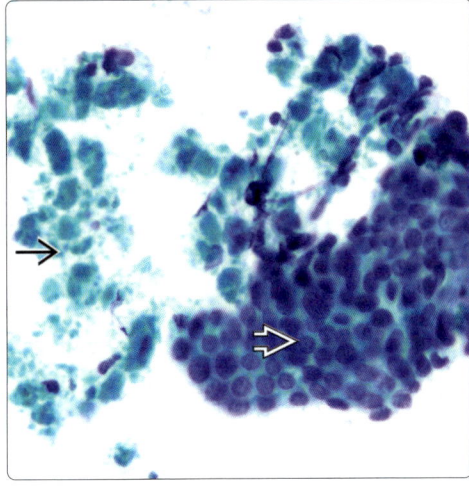

(Left) H&E-stained cell block section shows an infarcted papillary lesion ⇨. Note that the cellular details of the constituent cells are lost. The presence of fibrovascular cores in the lesion allows categorization as a papillary lesion. (Right) Pap-stained FNA smear in a case of papillary carcinoma shows necrosis ⇨ associated with a fragment of tumor cells ⇨. Note that the tumor cells demonstrate hyperchromatic, uniform nuclei and are not associated with myoepithelial cells.

Papillary Carcinoma, Loose Cohesion

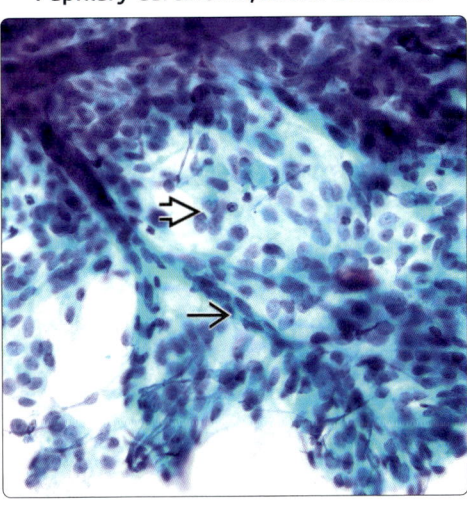

Papillary Carcinoma, Nuclear Features

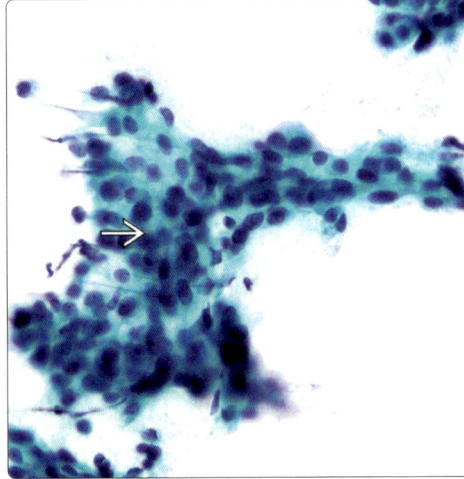

(Left) Pap-stained FNA smear in a case of solid papillary carcinoma shows loosely cohesive tumor cells ⇨ distributed around thin fibrovascular cores ⇨. Myoepithelial cells are absent in the lesion. (Right) Pap-stained FNA smear in a case of solid papillary carcinoma shows a fragment of tumor cells ⇨. The tumor cells demonstrate a vesicular nucleus without nucleolus associated with moderate amounts of delicate cytoplasm.

Myofibroblastoma, Mammary

KEY FACTS

CLINICAL ISSUES
- Benign, well-circumscribed mammary stromal tumor derived from mammary myofibroblasts
- Uncommon mammary neoplasm comprising < 1% of mammary tumors that typically occur in older patients (50-75 years); more commonly in males
- Palpable, painless, mobile, slow-growing, usually solitary mass

CYTOPATHOLOGY
- Fragments of spindle and plump, ovoid cells with insignificant atypia or mitotic activity
- Nuclear grooves and intranuclear inclusions may be present
- Positive for CD34, desmin, and vimentin
- Negative for S100, cytokeratin, and melanoma markers
- Positive for AR, ER, and PR

TOP DIFFERENTIAL DIAGNOSES
- Fibromatosis/nodular fascitis
  - Highly infiltrative lesions composed of myofibroblasts with markedly spindle-shaped nuclei that are CD34(-), unlike plump CD34(+) spindle cells of myofibroblastoma (MFB)
- Schwannoma
  - Spindle cells of MFB can be similar to schwannoma but immunophenotypic findings are different
    - Schwannoma are S100(+), CD34(-), and desmin (-)
- Spindle cell metaplastic carcinoma
  - Tumor mass with infiltrating edges composed of spindle and epithelioid tumor cells or spindle cells alone with varying degrees of cytologic atypia with evidence of positive cytokeratin expression
- Metastatic melanoma
  - Spindle cells of melanoma generally exhibit cytologic atypia and are positive for S100 and other melanoma markers, unlike MFB

Myofibroblastoma Spindle Cells
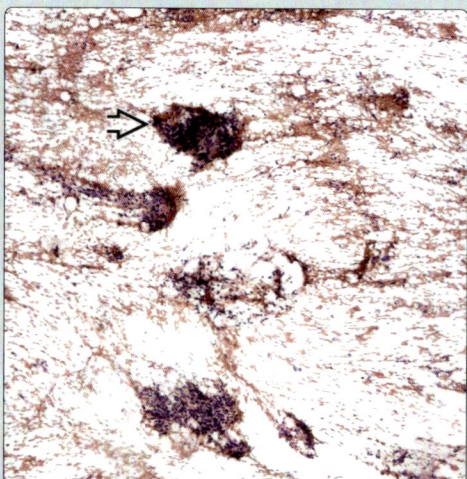

Loosely Cohesive Spindle Cells
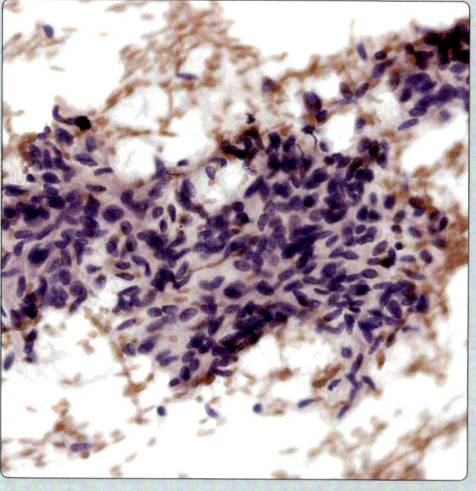

(Left) Pap-stained FNA smear of myofibroblastoma (MFB) shows fragments containing spindle cells of varying sizes ➡. (Right) Pap-stained FNA smear of MFB shows a single fragment comprised of loosely cohesive spindle cells.

Myofibroblastoma
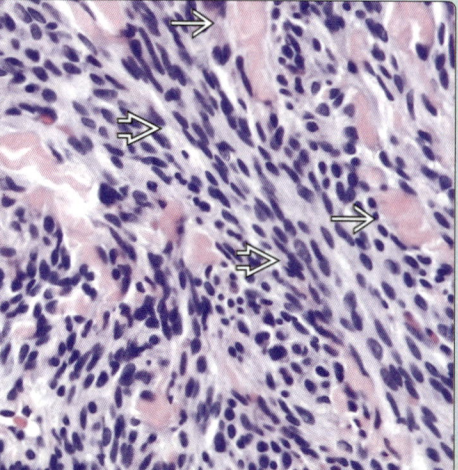

CD34 Positive in Myofibroblastoma
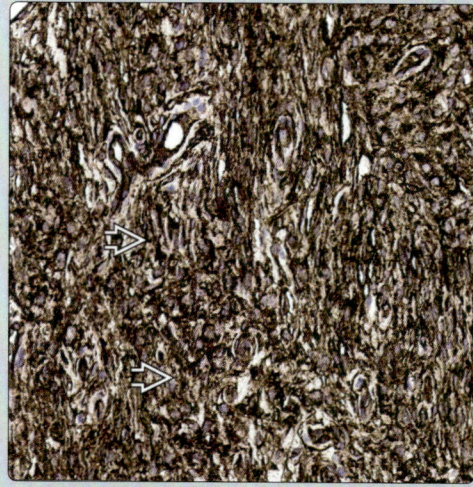

(Left) Core biopsy of MFB stained with H&E shows plump spindle cells ➡ without significant atypia associated with thick bands of collagen ➡. (Right) Core biopsy of MFB immunostained with CD34 shows the spindle tumor cells to be diffusely positive ➡, which is one of the defining features of this tumor.

Myofibroblastoma, Mammary

TERMINOLOGY

Abbreviations
- Myofibroblastoma (MFB)

Definitions
- Benign spindle cell mammary tumor derived from mammary myofibroblasts

ETIOLOGY/PATHOGENESIS

Hormonal and Genetic Factors
- Characteristically expresses AR, ER, and PR
  - Chromosome 13 rearrangements associated with loss of 13q14 and partial loss of 16q are commonly noted

CLINICAL ISSUES

Epidemiology
- Incidence
  - Uncommon mammary neoplasm comprising < 1% of mammary tumors that typically occur in older patients (50-75 years); majority of cases reported in males

Presentation
- Palpable, painless, mobile, slow-growing, solitary unilateral, bilateral, or multicentric mass; usually ~ 2 cm in size

Prognosis
- No recurrences following surgical excision

IMAGING

Mammographic, US, and MR Findings
- Well-demarcated, circumscribed, or lobulated mass with features similar to those seen in fibroadenoma

CYTOPATHOLOGY

Cells and Background
- Variable cellularity with fragments of loosely cohesive spindle cells and scattered single cells in background
  - Spindle cells may show palisading in some fragments
- Nuclear shape ranges from very spindle with condensed nuclear chromatin to plump and ovoid with vesicular chromatin
- Nuclear grooves and intranuclear inclusions can be present
- Tumor cells can exhibit mild pleomorphism
  - Mitotic activity is inconspicuous
- Rare types of MFB can show distinctly epithelioid cells or cells resembling decidual cells
- Mast cells, fibrotic or myxoid stromal fragments, and adipose tissue may be present
  - Epithelial cells are usually absent

ANCILLARY TESTS

Immunophenotype
- Positive: Vimentin, desmin, CD34, CD10; ER, PR, and AR
- Frequently positive for SMA, BCL2, CD99
- Negative for cytokeratin, EMA, S100, HMB-45, and C-kit

DIFFERENTIAL DIAGNOSIS

Fibromatosis/Nodular Fascitis
- Cells are CD34(-), unlike plump CD34(+) spindle cells of MFB

Schwannoma
- Schwannoma are S100(+), CD34(-), and desmin (-)

Spindle Cell Metaplastic Carcinoma
- Varying degrees of cytologic atypia with evidence of positive cytokeratin expression

Metastatic Melanoma
- Positive for S100 and other melanoma markers, unlike MFB

SELECTED REFERENCES
1. Yan M et al: Clinicopathological and radiological characterization of myofibroblastoma of breast: a single institutional case review. Ann Diagn Pathol. 48:151591, 2020

Ovoid Cells
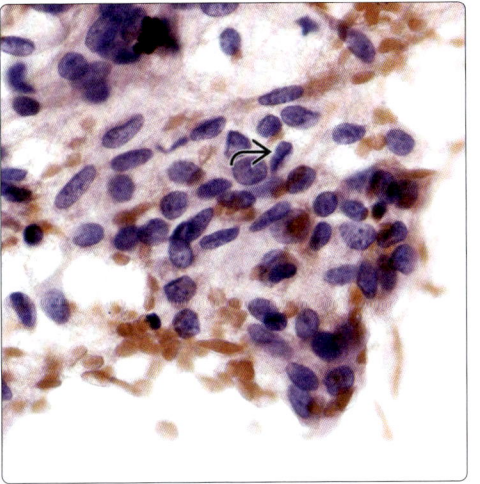

Spindle Cell Cytologic Features
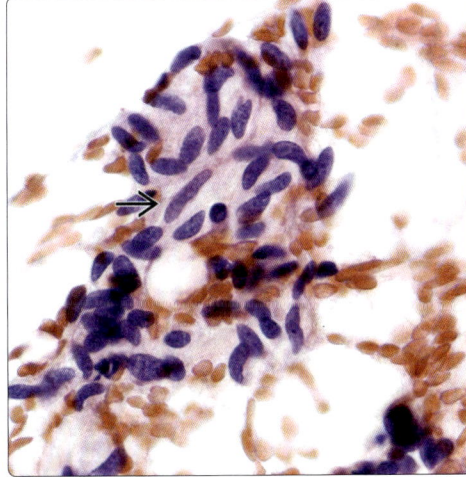

(Left) Pap-stained FNA smear of MFB shows plump, ovoid tumor cells with vesicular chromatin. Note the presence of nuclear grooves in some of the tumor cells ➔. (Right) Pap-stained FNA smear of MFB shows spindle cells with scant cytoplasm and condensed nuclear chromatin ➔.

Ductal Carcinoma and Variants of Invasive Mammary Carcinoma

TERMINOLOGY

Definitions

- Ductal carcinoma in situ (DCIS): Ductal carcinoma restricted within basement membrane of ducts and acini of breast lobules
- Invasive ductal carcinoma (IDC): Ductal carcinoma invading stroma
  - Tumors of no special histologies are referred to as IDC of no special type/not otherwise specified (NOS)

IDC Special Histologic Types

- Tubular carcinoma (TC)
- Invasive cribriform carcinoma (CC)
- Mucinous (colloid) carcinoma (MUC)
- Medullary carcinoma (MEC)
- Invasive micropapillary carcinoma (IMPC)
- Invasive papillary carcinoma (IPC)
- Invasive apocrine carcinoma (IAC)
- Neuroendocrine tumor
  - Tumor must express ≥ 1 neuroendocrine marker in > 50% of tumor cells
  - Carcinoma must have morphologic features similar to neuroendocrine tumors of lung and gastrointestinal tract
    - Solid neuroendocrine carcinoma
    - Small cell carcinoma
    - Large cell neuroendocrine carcinoma
- Metaplastic carcinoma (MPC)
  - Carcinomas with squamous &/or spindle cells
    - Squamous carcinoma
    - Spindle cell carcinoma
    - Adenosquamous carcinoma
    - Low-grade carcinoma with fibromatosis-like stroma
  - Matrix-producing MPC
  - Carcinosarcoma
- Lipid-rich carcinoma
- Glycogen-rich clear cell carcinoma
- Adenoid cystic carcinoma (ACC)
  - Correlate of more common salivary gland carcinoma
- Secretory carcinoma (SEC)
  - Correlate of salivary gland and thyroid carcinoma
  - Usually has t(12;15)(p13;q25) translocation, *ETV6::NTRK3* fusion gene

EPIDEMIOLOGY

Incidence

- Majority of breast cancers occur in women
  - 1 in 100 breast cancer cases occur in men
- DCIS: Comprises < 5% in populations without mammographic screening; with screening, 20-30% of carcinomas are detected as DCIS
- IDC: Highest incidence of invasive breast cancer is in White women and lowest is in Native American women
  - Black women have lower incidence than White women but have higher mortality rates
  - Hispanic women have lower incidence and lower mortality rates
- Majority of IDCs of special histologic types are very rare and occur in < 1% of all breast cancers except TC/CC and MUC
- TC/CC and MUC occur in 1-4% and up to 7% of all breast tumors, respectively

Age Range

- DCIS: Wide age range, including pre- and post menopause
- IDC: Median age at diagnosis is 61 years
  - < 15% of invasive breast cancers are diagnosed before age 44
  - MUC tends to occur in older women (66 years)
  - SEC occurs over wide age range: < 5 years to > 80 years (median: 25 years)

Presentation

- DCIS: Mammographic calcifications in 85%, palpable mass or radiologic density in 10%, nipple discharge in 5%, Paget disease of nipple in < 1%
- IDC: Patients present most commonly with palpable mass or abnormality on screening
  - For women < 40 years, 85% of carcinomas are detected as palpable mass and 15% on breast imaging

Ductal Carcinoma: 3D Clusters

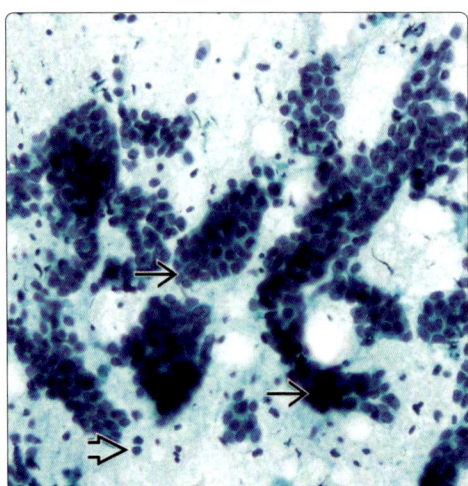

Invasive Ductal Carcinoma

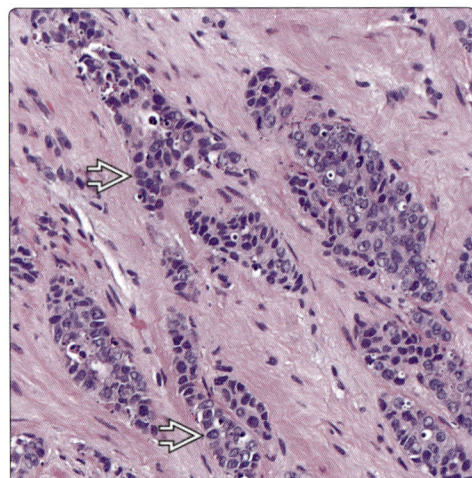

(Left) Pap-stained FNA smear of a low-grade ductal carcinoma shows high cellularity with many 3D clusters ➡ of different shapes and sizes, which contain many tumor cells, and single cells ➡. (Right) Core biopsy of invasive ductal carcinoma, stained with H&E, shows irregular clusters of tumor cells ➡ of varying sizes and shapes without lumen formation. The tumor cells demonstrate moderate nuclear pleomorphism without any evidence of myoepithelial cells surrounding the clusters.

Ductal Carcinoma and Variants of Invasive Mammary Carcinoma

- For women > 40 years, 60% are detected by screening and 15% on breast imaging
- Palpable cancers are larger (2-3 cm on average) than screen-detected cancers (1-2 cm on average)
- IDCs of special histologic types that present as well-circumscribed lobulated mass: MUC and MEC
- Uncommon presentations of IDCs include nipple discharge and Paget disease
- Axillary nodal or distant metastasis may be 1st sign, especially in women who have not undergone screening or in aggressive variants

Treatment

- DCIS: Surgery, either segmental mastectomy with clean margins or mastectomy, usually for widespread disease
  - Radiation therapy for patients treated with segmental mastectomy
  - Hormonal therapy for ER(+) DCIS
- Most patients with IDCs will be treated with multiple modalities
  - Surgery: Controls local disease and may be curative for localized cancers
  - Radiation therapy: Reduces local recurrences and has smaller effect on survival
  - Endocrine therapy: Improves survival for patients with hormone-sensitive tumors
  - Chemotherapy: Systemic therapy for selected patients with sensitive cancers; general correlation with higher proliferative rates
  - *HER2*-targeted therapy improves survival for carcinomas with overexpression

Prognosis

- DCIS
  - If treated with complete excision with radiation and hormonal therapy, risk of recurrence is < 10%
  - If treated by mastectomy, risk of recurrence is < 5%
- IDC: Depends on tumor stage, tumor grade, biomarker expression
  - TC and CC have excellent prognosis
  - MUC and MEC (when strictly defined by morphologic criteria) have favorable prognosis with 10-year survival rate > 80%
    - Patients with MUC have lower incidence, and those with IMPC have higher incidence of lymph node metastasis than those with IDC, NOS
  - IMPC: More aggressive clinical course and increased incidence of local recurrence compared with IDC, NOS
    - Strongly associated with lymphovascular invasion

ETIOLOGY/PATHOGENESIS

Pathogenesis

- DCIS: Biologically heterogeneous, belonging to 4 genomic types similar to IDC
  - *HER2* subtype is more frequent, and triple negative is less frequent than IDC
- IDC: Heterogeneous group of carcinomas with regard to pathologic features, prognosis, and clinical outcome
  - IDC, NOS forms 75% of invasive tumors
  - Remaining 25% fall under invasive carcinomas of special histologic types
- IDCs can be divided into 4 major types at genomic level
  - Luminal A (55%): ER(+), PR(+), HER2(-)
  - Luminal B (15%): ER(+), PR(+), HER2(+)
  - HER2 (15-20%): ER(-), PR(-), HER2(+)
  - Basal-like (10-15%): ER(-), PR(-), HER2(-); a.k.a. triple-negative
  - Gene expression profiling demonstrates that each type shares global expression patterns

CLINICAL IMPLICATIONS

Imaging Findings

- Mammographic findings
  - Majority of IDCs form irregular masses
  - Circumscribed or lobulated masses; basal-like/triple-negative cancers, MUC, MEC
  - Calcifications in DCIS and IDCs with associated DCIS; TC/CC commonly associated with calcifications
  - Architectural distortion is uncommon finding
- Ultrasonographic findings
  - Majority of IDCs present as hypoechoic masses with irregular edges
  - Round, oval, and lobulated circumscribed masses with MUC, MEC, and basal-like IDCs
  - MUC can be isoechoic to fat
  - Very rarely, cancers can be hyperechoic due to infiltrative pattern into adipose tissue with minimal stromal response
- MR findings
  - Carcinomas are detected by MR due to quick uptake of contrast agents resulting in rapid enhancement
  - MR is very sensitive but not very specific for detecting invasive tumors

CYTOPATHOLOGY

Ductal Carcinoma

- High cellularity with many loosely cohesive, disorganized, 3D clusters and sheets, including many single tumor cells
- Absence of myoepithelial cells in clusters; naked bipolar nuclei absent in backgrounds of smears
  - Sampling of associated benign epithelial elements may result in few benign clusters with some naked nuclei in background
- Tumor cells can have central or eccentric nucleus and show varying grades of nuclear atypia
- Nuclear membrane irregularity, coarse nuclear chromatin, and prominent nucleolus
  - Nuclear pleomorphism and mitotic activity increases with increasing grade of tumor
- Intracytoplasmic lumen with condensed mucin droplet may be present in tumor cells
- Necrosis may be noted in tumors, usually of high grade
- High-grade DCIS can exhibit pattern indistinguishable from invasive carcinoma
- Low-grade DCIS generally shows fragments of atypical epithelial cells with abnormal architectural pattern; punched-out, well-defined holes create cribriform pattern
- Myoepithelial cells present in fragments, and naked nuclei will be present in background in low- and intermediate-grade DCIS

Ductal Carcinoma and Variants of Invasive Mammary Carcinoma

- While diagnosis of ductal carcinoma can be rendered, overlapping features preclude accurate categorization as DCIS or IDC on FNA material
- Cell blocks containing stromal fragments with invasive carcinoma may aid in rendering specific diagnosis of invasive carcinoma in selected cases

IMPC

- Clusters of tumor cells forming pseudopapillary groups without any fibrovascular cores
  - Clusters are often angulated with smooth edges
- Luminal aspect of tumor cells faces outward rather than inward toward center of cluster
- Specific arrangement of tumor cells referred to as reversed polarity or inside-out pattern
  - Reversed polarity is best observed in cell blocks rather than smears
- Tumor cells have intermediate to high nuclear grade, prominent nucleolus, and usually conspicuous mitotic activity

IPC

- High cellularity, including fragments with fibrovascular cores
- Many 3D clusters and sheets associated with abundant single tumor cells
- Tumor cells may be columnar and exhibit varying grades of atypia
- Myoepithelial cells are absent from clusters and naked nuclei will not be present in background

TC/CC

- Usually low cellularity; cohesive clusters associated with few single tumor cells
- Tumor cells arranged as tubules with straight, parallel, and rigid edges
- Angular, twisted, or branched glands, often with pointed ends
- Tumor cells show low nuclear grade, minimal nuclear enlargement and pleomorphism, fine nuclear chromatin, and inconspicuous nucleoli
- Few tumor cells will show irregular nuclear membranes, and rare cells may show mitotic figures
- Naked bipolar nuclei can be present, derived from sampling of admixed/adjacent benign tissue
- Metachromatic stromal fragments can be seen
- CC shows cohesive sheets of tumor cells with features similar to TC with punched-out holes of equal size giving rise to cribriform pattern

MUC

- Slimy, mucinous material is aspirated
- Cellularity is usually moderate or high with tumor cells floating in abundant extracellular mucin; intracytoplasmic mucin is not common, however
- Branching capillaries commonly noted in mucin pool
- Tumor cells can demonstrate varying grades of atypia, usually low grade with small, uniform nucleus and fine nuclear chromatin without nucleolus
- Tumor cells can be present as 3D rounded or glandular clusters or cords and irregular strands
- Tumor cells can be plasmacytoid and show evidence of neuroendocrine differentiation on ancillary immunostains
- Neurosecretory granules can be seen as fine, red cytoplasmic granules in Romanowsky stains

MEC

- High cellularity with large tumor cells associated with abundant small lymphoid cells and plasma cells
- Lymphoglandular bodies can be present in backgrounds of smears
- Tumor cells are large with prominent nucleolus and irregular nuclear membranes
  - Demonstrate significant pleomorphism and mitotic activity
- Tumor cells arranged in syncytial groups
  - Single tumor cells can be present
- Cytologic features similar to MEC are usually noted with many basal-like/triple-negative breast carcinomas

SEC

- High cellularity with many large, irregular tissue fragments with loosely arranged tumor cells
- Nuclei are usually small, round, oval, relatively uniform with fine, granular chromatin and small nucleoli
  - Mitoses are rare
- Tumor cells demonstrate abundant foamy, vacuolated cytoplasm
  - Secretory material can be seen as intra- or extracellular hyaline globules

Neuroendocrine Tumor

- High cellularity with tumor cells generally arranged as loose monolayered sheets, rosette-like clusters, or trabecular and ribbon-like cords
- Tumor cells are also commonly distributed as single cells in background
- Tumor cells are usually small, uniform, often plasmacytoid or elongated, with stippled salt and pepper nuclear chromatin
- Nuclear membrane irregularity and pleomorphism is minimal, nucleoli are generally absent, and mitotic figures are rare
- Cytoplasm is variable in amount and can show red neurosecretory granules with Romanowsky stains
- Small cell carcinoma shows tumor cells with high nuclear:cytoplasmic ratio, fine nuclear chromatin without nucleolus, and scant cytoplasm
- Nuclear molding, increased mitotic activity, apoptotic bodies, and crush artifact are commonly present

MPC

- Squamous carcinoma
  - High cellularity with sheets and fragments of tumor cells associated usually with inflammation and necrosis in background
    - Cystic degeneration is common
  - Tumor cells show hyperchromatic, dark nucleus exhibiting pleomorphism with dense cytoplasm
  - Tumor cells commonly show evidence of keratinization, including presence of keratin pearls, keratohyalin granules, and intercellular bridges
- Spindle cell carcinoma
  - Spindle-shaped tumor cells with varying grades of atypia
    - Some spindle cells can be deceptively bland

Ductal Carcinoma and Variants of Invasive Mammary Carcinoma

- o Usually some epithelioid cells are seen with spindle tumor cells
- Matrix-producing MPC
  - o Spindle and epithelioid tumor cells with high nuclear grade, significant nuclear pleomorphism, and mitotic activity
  - o Associated with different types of matrix, including myxoid, chondromyxoid, or osteoid types
  - o Necrosis is commonly noted in these high-grade tumors
- Carcinosarcoma
  - o Fragments of distinctly epithelial and mesenchymal high-grade tumor
  - o Background may show myxoid, chondromyxoid, or osteoid matrix
  - o Sampling may result in presence of epithelial or mesenchymal component alone

IAC

- High cellularity with loosely cohesive clusters and abundant single tumor cells
- Tumor cells show centrally located large, round nucleus with coarsely granular chromatin, prominent large nucleolus, and significant mitotic activity
- Cytoplasm of tumor cells is abundant, well defined, and filled with mitochondria, which gives finely granular appearance

ACC

- Abundant loose clusters and single small basaloid tumor cells associated with metachromatic hyaline material
- Metachromatic extracellular material is usually distributed as hyaline spherules/globules
- Hyaline globules may or may not be bordered by tumor cells
- Hyaline globules are translucent in Pap stain and magenta in Romanowsky stain
- Tumor cells show hyperchromatic, irregular nuclei associated with scant cytoplasm; many naked tumor nuclei are commonly found in background

Lipid-Rich Carcinoma

- High cellularity with tumor cells, usually of high grade, exhibiting multivacuolated cytoplasm
- Vacuoles in cytoplasm caused by neutral lipid
- Special stains, such as oil red O, will be useful for making definite diagnosis

Glycogen-Rich Carcinoma

- High-grade tumor cells with abundant clear cytoplasm due to high glycogen content of cytoplasm material
- Disruption of friable tumor cells can result in many naked tumor nuclei and lacy, tigroid background

ANCILLARY TESTS

Immunohistochemistry

- Cytokeratins, including range of low and high molecular weight cytokeratins, for diagnosis of carcinoma
  - o Cytokeratins are particularly useful for making diagnosis of MPC and distinction of ductal carcinoma from mimics, such as lymphoma and melanoma
- Prognostic and predictive markers, including ER, PR, and HER2, are not recommended on cytologic material of primary index breast carcinoma
- Myoepithelial markers, including p63, SMA, SMMH, and calponin, for distinction of benign from malignant clusters of ductal epithelial cells
- Immunomarkers, including GCDFP-15, mammaglobin, and GATA3, to evaluate breast origin
  - o GCDFP-15 and mammaglobin have low sensitivity
  - o GATA3 is more sensitive but less specific; stains many other cell types, most notably urothelium
- Immunomarkers, such as vimentin, S100, and SMA, for evaluation of MPCs
- Gynecologic immunomarkers, including PAX8 and WT1, for distinction from müllerian primaries
  - o ER and PR often (+) in both tumor types
- Lung immunomarkers, including TTF-1 and napsin A, for distinction from lung primaries
- Gastrointestinal immunomarkers, including CDX2 and CK20, for distinction from gastrointestinal carcinoma (especially colon)
- Melanoma immunomarkers, including S100, HMB-45, and Melan-A, for distinction from melanoma
- Lymphocytic immunomarkers, including LCA, CD3, and CD20, for distinction of poorly differentiated ductal carcinoma from high-grade lymphoma

DIFFERENTIAL DIAGNOSIS

Radial Sclerosing Lesion/Sclerosing Adenosis

- Can demonstrate tubule-like, round, and angular clusters that can mimic TC
  - o Tubular clusters in TC have rigid parallel edges; myoepithelial cells are absent from clusters, unlike radial sclerosing lesion and sclerosing adenosis (SA)
  - o When distinction is problematic, additional sampling with core needle biopsy of lesion is recommended

Microglandular Adenosis

- Small clusters of tumor cells with low-grade nuclear features without associated myoepithelial cells in microglandular adenosis (MA) can mimic low-grade ductal carcinoma
- Imaging findings, presence of thick secretions in clusters of tumor cells, and ancillary immunostains will be useful
  - o ER(-), PR(-), S100(+), unlike low-grade ductal carcinoma

Myxoid Fibroadenoma

- Clusters of epithelial cells in background of abundant myxoid material in myxoid fibroadenoma can mimic MUC
- Presence of myoepithelial cells in clusters and abundant naked nuclei in background, unlike MUC

Mucocele-Like Tumor

- Shows low cellularity with few clusters of benign ductal cells with associated myoepithelial cells, unlike MUC
- Malignant mucocele-like tumors show features similar to MUC and cannot be distinguished on cytology

Metastatic Tumor

- Can mimic primary breast carcinomas

Ductal Carcinoma and Variants of Invasive Mammary Carcinoma

- Metastatic adenocarcinoma, squamous carcinoma, and neuroendocrine tumors from other sites can mimic primary breast carcinoma
- Close mimics are metastatic serous ovarian tumors, invasive micropapillary tumors from ovary, lung, and urinary bladder, and metastatic neuroendocrine tumors from gastrointestinal tract and lung
- Clinical history and pertinent immunostains are useful

Papilloma
- High cellularity, including presence of many single epithelial cells in background, may mimic low-grade ductal carcinoma
- Presence of fibrovascular cores in lesion, myoepithelial cells admixed with epithelial cells in clusters, unlike ductal carcinoma
- Naked nuclei in background along with single epithelial cells only in papilloma
- IPC shows fibrovascular cores, but myoepithelial cells in clusters and naked nuclei in background are absent

Primary/Metastatic Lymphoma
- Large cell lymphoma, primary or metastatic to breast, can mimic high-grade ductal carcinoma
- Lymphoglandular bodies are usually present in lymphomas, unlike ductal carcinoma; MEC may, however, show lymphoglandular bodies in background
- Ancillary immunostains can be useful for distinction

Intramammary Lymph Node Metastasis
- Imaging and cytologic features of metastatic carcinoma to intramammary lymph nodes can mimic MEC
- Presence of additional index lesion with proven invasive tumor is useful to avoid misinterpretation

Granular Cell Tumor/Apocrine Metaplasia
- Tumor cells of granular cell tumor (GCT) and apocrine cells aspirated from variety of benign lesions, such as SA, can mimic tumor cells of IAC
- IAC shows significant atypia of cells, demonstrating abundant granular cytoplasm usually with macronucleoli, mitotic activity, and necrosis
- Ancillary immunostain for cytokeratin and S100 is useful for distinction of GCT from IAC

Malignant Phyllodes/Primary Sarcoma/Metastatic Sarcoma
- Malignant spindle cells ± heterologous sarcomatous component in malignant phyllodes and any of primary or metastatic sarcomas of breast can mimic MPC
- Ancillary immunostains to evaluate cytokeratin expression in sarcomatous tumor cells is useful

SELECTED REFERENCES

1. Agrawal S et al: Accuracy of breast fine-needle aspiration biopsy using the International Academy of Cytology Yokohama system in clinico-radiologically indeterminate lesions: initial findings demonstrating value in lesions of low suspicion of malignancy. Acta Cytol. 65(3):220-6, 2021
2. Agrawal S et al: Prospective evaluation of accuracy of fine-needle aspiration biopsy for breast lesions using the International Academy of Cytology Yokohama System for reporting breast cytopathology. Diagn Cytopathol. 49(7):805-10, 2021
3. Verma P et al: Fine-needle aspiration cytology versus core-needle biopsy for breast lesions: a dilemma of superiority between the two. Acta Cytol. 65(5):411-6, 2021
4. Field AS et al: Breast fine needle aspiration biopsy cytology: the potential impact of the International Academy of Cytology Yokohama System for reporting breast fine needle aspiration biopsy cytopathology and the use of rapid on-site evaluation. J Am Soc Cytopathol. 9(2):103-11, 2020
5. Noda Y et al: Fine-needle aspiration cytology for the diagnosis of solid basaloid adenoid cystic carcinoma of the breast: its role, limitation, and perspective. Diagn Cytopathol. 48(7):652-6, 2020
6. Pinto D et al: The role of breast fine needle aspiration during and post-COVID-19 pandemic: a fast and safe alternative to needle core biopsy. Cytopathology. 31(6):627-9, 2020
7. Sakuma T et al: Fine-needle aspiration cytology of solid papillary carcinoma of the breast. Diagn Cytopathol. 48(1):53-6, 2020
8. Field AS et al: The International Academy of Cytology Yokohama system for reporting breast fine-needle aspiration biopsy cytopathology. Acta Cytol. 63(4):257-73, 2019
9. Michelow P et al: Spindle cell lesions of the breast on fine-needle aspiration biopsy: a miscellany of masses. Acta Cytol. 63(4):328-39, 2019
10. Wang M et al: A sensitivity and specificity comparison of fine needle aspiration cytology and core needle biopsy in evaluation of suspicious breast lesions: a systematic review and meta-analysis. Breast. 31:157-66, 2017
11. Aker F et al: Accuracy of fine-needle aspiration cytology in the diagnosis of breast cancer a single-center retrospective study from Turkey with cytohistological correlation in 733 cases. Diagn Cytopathol. 43(12):978-86, 2015
12. Mucha Dufloth R et al: Fine needle aspiration cytology of lobular breast carcinoma and its variants. Acta Cytol. 59(1):37-42, 2015
13. Brancato B et al: Accuracy of needle biopsy of breast lesions visible on ultrasound: audit of fine needle versus core needle biopsy in 3233 consecutive samplings with ascertained outcomes. Breast. 21(4):449-54, 2012
14. Abdel-Hadi M et al: Should fine-needle aspiration cytology be the first choice diagnostic modality for assessment of all nonpalpable breast lesions? The experience of a breast cancer screening center in Alexandria, Egypt. Diagn Cytopathol. 38(12):880-9, 2010
15. Lim KH et al: Metaplastic breast carcinoma: clinicopathologic features and prognostic value of triple negativity. Jpn J Clin Oncol. 40(2):112-8, 2010
16. Marginean F et al: Histological features of medullary carcinoma and prognosis in triple-negative basal-like carcinomas of the breast. Mod Pathol. 23(10):1357-63, 2010
17. Pal SK et al: Papillary carcinoma of the breast: an overview. Breast Cancer Res Treat. 122(3):637-45, 2010
18. Righi L et al: Neuroendocrine differentiation in breast cancer: established facts and unresolved problems. Semin Diagn Pathol. 27(1):69-76, 2010
19. Schnitt SJ: Molecular biology of breast tumor progression: a view from the other side. Int J Surg Pathol. 18(3 Suppl):170S-3S, 2010
20. Wei B et al: Invasive neuroendocrine carcinoma of the breast: a distinctive subtype of aggressive mammary carcinoma. Cancer. 116(19):4463-73, 2010
21. Yu JI et al: Differences in prognostic factors and patterns of failure between invasive micropapillary carcinoma and invasive ductal carcinoma of the breast: matched case-control study. Breast. 19(3):231-7, 2010
22. Da Silva L et al: Molecular and morphological analysis of adenoid cystic carcinoma of the breast with synchronous tubular adenosis. Virchows Arch. 454(1):107-14, 2009
23. Downs-Kelly E et al: Matrix-producing carcinoma of the breast: an aggressive subtype of metaplastic carcinoma. Am J Surg Pathol. 33(4):534-41, 2009
24. Laé M et al: Secretory breast carcinomas with ETV6-NTRK3 fusion gene belong to the basal-like carcinoma spectrum. Mod Pathol. 22(2):291-8, 2009
25. Lotan TL et al: Immunohistochemical panel to identify the primary site of invasive micropapillary carcinoma. Am J Surg Pathol. 33(7):1037-41, 2009
26. Di Saverio S et al: A retrospective review with long term follow up of 11,400 cases of pure mucinous breast carcinoma. Breast Cancer Res Treat. 111(3):541-7, 2008
27. Haji BE et al: Fine-needle aspiration cytologic features of four special types of breast cancers: mucinous, medullary, apocrine, and papillary. Diagn Cytopathol. 35(7):408-16, 2007
28. Lien HC et al: Molecular signatures of metaplastic carcinoma of the breast by large-scale transcriptional profiling: identification of genes potentially related to epithelial-mesenchymal transition. Oncogene. 26(57):7859-71, 2007
29. Rodríguez-Pinilla SM et al: Sporadic invasive breast carcinomas with medullary features display a basal-like phenotype: an immunohistochemical and gene amplification study. Am J Surg Pathol. 31(4):501-8, 2007
30. Carter MR et al: Spindle cell (sarcomatoid) carcinoma of the breast: a clinicopathologic and immunohistochemical analysis of 29 cases. Am J Surg Pathol. 30(3):300-9, 2006
31. Kasagawa T et al: Two cases of adenoid cystic carcinoma: preoperative cytological findings were useful in determining treatment strategy. Breast Cancer. 13(1):112-6, 2006

Ductal Carcinoma and Variants of Invasive Mammary Carcinoma

Ductal Carcinoma: Low Grade With Absence of Bipolar Naked Nuclei

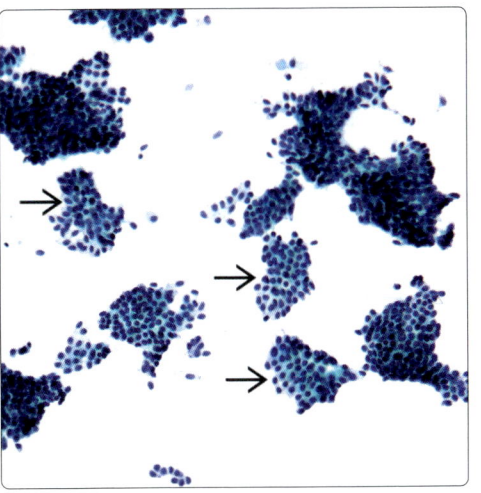

Ductal Carcinoma: High Grade With Coarse Chromatin and Irregular Nuclei

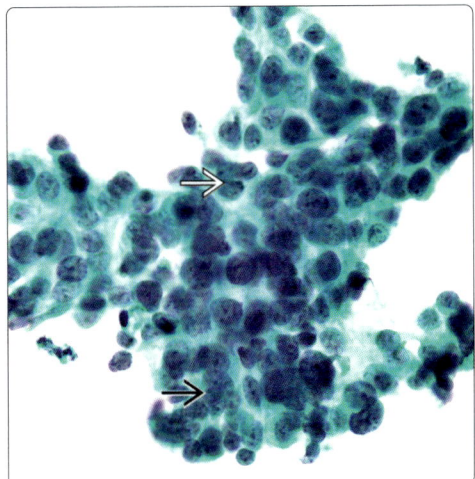

(Left) Pap-stained FNA smear of low-grade ductal carcinoma shows loose clusters of uniform, mildly atypical ductal epithelial cells ➡. Note that there are no bipolar naked nuclei in the background. (Right) Pap-stained FNA smear of high-grade ductal carcinoma shows a large, irregular fragment of tumor cells with large nuclei, coarse clumped nuclear chromatin ➡, and irregular nuclear membranes ➡.

Ductal Carcinoma: High Grade With Prominent Nucleoli

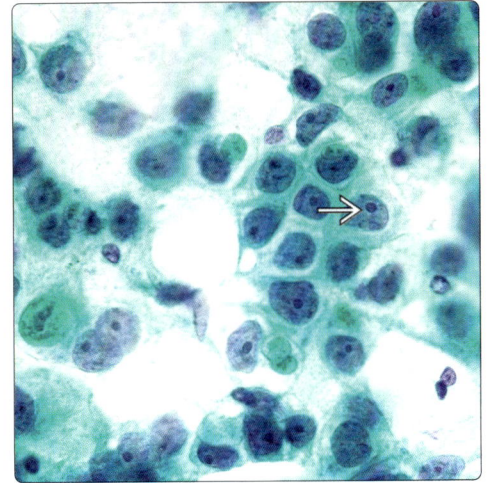

Tubular Carcinoma

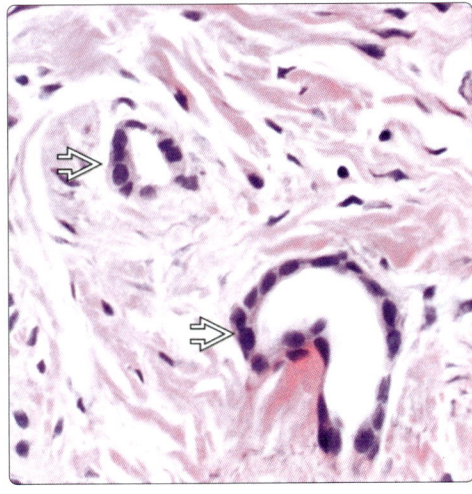

(Left) Pap-stained FNA smear of high-grade ductal carcinoma shows large tumor cells with prominent nucleoli ➡ associated with a moderate amount of cytoplasm. (Right) Core biopsy of tubular carcinoma of breast stained with H&E shows small glands with round and angular configuration ➡ and mild nuclear atypia without any myoepithelial cells surrounding them.

Tubular Carcinoma With Low-Grade Nuclei

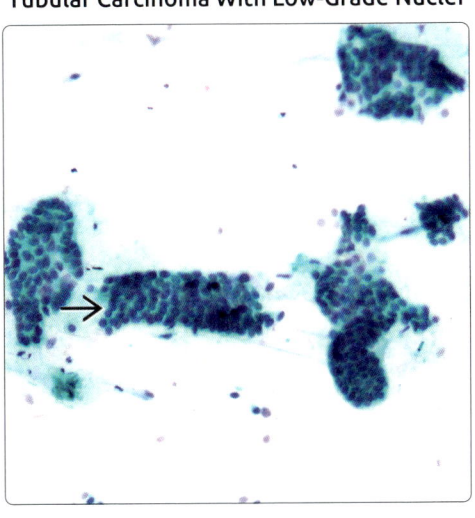

Tubular Carcinoma Architecture

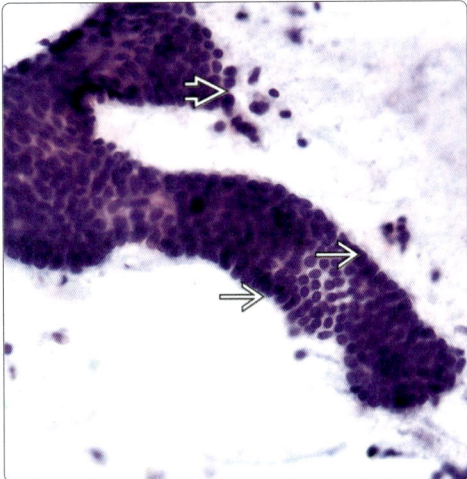

(Left) Pap-stained FNA smear of tubular carcinoma of the breast shows tubular clusters ➡ composed of uniform, cohesive, mildly atypical ductal epithelial cells of low nuclear grade. (Right) Pap-stained smear of tubular carcinoma of the breast shows a tubular arrangement of tumor cells ➡ without associated myoepithelial cells. Note that the tubule demonstrates parallel rigid edges and has an angular contour at one end ➡.

Ductal Carcinoma and Variants of Invasive Mammary Carcinoma

Mucinous Carcinoma: Low Power
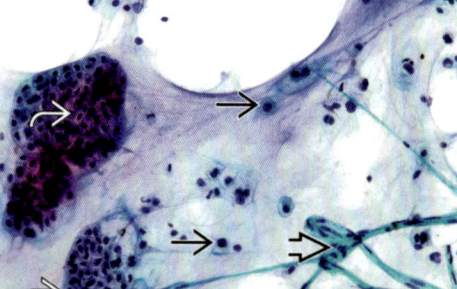

Mucinous Carcinoma
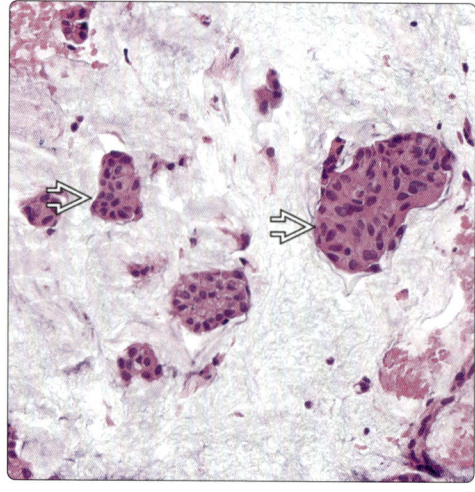

(Left) Pap-stained FNA smear of mucinous carcinoma shows clusters ⇨ and individual tumor cells ⇨ floating in mucin. Note the branching capillary network ⇨ in the mucin pool. (Right) Core biopsy of mucinous carcinoma stained with H&E shows clusters of tumor cells ⇨ with mild nuclear pleomorphism associated with abundant extracellular mucin.

Invasive Micropapillary Carcinoma Architecture
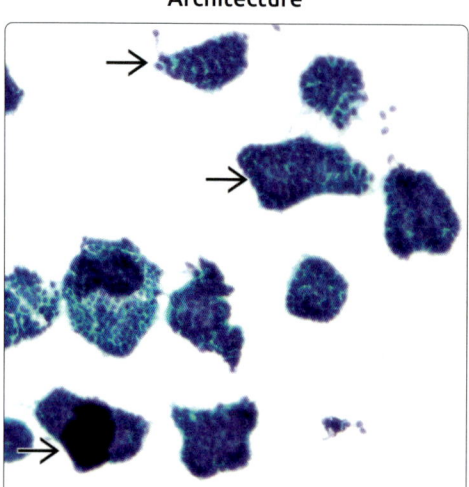

Invasive Micropapillary Carcinoma
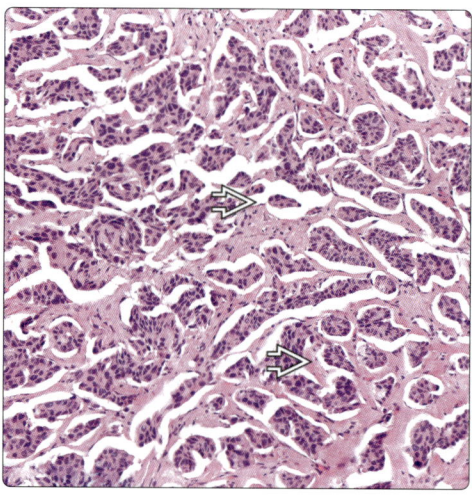

(Left) Pap-stained smear of invasive micropapillary breast carcinoma shows characteristic angular clusters of tumor cells ⇨ without any single cells in the background. (Right) Core biopsy of invasive micropapillary carcinoma shows small, angular clusters ⇨ of tumor cells with an inside-out pattern located within spaces. The tumor cells demonstrate moderate nuclear atypia.

Apocrine Carcinoma
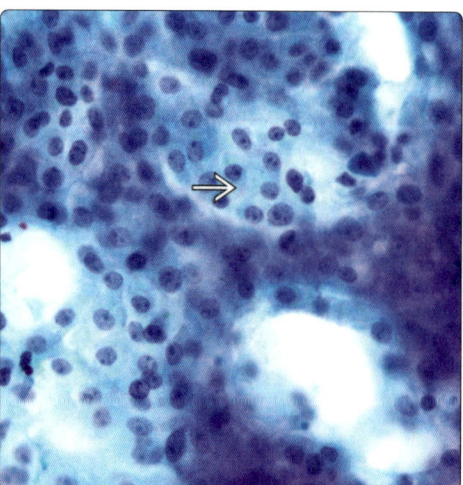

Secretory Carcinoma
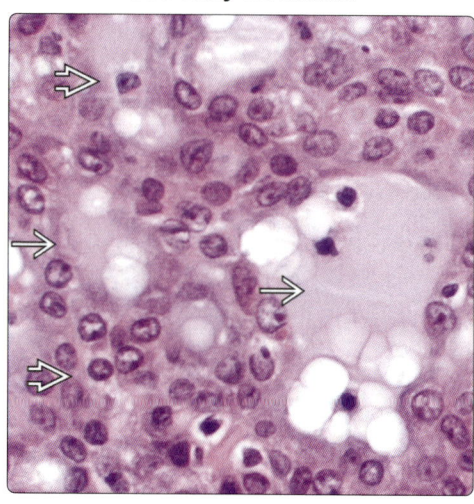

(Left) Pap-stained FNA smear of apocrine carcinoma of the breast shows a fragment of tumor cells with central round nuclei associated with abundant granular cytoplasm ⇨ due to the presence of increased numbers of mitochondria. (Right) Core biopsy of secretory carcinoma stained with H&E shows tumor cells ⇨ with vesicular nuclei, moderate amount of granular eosinophilic and vacuolated cytoplasm, including thin eosinophilic secretory material ⇨ amidst the tumor cells.

Ductal Carcinoma and Variants of Invasive Mammary Carcinoma

Secretory Carcinoma

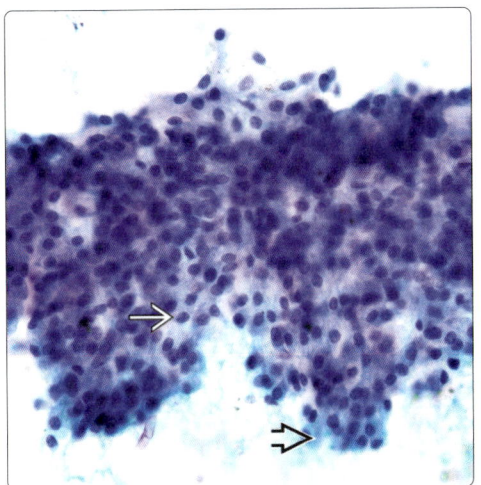

Neuroendocrine Carcinoma

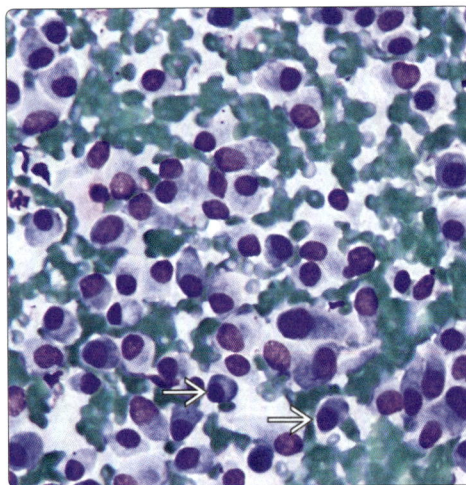

(Left) Pap-stained FNA smear of secretory carcinoma shows a fragment of tumor cells with round/oval nuclei of low nuclear grade ➡ associated with moderate amounts of delicate cytoplasm ➡. (Right) Diff-Quik-stained FNA smear of a case of invasive ductal carcinoma with neuroendocrine differentiation shows high cellularity with many plasmacytoid tumor cells ➡ with eccentrically placed nuclei and a moderate amount of cytoplasm.

Metaplastic Carcinoma Cytology

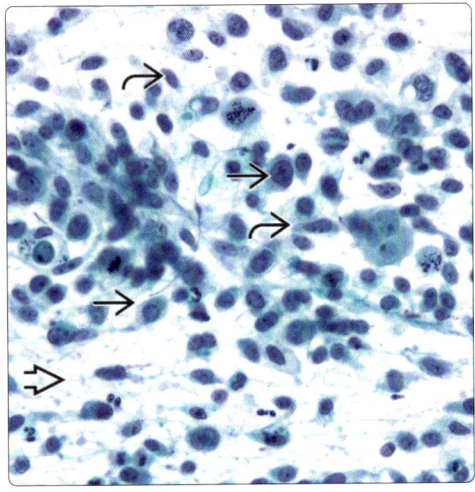

Metaplastic Carcinoma

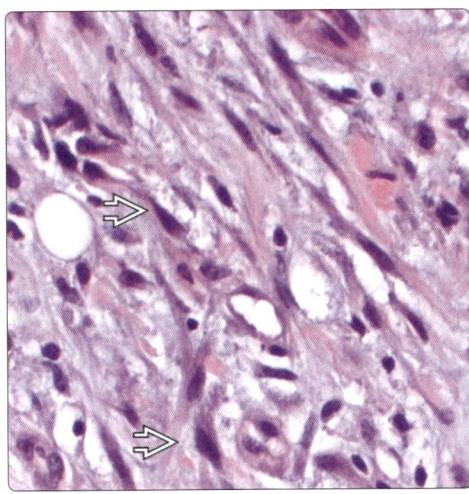

(Left) Pap-stained FNA smear of metaplastic carcinoma shows a poorly differentiated high-grade malignant tumor with spindle ➡ and epithelioid ➡ malignant tumor cells in a myxoid background ➡. (Right) Core biopsy of metaplastic carcinoma shows spindle tumor cells ➡ exhibiting nuclear hyperchromasia, moderate pleomorphism, and scant cytoplasm.

Metaplastic Carcinoma Histology

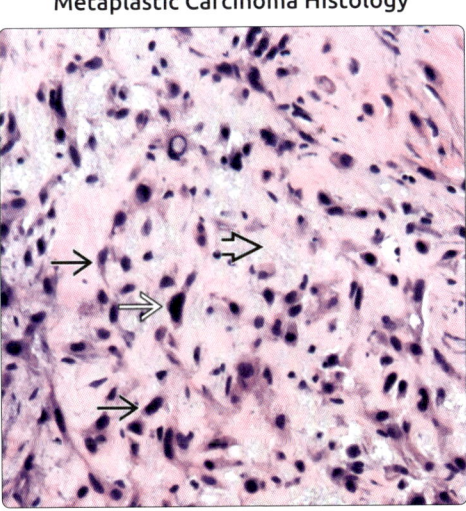

Metaplastic Carcinoma: CK5/6(+)

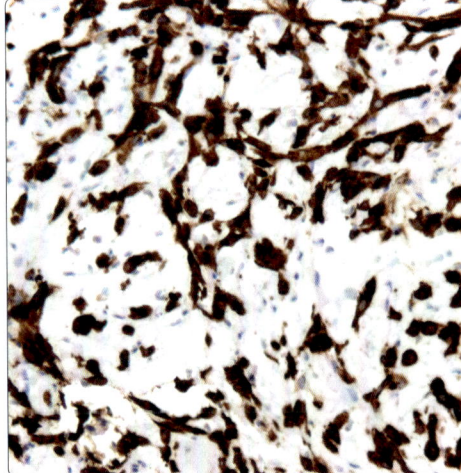

(Left) H&E-stained section of metaplastic carcinoma of the breast shows spindle tumor cells ➡ with hyperchromatic, dark nuclei ➡ associated with myxoid change in the stroma ➡. (Right) Metaplastic carcinoma of breast immunostained for CK5/6 shows diffuse and strong staining of the tumor cells, thereby confirming the diagnosis of sarcomatoid carcinoma.

Lobular Carcinoma

KEY FACTS

CLINICAL ISSUES
- Neoplastic proliferation of epithelial cells lacking cell adhesion

CYTOPATHOLOGY
- Classic type shows small, often plasmacytoid tumor cells
  - Cytoplasmic vacuoles with intracytoplasmic lumen containing mucin droplet
- Other types: Signet-ring cell, histiocytoid, and pleomorphic
  - Signet-ring cell variant shows single large mucin vacuole occupying most of cytoplasm with peripherally placed nucleus
  - Histiocytoid variant shows abundant cytoplasm
  - Pleomorphic variant shows large nuclei with pleomorphism, often with prominent nucleoli and evidence of mitotic activity
- Cytomorphologic findings similar for atypical lobular hyperplasia (ALH)/lobular carcinoma in situ (LCIS)/infiltrating lobular carcinoma (ILC)

ANCILLARY TESTS
- Absence of E-cadherin expression; ER(+), PR(+), mucicarmine (+)

TOP DIFFERENTIAL DIAGNOSES
- Ductal carcinoma
  - Classic and pleomorphic LC can mimic low- and high-grade ductal carcinoma
    - Usually LC shows dyscohesive E-cadherin (-) (unlike ductal carcinoma); LC is more often mucin (+)
- Metastatic carcinoid/metastatic melanoma/metastatic gastric carcinoma
  - Plasmacytoid tumor cells of LC can look similar to metastatic carcinoid, melanoma, or signet-ring cells of gastric carcinoma; ancillary immunostaining will be useful
- Histiocytes
  - Ancillary mucin staining and immunostaining may be useful

Lobular Carcinoma
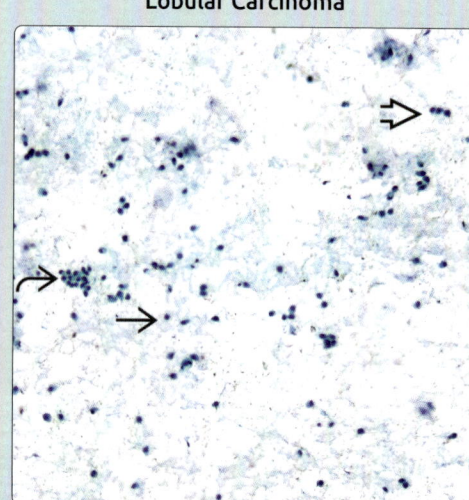

Lobular Carcinoma, Cytoplasmic Vacuoles
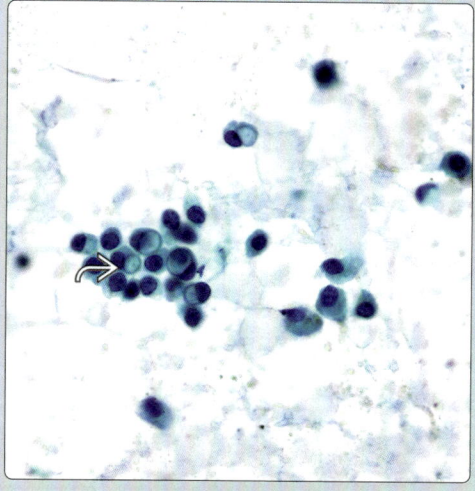

(Left) Pap-stained FNA smear of lobular carcinoma shows predominantly dispersed tumor cells ➡ with rare loose clusters ➡ and single-file cell chains ➡. (Right) Pap-stained FNA smear shows cytoplasmic vacuoles in some of the tumor cells ➡.

Lobular Carcinoma In Situ and Invasive Carcinoma
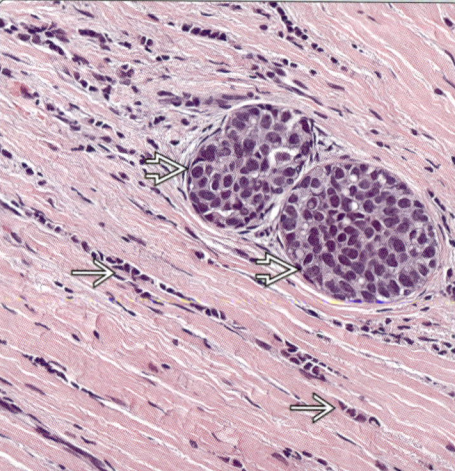

E-Cadherin in Lobular Carcinoma In Situ and Invasive Carcinoma
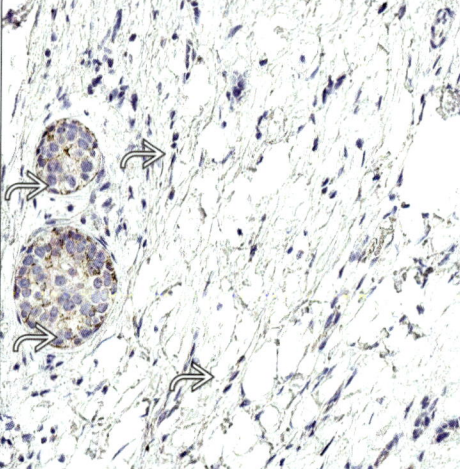

(Left) Core biopsy stained with H&E shows lobular carcinoma in situ and invasive carcinoma with tumor cells filling the lobules ➡ as well as infiltrating stroma in a striking single file pattern ➡. (Right) Core biopsy of lobular carcinoma in situ and invasive carcinoma immunostained with E-cadherin shows absence of membranous staining in the tumor cells ➡, which is the characteristic feature of lobular phenotype of mammary carcinoma.

Lobular Carcinoma

TERMINOLOGY

Abbreviations
- Lobular carcinoma (LC)

Definitions
- Neoplastic proliferation of epithelial cells lacking cell adhesion, confined to ducts and lobules, or invading stroma

ETIOLOGY/PATHOGENESIS

Molecular Pathology
- Hallmark molecular feature of all LC is loss of expression of E-cadherin (CDH11) located on chromosome 16q

CYTOPATHOLOGY

Cellularity
- Variable; low in classic LC and high in pleomorphic LC

Pattern
- Classic LC shows dispersed population of small tumor cells distributed singly, in loose clusters, or in single-file chains

Cells
- Cells of classic LC small and often plasmacytoid
  - Cytomorphologic findings similar for atypical lobular hyperplasia (ALH)/LC in situ (LCIS)/infiltrating LC (ILC)
- Other variants of LC include signet-ring cell, histiocytoid, and pleomorphic types

Nuclear Details
- Nuclei in classic LC are centrally or eccentrically placed and are usually small and round in shape; nuclear chromatin is fine with minimal hyperchromasia
- Tumor cells of pleomorphic LC have large nuclei with pleomorphism, often with prominent nucleoli and evidence of mitotic activity

Cytoplasmic Details
- Cytoplasmic vacuolization ranging from multiple small vacuoles to single sharply punched-out vacuole
- Single punched-out vacuole often shows centrally placed droplet of condensed mucin ("bull's-eye") representing intracytoplasmic lumen (ICL) formation
- Signet-ring cell variant shows single large mucin vacuole occupying most of cytoplasm with peripherally placed nucleus; histiocytoid variant of LC shows abundant cytoplasm

ANCILLARY TESTS

Immunohistochemistry
- Majority of LC are E-cadherin (-), ER(+), and PR(+)
  - Mucicarmine (+) in mucin vacuoles

DIFFERENTIAL DIAGNOSIS

Ductal Carcinoma
- Classic and pleomorphic LC can mimic low- and high-grade ductal carcinoma
  - Usually LC shows dyscohesive E-cadherin (-) (unlike ductal carcinoma); LC is more often mucin (+)

Metastatic Carcinoid/Metastatic Melanoma/Metastatic Gastric Carcinoma
- Plasmacytoid tumor cells of LC can look similar to metastatic carcinoid, melanoma, or signet-ring cells of gastric carcinoma
- Ancillary immunostains will be useful

Histiocytes
- Ancillary mucin staining and immunostaining will be useful

SELECTED REFERENCES

1. McCart Reed AE et al: Invasive lobular carcinoma of the breast: the increasing importance of this special subtype. Breast Cancer Res. 23(1):6, 2021
2. Sokolova A et al: Lobular carcinoma in situ: diagnostic criteria and molecular correlates. Mod Pathol. 34(Suppl 1):8-14, 2021
3. Calle C et al: Non-invasive lobular neoplasia of the breast: morphologic features, clinical presentation, and management dilemmas. Breast J. 26(6):1148-55, 2020
4. Harrison BT et al: Genomic profiling of pleomorphic and florid lobular carcinoma in situ reveals highly recurrent ERBB2 and ERRB3 alterations. Mod Pathol. 33(7):1287-97, 2020

Lobular Carcinoma, Dyscohesive Tumor Cells

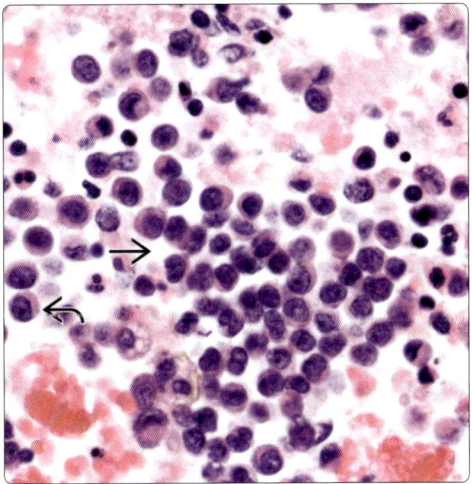

Lobular Carcinoma

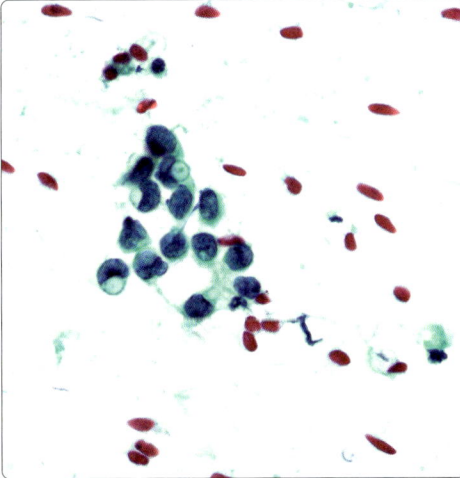

(Left) H&E-stained cell block of lobular carcinoma shows dyscohesive tumor cells ➡ with eccentrically placed nuclei ➡ in many tumor cells. (Right) Pap-stained FNA smear of lobular carcinoma shows tumor cells with centrally and eccentrically placed nucleus and vacuoles in the cytoplasm of some of the tumor cells. One of the tumor cells shows an inspissated mucin droplet within the intracytoplasmic vacuole.

Phyllodes Tumor

KEY FACTS

CLINICAL ISSUES

- Biphasic tumor with stromal component & benign epithelial component; classified as low, intermediate, or high grade based on extent of cellular atypia & stromal overgrowth; < 1% of breast tumors
- Complete excision of all phyllodes tumors (PTs) is recommended to avoid local recurrence, which increase from low grade to high grade
  - Whereas incomplete excision increases rates of recurrence, mastectomy can decrease them

CYTOPATHOLOGY

- Cellular stromal fragments & increased numbers of stromal cells in background; benign ductal epithelial fragments often exhibiting hyperplasia
- Extent of atypia of stromal cells, including nuclear pleomorphism & mitotic activity, increases with increasing grades of PT

TOP DIFFERENTIAL DIAGNOSES

- Fibroadenoma with cellular stroma
  - Cytologic features of low-grade PT & cellular FA overlap & cannot be distinguished on FNA
    - Significant atypia in stromal fragments & single stromal cells in high-grade PT, unlike fibroadenoma
- Spindle cell carcinoma/metaplastic carcinoma
  - Spindle cells in metaplastic carcinomas may show epithelioid cells in focal areas & demonstrate positivity for cytokeratins & p63, unlike spindle cells of high-grade PT
- Primary sarcoma of breast/metastatic spindle cell tumor
  - High-grade PT with stromal overgrowth can mimic primary sarcoma, metastatic spindle cell carcinoma, melanoma, & metastatic sarcoma
    - Presence of benign epithelial elements in high-grade PT at least in some foci; ancillary immunostaining & clinical history may be useful for distinction

Low-Grade Phyllodes Tumor Cytology
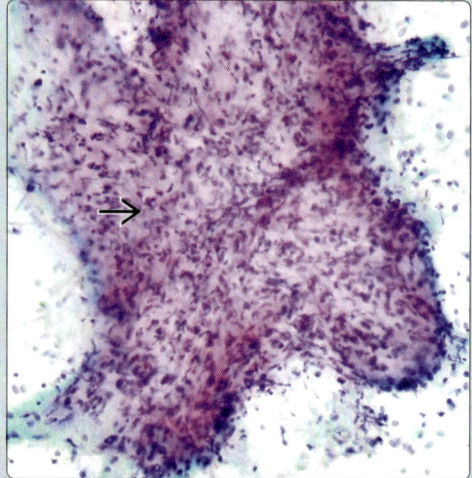

Low-Grade Phyllodes Tumor Histology
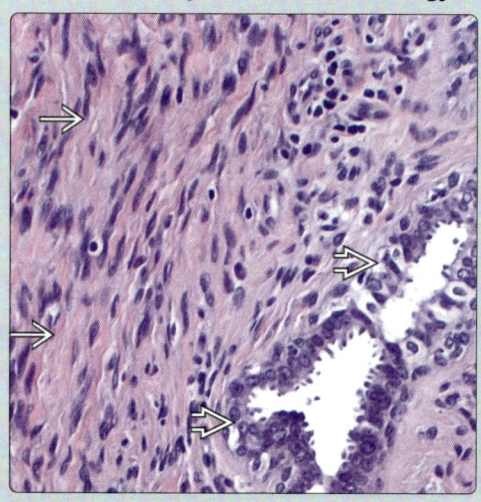

(Left) Pap-stained FNA smear of a low-grade phyllodes tumor shows a cellular stromal fragment composed of stromal cells without significant atypia ➡. (Right) Core biopsy of a low-grade phyllodes tumor stained with H&E shows a benign gland ➡ associated with increased stromal cellularity ➡. The stromal cells show mild nuclear pleomorphism without any mitotic figures.

High-Grade Phyllodes Tumor Cytology
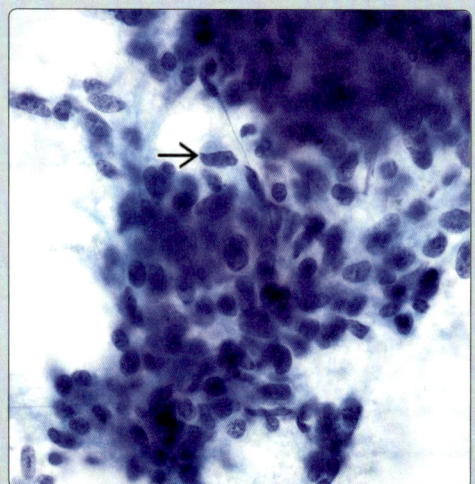

High-Grade Phyllodes Tumor Histology
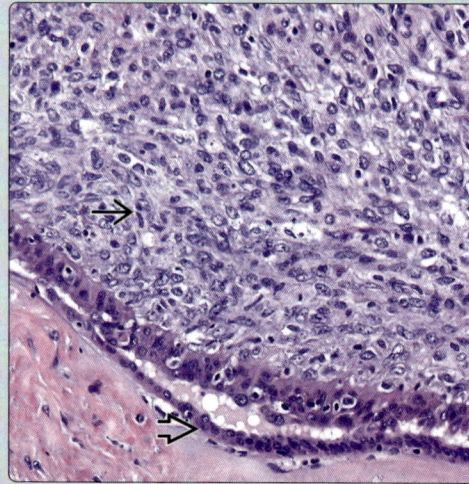

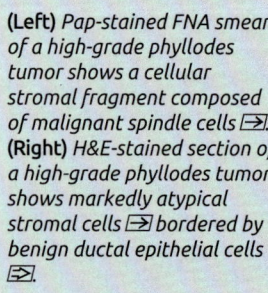

(Left) Pap-stained FNA smear of a high-grade phyllodes tumor shows a cellular stromal fragment composed of malignant spindle cells ➡. (Right) H&E-stained section of a high-grade phyllodes tumor shows markedly atypical stromal cells ➡ bordered by benign ductal epithelial cells ➡.

Phyllodes Tumor

TERMINOLOGY

Definitions
- Biphasic tumor consisting of intralobular-type stromal cells & benign epithelial cells classified into low-/benign, intermediate-/borderline, & high-grade/malignant based on extent of atypia & overgrowth of stroma

CLINICAL ISSUES

Epidemiology
- Incidence
  - Uncommon: < 1% of all breast tumors; more common in Asian populations (7% of breast tumors); peak age range: 35-55 years

Prognosis
- Complete excision of all phyllodes tumors (PTs) is recommended to avoid local recurrence, which ↑ from low grade to high grade; whereas, incomplete excision ↑ rates of recurrence, mastectomy can ↓ them

IMAGING

Mammographic Findings
- Circumscribed, lobulated mass with average size of 4-8 cm often with ill-defined edges

CYTOPATHOLOGY

Cellularity
- Cellularity & extent of atypia of spindle cells increases with increasing grade of PT

Pattern
- Cellular stromal fragments composed of spindle cells
- Fragments of benign ductal epithelium, usually exhibiting hyperplasia without atypia

Cells
- Increased numbers of individually distributed stromal cells with elongated nuclei & scant to moderate cytoplasm in backgrounds of smears
- Significant atypia in individually distributed stromal cells, including nuclear enlargement, pleomorphism, & mitotic figures in high-grade PT
- Heterologous differentiation of sarcomatous stroma in malignant PT exhibiting features of liposarcoma, osteosarcoma, chondrosarcoma, & rhabdomyosarcoma can be noted
- Squamous metaplasia & individual epithelial cells can be seen in background

DIFFERENTIAL DIAGNOSIS

Fibroadenoma With Cellular Stroma
- Cytologic features of low-grade PT & cellular fibroadenoma (FA) overlap & cannot be distinguished on FNA
  - Significant atypia in stromal fragments & single stromal cells in high-grade PT, unlike FA

Metaplastic Carcinoma
- Spindle cells in metaplastic carcinomas may show epithelioid cells in focal areas & demonstrate positivity for cytokeratins & p63, unlike spindle cells of high-grade PT

Primary Sarcoma/Metastatic Spindle Cell Tumor
- High-grade PT with stromal overgrowth can mimic primary sarcoma, metastatic spindle cell carcinoma, melanoma, & metastatic sarcoma
- Presence of benign epithelial elements in high-grade PT at least in some foci; ancillary immunostaining & clinical history may be useful for distinction

SELECTED REFERENCES
1. Tan PH: Fibroepithelial lesions revisited: implications for diagnosis and management. Mod Pathol. 34(Suppl 1):15-37, 2021
2. Yuniandini A et al: A retrospective review of phyllodes tumors of the breast from a single institution. Breast Dis. 40(S1):S63-70, 2021
3. Tan BY et al: Morphologic and genetic heterogeneity in breast fibroepithelial lesions-a comprehensive mapping study. Mod Pathol. 33(9):1732-45, 2020
4. Strode M et al: Update on the diagnosis and management of malignant phyllodes tumors of the breast. Breast. 33:91-6, 2017
5. Zhang Y et al: Phyllodes tumor of the breast: histopathologic features, differential diagnosis, and molecular/genetic ppdates. Arch Pathol Lab Med. 140(7):665-71, 2016

Low-Grade Phyllodes Tumor with Leaf-Like Architecture
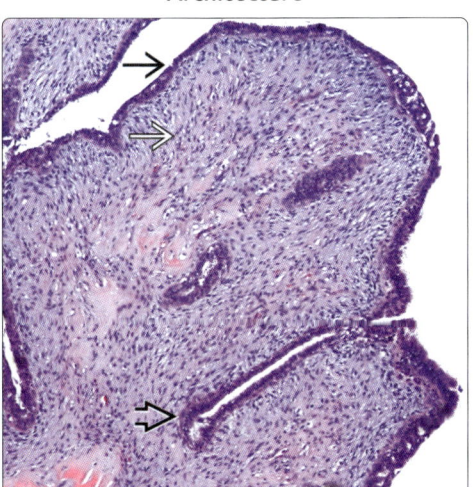

Low-Grade Phyllodes Tumor Infiltrating Adipose Tissue
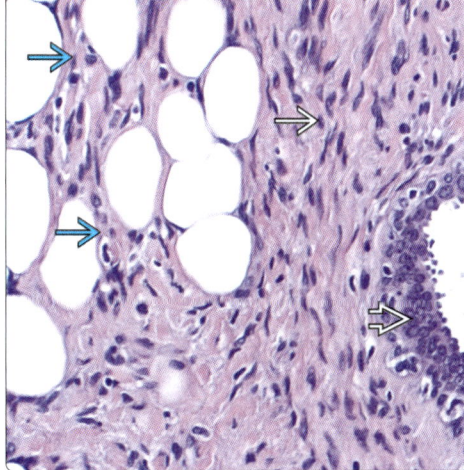

(Left) H&E-stained section of a low-grade phyllodes tumor with leaf-like proliferation ➡ of stromal cells shows increased cellularity without significant atypia ➡ bordered by benign ductal epithelial cells ➡. (Right) Core biopsy of a low-grade phyllodes tumor shows a benign gland ➡ associated with increased stromal cellularity ➡ and infiltration of the stromal spindle cells into adipose tissue ➡.

Angiosarcoma and Other Sarcomas

KEY FACTS

CLINICAL ISSUES
- Angiosarcoma (AS) is most common idiopathic primary breast sarcoma, followed by liposarcoma (LIS)
- Sarcomas associated with prior use of breast external beam radiation therapy: AS, malignant fibrous histiocytoma, fibrosarcoma; edema of arm following breast and axillary surgery increases risk of AS of skin, a.k.a. Stewart-Treves syndrome
- Patients with idiopathic sarcomas present with palpable mass; those with breast radiation-related or edema-related AS present with dark red or violaceous discoloration of skin

CYTOPATHOLOGY
- Primary sarcomas can demonstrate malignant spindle cells, round cells, &/or epithelioid cells with varying grades of atypia, pleomorphism, mitotic activity, and necrosis
- Special features include vasoformation, intracytoplasmic lumen containing RBCs in AS, lipoblasts in LIS, strap cells in rhabdomyosarcoma, cartilaginous matrix in chondrosarcoma, osteoid in osteosarcoma

ANCILLARY TESTS
- Panel of immunomarkers: Cytokeratin, S100, markers of endothelial cells, smooth and skeletal muscle (useful for specific diagnosis)

TOP DIFFERENTIAL DIAGNOSES
- Granulation tissue/mesenchymal repair/radiation change
- Hemangioma/angiolipoma/pseudoangiomatous stromal hyperplasia
  - Scant spindle cells with minimal atypia (unlike sarcomas)
- Mammary carcinoma
- Malignant phyllodes tumor
- Metaplastic carcinoma/metastatic sarcoma/melanoma

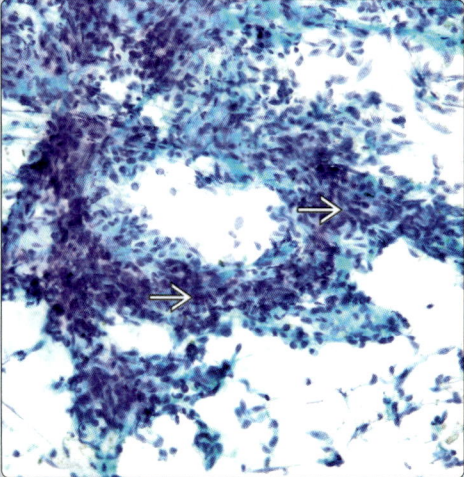

Angiosarcoma: Vascular Channel Formation

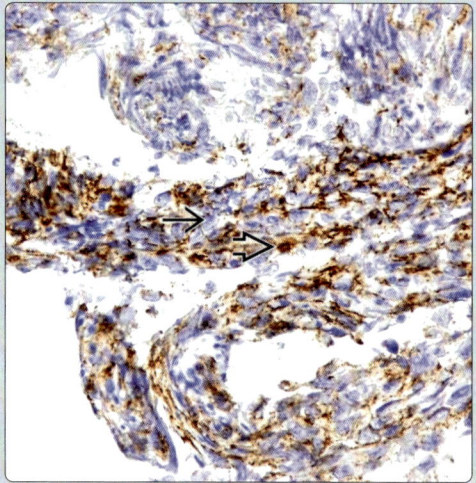

Angiosarcoma: CD31(+)

(Left) Pap-stained FNA smear of a high-grade angiosarcoma (AS) of the breast shows spindle-shaped tumor cells forming prominent vascular channels ➡. (Right) Immunostaining of a cell block for CD31 shows the tumor cells forming prominent vascular channels ➡ to be positive ➡, which supports the diagnosis of AS.

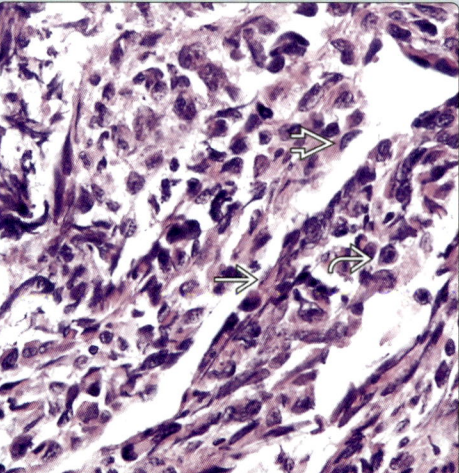

Angiosarcoma: Cell Block

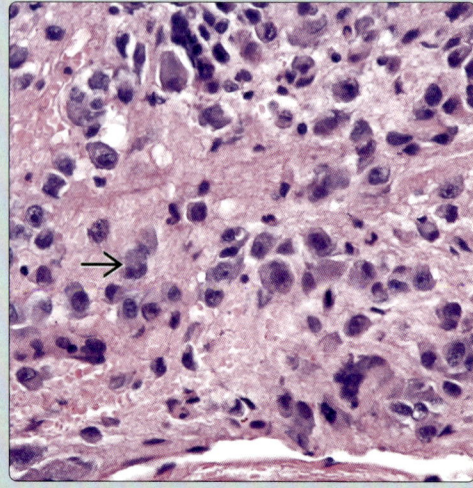

Angiosarcoma: Cell Block

(Left) H&E-stained tissue section of a cell block of AS shows vascular channels ➡ composed of spindle ➡ and epithelioid ➡ tumor cells. (Right) H&E-stained tissue section of a cell block of epithelioid AS with individually distributed epithelioid tumor cells ➡ is shown.

Angiosarcoma and Other Sarcomas

TERMINOLOGY

Definitions
- Angiosarcoma (AS): Malignant neoplasm arising from endothelial cells
- Other sarcomas: Malignant neoplasms arising from mesenchymal cells other than endothelial cells
- Liposarcoma (LIS): Malignant neoplasm arising from adipocytes
- Leiomyosarcoma (LES): Malignant neoplasm arising from smooth muscle
- Malignant peripheral nerve sheath tumor (MPNST): Malignant tumor arising from neural structures
- Osteogenic sarcoma (OS): Malignant neoplasm arising from osteoblasts
- Chondrosarcoma (CS): Malignant neoplasm arising from chondrocytes
- Malignant fibrous histiocytoma (MFH), fibrosarcoma (FS): Malignant neoplasm arising from fibroblasts
- Rhabdomyosarcoma (RMS): Malignant neoplasm arising from skeletal muscle
- Synovial sarcoma (SS): Malignant neoplasm that can arise from different types of soft tissue, such as muscle, ligaments, or from soft tissue in lung or abdomen

ETIOLOGY/PATHOGENESIS

Idiopathic
- Etiology of most soft tissue sarcomas of breast remains unknown
  - AS is most common sarcoma of breast, followed by LIS

Radiation
- Sarcomas associated with prior use of breast external beam radiation therapy
- Most common: AS, MFH, FS

Edema
- Women with markedly edematous arms after breast and axillary surgery for cancer are at increased risk for AS of skin, a.k.a. Stewart-Treves syndrome

CLINICAL ISSUES

Epidemiology
- Incidence
  - Mammary sarcomas: < 0.1% of breast malignancies
  - Primary sarcomas other than AS are exceedingly rare
- Age
  - Average age of women diagnosed with idiopathic sarcomas of breast: 40s
  - Average age of women diagnosed with radiation-related or edema-related AS: 60s

Site
- Idiopathic sarcomas generally arise deep in breast
- Radiation-related AS arises in skin
- Edema-related AS arises in skin of edematous area
  - Arm is most common site

Presentation
- Patients with idiopathic sarcomas present with rapidly enlarging palpable mass in breast
- Patients with radiation-related or edema-related AS present with dark red or violaceous discoloration of skin

Prognosis
- Primary mammary sarcomas have prognosis similar to that of their soft tissue counterparts
- Median survival is usually 3 years; same for idiopathic and treatment-related sarcomas
  - Many patients develop distant metastasis to sites such as lung, liver, bone, and contralateral breast
  - Metastasis to regional lymph nodes is rare

IMAGING

Mammographic Findings
- Lobulated or ill-defined mass
- AS may be difficult to image as desmoplastic response commonly associated with carcinomas is not present

CYTOPATHOLOGY

Angiosarcoma
- Aspirates are bloody, resulting in hemorrhagic background, very often including hemosiderin-laden macrophages
- Cellularity depends on degree of differentiation of AS
- Low-grade AS usually demonstrates few scattered, mildly atypical spindle cells
- High-grade AS shows abundant individual spindle &/or epithelioid cells with significant atypia
- Tumor cells can have elongated, round, or oval centrally or eccentrically placed nuclei
- Nuclear hyperchromasia, pleomorphism, prominent nucleoli, and conspicuous mitotic activity of tumor cells in high-grade tumors
- Tumor cells can form arborizing vascular channels, acinar-like, rosette-like, pseudopapillary clusters
- Tumor cells demonstrate moderate amounts of cytoplasm
  - Cytoplasmic borders are often wispy and frayed
- Cytoplasm can be vacuolated; intracytoplasmic lumen can be noted, which may contain red blood cells

Other Sarcomas
- Malignant spindle cells of varying grades of cytologic atypia can be encountered in FS, LES, RMS, monophasic SS, and MPNST
- Malignant spindle cells may show wavy, serpentine nuclei in MPNST
  - Malignant spindle nuclei with blunt ends in LES
- Malignant spindle cells with significant pleomorphism can be seen in pleomorphic variants of LIS, RMS, MPNST, and MFH
- Lipoblasts are characteristic feature of LS
- Lipoblasts have lipid vacuoles in cytoplasm, which cause scalloping of nuclei
- Myxoid background can be noted in sarcomas such as RMS, myxoid LIS, myxoid CS, MPNST, and myxofibrosarcoma
- Myxoid background with chicken-wire pattern of capillary network is characteristic feature of myxoid LIS
- Malignant cells in lacunar spaces associated with fibromyxoid matrix is noted in myxoid CS
- Malignant cells with small- to medium-sized round nucleus with dense or vacuolated cytoplasm can be seen in round cell LIS

Angiosarcoma and Other Sarcomas

- Small round blue cells often with strap cells noted in embryonal and alveolar RMS
- Small, round, ovoid, elongated cells associated with cartilaginous matrix noted in mesenchymal CS
- Presence of osteoid with hyaline, fibrillar material amidst tumor cells with plasmacytoid, spindle pleomorphic tumor cells is noted in OS
- Malignant cells with varying grades of atypia located within lacunar spaces and associated with chondromyxoid matrix in CS
- Sarcomas with epithelioid tumor cells are seen in addition to AS in epithelioid variants of LES, MPNST, and SS
- SS shows least cytologic atypia amongst all sarcomas

ANCILLARY TESTS

Immunohistochemistry
- Panel of pertinent immunomarkers should be performed and interpreted in conjunction with cytomorphologic features
  - AS: Factor VIII, CD34, CD31, ERG, MYC
  - LIS: Vimentin, S100, CDK4, MDM2
  - CS: S100; mesenchymal CS: CD57, CD99, S100
  - LES: Vimentin, SMA, desmin, caldesmon
  - RMS: Vimentin, desmin, myogenin, myoglobin
  - MPNST: S100, SOX10
  - SS, epithelioid variants of AS, LES, MPNST: Focal cytokeratin staining

Genetic Testing
- Availability of tissue for cytogenetic analysis may be useful in suspected primary sarcomas (e.g., SS, RMS, LS)

DIFFERENTIAL DIAGNOSIS

Hemangioma
- Benign proliferations of blood vessels; almost all < 2 cm in size; small perilobular or capillary hemangiomas are almost always incidental findings (0.1-0.2 cm) and usually not subject to aspiration biopsy
  - Larger (cavernous or venous) hemangiomas may be palpable or present as mass on imaging
  - Scant spindle cells with minimal atypia (unlike sarcomas) may be noted in hemorrhagic background

Pseudoangiomatous Stromal Hyperplasia
- Can present as palpable mass or radiologic density, is not associated with hemorrhage, and does not involve skin or cause hemorrhagic skin lesions
  - Shows benign ductal epithelial cells associated with increased numbers of naked nuclei and elongated spindle cells that do not exhibit cytologic atypia, unlike sarcomas

Angiolipoma
- Benign, well-circumscribed, usually small lesion (< 2 cm) composed of adipose tissue and small, round, capillary-sized blood vessels, which may have fibrin thrombi
  - Relatively few spindle cells without cytologic atypia in direct smears associated with fragments of adipose tissue without cellularity, cellular pleomorphism, and mitoses of sarcomas

Mammary Carcinoma
- Tumor cells of epithelioid sarcomas can mimic poorly differentiated ductal carcinoma
- Radiation- or edema-related AS is present with dark red/violaceous discoloration of skin, unlike carcinomas
- Ancillary immunostaining for epithelial and pertinent mesenchymal markers may be required to arrive at correct diagnosis

Malignant Phyllodes Tumor
- Sarcomatous stromal component of malignant phyllodes tumor can mimic any primary breast sarcoma
- Recognition of intimately admixed benign ductal epithelium in smears is useful

Metaplastic Carcinoma
- Malignant spindle cells of metaplastic carcinoma and heterologous elements in matrix-producing metaplastic carcinomas can be similar to any primary breast sarcoma
- Recognition of areas with epithelial features and ancillary immunostains for cytokeratins (particularly high molecular weight cytokeratins) and p63 are useful

Metastatic Sarcoma/Melanoma
- Breast involvement is usually part of disseminated spread; clinical history alone for sarcomas and, in addition, ancillary immunostains in case of melanomas are useful for distinction

Granulation Tissue/Mesenchymal Repair
- Vascular proliferation with reactive atypia of endothelial cells and myofibroblasts in lesion can mimic AS
- Clinical history accounting for tissue trauma, imaging features, and associated acute and chronic inflammation is useful

Radiation Change
- Atypical myofibroblasts and endothelial cells in radiated indurated areas can mimic sarcomas
- Cellularity is usually low for degree of nuclear atypia; cytoplasm is usually moderate to abundant

SELECTED REFERENCES

1. Al-Wiswasy M et al: Primary stromal sarcoma of breast: a case report and literature review. Breast Dis. 40(3):199-205, 2021
2. Friedrich AU et al: Characteristics and long-term risk of breast angiosarcoma. Ann Surg Oncol. 28(9):5112-8, 2021
3. Bonito FJP et al: Radiation-induced angiosarcoma of the breast: a review. Breast J. 26(3):458-63, 2020
4. Abdou Y et al: Primary and secondary breast angiosarcoma: single center report and a meta-analysis. Breast Cancer Res Treat. 178(3):523-33, 2019
5. Duncan MA et al: Sarcomas of the breast. Surg Clin North Am. 98(4):869-76, 2018
6. Yin M et al: Prognosis and treatment of non-metastatic primary and secondary breast angiosarcoma: a comparative study. BMC Cancer. 17(1):295, 2017
7. Masai K et al: Clinicopathological features of breast angiosarcoma. Breast Cancer. 23(5):718-23, 2016
8. Fraga-Guedes C et al: Angiosarcoma and atypical vascular lesions of the breast: diagnostic and prognostic role of MYC gene amplification and protein expression. Breast Cancer Res Treat. 151(1):131-40, 2015
9. Ginter PS et al: Diagnostic utility of MYC amplification and anti-MYC immunohistochemistry in atypical vascular lesions, primary or radiation-induced mammary angiosarcomas, and primary angiosarcomas of other sites. Hum Pathol. 45(4):709-16, 2014
10. des Guetz G et al: Postirradiation sarcoma: clinicopathologic features and role of chemotherapy in the treatment strategy. Sarcoma. 2009:764379, 2009

Angiosarcoma and Other Sarcomas

Angiosarcoma: Spindle Tumor Cells

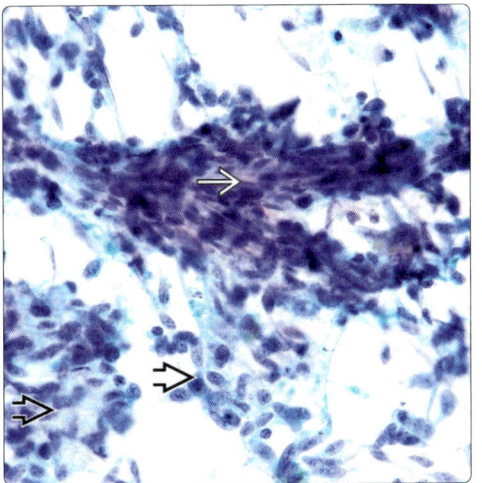

Angiosarcoma: Spindle Tumor Cells

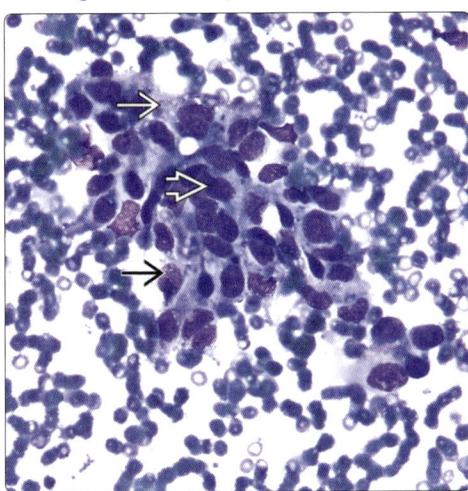

(Left) Pap-stained FNA smear of high-grade AS shows vascular channel formation ⇒ with plump spindle tumor cells emanating from the channels and forming loosely cohesive clusters ⇒. (Right) Diff-Quik-stained FNA smear of AS of the breast shows a loosely cohesive cluster ⇒ of plump spindle cells ⇒ with a moderate amount of delicate cytoplasm ⇒.

Angiosarcoma: Spindle Tumor Cells

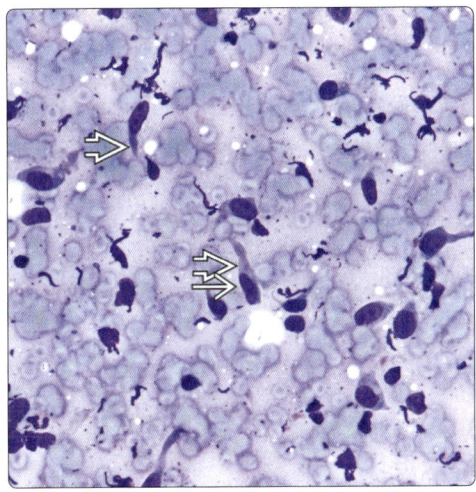

Angiosarcoma: Spindle Tumor Cells

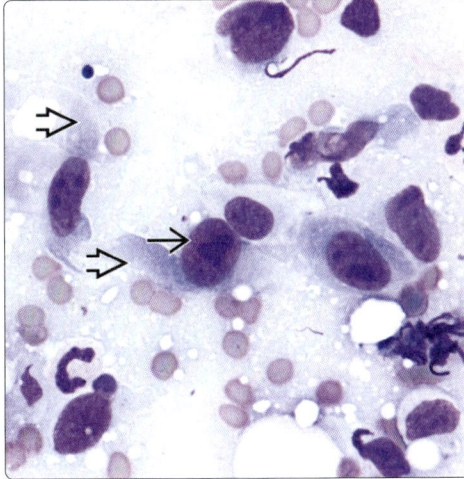

(Left) Diff-Quik-stained FNA smear of high-grade AS shows scattered single tumor cells ⇒, a common feature of these tumors. Note that many of the tumor cells show an eccentrically placed nucleus with a cytoplasmic tail ⇒. (Right) Diff-Quik-stained FNA smear of high-grade AS shows individual tumor cells ⇒ with oval and spindle-shaped nucleus, prominent nucleolus, and moderate amounts of delicate and wispy cytoplasm ⇒.

Angiosarcoma: Epithelioid Tumor Cells

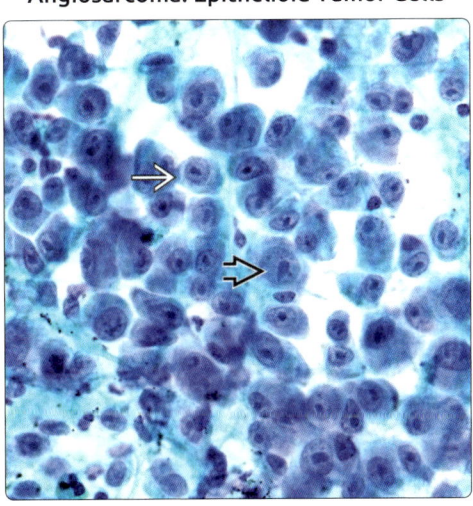

Angiosarcoma: CD31(+)

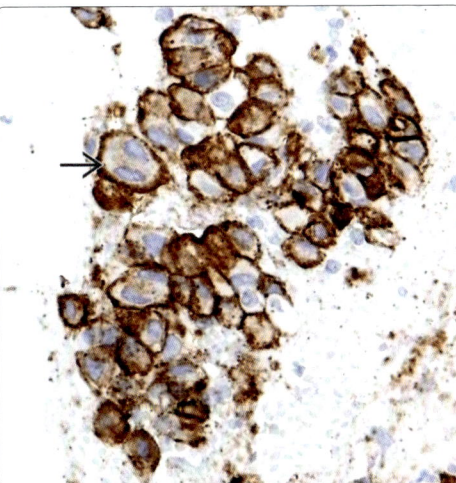

(Left) Pap-stained FNA smear shows high-grade AS with dyscohesive epithelioid tumor cells ⇒ with large nuclei ⇒, prominent nucleoli, and moderate amounts of cytoplasm. This tumor can be mistaken for poorly differentiated ductal carcinoma of the breast. (Right) CD31 immunostaining of a cell block section of the same case of epithelioid AS shows membranous staining ⇒ of all tumor cells, which confirms the diagnosis of AS.

Lymphomas and Metastatic Tumors

KEY FACTS

CLINICAL ISSUES

- **Lymphomas** of breast are rare; < 0.5% of all breast malignancies
  - Majority of breast lymphomas are non-Hodgkin B-cell lymphomas; diffuse large B-cell lymphoma is most common type of lymphoma involving breast
  - Breast implant-associated anaplastic large cell lymphoma is rare type of CD30(+) T-cell lymphoma
- **Metastases** to breast comprise 0.5-6.0% of all breast malignancies
  - Embryonal rhabdomyosarcoma: Most common type of metastasis to breast in children and adolescents
  - Malignant melanoma: Most common type of metastasis to breast in adults
  - Prostatic cancer: Most common type of metastasis in men

CYTOPATHOLOGY

- **Lymphoma**: Dispersed atypical lymphoid cells with lymphoglandular bodies in background; cytomorphology depends on type of lymphoma
- **Metastatic tumor**: Cytology depends on source of metastatic tumor; presence of cell types not usually seen in primary tumors raises possibility of metastasis

TOP DIFFERENTIAL DIAGNOSES

- **DDx of lymphoma**: Inflammatory myofibroblastic tumor (pseudolymphoma, plasma cell granuloma), carcinoma, leukemic breast involvement (granulocytic sarcoma), intramammary lymph node
- **DDx of metastases**: Primary breast carcinoma
  - Clinical history, comparison with extramammary primary tumor, and utilization of appropriate immunomarkers may be useful to confirm or exclude metastatic tumors in breast

Large Cell Lymphoma Morphology
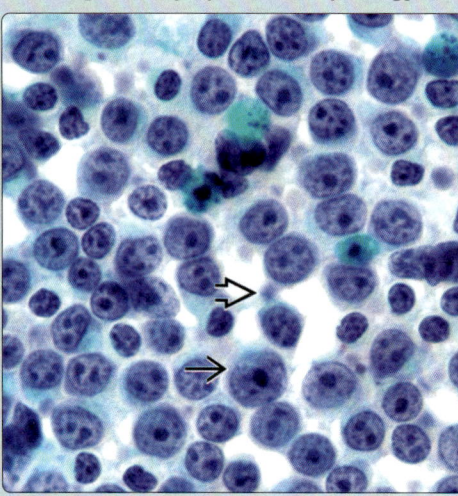

Large Cell Lymphoma, CD45 Positive
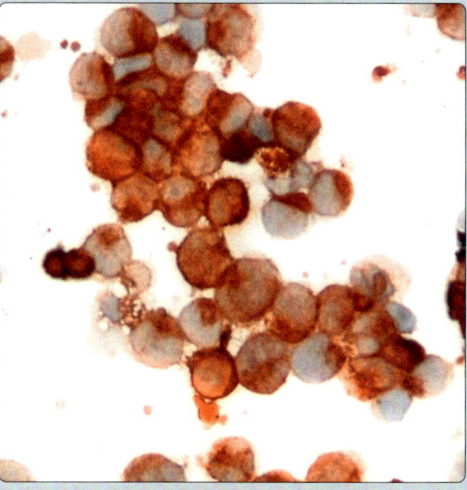

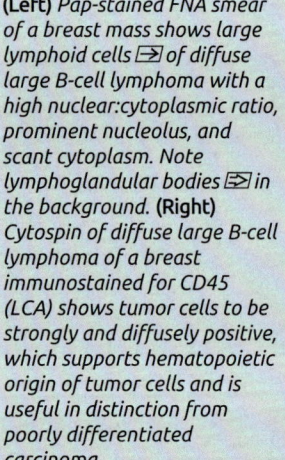

(Left) Pap-stained FNA smear of a breast mass shows large lymphoid cells ➡ of diffuse large B-cell lymphoma with a high nuclear:cytoplasmic ratio, prominent nucleolus, and scant cytoplasm. Note lymphoglandular bodies ➡ in the background. *(Right)* Cytospin of diffuse large B-cell lymphoma of a breast immunostained for CD45 (LCA) shows tumor cells to be strongly and diffusely positive, which supports hematopoietic origin of tumor cells and is useful in distinction from poorly differentiated carcinoma.

Metastatic Prostate Carcinoma
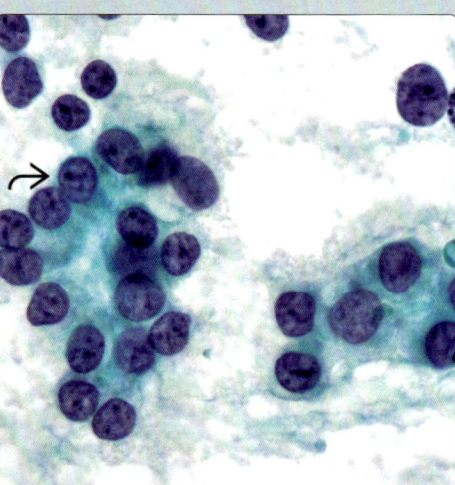

Metastatic Melanoma
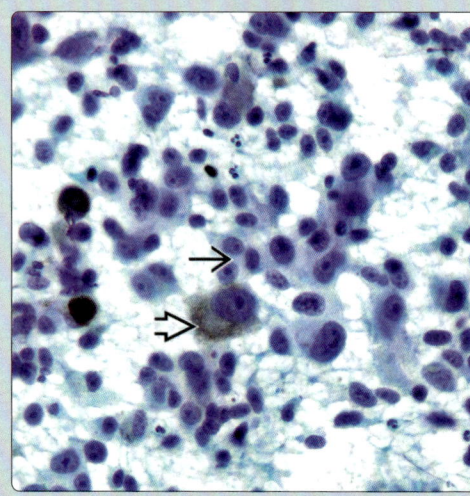

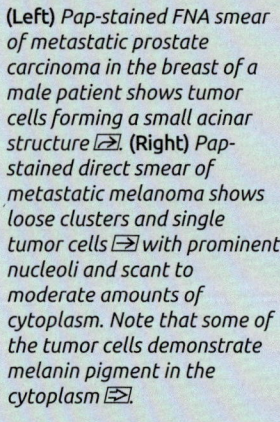

(Left) Pap-stained FNA smear of metastatic prostate carcinoma in the breast of a male patient shows tumor cells forming a small acinar structure ➡. *(Right)* Pap-stained direct smear of metastatic melanoma shows loose clusters and single tumor cells ➡ with prominent nucleoli and scant to moderate amounts of cytoplasm. Note that some of the tumor cells demonstrate melanin pigment in the cytoplasm ➡.

Lymphomas and Metastatic Tumors

TERMINOLOGY

Definitions

- **Lymphoma**: Clonal population of malignant lymphocytes involving breast
  - Primary breast lymphoma: Restricted to breast parenchyma and axillary nodes when initially diagnosed without any prior history of lymphoma or with concurrent involvement of other sites
  - Secondary breast lymphoma: Breast involvement in patients with systemic disease; very often, intramammary lymph node is involved by secondary lymphoma
- **Metastatic tumors**: Different primary tumors can metastasize to breast

CLINICAL ISSUES

Presentation

- **Lymphoma**
  - Rare tumors in breast; comprise < 0.5% of all breast malignancies; age range: 12-90 years with bimodal peaks in 30s and 40s
  - Usually present with palpable, circumscribed or irregular breast mass
    - Rarely, whole breast becomes edematous and enlarged due to lymphatic blockage by involved lymph nodes mimicking inflammatory breast carcinoma
  - Diffuse large B-cell lymphoma comprises 80% of primary breast lymphomas
    - Burkitt lymphoma can occur in young women, usually in Africa, who are often pregnant/lactating
  - Follicular lymphoma, extranodal marginal zone lymphoma, and T-cell lymphoma can rarely involve breast
  - Breast implant-associated anaplastic large cell lymphoma is rare type of CD30(+) T-cell lymphoma that arises around breast implants
- **Metastatic tumors**
  - Comprise 0.5-6.0% of all breast malignancies
    - Women are affected 5-6x more frequently than men
    - Patient is known to have another malignancy in 70-80% of cases
    - Metastases may be 1st presentation in 20-30% of cases

CYTOPATHOLOGY

Cellularity

- **Lymphoma**
  - Dispersed atypical lymphoid cells with lymphoglandular bodies in background
    - Cytomorphology of lymphoid cells depends on type of lymphoma involving breast
  - In diffuse large B-cell lymphoma, large lymphoid cells with round/oval, uniform, or pleomorphic nuclei with distinct single or multiple nucleoli and variable amounts of cytoplasm are noted
  - In Burkitt lymphoma, intermediate-sized lymphoid cells with round nuclei, multiple nucleoli, coarse chromatin, thick nuclear membrane, and moderate amounts of cytoplasm with fine vacuoles containing lipids are noted
  - Mitotic activity is significant in both types of high-grade lymphoma with presence of apoptotic bodies
    - Macrophages with ingested cellular debris results in starry-sky appearance in high-grade lymphomas
  - In breast implant-associated anaplastic large cell lymphoma, large pleomorphic lymphoid cells with irregular nuclei, dispersed chromatin, prominent nucleolus, and abundant pale to eosinophilic cytoplasm are noted
- **Metastatic tumors**
  - Cytology depends on source of metastatic tumor; comparison of cytomorphology of breast tumor with known extramammary primary tumor may be useful
  - Breast tumor with cells not commonly seen in primary tumors, such as presence of neuroendocrine small cells, squamoid cells, clear cells, or tumor cells with melanin pigment, raises possibility of metastatic tumor
  - Ancillary immunostaining can be useful to confirm or exclude metastatic tumor

DIFFERENTIAL DIAGNOSIS

DDx of Lymphoma

- Inflammatory myofibroblastic tumor
  - Consists of infiltrate of mixed inflammatory cells, often with prominent component of plasma cells and myofibroblasts, unlike predominant clonal population of lymphoid cells alone in lymphomas of breast
- Primary mammary carcinoma
  - Low-grade lymphomas can mimic lobular carcinomas, and high-grade lymphomas can mimic poorly differentiated carcinoma
  - Presence of dyscohesive cells with lymphoglandular bodies may be useful for distinction
    - Ancillary immunostaining for LCA and cytokeratins is useful
- Leukemic breast involvement (granulocytic sarcoma, chloroma)
  - Solid tumors composed of myeloid leukemia cells rarely present as breast mass without systemic acute myeloid leukemia; leukemia should be considered when B- or T-cell markers are negative in LCA(+) tumor cells
- Intramammary lymph node
  - Imaging features are usually characteristic for lymph node
    - Polymorphous population of lymphoid cells that are polyclonal by immunophenotyping

DDx of Metastatic Tumors

- Primary breast tumor: Clinical history, comparison with extramammary primary tumor, and utilization of appropriate immunomarkers may be useful to confirm or exclude metastatic tumors in breast

SELECTED REFERENCES

1. Elgaafary S et al: Molecular characterization of Burkitt lymphoma in the breast or ovary. Leuk Lymphoma. 62(9):2120-9, 2021
2. Evans MG et al: B-cell lymphomas associated with breast implants: report of three cases and review of the literature. Ann Diagn Pathol. 46:151512, 2020
3. de Leval L: Breast implant-associated anaplastic large cell lymphoma and other rare T-cell lymphomas. Hematol Oncol. 37 Suppl 1:24-9, 2019
4. Hoffmann J et al: Hematolymphoid lesions of the breast. Semin Diagn Pathol. 34(5):462-9, 2017

Cytology Specimens for Risk Assessment of Breast Cancer

TERMINOLOGY

Definition
- Breast cytology specimens for evaluating changes in breast parenchyma that can be utilized for risk assessment and chemoprevention of breast cancer
  - Investigational and not standard of care

NIPPLE ASPIRATION FLUID

Collection
- Nipple aspiration fluid (NAF) can be collected following breast massage ± use of breast pump for providing suction
- Volume of NAF: Variable; usually few µL

Factors Influencing NAF Production
- NAF production with volumes sufficient for analysis is positively correlated with age of 30-50 years, history of prior lactation, and non-Asian ethnicity
- NAF can be collected from 39-66% of women without regard to risk
- NAF can be collected from 50-95% of women at high risk for developing breast cancer

Utility of NAF for Risk Assessment
- NAF production
  - Women who produce NAF are at higher risk than women who do not produce NAF
- NAF cytology
  - Stepwise increase in risk for breast cancer based on cytologic changes
    - Women who do not produce NAF
    - NAF producers with nonproliferative changes of epithelial cells
    - NAF producers with proliferative changes of epithelial cells ± atypia

Criteria for Adequacy of NAF and Categorization of NAF Cytology
- Minimum of 10 epithelial cells necessary to qualify as adequate for evaluation
- Categorization
  - Unsatisfactory/nondiagnostic

Nipple Aspirate Fluid
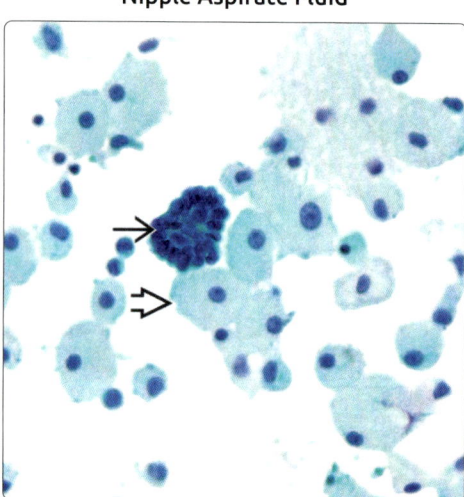

CD68(+) Foamy Macrophages
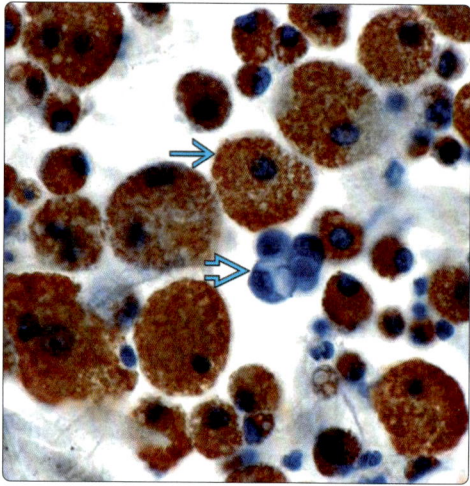

(Left) Pap-stained cytospin smear of nipple aspirate fluid shows a small, tight cluster of benign ductal cells ➡ associated with abundant foamy histiocytes in the background ➡. (Right) Nipple aspirate fluid smear shows abundant foamy macrophages that are positive for CD68 ➡. Note the cluster of ductal epithelial cells in the background ➡.

Ductal Lavage With Mild Atypia
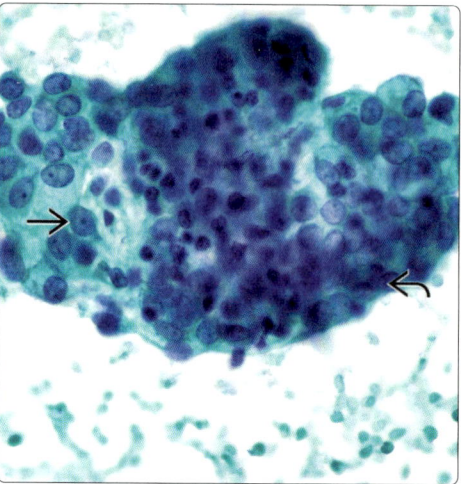

Atypical Cells Suspicious for Malignancy
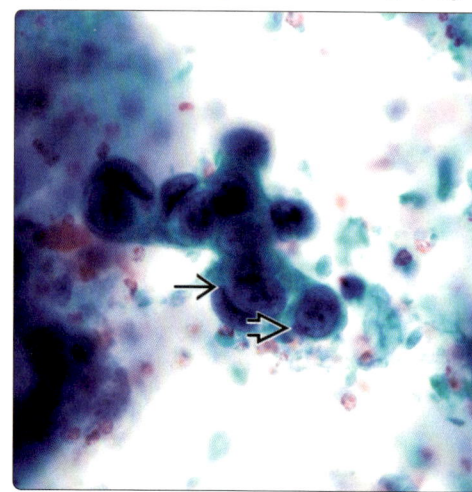

(Left) Pap-stained cytospin smear of ductal lavage cytology shows a fragment of mildly atypical ductal epithelial cells ➡ with enlarged nuclei ➡, mild nuclear pleomorphism, and moderate amount of cytoplasm. (Right) Pap-stained cytospin smear of ductal lavage cytology shows a cluster of markedly atypical cells ➡ with large, hyperchromatic nuclei ➡, very suspicious for malignancy.

Cytology Specimens for Risk Assessment of Breast Cancer

- ○ Mild atypia
- ○ Marked atypia/suspicious
- ○ Malignant
- Predominant component of NAF is foamy histiocytes with few epithelial cells
- Overall, 53-83% of NAF specimens will be adequate for evaluation
- Median number of epithelial cells in NAF is 120
- Up to 50% of high-risk women fail to produce NAF
- Up to 73% of high-risk women who produce NAF have nondiagnostic specimens with < 10 epithelial cells

Significance of NAF Cytology

- Relative risk for women producing NAF with atypia is reported to be 5x that of women who do not produce NAF
- Women producing NAF with proliferative epithelium ± atypia have 2.4-2.8x increased risk of breast cancer compared with those who do not produce NAF

DUCTAL LAVAGE

Sample Collection

- NAF-producing ducts are cannulated with microcatheter followed by infusion of saline or other physiologic solution
- Breast is massaged and effluent is collected in preservative solution

Specimen Preparation for Cytologic Examination

- Preservative solution with breast lavage fluid is used to prepare specimen
  - ○ Filter, monolayer, and cytospin preparations can be prepared for cytologic examination
  - ○ Median number of cells in ductal lavage (DL) is 1,200

Criteria for Adequacy of DL for Cytologic Examination

- Minimum of 10 epithelial cells necessary to qualify as adequate for evaluation
- Up to 56-60% of high-risk women will yield DL that will be adequate for cytologic examination

Categorization of DL Cytology

- Similar to NAF specimens

Significance of DL Cytology

- Women with atypia detected on DL cytology are presumed to be at higher risk for developing breast cancer
- Indirect evidence for significance of DL cytology based on follow-up studies of NAF and random periareolar fine-needle aspiration (RPFNA) cytology for risk assessment
- DL cytology is being utilized for clinical risk stratification, although magnitude of risk conferred by DL atypia is yet to be defined
- Impact of DL atypia on short-term risk for developing breast cancer is presently not known
- Sensitivity of DL cytology for breast cancer detection is very low (~ 13%) using marked atypia as deciding factor

Clinical Management of Atypia Detected on DL Cytology

- Experts have reported that women with atypia detected on DL cytology may be offered standard risk reduction options, such as antiestrogen therapy
- Marked atypia detected on DL cytology should lead to investigation of ducts yielding atypical cells using techniques such as ductoscopy &/or imaging studies for further investigation

RPFNA

Sample Collection

- Non-lesion-directed random 4-quadrant or 2-quadrant FNA of breast
- Generally, 4-5 aspirations are performed from each anesthetized site
- Specimen is generally pooled in preservative solution and processed for conventional cytomorphologic and biomarker examination

Sample Preparation for Cytologic Examination

- Filter, monolayer, or cytospin preparation

Specimen Categorization

- Unsatisfactory/insufficient cellularity
- Benign
- Atypical/indeterminate
- Suspicious
- Probably malignant
- Malignant

Significance of RPFNA

- Cytologic evidence of atypia confers 5x increase in risk for developing breast cancer
- RPFNA allows stratification of women with elevated Gail risk

SELECTED REFERENCES

1. Jiwa N et al: Diagnostic accuracy of nipple aspirate fluid cytology in asymptomatic patients: a meta-analysis and systematic review of the literature. Ann Surg Oncol. 28(7):3751-60, 2021
2. Patuleia SIS et al: The changing microRNA landscape by color and cloudiness: a cautionary tale for nipple aspirate fluid biomarker analysis. Cell Oncol (Dordr). 44(6):1339-49, 2021
3. Masood S: Development of a novel approach for breast cancer prediction and early detection using minimally invasive procedures and molecular analysis: how cytomorphology became a breast cancer risk predictor. Breast J. 21(1):82-96, 2015
4. Arun B et al: Comparison of ductal lavage and random periareolar fine needle aspiration as tissue acquisition methods in early breast cancer prevention trials. Clin Cancer Res. 13(16):4943-8, 2007
5. Zalles CM et al: Comparison of cytomorphology in specimens obtained by random periareolar fine needle aspiration and ductal lavage from women at high risk for development of breast cancer. Breast Cancer Res Treat. 97(2):191-7, 2006
6. Fabian CJ et al: Breast-tissue sampling for risk assessment and prevention. Endocr Relat Cancer. 12(2):185-213, 2005
7. Khan SA et al: Ductal lavage findings in women with known breast cancer undergoing mastectomy. J Natl Cancer Inst. 96(20):1510-7, 2004
8. Krishnamurthy S et al: Nipple aspirate fluid cytology in breast carcinoma. Cancer. 99(2):97-104, 2003

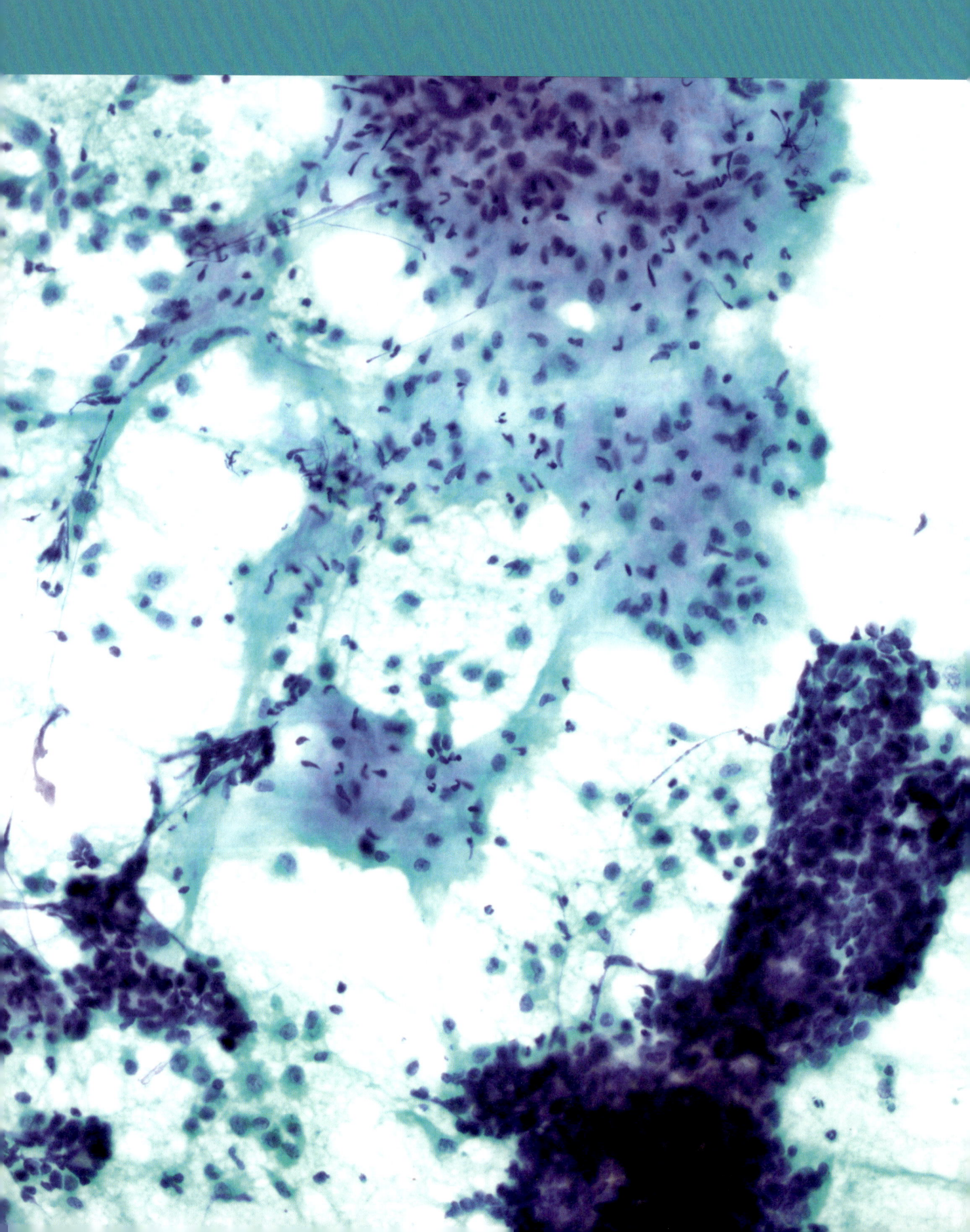

PART III
SECTION 7
Skin and Subcutaneous Cytology

Cutaneous and Adnexal Cytology 470

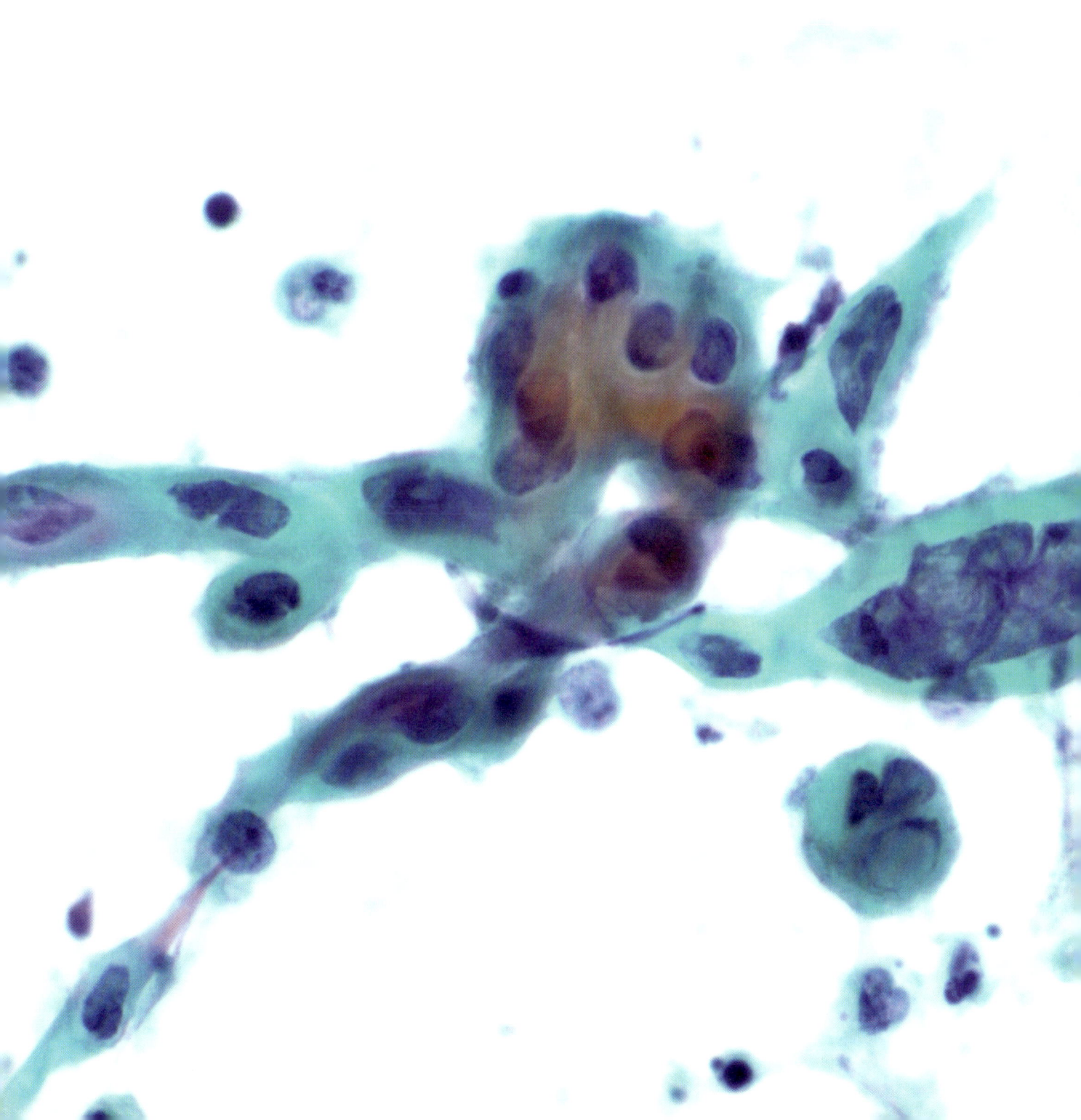

Cutaneous and Adnexal Cytology

TZANCK SMEARS

Herpes

- Clinical features
  - Herpes simplex virus type 1 (HSV1): Primary infections are usually mild and in childhood
    - Recurrences usually around lips
  - Herpes simplex virus type 2 (HSV2): Usually sexually transmitted and affects genital area
    - Usually presents as grouped clear vesicles
  - Herpes zoster (varicella zoster, shingles) typically presents as grouped erythematous papules in dermatomal distribution
    - Papules develop central vesiculation and may become pustular
    - Herpes zoster results from reactivation of latent varicella-zoster virus infection
    - May result in significant postherpetic neuralgia
- Cytologic findings
  - Herpes simplex, herpes/varicella zoster, and varicella are cytologically indistinguishable
    - Diagnosis can be confirmed with Tzanck preparation, which is unroofing of small vesicle followed by touch or scrape preparation
    - Multinucleated cells with margination of chromatin, nuclear molding, ground-glass chromatin
    - Cowdry A bodies: Intranuclear eosinophilic inclusions with surrounding chromatin clearing
    - May see neutrophils &/or necrosis

Molluscum contagiosum

- Clinical features
  - Occurs in children and adults
  - Generally transmitted by direct skin-to-skin contact
  - Some cases are sexually transmitted
  - Risk factors include immune suppression, especially in HIV patients and those receiving chemotherapy
  - Multiple discrete, 2- to 8-mm, flesh-colored or off-white, dome-shaped umbilicated papules and vesicles
  - Most lesions are self-limited and spontaneously regress in 6-12 months
  - Treatment: Curettage, cryotherapy, topical therapy, shave of solitary lesion
- Cytologic findings
  - Caused by pox virus, which is DNA virus
  - Large, intracytoplasmic inclusions occupy most of affected cells, pushing nucleus to periphery
    - These inclusions are spontaneously extruded at umbilication
  - Pasty material at umbilication can be squashed between 2 slides, which will extrude inclusions
  - Inclusions are dark purple on Romanowsky stains and usually eosinophilic on Pap stain
  - Differential diagnosis includes herpes, which shows multinucleation, molding, and intranuclear inclusions surrounded by halo
  - CMV inclusions are much smaller and intranuclear and cytoplasmic, with cytoplasmic inclusions being smaller and less well defined

FNA

Nonneoplastic Conditions

- Epidermal inclusion cyst
  - General features
    - Benign, unilocular cyst lined by squamoid epithelium
    - Can rupture or get inflamed
  - Cytology
    - Immediately under skin and difficult to separate from skin at time of aspiration
    - Sour smell as needle is withdrawn from lesion
    - Pasty yellow material that shows anucleate squames on cytology
    - Infected/ruptured cysts show inflammatory activity and giant cells
- Endometriosis
  - General features
  - Deposition of endometrial tissue outside endometrial cavity

Fat Necrosis

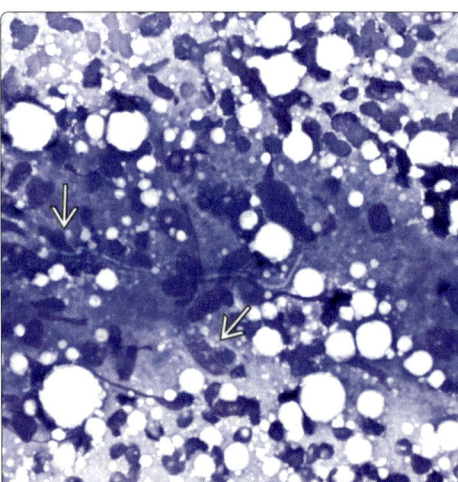

Diffuse Large B-Cell Lymphoma

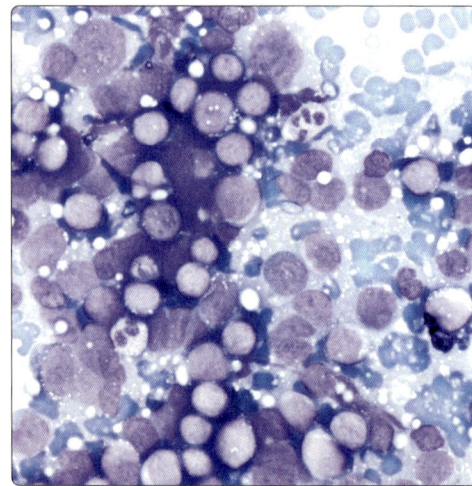

(Left) Diff-Quik-stained smear of a subcutaneous nodule shows a granulomatous response to saponified fat. Note the elongated and boomerang-shaped nuclei ➡. (Right) Diff-Quik-stained smear from a subcutaneous mass in a patient with known diffuse large B-cell lymphoma shows a population of large lymphocytes having an identical pattern to the patient's node-based diffuse large B-cell lymphoma.

Cutaneous and Adnexal Cytology

- Can be seen as nodule along or under C-section scar, as enlarging abdominal wall mass, or as palpable inguinal mass or under C-section flap as enlarging mass, and can be subject of aspiration
- Cytology
  - Biphasic population of tubular or geometric-shaped endometrial glands with accompanying bipolar stromal cells
  - Glandular elements can present as tubules or flat sheets with stromal cells that cling to periphery
  - Bipolar stromal cells in background with blood vessels cruising through stromal fragments, when present
  - Hemosiderin-laden macrophages, atypia, nuclear crowding, enlargement, and hyperchromasia may be seen in glandular component
  - Mitotic activity may be seen if in proliferative phase

Cutaneous and Adnexal Neoplasms

- **Pilomatrixoma**
  - General features
    - Benign tumor of follicular origin, a.k.a. calcifying epithelioma of Malherbe
    - Most common in head and neck, followed by upper extremities
    - > 1/2 occur in children and teens
  - Cytology
    - Aspirates are usually cellular
    - Small fragments of basaloid or basophilic cells with high nuclear:cytoplasmic ratio, evenly dispersed chromatin
    - May have prominent nucleoli
    - Clumps of refractile keratin may be seen
    - These tumors can have mitosis and hence could be misinterpreted as carcinomas
    - Ghost cells (a.k.a. eosinophilic shadow cells), which have no nuclear staining, are clue to correct diagnosis
    - Multinucleated giant cells are seen
    - Most have calcifications that may be associated with ghost cells
    - May have metaplastic bone formation
- **Clear cell hidradenoma**
  - General features
    - Benign cutaneous adnexal tumor showing apocrine or eccrine differentiation
    - Usually well-circumscribed dermal/subcutaneous nodule that classically does not connect to epidermis and is deep-seated
    - Composed of solid &/or cystic areas
  - Cytology
    - Clear or yellow-tinged fluid is obtained depending upon cystic component
    - 1st cellular component consists of clear cells with bland oval to round nuclei with small nucleoli
    - Cells are PAS(+) and diastase sensitive as they contain glycogen
    - Glycogen may give yellow tinge to cytoplasm on Pap stain
    - 2nd cellular component may consist of poroid cells, which are basaloid cells with scant cytoplasm
    - 3rd cellular component can be squamoid cells, which resemble keratinocytes with eosinophilic, well-demarcated cytoplasm
    - Differential is metastatic renal cell carcinoma, which is PAX8(+) and RCC(+)
    - Hidradenocarcinoma has necrosis, mitosis, and atypia
- **Basal cell carcinoma (BCC)**
  - General features
    - Most common skin malignancy
    - Most are slow growing; some are aggressive with deeply invasive recurrences and local destruction
    - Occur mainly in sun-exposed skin, especially in fair-skinned people
    - 80% occur in head and neck
  - Cytology
    - Lesions can be scraped or aspirated
    - Tightly cohesive crowded fragments of small basaloid cells with high nuclear:cytoplasmic ratio, small round to oval hyperchromatic nuclei, and usually inconspicuous nucleoli
    - Nuclear molding is not seen, distinguishing BCC from small cell carcinoma
    - May see peripheral palisading at edges of fragments, mainly in nodular and superficial BCCs
    - Some show focal keratinization (keratinizing or metaplastic BCC)
    - Differential diagnosis: Metastatic small cell carcinoma, poorly differentiated squamous cell carcinoma (SCCa), Merkel cell carcinoma (MCC)
- **SCCa**
  - General features
    - Common cutaneous malignancy related to sun, UV exposure, radiation, chronic wounds, and burn scars
    - Rare cases associated with high-risk HPV infection
  - Cytology
    - Usually not aspirated except in cases of recurrent subcutaneous nodule at previous excision site
    - Resembles SqCa in other sites but with easily recognizable keratinization
- **Eccrine carcinoma**
  - General features
    - Usually presents as solitary lesion
    - Some arise in preexisting benign eccrine neoplasm
  - Cytology
    - Adenocarcinomas of variable grade
    - Mitoses are clue to malignancy
    - Mitoses are rare in benign adnexal tumors except pilomatrixomas
    - Important to distinguish primary from metastasis
    - May express estrogen and progesterone receptor, hence not helpful in differential
    - Most express p63, whereas metastases from viscera, breast, and other sites rarely do
- **Melanoma**
  - General features
    - May present as macule, papule, patch, or nodule having irregular borders, irregular pigmentation, and asymmetry, often growing or changing
    - Most pigmented, some amelanotic
  - Cytology

Cutaneous and Adnexal Cytology

- Usually recurrences and nodular amelanotic melanoma are aspirated
- FNAs are cellular and dyshesive and usually have variable nonuniform population of cells
- Epithelioid &/or spindled cells
- Intracytoplasmic melanin pigment is good clue: Dark brown on Pap stain, dark blue on Diff-Quik
- Pigment is generally fine but occasionally coarser
- Commonly shows binucleated and sometimes multinucleated tumor cells
- Characteristic binucleated tumor cells with "mirror image" nuclei
- Often shows prominent nucleoli, intranuclear cytoplasmic inclusions, plasmacytoid cells, and mitosis
- Diff-Quik stain may show more cytoplasmic vacuoles than Pap stain

- **MCC**
  - General features
    - Occurs mainly in older White patients; slight male predominance
    - Most common in sun-exposed skin, especially head and neck; extremities are next most common site
    - Typically asymptomatic, rapidly growing, reddish-blue or flesh-colored papule or nodule
    - Clinical differential of BCC and amelanotic melanoma
    - Merkel cell polyoma virus (MCPyV), which is detected in 80% of MCC, is clonally integrated into tumor genome
    - MCCs that are polyoma virus (-) may have *RB1* or *TP3* inactivating mutations or other mutations
    - Truncation mutation in viral large T-antigen gene
  - Cytology
    - Dyshesive cellular aspirates with single cells, loose clusters, and rare rosette configuration
    - Small to intermediate cells, round to oval nuclei, finely granular to powdery chromatin, small nucleoli, delicate nuclear membrane, high nuclear:cytoplasmic ratio, focal molding, occasional DNA streaking
    - May show increased mitotic activity and increased apoptotic cells
    - Usually relatively monomorphous; occasional cases have mild to moderate nuclear pleomorphism
    - Immunohistochemistry: MCC expresses CK20 (paranuclear dot-like positivity) in 95%; synaptophysin, chromogranin, CD56, and TTF-1 (-)
    - Immunoreactive for CM2B4, which recognizes large T antigen of MCPyV

- **Cutaneous angiosarcoma**
  - General features
    - Most commonly occurs on skin, mainly in older patients, M > F, and present in head and neck, especially on scalp and forehead
    - May present as red, blue-black, or violet nodule, as bruise or as nonhealing ulcer
  - Cytology
    - Aspirates of low-grade tumors may be bloody and paucicellular
    - Higher grade lesions yield more cellular aspirates
    - Spindled &/or epithelioid tumor cells are bland to bizarre
    - Arranged singly in papillary clusters and vasoformative
    - Identifying vasoformation is clue to diagnosis
    - Can see tumor cells lined up along vascular spaces or along red blood cells, neoplastic vessels, whorls, rosette-like structures, intracytoplasmic lumina with red blood cells
    - Diagnostic pitfalls include cytologic features of epithelioid angiosarcoma that may be misinterpreted as adenocarcinoma: Epithelioid cells, pseudoacini, rosette-like structures, intracytoplasmic lumina, papillary configuration
    - Immunohistochemistry: CD31 [cytoplasmic/membranous (+)] and ERG [nuclear (+)]

- **Kaposi sarcoma**
  - 4 types
    - **Type 1**: Sporadic indolent form in older men, especially of Mediterranean and Eastern European origin
    - **Type 2** (endemic): African form involving children and adults
    - **Type 3**: Associated with immunosuppression
    - **Type 4** (AIDS-associated): Most aggressive variant; incidence has decreased with widespread use of HAART
  - Clinical appearance: Initially red-brown to purple patches and plaques, later develop nodules
  - Cytology
    - FNAs may be bloody and paucicellular, especially in early lesions
    - Loosely cohesive fragments of generally bland spindle cells with entrapped red blood cells
    - Also single cells, naked nuclei, focal crush artifact
    - Elongated nuclei with finely granular cytoplasm and inconspicuous nucleoli
    - Generally pale cytoplasm that may contain hemosiderin
    - May see intracellular and extracellular hyaline globules
    - Immunohistochemistry: CD34(+), often CD31(+) and HHV8(+)

- **Metastasis**
  - General findings
    - Metastasis can be hematogenous, lymphatic, or direct extension from primary tumor or unintended implantation during surgical procedure
    - Incidence ~ 2-10% in patients with internal malignancy
    - In most cases, primary is known; breast, lung, and kidney are 3 main primaries
  - Cytology
    - Cytologic features depend upon primary site
    - Immunohistochemical work-up and confirmation necessary

SELECTED REFERENCES

1. Kundu R et al: Phaeohyphomycosis: cytomorphologic evaluation in eleven cases. Acta Cytol. 64(5):406-12, 2020
2. Fernando A et al: Ultrasound-guided fine-needle aspiration biopsy in skin lesions. Skin Res Technol. 25(3):399-401, 2019
3. Viswanathan K et al: Fine needle aspiration of pilomatrixoma: cytologic features on thinprep and diagnostic pitfalls. Diagn Cytopathol. 46(5):452-5, 2018

Cutaneous and Adnexal Cytology

Plasma Cells in Multiple Myeloma

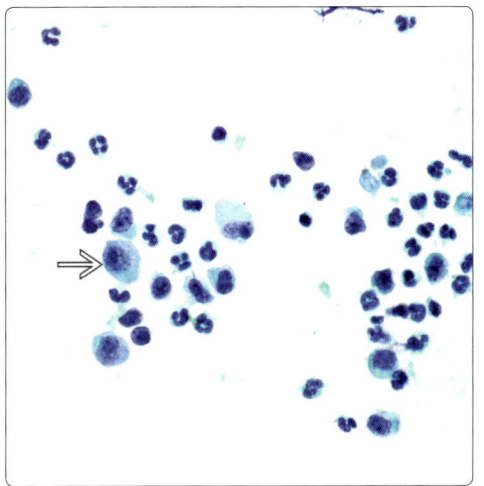

Pilomatrixoma Components

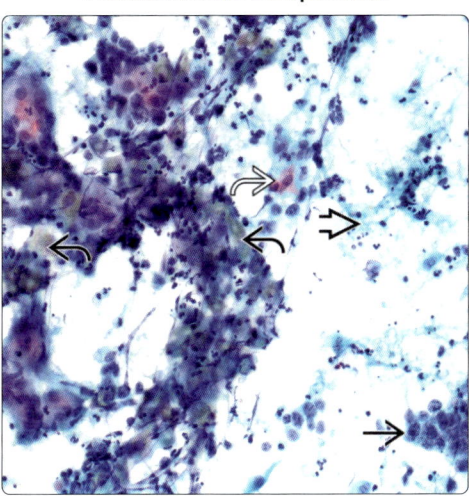

(Left) Pap-stained smear of a subcutaneous nodule in a patient with multiple myeloma shows many plasma cells ⇨, which on kappa/lambda in situ hybridization showed a lambda light chain restriction. (Right) Pap-stained smear of pilomatrixoma shows basaloid cells ⇨, ghosts of squamous cells ⇨, and keratinized cells ⇨ in a dirty background ⇨.

Endometriosis

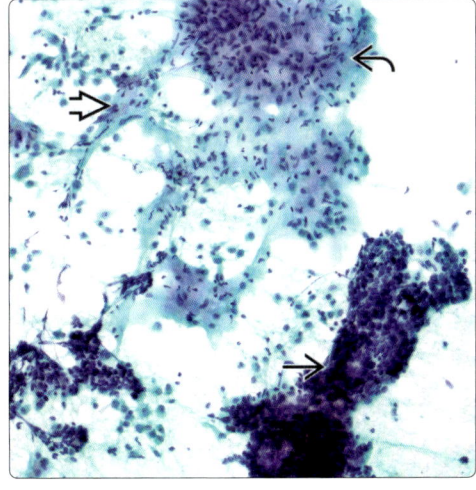

Clear Cell Hidradenoma

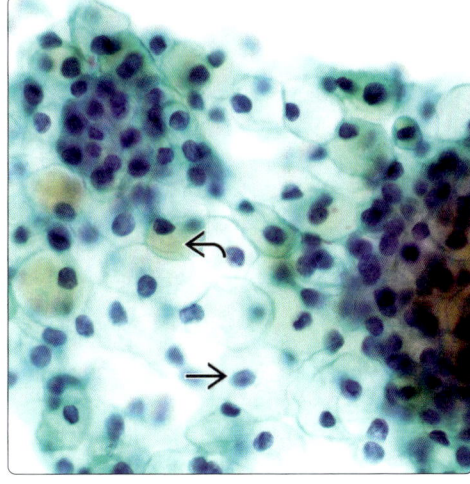

(Left) Pap-stained smear of endometriosis at a C-section line demonstrates a biphasic pattern of tubular endometrial glands ⇨ with spindle stromal cells and stromal fragments ⇨. Blood vessels ⇨ transgress the stroma and beyond. (Right) Pap-stained smear from an FNA of clear cell hidradenoma shows cells that have clear cytoplasm ⇨ with bland nuclei. The glycogen in the cells stains yellow ⇨. There is a lack of mitosis, necrosis, or atypia.

Basal Cell Carcinoma

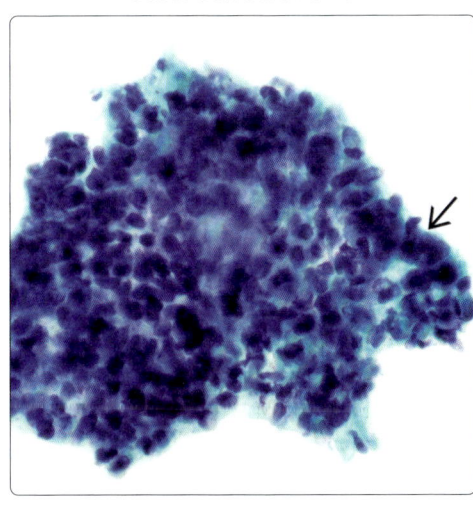

Cutaneous Angiosarcoma

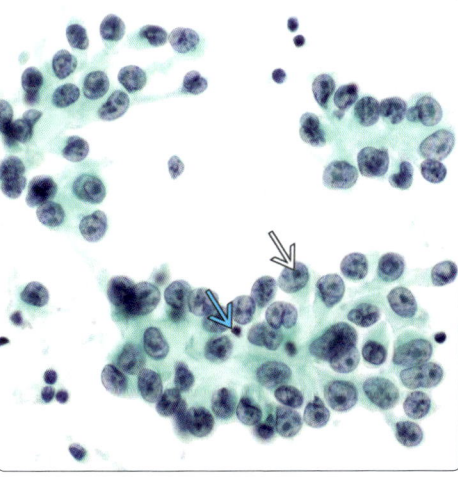

(Left) Pap stain shows tightly cohesive cells with peripheral palisading ⇨ from a basal cell carcinoma. The cells have scant cytoplasm and are hyperchromatic. (Right) Pap-stained smear of a violaceous skin nodule in a background of severe actinic keratosis shows a wreath-like arrangement of the cell groups. The nuclei are irregular with distinct nucleoli ⇨. Rare lymphocytes ⇨ are noted. The cells were CD31 positive, confirming the endothelial nature of the tumor. Clinical context is key to consideration of this diagnosis.

PART IV
Fine-Needle Aspiration, Deep Organs and Tissues

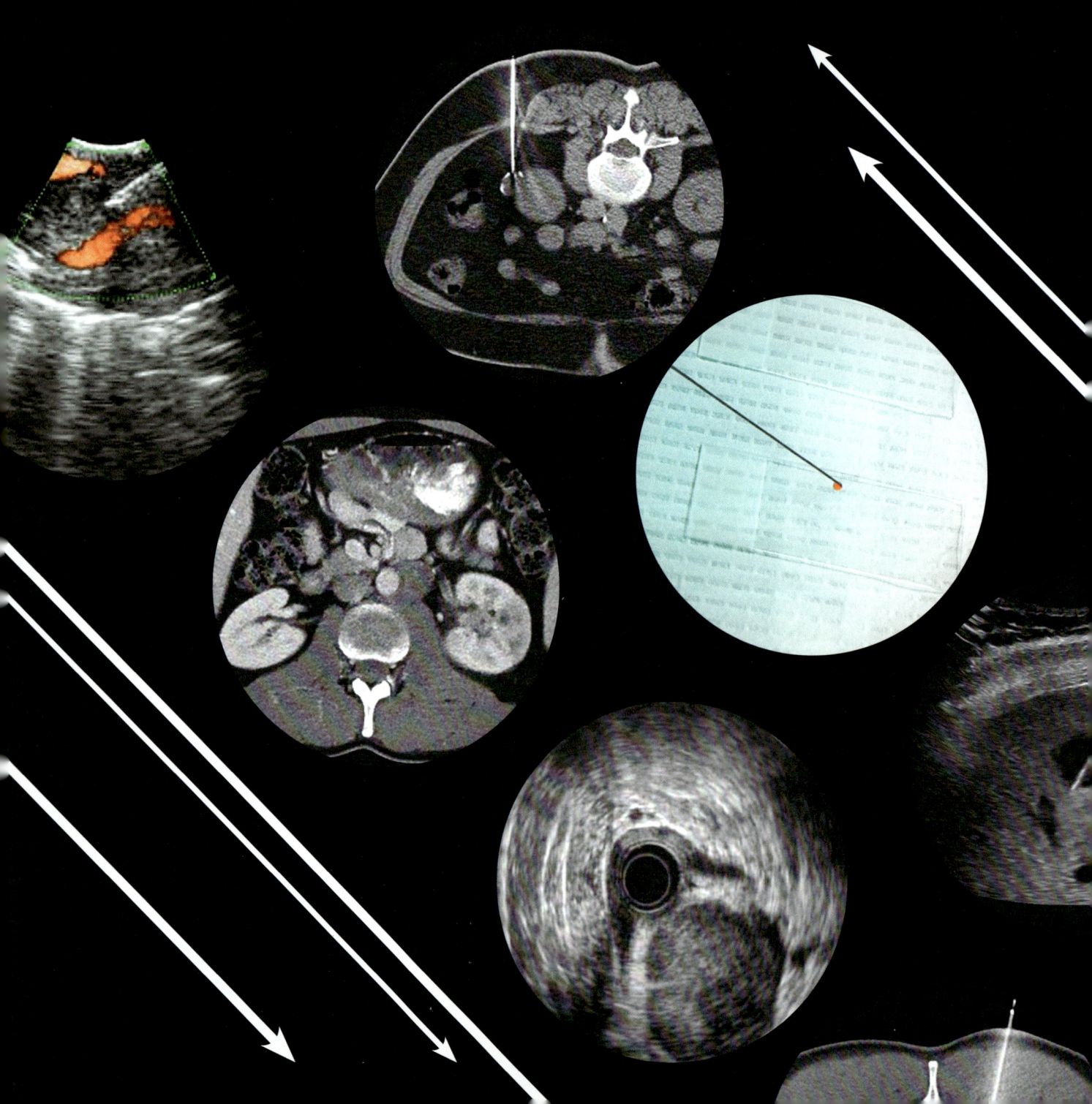

PART IV
SECTION 1
Overview

Techniques and Modalities of Deep Aspiration Biopsies   476

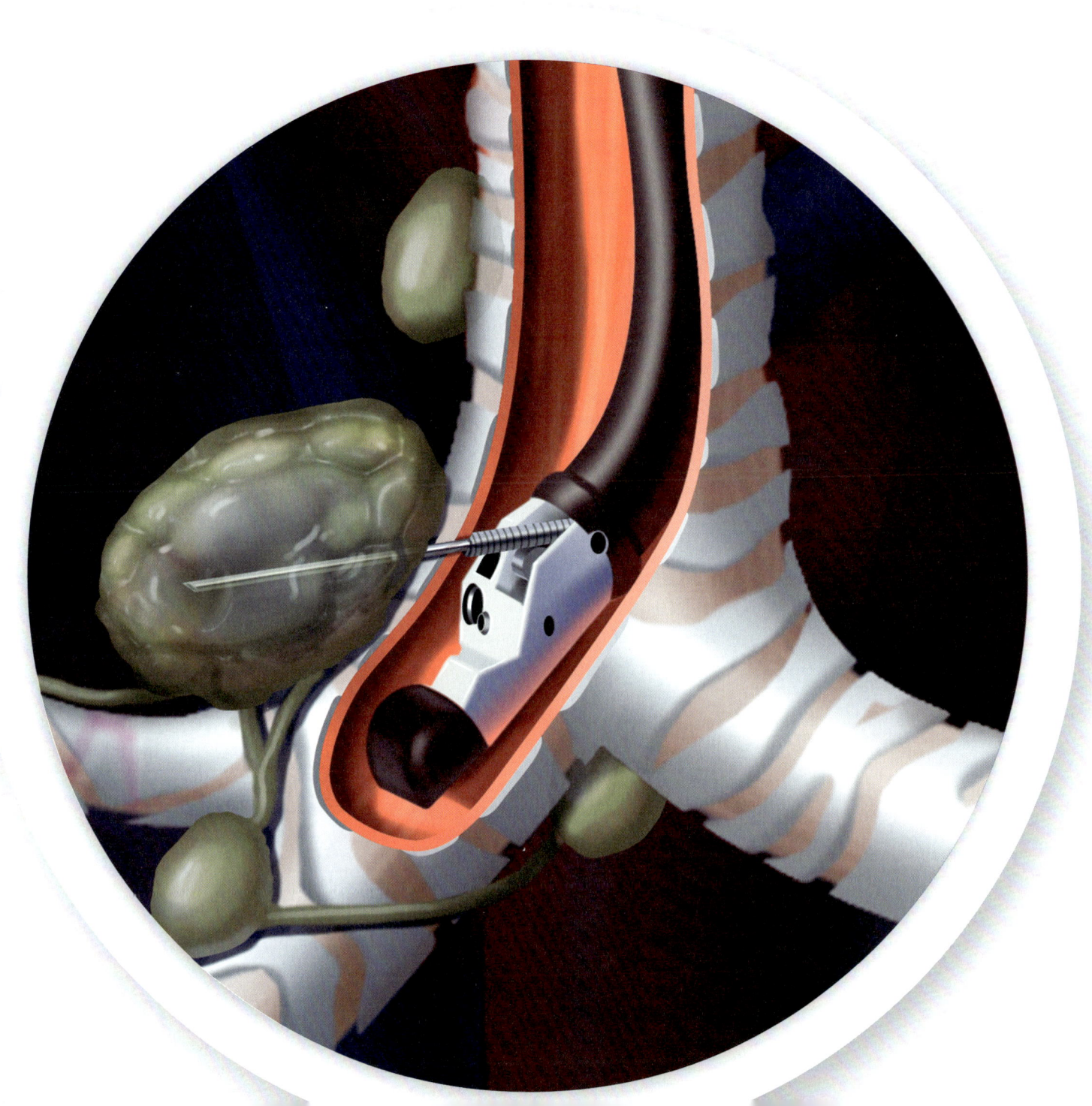

Techniques and Modalities of Deep Aspiration Biopsies

PREPROCEDURE

Indications
- Establish malignant or benign diagnosis in mass or nodule
- Determine nature/extent of diffuse parenchymal disease

Contraindications
- Uncorrectable bleeding diathesis
- Lack of safe access
  - Intervening bowel, vessels, or certain viscera

Review Imaging
- Decide on approach based on location
- Colon, esophageal, gastric, and proximal small bowel masses biopsied via colonoscopy or upper endoscopy
  - Double-balloon or push endoscopy may reach some jejunal masses but more distal masses may be inaccessible
- Endobronchial lesions &/or peribronchial nodes approached by bronchoscopy
- US is preferred modality for percutaneous biopsy but lesion is not always visible
  - US allows real-time evaluation of needle localization
  - Much faster and less expensive than CT
  - No ionizing radiation

Review Patient Chart
- Allergies and current medications, especially any anticoagulant or antiplatelet agents
- Laboratory parameters
  - Platelet count > 50,000/μL
  - International normalized ratio (INR) ≤ 1.5
  - Normal prothrombin time (PT), partial thromboplastin time (PTT)

Special Considerations
- Ascites: Preprocedure paracentesis may reduce postbiopsy hemorrhage risk
- Adnexal masses: Prior consultation with gynecologic oncology in suspected malignancy
  - Resection preferred to biopsy
- Lung lesion: Have chest tube ready to treat pneumothorax
- Liver and renal transplant: Consultation with transplant team regarding selection of preprocedure antibiotics

Mediastinal Adenopathy
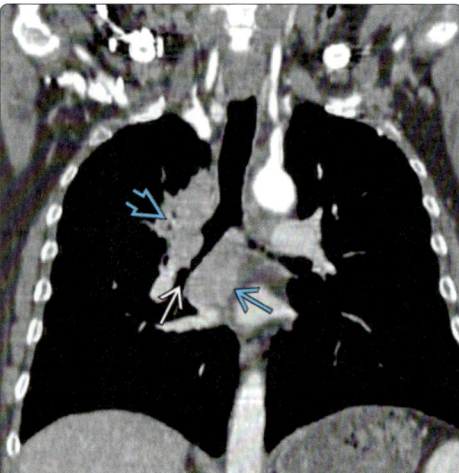

Endobronchial Biopsy
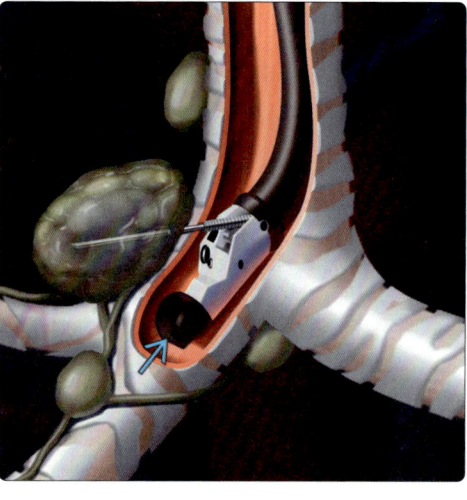

(Left) Coronal chest CT in a patient with a lung mass shows right hilar ➡ and subcarinal ➡ adenopathy with irregular narrowing of the right mainstem bronchus ➡. The safest route for biopsy would be via bronchoscopy. (Right) Graphic shows a bronchoscopic biopsy of a paratracheal lymph node. Both bronchoscopes and endoscopes may have a built-in US probe ➡ to allow real-time viewing during biopsy, improving diagnostic yield.

Endoscopy of Gastric Leiomyoma
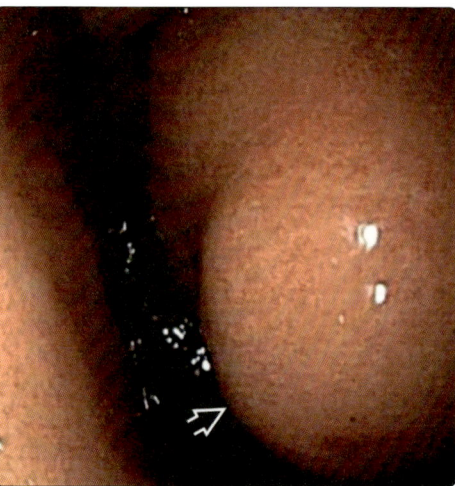

Endoscopic US of Gastric Leiomyoma
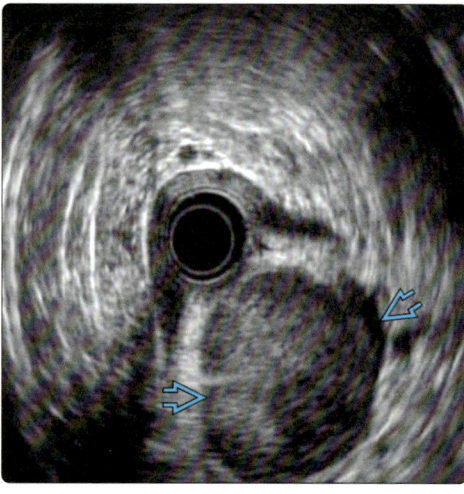

(Left) This patient with dysphagia underwent endoscopic examination and was found to have a gastric leiomyoma ➡ near the gastroesophageal junction. The tumor forms a smooth nodule surfaced by normal mucosa. (Right) Endoscopic US in the same patient demonstrates a well-circumscribed, hypoechoic mass ➡ with an apparent origin in the muscularis mucosae. FNA confirmed a diagnosis of leiomyoma. (From DP: Endoscopic.)

Techniques and Modalities of Deep Aspiration Biopsies

- Lesion suspicious for pheochromocytoma: At risk for hypertensive crisis with biopsy; need to be on α-blockers
- Possible echinococcal cyst: Risk of anaphylaxis is contraindication to biopsy

PROCEDURE

Biopsy Techniques

- **Bronchoscopic and endoscopic biopsy**
  - Can be performed with direct visualization of intraluminal mass or with US guidance
    - US-guided biopsy has improved diagnostic yield
    - Radial array probe produces axial images
      - Ideal for evaluating bronchial or gut wall structure, adjacent tissue, or lymph nodes
    - Curved linear array transducer at distal tip of bronchoscope/endoscope
      - Real-time imaging in craniocaudal plane; ideal to view needle as it is advanced into lesion
      - Color Doppler capability allows identification and avoidance of vascular structures
- **Solid organ biopsy**
  - Single-needle technique
    - Biopsy device (either needle or core biopsy device) is placed in lesion and biopsy is performed
    - Appropriate for superficial and easily accessed lesions
    - Generally done under US guidance
  - Coaxial-needle technique
    - 2 separate components: Introducer needle and biopsy needle(s)
      - 14- to 19-gauge introducer needle
      - 16- to 20-gauge core biopsy device
      - 22-gauge needle for FNA
    - Advance introducer needle to target
      - Remove stylet
      - Needle for aspiration or biopsy device fits through introducer
    - Better for deeper, less accessible lesions
      - Once appropriately positioned, introducer needle stays in place while multiple biopsies are attained
- **FNA technique**
  - Use specialized needle with beveled tip (e.g., Chiba, Franseen) especially designed for FNA
  - May try French technique
    - Capillary action alone, no aspiration
    - Does not work as well for deep lesions as it does for superficial lesions
  - Aspiration technique
    - Attach 10-cc syringe
    - Pull back plunger so there is 2-3 cc of air in hub, hence easier to express sample onto slide
    - Aspirate while performing biopsy
    - Use sharp "sewing machine" motion in fan-like pattern through lesion
    - Release suction before removing needle
    - Failure to release suction pulls sample into syringe rather than keeping it in needle; also increases likelihood of aspirating blood
  - Pass sample to cytopathologist for appropriate slide preparation
  - Based on evaluation by cytopathologist, may need additional FNA samples or core biopsy
- **Core biopsy technique**
  - Set desired specimen size, dependent on size of lesion
    - Most devices allow 1-3 cm
  - Set safety stop and position into lesion
    - Either using single-needle positioning technique or through coaxial introducer
  - Once appropriately placed, release safety and "fire"
    - Inner stylet with specimen notch fires first
    - Outer cannula then cuts core of tissue, trapping it in specimen notch
  - Pass specimen to cytopathologist
    - May perform touch prep if necessary
  - Usually at least 2 core biopsies are done
    - Must know what diagnosis is suspected for appropriate handling
    - For microscopic evaluation, put in formalin
    - If lymphoma is suspected, send sample either fresh or in saline for flow cytometry

POST PROCEDURE

Monitor for Complications

- Hemorrhage is most common after liver, kidney, and splenic biopsy
  - Consider tract embolization with Gelfoam
  - Hemodynamic support
- Postprocedure pain related to site biopsied
  - Intercostal approach is more painful
  - Bleeding may irritate liver capsule/peritoneum
- Delayed complications
  - Infection/sepsis
  - Pseudoaneurysm

Expected Outcome

- Reported diagnostic accuracy
  - Bronchoscopic/endoscopic sensitivity: 73-100%, depending on patient selection
  - Liver biopsy: 83-95%
  - Thoracic biopsy: 77-96%
  - Musculoskeletal biopsy: 76-93%
  - Other sites: 70-90%
- Diagnostic yield also depends on size and ease of accessing lesion
- Necrotic lesions are typically nondiagnostic
- Higher accuracy rate if both FNA and core sample are obtained
- Presence of on-site cytopathology is essential for increasing diagnostic biopsy rates

SELECTED REFERENCES

1. Heslop G et al: Modern approach to the neck mass. Surg Clin North Am. 102(2S):e1-6, 2022
2. Vieites Branco I et al: Fluoro-CT guided biopsy of lung nodules: a step by step revision. Port J Card Thorac Vasc Surg. 28(4):43-46, 2022
3. Rodriguez EF et al: Ultrasound-guided transthoracic fine-needle aspiration: a reliable tool in diagnosis and molecular profiling of lung masses. Acta Cytol. 64(3):208-15, 2020
4. Soltani AK et al: Current status of newer generation endoscopic ultrasound core needles in the diagnostic evaluation of gastrointestinal lesions. J Am Soc Cytopathol. 9(5):389-95, 2020

Techniques and Modalities of Deep Aspiration Biopsies

Preprocedure CT to Determine Optimal Approach for Biopsy

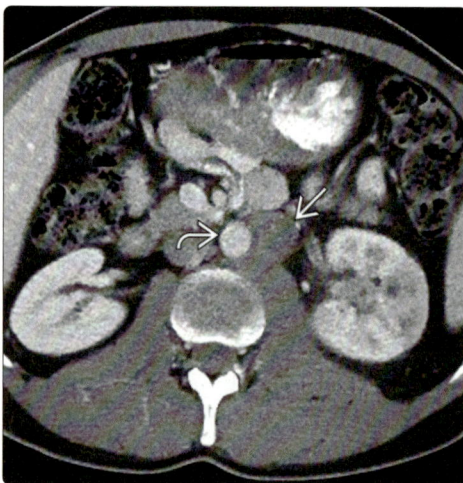

Localizing Grid on Skin

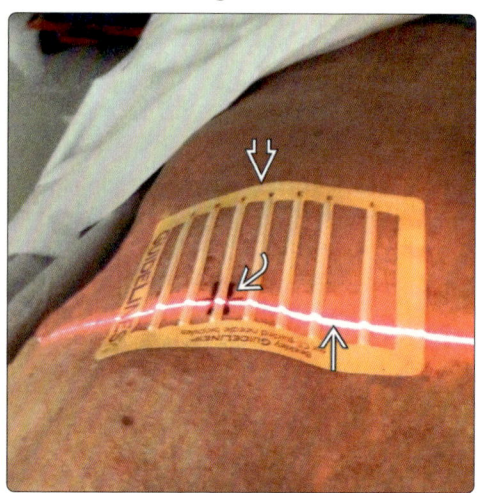

(Left) Preprocedure contrast-enhanced CT in a patient with colon cancer shows a new abnormal lymph node ➡ adjacent to the aorta ➡. A posterior approach was deemed safest, so the patient was placed in prone position. (Right) A localizing grid ➡ is placed, and a limited CT through the area is done to pick the best entry site. The laser line ➡ demarcates the slice position corresponding to CT selected for the entry site. The best spot along this line is marked ➡ and the grid removed.

Metallic Marker for Entry Site

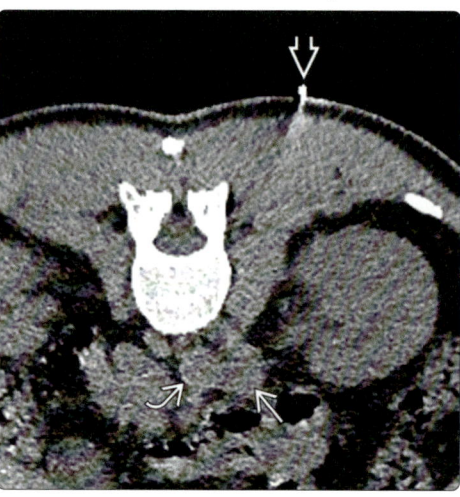

Anesthesia of Entry Site

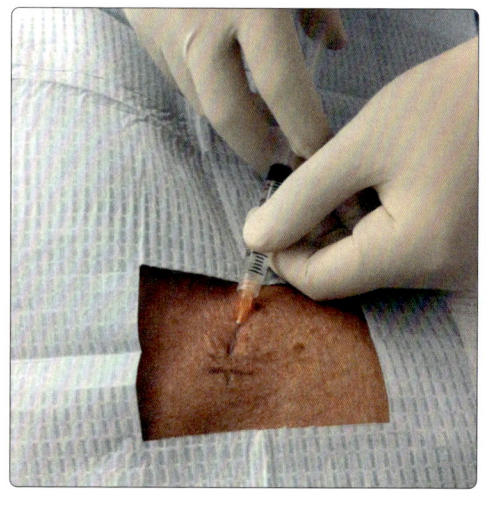

(Left) Prone CT shows a metallic marker at the entry site ➡. The needle tip will need to be angled medially toward the abnormal lymph node ➡. IV contrast only opacifies the vessels for a short time, so it is not used during the biopsy. Without contrast, the aorta ➡ has a very similar appearance to the lymph node. It is important to completely understand the landmarks before introducing the needle. (Right) Once the site is picked, the area is sterilely prepped and draped, and the skin anesthetized.

Coaxial Needle System Insertion

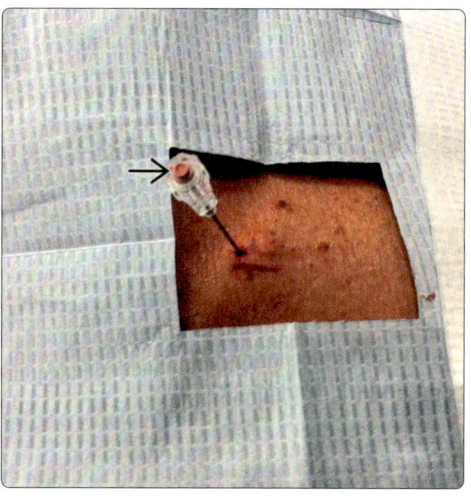

CT Confirmation of Correct Needle Placement

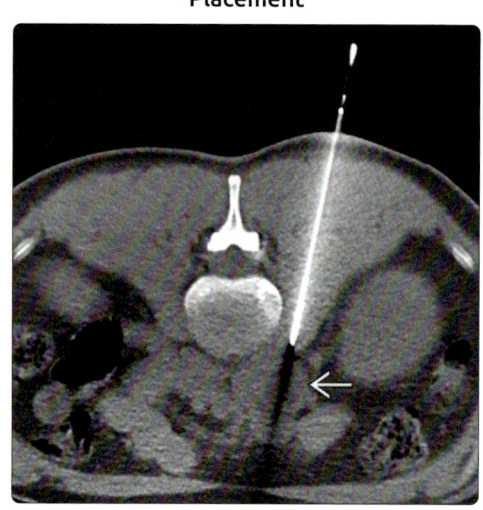

(Left) The coaxial system, with its sharp inner stylet ➡, is slowly introduced. Every few centimeters, a CT should be taken to ensure that the needle is on the correct trajectory. (Right) CT shows the needle appropriately placed with the tip adjacent to the lymph node ➡. The black streak is an artifact created by the tip of the needle, but it shows the trajectory the biopsy needle would take directly through the target. At this point, the stylet is removed and an FNA needle inserted.

Techniques and Modalities of Deep Aspiration Biopsies

Aspirate Slide Preparation

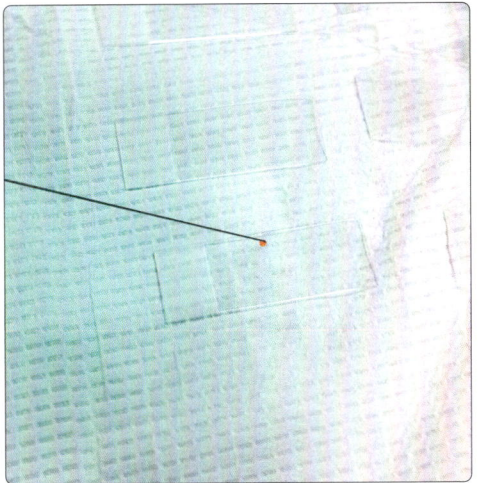

Core Biopsy

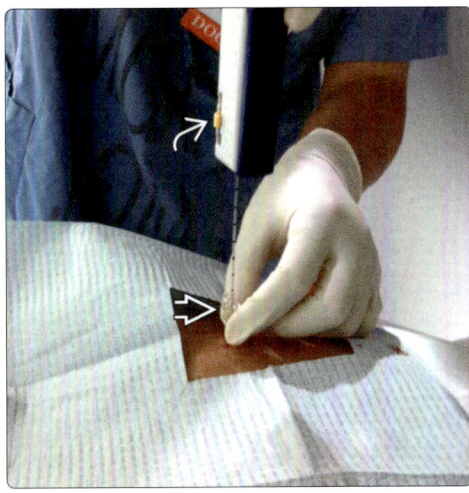

(Left) *FNA was performed with suction. It is important to stop suction before removing the needle to decrease chances of getting blood in the aspirate. The needle is passed to the cytopathologist for slide preparation.* (Right) *Core biopsy can also be performed by placing biopsy device through the introducer needle ⇨. These devices come with an adjustment ➡ to set the throw of the needle. Pick the largest throw that samples the lesion without damaging surrounding tissues. Typically 18- or 16-gauge needles are used.*

Biopsy Extrusion Into Container

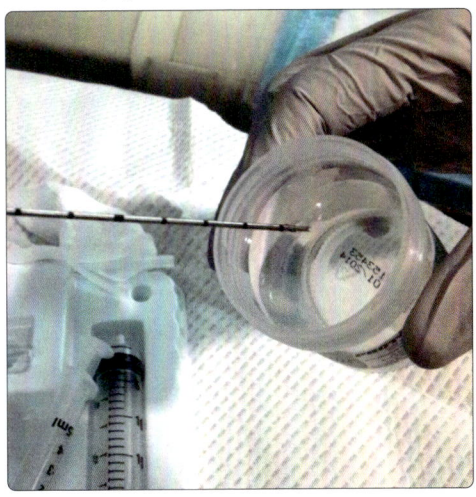

US Guidance of Needle

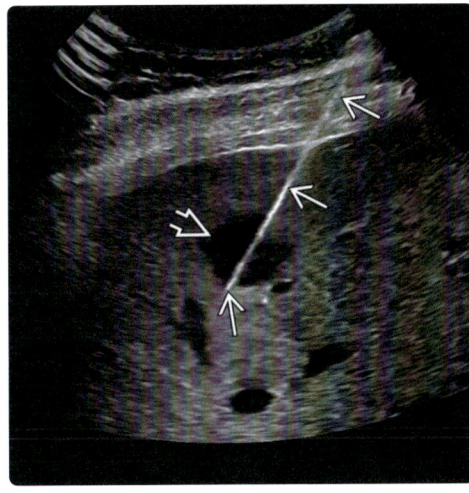

(Left) *The specimen is extruded from the core biopsy needle and is placed in a specimen container. It is imperative to know in advance what studies are needed so that samples can be put into saline or RPMI, in addition to formalin, if flow cytometry is needed.* (Right) *US in a patient with colon cancer shows a single hypoechoic liver lesion ⇨. When possible, biopsies should be performed using US as it is faster, less expensive, and the needle can be seen in real time. The entire course of the FNA needle ⇨ is seen.*

Introducer Needle With Stylet

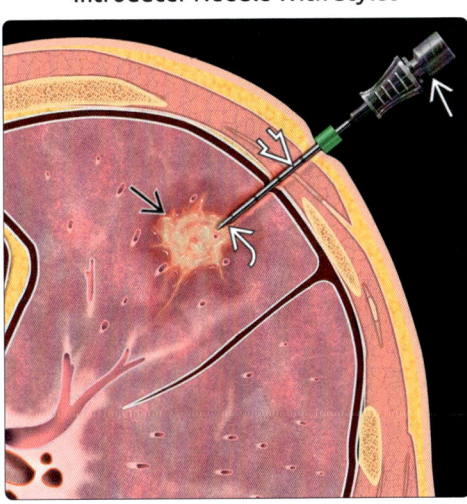

CT Showing Introducer Needle

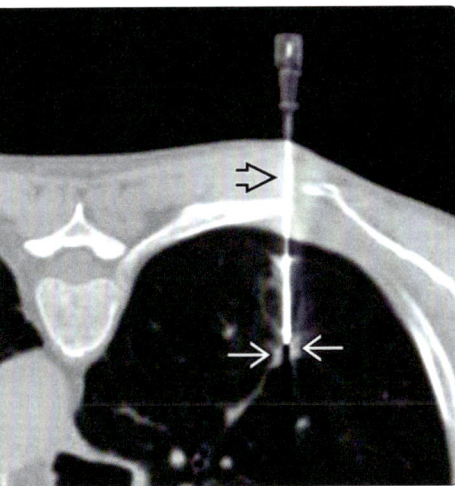

(Left) *Graphic shows an introducer needle ⇨ positioned with the tip ➡ at the edge of a lung mass ⇨. The sharp inner stylet ⇨ of the needle is still in place and will be removed to allow introduction of a biopsy needle into the mass.* (Right) *CT shows the introducer needle ⇨ in the target lung lesion ⇨. By using the coaxial technique, only a single puncture of the pleura is needed, yet multiple samples may be obtained.*

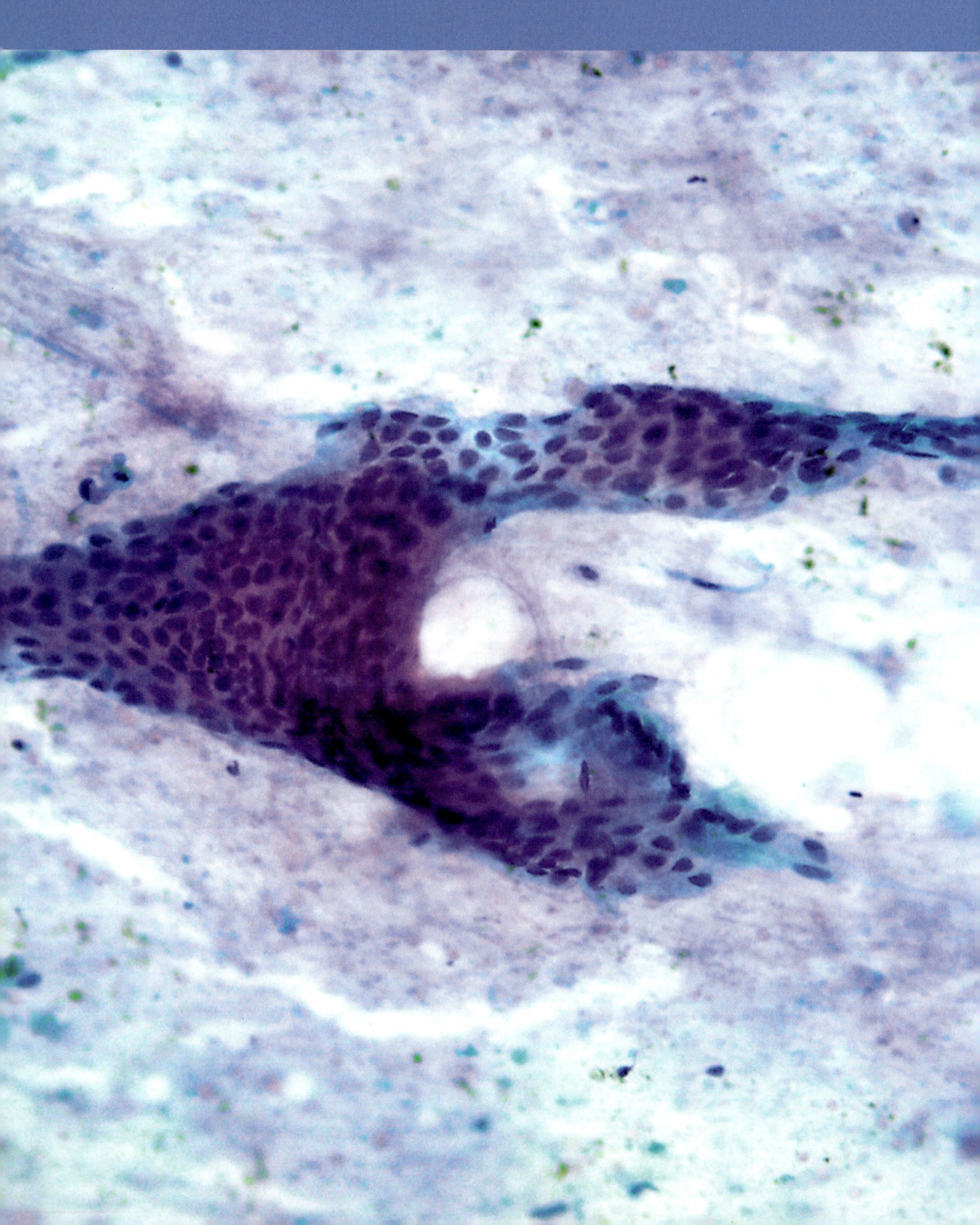

PART IV
SECTION 2
Mediastinum

Overview
Anatomic Compartments and Constituent Tumors   482

Nonneoplastic Lesions
Mediastinal Cysts and Inflammatory Lesions   484

Neoplasms
Thymoma   486
Thymic Carcinoma   488
Germ Cell Tumors   490
Neurogenic Tumors   492
Metastatic Tumors of Mediastinum   494

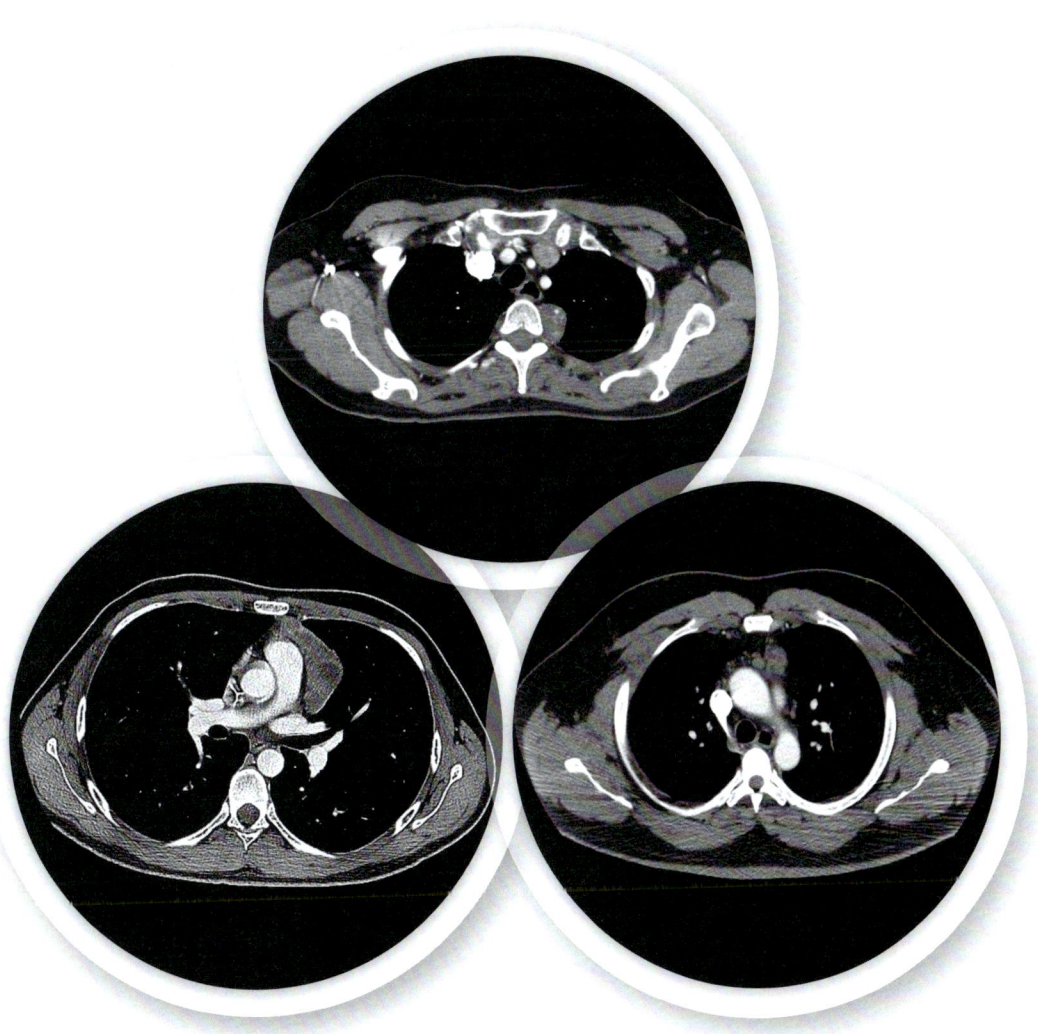

Anatomic Compartments and Constituent Tumors

TERMINOLOGY

Definitions
- Mediastinum is defined as potential space between thoracic cavities, confined anteriorly by sternum and posteriorly by thoracic spine; upper and lower limits are thoracic inlet and diaphragm, respectively
- Mediastinum is arbitrarily divided into superior, anterior, middle, and posterior compartments

EPIDEMIOLOGY

Age Range
- Children
    - Hodgkin and non-Hodgkin lymphoma
    - Neuroblastoma, ganglioneuroblastoma
    - Benign teratomas
    - Benign cysts
- Adults
    - Metastasis
    - Lymphoma
    - Neurogenic tumors
    - Thymoma
    - Germ cell tumors
    - Benign cysts

Incidence
- Anterior mediastinum
    - Metastasis
    - Lymphoma
    - Thymoma, thymic carcinoma, thymic cyst
    - Germ cell tumors
    - Mesenchymal tumors
    - Benign cysts
- Middle mediastinum
    - Metastasis
    - Lymphoma
    - Congenital cysts
    - Fibrosis
- Posterior mediastinum
    - Metastasis
    - Lymphoma

Enlarged Thymus, Anterior Mediastinum
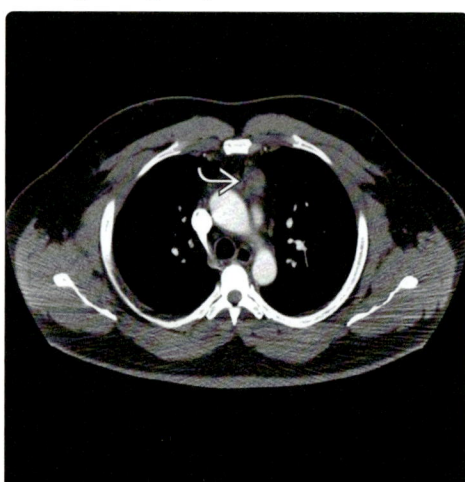

Malignant Teratoma, Anterior Mediastinum
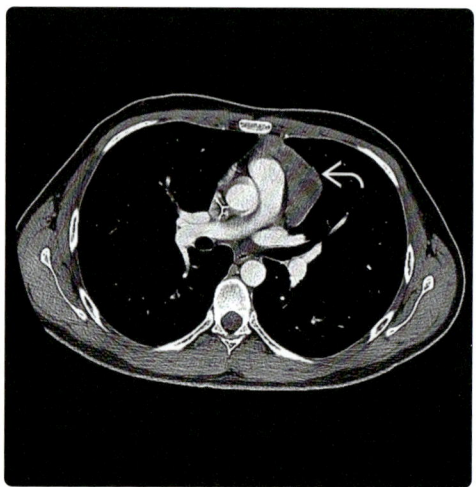

(Left) Chest CT scan shows a well-defined mass in the anterior mediastinum with features suggestive of an enlarged thymus, most likely representing thymic hyperplasia ⮕. (Right) Chest CT scan of a malignant teratoma shows a large mass in the anterior mediastinum ⮕.

Thymoma, Superior and Anterior Mediastinum
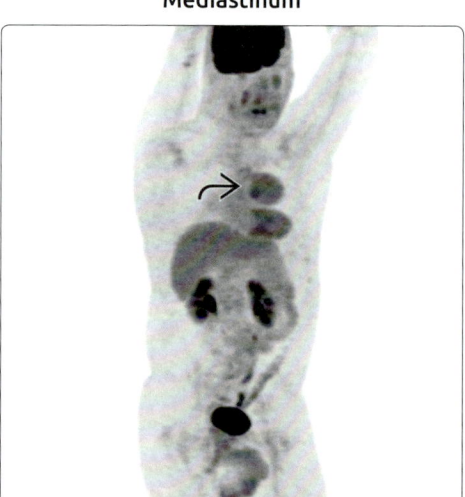

Thymoma, Superior and Anterior Mediastinum
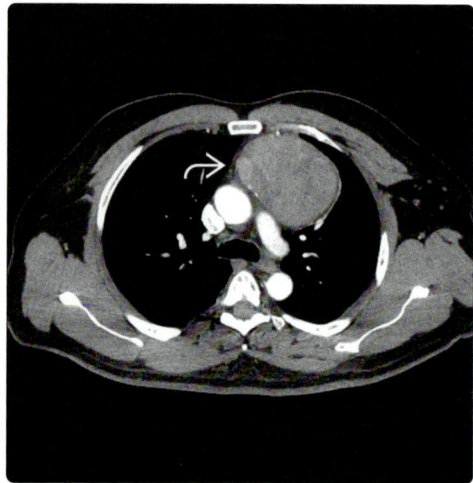

(Left) Chest PET/CT scan shows a well-defined mass ⮕ in the anterior mediastinum, consistent with thymoma. (Right) Chest CT scan shows a large, well-defined mass ⮕ in the anterior mediastinum, consistent with a thymoma.

Anatomic Compartments and Constituent Tumors

- Neurogenic tumors
  - Nerve sheath tumors
  - Neuroblastoma, ganglioneuroma
  - Paraganglioma
- Benign cysts
- Superior mediastinum
  - Metastasis
  - Lymphoma
  - Thyroid goiter or neoplasm
  - Thymoma
  - Benign cysts
  - Parathyroid cyst, hyperplasia or neoplasm

CLINICAL IMPLICATIONS

Imaging Findings

- Mediastinal mass or cyst
- CT scan is critical for differential diagnosis

CYTOPATHOLOGY

Cells

- Biphasic cellular pattern
  - Thymoma
- Lymphoid cells
  - Lymphoma
  - Thymic hyperplasia
  - Thymic cyst
- Overtly malignant cells
  - Metastasis, especially lung primary
  - Lymphoma
  - Melanoma
  - Thymic carcinoma
  - Germ cell tumors
  - Malignant neurogenic tumors
- Scant benign epithelial cells with cystic debris
  - Congenital cyst
  - Cystic teratoma
  - Thymic cyst
- Inflammatory cells
  - Hodgkin lymphoma
  - Granulomatous inflammation

SELECTED REFERENCES

1. Park JW et al: Pictorial review of mediastinal masses with an emphasis on magnetic resonance imaging. Korean J Radiol. 22(1):139-54, 2021
2. Jiajue R et al: Persistent hypercalcemia crisis and recurrent acute pancreatitis due to multiple ectopic parathyroid carcinomas: case report and literature review of mediastinal parathyroid carcinoma. Front Endocrinol (Lausanne). 11:647, 2020
3. Lott-Limbach AA et al: Mediastinal sarcomas: experience using fine needle aspiration cytopathology. Mediastinum. 4:14, 2020
4. Saad Abdalla Al-Zawi A et al: Posterior mediastinal paravertebral müllerian cyst (cyst of Hattori): literature review. Adv Respir Med. 88(2):134-41, 2020
5. Suster D et al: The role of needle core biopsies in the evaluation of thymic epithelial neoplasms. J Am Soc Cytopathol. 9(5):346-58, 2020
6. Marcus A et al: Sensitivity and specificity of fine needle aspiration for the diagnosis of mediastinal lesions. Ann Diagn Pathol. 39:69-73, 2019
7. Mishra MM et al: Diagnosis of mediastinal lesions unassociated with lung carcinoma diagnosed by endobronchial ultrasound transbronchial needle aspiration (EBUS-TBNA). J Am Soc Cytopathol. 5(4):189-95, 2016
8. Borak S et al: Metastatic inflammatory myofibroblastic tumor identified by EUS-FNA in mediastinal lymph nodes with ancillary FISH studies for ALK rearrangement. Diagn Cytopathol. 40 Suppl 2:E118-25, 2012
9. Stacchini A et al: Diagnosis of deep-seated lymphomas by endoscopic ultrasound-guided fine needle aspiration combined with flow cytometry. Cytopathology. 23(1):50-6, 2012
10. Zeppa P et al: Impact of endoscopic ultrasound-guided fine needle aspiration (EUS-FNA) in lymph nodal and mediastinal lesions: a multicenter experience. Diagn Cytopathol. 39(10):723-9, 2011
11. Monaco SE et al: Diagnostic difficulties and pitfalls in rapid on-site evaluation of endobronchial ultrasound guided fine needle aspiration. Cytojournal. 7:9, 2010
12. Skov BG et al: Cytopathologic diagnoses of fine-needle aspirations from endoscopic ultrasound of the mediastinum: reproducibility of the diagnoses and representativeness of aspirates from lymph nodes. Cancer. 111(4):234-41, 2007
13. Kramer H et al: Analysis of cytological specimens from mediastinal lesions obtained by endoscopic ultrasound-guided fine-needle aspiration. Cancer. 108(4):206-11, 2006
14. Pantidou A et al: Mediastinum thymoma diagnosed by FNA and ThinPrep technique: a case report. Diagn Cytopathol. 34(1):37-40, 2006
15. Ishikawa M et al: Diagnosis of nasopharyngeal carcinoma metastatic to mediastinal lymph nodes by endoscopic ultrasonography-guided fine-needle aspiration biopsy. Acta Otolaryngol. 125(9):1014-7, 2005
16. Kwon MS: Aspiration cytology of mediastinal seminoma: report of a case with emphasis on the diagnostic role of aspiration cytology, cell block and immunocytochemistry. Acta Cytol. 49(6):669-72, 2005
17. Shabb NS et al: Fine-needle aspiration of the mediastinum: a clinical, radiologic, cytologic, and histologic study of 42 cases. Diagn Cytopathol. 19(6):428-36, 1998

Schwannoma, Posterior Mediastinum

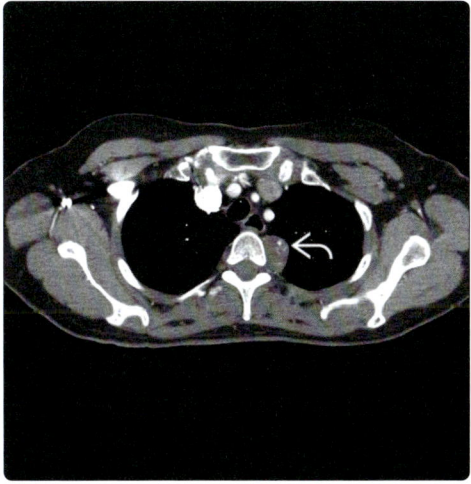

Ganglioneuroblastoma, Posterior Mediastinum

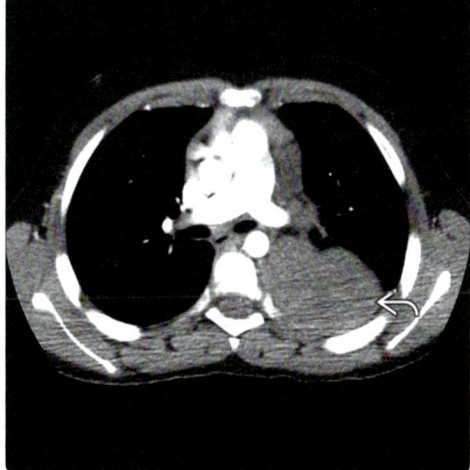

(Left) Chest CT scan shows a well-defined mass ➡ in the posterior mediastinum, consistent with a schwannoma. *(Right)* Chest CT scan of ganglioneuroblastoma shows a large, relatively well-circumscribed mass ➡ in the posterior mediastinum.

Mediastinal Cysts and Inflammatory Lesions

KEY FACTS

CLINICAL ISSUES
- Cystic or mass lesions in mediastinum
- Most common mediastinal cysts: Foregut cysts (bronchogenic cysts, gastroenteric cysts)
- Occasionally symptomatic in patients with benign mediastinal cyst
- Incidental radiographic finding for most cystic lesions
- Inflammatory lesion usually as part of systemic inflammatory disease
- Clinical and radiologic correlation is critical

CYTOPATHOLOGY
- Scant cellularity
- Variable amounts of benign epithelial cells (squamous, respiratory, &/or gastroenteric) with cystic debris
- Epithelioid granulomas ± necrosis
- Background can be proteinaceous, necrotic, or comprised of inflammatory cells

ANCILLARY TESTS
- Special stains for mycobacteria and fungal forms in specimens with granuloma and necrosis
- Bacterial, fungal cultures
- Flow cytometry analysis to rule out lymphoma

TOP DIFFERENTIAL DIAGNOSES
- Cystic lesions
  - Cystic thymoma
    - Features indistinguishable from thymic cysts
    - More common than thymic cyst
  - Mature cystic teratoma
    - Features indistinguishable from bronchogenic or gastroenteric cysts
- Granulomatous inflammation
  - Infection
  - Sarcoidosis
  - Malignancy: Hodgkin lymphoma, seminoma

Bronchogenic Cyst
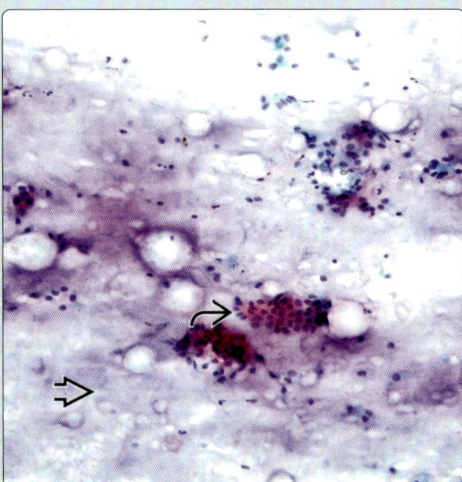

Columnar Epithelium
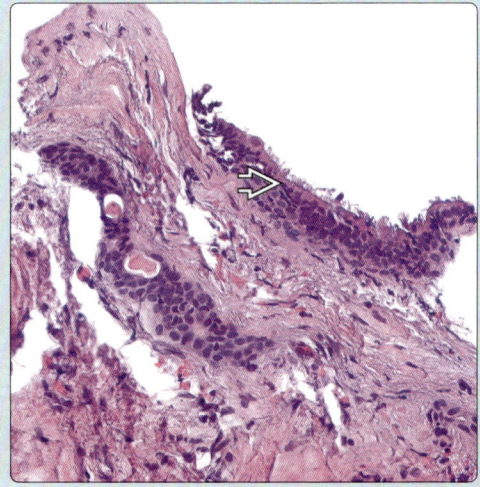

(Left) Pap-stained FNA smear shows a bronchogenic cyst with groups of benign respiratory epithelial cells ➡ in a background of proteinaceous material ➡. *(Right)* Core biopsy of bronchogenic cyst stained with H&E shows ciliated columnar epithelium ➡ lining the cyst.

Thymic Cyst Contents
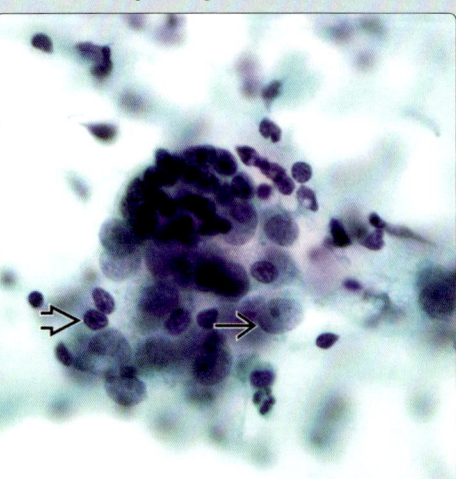

Columnar Epithelium
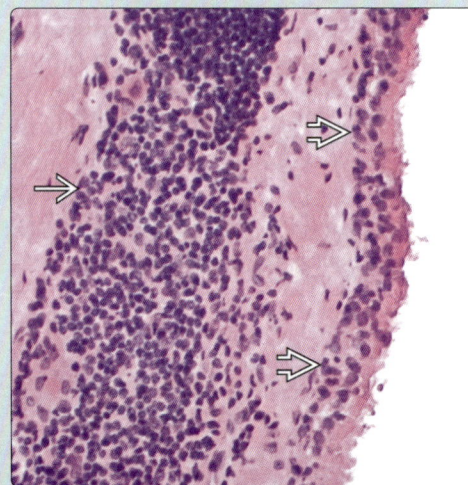

(Left) Pap-stained FNA smear shows contents of a thymic cyst, including epithelial cells ➡ and lymphocytes ➡. *(Right)* Surgical resection of a thymic cyst stained with H&E shows benign, ciliated columnar epithelium ➡ lining the cyst with thymic tissue ➡ in the wall.

Mediastinal Cysts and Inflammatory Lesions

ETIOLOGY/PATHOGENESIS

Developmental Anomaly
- Most common mediastinal cysts: Foregut cysts (bronchogenic cysts, gastroenteric cysts)
- Neurogenic cysts
- Pericardial cysts
- Thymic cysts

CLINICAL ISSUES

Presentation
- Occasionally symptomatic in patients with benign mediastinal cyst
- Incidental radiographic finding for most cystic lesions
- Inflammatory lesion usually as part of systemic inflammation disease

CYTOPATHOLOGY

Cellularity
- Usually low

Background
- Proteinaceous or necrosis

Cells
- Foregut cysts
  o Bronchogenic cysts: Respiratory ciliated columnar cells and squamous cells
  o Gastroenteric cysts: Gastroenteric epithelial cells and squamous cells
- Pericardial cysts
  o Mesothelial cells
- Thymic cysts
  o Squamous or glandular epithelial cells
  o Lymphocytes
- Granulomatous inflammation
  o Histiocytes, multinucleated giant cells, and inflammatory cells

DIFFERENTIAL DIAGNOSIS

Cystic Lesions
- Cystic thymoma
  o More common than thymic cyst
  o Can be indistinguishable in FNA
- Mature cystic teratoma
  o Calcification radiographically
  o Benign epithelial cells; can be indistinguishable from other cysts
- Seminoma
  o Paucicellular with atypical cells and cystic debris
- Benign peripheral nerve sheath tumors
  o Paucicellular with spindle cells and debris

Granulomatous Inflammation
- Infection
  o Mycobacterial infection
  o Fungal infection
- Sarcoidosis
  o Usually noncaseating granuloma
- Hodgkin lymphoma
  o Most commonly seen in young women
  o Epithelioid granulomas associated with features of Hodgkin lymphoma
- Seminoma
  o Epithelioid granulomas associated with features of seminoma

Metastatic Malignant Neoplasm
- Atypical cells with extensive necrosis

SELECTED REFERENCES
1. Pan F et al: Utility and safety of endobronchial ultrasound-guided transbronchial needle aspiration in the diagnosis of isolated mediastinal masses. J Multidiscip Healthc. 14:2047-52, 2021
2. Syred K et al: Non-neoplastic mediastinal cysts. Adv Anat Pathol. 27(5):294-302, 2020
3. Liu T et al: Mediastinal lesions across the age spectrum: a clinicopathological comparison between pediatric and adult patients. Oncotarget. 8(35): 59845-53, 2017

Bronchogenic Cyst

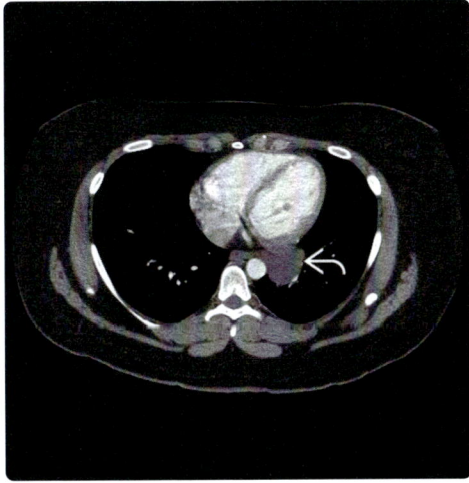

Fungal Infection, *Aspergillus*

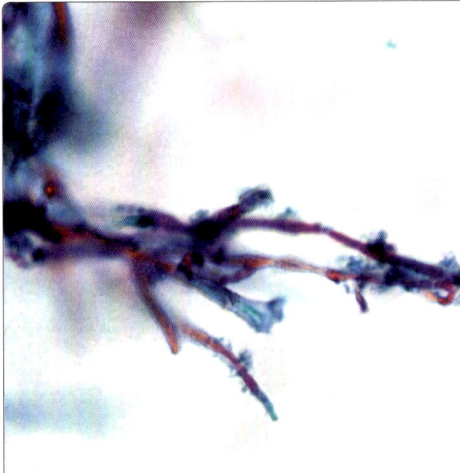

(Left) Chest CT scan shows a bronchogenic cyst ➤ in the posterior mediastinum. Most mediastinal cysts are discovered incidentally by radiologic studies. *(Right)* Pap-stained smear shows fungal forms of an Aspergillus species with branching hyphae.

Thymoma

KEY FACTS

CLINICAL ISSUES
- Primary thymic epithelial neoplasm associated with nonneoplastic T lymphocytes
- Accounts for ~ 25% of all primary mediastinal neoplasms
- Usually in adults; average: 50 years old
- Round or oval lobulated mass in anterior mediastinum
- Low-grade malignant neoplasms with generally indolent behavior in majority of patients
- Poor prognosis for stages III and IV tumors compared with stages I and II tumors
- Cystic changes and necrosis are common in large tumors

CYTOPATHOLOGY
- Biphasic pattern of epithelial cells and small lymphocytes
- 2 types of epithelial cells identified
  - Epithelioid cells with smooth or slightly irregular nuclear contours, scant to moderate cytoplasm, and indistinct cell borders
  - Spindle cells with elongated nuclei, fine nuclear chromatin, and inconspicuous nucleoli
- Cellular atypia seen in type B3 thymoma (atypical thymoma)
- Variable numbers of T cells; predominantly small and mature but may be immature

ANCILLARY TESTS
- Immunohistochemistry
  - Expression of cytokeratins and p63, p40 in epithelial cells
  - CD5 usually negative in epithelial cells except for atypical thymoma or thymic carcinoma
  - TdT, CD1a, and CD99 expression in T lymphocytes

TOP DIFFERENTIAL DIAGNOSES
- Lymphoblastic lymphoma
- Thymic carcinoid tumor
- Seminoma
- Spindle cell tumors

Biphasic Pattern

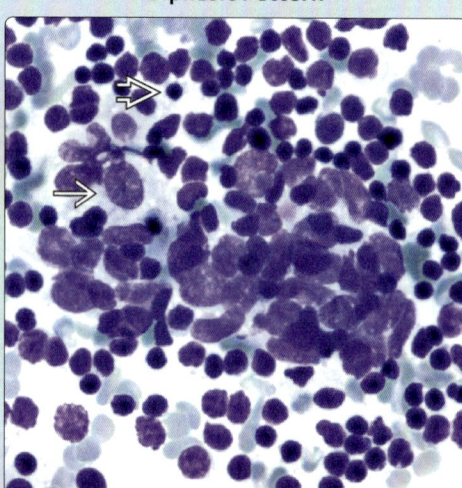

Epithelioid Cells

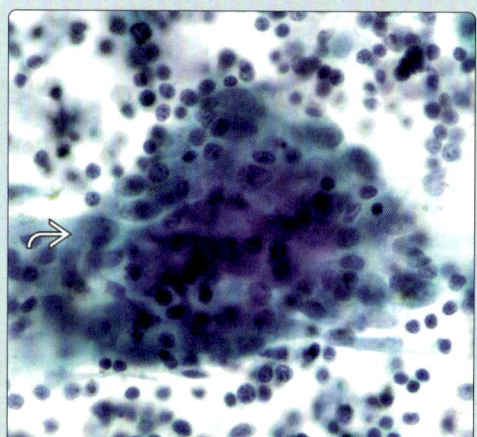

(Left) Diff-Quik-stained FNA smear of thymoma shows a biphasic pattern with the presence of epithelioid tumor cells ➡ and lymphocytes ➡. (Right) Pap-stained FNA smear shows epithelioid tumor cells with moderate cytoplasm ➡ in a background of small lymphocytes.

Thymoma

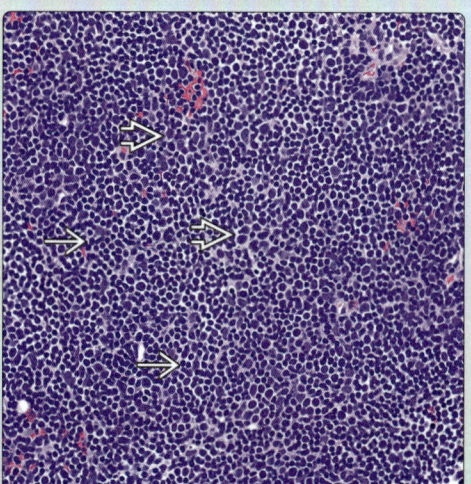

Thymoma

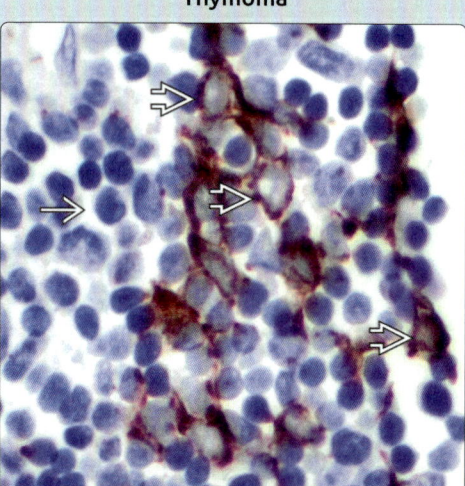

(Left) Core biopsy of thymoma stained with H&E shows a biphasic pattern, including epithelial cells ➡ interspersed amidst abundant small lymphocytes ➡. (Right) Core biopsy of thymoma immunostained with pancytokeratin highlights the network of positively stained epithelial cells ➡ amidst the negatively stained small lymphocytes ➡.

Thymoma

TERMINOLOGY

Definitions
- Primary thymic epithelial neoplasm associated with nonneoplastic T lymphocytes

CLINICAL ISSUES

Natural History
- Low-grade malignant neoplasms with generally indolent behavior in majority of patients

IMAGING

Radiographic Findings
- Round or oval lobulated mass in anterior mediastinum

CYTOPATHOLOGY

Pattern
- Biphasic pattern with epithelial cells and small lymphocytes

Cells
- 2 types of epithelial cells identified
  - Epithelioid cells
    - Variable in size and morphology
    - Smooth or slightly irregular nuclear contour
    - Fine chromatin with inconspicuous nucleoli
    - Scant to moderate cytoplasm with delicate or dense texture
    - Indistinct cell borders
  - Spindle cells
    - Arranged in loose groups or in bundles
    - Slender nuclei with fine chromatin and inconspicuous nucleoli
- Cellular atypia seen in type B3 thymoma (atypical thymoma)
- Lymphocytes
  - Present in different proportions
  - Predominantly small mature T lymphocytes
  - Immature T cells, especially in type B1 thymoma

ANCILLARY TESTS

Immunohistochemistry
- Epithelial components positive for pancytokeratin and p63, p40
- Epithelial components usually negative for CD5 except for atypical thymoma or thymic carcinoma
- T cells with expression of CD3, TdT, CD1a, and CD99
  - Similar to thymic cortical lymphocytes

DIFFERENTIAL DIAGNOSIS

Lymphoblastic Lymphoma
- Usually in pediatric patients
- T-cell gene rearrangement analysis to demonstrate clonal proliferation of T cells

Thymic Carcinoid Tumor
- May have spindled morphology
- Expression of neuroendocrine markers

Seminoma
- Biphasic pattern but with malignant germ cell tumor cells admixed with lymphocytes

Spindle Cell Tumor
- Carcinoma, neural tumors, solitary fibrous tumor, mesothelioma, and melanoma

SELECTED REFERENCES

1. Oramas DM et al: Thymoma: challenges and pitfalls in biopsy interpretation. Adv Anat Pathol. 28(5):291-7, 2021
2. Illei PB et al: Fine needle aspiration of thymic epithelial neoplasms and non-neoplastic lesions. Semin Diagn Pathol. 37(4):166-73, 2020
3. Suster D et al: The role of needle core biopsies in the evaluation of thymic epithelial neoplasms. J Am Soc Cytopathol. 9(5):346-58, 2020
4. Wang M et al: Pitfalls of FNA diagnosis of thymic tumors. Cancer Cytopathol. 128(1):57-67, 2020
5. Weissferdt A et al: Thymoma: a clinicopathological correlation of 1470 cases. Hum Pathol. 73:7-15, 2018
6. Tseng YC et al: Long term oncological outcome of thymoma and thymic carcinoma - an analysis of 235 cases from a single institution. PLoS One. 12(6):e0179527, 2017

Mild Cellular Atypia
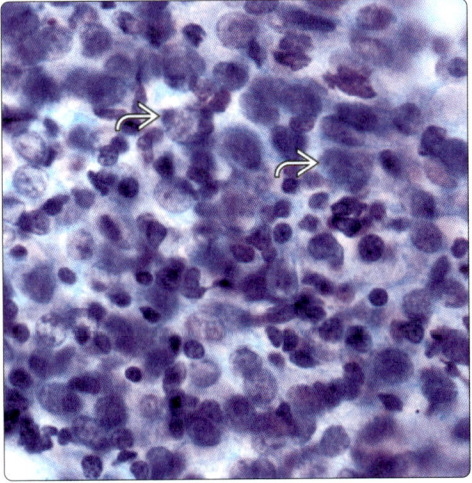

Epithelioid and Spindled Atypical Cells
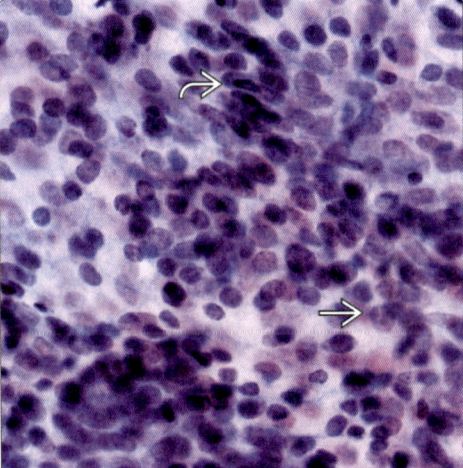

(Left) Diff-Quik-stained FNA smear shows epithelioid tumor cells ➔ with mild cellular atypia in atypical thymoma. (Right) Pap-stained FNA smear shows mixed epithelioid ➔ and spindle ➔ tumor cells with mild cellular atypia in atypical thymoma.

Thymic Carcinoma

KEY FACTS

CLINICAL ISSUES
- Primary thymic epithelial neoplasm with cytologic features of malignancy without thymic differentiation
- Lobulated, marginated, anterior mediastinal mass
- Accounts for < 1% of thymic tumors
- Most frequent in patients aged 30-60 years
- Highly aggressive neoplasm with poor prognosis
- Usual sites of metastases include lymph nodes, bone, lung, pleura, liver, and brain

CYTOPATHOLOGY
- Clearly malignant cells with variety of cytomorphologic features
  - Squamous carcinoma with keratinizing or nonkeratinizing types
  - Other types
    - Lymphoepithelioma-like with biphasic pattern resembling thymoma
    - Mucoepidermoid, resembling salivary gland carcinoma
  - Clear cell, basaloid, or sarcomatoid
- Necrosis, blood, and inflammatory cells in background
- Mature T cells and B cells

ANCILLARY TESTS
- Tumor cells positive for CD5, CD70, and CD117
- Tumor cells negative for CD57

TOP DIFFERENTIAL DIAGNOSES
- Atypical thymoma (WHO type B3)
  - Tumor cells with cellular atypia but not clearly malignant
  - Lack of necrosis
  - Immature T lymphocytes
- Metastatic carcinoma of lung and other organs
  - Clinical and radiological findings and pertinent immunostains useful

Single Population of Cells
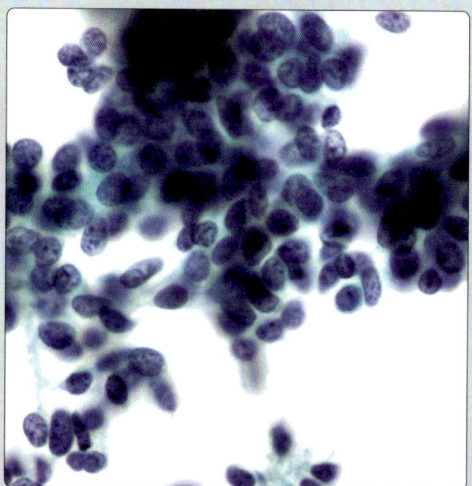

Pleomorphic Malignant Cells
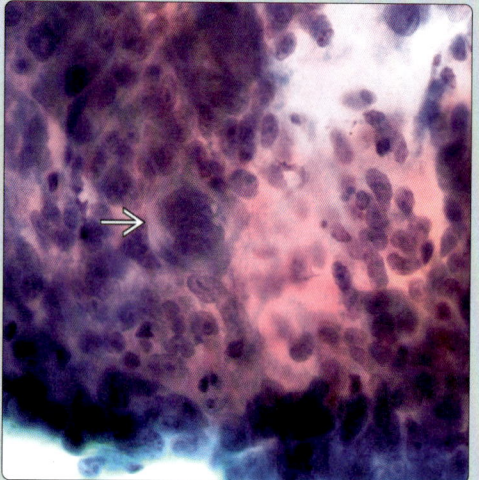

(Left) Pap-stained FNA smear of thymic carcinoma shows a single population of epithelial tumor cells without the biphasic pattern of thymoma. (Right) Pap-stained smear shows thymic carcinoma with markedly pleomorphic malignant cells ⇒.

Thymic Carcinoma
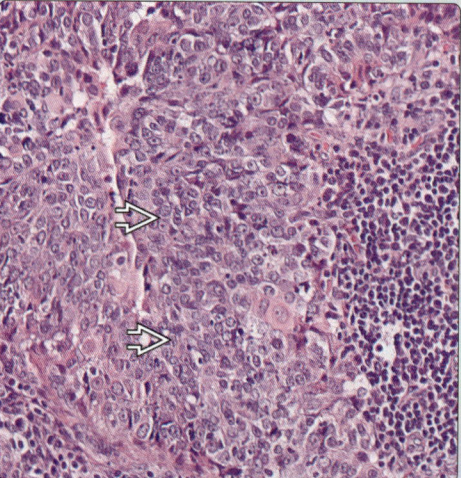

CD5 Positive in Thymic carcinoma
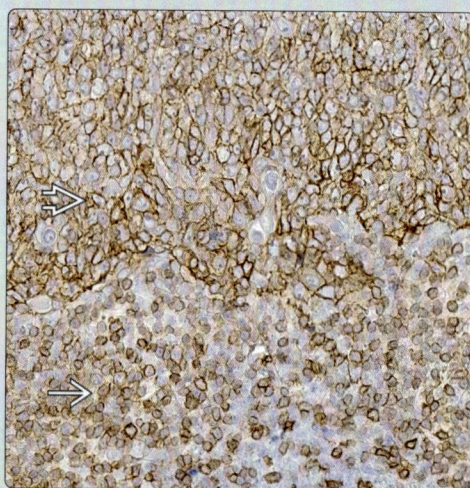

(Left) Core biopsy stained with H&E shows sheets of malignant cells with a large nucleus, prominent nucleolus, and a small amount of cytoplasm ⇒. (Right) Core biopsy of thymic carcinoma immunostained with CD5 shows positive staining in the tumor cells ⇒. Many of the small lymphocytes associated with the tumor are also CD5 positive ⇒.

Thymic Carcinoma

TERMINOLOGY

Synonyms
- WHO type C thymoma
- Poorly differentiated (high-grade) thymic epithelial neoplasm

Definitions
- Primary thymic epithelial neoplasm with cytologic features of malignancy without thymic differentiation

CLINICAL ISSUES

Natural History
- Highly aggressive neoplasm

Prognosis
- Poor prognosis with metastases to lymph nodes, lung, pleura, bone, liver, and brain

IMAGING

CT Findings
- Anterior mediastinal mass with heterogeneous enhancement and areas of necrosis

CYTOPATHOLOGY

Cellularity
- Varies from paucicellular to highly cellular

Pattern
- No biphasic pattern of thymoma except for lymphoepithelioma-like thymic carcinoma

Background
- Necrosis, blood, and inflammatory cells

Cells
- Clearly malignant cells with variety of cytomorphologic features
  - Squamous carcinoma with keratinizing or nonkeratinizing types
  - Lymphoepithelioma-like carcinoma similar to nasopharyngeal carcinoma
  - Mucoepidermoid carcinoma similar to salivary gland tumor
  - Clear cell carcinoma
  - Basaloid carcinoma
  - Sarcomatoid carcinoma

ANCILLARY TESTS

Immunohistochemistry
- Tumor cells
  - CK(+)
  - CD5(+)
  - CD70(+)
  - CD117(+)
  - CD57(-)

DIFFERENTIAL DIAGNOSIS

Atypical Thymoma (WHO Type B3)
- Tumor cells with cellular atypia but not clearly malignant
- Lack of necrosis
- Immature T lymphocytes

Metastatic Carcinomas of Lung and Other Organs
- Diagnosis of exclusion, must rule out lung and other metastasis

SELECTED REFERENCES

1. Smith AP et al: A diagnostic review of carcinomas and sarcomas of the mediastinum: making the diagnosis on fine-needle aspiration and core needle biopsy specimens. Semin Diagn Pathol. 37(4):187-98, 2020
2. Suster D et al: The role of needle core biopsies in the evaluation of thymic epithelial neoplasms. J Am Soc Cytopathol. 9(5):346-58, 2020
3. Berghmans T et al: Systemic treatments for thymoma and thymic carcinoma: a systematic review. Lung Cancer. 126:25-31, 2018
4. Lesueur P et al: Review of the mechanisms involved in the abscopal effect and future directions with a focus on thymic carcinoma. Tumori. 103(3):217-22, 2017
5. Tseng YC et al: Long term oncological outcome of thymoma and thymic carcinoma - an analysis of 235 cases from a single institution. PLoS One. 12(6):e0179527, 2017

Prominent Nucleoli

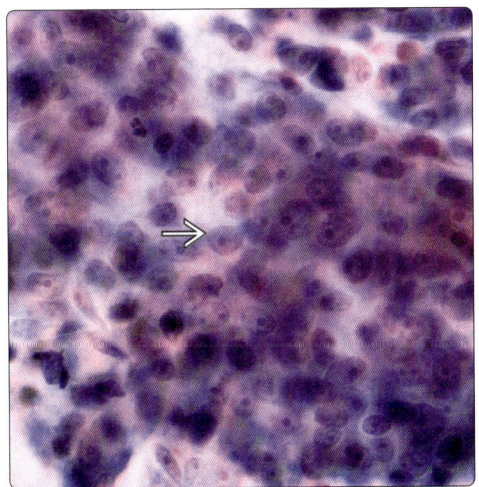

Nuclear Features

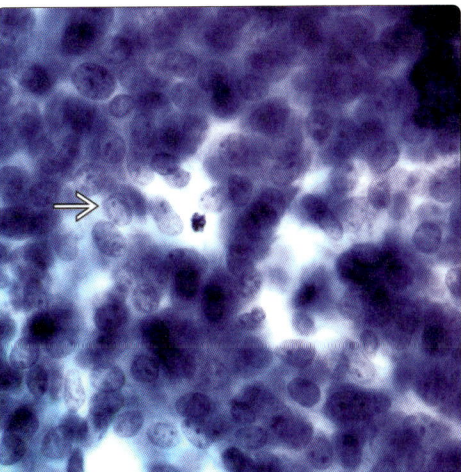

(Left) Pap-stained smear of thymic carcinoma shows tumor cells with prominent nucleoli ➡. (Right) Pap-stained FNA smear of thymic carcinoma shows tumor cells with a large nuclei and irregularly clumped chromatin ➡.

Germ Cell Tumors

KEY FACTS

CLINICAL ISSUES

- Extragonadal germ cell tumors arising in anterior mediastinum
- Most common benign germ cell tumor: Mature cystic teratoma
- Most common malignant germ cell tumor: Seminoma
- Yolk sac tumors are more common in young children than in other age groups with female predilection

CYTOPATHOLOGY

- Seminoma: Dyscohesive tumor cells with prominent nucleoli associated with lymphocytes
  - Tigroid background: Lacy interwoven PAS(+) glycogen-rich material, best seen on Diff-Quik
- Mature cystic teratoma: Benign epithelial cells in background of cystic contents
  - Immature teratoma will contain cytologically malignant cells
- Embryonal carcinoma: High-grade, poorly differentiated, cohesive malignant cells
- Yolk sac tumor: High-grade malignant cells
  - Malignant cells with irregular nuclear contour, coarse chromatin, and vacuolated cytoplasm
  - Schiller-Duval bodies: Glomerular-like structures
  - Hyaline globules: α-fetoprotein

TOP DIFFERENTIAL DIAGNOSES

- Seminoma: Thymoma, thymic carcinoma, anaplastic lymphoma, metastatic large cell carcinoma
- Mature cystic teratoma: Thymic cyst and other benign cysts
  - Immature teratoma: Poorly differentiated sarcoma or carcinoma
- Embryonal carcinoma: Poorly differentiated adenocarcinoma
- Yolk sac tumor: Poorly differentiated adenocarcinoma

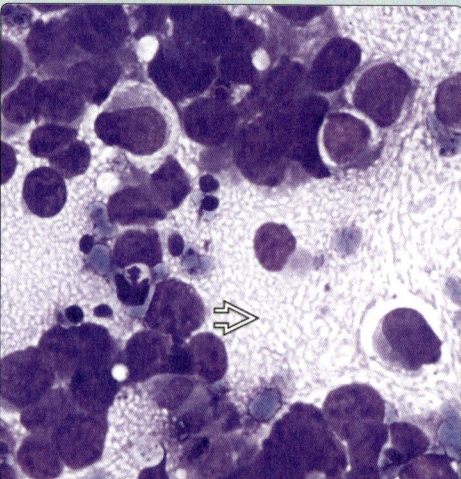

Seminoma, Tigroid Background

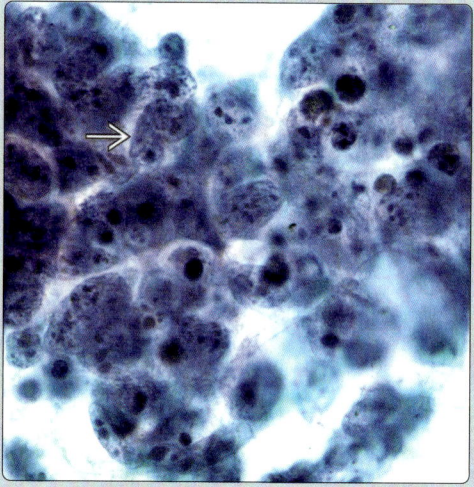

Embryonal Carcinoma

(Left) Diff-Quik-stained FNA smear of seminoma shows tumor cells with a lacy reticular tigroid background ⇨ resulting from the disrupted glycogen-rich cytoplasm of the tumor cells. (Right) Pap-stained FNA smear of embryonal carcinoma shows high-grade tumor cells ➡.

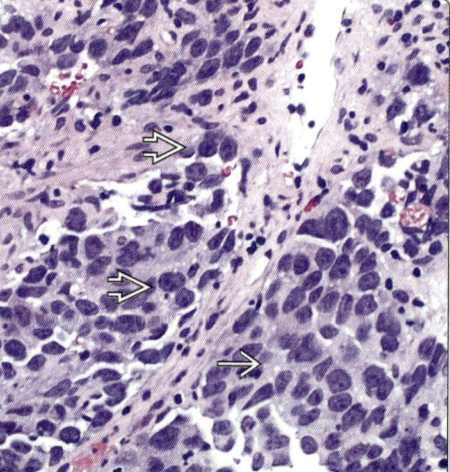

Seminoma

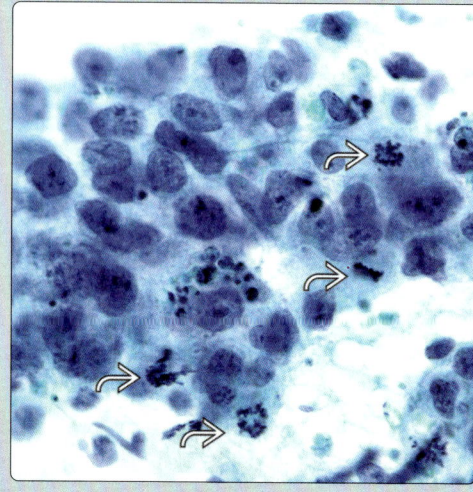

Yolk Sac Tumor, High Mitotic Rate

(Left) Core biopsy of metastatic seminoma stained with H&E shows nests of large tumor cells ➡ with variable nuclear shapes, prominent nucleolus, and a moderate amount of delicate cytoplasm ➡. (Right) Pap-stained FNA smear of a yolk sac tumor shows poorly differentiated tumor cells with scattered mitotic figures ➡.

Germ Cell Tumors

TERMINOLOGY

Definitions
- Extragonadal germ cell tumors arising in anterior mediastinum

CYTOPATHOLOGY

Background
- Seminoma: Lymphoid cells and tigroid background
- Mature cystic teratoma: Proteinaceous background

Cells
- Seminoma (germinoma)
  - Dual cell population with malignant germinoma cells and reactive lymphoid cells
    - Seminoma cells: Dyscohesive, uniform, and large with hyperchromatic nuclei, fine chromatin, and prominent nucleoli; cytoplasm usually clear and fragile; syncytiotrophoblast-like cells may be present
    - Background: Tigroid [lacy, interwoven, PAS(+), glycogen-rich material], best seen in Diff-Quik slides
- Teratomas
  - Mature cystic teratoma
    - Fragments of benign epithelium (squamous, respiratory, gastrointestinal) ± mesenchymal tissue (nerve, cartilage, adipose tissue)
  - Immature teratoma: Malignant cells
- Embryonal carcinoma
- Yolk sac (endodermal sinus) tumor
  - Malignant cells with irregular nuclear contour, coarse chromatin, and vacuolated cytoplasm
  - Schiller-Duval bodies: Glomerular-like structures
  - Hyaline globules: α-fetoprotein
- Choriocarcinoma
  - Syncytiotrophoblasts and cytotrophoblasts

ANCILLARY TESTS

Immunohistochemistry
- Seminoma
  - Positive for placental-like alkaline phosphatase (PLAP), OCT3/4, SALL4, CD117, SOX17, and CD57; negative for CD5
- Embryonal carcinoma
  - Positive for cytokeratin, SALL4, CD30, PLAP, OCT3/4, CD57, SOX2, and CD5; negative for α-fetoprotein
- Yolk sac tumor
  - Positive for cytokeratin, glypican 3, AFP, and SALL4; negative for CD30, CD117, and CD5; variable for α-fetoprotein
- Choriocarcinoma
  - Positive for β-HCG, GATA3, PLAP, SALL4; negative for OCT3/4, glypican 3 (+/-)

DIFFERENTIAL DIAGNOSIS

Seminoma
- Thymic carcinoma, large cell lymphoma, poorly differentiated carcinoma; thoracic SMARCA4-deficient undifferentiated tumor; NUT carcinoma

Embryonal Carcinoma
- Poorly differentiated adenocarcinoma; thoracic SMARCA4-deficient undifferentiated tumor; NUT carcinoma

Yolk Sac Tumor
- Poorly differentiated adenocarcinoma; thoracic SMARCA4-deficient undifferentiated tumor; NUT carcinoma

Teratoma
- Thymic cysts and other benign cysts can mimic mature cystic teratoma

SELECTED REFERENCES
1. Marx A et al: The 2021 WHO Classification of Tumors of the Thymus and Mediastinum: what is new in thymic epithelial, germ cell, and mesenchymal tumors? J Thorac Oncol. 17(2):200-13, 2022
2. El-Zaatari ZM et al: Mediastinal germ cell tumors: a review and update on pathologic, clinical, and molecular features. Adv Anat Pathol. 28(5):335-50, 2021

Teratoma, Benign Glandular Epithelium

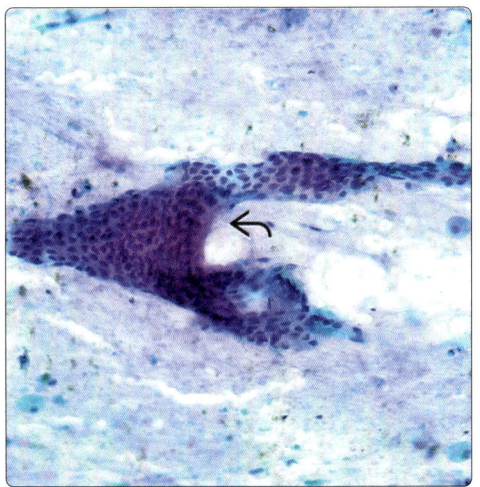

Teratoma, Benign Respiratory Epithelium

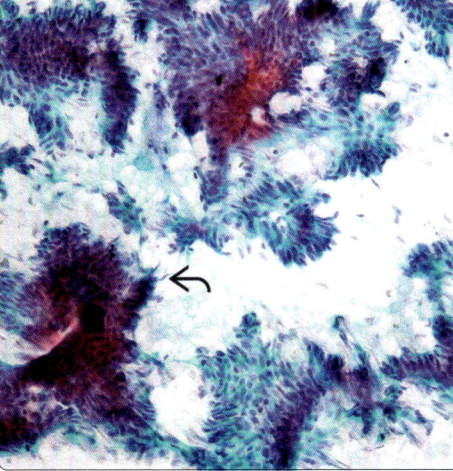

(Left) Pap-stained FNA smear of a mature cystic teratoma shows benign glandular epithelium ➡ in a background of proteinaceous material. **(Right)** Pap-stained FNA smear of a mature cystic teratoma shows respiratory-type epithelium ➡.

Neurogenic Tumors

KEY FACTS

CLINICAL ISSUES

- Neoplasms derived from neural crest (paraganglionic, autonomic/sympathetic, and peripheral nervous systems)
- Most commonly seen in posterior mediastinum
- Malignant tumors of sympathetic nervous system, such as neuroblastomas, are common in children
- Peripheral nerve sheath tumors and paragangliomas are common in adults

CYTOPATHOLOGY

- Neuroblastoma/ganglioneuroblastoma: Neuroblasts ± ganglion cells
- Ganglioneuroma: Ganglion cells with spindle cells without neuroblasts
- Peripheral nervous system tumor
  - Schwannoma/neurofibroma: Spindle cells with wavy nuclei and fine chromatin without significant atypia
- Malignant peripheral nerve sheath tumor: Tumor cells are spindled, epithelioid, or pleomorphic with cytologic atypia
- Paraganglioma: Round and oval tumor cells with neuroendocrine features and frequent intranuclear inclusions

TOP DIFFERENTIAL DIAGNOSES

- Neuroblastoma
  - Ewing sarcomas: Positive for CD99, *EWSR1* gene rearrangement by FISH
- Peripheral nervous system tumor: Spindle cell neoplasm
  - Spindle cell thymoma: Positive for cytokeratins and p63; negative for S100
  - Spindle cell carcinoid tumor: Positive for synaptophysin and chromogranin
  - Spindle cell melanoma: Positive for melanoma markers
- Paraganglioma
  - Carcinoid tumors: Usually positive for cytokeratin

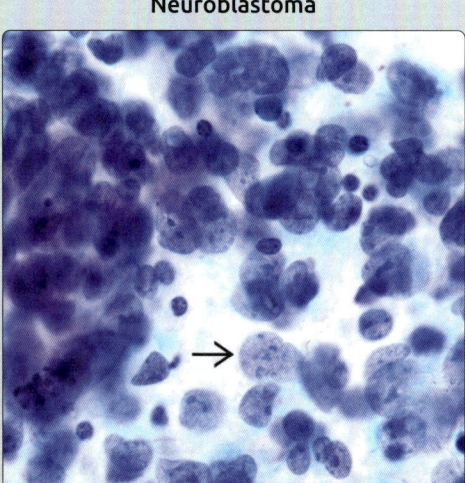

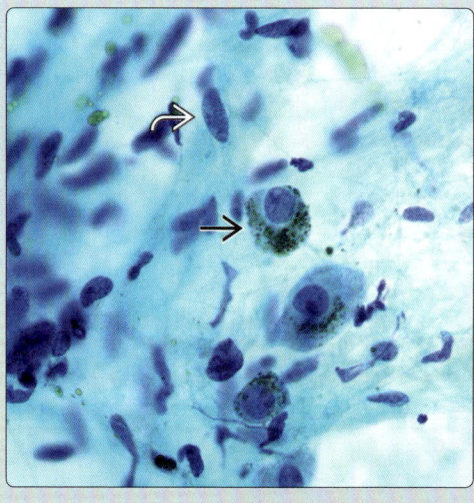

(Left) Pap-stained FNA smear of neuroblastoma shows tumor cells with coarsely granular chromatin and scant cytoplasm ➡. (Right) Pap-stained FNA smear shows a mixture of ganglion cells ➡ and spindle cells ➡ typical of ganglioneuroma.

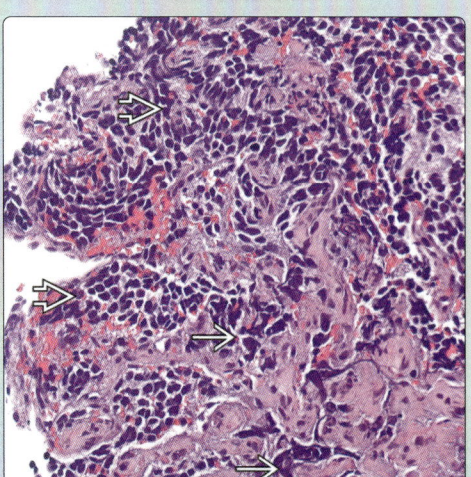

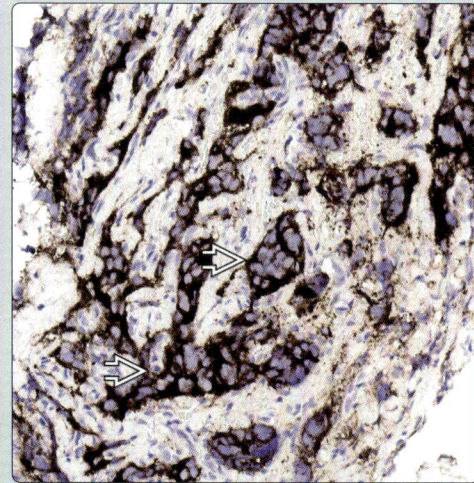

(Left) Core biopsy of a metastatic neuroblastoma shows small round blue tumor cells ➡ with scant cytoplasm. Some of the tumor cells demonstrate crush artifacts ➡. (Right) Core biopsy of neuroblastoma immunostained for synaptophysin shows diffuse and strong positivity in all the tumor cells ➡.

Neurogenic Tumors

TERMINOLOGY

Definitions
- Neoplasms derived from neural crest (paraganglionic, autonomic/sympathetic, and peripheral nervous systems) and located predominantly in posterior mediastinum

CLINICAL ISSUES

Epidemiology
- Incidence
  - Adults: 20% of mediastinal neoplasms
  - Children: 40% of mediastinal neoplasms
- Age
  - Adults: Paragangliomas and peripheral nerve sheath tumors, such as schwannomas, are common
  - Children: Malignant tumors of sympathetic nervous system, such as neuroblastomas, are common

CYTOPATHOLOGY

Cells
- Neuroblastoma
  - Neuroblast: Small blue cell tumor with monomorphic hyperchromatic nuclei, granular chromatin, and scant cytoplasm
  - Homer Wright rosettes, cytoplasmic process, and fibrillary material
  - Frequent mitoses and necrosis
- Ganglioneuroblastoma
  - Neuroblasts present
  - Ganglion cell proliferation: Large ganglion cells with prominent nucleoli and abundant granular cytoplasm
- Ganglioneuroma
  - Ganglion cells with benign spindle cells without neuroblasts
- Malignant peripheral nerve sheath tumor
  - Tumor cells are spindled, epithelioid, or pleomorphic with cytologic atypia
  - Mitoses and necrosis
- Schwannoma/neurofibroma
  - Spindle cells with wavy nuclei and fine chromatin
  - Alternating cellular areas (Antoni A) and hypocellular areas (Antoni B) in schwannoma
  - Myxoid or cystic background in schwannoma
- Paraganglioma
  - Round and oval tumor cells with neuroendocrine features and frequent intranuclear inclusions

ANCILLARY TESTS

Immunohistochemistry
- Neuroblastoma: Positive for CD56; negative for CD99
- Schwannoma/ganglioneuroma: Positive for S100
- Paraganglioma: Positive for synaptophysin and chromogranin; usually negative for cytokeratin

Genetic Testing
- Neuroblastoma: Negative for *EWSR1* gene rearrangement by FISH

DIFFERENTIAL DIAGNOSIS

Neuroblastoma
- Ewing sarcomas: CD99(+), *EWSR1* gene rearrangement by FISH

Peripheral Nervous System Tumors
- Spindle cell neoplasm
  - Spindle cell thymoma: Positive for cytokeratins and p63; negative for S100
  - Spindle cell carcinoid tumor: Positive for synaptophysin and chromogranin
  - Spindle cell melanoma: Positive for melanoma markers

Paraganglioma
- Carcinoid tumors: Usually positive for cytokeratin

SELECTED REFERENCES
1. Galetta D et al: Primary intrathoracic neurogenic tumors: clinical, pathological, and long-term outcomes. Thorac Cardiovasc Surg. 69(8):749-55, 2020
2. Rodriguez EF et al: Neurogenic tumors of the mediastinum. Semin Diagn Pathol. 37(4):179-86, 2020

Malignant Peripheral Nerve Sheath Tumor

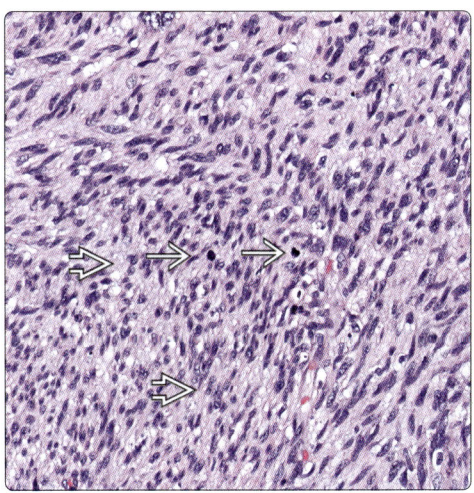

Malignant Peripheral Nerve Sheath Tumor

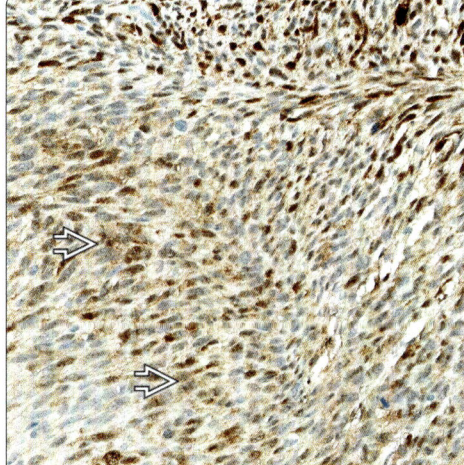

(Left) Core biopsy of a malignant peripheral nerve sheath tumor (MPNST) shows hyperchromatic malignant spindle cells ➡ with moderate nuclear pleomorphism and scattered mitotic figures ➡ in the tumor cells. *(Right)* Core biopsy of MPNST immunostained for S100 shows positivity in the spindle tumor cells ➡.

Metastatic Tumors of Mediastinum

KEY FACTS

CLINICAL ISSUES

- Metastases are more common than primary tumors
- Predominantly in adults
- Radiology correlation is critical, especially in patients with lung nodules
- Presentation
  - Mediastinal lymphadenopathy
  - Mediastinal mass

CYTOPATHOLOGY

- Variable cellularity, usually high
- Necrotic debris or lymphoid tissue may be present in background

TOP DIFFERENTIAL DIAGNOSES

- Small cell tumors
  - Metastasis: Small cell carcinoma of lung, small round blue cell tumors, lymphoma
  - Primary: Neuroblastoma, predominantly in children
- Squamous cell carcinoma
  - Metastases from lung and head and neck
  - Primary: Thymic carcinoma
- Other carcinomas and epithelioid tumors
  - Metastases from lung, breast, upper gastrointestinal tract, thyroid, melanoma
  - Primary: Thymoma, germ cell tumor
- Neuroendocrine tumors
  - More frequently lung primary
  - Primary: Neuroblastoma, paraganglioma
- Spindle cell tumors
  - Carcinoid, melanoma, carcinoma, sarcoma, neural tumor, thymoma/thymic carcinoma
  - Primary: Thymoma, thymic carcinoma, peripheral nervous system tumor
- Pleomorphic tumors
  - Metastases: Large cell carcinoma of lung, anaplastic thyroid carcinoma, sarcoma
  - Primary: Embryonal carcinoma

Metastatic Renal Cell Carcinoma

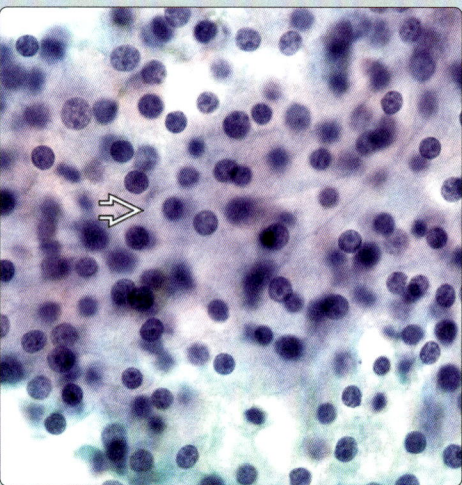

Metastatic Signet-Ring Cell Adenocarcinoma

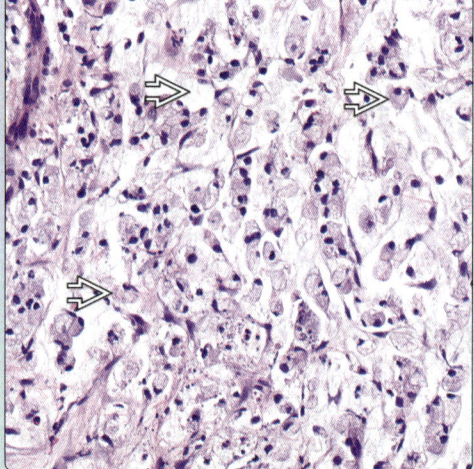

(Left) Pap-stained smear shows metastatic renal cell carcinoma with clear cell features ➡. (Right) Core biopsy of metastatic signet-ring cell adenocarcinoma from a gastroesophageal primary, stained with H&E, shows tumor cells ➡ with eccentrically placed nuclei and abundant, vacuolated, mucin-filled cytoplasm.

Metastatic Melanoma

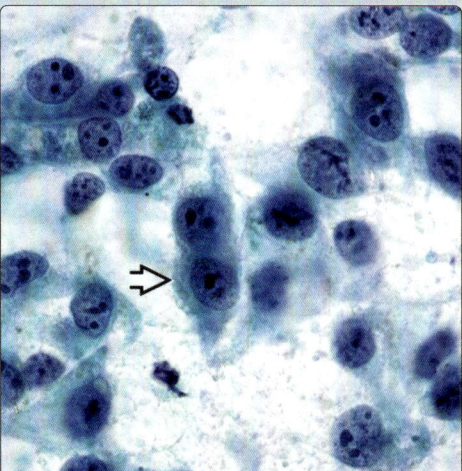

Metastatic Lung Carcinoma

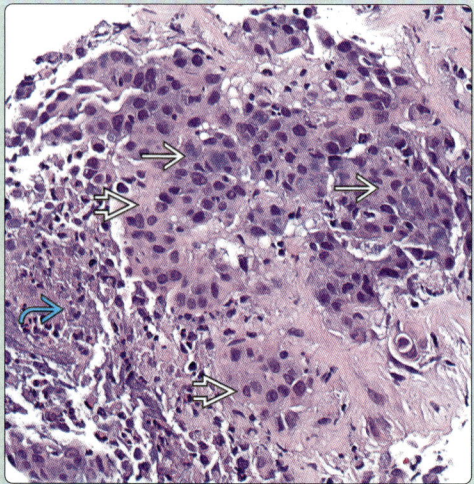

(Left) Pap-stained smear shows metastatic melanoma with prominent nucleoli and delicate cytoplasm ➡. (Right) Core biopsy of metastatic lung carcinoma in a mediastinal lymph node, stained with H&E, shows tumor cells ➡ with a moderate amount of cytoplasm, which is bluish-gray in some tumor cells ➡, indicating the presence of mucin and associated with necrosis ➡.

Metastatic Tumors of Mediastinum

CLINICAL ISSUES

Epidemiology
- Incidence
  - Metastatic tumors are more common than primary mediastinal tumors
  - Common primaries include carcinomas of lung, breast, head and neck, thyroid, kidney, upper gastrointestinal tract, and prostate as well as melanoma

Presentation
- Mediastinal lymphadenopathy
- Mediastinal mass

CYTOPATHOLOGY

Pattern
- Malignant cells ± lymphoid tissue

Background
- Lymphoid or necrotic

ANCILLARY TESTS

Immunohistochemistry
- Thymoma: Cytokeratins (+), p63(+), WT1(-), CD5(-)
- Thymic carcinoma: CD5(+), CD70(+), CD117(+), CD57(-)
- Seminoma: SALL4(+), PLAP(+), OCT3/4(+), CD57(+), CD5(-)
- Embryonal carcinoma: SALL4(+), OCT3/4(+), CD57(+), CD5(+), CD30(+)
- Neuroblastoma: CD56(+), CD99(-)
- Melanoma: HMB-45(+), Melan-A (+), pan-melanoma marker (+), SOX10(+)
- Thyroid carcinoma: PAX8(+), TTF-1(+)

DIFFERENTIAL DIAGNOSIS

Small Cell Tumors
- Small cell carcinoma of lung
- Non-Hodgkin lymphoma: Large B-cell lymphoma, lymphoblastic lymphoma
- Small blue round cell tumors
- Primary: Neuroblastoma, predominantly in children

Squamous Cell Carcinomas
- Lung and head and neck
- Primary: Thymic carcinoma

Other Carcinomas and Epithelioid Tumors
- Carcinomas of lung, breast, upper gastrointestinal tract, thyroid, urothelial, or prostate origin
- Melanoma, mesothelioma, germ cell tumors
- Primary: Thymoma, germ cell tumor

Spindle Cell Tumors
- Carcinoid tumor, melanoma, sarcoma, carcinoma
- Primary: Thymoma, thymic carcinoma, peripheral nervous system tumor

Clear Cell Tumors
- Renal cell carcinoma
- Non-small cell lung carcinoma
- Primary: Thymoma

Neuroendocrine Tumors
- Large cell, low- and intermediate-grade neuroendocrine carcinoma of lung
- Primary: Neuroblastoma, paraganglioma

Pleomorphic Tumors
- Large cell carcinoma of lung
- Anaplastic carcinoma of thyroid
- Sarcoma
- Primary: Embryonal carcinoma

SELECTED REFERENCES

1. Shiraishi O et al: Risk factors and prognostic impact of mediastinal lymph node metastases in patients with esophagogastric junction cancer. Ann Surg Oncol. 27(11):4433-40, 2020
2. Nambirajan A et al: Endobronchial ultrasound-guided transbronchial needle aspiration cytology in patients with known or suspected extra-pulmonary malignancies: a cytopathology-based study. Cytopathology. 30(1):82-90, 2019

Metastatic Small Cell Carcinoma

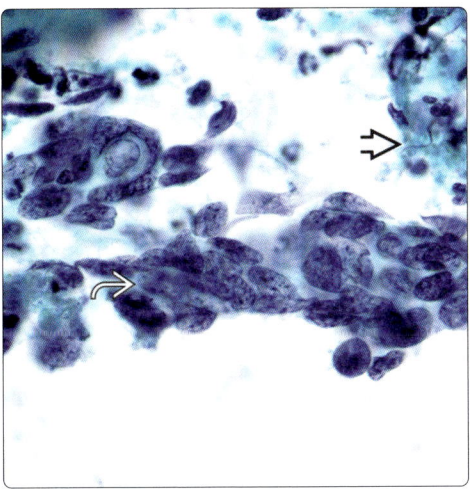

Metastatic Urothelial Carcinoma

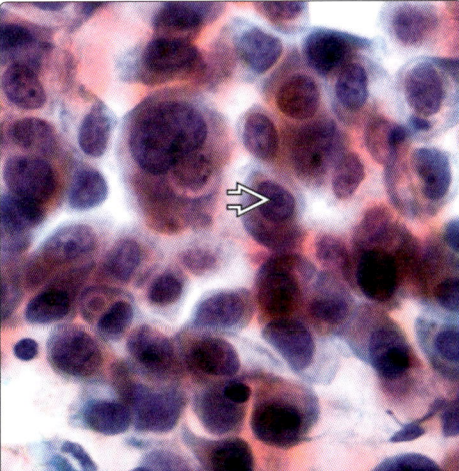

(Left) Pap-stained smear shows small cell carcinoma with scant cytoplasm and stippled chromatin ➡ in a background of necrosis ➡. **(Right)** Pap-stained smear shows metastatic urothelial carcinoma with a high nuclear:cytoplasmic ratio, irregular chromatin, and prominent nucleoli ➡.

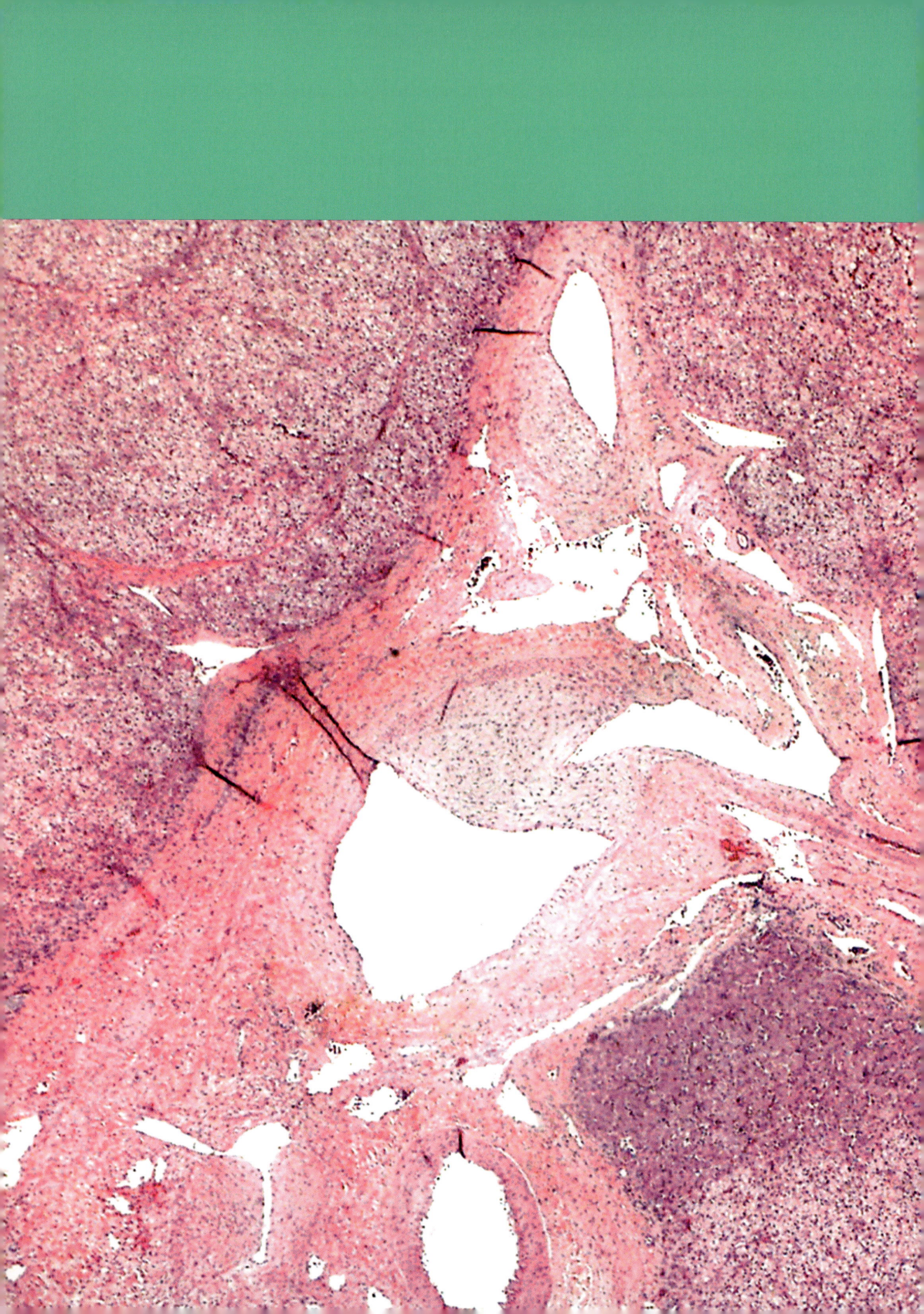

PART IV
SECTION 3
Liver

Overview
Cytology of Normal Liver 498
Inflammatory and Infectious Conditions of Liver 500

Benign Hepatic Neoplasms
Hepatocellular Adenoma 502
Focal Nodular Hyperplasia 504
Hemangioma, Liver 506

Malignant Neoplasms
Hepatocellular Carcinoma 508
Hepatoblastoma 510
Liver Metastasis 512

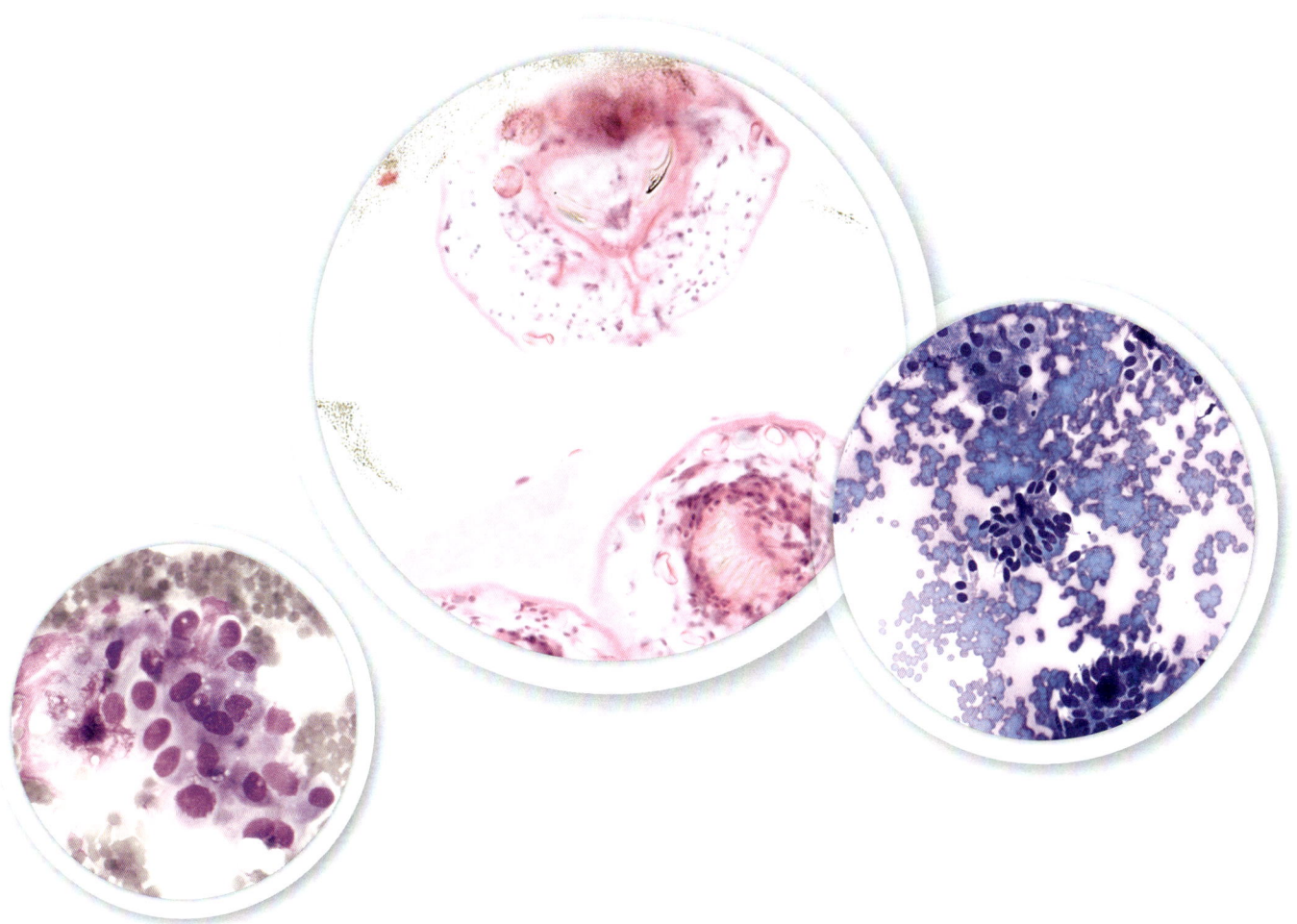

Cytology of Normal Liver

CLINICAL IMPLICATIONS

Clinical Presentation
- Symptoms associated with liver mass
- May be asymptomatic
- Aspiration is usually performed on nodular liver lesions to rule out neoplasm, but recognition of normal or nonneoplastic liver is essential for proper evaluation at time of adequacy check and final diagnosis

Imaging Findings
- General features
  o Mass/lesion must be visible on imaging studies for FNA to be performed
  o Mass may be cystic or solid, multiple or solitary
  o Certain liver lesions have characteristic imaging features

CYTOLOGIC FEATURES

Hepatocytes
- Polygonal shape; round, centrally located nuclei, low nuclear:cytoplasmic ratio
- Binucleation may occur
- Nucleoli may be prominent
- Abundant granular cytoplasm
- Some nuclear size variation may occur
- Cells arranged singly, in small sheets, or in trabeculae 2-3 cells thick
- Alterations that may occur and are within range of normal liver findings
  o Lipofuscin (yellow-brown, fine) accumulates within cytoplasm with increasing age over lifetime of patient
  o Iron (golden yellow, often clumpy) may be within hepatocytes and extracellular locations
    – Abundant in hemochromatosis
  o Bile (green-yellow, clumpy, or ropy) within cytoplasm or in adjacent sinusoidal channels
  o Mallory-Denk bodies (blue-green on Pap stain, ropy) are intracytoplasmic and infrequently seen
  o Nuclear glycogenation (nuclear holes) related to diabetes, obesity
  o Steatosis (cytoplasmic vacuoles) secondary to numerous conditions

Normal Liver Components

Normal Liver Components

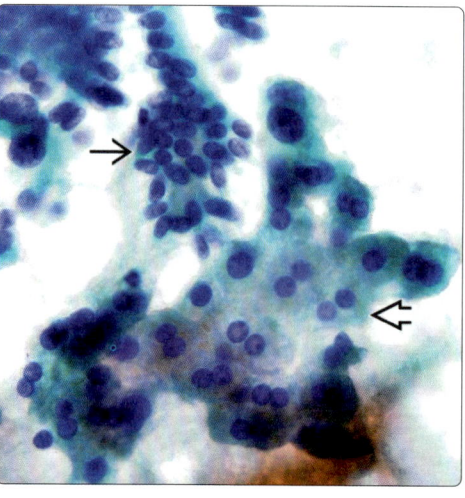

(Left) Diff-Quik stain shows a benign sheet of bile ductal epithelial cells ⇨ and adjacent hepatocytes ⇨. (Right) Pap stain shows a sheet of hepatocytes 2-3 cells thick ⇨ with an adjacent bile duct ⇨. The differences in the cell size and architecture usually make distinguishing these cell types straightforward.

Steatosis in Normal Hepatocytes

Mesothelial Cells With Pap Stain

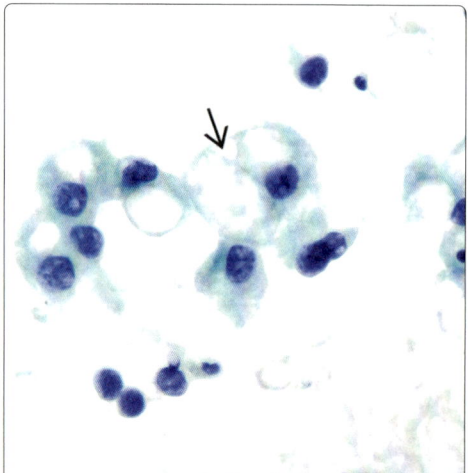
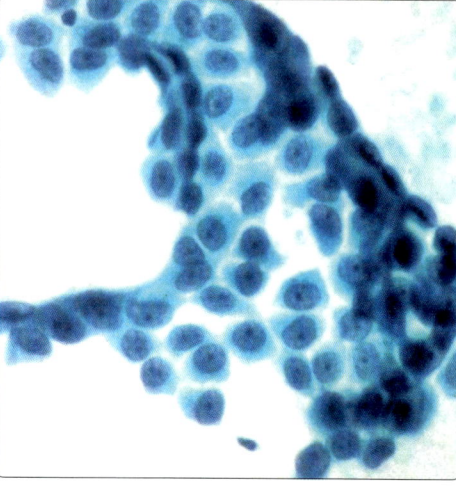

(Left) Steatosis ⇨, as seen on Pap stain, is usually a nonneoplastic finding but does not rule out the possibility of hepatocellular carcinoma. (Right) A sheet of mesothelial cells on Pap stain resembles hepatocytes but has a slightly higher nuclear:cytoplasmic ratio and lacks the characteristic features of normal liver.

Cytology of Normal Liver

Biliary Epithelium
- Cuboidal to low columnar cells
- Arranged in flat sheets with honeycomb pattern
- Round nuclei with inconspicuous nucleoli
- Fine chromatin
- Scant amount of associated cytoplasm
- Some nuclear size variation may occur

Kupffer Cells
- Oval to elongated nuclei
- Fine chromatin
- Scant cytoplasm
- Intermingle with hepatocytes
- Not usually prominent but may become more visible with certain disease processes

Endothelial Cells
- Elongated nuclei wrapping around hepatocytes
- No visible cytoplasm

DIFFERENTIAL DIAGNOSIS

Normal Mesothelial Cells
- May indicate that FNA sample was not taken from liver/lesion
- Arranged in cohesive sheets
- Round nuclei; nucleoli may be visible
- Fair amount of associated cytoplasm but not as much or as granular as hepatocytes
- Empty spaces between cells ("windows")
- Hepatocyte nuclei are centrally located, whereas nuclei of mesothelial cells are more peripheral within cytoplasm

Hepatocellular Adenoma
- Cytologic features similar to those of normal liver
- Radiographic-guided FNA placement in mass/lesion is required to confirm diagnosis

Hepatocellular Carcinoma
- Well-differentiated carcinomas resemble nonneoplastic hepatocytes
- Presence of transgressing vessels and thickened trabeculae of hepatocytes (> 3 cells thick) lined by endothelial cells is required for malignancy

Metastatic Malignancies
- Often more cellular than nonneoplastic liver
- Usually cytologic features of malignancy are present
- Bile or Mallory-Denk bodies indicate hepatic origin

Other
- Even experienced radiologists may inadvertently sample another organ in vicinity of liver
- Recognition of normal and neoplastic extrahepatic tissue is imperative at time of adequacy check to raise possibility of sampling discrepancy
  - Right lung: Needle may go through diaphragm or be placed superior in pleural cavity above diaphragm
    - Columnar cells (with terminal bars and cilia) and macrophages; usually low cellularity
  - Right kidney: Needle may be inferior to liver and sample kidney instead
    - Normal kidney shows low cellularity, scattered small tubules, rare glomeruli (rounded mass of capillaries and spindled cells)
  - Right adrenal: Inferiorly located needle
    - Normal adrenal shows low cellularity, cells with round (often bare) nuclei, and little vacuolated cytoplasm
    - Tumors (adrenal adenoma/pheochromocytoma) show endocrine atypia (varying size of nuclei and lack of pleomorphism)
    - Endocrine tumors often associated with endothelial cells simulating hepatic trabeculae

SELECTED REFERENCES
1. Shyu S et al: Significance of hepatocyte atypia in liver fine needle aspiration. Diagn Cytopathol. 50(4):186-95, 2022
2. Rai SPV et al: Efficacy and validity of image-guided percutaneous fine needle aspiration and core biopsy of liver pathologies: saga of focal hepatic lesions from the nodule to the needle to the slide. J Cytol. 38(1):21-30, 2021
3. Lew M et al: Optimizing small liver biopsy specimens: a combined cytopathology and surgical pathology perspective. J Am Soc Cytopathol. 9(5):405-41, 2020

Normal Hepatocytes
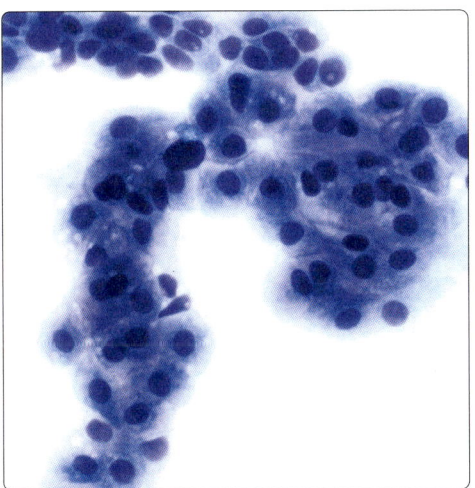

Adrenal Adenoma
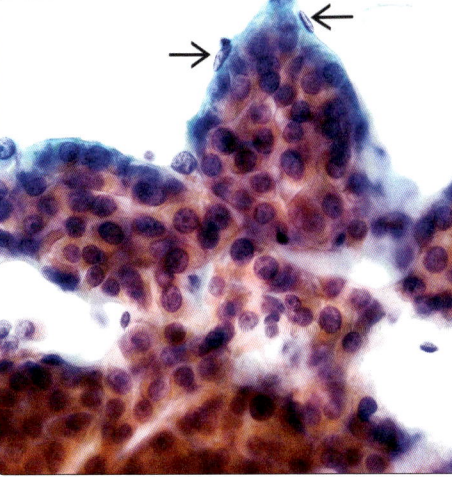

(Left) Diff-Quik stain shows normal hepatocytes arranged singly and in thin trabeculae (2-3 cells thick) with centrally located nuclei, some binucleate. (Right) Pap stain shows adrenal adenoma resembling hepatocellular carcinoma lined by endothelial cells ➡. Recognition that the needle is actually in the adrenal and not the liver is extremely helpful in rendering the correct diagnosis.

Inflammatory and Infectious Conditions of Liver

EPIDEMIOLOGY

Age
- Usually seen in adults but can affect all ages

Natural History
- Organisms may gain access to liver through hepatic artery, portal vein, ascension through biliary tract, or direct extension

ETIOLOGY/PATHOGENESIS

Hepatic Abscess
- Bacterial causes
  - *Streptococcus, Klebsiella, Staphylococcus, Salmonella, Mycobacterium*, others
- Fungal causes
  - *Aspergillus, Candida, Cryptococcus, Histoplasma*, Mucorales, others
- Parasitic causes
  - *Entamoeba histolytica, Fasciola hepatica, Schistosoma, Toxocara, Echinococcus granulosus*, others
- Viral causes
  - Adenovirus, cytomegalovirus (CMV), herpes simplex virus (HSV), others

Granuloma
- Infectious causes
  - Associated with numerous bacteria, fungi, and viruses
- Noninfectious causes
  - Lipogranuloma, primary biliary cirrhosis, sarcoidosis, malignancy, metals, drugs, immunological diseases, and foreign material
    - Obtain liver enzymes and additional history

Hydatid Cyst
- *Echinococcosis* species endemic in certain areas
  - Most commonly Middle East and Africa
- Often clinical diagnosis, but atypical presentation may result in cytologic aspirate
- Possibility of anaphylactic shock militates against aspiration, though this has been disputed with use of smaller gauge needles

Amoebic Abscess
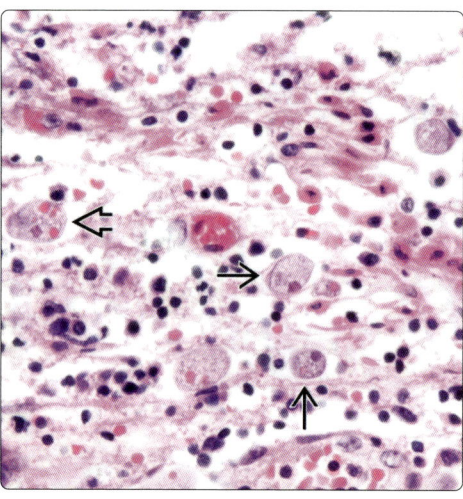

Histoplasma in Hepatocytes
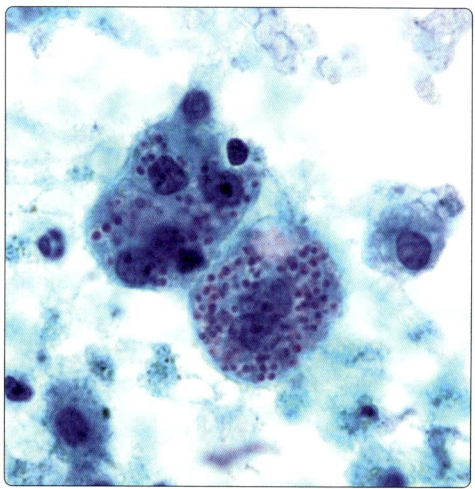

(Left) *Entamoeba histolytica* on H&E stain is represented by numerous trophozoites ➔ with a round, regular, dark nucleus the size of a red blood cell. Some trophozoites have ingested red blood cells ➔. (Right) Pap stain shows benign hepatocytes filled with small, intracellular, yeast-like organisms with uniform size, consistent with *Histoplasma* organisms.

Charcot-Leyden Crystals
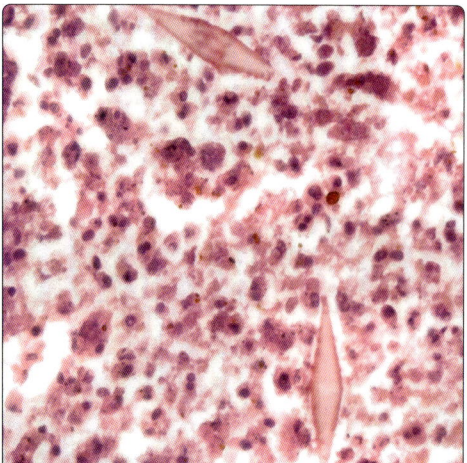

Lipogranuloma
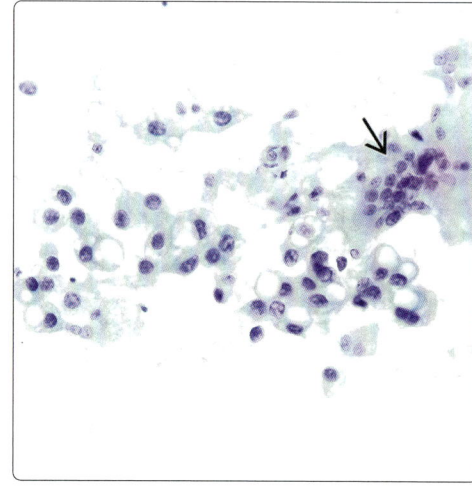

(Left) Toxocariasis (visceral larva migrans) on H&E shows Charcot-Leyden crystals with a hexagonal bipyramidal structure associated with eosinophils. Larvae are rarely seen. (Right) A lipogranuloma on Pap stain shows hepatocytes with steatotic vacuoles and a multinucleated giant cell ➔.

Inflammatory and Infectious Conditions of Liver

CLINICAL IMPLICATIONS

Clinical Presentation
- Abdominal/right upper quadrant pain, fever, or hepatomegaly
- May be asymptomatic

Clinical Risk Factors
- Immunosuppression (e.g., organ transplant, genetic defect, drug, viral infection, autoimmune disease, cancer, others)

CYTOLOGIC FEATURES

Abscess
- Abundant polymorphonuclear leukocytes
- Some macrophages may be included
- Hepatocytes are often absent
- Organisms (bacterial, fungal, parasitic, or viral) may not be evident on smears
  o Cell block for special stains (GMS, AFB, Fite, PAS, Gram) or immunocytochemistry (CMV, HSV)
  o PCR-based techniques for identifying infectious organisms in liver abscess is another option using fresh, fixed/cell block, or smeared material
  o Certain infectious organisms (e.g., such as *E. histolytica*) may produce little inflammation
  o Charcot-Leyden crystals formed from degenerating eosinophils may be sign of parasite

Granulomas
- Lipogranuloma
  o Steatosis
  o Multinucleated giant cells
- Sarcoidosis
  o Nonnecrotizing, tightly cohesive epithelioid histocytes
  o Multinucleated giant cells may be seen
- Infectious (e.g., tuberculous)
  o Epithelioid histocytes
  o Mononuclear inflammatory cells (mostly lymphocytes)
  o Multinucleated giant cells
  o Necrosis

- Drug related
  o Eosinophils present
  o In cases of intravenous recreational drugs, there may be polarizable crystals

Hydatid Cyst
- Diagnosis rests on presence of hooklets or protoscolices
- Acellular laminated membrane may be present

DIFFERENTIAL DIAGNOSIS

Benign and Malignant Neoplasms
- Necrotic material from carcinomas, such as squamous cell carcinoma, may be misinterpreted as abscess
  o Obtain cell block and examine background for viable malignant cells
- Presence of granulomas does not exclude neoplastic process
  o Granulomas are associated with hepatocellular adenoma, Hodgkin and non-Hodgkin lymphomas, carcinomas (e.g., squamous cell carcinoma), and sarcomas (e.g., synovial sarcoma)

DIAGNOSTIC CHECKLIST

Pathologic Interpretation Pearls
- At time of adequacy check, request additional material to be submitted for cultures

SELECTED REFERENCES

1. He S et al: Percutaneous fine-needle aspiration for pyogenic liver abscess (3-6cm): a two-center retrospective study. BMC Infect Dis. 20(1):516, 2020
2. Devi S et al: Isolated tubercular liver abscess in a non-immunodeficient patient: a rare case report. Cureus. 11(12):e6282, 2019
3. Dinoop KP et al: Comparison of nested-multiplex, Taqman & SYBR Green real-time PCR in diagnosis of amoebic liver abscess in a tertiary health care institute in India. Indian J Med Res. 143(1):49-56, 2016
4. Desoubeaux G et al: Unusual multiple large abscesses of the liver: interest of the radiological features and the real-time PCR to distinguish between bacterial and amebic etiologies. Pathog Glob Health. 108(1):53-7, 2014
5. Mokhtari M et al: Amebic liver abscess: fine needle aspiration diagnosis. Acta Cytol. 58(3):225-8, 2014
6. Kim AR et al: Fine needle aspiration cytology of hepatic hydatid cyst: a case study. Korean J Pathol. 47(4):395-8, 2013

Hydatid Cyst Protoscolices and Hooklets

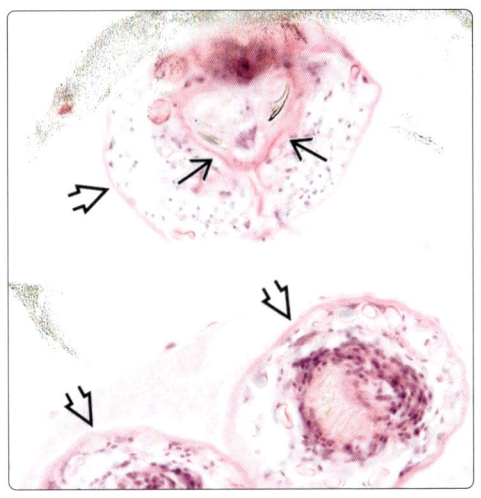

***Echinococcus* Hooklets on Cell Block**

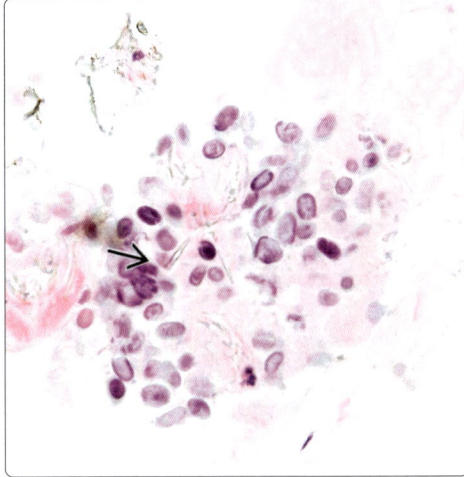

(Left) This aspirate of a hydatid cyst (Echinococcus) contains several protoscolices ➡ and refractile hooklets ➡ in the H&E-stained cell block. (Right) Detached fragments of hooklets of Echinococcus ➡ are present in the cell block on H&E stain. The identification of either the protoscolices or hooklets is required for a definitive diagnosis of a hydatid cyst.

Hepatocellular Adenoma

KEY FACTS

TERMINOLOGY
- Benign liver neoplasm composed of cells of hepatocyte origin

ETIOLOGY/PATHOGENESIS
- Sex hormones appear to play role
- Almost always associated with oral contraceptive or long-term steroid use
- Also associated with glycogen storage disease types I and III, galactosemia, tyrosinemia, vascular diseases, familial polyposis syndrome, and β-thalassemia

CLINICAL ISSUES
- Typically seen in women of reproductive age
- Complications
  o Bleeding
  o Rupture; pregnancy is risk factor
  o Slight chance of malignant transformation

CYTOPATHOLOGY
- Normal-appearing hepatocytes
  o Low nuclear:cytoplasmic ratio
  o No nuclear atypia
  o No large, prominent nucleoli
  o Hepatocytes 1-3 cells thick
  o No endothelial wrapping of thickened cords
- Lack of biliary epithelium and fibrosis in background
- Ancillary tests
  o Immunohistochemical staining for glypican-3, heat shock protein 70, and glutamine synthetase can help differentiate from hepatocellular carcinoma

TOP DIFFERENTIAL DIAGNOSES
- Hepatocellular carcinoma
- Focal nodular hyperplasia
- Nodular regenerative hyperplasia
- Nonneoplastic liver

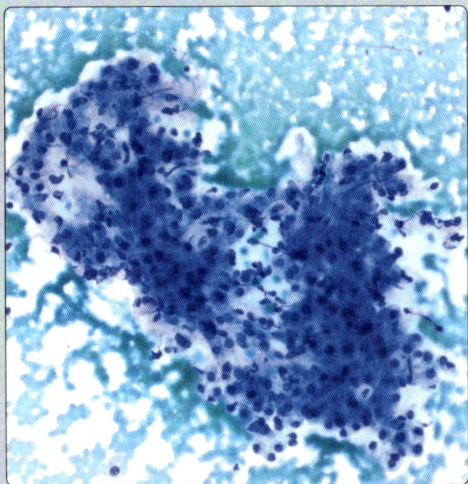

Hepatocytes in Hepatocellular Adenoma

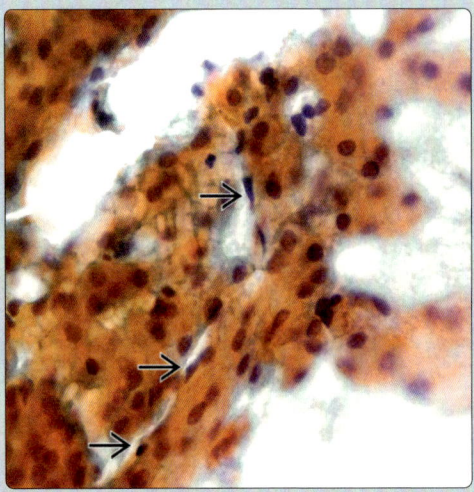

Hepatocellular Adenoma Endothelial Cells

(Left) Diff-Quik stain shows a sheet of benign hepatocytes without thickened trabecula (1-3 cells thick). (Right) Higher power Pap stain demonstrates cords of hepatocytes with associated sinusoidal endothelial cells ➔. The cords of hepatocytes are < 3 cells thick and may show focal endothelial cells.

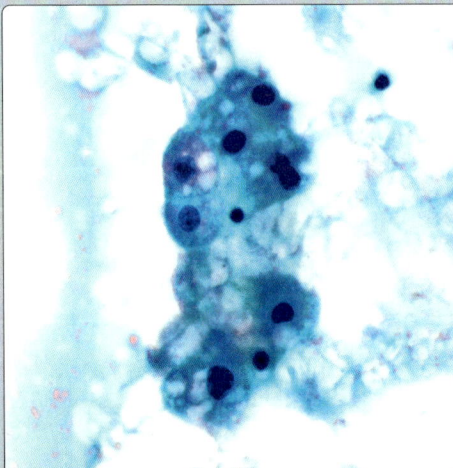

Hepatocellular Adenoma With Steatosis

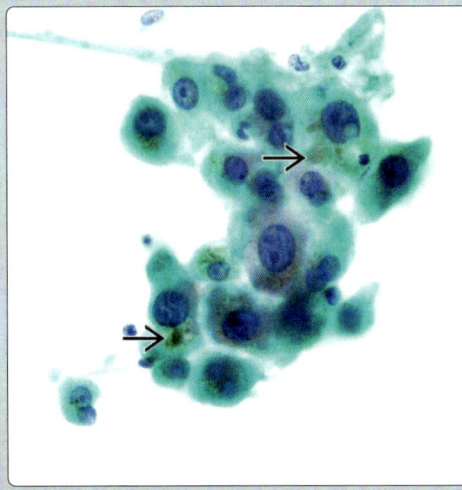

Hepatocellular Adenoma Cytoplasmic Bile

(Left) Pap stain shows benign hepatocytes with steatotic changes. (Right) Pap stain shows some nuclear size variation, but overall, the hepatocytes have a low nuclear:cytoplasmic ratio and small nucleoli. Again, the cords are not thickened. Intracytoplasmic bile ➔ may be seen.

Hepatocellular Adenoma

CLINICAL ISSUES

Presentation
- Liver mass
  - Arising in noncirrhotic liver
  - Often without underlying liver disease
  - Associated with oral contraceptive use
    - May regress after withdrawal of oral contraceptives
- Symptoms
  - May be asymptomatic
    - Found on imaging in 20% of cases
  - Palpable mass
  - Abdominal pain
    - Acute (indicative of rupture), intermittent, or chronic

Treatment
- Stop oral contraceptives
- Embolization
- Surgical resection to prevent bleeding and rupture

CYTOPATHOLOGY

Cells
- Normal-appearing hepatocytes
  - Low nuclear:cytoplasmic ratio
  - No nuclear atypia
  - No large, prominent nucleoli
  - Hepatocytes 1-3 cells thick
    - No/minimal endothelial wrapping of thickened cords
  - Rare transgressing vessels
  - May have glycogen, fat, bile, or Mallory-Denk bodies in cytoplasm
- Lack of biliary epithelium and fibrosis in background

MACROSCOPIC

General Features
- Unencapsulated, well-demarcated mass
  - Typically solitary but may be multiple
  - Tan to brown; may have hemorrhage or necrosis

Size
- Typically 5-15 cm but may be up to 30 cm

MICROSCOPIC

Histologic Features
- Background of noncirrhotic liver
- Cords or sheets of benign hepatocytes

DIFFERENTIAL DIAGNOSIS

Hepatocellular Carcinoma
- Cytologic atypia with increased nuclear:cytoplasmic ratio and prominent nucleoli
- Thickened trabecula and pseudoglandular formation
- Often arises in background of cirrhosis &/or chronic liver disease
- More common in men and older individuals

Focal Nodular Hyperplasia
- Bile duct cells and fibrosis in background

DIAGNOSTIC CHECKLIST

Clinically Relevant Pathologic Features
- Liver mass in woman on oral contraceptives

Pathologic Interpretation Pearls
- May be indistinguishable from nonneoplastic liver
  - Radiographic confirmation that needle tip is in mass lesion required for diagnosis
- May be indistinguishable from dysplastic &/or regenerative nodules, focal nodular hyperplasia, or well-differentiated hepatocellular carcinoma by cytomorphology alone
  - Correlate with clinical history and laboratory data, radiologic findings, histopathology (i.e., core needle biopsy when available), and ancillary studies

SELECTED REFERENCES
1. Renzulli M et al: Hepatocellular adenoma: an unsolved diagnostic enigma. World J Gastroenterol. 25(20):2442-9, 2019

Hepatocellular Adenoma Histology

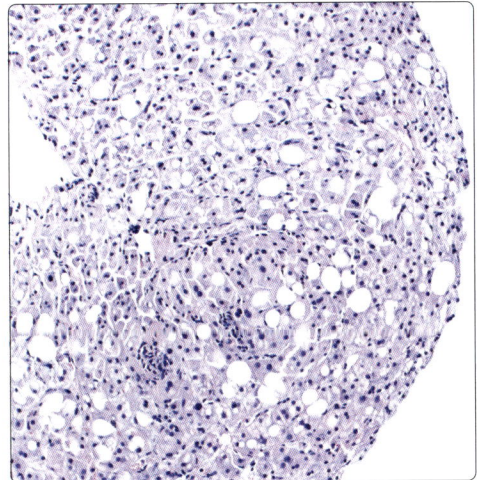

Hepatocellular Adenoma Reticulin Stain

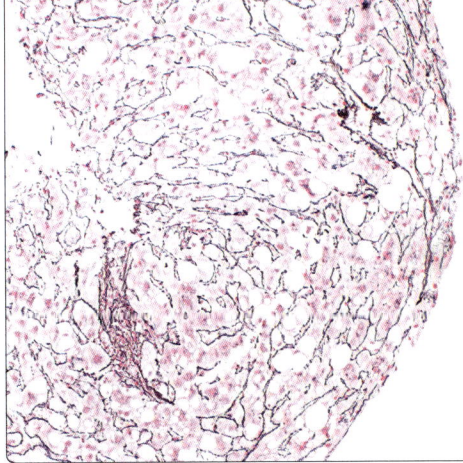

(Left) H&E-stained section shows cords of benign hepatocytes 1-2 cells thick, some steatosis, unpaired arteries, and no portal tracts. *(Right)* Corresponding reticulin stain shows intact reticulin framework.

Focal Nodular Hyperplasia

KEY FACTS

ETIOLOGY/PATHOGENESIS
- Exact mechanism is unclear
  - Likely caused by hyperplastic response to localized vascular abnormality/response to abnormal blood flow
- Contraceptives are thought not to play role (in contrast to hepatic adenomas)
- Hepatocytes polyclonal, unlike hepatocytic adenomas

CLINICAL ISSUES
- Mostly incidental finding on imaging studies
- Most common in women

IMAGING
- Bright, homogeneously enhancing mass in arterial-phase CT or MR with delayed enhancement of central scar
- Peripheral lobulation

CYTOPATHOLOGY
- Bland hepatocytes
- Fragments of fibrous stroma may be seen
- Hemorrhage &/or necrosis rare
- Benign ductular epithelium may be present
  - May help to distinguish from hepatic adenoma

MICROSCOPIC
- Hyperplastic hepatocytes arranged into plates 2 cells thick
- Subdivided into nodules by fibrous septa
- Intact reticulin framework

TOP DIFFERENTIAL DIAGNOSES
- Hepatocellular adenoma
  - No ductular epithelium or fibrous tissue
- Well-differentiated hepatocellular carcinoma
  - Cytologic atypia of thickened cords of hepatocytes is present
- Nodular regenerative hyperplasia
- Cirrhosis
- Adenocarcinoma

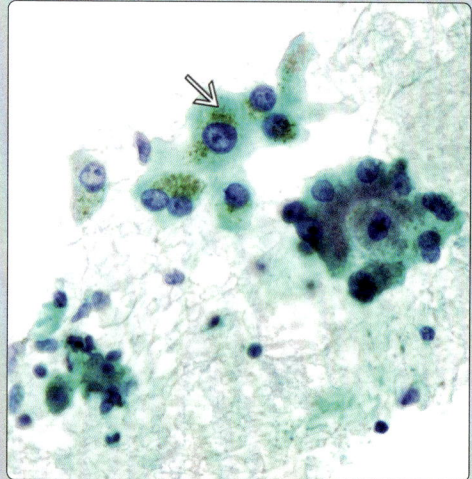

Focal Nodular Hyperplasia Hepatocytes

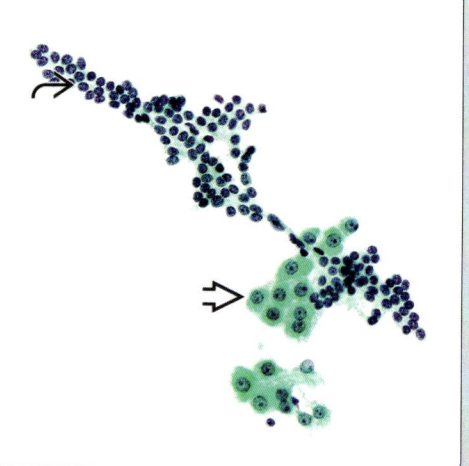

Focal Nodular Hyperplasia

(Left) Pap-stained aspirate shows unremarkable-appearing hepatocytes with lipofuscin pigment within the cytoplasm ➡. There is no way to differentiate it from normal liver other than by evidence of needle placement in the mass. Correlation with radiographic vascular findings is key to diagnosis on small biopsy and cytology. (Right) Pap stain shows smears contain hepatocytes ➡ and ductular epithelium ➡.

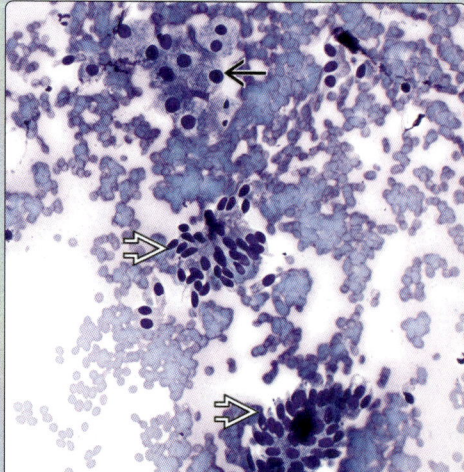

Ductular Reaction in Focal Nodular Hyperplasia

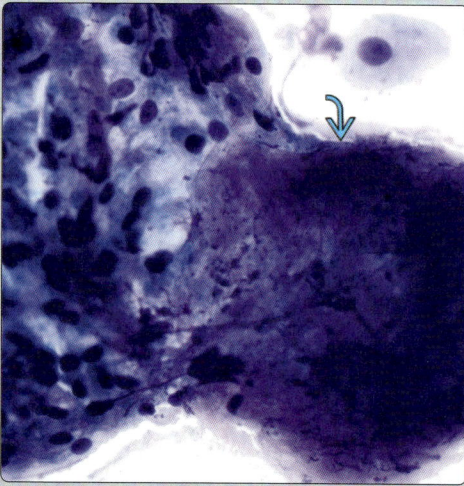

Fibrous Tissue in Focal Nodular Hyperplasia

(Left) Diff-Quik stain shows increased ductal epithelial elements ➡ and benign hepatocytes ➡. (Right) Diff-Quik stain shows an unremarkable sheet of hepatocytes adjacent to fibrous stroma ➡.

Focal Nodular Hyperplasia

CLINICAL ISSUES

Presentation
- Mostly incidental finding on imaging studies
- If large, may present as abdominal mass &/or compress surrounding structures
- More common in adult women of reproductive age (20s-40s)
- Normal liver biochemical tests

Treatment
- Most cases do not require any treatment
- Surgery performed for large and symptomatic lesions

Prognosis
- Benign lesion
- Rupture, bleeding rare

IMAGING

General Features
- Bright, homogeneously enhancing mass in arterial-phase CT or MR with delayed enhancement of central scar
- Peripheral lobulation

CYTOPATHOLOGY

Background
- Fragments of fibrous stroma may be seen

Cells
- Bland hepatocytes
- Benign ductular epithelium may be present (may help to distinguish from hepatic adenoma)

MACROSCOPIC

General Features
- Unencapsulated, lobulated, well-circumscribed lesion
  - ~ 20% are multiple
- Central stellate scar with radiating septa
- Noncirrhotic background liver

Size
- Most < 5 cm

MICROSCOPIC

Histologic Features
- Classic triad
  - Fibrous septa, usually with large, central stellate scar
    - Scar contains numerous, thick-walled arteries
    - Fibrous septa contain large, dystrophic vessels with eccentrically thickened walls; some may be thrombosed
  - Ductular reaction (not true ducts) at junction between septa and parenchyma
  - Mononuclear inflammatory infiltrate in fibrous septa

DIFFERENTIAL DIAGNOSIS

Hepatocellular Adenoma
- Absence of ductular fragments and fibrous septa

Cirrhosis
- Requires radiographic correlation

Hepatocellular Carcinoma
- Lack of portal structures
- Thickened hepatic trabecula or pseudoacini
- Cytologic atypia with increased nuclear:cytoplasmic ratio and prominent nucleoli
- Fibrolamellar type has fibrous tissue, but malignant hepatocytes show abundant eosinophilic granular cytoplasm

Adenocarcinoma
- Ductular fragments may be misinterpreted as malignant
- Look for overt cytologic features of malignancy

SELECTED REFERENCES
1. Lew M et al: Optimizing small liver biopsy specimens: a combined cytopathology and surgical pathology perspective. J Am Soc Cytopathol. 9(5):405-21, 2020

Focal Nodular Hyperplasia Central Scar

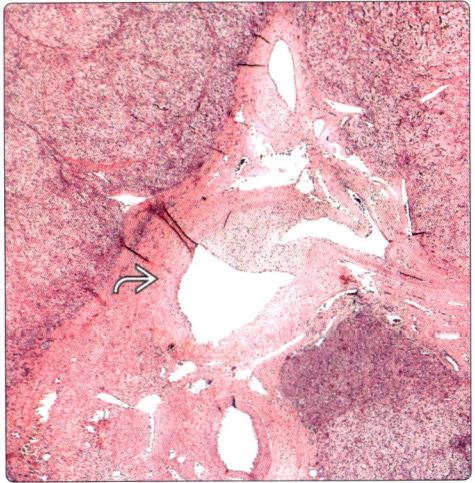

Fibrolamellar Hepatocellular Carcinoma

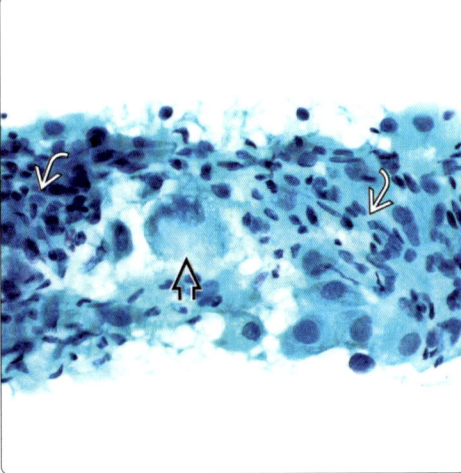

(Left) H&E-stained tissue section shows prominent fibrous septa, which contain abnormal vessels ➡. *(Right)* Pap stain shows fragments of fibrous tissue ➡, but the associated hepatocytes are malignant with abundant granular cytoplasm ➡ and prominent nucleoli.

Hemangioma, Liver

KEY FACTS

CLINICAL ISSUES
- Ranges from 1-20% in autopsy studies
  - Most common primary tumor of liver
- Majority are clinically silent, discovered incidentally
  - Tumors < 4 cm are rarely symptomatic
- Vague abdominal pain, hepatomegaly, palpable mass in large lesions
- Complications rare
  - Spontaneous rupture, consumptive coagulopathy
- Surgical resection or ablative therapy if symptomatic
- Core needle biopsy may be contraindicated because of bleeding
- FNA is relatively safe
  - Needle fills with blood without aspirating

IMAGING
- Heterogeneous appearance that is virtually diagnostic on MR scans; biopsy is rarely necessary
- Atypical imaging features prompt biopsy

CYTOPATHOLOGY
- Paucicellular
- Bloody smears
- Bland oval- to spindle-shaped cells in small groups or as single cells
- Fine chromatin, may show nuclear grooves

TOP DIFFERENTIAL DIAGNOSES
- Angiosarcoma
  - Malignant endothelial cells with irregular nuclear shape, chromatin, vasoformative features
- Normal liver (false-negative)
  - Bland spindled cells of hemangioma may be overlooked since smears are often paucicellular
  - Bloody background, radiographic suspicion, and cell block to increase sensitivity are helpful
- Hemangioendothelioma
  - Larger epithelioid cells with nuclear pseudoinclusions and vasoformative features

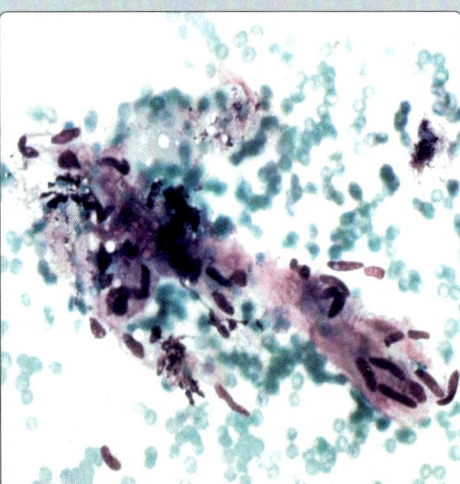

Hemangioma Spindled Cells

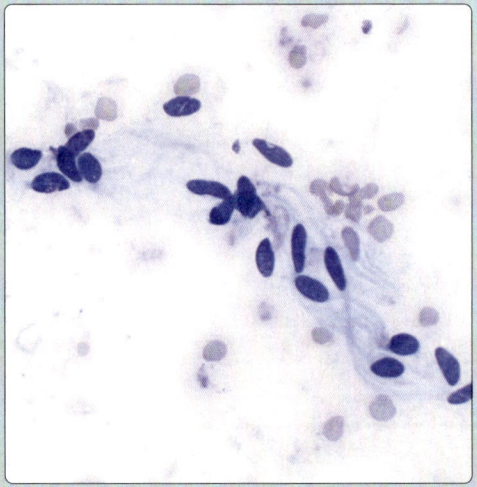

Hemangioma Spindled Cells

(Left) In this Diff-Quik-stained smear, several elongated, bland spindled cells are present. Overall, the cellularity is low with abundant blood in the background. (Right) Diff-Quik stain, hypocellular aspirate, shows a cluster of bland spindled cells in a background of abundant blood.

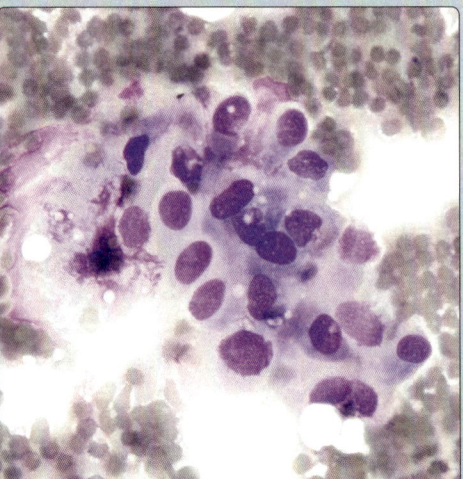

Hemangioma Epithelioid Cells

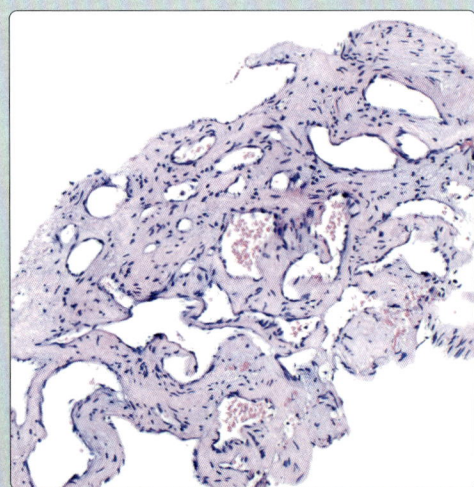

Hemangioma Histology

(Left) In some cases, the cells may appear more rounded and epithelioid, as seen in this Diff-Quik stain. (Right) Core needle biopsy stained with H&E shows dilated vascular spaces lined by bland, flattened endothelial cells. The variably thick intervening fibrous bands are paucicellular.

Hemangioma, Liver

TERMINOLOGY

Definitions
- Benign vascular tumor
  - Most common primary tumor of liver

ETIOLOGY/PATHOGENESIS

Unknown
- Postulated but unproven role of sex hormones

CLINICAL ISSUES

Epidemiology
- Age
  - All ages
- Sex
  - More common in women

Presentation
- Majority are clinically silent, discovered incidentally
  - Larger tumors may be symptomatic

IMAGING

MR Findings
- Heterogeneous appearance that is virtually diagnostic
- Atypical imaging features prompt biopsy

CYTOPATHOLOGY

Background and Cellularity
- Bloody and paucicellular; blood in needle without aspiration

Cells
- Bland oval- to spindle-shaped cells in small groups or as single cells

Nuclear Details
- Fine chromatin; may show nuclear grooves

Cytoplasmic Details
- Fair amount of associated cytoplasm

MACROSCOPIC

General Features
- Usually solitary and subcapsular

Size
- Most < 4 cm
  - Tumors up to 30 cm have been described

MICROSCOPIC

Histologic Features
- Well demarcated from surrounding liver
- Dilated, variably sized vascular spaces
  - Spaces lined by flat, bland endothelial cells

DIFFERENTIAL DIAGNOSIS

Angiosarcoma
- Malignant endothelial cells with irregular nuclear shape, irregular chromatin, vasoformative features

Normal Liver (False-Negative)
- Bland spindled cells of hemangioma may be overlooked since smears are often paucicellular
- Bloody background, radiographic suspicion, and cell block to increase sensitivity are helpful

Epithelioid Hemangioendothelioma
- Larger epithelioid cells with nuclear pseudoinclusions, abundant vacuolated cytoplasm ("blister" cells), and vasoformative features
- May see fragments of myxohyaline stroma

SELECTED REFERENCES

1. Li T et al: Hepatic sclerosing hemangioma mimicking malignancy: a case and literature review. Am J Med Case Rep. 9(3):144-6, 2021
2. Alimoradi M et al: Massive liver haemangioma causing Kasabach-Merritt syndrome in an adult. Ann R Coll Surg Engl. 102(9):e1-4, 2020
3. Patacsil SJ et al: A review of benign hepatic tumors and their imaging characteristics. Cureus. 12(1):e6813, 2020

Epithelioid Hemangioendothelioma

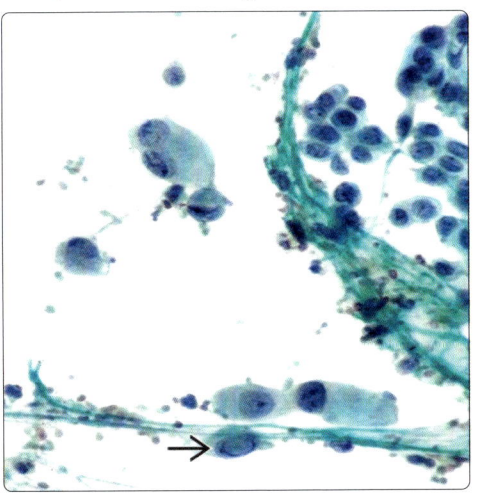

Angiosarcoma

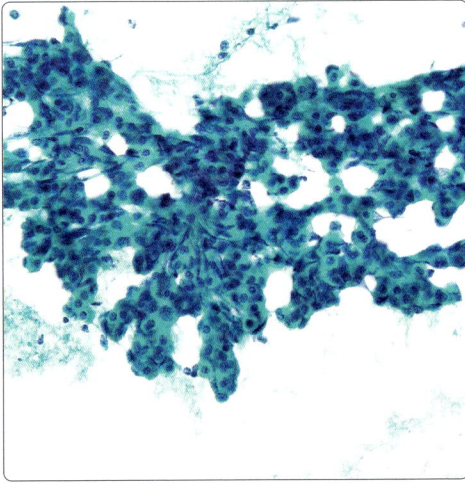

(Left) Epithelioid hemangioendothelioma shows epithelioid cells with round nuclei and abundant cytoplasm, as seen in this Pap-stained smear. Intranuclear pseudoinclusions ⇒ may be present. *(Right)* In this Pap-stained smear of an angiosarcoma, vasoformative features are evident. The cells appear to be extending, trying to form a vascular structure.

Hepatocellular Carcinoma

KEY FACTS

TERMINOLOGY
- Hepatocellular carcinoma (HCC)
- Primary malignant neoplasm of liver with hepatocytic differentiation

CLINICAL ISSUES
- Associated with cirrhosis; in USA incidence is ~ 4 per 100,000; up to 150 per 100,000 in parts of Asia and Africa
- Fibrolamellar variant: 5% of HCC, arises in noncirrhotic livers, better prognosis

CYTOPATHOLOGY
- Well-differentiated carcinomas resemble hepatocytes but with larger nuclei, macronucleoli
  - Thick, disordered plates or balls of neoplastic cells, focally lined by sinusoidal endothelial cells (endothelial wrapping)
  - Large tissue fragments traversed by blood vessels (transgressing vessels)
  - May show presence of bile, Mallory-Denk bodies, hyaline inclusions, or fat in cytoplasm
- Poorly differentiated carcinomas show no resemblance to hepatocytes
  - Numerous dyshesive, bare nuclei in background
- Fibrolamellar variant neoplastic cells are larger with oncocytic cytoplasm and sometimes fragments of fibrous stroma in background

ANCILLARY TESTS
- Positive for Hep-Par1, glypican-3, arginase-1, glutamine synthetase, CAM5.2 (keratins 8 and 18), and monoclonal CEA with canalicular pattern
- *DNAJB1::PRKACA* fusion reported as specific recurrent abnormality in fibrolamellar subtype

TOP DIFFERENTIAL DIAGNOSES
- Cholangiocarcinoma
- Metastatic adenocarcinoma
- Benign hepatic lesions

Well-Differentiated Hepatocellular Carcinoma

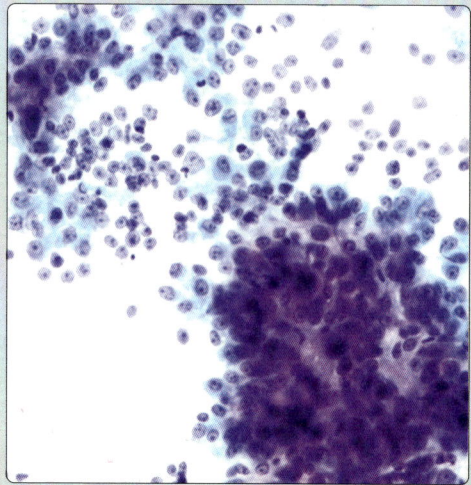

Moderately Differentiated Hepatocellular Carcinoma

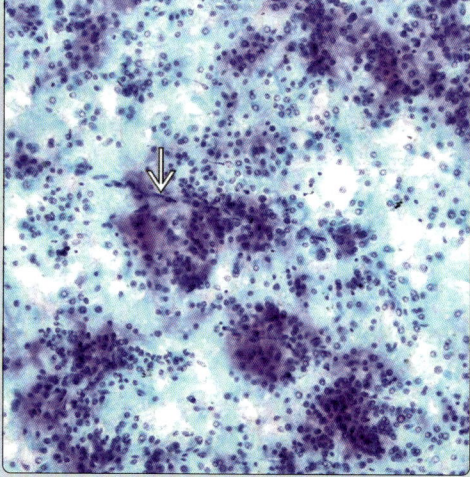

(Left) Pap stain shows hepatocytes with enlarged, irregular nuclei, prominent nucleoli, and increased nuclear:cytoplasmic ratio. (Right) Pap stain shows sheets and singly dispersed malignant hepatocytes with a transgressing vessel ➡.

Poorly Differentiated Hepatocellular Carcinoma

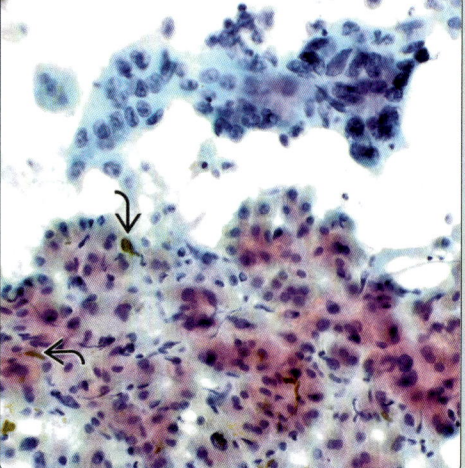

Thickened Cell Plates of Hepatocellular Carcinoma

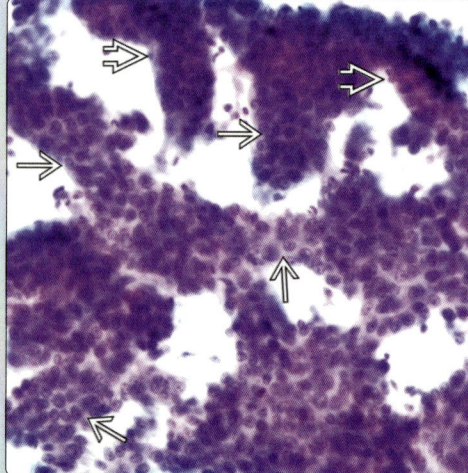

(Left) Pap stain shows malignant hepatocytes with pleomorphic nuclei and intracytoplasmic bile ➡. (Right) Pap stain shows thickened trabeculae (> 3 cells) ➡ of malignant hepatocytes lined by endothelial cells ➡.

Hepatocellular Carcinoma

TERMINOLOGY

Abbreviations
- Hepatocellular carcinoma (HCC)

ETIOLOGY/PATHOGENESIS

Environmental Exposure
- Aflatoxin B1 is major cause in China/southern Africa
- Alcoholic cirrhosis is major cause in West
- Anabolic steroids, Thorotrast, oral contraceptives, smoking

Infectious Agents
- Chronic viral hepatitis (hepatitis B and hepatitis C)

Metabolic Disorders
- Hemochromatosis, tyrosinemia, hypercitrullinemia, α-1-antitrypsin deficiency, fructosemia

Cirrhosis
- 70-90% arise in cirrhosis

CLINICAL ISSUES

Epidemiology
- Incidence
  - Varies widely depending on geography in parallel with prevalence of hepatitis B and C and aflatoxin exposure
    - East Asia and southern Africa have highest incidence worldwide (up to 150 per 100,000)
    - In USA, annual incidence ~ 4 per 100,000
- Age
  - Older age in West, more common in men
- Fibrolamellar variant
  - 5% of HCC arises in younger patients (usually < 35 years) in noncirrhotic livers

CYTOPATHOLOGY

Cells
- Well-differentiated carcinomas resemble hepatocytes but with larger nuclei, macronucleoli, and absent bile ducts
- Poorly differentiated carcinomas show no resemblance to hepatocytes
  - Numerous dyshesive, bare nuclei in background
- Thick, disordered plates or balls of neoplastic cells, focally lined by sinusoidal endothelial cells (endothelial wrapping)
- Large tissue fragments traversed by blood vessels (transgressing vessels)
- May show presence of bile, Mallory-Denk bodies, hyaline inclusions, or fat in cytoplasm
- Fibrolamellar variant has neoplastic cells that are larger with oncocytic cytoplasm
  - Background fragments of fibrous stroma may be seen

ANCILLARY TESTS

Immunohistochemistry
- Positive for Hep-Par1, glypican-3, arginase-1, glutamine synthetase, and CAM5.2 (keratins 8 and 18)
- AFP staining highly specific but insensitive (25%)
- Polyclonal CEA and CD10 demonstrate canalicular pattern
- Sinusoidal capillarization demonstrated with CD34

DIFFERENTIAL DIAGNOSIS

Cholangiocarcinoma
- Mucicarmine (+); expresses CK7, CK19, and CA19-9

Metastatic Adenocarcinoma
- Hep-Par1 and arginase-1 (-); MOC-31(+)

Benign Hepatic Lesions
- Hepatic cords 2-3 cells in thickness
- No "transgressing vessels"
- Glypican-3(-)

SELECTED REFERENCES

1. Zhang L et al: Fine needle biopsy of malignant tumors of the liver: a retrospective study of 624 cases from a single institution experience. Diagn Pathol. 15(1):43, 2020
2. El Jabbour T et al: Update on hepatocellular carcinoma: pathologists' review. World J Gastroenterol. 25(14):1653-65, 2019
3. WHO Classification of Tumours Editorial Board. Digestive System Tumors: WHO Classification of Tumours, 5th Edition. IARC Press. 2019

Fibrolamellar Variant of Hepatocellular Carcinoma

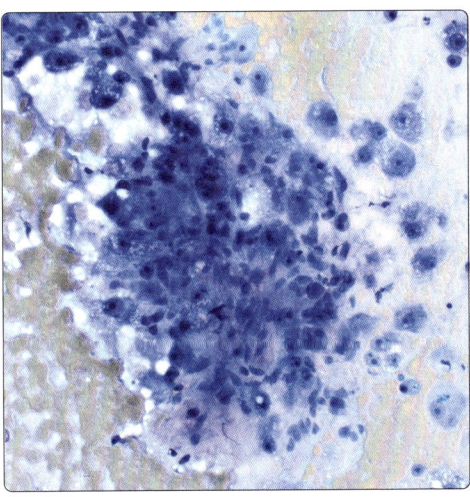

Fibrolamellar Variant of Hepatocellular Carcinoma

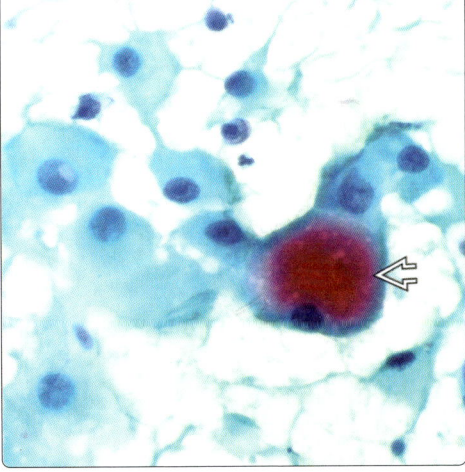

(Left) Diff-Quik stain shows fibrous stroma admixed with malignant hepatocytes with large, prominent nucleoli and abundant granular cytoplasm. (Right) Pap stain shows malignant hepatocytes with abundant granular cytoplasm and hyaline inclusion bodies ⇨.

Hepatoblastoma

KEY FACTS

TERMINOLOGY
- Predominantly pediatric liver tumor that mimics developing fetal or embryonal liver histologically

CLINICAL ISSUES
- Most common malignant liver neoplasm in children
- Typically presents with abdominal mass
- Serum α-fetoprotein is markedly elevated in 90% of cases
- Key prognostic factor of survival is tumor stage
- Is 2.1% of all pediatric cancers in patients 1-19 years old
- 88% in children ≤ 5 years and 3% > 15 years
- Mean age at diagnosis: 19 months; M:F = 3:2

CYTOPATHOLOGY
- Hepatoblastoma (HB) may be composed of different cell types
- Fetal epithelial cells are smaller than normal hepatocytes
- Embryonal cells: Primitive cells in sheets, pseudorosettes, acini, or tubules
- Small cell, mesenchymal cell patterns

ANCILLARY TESTS
- Nuclear β-catenin staining in epithelial and mesenchymal components (70% of HB)
- Positive glypican-3 and Hep-Par1 staining in fetal and embryonal epithelial cells
- Positive glutamine synthetase staining in fetal and variably in embryonal cells

TOP DIFFERENTIAL DIAGNOSES
- Normal liver parenchyma
  - Positive nuclear &/or cytoplasmic β-catenin staining in HB
- Hepatocellular carcinoma
  - Unusual in pediatric age group
- Other small blue cell tumors
  - History, immunocytochemistry, and molecular testing needed to differentiate from other pediatric tumors with similar morphology

Hepatoblastoma Rosette

Hepatoblastoma, Fetal Type

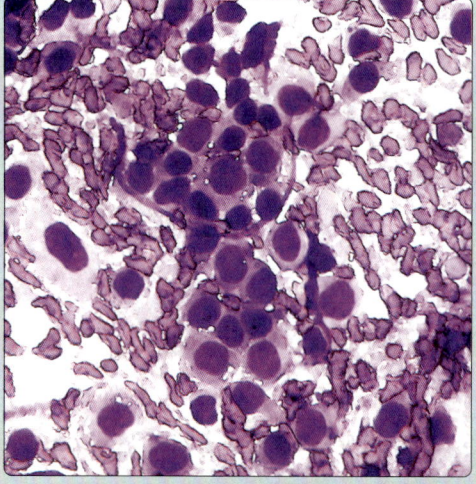

(Left) This Diff-Quik smear shows immature small blue cells with oval nuclei and scant cytoplasm forming a rosette-like structure. (Courtesy M. Feingold, MD.) (Right) These fetal-type cells on Diff-Quik are smaller than nonneoplastic hepatocytes and have round nuclei and inconspicuous nucleoli. (Courtesy N. Quintanilla, MD.)

Hepatoblastoma With Elongated Nuclei

Hepatoblastoma Histology

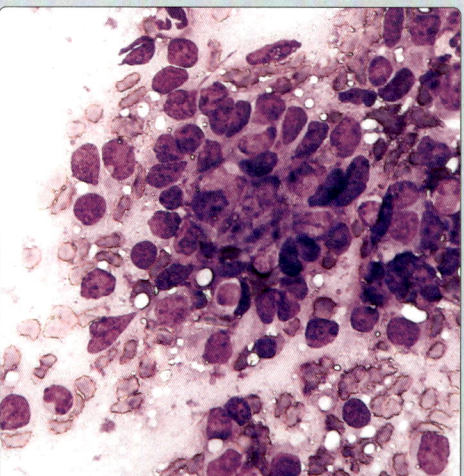
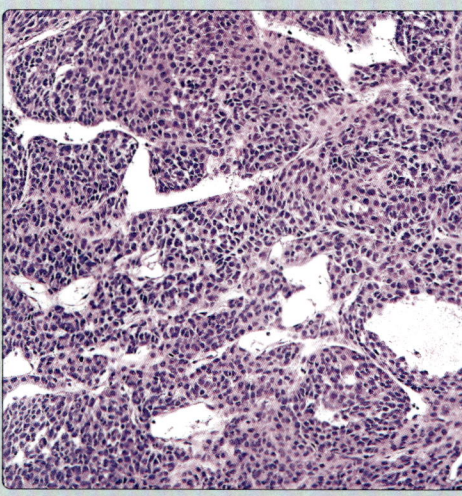

(Left) This is another Diff-Quik stain of a hepatoblastoma. The nuclei are more elongated in this example. (Courtesy N. Quintanilla, MD.) (Right) Macrotrabecular hepatoblastoma, as seen in this H&E-stained tissue section, superficially resembles a hepatocellular carcinoma. (Courtesy N. Quintanilla, MD.)

Hepatoblastoma

CLINICAL ISSUES

Laboratory Tests
- Increased serum α-fetoprotein in 75-96% of patients
  - Often ≥ 100,000 ng/mL
    - Caveat: Neonates < 6 months of age normally have elevated α-fetoprotein
  - Useful marker of response to therapy and recurrence

Conditions Associated With Hepatoblastoma
- Familial adenomatous polyposis, Beckwith-Wiedemann, Li-Fraumeni, and Simpson-Golabi-Behmel syndromes, trisomy 18, glycogen storage disease types I-IV, and hemihypertrophy

CYTOPATHOLOGY

Cells
- Hepatoblastoma (HB) may be composed of different cell types
- Fetal cells
  - Uniform cells arranged in slender cords (2-3 cells thick) and thin trabeculae
  - Fetal epithelial cells are smaller than normal hepatocytes
  - Central round to oval nuclei, inconspicuous nucleolus, and abundant clear to pink cytoplasm with distinct membrane
- Embryonal
  - Primitive cells in sheets, pseudorosettes, acini, or tubules
  - Small, angulated nuclei (larger than fetal nuclei) with coarse nuclear chromatin, prominent nucleoli, scant cytoplasm, indistinct membranes
  - Mitotic figures are more frequent
- Small cell
  - Resembles neuroblast, blastemal cells, or cells found in small round blue cell neoplasms
  - High nuclear:cytoplasmic ratio with almost no cytoplasm, hyperchromatic nuclei, inconspicuous nucleoli
- Mesenchymal
  - Primitive mesenchymal cells (immature spindle cells) with scant cytoplasm and elongated, plump nuclei
  - High cellularity
  - Osteoid-like areas, cartilage, more rarely other elements

MACROSCOPIC

Size
- Large; can be > 15 cm

ANCILLARY TESTS

Immunohistochemistry
- Nuclear β-catenin staining in epithelial and mesenchymal components (70% of HB)
- Positive glypican-3 and Hep-Par1 staining in fetal and embryonal epithelial cells
- Positive glutamine synthetase staining in fetal cells and variably in embryonal cells
- INI1/BAF47 loss in some small undifferentiated cells, especially if rhabdoid phenotype
- SALL4 expressed in embryonal component and less in fetal component; high levels of expression may be associated with worse prognosis

DIFFERENTIAL DIAGNOSIS

Normal Liver Parenchyma
- Must distinguish fetal epithelial cells of HB from normal hepatocytes, particularly near margin
  - HB is nuclear &/or cytoplasmic β-catenin positive
  - Fetal cells are smaller than normal hepatocytes

Other Small Blue Cell Tumors
- History and immunocytochemistry are required

Hepatocellular Carcinoma
- Biphasic pattern with both fetal and embryonal cells points to HB
- Clinical picture is different and most helpful

SELECTED REFERENCES
1. Chen T et al: A comprehensive genomic analysis constructs miRNA-mRNA interaction network in hepatoblastoma. Front Cell Dev Biol. 9:655703, 2021

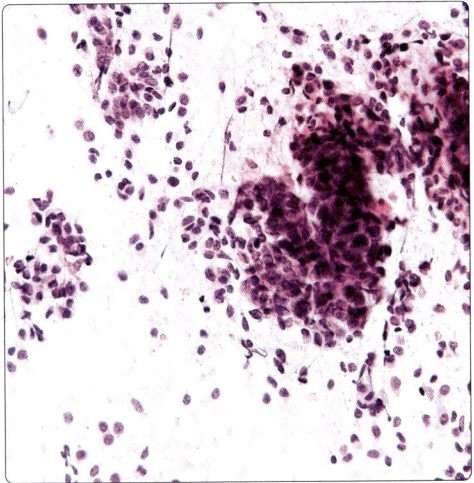

Hepatoblastoma, Embryonal Type

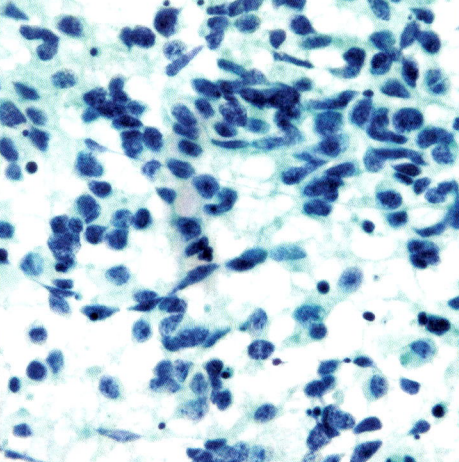

Hepatoblastoma, Small Blue Cells

(Left) H&E-stained smear of an embryonal hepatoblastoma shows elongated, hyperchromatic nuclei with scant associated cytoplasm. (Courtesy N. Quintanilla, MD.) *(Right)* Hepatoblastoma is in the differential of any small blue cell tumor of childhood, as seen in this Pap stain. If originating in the liver, the findings can be consistent with hepatoblastoma.

Liver Metastasis

KEY FACTS

CLINICAL ISSUES

- Most common liver malignancy
- Gastrointestinal, lung, breast, and genitourinary origins most common

CYTOPATHOLOGY

- Usually cellular smears, ± background necrosis
  - Carcinomas show cohesive cell pattern, whereas lymphomas, melanomas, and usually neuroendocrine tumors, are dyshesive
  - Hematopoietic neoplasms will usually show lymphoglandular bodies in background, indicating lymphoid nature of cells
- Large bowel primaries have hyperchromatic, elongated, cigar-shaped nuclei, necrosis, and are CK20(+), CK7(-), and CDX2(+)
- Prostate primaries usually show little nuclear pleomorphism but prominent nucleoli; PSA(+)
- Breast primaries may be quite bland and mimic neuroendocrine or lymphocytic neoplasms with eccentrically placed nuclei
- Metastatic gastrointestinal stromal tumor is most common liver metastasis to show spindle morphology; c-kit and DOG1 (+)
- Melanoma is great mimicker with variable morphology; S100, Melan-A, SOX10, HMB45 (+)
- Small cells with signet-ring morphology or intracytoplasmic mucin: Think stomach or breast

TOP DIFFERENTIAL DIAGNOSES

- Hepatocellular carcinoma
  - "Transgressing vessels," endothelial wrapping

DIAGNOSTIC CHECKLIST

- Correlate clinically and with imaging
- Molecular testing for unknown primary also available
- Metastatic adenocarcinoma vs. cholangiocarcinoma cannot be determined by cytomorphology alone

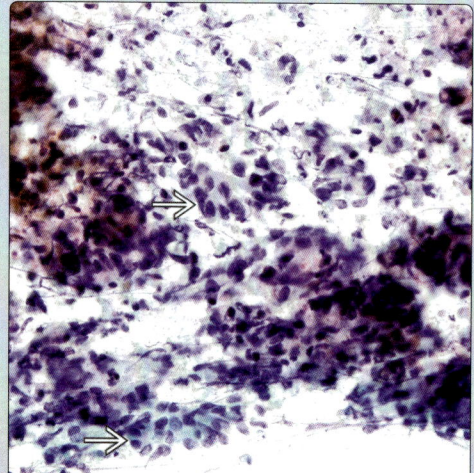

Metastatic Colonic Adenocarcinoma

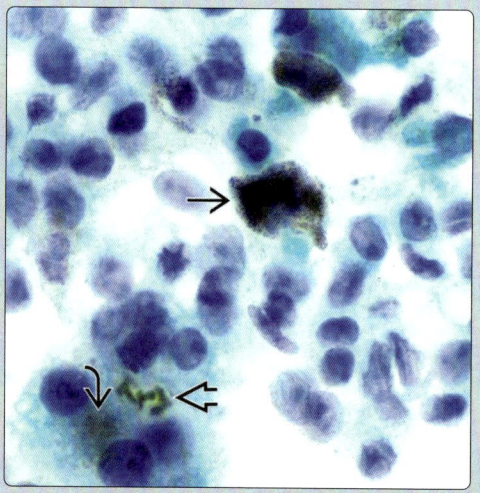

Metastatic Melanoma

(Left) This metastatic adenocarcinoma on Pap stain is suggestive of large bowel origin. Malignant epithelial cells ➡ show elongated hyperchromatic nuclei in a background of necrosis. **(Right)** *The melanin pigment of metastatic melanoma ➡ must be distinguished from lipofuscin ➡ and bile ➡, as seen in this Pap stain.*

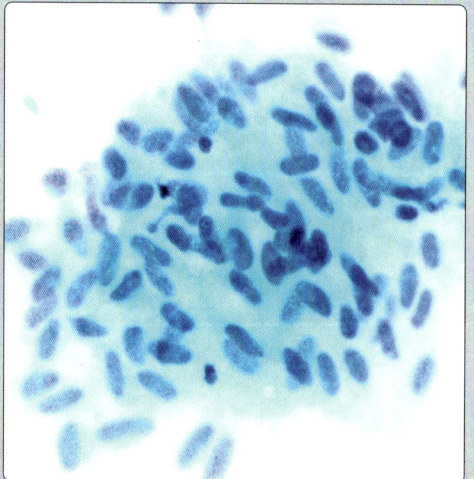

Metastatic Gastrointestinal Stromal Tumor

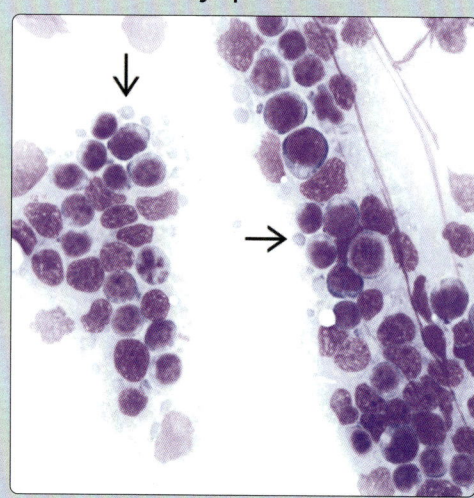

Lymphoma

(Left) Pap stain shows bland, elongated spindled nuclei in a metastatic gastrointestinal stromal tumor. **(Right)** *Lymphoglandular bodies ➡, seen on this Diff-Quik stain, are indicative of the presence of a lymphocytic population and, in the presence of dyshesive cells, strongly suggest a lymphoma.*

Liver Metastasis

CLINICAL ISSUES

Epidemiology
- Incidence
  - Most common liver malignancy
  - Gastrointestinal, lung, breast, and genitourinary origins are most common

CYTOPATHOLOGY

Cellularity
- Highly cellular smears

Pattern
- Carcinomas show cohesion, but neuroendocrine tumors can be quite dyshesive
- Lymphoma and melanoma are dyshesive

Nuclear Details
- Adenocarcinomas show vesicular nuclei with prominent nucleoli
  - Large bowel primaries have hyperchromatic, elongated, cigar-shaped nuclei, and background necrosis
  - Prostate primaries usually show little nuclear pleomorphism but prominent nucleoli
  - Breast primaries may be quite bland and mimic neuroendocrine or lymphocytic neoplasms with eccentrically placed nuclei
- Squamous cell carcinomas have hyperchromatic nuclei, often with sharp angulation
- Pancreas, lung, and urothelial carcinomas may show features of glandular and squamous differentiation
- Sarcomas have spindle morphology
  - Metastatic gastrointestinal stromal tumor (GIST) most common liver metastasis to show spindle morphology
- Melanoma is great mimicker
  - May be cohesive or dyshesive
  - May be epithelioid, plasmacytoid, lymphoid, or spindle-shaped
  - May be binucleated
  - May have prominent or no nucleoli
  - Have nuclear "holes"
  - Cytoplasmic pigment may be absent

Cytoplasmic Details
- If small cells with signet-ring morphology or intracytoplasmic mucin present, think stomach or breast

DIFFERENTIAL DIAGNOSIS

Hepatocellular Carcinoma
- "Transgressing vessels," endothelial wrapping
  - Other tumors, such as renal cell carcinomas and adrenal cortical carcinomas, can show association with vessels
- Intracytoplasmic bile or Mallory-Denk bodies indicative of hepatocellular origin
- Hep-Par1, arginase, and glypican-3 (+); MOC-31(-)

Adenocarcinoma
- MOC-31(+)
- Other markers based on suspicion; rule out unknown primary
  - Prostate: PSA, NKX3.1; lung, thyroid: TTF-1; breast: GATA3, mammaglobin, ER; gastrointestinal tract: CDX2

Lymphoma
- Obtain flow cytometry at time of adequacy check, lymphoma panel

Melanoma
- Melan-A, S100 (most sensitive but least specific), HMB-45, SOX-10

Sarcoma
- Cytokeratin negative
- C-kit (CD117), CD34, and DOG1 positive in GIST

SELECTED REFERENCES
1. Bellizzi AM: An algorithmic immunohistochemical approach to define tumor type and assign site of origin. Adv Anat Pathol. 27(3):114-63, 2020
2. Gan Q et al: Small but powerful: the promising role of small specimens for biomarker testing. J Am Soc Cytopathol. 9(5):450-60, 2020

Metastatic Renal Cell Carcinoma
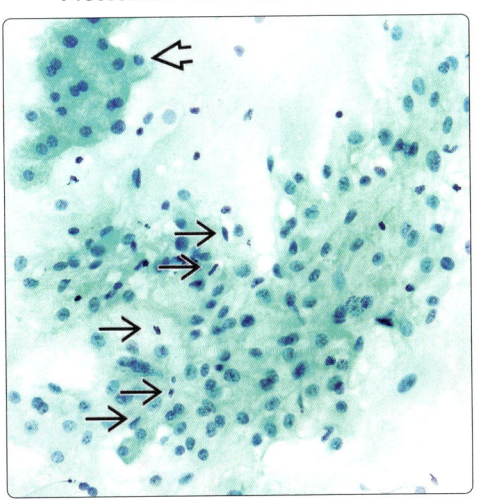

Metastatic Breast Carcinoma
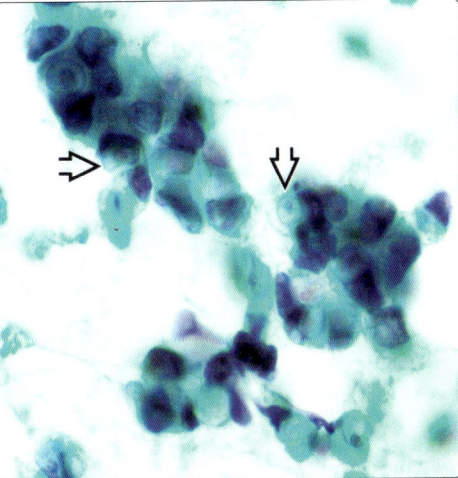

(Left) Hepatocellular carcinoma is not the only malignancy associated with endothelial cells ⇒. This Pap stain shows a metastatic renal cell carcinoma. Note hepatocytes in the background ⇒. **(Right)** Some metastatic adenocarcinomas, such as this breast primary on Pap stain, may show intracytoplasmic mucin ⇒. Stomach primaries can also show such features.

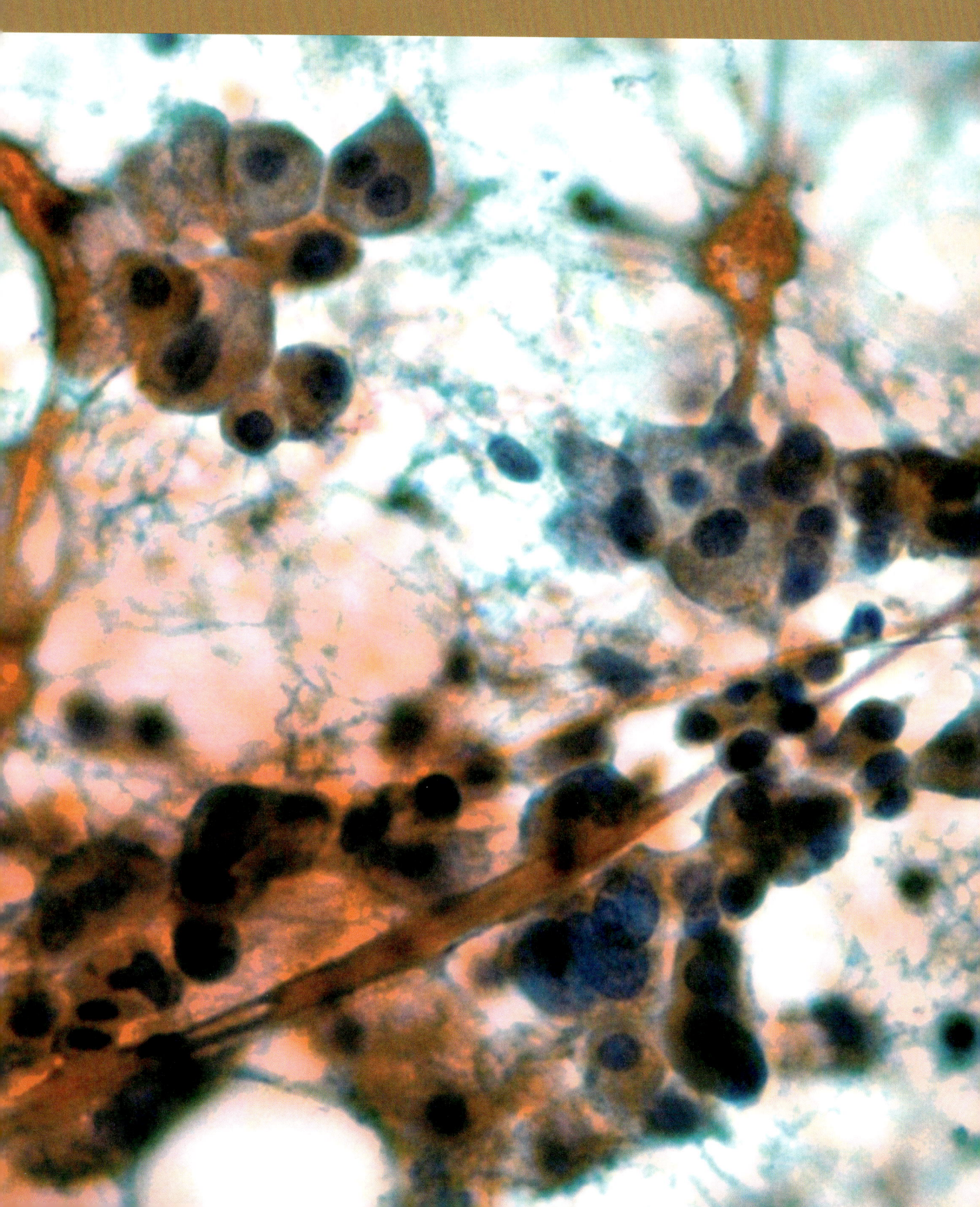

PART IV
SECTION 4
Kidney

Overview

Cytology of Normal Kidney	516

Benign Lesions and Neoplasms

Renal Cysts	518
Angiomyolipoma	520
Oncocytoma, Kidney	522
Metanephric Adenoma	524
Metanephric Stromal Tumor	526
Xanthogranulomatous Pyelonephritis/Malakoplakia	527

Malignant Neoplasms

Clear Cell Renal Cell Carcinoma	528
Papillary Renal Cell Carcinoma	532
Clear Cell Papillary Renal Cell Carcinoma	534
Chromophobe Renal Cell Carcinoma	536
TFE3- and *TFEB*-Rearranged Renal Cell Carcinomas	538
Collecting Duct Carcinoma	540
Renal Medullary Carcinoma	541
Mucinous Tubular and Spindle Cell Carcinoma of Kidney	542
Carcinoid Tumor	543
Primary Renal Sarcomas in Adults	544
Renal Lymphomas	545
Nephroblastoma (Wilms Tumor)	546
Clear Cell Sarcoma of Kidney	548
Congenital Mesoblastic Nephroma	550
Rhabdoid Tumor of Kidney	552
Metastatic Tumors to Kidney	553

Tumors of Renal Pelvis

Urothelial Carcinoma	554

Cytology of Normal Kidney

ANATOMIC FEATURES

Shape and Size
- Kidneys are paired, bean-shaped organs
- Surrounded by Gerota fascia and abdominal organs
- Each kidney weighs ~ 150 g and measures ~ 11 x 5 x 3 cm

ARCHITECTURAL ORGANIZATION

Cortex
- Consists of glomeruli, proximal tubules, distal tubules, and initial portions of collecting ducts

Medulla
- Composed of straight portions of proximal tubule, loops of Henle, and collecting ducts

Functional Unit
- Nephron is functional unit of kidney consisting of glomerulus and associated renal tubules

RENAL FNA

Clinical Indications
- Modern imaging technology is remarkably accurate for diagnosis of renal masses; however, renal FNA plays vital role in managing patients in certain circumstances
  - Confirming primary renal tumor in patients with inoperable disease
  - Suspicious for metastatic tumor or infection of kidney
  - When partial nephrectomy is considered (young patients, small lesion, poor renal function, or certain types of tumor)
  - Suspicious for urothelial carcinoma that may require ureterectomy
  - Lesions with equivocal radiology findings
  - Diagnosis for evacuated renal cysts

Accuracy of Diagnosis
- Accuracy of renal FNA in distinguishing benign and malignant lesions is 73-94%

Renal Tubular Cells and Glomerulus

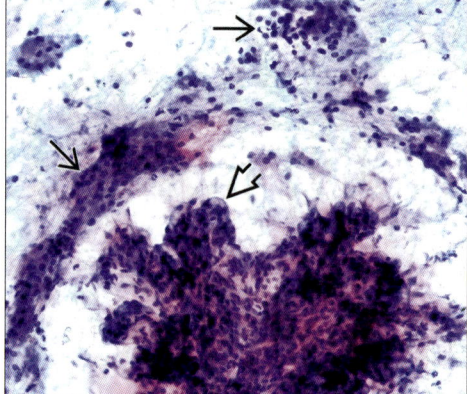

Distorted Renal Glomerulus

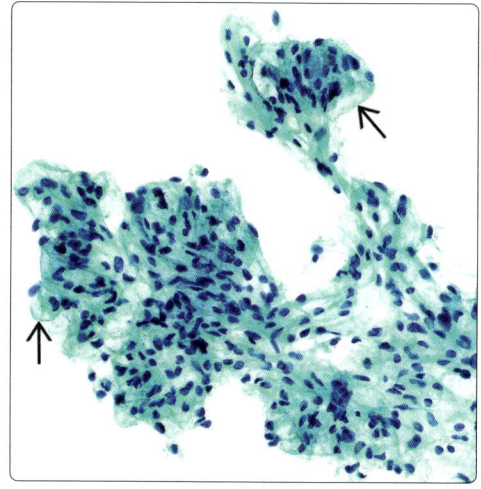

(Left) Aspiration of normal kidney shows normal renal tubular cells ⇨ and a renal glomerulus that appears as a densely cellular complex capillary network ⇨, as seen on this Pap stain. **(Right)** A smear-distorted renal glomerulus may simulate papillary lesions of the kidney. Identifying capillary loops around the edges ⇨ is helpful for the distinction, as seen in this Pap stain.

Proximal Tubular Cells

Cells of Distal Tubules and Loops of Henle

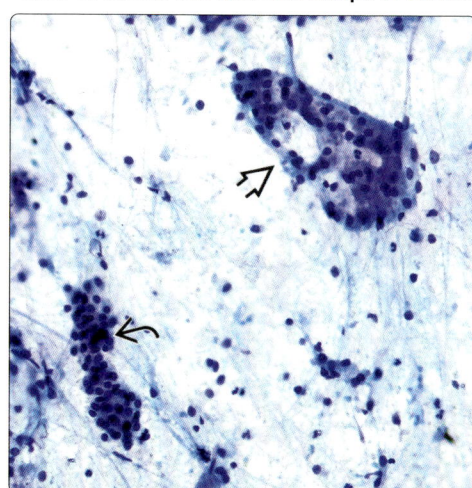

(Left) Proximal tubular cells are arranged in small flat sheets or isolated cells with uniform central nuclei and abundant granular cytoplasm ⇨ (Pap stain). **(Right)** Cells of distal tubules and loops of Henle are in small sheets ⇨ or tubular segments ⇨ with scant, dense cytoplasm and small nuclei, as seen in this Pap stain.

Cytology of Normal Kidney

- Diagnostic sensitivity of 86% and specificity of 98% reported for malignant tumors
- Common causes of false-negative diagnoses: Insufficient cells in cystic tumors, small tumors, or extensive necrosis
- False-positive diagnoses reported in angiomyolipoma, inflammatory lesions, regenerative atypia, and infarct
- Nondiagnostic rates up to 30% have been reported

Specimen Collection and Preparation
- Procedure
  - Renal FNA or cores are commonly performed by radiologists under image guidance to ensure adequate sampling
- Cytology preparation
  - Simultaneous air-dried (for Diff-Quik stain) and wet-fixed (for Pap stain) preparations are recommended
  - Diff-Quik stain may provide valuable diagnostic features that complement those identified on Pap stain
  - Intraprocedure adequacy check is essential to ensure adequate diagnostic material
  - When feasible, cell block should be obtained in case ancillary tests are needed

Complications and Contraindications
- Subcapsular hematoma rate up to 40% has been reported
- Anticoagulation medication (such as aspirin) should be discontinued 7-10 days before procedure

CYTOLOGY

Cellularity
- Usually low to moderate cellularity

Pattern
- Small flat sheets of tubular cells from various levels
- Densely cellular glomeruli may be seen

Background
- Stripped round nuclei of tubular cells
- No necrosis or hemorrhage

Cells
- Renal tubular cells
  - Proximal convoluted tubular cells are arranged in small, flat sheets, tubules, or single cells
  - Cells of distal convoluted tubules and loops of Henle are arranged in tubules or small sheets with less voluminous cytoplasm
- Glomeruli appear as compact, rounded, cellular structures with complex network of capillaries

Nuclear Details
- Renal tubular cells have uniform, small, round, central nuclei with indistinct small nucleoli
- Glomeruli consist of evenly distributed endothelial and mesangial cells with elongated or oval nuclei

Cytoplasmic Details
- Proximal convoluted tubular cells have abundant granular cytoplasm with irregular, torn cell borders
- Cells of distal convoluted tubules and loops of Henle have scant, dense cytoplasm with occasional cytoplasmic pigment (probably lipofuscin)

ANCILLARY STUDIES

Immunohistochemistry
- Proximal tubular cells: AE1/AE3(+), CD10(+), RCC(+), PAX2(+), PAX8(+), Ksp-cadherin [(-) or focal (+)]
- Distal tubular cells: AE1/AE3(+), CD10(-), RCC(-), PAX2(+), PAX8(+), Ksp-cadherin (+)

Flow Cytometry
- Essential for diagnosing and phenotyping non-Hodgkin lymphomas

Cytogenetic and Molecular Tests
- Helpful in diagnosis of familial renal cancers and differential diagnosis of certain types of renal malignancy

DIFFERENTIAL DIAGNOSIS

Oncocytoma and Chromophobe Renal Cell Carcinoma
- Cells mimic proximal tubular cells with granular cytoplasm
- Tumors have high cellularity, binucleation or variation of nuclear size, and well-defined cell borders
- Chromophobe renal cell carcinoma has significant nuclear atypia

Low-Grade Clear Cell Renal Cell Carcinoma
- Cells mimic proximal tubular cells or adrenal cortical cells
- Hypercellular aspirate, larger sheets of tumor cells, nuclear atypia, and tortuous vasculature

Papillary Renal Cell Carcinoma
- Tumor cells are often low grade and may mimic distal tubular cells or distorted glomeruli
- Mild nuclear atypia with foamy macrophages
- No capillary loops, as seen in peripheral of distorted glomeruli

Other Misinterpretations of Benign Elements
- Distorted glomeruli may resemble vascular tumors or granuloma
- Inadvertently sampled adrenal cortical cells or hepatocytes may be misinterpreted as tumor cells
- Normal cells from other abdominal organs as well as benign mesothelial cells may also be sampled

SELECTED REFERENCES

1. Chen HI et al: Accuracy of subclassification and grading of renal tumors on fine needle aspiration cytology alone. Acta Cytol. 65(2):140-9, 2021
2. Trpkov K et al: New developments in existing WHO entities and evolving molecular concepts: the Genitourinary Pathology Society (GUPS) update on renal neoplasia. Mod Pathol. 34(7):1392-424, 2021
3. Bazaga S et al: Endoscopic ultrasound-guided fine-needle aspiration of renal lesions: experience in a tertiary center. Rev Esp Enferm Dig. 112(11):838-42, 2020
4. Gupta R et al: Pediatric fine-needle aspiration cytology: an audit of 266 cases of pediatric tumors with cytologic-histologic correlation. Cytojournal. 17:25, 2020
5. Ponce-Zepeda J et al: Touch preparation for rapid onsite evaluations of renal mass biopsies: concordance rate, pearls, and pitfalls. J Am Soc Cytopathol. 9(5):422-8, 2020
6. Lau HD et al: Evaluation of diagnostic accuracy and a practical algorithmic approach for the diagnosis of renal masses by FNA. Cancer Cytopathol. 126(9):782-96, 2018
7. Perrino CM et al: World Health Organization (WHO)/International Society of Urological Pathology (ISUP) grading in fine-needle aspiration biopsies of renal masses. Diagn Cytopathol. 46(11):895-900, 2018

Renal Cysts

KEY FACTS

CLINICAL ISSUES
- Common (in 50% of people > 50 years old)
- May represent benign and neoplastic lesions
- Radiology Bosniak classification: Categories 1 and 2 (benign), 2F and 3 (indeterminate), and 4 (malignant)

CYTOPATHOLOGY
- FNA often performed on cysts of indeterminate categories 2F (F for follow-up needed) and 3
- Usually hypocellular aspirate
- Macrophages, degenerated cells, Liesegang rings (lamellated concretions)
- Specific cytology features depend on underlying lesion

TOP DIFFERENTIAL DIAGNOSES
- Simple cyst
  - Unilocular, thin-walled cyst with isolated or small, flat sheets of bland lining cells and macrophages
- Cystic renal cell carcinoma (RCC)
  - Often multilocular thick-walled cysts with cytologic and immunohistochemical features of RCC
- Cystic partially differentiated nephroblastoma
  - Multilocular cysts in children with polygonal lining cells and diagnostic blastemal cells [WT1(+)/cytokeratin (-)]
- Cystic nephroma
  - Benign multicystic tumor with rare polygonal epithelial cells and clean background

DIAGNOSTIC CHECKLIST
- Correlation with imaging findings is critical
- Interpretation of atypical cells in categories 1 and 2 cysts should be conservative
- Suspicious for malignancy is used for atypical cells mainly in indeterminate cysts (categories 2F and 3)
- FNA has low sensitivity and low negative predictive value for category 2F and 3 cysts
- Possibility of unsampled tumor should be considered for macrophage-only specimens

Bland Cyst-Lining Cells in Benign Renal Cyst
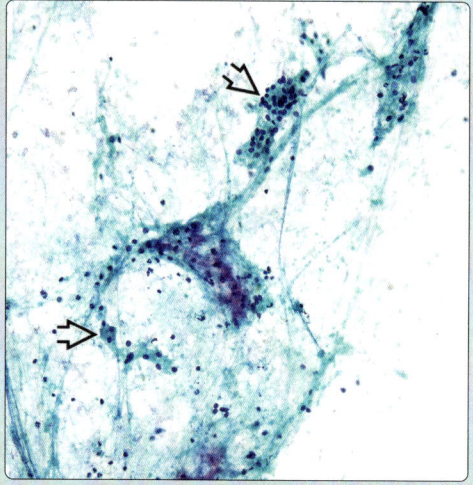

Macrophages in Benign Renal Cyst
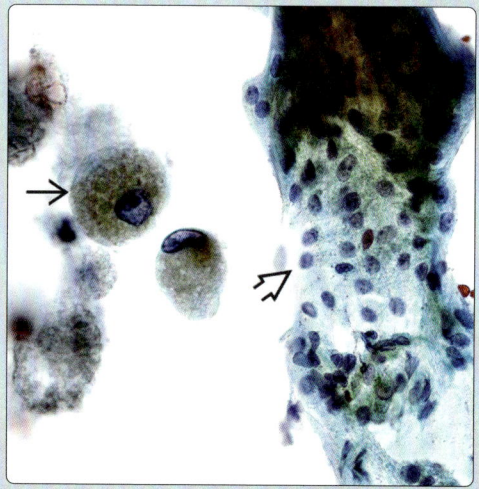

(Left) Pap stain of aspirate from a benign renal cyst shows small monolayer clusters of bland cyst-lining cells/renal tubular cells ⇨ in a background of degenerated cells and debris. (Right) High magnification of Pap stain on a benign renal cyst shows macrophages ⇨ and benign tubular epithelium ⇨. (Courtesy V. Schnadig, MD.)

Histology of Multilocular Cystic Renal Cell Carcinoma
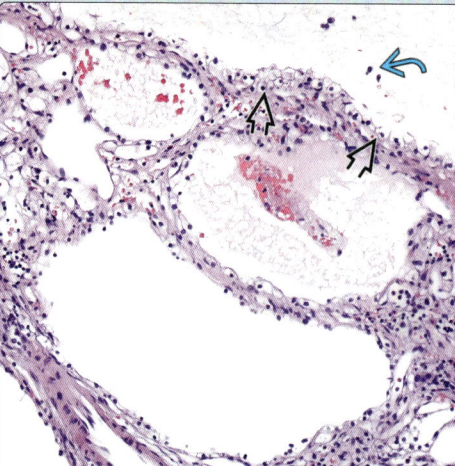

Tumor Cells in Multilocular Cystic Renal Cell Carcinoma
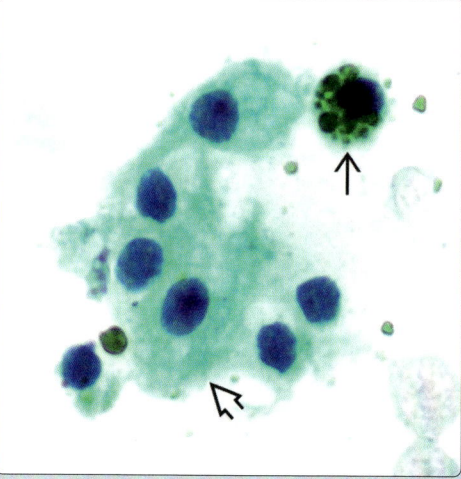

(Left) H&E stain of a multilocular cystic renal cell carcinoma shows cystic spaces lined by low-grade clear cells ⇨ with a few intracystic floating tumor cells ⇨. (Right) The tumor cells in multilocular cystic renal cell carcinoma demonstrate abundant vacuolated or clear cytoplasm ⇨ and occasional nucleoli on Pap stain. A hemosiderin-laden macrophage ⇨ is seen.

Renal Cysts

CLINICAL ISSUES

Epidemiology
- Incidence
  - Renal cysts are common and include benign and neoplastic lesions from simple cyst to cystic renal cell carcinoma (RCC)
  - Occur in 50% of people > 50 years
  - ~ 70-85% of renal lesions are cystic

IMAGING

Bosniak Classification System
- Categories 1 and 2 (benign)
  - Most common
  - FNA is not required, though fluid is sometimes sent to cytology lab
- Categories 2F and 3 (indeterminate)
  - 5% (2F) to 57% (3) found to be malignant
  - Evaluation is required, often FNA
- Category 4 (malignant)
  - Managed surgically
  - FNA is not required

CYTOPATHOLOGY

Cellularity
- Usually hypocellular

Background
- Degenerated cells, inflammatory cells (infected cysts), reactive stromal cells, and crystals may be seen

Common Cytologic Features
- Macrophages are most commonly seen; may mimic tumor by forming clusters with cytologic atypia
- Benign renal tubular cells may be present
- Liesegang rings (lamellated concretions) are often seen in chronic cystic lesions

Specific Cytologic Features
- Vary among specific lesions

DIFFERENTIAL DIAGNOSIS

Simple Cyst
- Most common and typical category 1 cyst: Unilocular, thin wall and no mural nodule or intracystic density
- Cyst wall cells: Isolated or small, flat sheets (< 10 cells) of bland cells with variable cytoplasm
- Macrophages (can be atypical) and Liesegang rings

Cystic Renal Cell Carcinoma
- ~ 15% of RCCs are predominantly cystic
- Histology types: Multilocular cystic RCC (low-grade ccRCC), unilocular (often papillary RCC), acquired cystic kidney disease-associated RCC, and necrotic RCC (often ccRCC)
- Imaging often shows multilocular cysts, thick/calcified wall, mural nodules, or dense intracystic content
- Cytology and immunohistochemistry features of RCC
- Obtaining diagnostic cells in cystic RCC is challenging

Cystic Partially Differentiated Nephroblastoma
- Children (< 2 years) with multilocular cystic tumor
- Cyst lining epithelial cells: Polygonal cells with variable cytoplasm and mildly atypical nuclei
- Blastemal cells: Isolated or loose clusters of hyperchromatic cells with scant cytoplasm (diagnostic feature)
- Blastemal and epithelial cells: WT1(+), PAX8(+), CD56(+)

Cystic Nephroma
- Rare benign multicystic tumor, mainly in females
- Hypocellular aspirate containing few polygonal epithelial cells with variable cytoplasm (ample, granular, or clear) and nuclear enlargement, irregular contours, or hyperchromasia
- Cystic background without necrosis or inflammation

SELECTED REFERENCES

1. Schieda N et al: Bosniak classification of cystic renal masses, version 2019: a pictorial guide to clinical use. Radiographics. 41(3):814-88, 2021
2. Sigmon DF et al: Renal Cyst. StatPearls, 2021
3. Matoso A et al: Atypical renal cysts: a morphologic, immunohistochemical, and molecular study. Am J Surg Pathol. 40(2):202-11, 2016
4. Ellimoottil C et al: New modalities for evaluation and surveillance of complex renal cysts. J Urol. 192(6):1604-11, 2014

Cystic Chromophobe Renal Cell Carcinoma

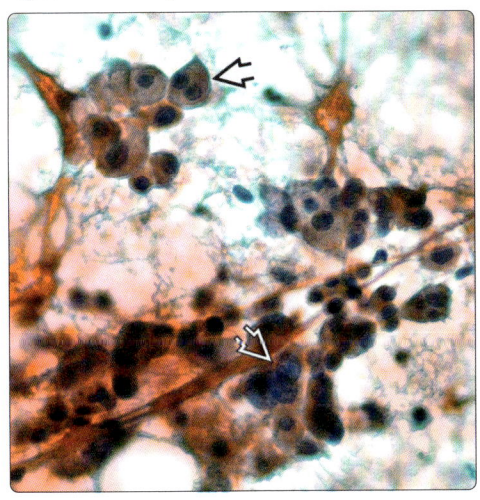

Cystic Papillary Renal Cell Carcinoma

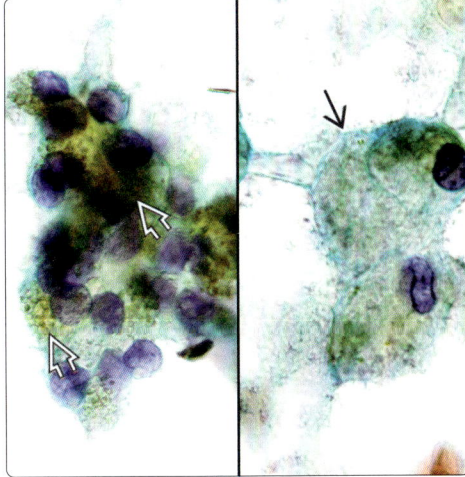

(Left) Pap stain of cystic chromophobe renal cell carcinoma shows sharp cell borders ⇨, anisonucleosis, and irregular nuclear membranes ⇨. *(Courtesy S. Lai, MD.)* *(Right)* Pap stain of cystic papillary renal cell carcinoma shows clusters of bland epithelial cells with intracytoplasmic hemosiderin ⇨ and foamy macrophages ⇨. *(Courtesy V. Schnadig, MD.)*

Angiomyolipoma

KEY FACTS

TERMINOLOGY
- Mesenchymal tumor believed to originate from perivascular epithelioid cells

CLINICAL ISSUES
- Associated with tuberous sclerosis (~ 50%, often multifocal/bilateral) or sporadic (often solitary)
- Often asymptomatic with incidental finding of renal mass with intratumoral fat on CT
- Majority with benign clinical behavior

CYTOPATHOLOGY
- Syncytial tissue fragments with bloody background
- Bland spindle cells admixed with fat droplets
- Blood vessels rarely seen
- Epithelioid variant: Round pleomorphic cells
- Triphasic elements on cell block: Fat, smooth muscle, and thick hyalinized vessels

MACROSCOPIC
- Well-circumscribed mass (mean size: 6 cm)

MICROSCOPIC
- Triphasic tumor: Adipose tissue, smooth muscle, and dystrophic vessels in variable proportions

ANCILLARY TESTS
- Immunohistochemistry: Expresses melanocytic and smooth muscle markers: HMB-45(+), Melan-A (+), and SMA(+)

TOP DIFFERENTIAL DIAGNOSES
- Retroperitoneal low-grade liposarcoma
  - Extrarenal tumor, lack of dysmorphic vessels, HMB-45(-)
- Clear cell renal cell carcinoma (RCC)
  - Vacuolated or granular cytoplasm, HMB-45(-)
- Sarcomatoid RCC or primary renal sarcomas
  - Marked atypia, lack of triphasic elements, HMB-45(-)

Classic Triphasic Tumor Elements of Angiomyolipoma
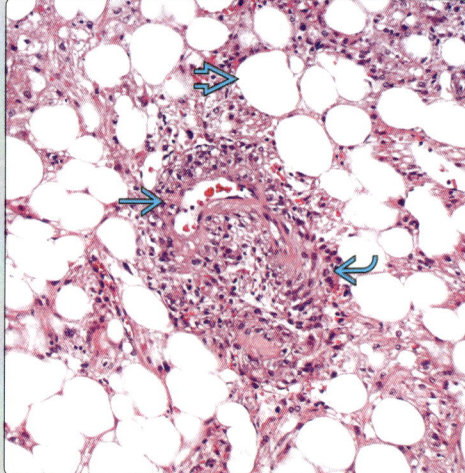

FNA Cytology With Triphasic Elements
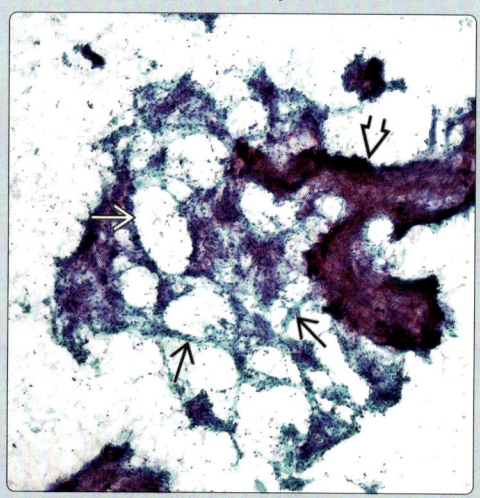

(Left) Typical H&E-stained histology of angiomyolipoma (AML) includes mature fat ➡, thick blood vessels ➡, and perivascular proliferation of smooth muscle ➡. **(Right)** Pap stain of AML aspirate shows a triphasic tumor consisting of thick hyalinized vessels ➡, adipose tissue ➡, and smooth muscle cells ➡.

Bland Syncytial Smooth Muscle Cells
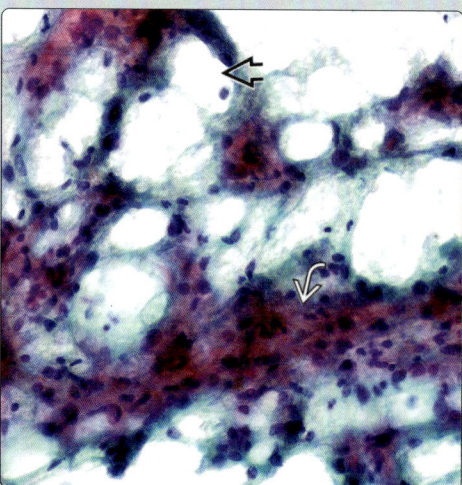

Epithelioid Angiomyolipoma
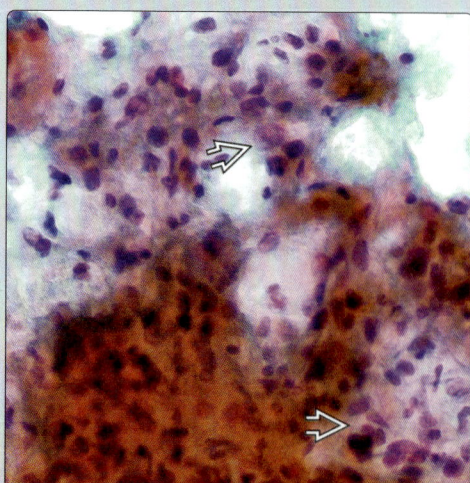

(Left) High magnification shows syncytial smooth muscle cells with bland oval to spindled nuclei, abundant eosinophilic cytoplasm ➡, and intimate association with mature fat ➡. No necrosis or mitotic activity is seen. **(Right)** Pap stain of epithelioid AML displays round tumor cells with abundant cytoplasm, pleomorphism, and prominent nucleoli ➡.

Angiomyolipoma

TERMINOLOGY

Abbreviations
- Angiomyolipoma (AML)

Definitions
- Mesenchymal tumor believed to originate from perivascular epithelioid cells (PEC)

ETIOLOGY/PATHOGENESIS

Genetic and Clinical Features
- Tuberous sclerosis complex (~ 50%): Median age: 25 years; often multifocal/bilateral; larger tumors that grow faster; alterations in *TSC1* (9q34) and *TSC2* (16p13.3)
- Sporadic cases (~ 50%): Often in women; median age: 45 years; solitary tumor; more with *TSC2* alterations

CLINICAL ISSUES

Presentation
- Often asymptomatic with incidental finding of renal mass with intratumoral fat on CT

Prognosis
- Overwhelming majority with benign clinical behavior

CYTOPATHOLOGY

Cellularity
- Usually hypocellular

Pattern
- Syncytial tissue fragments

Background
- Blood and fat droplets

Cells
- Spindle cells with fat droplets; vessels rarely seen
- Epithelioid variant: Round cells, abundant cytoplasm, pleomorphism, macronucleoli (mimic ganglion cells)

Nuclear Details
- Usually bland, round to spindle nuclei with truncated ends; mitoses uncommon

Cell Block Findings
- Triphasic elements: Fat, smooth muscle, and thick vessels

MACROSCOPIC

Key Findings
- Often well-circumscribed mass (mean: 6 cm)

MICROSCOPIC

Histologic Features
- Typically contains adipose tissue, smooth muscle, and dystrophic vessels in variable proportions

ANCILLARY TESTS

Immunohistochemistry
- Expresses melanocytic and smooth muscle markers: HMB-45, Melan-A (+), MITF, tyrosinase, SMA

DIFFERENTIAL DIAGNOSIS

Retroperitoneal Low-Grade Liposarcoma
- No dysmorphic vessels or smooth muscle, HMB-45(-)

Sarcomatoid Renal Cell Carcinoma
- Marked atypia, no triphasic elements, HMB-45(-)

Clear Cell Renal Cell Carcinoma
- Mimics epithelioid AML, vacuolated cytoplasm, HMB-45(-)

SELECTED REFERENCES
1. Anthony ML et al: Diagnostic pitfall of a rare variant of angiomyolipoma, epithelioid angiomyolipoma - a case report. Pan Afr Med J. 37:210, 2020
2. Boudaouara O et al: Renal angiomyolipoma: clinico-pathologic study of 17 cases with emphasis on the epithelioid histology and p53 gene abnormalities. Ann Diagn Pathol. 47:151538, 2020
3. Zhou H et al: Challenge of FNA diagnosis of angiomyolipoma: a study of 33 cases. Cancer. 125(4):257-66, 2017

Radiologic Features of Angiomyolipoma

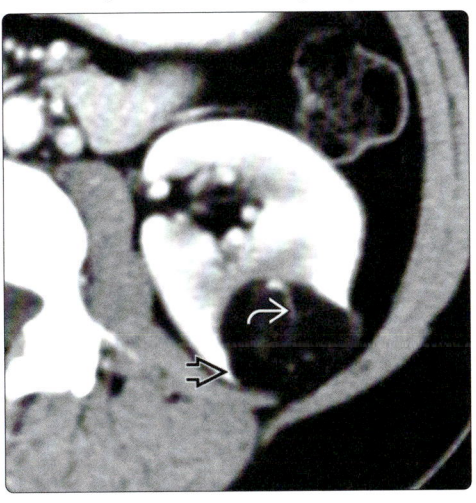

Gross Features of Angiomyolipoma

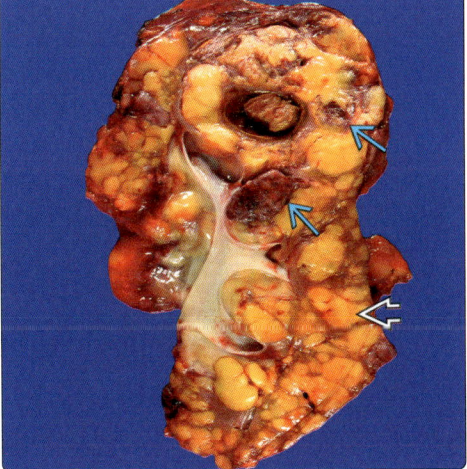

(Left) Axial CECT shows diagnostic features of angiomyolipoma: A spherical renal mass ➡ with a large fat component and prominent vessels ➡. (Courtesy M. Federle, MD.) **(Right)** *Variegated gross appearance of angiomyolipoma reflects fat ➡ and vessels with surrounding smooth muscle ➡.*

Oncocytoma, Kidney

KEY FACTS

CLASSIFICATION
- Benign neoplasm of kidney composed of cells with mitochondria-rich eosinophilic cytoplasm

CLINICAL ISSUES
- Majority are asymptomatic
- Few with hematuria, flank pain, or dysuria

CYTOPATHOLOGY
- Hypercellular aspirate with granular background
- Loosely cohesive clusters and isolated cells with distinct cytoplasmic membranes
- Abundant granular cytoplasm and uniform round nuclei
- Absent or scant mitoses
- Cell block: Rounded nests of uniform eosinophilic cells

MACROSCOPIC
- Circumscribed mahogany brown mass (mean: 4.4 cm) with central stellate scar, often unifocal

MICROSCOPIC
- Nests of uniform cells with eosinophilic, granular cytoplasm and loose reticular stroma

ANCILLARY TESTS
- Immunohistochemistry: AE1/AE3(+), PAX(+), CD117(+), vimentin (-), RCC(-), CK7(-)/focal (+)

TOP DIFFERENTIAL DIAGNOSES
- Inadvertent sampling of liver
  - Occurs in right kidney FNA, more nuclear variation, lipofuscin granules
  - Arginase-1 (+), PAX(-)
- Chromophobe renal cell carcinoma
  - Prominent nuclear irregularities with perinuclear halos
  - CK7(+), Hale colloidal iron stain (+)
- Clear cell renal cell carcinoma (eosinophilic variant)
  - Prominent nuclear atypia with intricate vessels
  - RCC(+), CD10(+), vimentin (+), CK7(-)

Mahogany Brown Mass With Central Scar
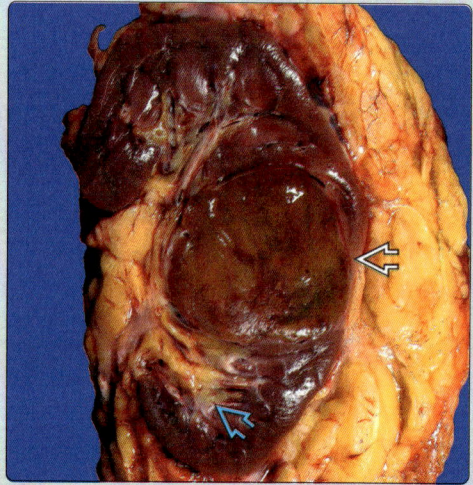

Oncocytoma Core Needle Biopsy
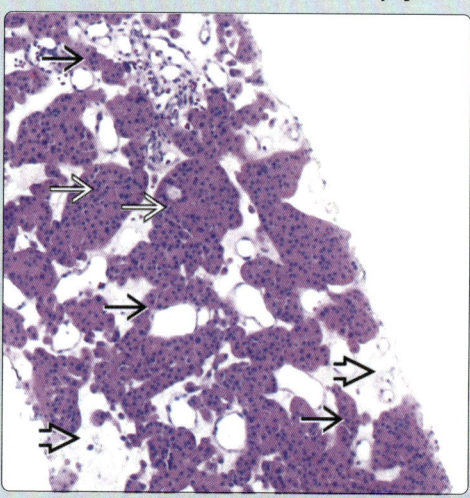

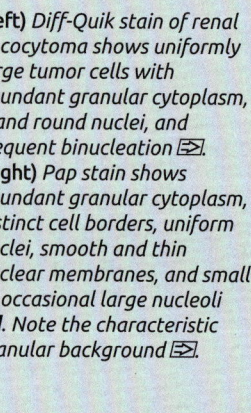

(Left) Gross photograph of renal oncocytoma shows a circumscribed mass ➡ with mahogany brown color and a central stellate scar ➡. (Right) H&E-stained core needle biopsy of oncocytoma shows solid nests ➡ and trabeculae ➡ of cells with pink (oncocytic) cytoplasm in a loose edematous stroma ➡.

Touch Preparation of Oncocytoma
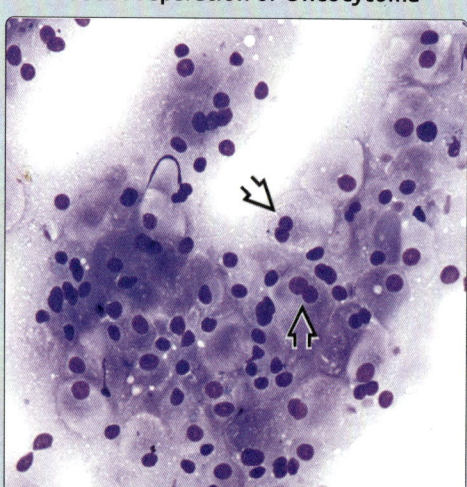

Bland Nuclei and Granular Background
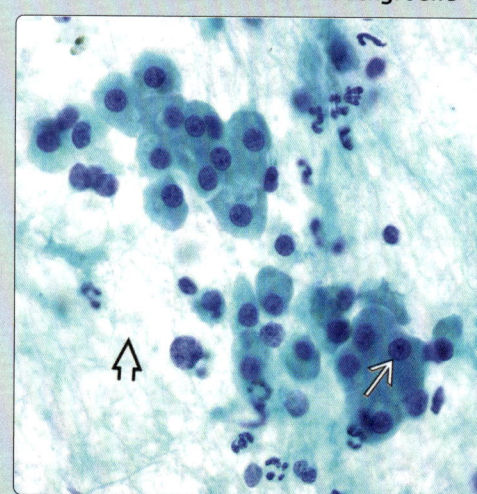

(Left) Diff-Quik stain of renal oncocytoma shows uniformly large tumor cells with abundant granular cytoplasm, bland round nuclei, and frequent binucleation ➡. (Right) Pap stain shows abundant granular cytoplasm, distinct cell borders, uniform nuclei, smooth and thin nuclear membranes, and small to occasional large nucleoli ➡. Note the characteristic granular background ➡.

Oncocytoma, Kidney

ETIOLOGY/PATHOGENESIS

Molecular Abnormalities
- Mixed normal and abnormal karyotypes, loss of chromosomes Y and 1

CLINICAL ISSUES

Epidemiology
- Accounts for 6-9% of renal tumors
- Age: 24-91 years (mean: 62 years)
- M:F = 2:1

IMAGING

Radiographic Findings
- Sharp demarcation, central scar, spoke-wheel feeding vessels
- Often incidental finding on imaging studies

CYTOPATHOLOGY

Cellularity
- Hypercellular

Pattern
- Loosely cohesive clusters and isolated cells

Background
- Granular background, no necrosis

Cells
- Uniformly large cells with abundant granular cytoplasm and distinct cell borders

Nuclear Details
- Small round nuclei with mild size variation, binucleation, and small nucleoli
- Absent or scant mitoses
- Rare pleomorphic nuclei and large nucleoli can be seen

Cytoplasmic Details
- Abundant, eosinophilic, and granular cytoplasm

Cell Block Findings
- Rounded nests of uniform cells with abundant eosinophilic and granular cytoplasm

ANCILLARY TESTS

Immunohistochemistry
- AE1/AE3, PAX8, CD117 (+)
- Vimentin, RCC (-); CK7(-)/focal (+)

Electron Microscopy
- Packed mitochondria showing mostly lamellar cristae

DIFFERENTIAL DIAGNOSIS

Inadvertent Sampling of Liver
- More nuclear variation with cytoplasmic lipofuscin granules
- Arginase-1 (+), Hep-Par1(+), PAX8(-)

Chromophobe Renal Cell Carcinoma
- Prominent nuclear irregularities with perinuclear halos
- CK7(+), Hale colloidal iron stain (+), microvesicles on EM

Clear Cell Renal Cell Carcinoma (Eosinophilic Variant)
- Prominent nuclear atypia with intricate vessels
- RCC(+), CD10(+), vimentin (+), CK7(-)

Hybrid Oncocytic/Chromophobe Tumor
- Sporadic or associated with oncocytomatosis or Birt-Hogg-Dubé syndrome
- Scattered chromophobe cells in background of typical oncocytoma

SELECTED REFERENCES

1. An J et al: HNF-1β as an immunohistochemical marker for distinguishing chromophobe renal cell carcinoma and hybrid oncocytic tumors from renal oncocytoma. Virchows Arch. 478(3):459-70, 2021
2. Abouhashem NS et al: Diagnostic utility of amylase α-1A, MOC 31, and CD 82 in renal oncocytoma versus chromophobe renal cell carcinoma. Indian J Pathol Microbiol. 63(3):405-11, 2020
3. Zhu B et al: Cytomorphology, immunoprofile, and management of renal oncocytic neoplasms. Cancer Cytopathol. 128(12):962-70, 2020
4. Iczkowski KA et al: Eosinophilic kidney tumors: old and new. Arch Pathol Lab Med. 143(12):1455-63, 2019

Focal Nuclear Pleomorphism

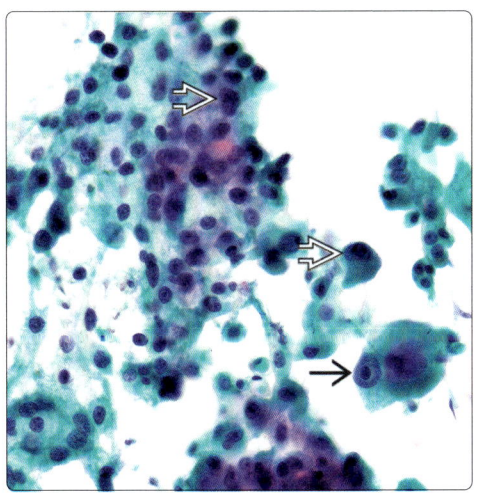

Focal CK7 Positive

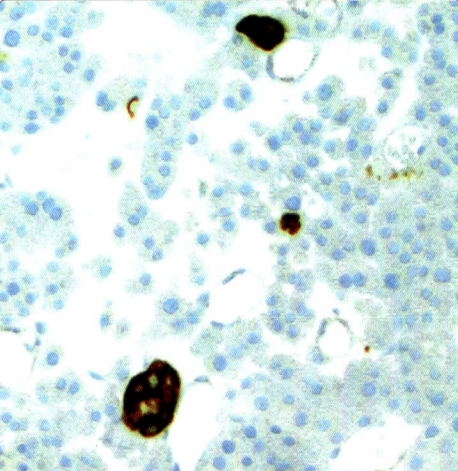

(Left) Pap stain displays mild nuclear size variation with smooth contours and small nucleoli. Rare pleomorphic nuclei ⇨ and macronucleoli ⇨ can be seen. **(Right)** Renal oncocytoma shows focal CK7(+) cells in this core needle biopsy.

Metanephric Adenoma

KEY FACTS

TERMINOLOGY
- Synonyms: Embryonal adenoma or nephrogenic nephroma
- Benign neoplasm composed of small primitive cells resembling early metanephric tubular differentiation
- Related tumors: Metanephric adenofibroma and metanephric stromal tumor

CLINICAL ISSUES
- Mean age: 41 years
- Female predominance (M:F = 1:2)
- Asymptomatic in 50% cases
- May have flank pain, hematuria, or polycythemia
- Imaging shows calcifications in up to 43% of cases

CYTOPATHOLOGY
- Tight clusters, papillae, tubules, or rosettes
- Small, round to oval cells with scant cytoplasm
- Uniform round nuclei with fine delicate chromatin
- Mitosis is rare to absent
- Closely packed tubules composed of small epithelial cells with little cytoplasm in cell block

ANCILLARY TESTS
- WT1(+), CD57(+), PAX8(+)
- Usually CK7(-), AMACR(-), EMA(-)
- No gain of chromosome 7 or 17, or loss of chromosome Y (common in papillary renal cell carcinoma)
- *BRAF* V600E mutations reported in 90% of cases

TOP DIFFERENTIAL DIAGNOSES
- Papillary renal cell carcinoma
  - Often multifocal, more cytoplasm, higher nuclear grade, more pleomorphic, prominent nucleoli
  - CK7(+), WT1(-), CD57(-)
- Epithelial predominant nephroblastoma (Wilms tumor)
  - Hyperchromatic, brisk mitoses, stromal or blastemal components
  - CD57 usually (-) or focal (+)

Well-Circumscribed Homogeneous Tumor

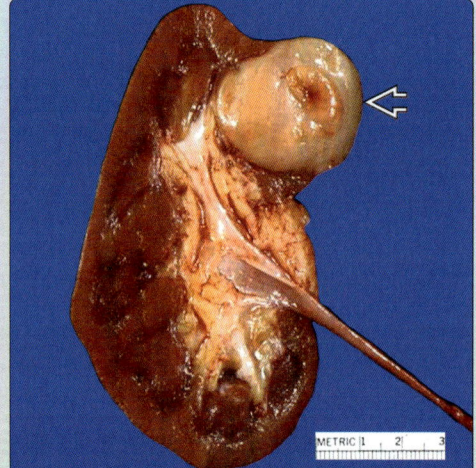

Small Round to Oval Epithelial Cells

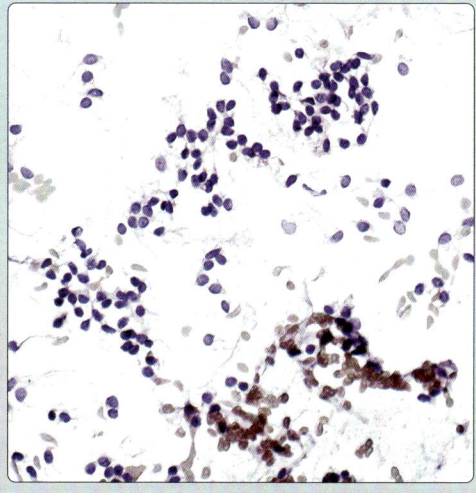

(Left) *Typical gross appearance of a metanephric adenoma shows a well-circumscribed tumor with a homogeneous tan-yellow cut surface ➡.* (Right) *FNA of the tumor shows clusters of small round to oval epithelial cells on Pap stain.*

Uniform Nuclei With Smooth Contours

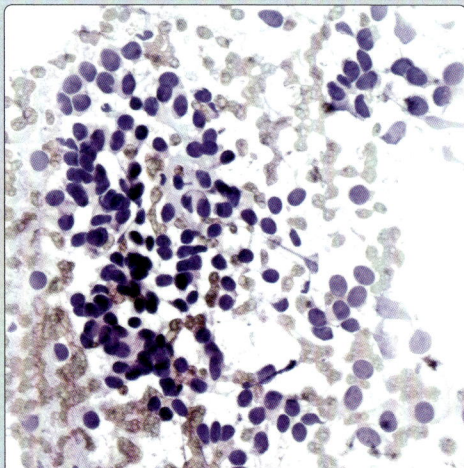

Delicate Chromatin and Small Nucleoli

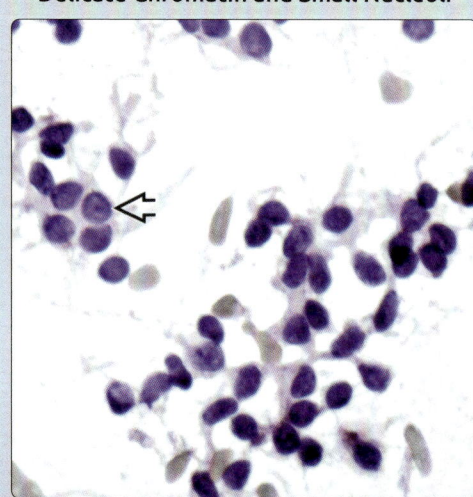

(Left) *Medium-power magnification of a Pap stain shows small, round to oval cells with scant cytoplasm, uniform nuclei, fine chromatin, and inconspicuous nucleoli.* (Right) *High-power magnification demonstrates tumor cells with scant cytoplasm, uniform nuclei, smooth nuclear contours, fine delicate chromatin, and occasional small nucleoli ➡. Mitosis is not seen in this Pap stain.*

Metanephric Adenoma

TERMINOLOGY

Definitions
- Benign neoplasm composed of small primitive cells resembling early metanephric tubular differentiation
  - Related tumors: Metanephric adenofibroma and metanephric stromal tumor

CLINICAL ISSUES

Epidemiology
- Mean age: 41 years; range: 11 months to 83 years
- Female predominance (M:F = 1:2)

Presentation
- Asymptomatic in 50% cases
- May have flank pain, hematuria, or polycythemia
- Calcifications in up to 43% of cases

CYTOPATHOLOGY

Cellularity
- Moderately cellular aspirate

Pattern
- Tight clusters, papillae, tubules, or rosettes

Background
- Clean

Cells
- Small, round/oval epithelial cells with scant cytoplasm

Nuclear Details
- Uniform round nuclei with fine delicate chromatin and inconspicuous nucleoli; mitosis rare to absent

Cytoplasmic Details
- Small amount of finely granular cytoplasm

Cell Block Findings
- Closely packed tubules composed of small epithelial cells with little cytoplasm

MACROSCOPIC

General Features
- Solitary circumscribed mass (mean: 5.5 cm), often with calcifications, hemorrhage, or necrosis

MICROSCOPIC

Histologic Features
- Crowded small acini of primitive blue cells
- Papillary/glomeruloid structures or cysts can be seen
- Hyalinization, calcifications, necrosis, and hemorrhage are common

ANCILLARY TESTS

Immunohistochemistry
- Positive for WT1, CD57, PAX8, p16
- Negative for CK7, EMA, AMACR
- No gain of chromosome 7 or 17, or loss of chromosome Y
- BRAF V600E mutations reported in 82-90% of cases
- Less common mutations: NF1, NOTCH1, SPEN, AKT2, APC, ATRX, and ETV4

DIFFERENTIAL DIAGNOSIS

Papillary Renal Cell Carcinoma
- Often multifocal, more cytoplasm, higher nuclear grade, more pleomorphic, prominent nucleoli
- CK7(+), WT1(-), CD57(-)

Epithelial Predominant Wilms Tumor
- Hyperchromatic, brisk mitoses, stromal or blastemal components, CD57 usually (-) or focal (+)

SELECTED REFERENCES

1. de Jel DVC et al: Paediatric metanephric tumours: a clinicopathological and molecular characterisation. Crit Rev Oncol Hematol. 150:102970, 2020
2. Treece AL: Pediatric renal tumors: updates in the molecular Era. Surg Pathol Clin. 13(4):695-718, 2020
3. Ding Y et al: Novel clinicopathological and molecular characterization of metanephric adenoma: a study of 28 cases. Diagn Pathol. 13(1):54, 2018

Compact Primitive Blue Cells

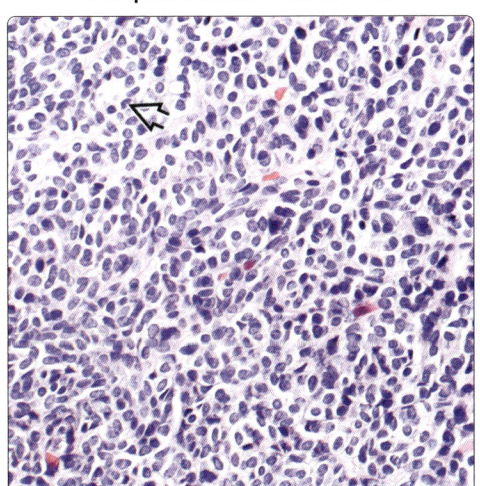

Diffuse Expression of WT1

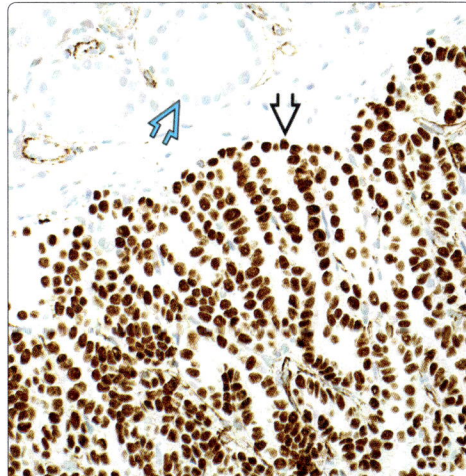

(Left) Histologically, metanephric adenoma is composed of compact primitive blue cells forming crowded small acini ➡, as seen in this H&E stain. (Right) Immunostain for WT1 demonstrates diffuse nuclear stain in tumor cells ➡ and negative stain in normal renal tubules ➡.

Metanephric Stromal Tumor

KEY FACTS

CLASSIFICATION
- Very rare benign tumor composed exclusively of metanephric stromal elements

CLINICAL ISSUES
- Age range: Up to 15 years (mean: 2 years)
- Presents with abdominal mass; rarely hypertension and hematuria
- Complete surgical excision is curative

CYTOPATHOLOGY
- Hypercellular aspirate
- Alternating hypercellular cohesive clusters and loose hypocellular areas
- Spindled to stellate, bland and uniform stromal cells
- Oval hyperchromatic nuclei, inconspicuous nucleoli

MACROSCOPIC
- Medullary mass with tan lobulated cut surface (mean: 5 cm)

MICROSCOPIC
- Spindle to stellate stromal cells surround and entrap renal tubules and blood vessels
- Frequent juxtaglomerular apparatus hyperplasia (JGAH) within entrapped glomeruli
- Epithelioid smooth muscle of intratumoral arterioles (angiodysplasia of vessels)

ANCILLARY TESTS
- CD34(+); keratins, WT1, desmin, S100 (-)
- Ch 17q rearrangement and *BRAF* V600E mutations

TOP DIFFERENTIAL DIAGNOSES
- Congenital mesoblastic nephroma, classic variant
  - Lack of angiodysplasia, concentric peritubular growth pattern, or JGAH; CD34(-)
- Metanephric adenofibroma
  - Biphasic tumor with epithelial and metanephric stromal tumor-like stromal components; WT1(+)

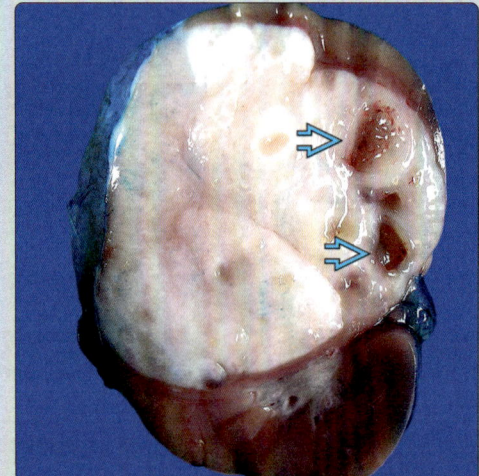

Lobulated Fibrous Mass of Metanephric Stromal Tumor

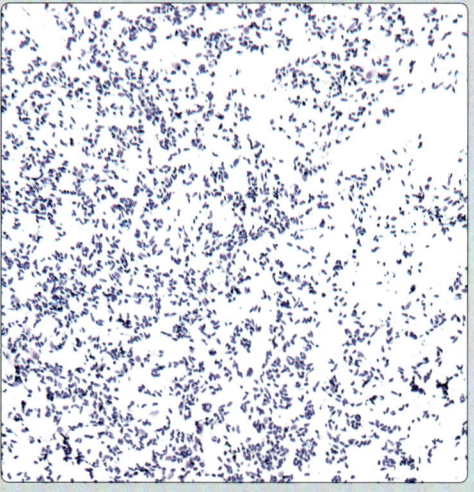

Hypercellular Monotonous Spindled Cells

(Left) Gross photograph of a metanephric stromal tumor shows a tan, lobulated, and fibrous mass with cyst formation ⟹. The tumor is centered in the renal medulla. *(Right)* Low magnification of an H&E stain shows a hypercellular smear composed of loose and monotonous spindled stromal cells.

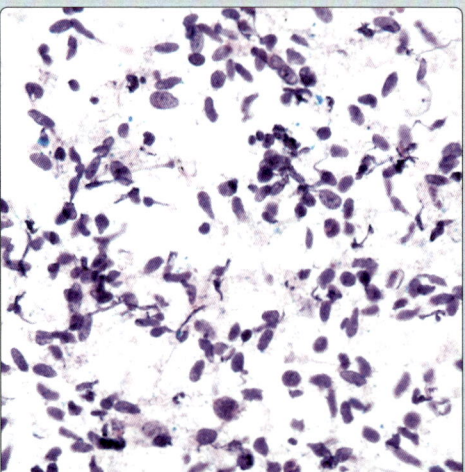

Spindle Nuclei and Wispy Cytoplasm

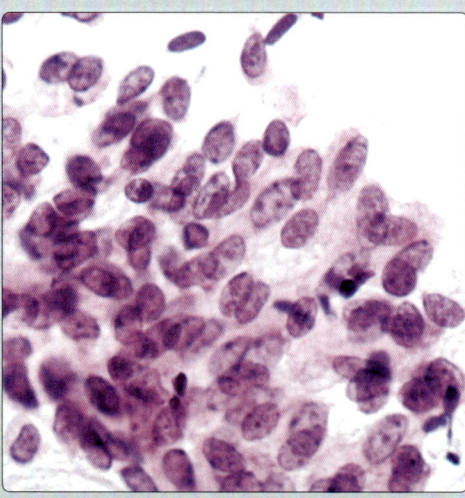

Oval Nuclei With Smooth Contours

(Left) H&E stain shows spindled to stellate cells with hyperchromatic nuclei and wispy cytoplasm. *(Right)* High magnification of an H&E stain shows oval nuclei, smooth nuclear contours, and inconspicuous nucleoli. There is no significant atypia.

Xanthogranulomatous Pyelonephritis/Malakoplakia

KEY FACTS

TERMINOLOGY
- Variants of chronic pyelonephritis characterized by mass lesion
- Xanthogranulomatous pyelonephritis (XPN) contains abundant foamy macrophages
- Michaelis-Gutmann bodies may be seen in renal malakoplakia (RMP)

ETIOLOGY/PATHOGENESIS
- Urinary tract obstruction with recurrent infection

CLINICAL ISSUES
- Most common in female patients in 5th and 6th decades
- Present with fever, flank pain, abdominal mass

CYTOPATHOLOGY
- Usually low cellularity
- Inflammatory/necrotic background
- XPN: Macrophages with abundant foamy cytoplasm
- RMP: Granular cytoplasm; Michaelis-Gutmann body is pathognomonic (2- to 5-μm, concentrically lamellar, targetoid, basophilic, or calcified cytoplasmic inclusions; positive for PAS and GMS stains)

MACROSCOPIC
- Large, yellow nodules with perirenal adhesions and dilated pelvicalyceal system

TOP DIFFERENTIAL DIAGNOSES
- Clear cell renal cell carcinoma
  - Simulating XPN/RMP on clinical, radiologic, gross, and cytologic examinations
  - Featured with vacuolated cytoplasm, prominent eosinophilic nucleoli, intricate vasculature
  - AE1/AE3(+) and CD68(-)
- Spindle cell neoplasms
  - May resemble reactive fibroblasts in XPN/RMP
  - Foamy macrophages, multinucleated giant cells, and inflammatory background favor XPN

Yellow Mass Lesion in Xanthogranulomatous Pyelonephritis
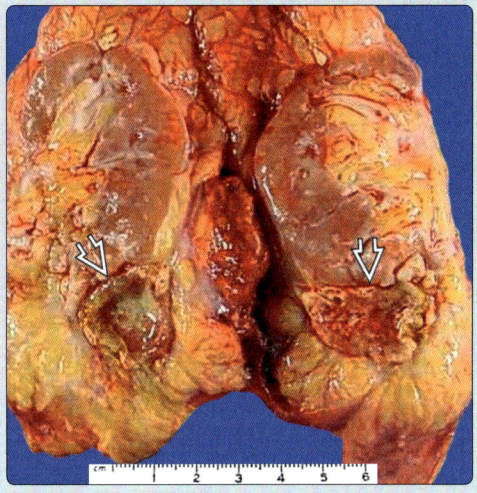

Xanthogranulomatous Pyelonephritis With Foamy Macrophages
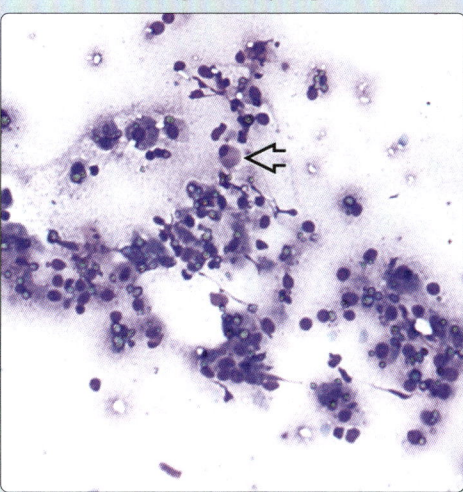

(Left) Gross photograph of xanthogranulomatous pyelonephritis shows a yellow nodular lesion extending into perirenal fat ➡. *(Right)* Macrophages ➡ can be distinguished from clear cell renal cell carcinoma by absence of nuclear atypia, prominent nucleoli, or intricate blood vessels, as seen in this Diff-Quik-stained smear.

Cytologic Features of Renal Malakoplakia
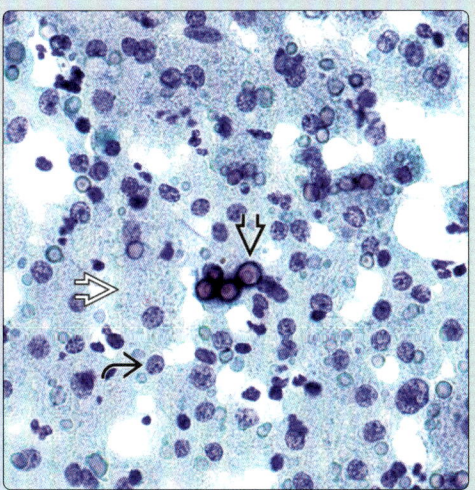

Michaelis-Gutmann Bodies
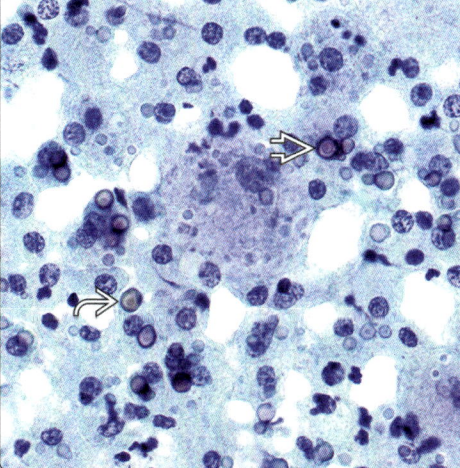

(Left) Pap-stained aspiration of malakoplakia reveals macrophages with abundant granular cytoplasm ➡, round nuclei, small nucleoli ➡, and Michaelis-Gutmann bodies ➡. *(Right)* Michaelis-Gutmann bodies are diagnostic for renal malakoplakia; they show classic targetoid ➡ or lamellar configurations ➡ of intracytoplasmic inclusions, as seen in this Pap stain.

Clear Cell Renal Cell Carcinoma

KEY FACTS

ETIOLOGY/PATHOGENESIS
- Mutations in *VHL* gene (3p25-26) or chromosome 3p losses seen in both familial and sporadic tumors

CLINICAL ISSUES
- Clear cell renal cell carcinoma (CC-RCC) accounts for 65-70% of all RCC
- Usually asymptomatic (60-80%)

CYTOPATHOLOGY
- Hypercellular aspirates with bloody or necrotic background
- Intricate and branching blood vessels
- Abundant delicate or finely vacuolated cytoplasm
- Eccentric nuclei with prominent nucleoli
- Cell block: Clear tumor cells associated with intricate and branching blood vessels

MACROSCOPIC
- Golden-yellow masses with necrosis and hemorrhage

ANCILLARY TESTS
- Positive: AE1/AE3, PAX8, vimentin, RCC, CD10, CA9
- Negative: CK7, AMACR, CD117
- Deletion of 3p is characteristic for CC-RCC and can be useful in challenging cases

TOP DIFFERENTIAL DIAGNOSES
- Benign renal tubular cells
- Papillary renal cell carcinoma
- Chromophobe renal cell carcinoma
- Translocation-associated renal cell carcinoma
- Adrenal cortical tumors
- Metastatic tumors

DIAGNOSTIC CHECKLIST
- Cytologic findings vary depending on tumor grade
- 2-tier grading system for FNA specimens: Low grade (Fuhrman grades 1-2) and high grade (Fuhrman grades 3-4)

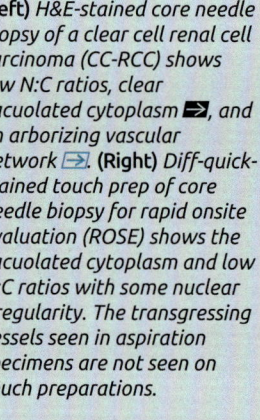

(Left) H&E-stained core needle biopsy of a clear cell renal cell carcinoma (CC-RCC) shows low N:C ratios, clear vacuolated cytoplasm ➡, and an arborizing vascular network ➡. (Right) Diff-quick-stained touch prep of core needle biopsy for rapid onsite evaluation (ROSE) shows the vacuolated cytoplasm and low N:C ratios with some nuclear irregularity. The transgressing vessels seen in aspiration specimens are not seen on touch preparations.

Core Needle Biopsy of Clear Cell Renal Cell Carcinoma

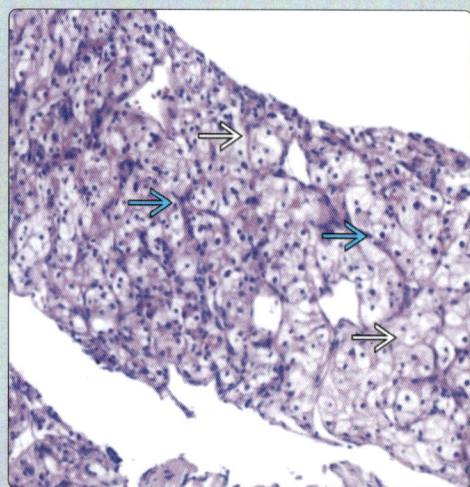

Touch Prep of Core for ROSE

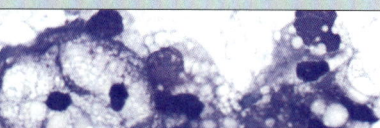
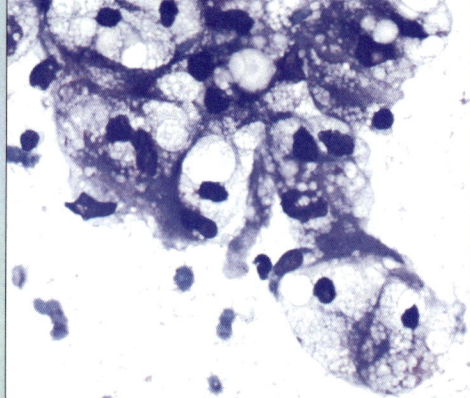

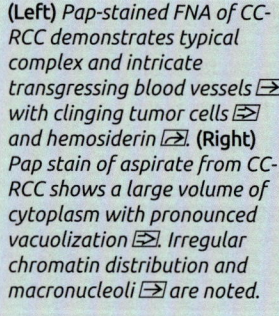

(Left) Pap-stained FNA of CC-RCC demonstrates typical complex and intricate transgressing blood vessels ➡ with clinging tumor cells ➡ and hemosiderin ➡. (Right) Pap stain of aspirate from CC-RCC shows a large volume of cytoplasm with pronounced vacuolization ➡. Irregular chromatin distribution and macronucleoli ➡ are noted.

Typical Intricate Blood Vessels

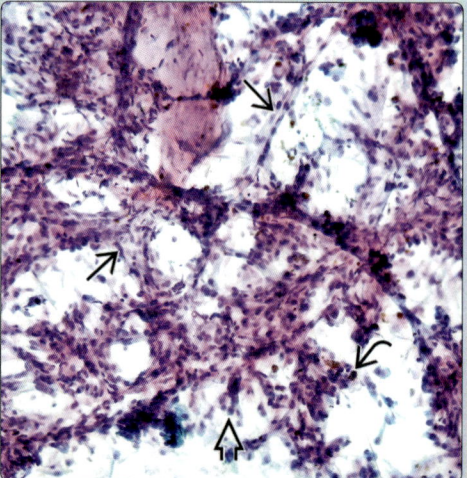

Pronounced Cytoplasmic Vacuolization

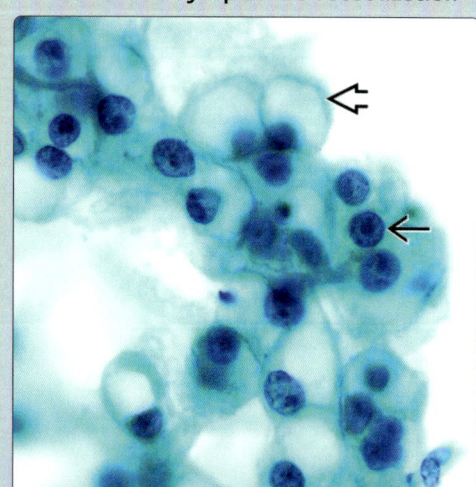

Clear Cell Renal Cell Carcinoma

TERMINOLOGY

Abbreviations
- Clear cell renal cell carcinoma (CC-RCC)

CLINICAL ISSUES

Epidemiology
- CC-RCC accounts for 65-70% of all RCC
- Majority occur in adults > 40 years; rare in children
- M:F ~ 3:1

Presentation
- Most cases are asymptomatic with incidental findings on imaging studies
- Classic triad of hematuria, mass lesion, and pain is present in < 30% of cases

Treatment
- Nephrectomy or partial nephrectomy
- Limited response to chemotherapy, radiation, and immunotherapy

Prognosis
- Aggressive; overall 5-year survival: 75%

CYTOPATHOLOGY

Cellularity
- Usually hypercellular

Pattern
- Large clusters of tumor cells intimately associated with tortuous blood vessels

Background
- Often bloody or necrotic with stromal components

Cells
- Large, round cells with eccentric nuclei and visible cell borders

Nuclear Details
- Fuhrman grade 1: Round nuclei with hyperchromasia and inconspicuous nucleoli
- Fuhrman grade 2: Enlarged nuclei with uneven chromatin, irregular nuclear contours, and small nucleoli
- Fuhrman grade 3: Pronounced irregular nuclear contours with large eosinophilic nucleoli
- Fuhrman grade 4: Marked nuclear atypia or spindle morphology, prominent macronucleoli

Cytoplasmic Details
- Abundant wispy cytoplasm, finely vacuolated or granular

Cell Block Findings
- Clear tumor cells associated with intricate and branching blood vessels
- Nuclear grading can be preliminarily performed on cell block, knowing that undergrading may occur

Cytology-Histology Correlation
- 2-tier grading system has been recommended for FNA specimens that accurately correlates with Fuhrman grading on histology: Low grade (Fuhrman grade 1 or 2) and high grade (Fuhrman grade 3 or 4)

MACROSCOPIC

Gross Features
- Typically golden-yellow masses with necrosis and hemorrhage
- Solid, tan-white to fleshy-appearing in high-grade or sarcomatoid areas

ANCILLARY TESTS

Immunohistochemistry
- Positive: AE1/AE3, PAX8, vimentin, RCC, CD10, CA9
- Negative: CK7, CD117, AMACR

Genetic Testing
- Deletion of 3p is characteristic and can be used in challenging cases

DIFFERENTIAL DIAGNOSIS

Benign Renal Tubular Cells
- Abundant pale cytoplasm simulating low-grade CC-RCC
- Usually in small, flat groups
- No vacuolated cytoplasm or branching vessels

Papillary Renal Cell Carcinoma
- Abundant papillary structures with foamy macrophages
- Usually low-grade atypia, lack of branching vessels
- Usually CK7(+), AMACR(+), and CA9(-)

Chromophobe Renal Cell Carcinoma
- Pronounced irregular nuclei with perinuclear haloes
- Less prominent vasculature
- CK7(+), CD117(+), Hale colloidal iron stain (+), vimentin (-), RCC(-), CD10(-) or weak (+)

Translocation-Associated Renal Cell Carcinoma
- Prominent papillary architecture and high-grade clear cells
- Strong nuclear stain for TFE3 or TFEB; AE1/AE3(-)

Adrenal Cortical Tumors
- Difficult to distinguish from low-grade CC-RCC
- Fine, bubbly cytoplasm and foamy lipid background
- Inhibin (+), Melan-A (+), AE1/AE3(-), RCC(-)

Metastatic Tumors
- May have clear cells or cytoplasmic vacuoles
- Intimate association of branching vessels with large low N:C ratio tumor cells favors primary
- Accurate history and immunohistochemistry is essential

SELECTED REFERENCES

1. Chen HI et al: Accuracy of subclassification and grading of renal tumors on fine needle aspiration cytology Alone. Acta Cytol. 65(2):140-9, 2021
2. Ponce-Zepeda J et al: Touch preparation for rapid onsite evaluations of renal mass biopsies: concordance rate, pearls, and pitfalls. J Am Soc Cytopathol. 9(5):422-8, 2020

Clear Cell Renal Cell Carcinoma

Classic Golden-Yellow Masses

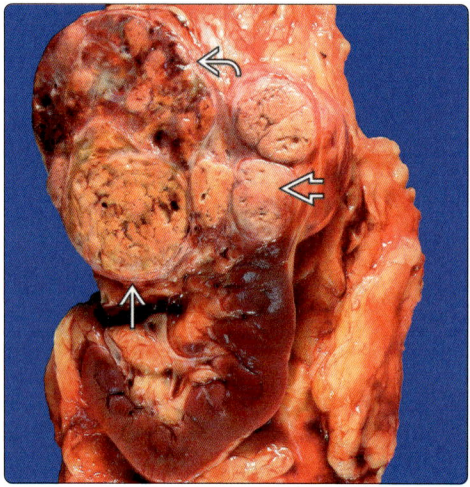

Clear Cells With Vascular Framework

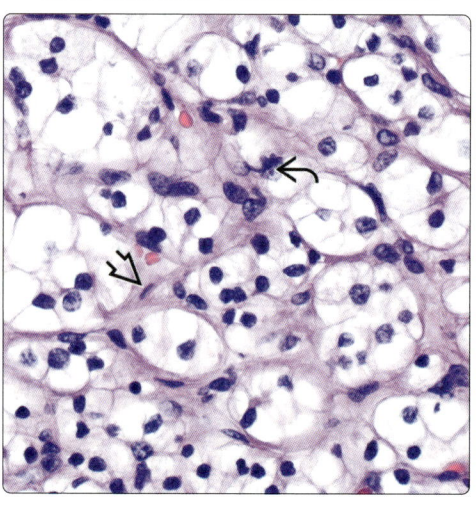

(Left) Gross photograph of CC-RCC shows multiple renal masses with classic golden-yellow color ➡, areas of hemorrhage ➡, and tan-white fleshy areas indicating sarcomatoid differentiation ➡. **(Right)** H&E-stained section shows nests of clear cells surrounded by delicate, prominent, interconnecting vascular framework ➡. Nuclear atypia and prominent nucleoli ➡ can be seen.

Complex Vasculature and Tumor Cells

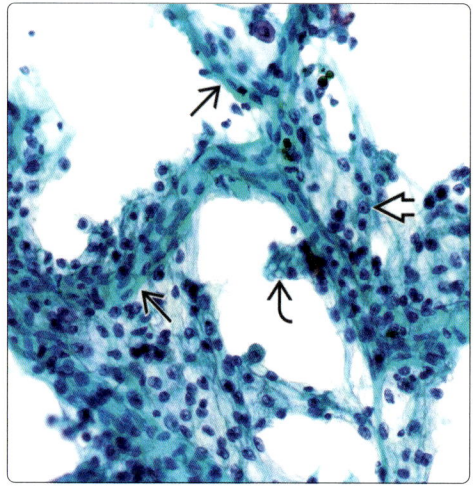

CD31 Highlights Complex Vasculature

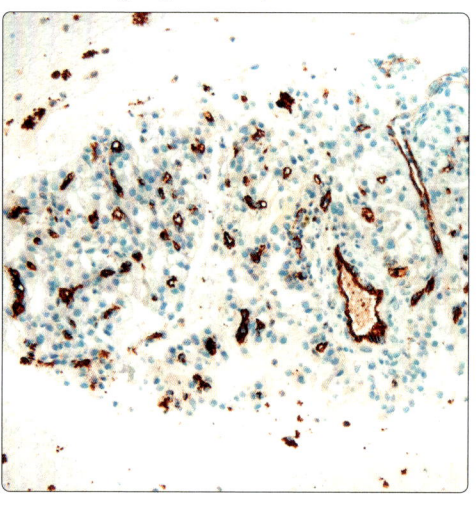

(Left) Pap-stained FNA reveals features reflecting the histologic findings with complex vasculature ➡ and closely associated tumor cells. Abundant clear to vacuolated cytoplasm ➡, eccentric nuclei, and prominent nucleoli ➡ are typical for tumor cells in CC-RCC. **(Right)** The complex vasculature is highlighted by immunostain of CD31 on a cell block section.

Low-Grade Clear Cell Renal Cell Carcinoma

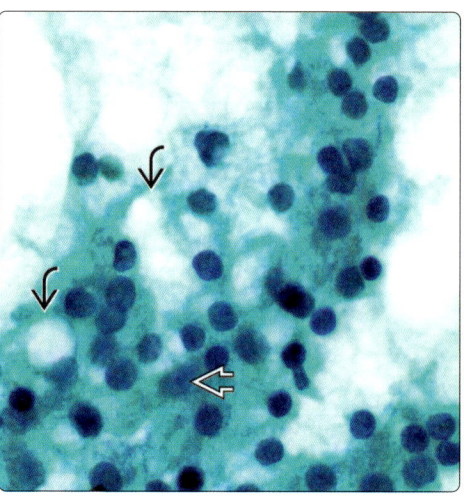

High-Grade Clear Cell Renal Cell Carcinoma

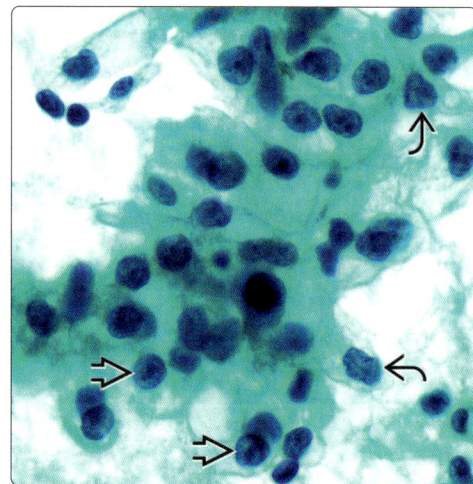

(Left) Pap stain of low-grade CC-RCC demonstrates abundant clear to vacuolated cytoplasm ➡, enlargement of nuclei, mild irregularity of nuclear membranes, slightly uneven chromatin, and occasional small nucleoli ➡. **(Right)** Pap stain of high-grade CC-RCC demonstrates more prominent nuclear enlargement, irregular nuclear contours ➡, and prominent macronucleoli ➡.

Clear Cell Renal Cell Carcinoma

Touch Prep of Core for ROSE

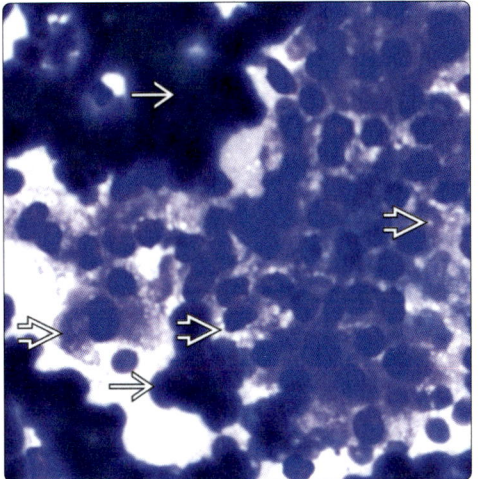

Occasional Signet-Ring Cells

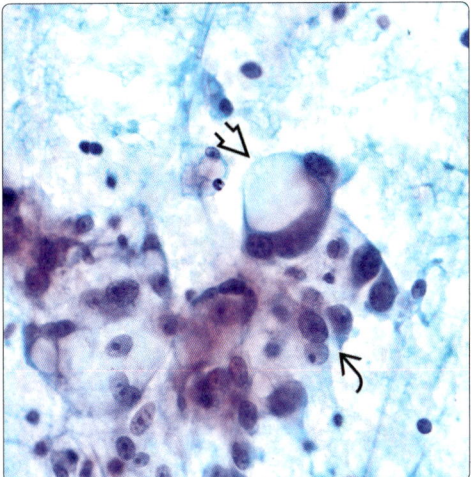

(Left) Diff-Quik-stained touch prep for ROSE is shown. The vacuolated cytoplasm ➡ is easily seen. Other details are difficult to visualize in this blood-obscured ➡ sample. Unlike FNAs, the transgressing vessels are not usually seen on touch preparations. (Right) Pap stain shows a signet-ring tumor cell with a single large, cytoplasmic vacuole indenting the nucleus ➡. The tumor can be separated from other tumors with signet-ring morphology by the presence of typical CC-RCC cytologic features in surrounding tumor cells ➡.

Clear to Finely Granular Cytoplasm

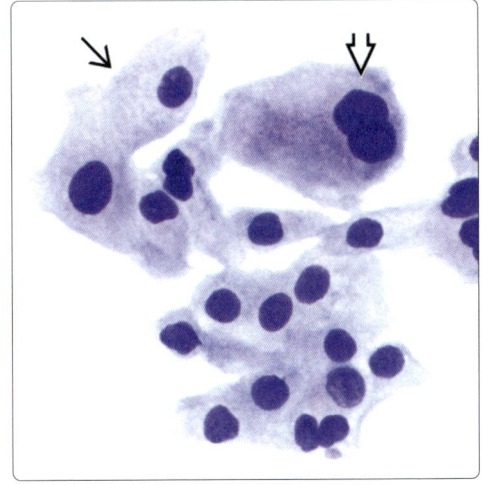

Coarsely Granular Cytoplasm

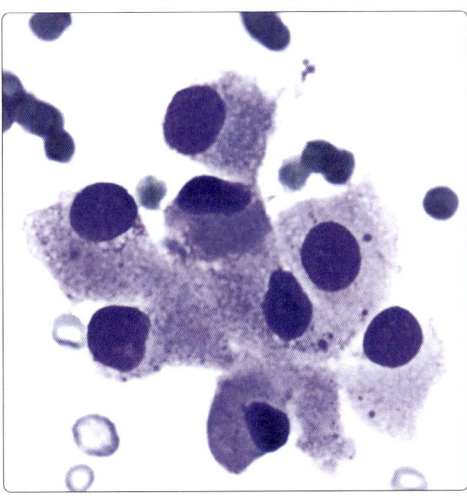

(Left) Diff-Quik stain shows clear to finely granular cytoplasm ➡. The eccentrically located nuclei ➡ and absence of background lipid help to distinguish clear cell carcinoma from adrenal cortical neoplasms. (Right) Coarsely granular cytoplasm is seen in Diff-Quik-stained high-grade CC-RCC. The eccentric nuclei and absence of background granules or perinuclear clearing distinguish this from oncocytoma and chromophobe carcinoma, respectively.

Sarcomatoid Differentiation

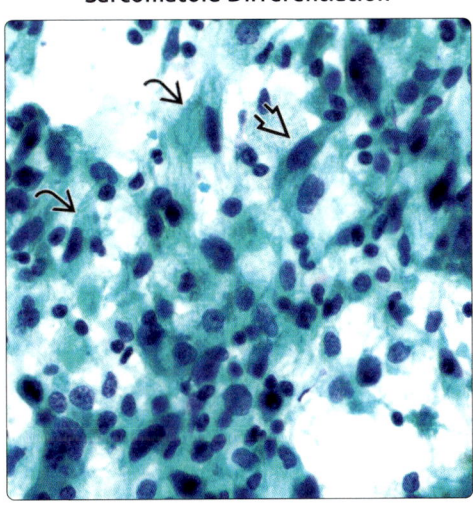

Sarcomatoid Differentiation

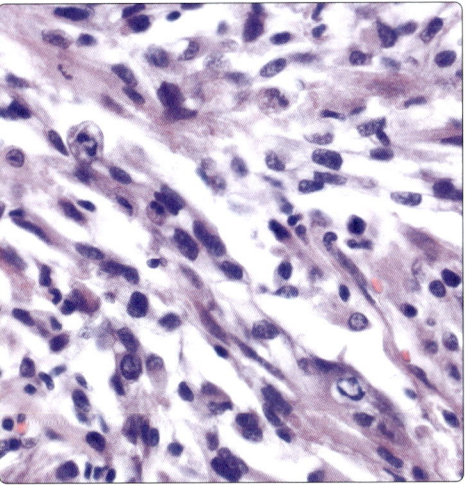

(Left) Pap stain of high-grade CC-RCC shows marked pleomorphism with spindle cell morphology ➡, typical for CC-RCC with sarcomatoid differentiation. Despite the pronounced nuclear atypia, classic features of clear cell carcinoma (relatively low N:C ratio and clear/vacuolated cytoplasm ➡) are still preserved. (Right) H&E-stained section from the same tumor shows a component of sarcomatoid differentiation adjacent to a component of conventional renal cell carcinoma.

Papillary Renal Cell Carcinoma

KEY FACTS

CLASSIFICATION
- Malignant tumor derived from renal tubular epithelium with papillary or tubulopapillary architecture
- Most common genetic abnormalities: Trisomies 7 and 17 and loss of chromosome Y

CLINICAL ISSUES
- Age 59-63 years, male predominant
- Triad: Abdominal mass, flank pain, hematuria

CYTOPATHOLOGY
- Hypercellular aspirate with abundant papillary structures or round spherules
- Type 1: Small, bland cuboidal cells with uniform, round nuclei and grooves, single layer
- Type 2: Larger eosinophilic cells with enlarged nuclei, prominent nucleoli, and pseudostratification
- Cytoplasm: Clear, eosinophilic, granular; ± hemosiderin
- Foamy macrophages or psammoma bodies may present

ANCILLARY TESTS
- Positive: CK7, AMACR, RCC, CD10, PAX8
- Negative: CA9, 34betaE12, *Ulex europaeus*, WT1, TFE3, CAIX23, p63

TOP DIFFERENTIAL DIAGNOSES
- Clear cell renal cell carcinoma with focal papillary growth
  - Intricate and branching blood vessels
  - Lacks foamy macrophages or hemosiderin
  - Usually CK7(-), AMACR(-), CA9(+)
- Clear cell papillary renal cell carcinoma (CCP RCC)
  - Distinct entity with low nuclear grade and clear cytoplasm
  - Lacks chromosome 7 and 17 gains or 3p deletions
  - CK7(+), CAIX23(+, basolateral pattern), RCC(-), CD10(-), AMACR(-)
- Distorted benign glomeruli (mimic spherules)
  - Identifying capillary loops on edge often helpful
- Papillary adenoma: Cytologically indistinguishable P-RCC

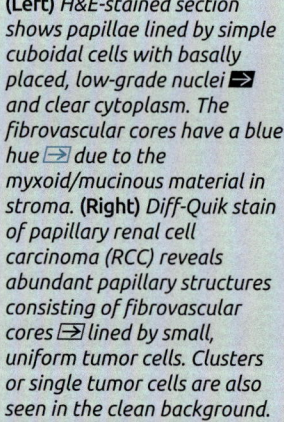

(Left) H&E-stained section shows papillae lined by simple cuboidal cells with basally placed, low-grade nuclei ➡ and clear cytoplasm. The fibrovascular cores have a blue hue ➡ due to the myxoid/mucinous material in stroma. (Right) Diff-Quik stain of papillary renal cell carcinoma (RCC) reveals abundant papillary structures consisting of fibrovascular cores ➡ lined by small, uniform tumor cells. Clusters or single tumor cells are also seen in the clean background.

Core Needle Biopsy Papillary Renal Cell Carcinoma, Type 1

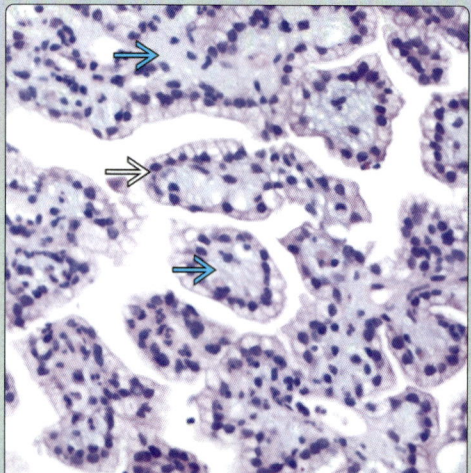

Papillae With Fibrovascular Cores

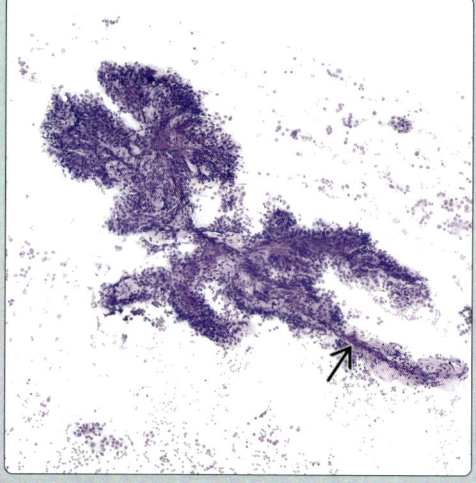

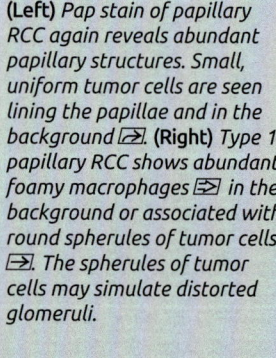

(Left) Pap stain of papillary RCC again reveals abundant papillary structures. Small, uniform tumor cells are seen lining the papillae and in the background ➡. (Right) Type 1 papillary RCC shows abundant foamy macrophages ➡ in the background or associated with round spherules of tumor cells ➡. The spherules of tumor cells may simulate distorted glomeruli.

Papillae Lined by Small Tumor Cells

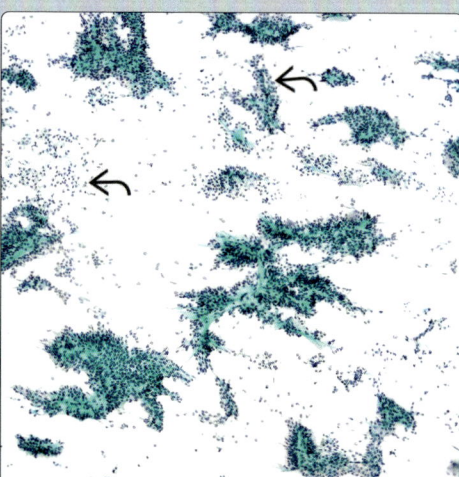

Foamy Macrophages and Spherules

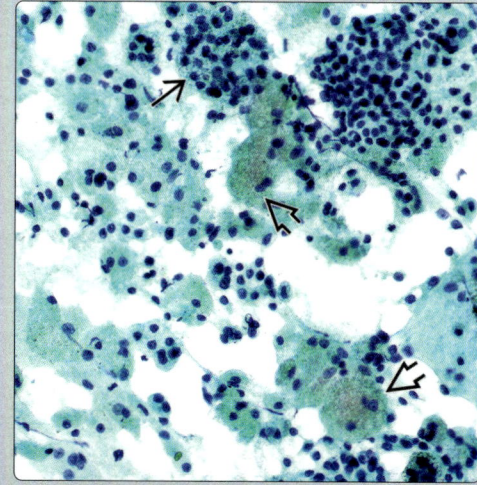

Papillary Renal Cell Carcinoma

ETIOLOGY/PATHOGENESIS

Molecular Characteristics
- Trisomies 7 and 17 loss of chromosome Y most common
- Tumors with trisomies 12, 16, and 20, or loss of 9p13 behave aggressively
- MET mutations seen in hereditary papillary renal carcinoma syndrome

CLINICAL ISSUES

Epidemiology
- Comprises 11-18.5% of renal cell carcinomas (RCCs)
- Range: 3rd-8th decades; peak: 59-63 years
- M:F = 1.8-4:1

Presentation
- Triad: Abdominal mass, flank pain, hematuria
- 50% asymptomatic with incidental masses on imaging

CYTOPATHOLOGY

Cellularity
- Usually hypercellular

Pattern
- Papillae with fibrovascular cores (present as round spherules on smears)

Background
- Usually clean, rarely necrotic or hemorrhagic

Cells
- Type 1: Small, bland cuboidal cells, single layer
- Type 2: Larger eosinophilic cells, pseudostratified

Nuclear Details
- Type 1: Uniform round nuclei with grooves
- Type 2: Enlarged nuclei with prominent nucleoli

Cytoplasmic Details
- Clear to eosinophilic/granular cytoplasm
  - May have intracytoplasmic hemosiderin

MACROSCOPIC

General Features
- Often well-circumscribed cortical mass with variable amount of hemorrhage or necrosis

ANCILLARY TESTS

Immunohistochemistry
- Positive: CK7, AMACR, RCC, CD10, PAX8
- Negative: CA9, 34betaE12, *Ulex europaeus*, WT1, TFE3, CAIX23, p63

DIFFERENTIAL DIAGNOSIS

Clear Cell RCC With Focal Papillary Growth
- Intricate blood vessels, lack of foamy macrophages or hemosiderin, usually CK7(-), AMACR(-), CA9(+)

Clear Cell Papillary RCC (CCP RCC)
- Distinct entity with low nuclear grade, lacks chromosome 7 and 17 gains or 3p deletions, CK7(+), CAIX23(+, basolateral pattern), RCC(-), AMACR(-), CD10(-)

Papillary Adenoma
- Similar lesion ≤ 15 mm, indistinguishable on cytology

Distorted Benign Glomeruli
- Mimic papillary RCC due to spherical or papillary arrangement but show capillary loops on edge

Other Differentials
- Papillary hyperplasia within renal cysts, papillary urothelial carcinoma

SELECTED REFERENCES

1. Griffin BB et al: Cytomorphologic analysis of clear cell papillary renal cell carcinoma: distinguishing diagnostic features. Cancer Cytopathol. 129(3):192-203, 2020
2. Magers MJ et al: Cytomorphologic comparison of type 1 and type 2 papillary renal cell carcinoma: a retrospective analysis of 28 cases. Cancer Cytopathol. 127(6):370-6, 2019

Low-Grade Nuclear Atypia

Papillary Renal Cell Carcinoma Type 2

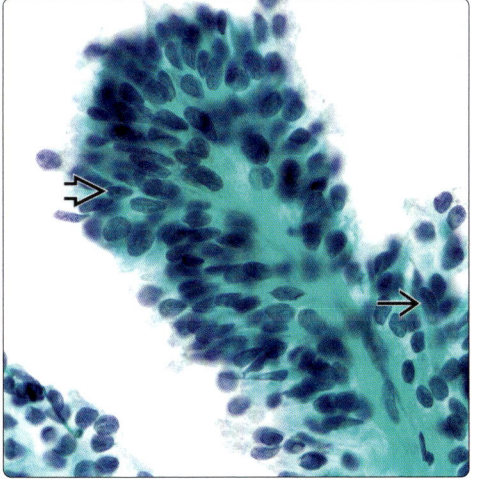
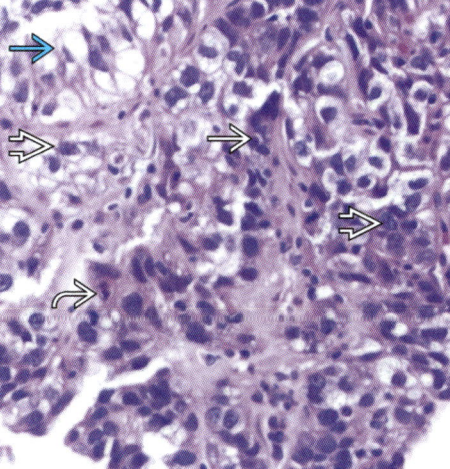

(Left) On high magnification of Pap stain, the tumor cells have fine and evenly distributed chromatin, inconspicuous nucleoli ➡, and occasional nuclear grooves ➡. *(Right)* H&E-stained core needle biopsy of a circumscribed renal mass shows a papillary architecture ➡. However, unlike type 1, the cells are stratified ➡ and have a higher nuclear grade ➡ and a more eosinophilic cytoplasm ➡.

Clear Cell Papillary Renal Cell Carcinoma

KEY FACTS

CLINICAL ISSUES
- Usually incidental renal mass, often in setting of end-stage renal disease or acquired cystic disease
- Low metastatic potential and good prognosis

CYTOPATHOLOGY
- Nests and 3D clusters most common architecture
  - Usually papillary; tubular/acinar patterns can be seen
  - Individual cells also often seen
- Columnar configuration with polarized nuclei
  - Cell blocks may help to identify this feature
- Low-grade, small, oval to round nuclei
  - Even chromatin without prominent nucleoli (grade 1 or 2)
- Delicate vacuolated cytoplasm, sometimes with granules or pigment
  - May have scant cytoplasm in some cases

MACROSCOPIC
- Small, well circumscribed, often encapsulated, usually with cystic component

ANCILLARY TESTS
- Positive: CK7, CA IX, HMCK (34βE12)
- Negative: AMACR, CD10
- No 3p deletions, gain of chromosome 7, or loss of Y chromosome

TOP DIFFERENTIAL DIAGNOSES
- Clear cell renal cell carcinoma
  - Lacks polarized nuclei, usually not papillary
  - CD10(+), CK7(-)
- Papillary renal cell carcinoma
  - Few cytoplasmic vacuoles, often many macrophages and necrotic debris in background
  - AMACR(+), CA IX(-) or focally (+)

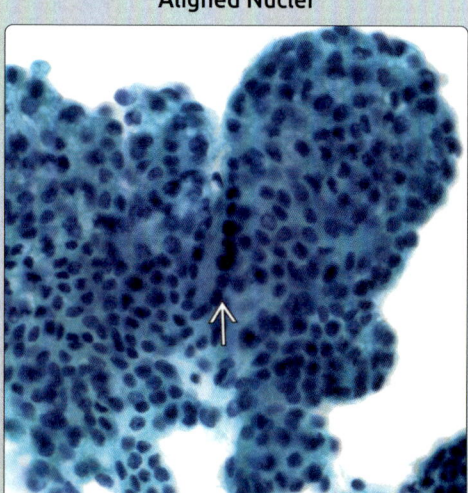

Aligned Nuclei

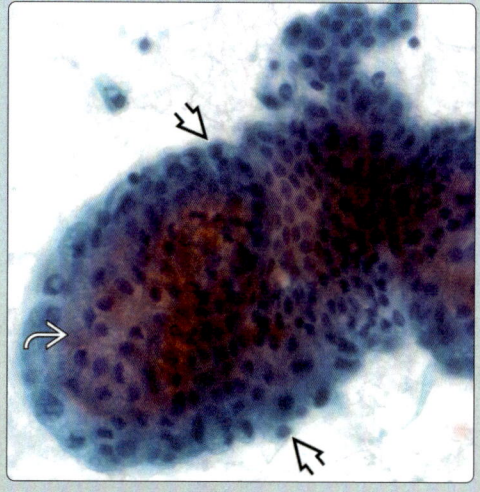

Vacuolated Cytoplasm

(Left) Pap-stained FNA of clear cell papillary renal cell carcinoma shows a complex 3D structure in which there are areas with obvious nuclear alignment ➡, a feature characteristic of this entity. (Right) Pap-stained rounded cluster of cells demonstrates the numerous cytoplasmic vacuoles ➡ corresponding to the histologic clear cell appearance. Also note that many nuclei are peripherally located ➡.

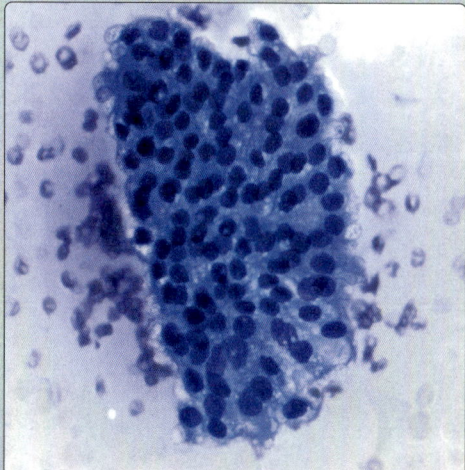

Diff-Quik Appearance

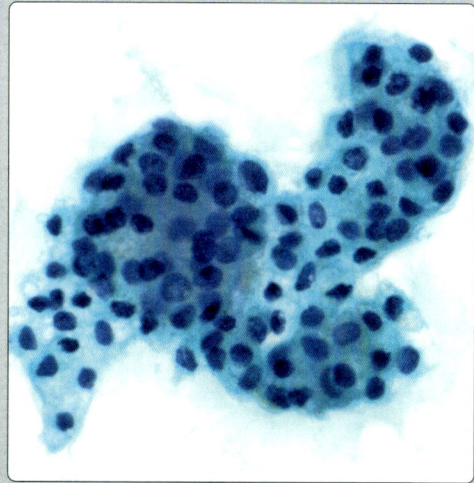

High-Power Appearance

(Left) Diff-Quik stain highlights the cytoplasmic vacuoles. The nuclei are oval to round and uniform. Cytoplasmic borders are indistinct. (Right) High-power view of a typical cluster of cells shows bland nuclei and abundant vacuolated and wispy cytoplasm on Pap stain. Although these features fit the diagnosis of clear cell papillary renal cell carcinoma, other low-grade carcinomas could look similar.

Clear Cell Papillary Renal Cell Carcinoma

CLINICAL ISSUES

Epidemiology
- 4th most common renal cell carcinoma

Presentation
- Sometimes in setting of end-stage renal disease or acquired cystic disease

Prognosis
- Low metastatic potential and good prognosis

CYTOPATHOLOGY

Pattern
- Nests and 3D clusters most common
- Papillary or tubular/acinar patterns can be seen

Cells
- Columnar configuration with polarized nuclei

Nuclear Details
- Low-grade, small, oval to round nuclei

Cytoplasmic Details
- Delicate cytoplasm with small vacuoles, sometimes with granules or pigment

Cell Block Findings
- Nuclei polarized away from basement membrane are characteristic; cell blocks may help to identify this feature

MACROSCOPIC

General Features
- Well circumscribed, often encapsulated and partially cystic
- Usually small, rarely invade perinephric fat

MICROSCOPIC

Histologic Features
- Usually prominent papillary architecture
  - Tubular/acinar and solid architecture may also be seen
- Clear cytoplasm
  - Solid areas may have scant cytoplasm that appears amphophilic
- Nuclei line up away from basement membrane
  - Low nuclear grade (1 or 2)
- Variable smooth muscle stroma
  - Abundant stroma seen in related entity, renal angioadenomyomatous tumor (RAT)

ANCILLARY TESTS

Immunohistochemistry
- Positive: CK7, CA IX, HMCK (34βE12)
  - CA IX has cup-shaped pattern of staining
- Negative: AMACR, CD10

Genetic Testing
- No 3p deletions, gain of chromosome 7, or loss of Y chromosome

DIFFERENTIAL DIAGNOSIS

Clear Cell Renal Cell Carcinoma
- Lacks polarized nuclei, usually not papillary
- CD10(+), CK7(-)

Papillary Renal Cell Carcinoma
- Few cytoplasmic vacuoles, more nuclear grooves and inclusions, often many macrophages and necrotic debris in background
- AMACR(+), CA IX(-) or focally (+)

Translocation-Associated Renal Cell Carcinoma
- Usually high nuclear grade
- Cytokeratin (-) or focally (+), TFE(+)

SELECTED REFERENCES
1. Griffin BB et al: Cytomorphologic analysis of clear cell papillary renal cell carcinoma: distinguishing diagnostic features. Cancer Cytopathol. 129(3):192-203, 2021
2. Zhao J et al: Clear cell papillary renal cell carcinoma. Arch Pathol Lab Med. 143(9):1154-58, 2019

Papillary Structure in Cell Block
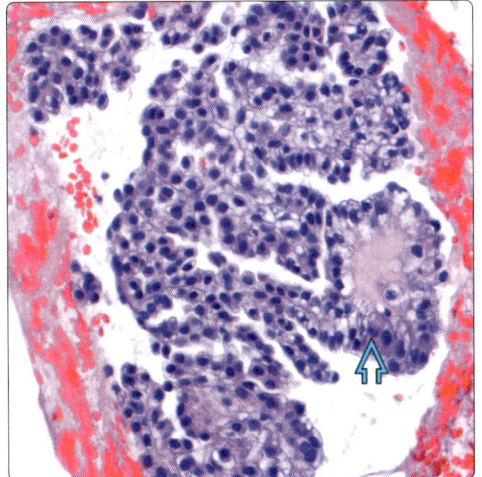

Clear Cells in Cell Block
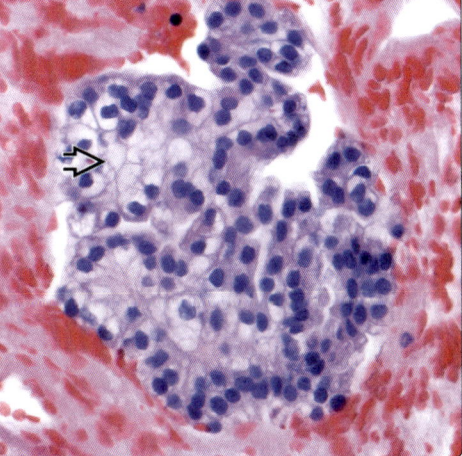

(Left) Cell blocks are crucial to the diagnosis of clear cell papillary renal cell carcinoma. This H&E-stained section contains a papillary structure ⇨ lined by cells with clear cytoplasm and nuclei oriented away from the basement membrane. Immunohistochemistry on the cell block is also very helpful for confirmation. (Right) H&E-stained cell blocks help to demonstrate the clear cell morphology ⇨ of the tumor. This finding, along with papillary-like architecture and bland nuclear features, helps to bring to mind the diagnosis.

Chromophobe Renal Cell Carcinoma

KEY FACTS

CLASSIFICATION
- RCC subtype with prominent cell membranes, wrinkled nuclei, perinuclear haloes, and eosinophilic cytoplasm

CLINICAL ISSUES
- 3rd most common subtype of RCC
- Age range: 26-62 years (mean: 58 years)
- M:F = 1.5:1
- Often incidental renal mass on imaging studies

CYTOPATHOLOGY
- Hypercellular aspirate
- Trabecular arrangement, loosely cohesive
- Large, round or polygonal cells with sharply defined cell borders (plant cell appearance)
- Hyperchromatic and wrinkled nuclei with perinuclear clearing (koilocytoid cells)
- Binucleation, pseudoinclusions, and indistinct nucleoli
- Usually clean background

- Cell block: Cords of tumor cells with distinct cytoplasmic borders, abundant granular cytoplasm, perinuclear clearing, and hyperchromatic and wrinkled nuclei

MACROSCOPIC
- Circumscribed mass (mean: 7 cm), tan to brown cut surface

ANCILLARY TESTS
- Positive immunohistochemistry: CK7, CD117
- Negative immunohistochemistry: CD10, vimentin, RCC
- Hale colloidal iron stain: Cytoplasmic staining
- Extensive chromosomal loss: 1, 6, 10, 13, 17, and 21

TOP DIFFERENTIAL DIAGNOSES
- Renal oncocytoma
  - Uniform round nuclei, no koilocytoid change
  - CK7(-) or focal (+), Hale colloidal iron stain (-)
- Clear cell RCC, eosinophilic variant
  - High nuclear grade with intricate vessels
  - CK7(-), CD117(-), CD10(+), vimentin (+), RCC (+)

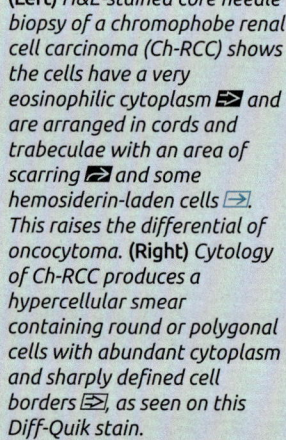

(Left) H&E-stained core needle biopsy of a chromophobe renal cell carcinoma (Ch-RCC) shows the cells have a very eosinophilic cytoplasm ➡ and are arranged in cords and trabeculae with an area of scarring ➡ and some hemosiderin-laden cells ➡. This raises the differential of oncocytoma. (Right) Cytology of Ch-RCC produces a hypercellular smear containing round or polygonal cells with abundant cytoplasm and sharply defined cell borders ➡, as seen on this Diff-Quik stain.

Core Needle Biopsy of Chromophobe Renal Cell Carcinoma

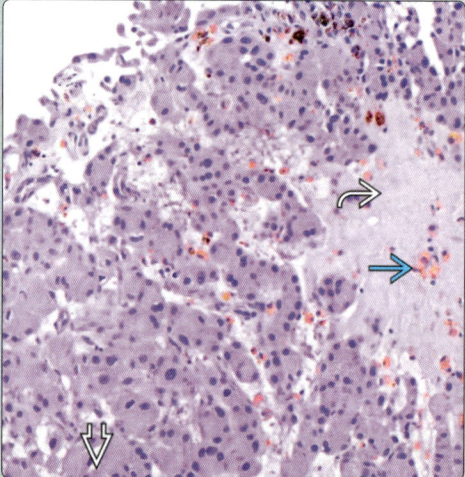

Sharply Defined Cell Borders

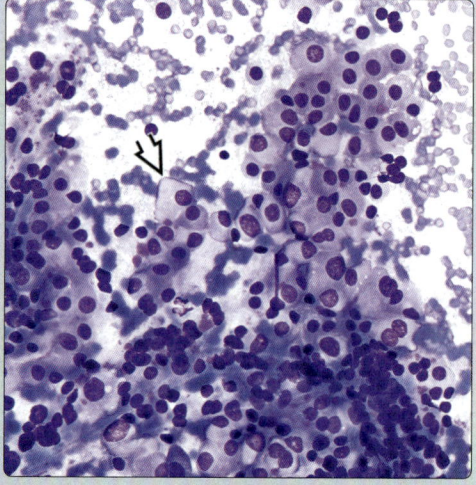

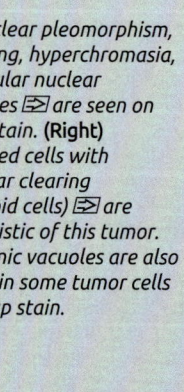

(Left) Nuclear pleomorphism, overlapping, hyperchromasia, and irregular nuclear membranes ➡ are seen on this Pap stain. (Right) Binucleated cells with perinuclear clearing (koilocytoid cells) ➡ are characteristic of this tumor. Cytoplasmic vacuoles are also observed in some tumor cells on this Pap stain.

Prominent Nuclear Atypia

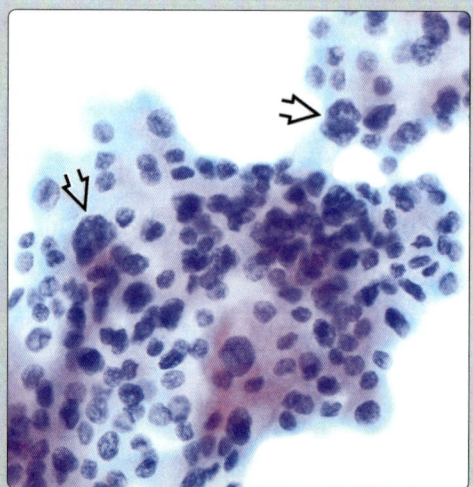

Koilocytoid Tumor Cells

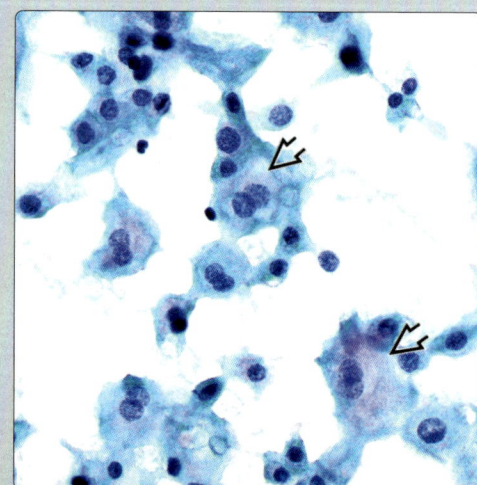

Chromophobe Renal Cell Carcinoma

CLINICAL ISSUES

Epidemiology
- 3rd most common subtype of renal cell carcinoma (RCC)
- Age range: 26-62 years (mean: 58 years)
- M:F = 1.5:1

Presentation
- Often incidental renal mass on imaging studies

Prognosis
- 5-year survival rate: 95%, better than clear cell RCC (CC-RCC) or papillary RCC

IMAGING

Radiographic Findings
- Circumscribed, hypovascular mass with central scar

CYTOPATHOLOGY

Cellularity
- Hypercellular aspirate

Pattern
- Trabecular arrangement, less cohesive than CC-RCC

Background
- Usually clean

Cells
- Large, round or polygonal cells with sharply defined cell borders (plant cell appearance)

Nuclear Details
- Central nuclei with prominent anisokaryosis, hyperchromasia, irregular outlines, grooves, binucleation, and small, indistinct nucleoli

Cytoplasmic Details
- Abundant vacuolated (fluffy) to granular cytoplasm
- Perinuclear vacuolated zone

Cell Block Findings
- Cords of tumor cells with well-delineated cytoplasmic borders, abundant granular cytoplasm, perinuclear clearing, and hyperchromatic and wrinkled nuclei

MACROSCOPIC

General Features
- Circumscribed mass, homogeneous beige cut surface

ANCILLARY TESTS

Histochemistry
- Hale colloidal iron: Diffuse cytoplasmic staining

Immunohistochemistry
- Positive: CK7, CD117, DOG1, MOC-31, PAX8, claudin-7
- Negative: RCC, CD10, vimentin, CA9, cyclin-D1, GST-α

Electron Microscopy
- Cytoplasmic microvesicles concentrated in perinuclear location; abundant mitochondria in eosinophilic cells

DIFFERENTIAL DIAGNOSIS

Renal Oncocytoma
- Uniform round nuclei, no koilocytoid change
- CK7[(-)/weak(+)], cyclin-D1(+), Hale colloidal iron stain (-)

Clear Cell Renal Cell Carcinoma, Eosinophilic Variant
- High nuclear grade with intricate vessels
- CK7(-), CD117(-), CD10(+), vimentin (+), RCC (+)

SELECTED REFERENCES
1. Moch H et al: Chromophobe renal cell carcinoma: current and controversial issues. Pathology. 53(1):101-8, 2021
2. Kucuk S et al: The diagnostic value of immunohistochemistry in the typing of renal tumors with eosinophylic cytoplasma. Bratisl Lek Listy. 121(9):663-9, 2020
3. Zhou J et al: Combined immunohistochemistry for the "three 7" markers (CK7, CD117, and claudin-7) is useful in the diagnosis of chromophobe renal cell carcinoma and for the exclusion of mimics: diagnostic experience from a single institution. Dis Markers. 2019:4708154, 2019

Anisokaryosis and Vacuolated Cytoplasm

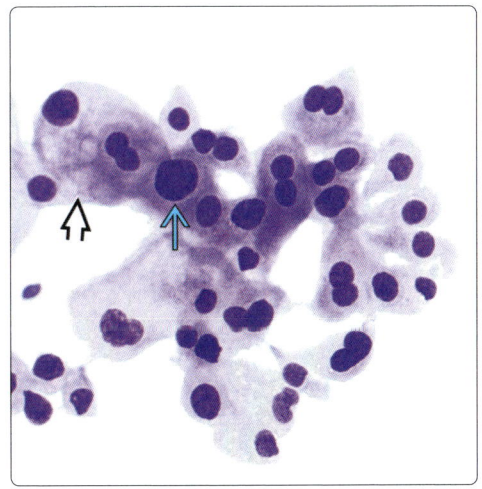

Diffusely Positive CK7

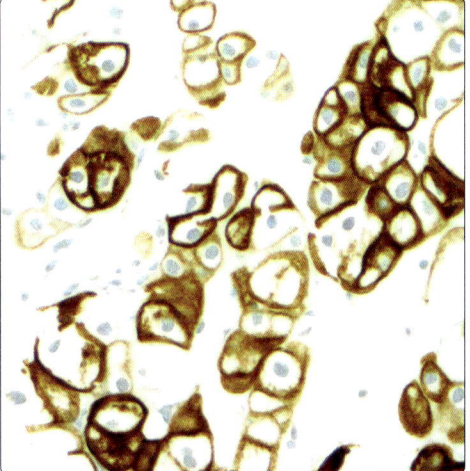

(Left) Diff-Quik stain demonstrates prominent anisokaryosis ⇨, sharply defined cell borders, and abundant granular to vacuolated cytoplasm ⇨. (Right) Diffusely positive CK7 helps differentiate this Ch-RCC from an oncocytoma.

TFE3- and TFEB-Rearranged Renal Cell Carcinomas

KEY FACTS

TERMINOLOGY
- Renal cell carcinoma (RCC) type defined by translocations involving *TFE3* or *TFEB*

CLINICAL ISSUES
- Comprises large percentage of pediatric RCC
- Much lower percentage of adult RCC (<4%)
- Overall, *TFE3* (Xp11) translocated tumors behave similarly to conventional RCC and are worse than papillary RCC
- *TFEB* translocated tumors are more indolent and typically organ confined

CYTOPATHOLOGY
- Loose cell aggregates or individual cells with papillary architecture including fibrovascular cores in some cases
- Focal tigroid background seen in Diff-Quik stains
- Psammoma bodies and hyaline globules may be seen
- Large cells with abundant coarsely vacuolated cytoplasm
- Irregular nuclei with nucleoli

ANCILLARY TESTS
- Pancytokeratin and EMA (-) or only focal (+)
- TFE3, CD10, RCC, AMACR usually (+) in Xp11 tumors
  - TFE3 nuclear stain may be difficult to interpret
- CD10 and RCC usually (-) or only focal (+) in *TFEB* tumors
- FISH testing to confirm translocations is key to diagnosis

TOP DIFFERENTIAL DIAGNOSES
- Conventional Clear Cell RCC
  - Pancytokeratin and EMA (+), AMACR and TFE3(-)
- Papillary RCC
  - Pancytokeratin (+) and TFE3 (-)
- Epithelioid Angiomyolipoma/PEComa
  - PAX8(-), CD68(+)

DIAGNOSTIC CHECKLIST
- Consider this entity in young patients
- Pancytokeratin is a useful screen: (-) or focal should prompt further investigation

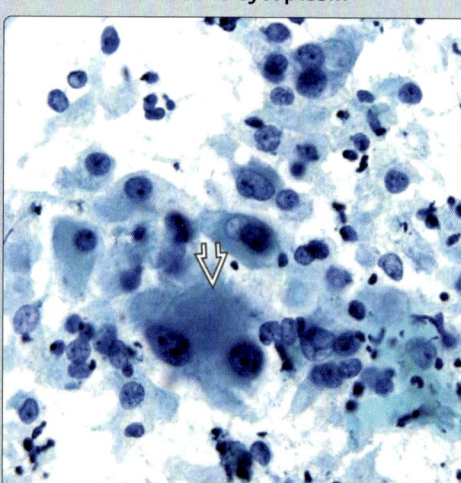

Abundant Cytoplasm

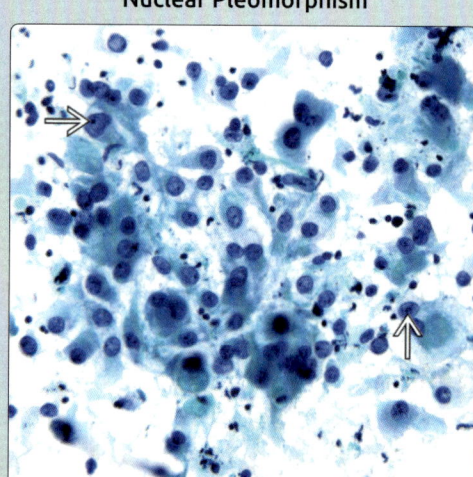

Nuclear Pleomorphism

(Left) This Pap-stained image of an Xp11 translocation renal cell carcinoma (RCC) shows loosely cohesive tumor cells with voluminous cytoplasm ➡ that exceeds what is typically seen in conventional RCC. (Courtesy P. Wakely, MD.) (Right) This Pap-stained low-power view of a cluster of Xp11 translocation RCC tumor cells highlights the nuclear size variability. The nuclei are round to oval with visible nucleoli ➡. The cytologic features extensively overlap with other more common types of RCC. (Courtesy P. Wakely, MD.)

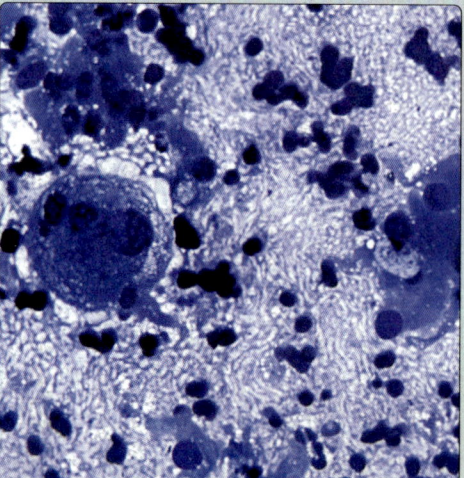

Tigroid Background

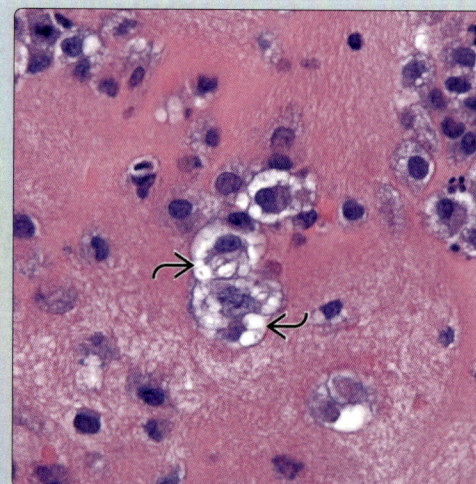

Vacuolated Cytoplasm on Cell Block

(Left) The stripe-like "tigroid" background that may be seen in Xp11 translocation RCC due to rupture of tumor cell cytoplasm is highlighted by the Diff-Quik stain, as in this example. (Courtesy P. Wakely, MD.) (Right) This H&E-stained cell block contains Xp11 translocation RCC tumor cells with abundant vacuolated cytoplasm ➡. The tumor cells are dyscohesive in the cell block, making identification of the characteristic architecture of this tumor type difficult in many cases. (Courtesy P. Wakely, MD.)

TFE3- and TFEB-Rearranged Renal Cell Carcinomas

TERMINOLOGY

Definitions
- Renal cell carcinoma (RCC) type defined by translocations involving *TFE3* or *TFEB*

CLINICAL ISSUES

Epidemiology
- Comprises large percentage of pediatric renal cell carcinomas (~ 40%)
- Much lower percentage of adult RCC (< 4%)

Prognosis
- Overall, *TFE3* (Xp11) translocated tumors behave similarly to conventional RCC; prognosis worse than papillary RCC
  - Specific translocation *ASPSCR1::TFE3* is associated with worst prognosis
- *TFEB* translocated tumors are more indolent and typically organ-confined

CYTOPATHOLOGY

Pattern
- Loose cell aggregates or individual cells with papillary architecture including fibrovascular cores in some cases

Background
- Focal tigroid background seen in Diff-Quik stains
- Psammoma bodies and hyaline globules may be seen

Cells
- Large cells with abundant coarsely vacuolated cytoplasm

Nuclear Details
- Irregular nuclei with nucleoli

MICROSCOPIC

Histologic Features
- *ASPSCR1::TFE3* carcinoma subset of Xp11 tumors
  - Voluminous cytoplasm with discrete cell borders
  - Psammoma bodies and hyaline globules common
- *PRCC::TFE3* carcinoma subset of Xp11 tumors
  - Less abundant cytoplasm
  - Few psammoma bodies or hyaline globules
- *TFEB* tumors
  - Abundant clear cytoplasm and well-defined cell borders
  - Often biphasic with a minor component of smaller cells clustered around hyaline basement membrane material
- Other rare types not as well defined, and features overlap even among more common types

ANCILLARY TESTS

Immunohistochemistry
- Pancytokeratin and EMA (-) or only focal (+)
- TFE3, CD10, RCC, AMACR usually (+) in Xp11 tumors
- CD10 and RCC usually (-) or only focal (+) in *TFEB* tumors

In Situ Hybridization
- FISH testing to confirm translocations is key to diagnosis

DIFFERENTIAL DIAGNOSIS

Conventional Clear Cell RCC
- Pancytokeratin and EMA (+); AMACR and TFE3(-)

Papillary RCC
- Pancytokeratin (+) and TFE3(-)

Epithelioid Angiomyolipoma/PEComa
- PAX8(-), CD68(+)

DIAGNOSTIC CHECKLIST

Pathologic Interpretation Pearls
- Consider this entity in young patients
- Pancytokeratin is useful screen: Focal or negative results should prompt further investigation

SELECTED REFERENCES
1. Akgul M et al: Diagnostic approach in TFE3-rearranged renal cell carcinoma: a multi-institutional international survey. J Clin Pathol. 74(5):291-9, 2021
2. Jin M et al: Cytopathology of Xp11 translocation renal cell carcinoma: a report of 5 cases. J Am Soc Cytopathol. 9(2):95-102, 2020

Histology of Xp11 Translocation Tumor
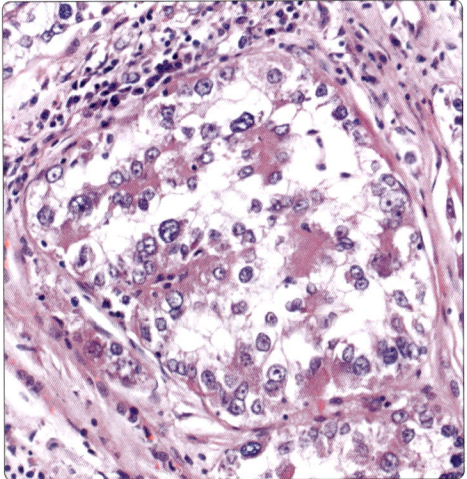

Histology of *TFEB* Translocation Tumor
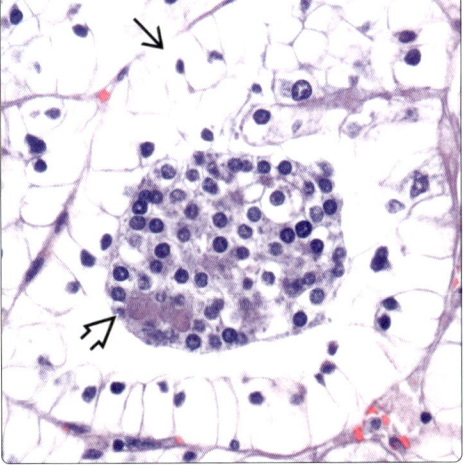

(Left) This histologic example of an Xp11 translocation RCC stained with H&E shows the voluminous clear cytoplasm and anisonucleosis also seen in corresponding cytology specimens. **(Right)** This H&E-stained histology example of a TFEB translocation RCC highlights the biphasic nature of the tumor with a mix of smaller, higher nuclear:cytoplasmic ratio cells ➡ and larger cells with abundant clear cytoplasm ➡. This biphasic pattern can sometimes be seen on corresponding cytology samples.

Collecting Duct Carcinoma

KEY FACTS

TERMINOLOGY
- a.k.a. carcinoma of collecting ducts of Bellini

CLINICAL ISSUES
- < 1% of malignant renal tumors; M:F ratio = 2:1
- Age range: 13-85 years (mean: < 50 years)
- Very aggressive; metastasis at diagnosis often
- Monosomies of chromosomes 1, 6, 14, 15, and 22

CYTOPATHOLOGY
- Hypercellular aspirate with necrotic background
- Dispersed small clusters, papillae, or tubules
- Marked pleomorphism, prominent nucleoli, irregular nuclear contours, and brisk mitoses
- Cytoplasmic vacuolization or mucin [Alcian blue or mucicarmine stains (+)]

MACROSCOPIC
- Medullary mass with necrosis and hemorrhage (1-15 cm)

MICROSCOPIC
- High-grade adenocarcinoma with predominant tubular morphology and marked desmoplasia

ANCILLARY TESTS
- Positive: PAX8, CK7, CEA, 34βE12, UEA-1
- Negative: CK20, AMACR, CA9, often p40/p63 and CD10

TOP DIFFERENTIAL DIAGNOSES
- Papillary renal cell carcinoma
  - Low-grade cytology with foamy macrophages
  - AMACR(+); 34βE12(-)
- Urothelial carcinoma with glandular features
  - Multilayered sheets with dense cytoplasm
  - PAX8 (-); p40/p63, GATA3 (+)
- Renal medullary carcinoma
  - Younger age (mean: 22 years); sickle cell trait
- Metastatic carcinomas
  - Clinical history and immunohistochemistry essential

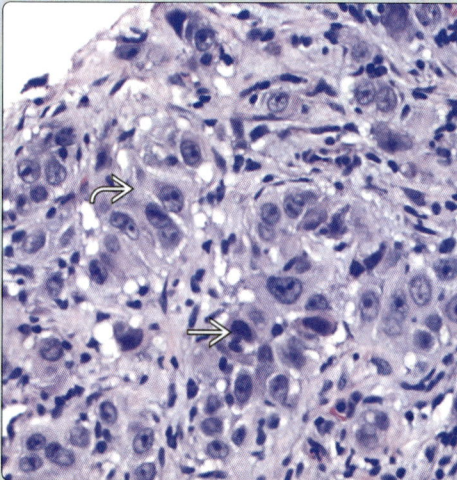

Core Needle Biopsy of Collecting Duct Carcinoma

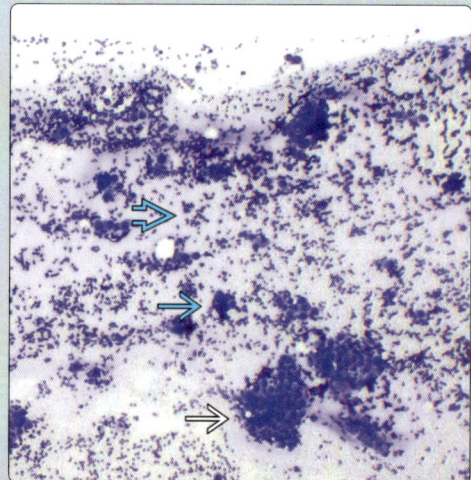

Touch Prep of Collecting Duct Carcinoma

(Left) H&E-stained section of CT-guided core needle biopsy shows highly malignant cells arranged in acini/tubules ➡ and cords ➡. (Right) Diff-Quik-stained touch prep of a core needle biopsy of a large renal mass at time of rapid onsite evaluation shows a cellular specimen with malignant cells arranged in large clusters ➡, acini ➡, and single malignant cells ➡.

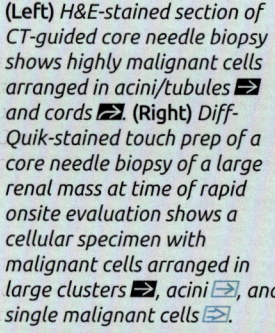

Pleomorphic Cells With Myxoid Stroma

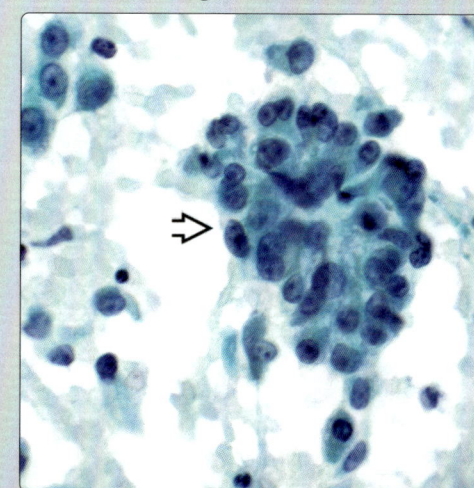

Tubular Configuration of Tumor Cells

(Left) Pap-stained FNA shows high-grade tumor cells arranged in small clusters ➡ and individual cells with myxoid stroma ➡ and a bloody background. (Right) Pap stain of an aspiration of a collecting duct carcinoma reveals a tubular structure ➡.

Renal Medullary Carcinoma

KEY FACTS

TERMINOLOGY
- Rapidly growing medullary tumor associated almost exclusively with sickle cell trait

CLINICAL ISSUES
- Rare renal tumor; occurs predominantly in young male patients of African descent
- Very aggressive tumor with mean survival of 4 months

CYTOPATHOLOGY
- Moderate cellularity with necrotic background
- Single cells, small loose clusters, or tubular pattern
- Uniformly high-grade cells with scant cytoplasm
- Hyperchromatic nuclei with irregular contours and prominent central nucleoli
- Occasional cytoplasmic granules or vacuoles

MACROSCOPIC
- Medulla-centered tumor (4-12 cm) often with satellite nodules, perihilar fat invasion, or tumor thrombi

MICROSCOPIC
- High-grade carcinoma with reticular or cribriform glands, desmoplasia, and inflammatory infiltrate

ANCILLARY TESTS
- Negative: SMARCB1 (INI1)
- Positive: PAX8, often CK7, pCEA, OCT3/4

TOP DIFFERENTIAL DIAGNOSES
- Wilms tumor
  - Sharply demarcated mass with triphasic pattern; WT1(+)
  - No hemoglobinopathy
- Yolk sac tumor
  - AFP, glypican-3, PAS-D (+)
  - No hemoglobinopathy
- Other high-grade malignancies
  - Difficult on cytology alone
  - Usually older age, no hemoglobinopathy

High-Grade Tumor Cells

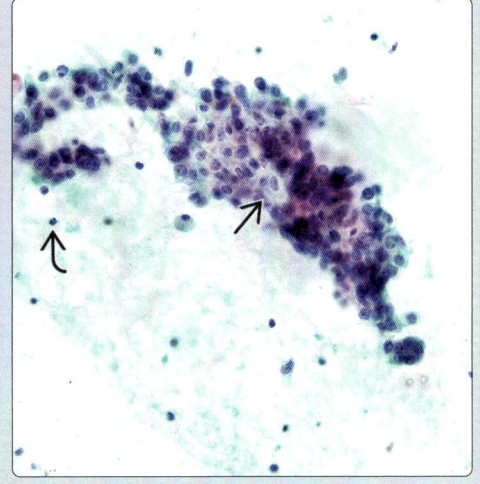

Cytoplasmic Vacuoles

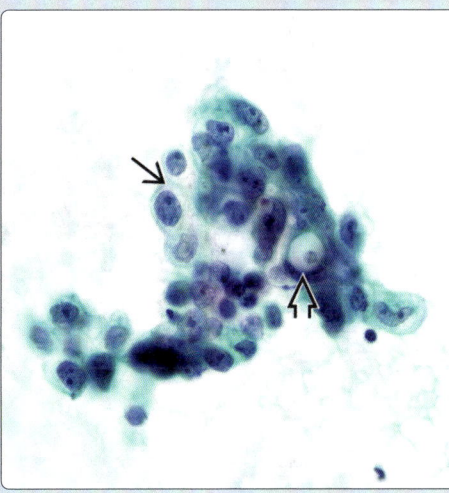

(Left) Medium magnification of a Pap-stained smear of renal medullary carcinoma demonstrates high nuclear:cytoplasmic ratio, round to oval nuclei, and prominent central nucleoli. Gland-like architecture ➡ and background neutrophils ➡ are seen. **(Right)** High magnification of Pap stain reveals clear cytoplasm ➡ with occasional cytoplasmic vacuoles ➡.

Intratumoral Neutrophils

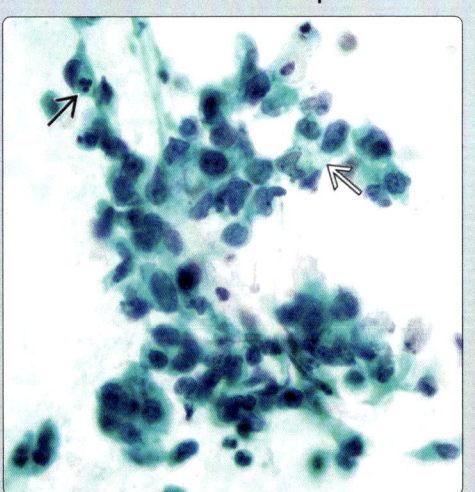

Pleomorphic Nuclei With Central Nucleoli

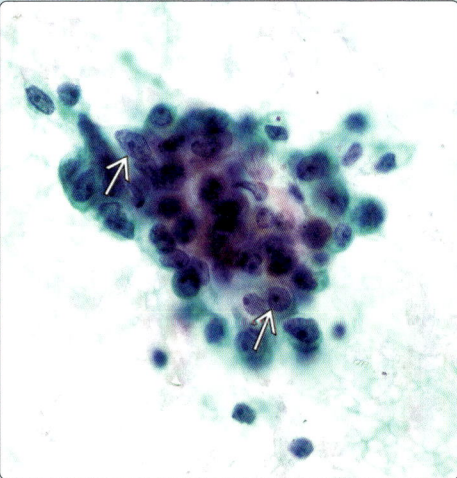

(Left) Renal medullary carcinoma on a Pap stain demonstrates pleomorphic tumor cells with clear to vacuolated cytoplasm ➡ and occasional intracytoplasmic neutrophils ➡. **(Right)** Typical nuclear features include round to oval nuclei with irregular nuclear membranes and prominent central nucleoli ➡, as seen on this Pap stain.

Mucinous Tubular and Spindle Cell Carcinoma of Kidney

KEY FACTS

TERMINOLOGY
- Renal epithelial neoplasm characterized by tubular formation merging with spindle cells and myxoid stroma

CLINICAL ISSUES
- < 1% of renal neoplasms
- Age: 13-81 years (mean: 58 years); M:F = 1:3
- Most patients have indolent clinical course

CYTOPATHOLOGY
- Hypercellular aspirate
- Clusters of relatively uniform round to spindled cells
- Bland nuclei with inconspicuous nucleoli
- Granular or clear cytoplasm, rarely vacuolated
- Abundant metachromatic myxoid matrix

MACROSCOPIC
- Well-circumscribed cortical mass with gray-yellow cut surface; 2-18 cm (mean: 4.2 cm)

MICROSCOPIC
- Slit-like tubules and bland spindle cells with basophilic extracellular mucin
- Typically low-grade, rarely high-grade tumors
- Metastasis or sarcomatoid transformation reported

ANCILLARY TESTS
- CK7, AMACR, PAX8 (+); CK20, CD10, RCC (-)
- Significant overlap with papillary renal cell carcinoma

TOP DIFFERENTIAL DIAGNOSES
- Sarcomatoid renal cell carcinoma
  - Usually high nuclear grade with epithelial component of specific type of renal cell carcinoma
- Primary renal sarcomas
  - Marked nuclear atypia without epithelial component
- Papillary renal cell carcinoma
  - Papillary architecture with foamy macrophages
  - Necrosis and hemorrhage; no stromal mucin

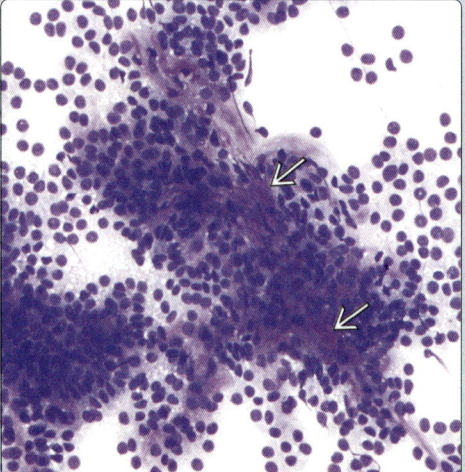

Epithelial Cells With Myxoid Stroma

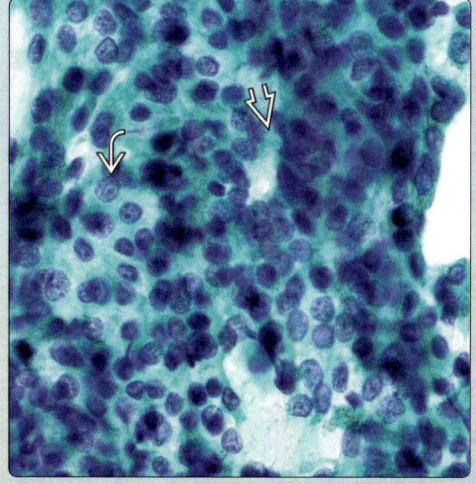

Epithelial (Tubular) Component

(Left) Diff-Quik stain shows cohesive clusters of round bland epithelial cells with abundant myxoid matrix ➡. *(Right)* Epithelial cells demonstrate round nuclei with smooth contours, finely granular chromatin, and small central nucleoli ➡. A vaguely glandular structure ➡ can also be seen on this Pap stain.

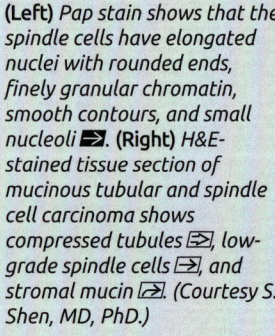

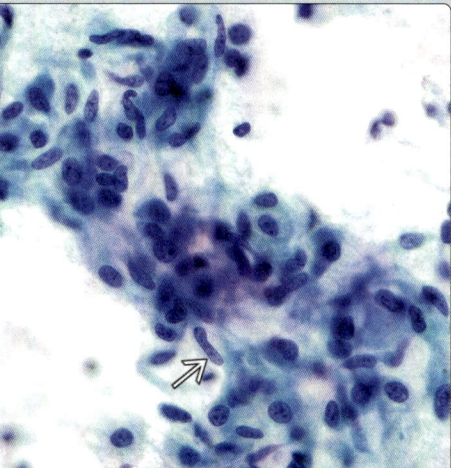

Spindle Cell Component

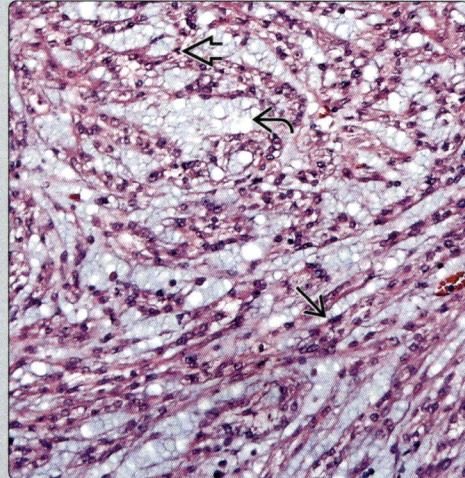

Histologic Features

(Left) Pap stain shows that the spindle cells have elongated nuclei with rounded ends, finely granular chromatin, smooth contours, and small nucleoli ➡. *(Right)* H&E-stained tissue section of mucinous tubular and spindle cell carcinoma shows compressed tubules ➡, low-grade spindle cells ➡, and stromal mucin ➡. (Courtesy S. Shen, MD, PhD.)

Carcinoid Tumor

KEY FACTS

CLINICAL ISSUES
- Exceedingly rare primary tumor of kidney
- Up to 20% arise in horseshoe kidneys
- Age range: 27-78 years (mean: 52 years)
- Flank pain, hematuria, or abdominal mass
- Not associated with carcinoid syndromes
- Protracted clinical course even with metastasis

CYTOPATHOLOGY
- Hypercellular aspirate with dispersed uniform cells
- Bloody background
- Plasmacytoid tumor cells often cling on blood vessels
- Moderate amount of granular cytoplasm
- Monotonous nuclei with finely stippled chromatin
- Mitoses are scant or absent

MACROSCOPIC
- Circumscribed solitary tumor; 2-17 cm (mean: 6.4 cm)
- Yellow cut surface, often with hemorrhage, no necrosis

- Perinephric fat invasion in 40% and lymph node metastasis in 1/3 of reported cases

ANCILLARY TESTS
- AE1/AE3, chromogranin, synaptophysin, CD56 (+); PAX8, WT1 (-)

TOP DIFFERENTIAL DIAGNOSES
- Renal oncocytoma
  - Coarsely granular cytoplasm with distinct cell borders; PAX8(+), neuroendocrine markers (-)
- Chromophobe renal cell carcinomas
  - Prominent nuclear irregularities, perinuclear halos; PAX8(+), neuroendocrine markers (-)
- Low-grade clear cell renal cell carcinomas
  - Prominent nuclear atypia, vacuolated cytoplasm; PAX8(+), neuroendocrine markers (-)
- Carcinoid tumor metastatic to kidney
  - Pertinent clinical history, often multifocal or lymphovascular tumor emboli

Dispersed Population of Uniform Cells
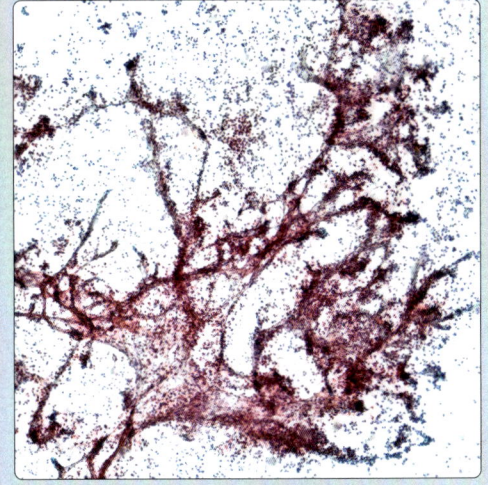

Tumor Cells Cling on Blood Vessels
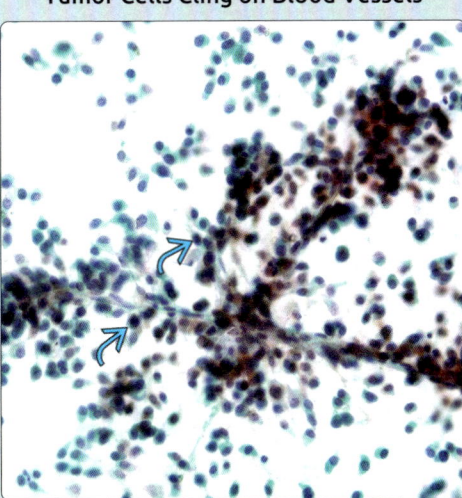

(Left) This Pap-stained aspirate of a renal carcinoid tumor shows a hypercellular smear with a dispersed population of uniform cells and abundant blood vessels. *(Right)* Tumor cells tend to cling on blood vessels ➡ with isolated cells spreading in the background, as displayed here with a Pap stain.

Plasmacytoid Tumor Cells
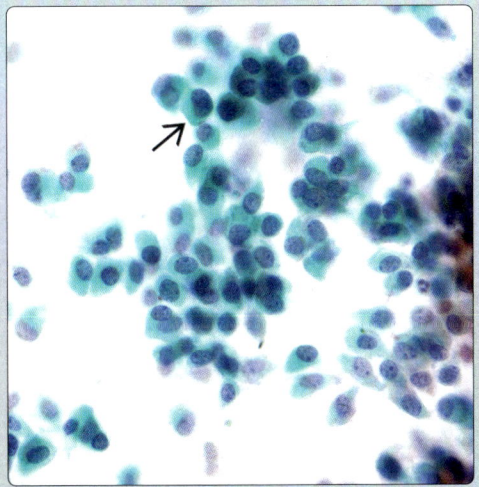

Typical Finely Stippled Chromatin
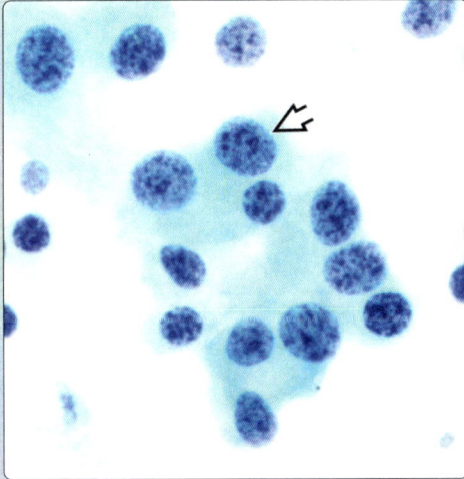

(Left) This Pap-stained smear contains numerous plasmacytoid tumor cells ➡ with a moderate amount of granular cytoplasm and eccentric, monotonous, round to oval nuclei. *(Right)* High magnification of a Pap-stained smear shows classic finely stippled chromatin and small nucleoli ➡. No mitosis or necrosis is seen.

Primary Renal Sarcomas in Adults

KEY FACTS

CLINICAL ISSUES
- Exceedingly rare (< 1% of primary renal neoplasms)
- Most common: Leiomyosarcoma (50-60% of cases)
- Uncommon: Synovial sarcoma, undifferentiated pleomorphic sarcoma, angiosarcoma

CYTOPATHOLOGY
- Cytologic features generally replicate their counterparts in soft tissue
- Atypical spindle cells are commonly seen in leiomyosarcoma, synovial sarcoma, and angiosarcoma
- Marked pleomorphism is observed in high-grade or dedifferentiated sarcomas

ANCILLARY TESTS
- Usually negative for cytokeratin and positive for specific markers of mesenchymal differentiation

TOP DIFFERENTIAL DIAGNOSES
- Sarcomatoid renal cell carcinoma
  - More common than primary sarcomas, presence of nonspindle neoplastic component; AE1/AE3, PAX8 (+)
- Angiomyolipoma
  - Triphasic elements: Adipocytes, smooth muscle, and dystrophic vessels; HMB-45, SMA (+)
- Mucinous tubular and spindle cell carcinoma
  - Low-grade, oval to spindle cells with myxoid matrix; CK7, AMACR, PAX8 (+); CK20, CD10, RCC (-)
- Metastatic malignant melanoma
  - Macronucleoli, pseudoinclusions, cytoplasmic projections, melanin pigment; Melan-A (+), AE1/AE3 (-)
- Poorly differentiated carcinomas
  - Cohesive epithelial component; AE1/AE3(+)

DIAGNOSTIC CHECKLIST
- Sarcomatoid differentiation in carcinoma is far more common than primary renal sarcomas
- Identifying epithelial component is critical in differential diagnosis

Renal Leiomyosarcoma
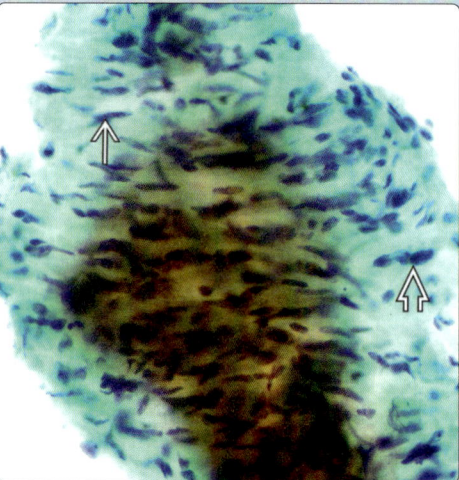

Renal Synovial Sarcoma
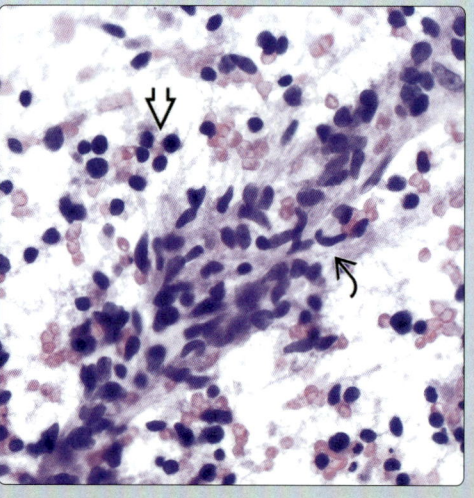

(Left) Leiomyosarcoma is the most common primary renal sarcoma and shows fascicular fragments of pleomorphic spindle cells ⇨ with cigar-shaped nuclei ⇨, as seen in this Pap-stained aspirate. (Right) This Diff-Quik-stained aspirate of a renal synovial sarcoma shows a loose fascicle of short, bland spindle cells ⇨ with naked nuclei in the background ⇨.

Renal Ewing Sarcoma
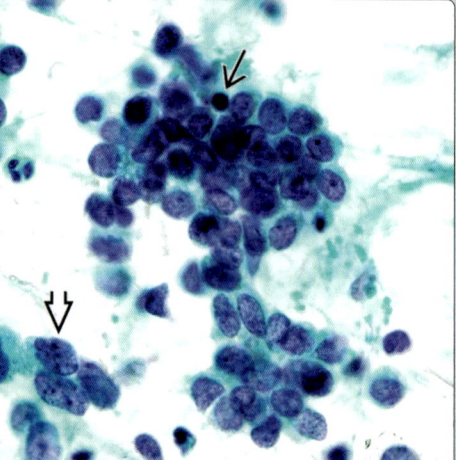

Renal Undifferentiated Pleomorphic Sarcoma
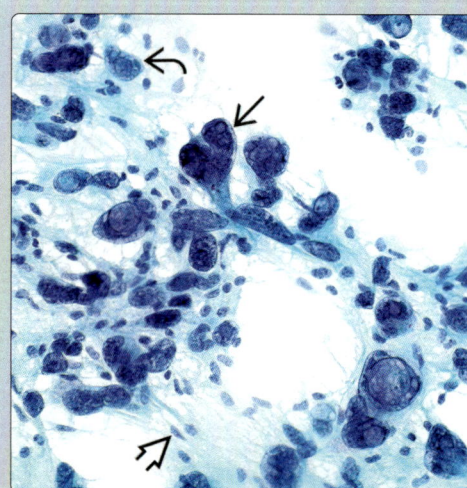

(Left) Pap-stained aspirate of Ewing sarcoma shows a mixed population of smaller dark cells ⇨ and larger pale cells ⇨ with nuclear molding. (Right) Pap-stained aspirate of renal undifferentiated pleomorphic sarcoma (malignant fibrous histiocytoma) shows bland fibroblasts ⇨, bizarre histiocyte-like cells ⇨, and anaplastic giant cells ⇨ in a myxoid background.

Renal Lymphomas

KEY FACTS

CLINICAL ISSUES
- Primary renal lymphoma (PRL) accounts for 1% of all renal lesions and 0.7% of all extranodal lymphomas
- Common PRL is Epstein-Barr virus (EBV)-associated posttransplant lymphoproliferative disorders (PTLD)
- Secondary renal lymphoma is 30x more common than PRL

CYTOPATHOLOGY
- Hypercellular aspirate
- Dispersed and uniform population of lymphocytes with scant cytoplasm
- Lymphoglandular bodies in background
- Nuclear atypia varies with lymphoma types

MACROSCOPIC
- Usually multiple, firm, homogeneous, pale nodules

MICROSCOPIC
- Diffuse infiltration, mass-forming, or intravascular patterns

ANCILLARY TESTS
- Flow cytometry is essential to confirm and subclassify lymphomas
- IHC on cell blocks may also be useful
- EBV in situ hybridization often positive in PTLD

TOP DIFFERENTIAL DIAGNOSES
- Infection and inflammation
  - Polymorphous population of inflammatory cells
  - No light chain restriction on flow cytometry or IHC
- Primary or metastatic epithelial tumors
  - Epithelial tumor cells usually dominant in specimen
  - Lack of background atypical lymphocytes or lymphoglandular bodies

DIAGNOSTIC CHECKLIST
- Key to correct diagnosis is to recognize atypical lymphocytes and lymphoglandular bodies
- Specimen should be prioritized for flow cytometry

Renal Follicular Lymphoma
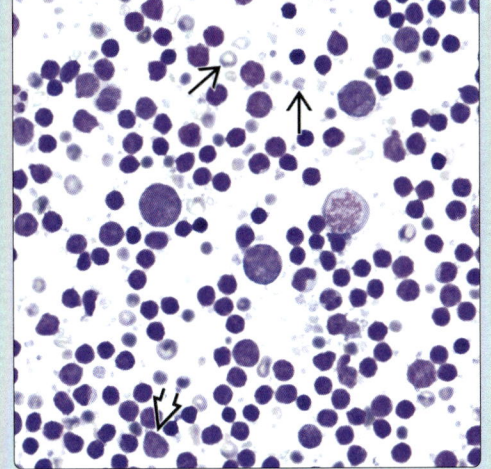

Renal Small Lymphocytic Lymphoma
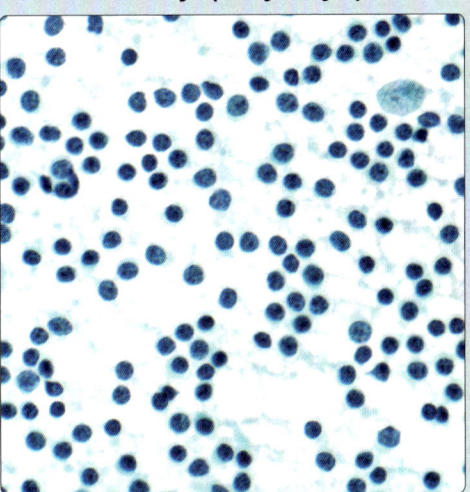

(Left) Diff-Quik-stained FNA of a renal follicular lymphoma shows medium-sized cells with irregular or cleaved nuclei ➡ and lymphoglandular bodies in the background ➡. (Right) Pap-stained small lymphocytic lymphoma shows monotonous population of slightly enlarged lymphocytes with coarse chromatin.

Renal Diffuse Large B-Cell Lymphoma
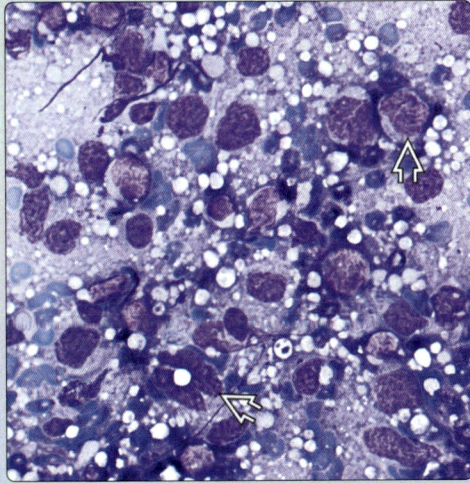

Ancillary Studies in Renal Posttransplant Lymphoproliferative Disorder
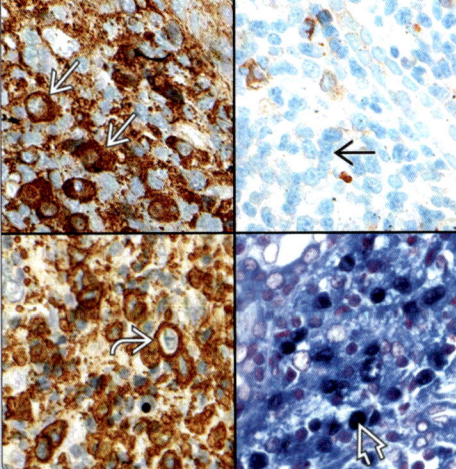

(Left) Diff-Quik-stained diffuse large B-cell lymphoma demonstrates large lymphocytes with pronounced nuclear irregularity ➡ and pleomorphism. (Right) Immunohistochemistry and in situ hybridization studies show the tumor cells in renal posttransplant lymphoproliferative disorder (PTLD) diffusely express κ-light chain ➡ with absence of λ-light chain stain ➡ and are positive for CD20 ➡ and Epstein-Barr virus in situ hybridization ➡.

Nephroblastoma (Wilms Tumor)

KEY FACTS

CLASSIFICATION
- Nephroblastoma (Wilms tumor) is malignant embryonal neoplasm derived from nephrogenic blastemal cells

CLINICAL ISSUES
- Affects 1 in 8,000 children; peak age: 2-3 years
- Accounts for 85% of pediatric renal malignancies
- 10% associated with syndromic conditions
- Overall survival > 90% with therapy

CYTOPATHOLOGY
- Hypercellular aspirate
- Chondromyxoid, necrotic, or inflammatory background
- Classically demonstrate triphasic components
  - Blastemal cells: Isolated or loose clusters of small round cells with scant cytoplasm and hyperchromatic nuclei
  - Epithelial cells: Tight clusters or tubules with moderate amount of cytoplasm, central nuclei, and fine chromatin
  - Stromal cells: Tight clusters of short spindle cells
- Anaplasia in 5%: Large pleomorphic cells, atypical mitoses

ANCILLARY TESTS
- Blastemal and epithelial cells: WT1(+), PAX8(+), CD56(+)

TOP DIFFERENTIAL DIAGNOSES
- Neuroblastoma
  - Pseudorosettes with fibrillar center (not true glands)
  - Neuropil background without triphasic pattern
- Clear cell sarcoma of kidney
  - Monotonous population, pale cytoplasm; no triphasic components; BCOR(+), WT1(-)
- Metanephric adenoma
  - Occurs in adults; no triphasic components; tight clusters, papillae, tubules, or rosettes; CD57 usually (-)

DIAGNOSTIC CHECKLIST
- FNA evaluation is reserved for patients with uncertain diagnosis or unresectable tumors
- Assessment of anaplasia is critical

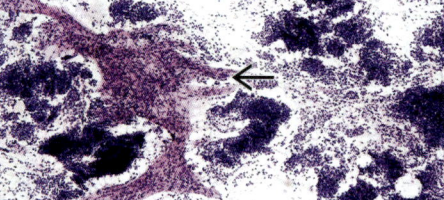

Mixed Blastemal and Stromal Cells

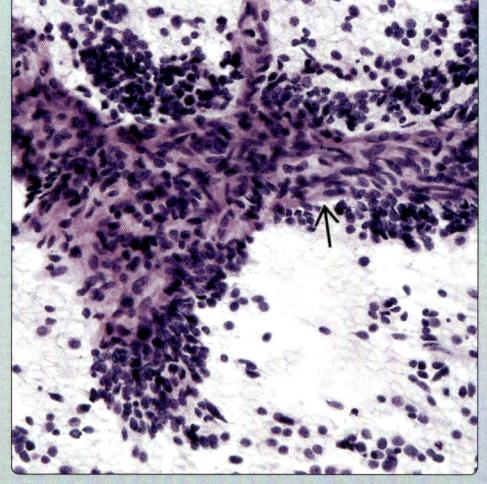

Short Spindled Stromal Cells

(Left) *FNA smear of a Wilms tumor is hypercellular and shows mixed blastemal ➡ and stromal ➡ components on a Diff-Quik stain.* (Right) *High magnification of the stromal component demonstrates closely packed, short spindle cells ➡ within a collagenous matrix on a Diff-Quik stain.*

Small Hyperchromatic Blastemal Cells

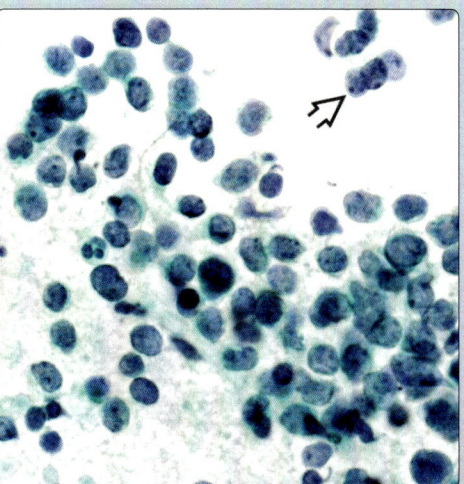

Epithelial Cells Forming Tubules

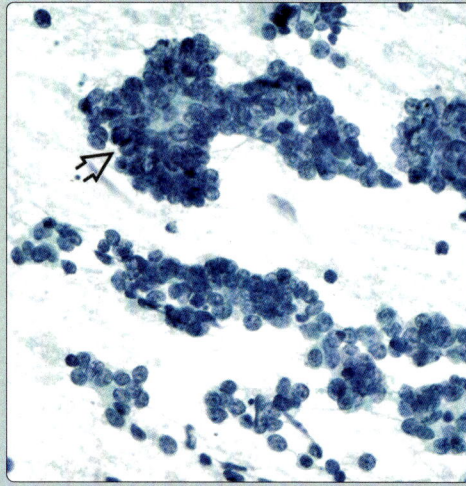

(Left) *Pap stain shows blastemal cells with scant cytoplasm, small round nuclei, fine chromatin, and inconspicuous nucleoli ➡.* (Right) *Pap stain shows an epithelial component forming a tubular structure ➡.*

Nephroblastoma (Wilms Tumor)

ETIOLOGY/PATHOGENESIS

Developmental Anomaly
- Malignant embryonal neoplasm derived from nephrogenic blastemal cells with divergent patterns of differentiation
- 10% associated with syndromic conditions
  - Denys-Drash, Beckwith-Wiedemann, Wilms tumor (WT), aniridia, genitourinary anomalies, and intellectual disability (WAGR) syndromes, and familial nephroblastoma
- Genetic abnormalities: *WT1* gene deletions or point mutations or *WT2* gene alterations

CLINICAL ISSUES

Epidemiology
- Affects 1 in 8,000 children
- Accounts for 85% of pediatric renal malignancies
- 98% aged < 10 years (peak: 2-3 years); very rare in adults

Presentation
- Abdominal mass, pain, hematuria, hypertension

Prognosis
- Excellent; overall survival > 90% with surgery and chemotherapy
- Unfavorable factors
  - High stage, diffuse anaplasia, presence of blastemal component in posttherapy tumor
  - Anaplasia (rare < 2 years of age)

CYTOPATHOLOGY

Cellularity
- Hypercellular aspirate

Pattern
- Typical triphasic tumor in 40%

Background
- Chondromyxoid matrix, necrosis, or inflammation

Cells
- **Blastemal cells** (most common): Isolated or loose clusters of small, round to oval cells
  - Cells with scant cytoplasm, hyperchromatic nuclei, fine chromatin, and inconspicuous nucleoli
- **Epithelial cells**: Tight clusters or tubules
  - Cells with moderate amount of cytoplasm, central nuclei, and fine chromatin
- **Stromal cells**: Tight clusters of short spindle cells
  - May differentiate into skeletal or smooth muscle
  - Rhabdomyoblasts may be seen
- Anaplasia seen in 5% of WT with pleomorphic cells, marked hyperchromasia, and atypical mitoses

ANCILLARY TESTS

Immunohistochemistry
- Blastemal and epithelial cells: WT1(+), PAX8(+), CD56(+)
- Epithelial cells: AE1/AE3 (+), vimentin (-)

DIFFERENTIAL DIAGNOSIS

Neuroblastoma
- Pseudorosettes with fibrillar center (not true glands)
- Neuropil background, lack of triphasic components

Clear Cell Sarcoma of Kidney
- Monotonous population, pale wispy cytoplasm, no triphasic components, BCOR(+), WT1(-)

Metanephric Adenoma
- Occurs in adults; no triphasic components; tight clusters, papillae, tubules, or rosettes; CD57 usually (-)

SELECTED REFERENCES
1. Gupta S et al: Diagnostic accuracy and cytomorphological spectrum of Wilms tumour in fine needle aspiration biopsy cytology samples supplemented with cell blocks. Pediatr Blood Cancer. 68(7):e28996, 2021
2. Parsons LN: Wilms tumor: challenges and newcomers in prognosis. Surg Pathol Clin. 13(4):683-93, 2020
3. Treece AL: Pediatric renal tumors: updates in the molecular Era. Surg Pathol Clin. 13(4):695-718, 2020

WT1 Expression in Nephroblastoma

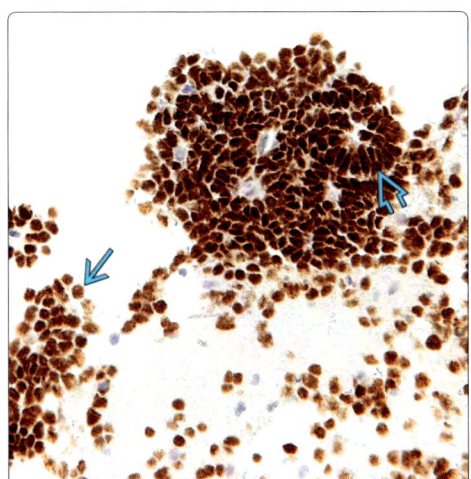

Anaplastic Nephroblastoma With *TP53* Overexpression

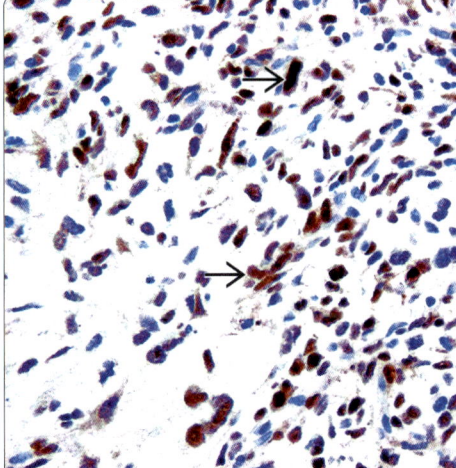

(Left) Both the epithelial ➡ and blastemal ➡ components are WT1 positive on immunostaining. (Right) Anaplastic nephroblastomas often show TP53 gene mutations, corresponding to immunohistochemical overexpression ➡. Mutations of TP53 gene have been associated with resistance to chemotherapy.

Clear Cell Sarcoma of Kidney

KEY FACTS

CLASSIFICATION
- Rare pediatric sarcoma of uncertain histogenesis with aggressive behavior and frequent bone metastasis

CLINICAL ISSUES
- Peak at 2-3 years of age; M:F = 2:1
- Comprises 3% of pediatric renal tumors
- Large renal mass; hematuria, hypertension
- Aggressive tumor; 70% survival with combined therapy

CYTOPATHOLOGY
- Cellular smear with dyscohesive cells
- Scant to abundant pale, wispy cytoplasm
- Round to oval nuclei with fine chromatin and small nucleoli
- Loose myxoid matrix may be present

MICROSCOPIC
- Classic pattern (90%): Chicken-wire vasculature, cords of polygonal cells, pale mucopolysaccharide-like material
- Variants: Myxoid, sclerosing, trabecular, anaplastic

ANCILLARY TESTS
- Positive: BCL6 corepressor (BCOR), vimentin, BCL2, cyclin-D1, NGFR
- Negative: AE1/AE3, EMA, WT1, CD99, CD34, S100
- BCOR ITD (85%); *YWHAE::NUTM2B/E* fusion (12%)

TOP DIFFERENTIAL DIAGNOSES
- Blastema-predominant Wilms tumor
  - Scant cytoplasm, hyperchromasia, coarse chromatin, WT1(+)
- Primitive neuroectodermal tumor
  - Small blue cells, pseudorosettes, CD99(+), FLI-1(+)
- Congenital mesoblastic nephroma
  - Spindle or polygonal cells with small nucleoli, SMA(+)
- Rhabdoid tumor of kidney
  - Large cells, abundant dense cytoplasm, macronucleoli, brisk mitoses, loss of SNF5 (INI1)

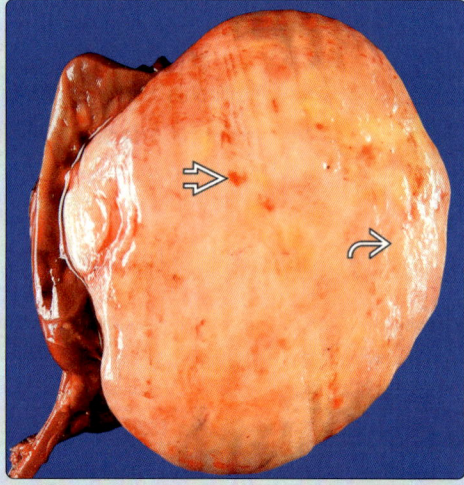
Large Well-Circumscribed Renal Mass

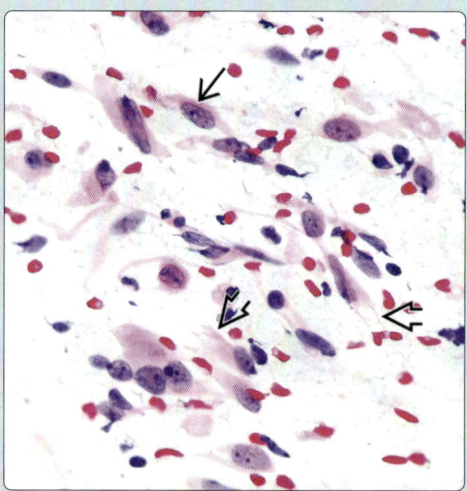
Tumor Cells With Pale Wispy Cytoplasm

(Left) Gross photograph of clear cell sarcoma of the kidney (CCSK) shows a large, well-circumscribed renal mass with a solid, tan-gray, glistening, and gelatinous cut surface ⇨ with focal hemorrhage ⇨. **(Right)** Touch imprint shows tumor cells with round to oval nuclei, fine chromatin, small nucleoli ⇨, and pale, wispy cytoplasm ⇨. (Courtesy V. Singh, MD.)

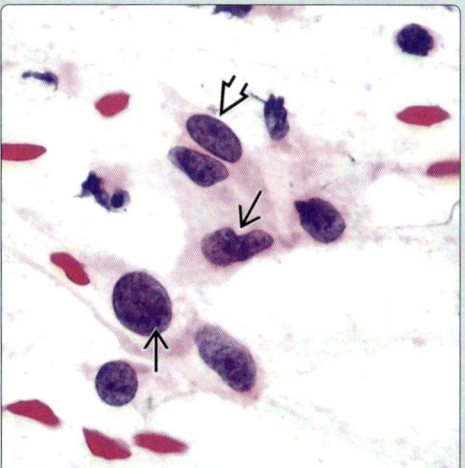
Nuclear Membrane Irregularity

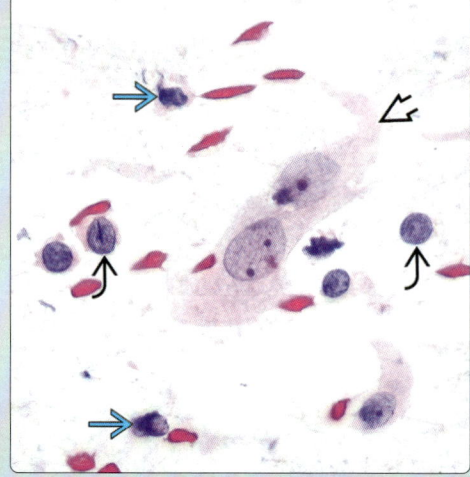
Delicate Cytoplasm and Nuclear Grooves

(Left) High magnification shows round to oval nuclei, occasional nuclear notches or grooves ⇨, fine chromatin, and inconspicuous to small nucleoli ⇨. **(Right)** Touch imprint of CCSK demonstrates tumor cells with delicate and pale cytoplasm ⇨. Small pyknotic cells (probably degenerated tumor cells) ⇨ and occasional stripped nuclei (some with nuclear grooves) ⇨ are seen in the background.

Clear Cell Sarcoma of Kidney

TERMINOLOGY

Abbreviations
- Clear cell sarcoma of kidney (CCSK)

ETIOLOGY/PATHOGENESIS

Molecular Genetics
- Internal tandem duplications (ITD) in BCL6 corepressor (*BCOR*) in 85%; t(10;17)(q22;p13) translocation creating fusion gene *YWHAE::NUTM2B/E* (12%)

CLINICAL ISSUES

Epidemiology
- CCSK comprises 3% of pediatric renal tumors
- Age: 2 months to 14 years (peak: 2-3 years); M:F = 2:1

Presentation
- Large, unicentric renal mass; hematuria, hypertension

Treatment
- Combined therapy: Unilateral nephrectomy, adjuvant chemotherapy, and tumor bed radiation therapy

Prognosis
- Aggressive tumor; 70% survival with combined therapy
- Metastasize to renal hilar lymph node, bone, lung, and brain

CYTOPATHOLOGY

Cellularity
- Variable cellularity

Pattern
- Tumor cells arranged singly or in small, perivascular clusters

Background
- Loose myxoid matrix may be present

Cells
- Cord cells: Large, polygonal tumor cells with abundant wispy cytoplasm and eccentric nuclei
- Septal cells: Spindle stromal cells
- Pyknotic cells: Degenerating tumor cells

Nuclear Details
- Round, oval, or bean-shaped nuclei with fine chromatin and inconspicuous to small nucleoli

MACROSCOPIC

General Features
- Well-circumscribed, tan-gray, glistening or gelatinous mass (2.3-24 cm) with occasional cystic changes or necrosis

MICROSCOPIC

Microscopic Features
- Classic pattern (90%): Chicken-wire vasculature, cords of polygonal cells, pale mucopolysaccharide-like material

ANCILLARY TESTS

Immunohistochemistry
- Positive: BCOR, vimentin, BCL2, cyclin-D1, NGFR
- Negative: AE1/AE3, EMA, WT1, CD99, CD34, desmin, S100

DIFFERENTIAL DIAGNOSIS

Blastema-Predominant Wilms Tumor
- Scant cytoplasm, hyperchromatic nuclei, molding, WT1(+)

Ewing/Primitive Neuroectodermal Tumor
- Small blue cells, pseudorosettes, CD99(+), FLI-1(+)

Congenital Mesoblastic Nephroma
- Spindle or polygonal cells with small nucleoli, SMA(+)

Rhabdoid Tumor of Kidney
- Abundant dense cytoplasm, brisk mitoses, SNF5 (INI1) (-)

SELECTED REFERENCES
1. Aldera AP et al: Clear cell sarcoma of the kidney. Arch Pathol Lab Med. 144(1):119-23, 2020

Histologic Features
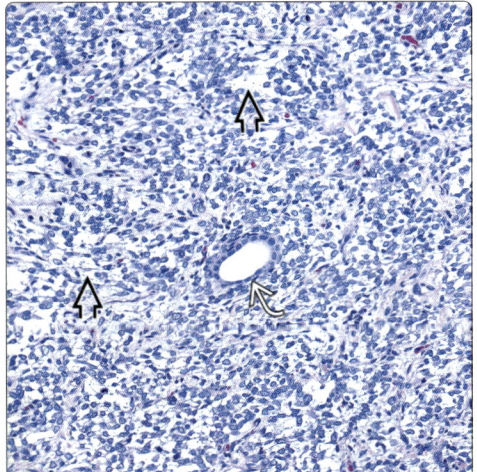

BCOR Immunohistochemistry
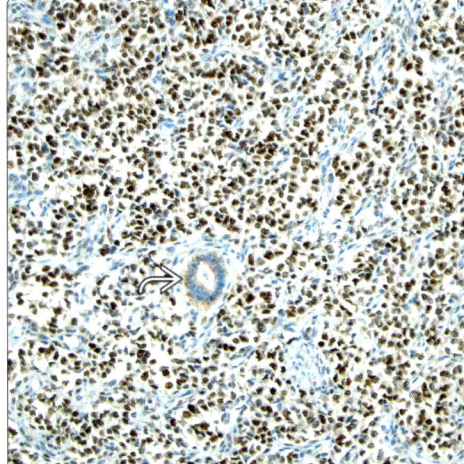

(Left) H&E-stained CCSK section shows cords of polygonal cells surrounded by abundant pale mucopolysaccharide material, simulating clear cytoplasm ➡. An entrapped renal tubule is seen in this field ➡. (Courtesy M. Reyes-Múgica, MD.) **(Right)** BCOR shows diffuse nuclear staining in tumor cells of CCSK. As internal control, an entrapped renal tubule is negative ➡. (Courtesy M. Reyes-Múgica, MD.)

Congenital Mesoblastic Nephroma

KEY FACTS

CLASSIFICATION
- Low-grade fibroblastic neoplasm of infantile kidney
- 3 types: Classic (24%), cellular (66%), and mixed (10%)

CLINICAL ISSUES
- Most common renal tumor in first 3 months of life
- Abdominal mass; may have hypertension
- Surgical resection leads to cure in most patients

CYTOPATHOLOGY
- Dyscohesive cells or loose clusters
- Clean background with naked nuclei in classic type
- Plump spindle cells or tadpole-shaped cells
- Oval nuclei with smooth contours and small nucleoli
- Delicate and fragile cytoplasm

MACROSCOPIC
- Classic type: Firm, whorled, gray-white
- Cellular type: Soft, fleshy, hemorrhagic, cystic

MICROSCOPIC
- Classic type: Intersecting spindle cells with minimal atypia
- Cellular variant: Dense cellular spindle cells with pushing border and active mitosis

ANCILLARY TESTS
- Vimentin (+), SMA(+), CD34(-), WT1(-), pan-CK(-), BCOR(-)

TOP DIFFERENTIAL DIAGNOSES
- Metanephric stromal tumor
  - Bland spindle cells with wispy cytoplasm, CD34(+)
- Clear cell sarcoma of kidney
  - Delicate cytoplasm, fine chromatin, small nucleoli, BCOR(+), SMA(-)
- Wilms tumor (particularly post therapy)
  - Rare in infants, triphasic components, necrosis, WT1(+)
- Rhabdoid tumor of kidney
  - Large tumor cells, abundant cytoplasm, macronucleoli, brisk mitoses, loss of SNF5 (INI1) (-)

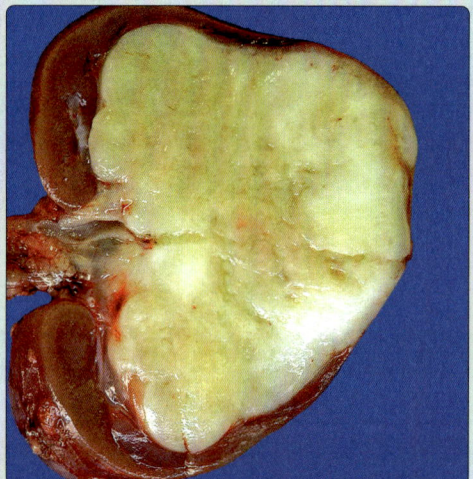

Lobulated Fibrous Renal Mass

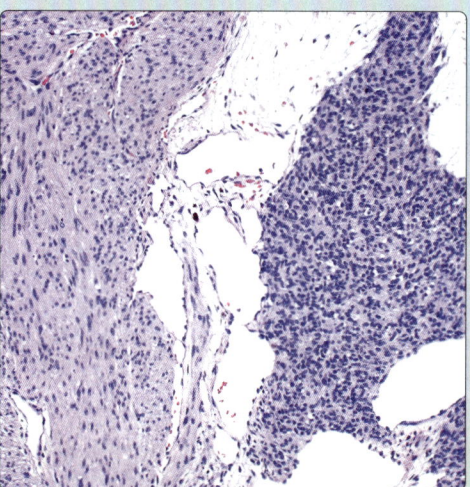

Histologic Features of Congenital Mesoblastic Nephroma

(Left) Gross photograph of classic-type congenital mesoblastic nephroma shows a solitary and lobulated renal mass with gray-white fibrous cut surface. *(Right)* Mixed classic (left) and cellular (right) congenital mesoblastic patterns are seen on this intermediate power.

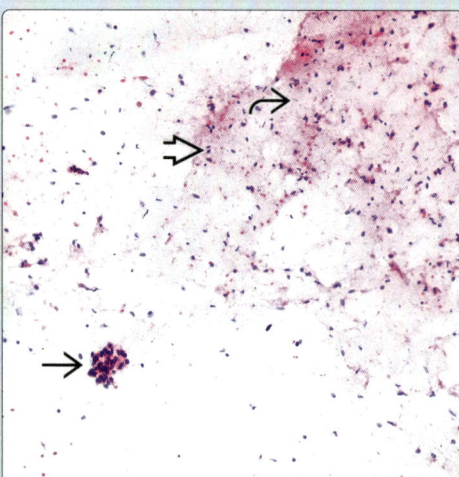

Bland Oval Cells

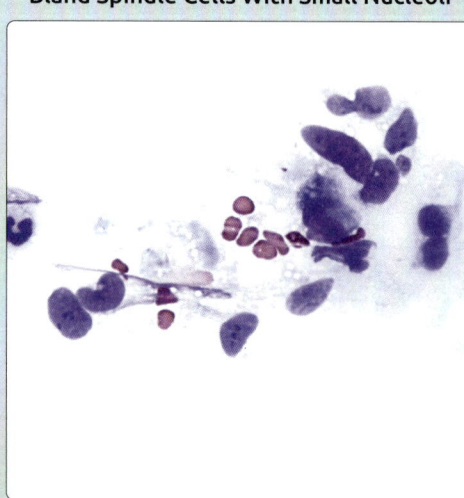

Bland Spindle Cells With Small Nucleoli

(Left) H&E-stained touch imprint shows a cluster of oval cells ➡ and many single cells ➡ in a granular background ➡, consistent with necrosis. (Courtesy V. Singh, MD.) *(Right)* Diff-Quik-stained aspirate smear shows bland spindle cells, isolated or in small clusters, with evenly dispersed chromatin and small nucleoli.

Congenital Mesoblastic Nephroma

TERMINOLOGY

Definitions
- Low-grade fibroblastic neoplasm of infantile kidney

ETIOLOGY/PATHOGENESIS

Genetic Features
- Cellular type: t(12;15)(p13;q25) resulting in *ETV6::NTRK3* gene fusion (similar to infantile fibrosarcoma)
- Classic type: *EGFR* internal tandem duplications

CLINICAL ISSUES

Epidemiology
- Most common renal tumor in first 3 months of life
- ~ 90% of tumors occur within 1 year of age

Presentation
- Abdominal mass; may have hypertension
- May be associated with polyhydramnios, premature delivery, and nonimmune hydrops
- Excellent outcome with tumor resection in most patients

CYTOPATHOLOGY

Cellularity
- Classic type is hypocellular with naked nuclei
- Cellular type shows richly cellular smears
- Dyscohesive cells or loose clusters

Cells
- Plump spindle cells or tadpole-shaped cells
- Oval nuclei with smooth contours and small nucleoli
- Delicate and fragile cytoplasm
- Active mitoses in cellular type

MACROSCOPIC

General Features
- Classic type: Firm, whorled, gray-white cut surface
- Cellular type: Soft, fleshy, hemorrhagic, or cystic

MICROSCOPIC

Histologic Features
- Classic type (24%): Intersecting spindle cells with extensive infiltration, minimal atypia, and rare mitoses (resembles fibromatosis)
- Cellular variant (66%): Dense cellularity with pushing border and numerous mitoses (resembles infantile fibrosarcoma)
- Mixed (10-20%): Shows combined features

ANCILLARY TESTS

Immunohistochemistry
- Vimentin (+), SMA(+), CD34(-), WT1(-), pan-CK(-), BCOR(-)

DIFFERENTIAL DIAGNOSIS

Metanephric Stromal Tumor
- Spindled to stellate, bland and uniform stromal cells with wispy cytoplasm; CD34(+)

Clear Cell Sarcoma of Kidney
- Delicate pale cytoplasm, round to oval nuclei, fine chromatin, and inconspicuous nucleoli; BCOR(+), SMA(-)

Nephroblastoma (Wilms Tumor)
- Very rare in infants; triphasic components; often necrosis; rare anaplasia; WT1(+)

Rhabdoid Tumor of Kidney
- Large tumor cells with abundant cytoplasm, macronucleoli, and brisk mitoses; SNF5 (INI1) (-)

SELECTED REFERENCES

1. Treece AL: Pediatric renal tumors: updates in the molecular era. Surg Pathol Clin. 13(4):695-718, 2020
2. Zhao M et al: Congenital mesoblastic nephroma is characterized by kinase mutations including EGFR internal tandem duplications, ETV6-NTRK3 fusion, and rare KLHL7-BRAF fusion. Histopathology. ;77(4):611-21, 2020
3. Lau HD et al: Evaluation of diagnostic accuracy and a practical algorithmic approach for the diagnosis of renal masses by FNA. Cancer Cytopathol. 126(9):782-96, 2018

Plump Naked Nuclei
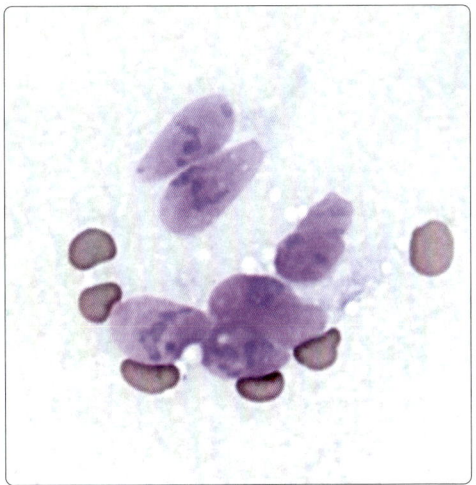

FISH Demonstrates t(12;15) Translocation
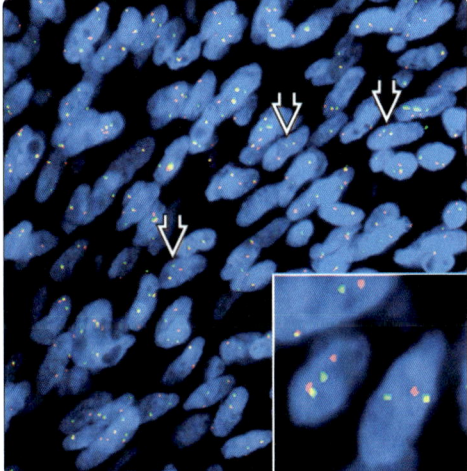

(Left) Diff-Quik-stained aspirate smear shows a clean background and plump naked nuclei with relatively smooth nuclear membranes and small nucleoli. **(Right)** FISH assay on smear demonstrates ETV6 gene break-apart pattern ➡ resulting from the t(12;15) in a mesoblastic nephroma. (Courtesy D. Lopez-Terrada, MD, PhD.)

Rhabdoid Tumor of Kidney

KEY FACTS

ETIOLOGY/PATHOGENESIS
- Inactivation or loss of *SMARCB1* (SNF5/INI1) tumor suppressor gene

CLINICAL ISSUES
- Epidemiology
  - Accounts for 2% of pediatric renal tumors
  - Most patients younger than 2 years (80%)
- Presentation
  - Highly aggressive pediatric renal tumor
  - Abdominal mass, hematuria, fever, hypercalcemia
  - Frequent metastases and 75% present with high stage
  - Mortality rate > 80% within 2 years of diagnosis

CYTOPATHOLOGY
- Hypercellular smear with dispersed monomorphic population of large cells and brisk mitoses
- Large, eccentric, round to oval nuclei
- Vesicular chromatin and macronucleoli
- Abundant dense cytoplasm with eosinophilic hyaline inclusions
- Background necrosis is common

MACROSCOPIC
- Large tumors with hemorrhage and necrosis (mean: 9.6 cm)

ANCILLARY TESTS
- Cytokeratin, vimentin (+); SNF5 (INI1) (-)

TOP DIFFERENTIAL DIAGNOSES
- Renal medullary carcinoma
  - Mean age: 22 years; sickle cell trait, inflammatory background
- Clear cell sarcoma of kidney
  - Pale cytoplasm, no cytoplasmic hyaline inclusions or macronucleoli; SNF5 (INI1), BCOR (+)
- Cellular mesoblastic nephroma
  - Spindle cells, no cytoplasmic hyaline inclusions or macronucleoli; SNF5 (INI1) (+)

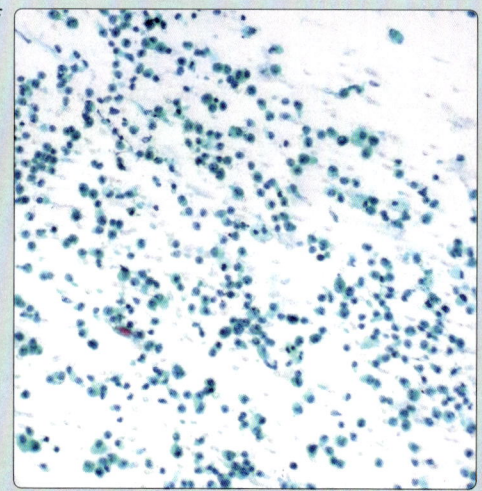
Hypercellular Aspirate

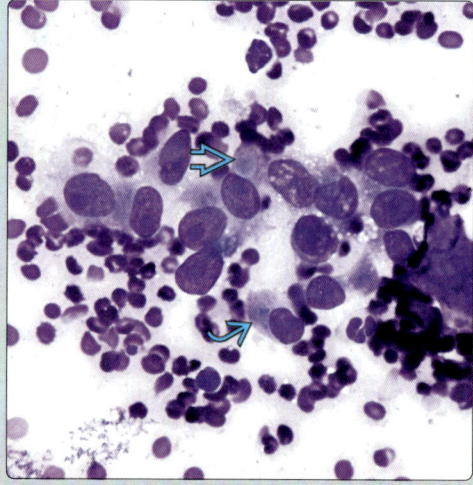
Intracytoplasmic Hyaline Inclusions

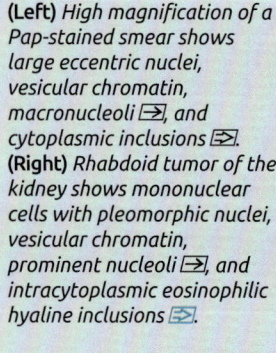

(Left) Fine-needle aspiration of rhabdoid tumor is hypercellular with a homogeneous population of large tumor cells, as seen in this Pap-stained smear. (Right) Diff-Quik stain demonstrates nuclei with macronucleoli, dense eccentric cytoplasm ➡, and intracytoplasmic inclusions with hyaline appearance ➡.

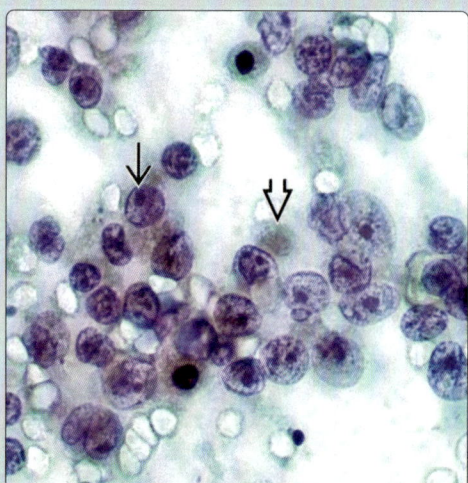
Eccentric Nuclei With Macronucleoli

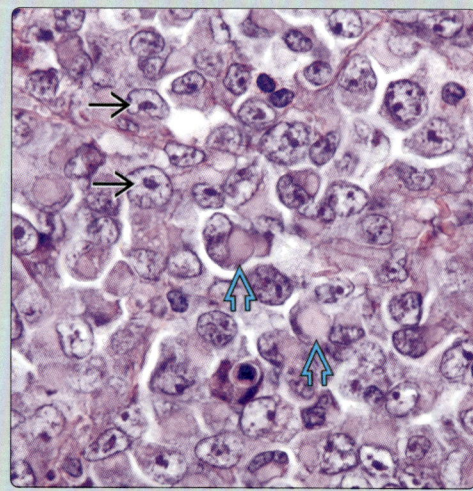
Histology Features

(Left) High magnification of a Pap-stained smear shows large eccentric nuclei, vesicular chromatin, macronucleoli ➡, and cytoplasmic inclusions ➡. (Right) Rhabdoid tumor of the kidney shows mononuclear cells with pleomorphic nuclei, vesicular chromatin, prominent nucleoli ➡, and intracytoplasmic eosinophilic hyaline inclusions ➡.

Metastatic Tumors to Kidney

KEY FACTS

CLINICAL ISSUES
- Up to 21% of malignant renal tumors on FNA are metastatic
- Lung is most common primary site

CYTOPATHOLOGY
- Common tumors: Adenocarcinoma, squamous cell carcinoma, small cell carcinoma, and melanoma
- Often high-grade tumor cells but lack usual features of renal cell carcinoma (RCC) or urothelial carcinoma

TOP DIFFERENTIAL DIAGNOSES
- Tumors with clear or oncocytic cells
  - Tumors of lung, breast, or salivary gland tumors
  - Lack of complex vasculatures, often higher nuclear:cytoplasmic ratios
- Tumors with low nuclear:cytoplasmic ratio
  - Adrenal cortical carcinoma, hepatocellular carcinoma, and anaplastic carcinoma of lung or pancreas
  - Distinction is challenging; pertinent history and immunohistochemistry is essential
- Collecting duct carcinoma
  - Desmoplasia and glandular structures simulate metastatic tumors
  - Clinical history and typical immunoprofile helpful

DIAGNOSTIC CHECKLIST
- Clinical history and radiologic findings are essential during cytologic evaluation
- Review of previous cytology and histology material (if available) can be helpful
- Unusual cytologic features for RCC or urothelial carcinoma should always alert one to consider metastatic tumors
- Primary renal tumors usually have unique immunoprofiles, as do many metastatic tumors, which can be very useful
- Cell block should be obtained whenever feasible for possible immunohistochemistry and molecular testing

Metastatic Squamous Carcinoma of Lung
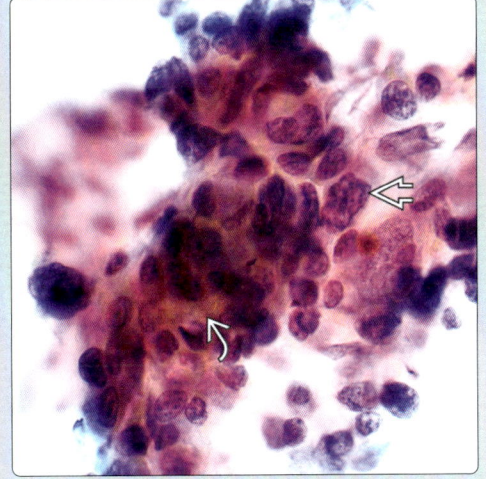

Metastatic Adenocarcinoma of Colon
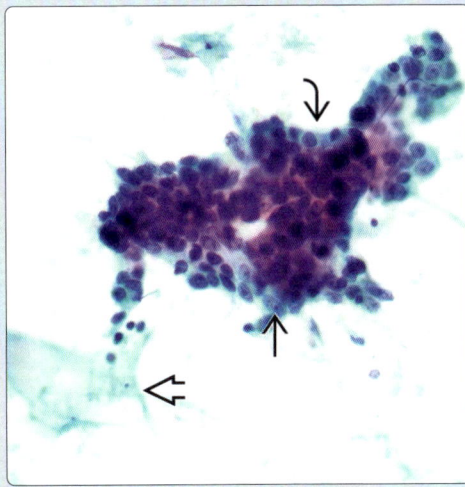

(Left) Pap stain of a metastatic lung squamous cell carcinoma shows cohesive tumor cells with marked nuclear atypia ➔ and dense orangeophilic cytoplasm ➔. Urothelial carcinoma with squamous differentiation could look similar; history is essential. (Right) Pap stain of a metastatic colon adenocarcinoma shows a 3D cluster with community borders ➔, glandular formation, prominent nucleoli ➔, and background mucin ➔.

Metastatic Melanoma
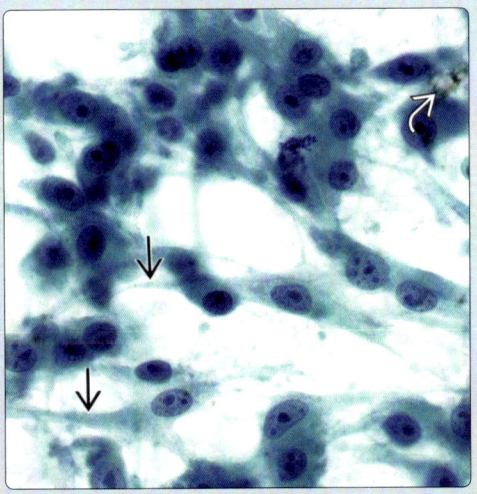

Metastatic Papillary Thyroid Carcinoma
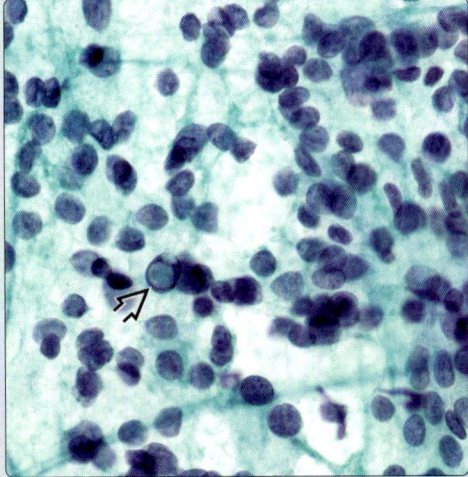

(Left) Pap stain of a metastatic melanoma shows neuron-like cytoplasmic projections ➔, macronucleoli, mitoses, and melanin pigment ➔. (Right) Pap stain of a metastatic papillary thyroid carcinoma shows nuclear overlapping, grooving, powdery chromatin, and intranuclear pseudoinclusions ➔.

Urothelial Carcinoma

KEY FACTS

CLINICAL ISSUES
- 5-10% of renal tumors, 90% of pelvicalyceal tumors
- Mean age: 67-70 years
- More common in male patients (M:F = 1.7-2:1)

IMAGING
- Obstructive mass with filling defect

CYTOPATHOLOGY
- Hypercellular aspirate
- Dense or squamoid cytoplasm, well-defined borders
- Low-grade urothelial carcinoma
  - Multilayered sheets or papillae
  - Nuclei with granular chromatin, small nucleoli
- High-grade urothelial carcinoma
  - Isolated markedly atypical cells
  - Nuclei with dark, clumpy chromatin, irregular contours, and prominent nucleoli
  - Necrosis in background

MOLECULAR
- Chromosome 9 deletions, *FGFR3* mutations

ANCILLARY TESTS
- Positive for GATA3, p40, p63, CK7, CK20 (focal), 34βE12
- Negative for PAX8, RCC, vimentin

TOP DIFFERENTIAL DIAGNOSES
- Collecting duct carcinoma
  - High-grade cytology, absent of multilayer sheets or dense cytoplasm
  - PAX8(+), GATA3(-), p40/p63(-)
- High-grade renal cell carcinoma
  - Abundant vacuolated cytoplasm, relatively low nuclear:cytoplasm ratio
  - PAX8(+), RCC(+), GATA3(-), p40/p63(-)
- Metastatic carcinoma
  - Often multifocal tumor with interstitial growth
  - Clinical history and immunohistochemistry essential

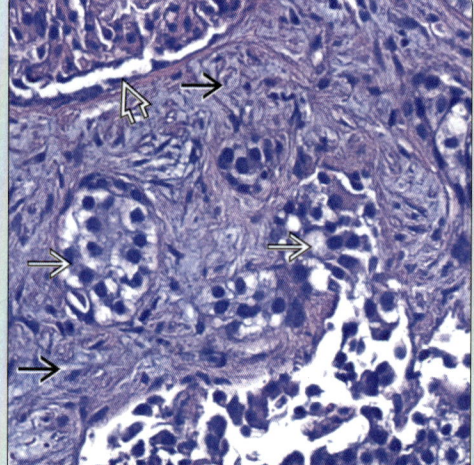

Urothelial Carcinoma and Normal Glomerulus

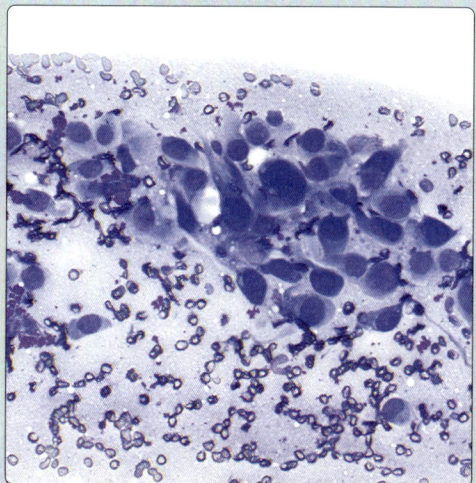

Dense Cytoplasm With Defined Border

(Left) H&E-stained section of a renal mass core needle biopsy shows infiltrating nests of malignant cells ➡ in the renal cortex. Note the bluish, desmoplastic stromal response ➡ and the intact glomerulus ➡. (Right) High magnification demonstrates polygonal cells with well-defined borders, dense cytoplasm, round to oval nuclei, and small nucleoli, as seen on this Diff-Quik stain. (Courtesy of B. Gorman, MD.)

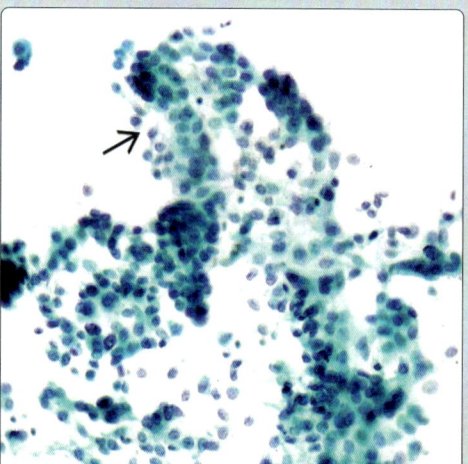

Papillary Configuration in Low-Grade Urothelial Carcinoma

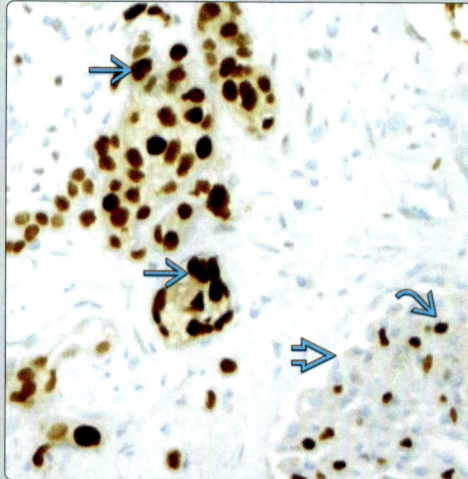

GATA3(+) Urothelial Carcinoma in Kidney

(Left) Aspiration of a low-grade urothelial carcinoma shows loosely cohesive clusters of tumor cells with vague papillary configurations ➡, as seen on this Pap stain. (Right) Immunohistochemistry shows GATA3(+) (nuclear) stain in the tumor cells ➡. The background glomerular cells are negative ➡ with the exception of lymphocytes in glomeruli ➡.

Urothelial Carcinoma

ETIOLOGY/PATHOGENESIS

Risk Factors
- Associated with toxin exposure (e.g., aromatic amines, tobacco, phenacetin) and lower urinary tract cancers

Molecular Features
- Chromosome 9 deletions, *FGFR3* mutations
- Microsatellite instability (loss of MLH1 and MSH2) associated with high-grade urothelial carcinoma in male patients

CLINICAL ISSUES

Epidemiology
- 5-10% of renal tumors, 90% of pelvicalyceal tumors
- Age: 34-93 years (mean: 67-70 years)
- More common in male patients (M:F = 1.7-2:1)

Presentation
- Flank pain, hematuria

Treatment
- Nephroureterectomy in high-grade or high-stage tumors

Prognosis
- 5-year survival: > 99% for pTa, 91% for pT1, 72% for pT2, 40% for pT3, and 16% for those with metastasis

IMAGING

Radiographic Findings
- Obstructive mass with filling defect

CYTOPATHOLOGY

Cellularity
- Hypercellular aspirate

Pattern
- Multilayered sheets or papillae (often in low-grade) or isolated high-grade tumor cells

Background
- Necrosis seen in high-grade tumors

Cells
- Polygonal or elongated cells with well-defined borders

Nuclear Details
- Low grade: Granular chromatin, small nucleoli
- High grade: Irregular nuclei, coarse chromatin, pleomorphism, prominent nucleoli, or sarcomatoid change

Cytoplasmic Details
- Dense, eosinophilic, or squamoid appearance

ANCILLARY TESTS

Immunohistochemistry
- Positive: GATA3, p40, p63, CK7, CK20 (focal), 34βE12, CEA
- Negative: PAX8, RCC, vimentin

DIFFERENTIAL DIAGNOSIS

Collecting Duct Carcinoma
- High grade, no multilayer sheets or dense cytoplasm
- PAX8(+), GATA3(-), p40(-), p63(-)

High-Grade Renal Cell Carcinoma
- Abundant vacuolated cytoplasm with low nuclear:cytoplasmic ratio
- PAX8(+), RCC(+), CD10(+); GATA3(-), p40/p63(-)

Metastatic Carcinomas
- Multifocality, interstitial growth, often high-grade tumors
- Clinical history and immunohistochemistry can be helpful

SELECTED REFERENCES

1. Agaimy A et al: Undifferentiated and dedifferentiated urological carcinomas: lessons learned from the recent developments. Semin Diagn Pathol. 38(6):152-62, 2021
2. Joseph JP et al: Percutaneous image-guided core needle biopsy for upper tract urothelial carcinoma. Urology. 135:95-100, 2020
3. Ponce-Zepeda J et al: Touch preparation for rapid onsite evaluations of renal mass biopsies: concordance rate, pearls, and pitfalls. J Am Soc Cytopathol. 9(5):422-8, 2020

Nuclear Atypia in High-Grade Urothelial Carcinoma

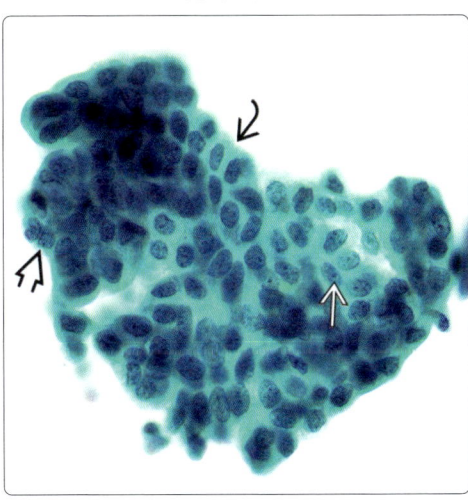

Sarcomatoid Change in High-Grade Urothelial Carcinoma

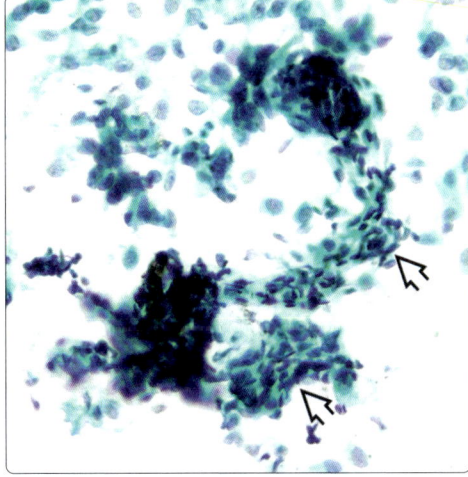

(Left) Pap stain of a high-grade urothelial carcinoma shows dense cytoplasm, well-defined cell borders ➡, high nuclear:cytoplasmic ratio, nuclear hyperchromasia, irregular nuclear contours ➡, and prominent nucleoli ➡. *(Right)* Spindle cell morphology (sarcomatoid change) ➡ can be observed in high-grade tumors, as seen on this Pap stain.

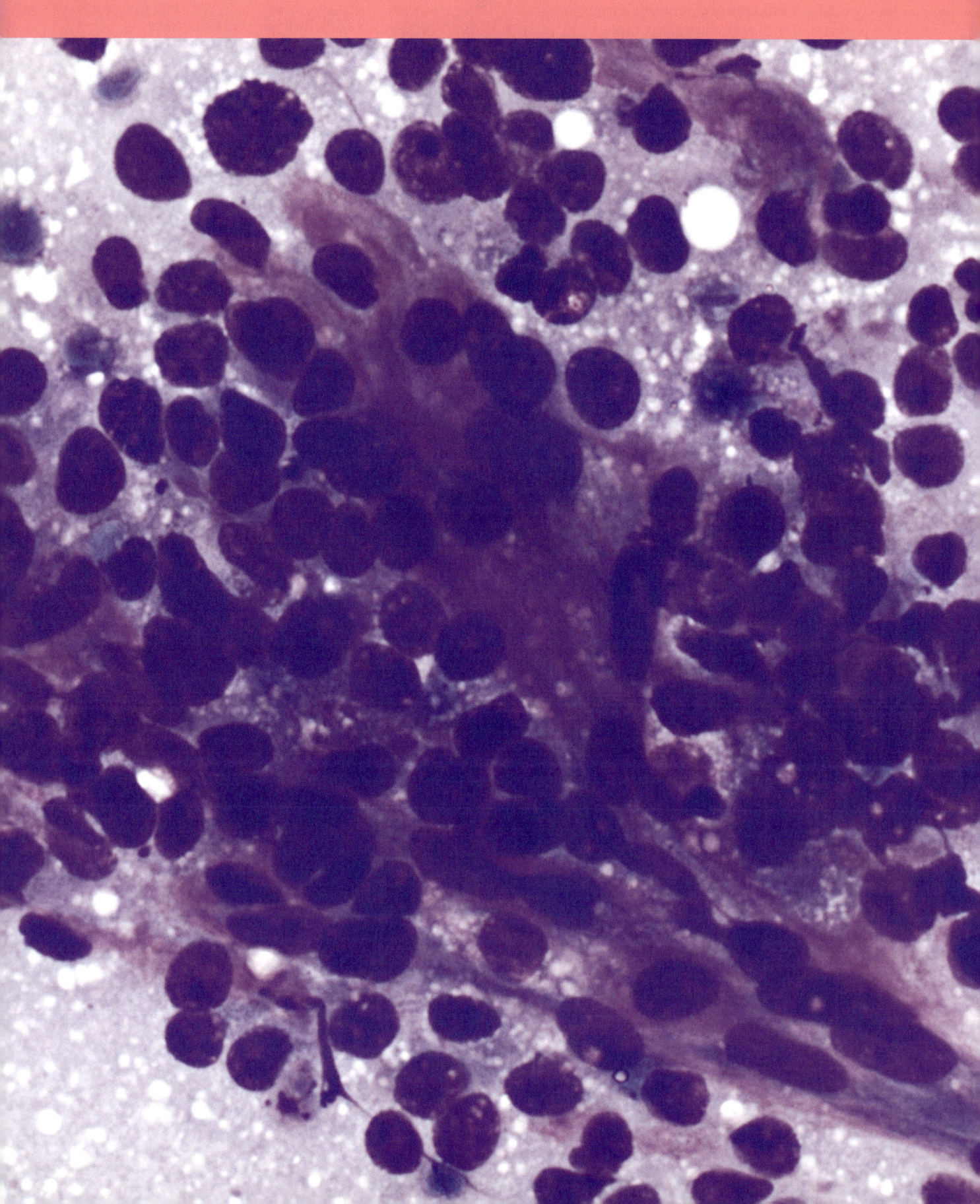

PART IV
SECTION 5
Adrenal Gland

Overview
Cytology of Normal Adrenal Gland 558

Adrenal Cortical Lesions
Adrenal Cortical Adenoma 560
Adrenal Cortical Carcinoma 562
Metastatic Tumors to Adrenal Gland 564

Adrenal Medullary Lesions
Pheochromocytoma 566

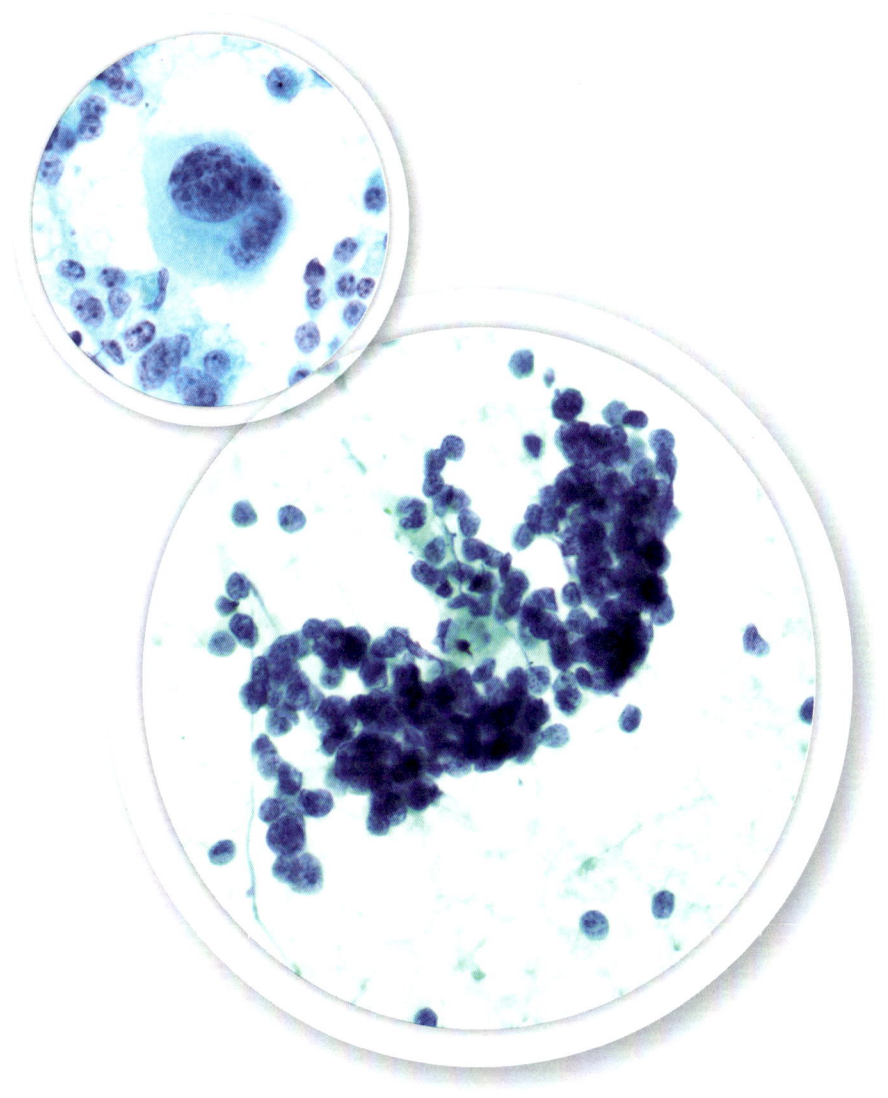

Cytology of Normal Adrenal Gland

MACROSCOPIC

General Features

- Weight
  - Combined weight of adrenal glands in adults is 4-8 grams
- Shape
  - In adults, right adrenal gland is pyramidal and left is crescentic

MICROSCOPIC

General Features

- Cortex in adult adrenal gland has 3 zones
  - Zona glomerulosa: Outer zone with lobular clusters of lipid-rich cells that produce mineralocorticoid hormones
  - Zona fasciculata: Largest zone with radial cords of lipid-rich cells that produce glucocorticoid
  - Zona reticularis: Inner zone consisting of small lipid-depleted cells that produce sex steroid
- Medulla consists of chromaffin cells arranged in nests, anastomosing cords, or solid sheets

ADRENAL FNA BIOPSY

Clinical Indications for Adrenal FNA

- Tumor staging for patients with known malignant tumor of other organs, mostly lung carcinomas
- Diagnosis of adrenal masses incidentally detected by imaging studies (incidentalomas)
- Investigate adrenal lesions suggested by clinical and radiologic presentations

Accuracy of Diagnosis

- Accuracy for primary adrenal lesions has been reportedly as high as 97-98%
- Specificity for malignancy is nearly 100% (excellent negative predictive value)

Specimen Collection and Preparation

- Procedure
  - Adrenal FNA is commonly performed by radiologists under CT or ultrasound guidance to ensure adequate sampling

Uniform Cells With Bubbly Background

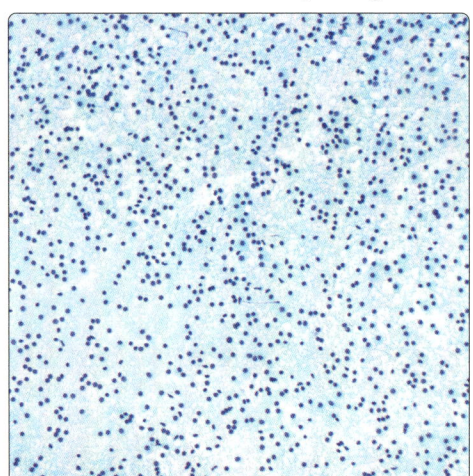

Cells of Zona Glomerulosa and Fasciculata

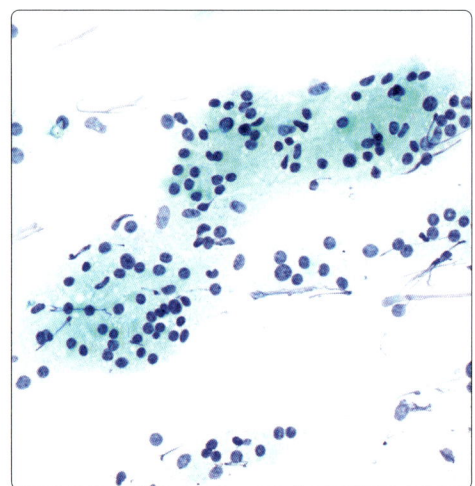

(Left) Pap-stained FNA of a normal adrenal gland shows dispersed uniform cells with stripped nuclei. The bubbly background containing abundant lipid-rich material is characteristic. (Right) Pap stain shows cells of zona glomerulosa and fasciculata with foamy or clear cytoplasm and indistinct cell borders.

Cells of Zona Reticularis

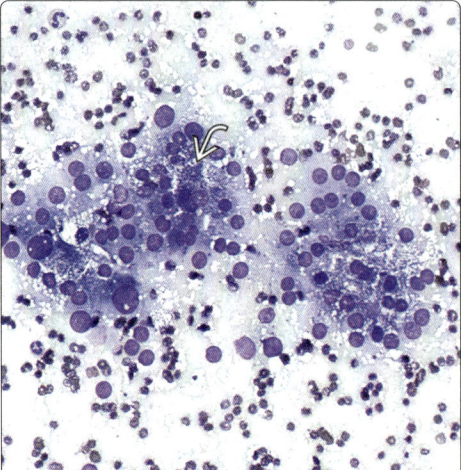

Stripped Nuclei of Adrenal Cortical Cells

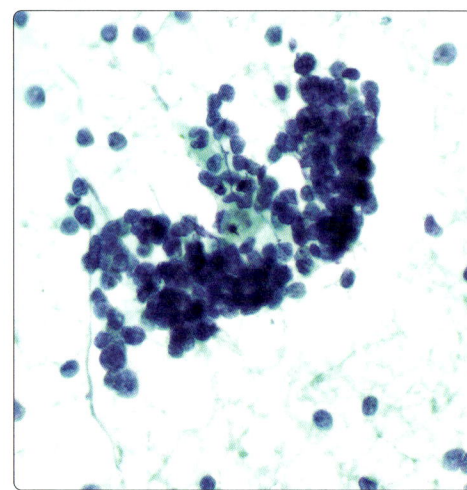

(Left) Diff-Quik stain displays cells from zona reticularis with less voluminous cytoplasm containing lipofuscin pigment 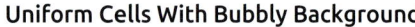. (Right) Pap stain shows clusters of stripped nuclei of adrenal cortical cells with nuclear crowding and overlapping, simulating malignant tumors, such as metastatic small cell carcinoma.

Cytology of Normal Adrenal Gland

- Endoscopic ultrasound (EUS)-guided FNA of adrenal glands is alternative modality
  - Left adrenal gland can be sampled via stomach
  - Right adrenal gland can be sampled via duodenum
- Cytology preparation
  - Simultaneous air-dried (for Diff-Quik stain) and wet-fixed (for Pap stain) preparations are recommended
  - Diff-Quik stain provides valuable background cytologic information that is often absent on Pap stain
  - Intraprocedure adequacy check is essential to ensure sufficient diagnostic material
  - Whenever feasible, cell block should be obtained for possible immunohistochemical or molecular testing

Complications and Contraindications

- Pheochromocytoma
  - Hypertensive crisis has been reported during aspiration of adrenal pheochromocytoma
  - Expert emergency personnel and facilities should be available at procedure site
- Anticoagulation medication (such as aspirin) should be discontinued 7-10 days before procedure
- Rare complications
  - Hematuria, bradycardia, hypotension, pneumothorax, and hemothorax

CYTOPATHOLOGY

Cellularity

- FNA of normal adrenal gland produces scattered, small clusters of uniform cells

Pattern

- Small clusters or cords
- Bare nuclei can be seen

Background

- Usually bloody
- Background of bubbly lipid material
  - Diff-Quik stain highlights lipid
- No necrosis

Cells

- Commonly from zona glomerulosa and zona fasciculata
  - Uniform polygonal cells with foamy, lipid-rich cytoplasm
- Cells from zona reticularis
  - Compact cyanophilic cytoplasm often containing lipofuscin pigment

Nuclear Details

- Centrally located, uniform, round to oval nuclei with fine chromatin and distinct nucleoli
  - Endocrine atypia consisting of focal nuclear enlargement, pleomorphism, and prominent nucleoli can be seen
- Stripped nuclei are often seen
- Mitoses are rare or absent

Cytoplasmic Details

- Foamy or clear cytoplasm with delicate frayed cytoplasmic membranes is characteristic
- Compact cyanophilic cells from zona reticularis may have lipofuscin pigment

ANCILLARY STUDIES

Immunohistochemistry

- Adrenal cortical cells
  - Positive: Inhibin, Melan-A, calretinin, vimentin, synaptophysin
  - Negative: AE1/AE3, PAX8
- Adrenal medullary chromaffin cells
  - Positive: Chromogranin, synaptophysin, S100
  - Negative: AE1/AE3

Molecular Tests

- Molecular tests may be needed for diagnosis or clinical management

DIFFERENTIAL DIAGNOSIS

Inadvertently Sampled Liver Tissue

- During FNA of right adrenal gland, be aware of possibility of inadvertent sampling of hepatocytes to avoid misinterpretation
- Hepatocytes usually do not have markedly vacuolated cytoplasm or delicate frayed cytoplasmic borders
- Lack of bubbly lipid-rich background
- Immunohistochemistry: AE1/AE3(+), Hep-Par1(+), Arginase-1(+), inhibin (-), Melan-A (-)

Metastatic Small Cell Carcinoma

- Stripped nuclei of adrenal cortical cells may form clusters with nuclear crowding and overlapping, simulating small cell carcinoma
- Important clue for adrenal origin is bubbly background of lipid material
- Small cell carcinoma has larger nuclei, prominent nuclear molding, more coarse chromatin, active mitosis or apoptosis, and necrosis
- Immunohistochemistry: AE1/AE3(+), CD56(+), inhibin (-), Melan-A (-)

Well-Differentiated Adrenal Cortical Carcinoma

- Usually present with large adrenal mass
- Hypercellular aspirate consisting of abundant isolated cells with intact cytoplasm
- Mild nuclear atypia with occasional mitoses
- Necrosis may be seen

SELECTED REFERENCES

1. Point du Jour KS et al: Adrenal gland fine needle aspiration: a multi-institutional analysis of 139 cases. J Am Soc Cytopathol. 10(2):168-74, 2021
2. Christiansen IS et al: EUS-B for suspected left adrenal metastasis in lung cancer. J Thorac Dis. 12(3):258-63, 2020
3. Kiseljak-Vassiliades K et al: American Association of Clinical Endocrinology disease state clinical review on the evaluation and management of adrenocortical carcinoma in an adult: a practical approach. Endocr Pract. 26(11):1366-83, 2020
4. Martin-Cardona A et al: EUS-guided tissue acquisition in the study of the adrenal glands: results of a nationwide multicenter study. PLoS One. 14(6):e0216658, 2019
5. Novotny AG et al: Fine-needle aspiration of adrenal lesions: a 20-year single institution experience with comparison of percutaneous and endoscopic ultrasound guided approaches. Diagn Cytopathol. 47(10):986-92, 2019
6. Patel S et al: Performance characteristics of EUS-FNA biopsy for adrenal lesions: a meta-analysis. Endosc Ultrasound. 8(3):180-7, 2019
7. Mete O et al: Immunohistochemical biomarkers of adrenal cortical neoplasms. Endocr Pathol. 29(2):137-49, 2018

Adrenal Cortical Adenoma

KEY FACTS

CLASSIFICATION
- Adrenal cortical adenoma (ACA) is benign epithelial tumor of adrenal cortical cells

CLINICAL ISSUES
- Occurs in 5% in adults; incidence increased with age
- 85% of ACA are nonfunctional (incidentaloma)
- Functional ACA: Conn syndrome (most common), Cushing syndrome, virilization, or feminization
- FNA is usually performed to rule out metastasis in patients with resectable cancer

CYTOPATHOLOGY
- Hypercellular smear
- Bubbly/frothy background with stripped nuclei
- Coarsely vacuolated with frayed cell borders
- Small round nuclei with smooth contours, even granular chromatin, and small nucleoli
- No nuclear pleomorphism, mitoses, or necrosis

MACROSCOPIC
- Often unilateral, small, and solitary mass with golden yellow cut surface

ANCILLARY TESTS
- Positive: Inhibin, Melan-A, calretinin, synaptophysin
- Negative: AE1/AE3, chromogranin

TOP DIFFERENTIAL DIAGNOSES
- Well-differentiated adrenal cortical carcinoma
  - Fast growing and infiltrative mass on radiology
  - Larger sheets of cells with necrosis and mitoses
- Adrenal nodular hyperplasia
  - Usually multiple and bilateral nodules
  - Indistinguishable from ACA on cytologic basis alone
- Metastatic small cell carcinoma
  - Nuclear molding with active mitosis and necrosis
  - Lack of frayed cell borders and bubbly background
  - AE1/AE3 (+), inhibin (-), Melan-A (-)

Radiographic Features
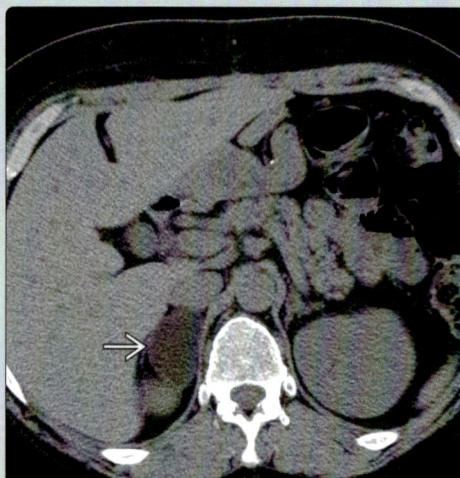

Core Needle biopsy of Adrenal Cortical Adenoma
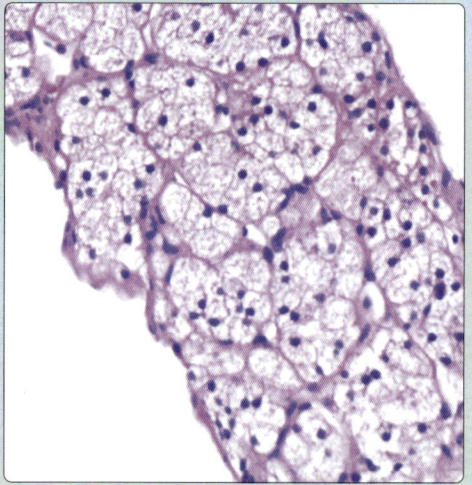

(Left) Axial NECT shows a well-circumscribed, oval mass of homogeneously low attenuation ⇨, diagnostic of a typical lipid-rich adrenal cortical adenoma (ACA). (Courtesy M. Federle, MD.) (Right) H&E-stained CT-guided core needle biopsy of a well-circumscribed adrenal lesion in a patient with history of lung cancer shows the trabecular or clustered arrangement of cells. The cytoplasm is vacuolated and eosinophilic. Nuclei are regular with low nuclear:cytoplasmic ratios. Note the lack of necrosis or mitosis.

Vacuolated Cells and Bubbly Background
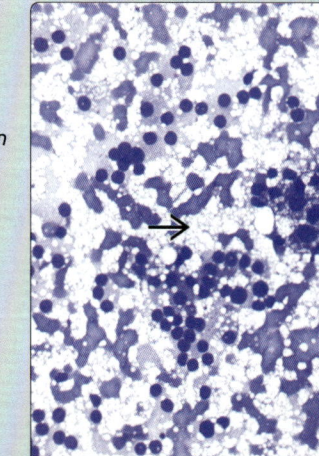

Nuclear and Cytoplasmic Details
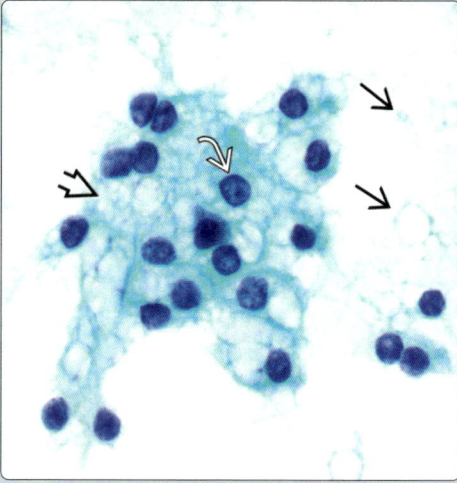

(Left) Aspiration of ACA demonstrates uniform cells with abundant coarsely vacuolated cytoplasm ⇨, frayed cytoplasmic borders, and bubbly background ⇨ on Diff-Quik stain. (Right) Pap stain shows a frothy background ⇨ and tumor cells with abundant vacuolated cytoplasm ⇨, round nuclei, and small nucleoli ⇨.

Adrenal Cortical Adenoma

TERMINOLOGY

Abbreviations
- Adrenal cortical adenoma (ACA)

CLINICAL ISSUES

Epidemiology
- Occurs in 5% of adults; increases with age

Presentation
- 85% of ACA are nonfunctional (incidentaloma)
- Functional ACA: Conn syndrome (most common), Cushing syndrome, virilization, or feminization
- On CT, shows slow-growing, round to oval mass with well-circumscribed and smooth contour, often lipid rich

CYTOPATHOLOGY

Cellularity
- Hypercellular aspirate

Pattern
- Dyscohesive cells or loose monolayer sheets

Background
- Bubbly/frothy lipid material (best seen on Diff-Quik stain)
- Many stripped nuclei, no necrosis

Cells
- Uniform bland epithelial cells

Nuclear Details
- Small, round nuclei with smooth contours, even granular chromatin, and small nucleoli
- Anisonucleosis can be prominent but no nuclear pleomorphism or mitoses

Cytoplasmic Details
- Coarsely vacuolated with frayed cell borders
- Oncocytic change and lipofuscin granules rarely seen

ANCILLARY TESTS

Immunohistochemistry
- Positive: Inhibin, Melan-A, calretinin, synaptophysin
- Negative: AE1/AE3, chromogranin

DIFFERENTIAL DIAGNOSIS

Well-Differentiated Adrenal Cortical Carcinoma
- Large, fast growing, and infiltrative mass on radiology
- Larger sheets of cells with necrosis and mitoses
- Distinguishing from ACA can be extremely difficult

Adrenal Nodular Hyperplasia
- Usually multiple and bilateral nodules
- Indistinguishable from ACA on cytologic basis alone

Metastatic Small Cell Carcinoma
- May simulate clusters of stripped nuclei in ACA
- Nuclear molding with active mitosis and necrosis
- Lack of frayed cell borders and bubbly background
- AE1/AE3(+), inhibin (-), Melan-A (-)

Other Metastatic Carcinomas
- Most often metastasize from kidney and lung
- Usually AE1/AE3 +), inhibin (-), and Melan-A (-)

Inadvertent Sampling of Liver Tissue
- May occur during FNA of right adrenal gland
- Granular cytoplasm and prominent nucleoli
- Lack of frayed cell borders and bubbly background
- AE1/AE3 +), Hep-Par1(+), inhibin (-), and Melan-A (-)

SELECTED REFERENCES

1. Point du Jour KS et al: Adrenal gland fine needle aspiration: a multi-institutional analysis of 139 cases. J Am Soc Cytopathol. 10(2):168-74, 2021
2. Hodgson A et al: A diagnostic approach to adrenocortical tumors. Surg Pathol Clin. 12(4):967-95, 2019
3. Lam AK: Update on adrenal tumours in 2017 World Health Organization (WHO) of endocrine tumours. Endocr Pathol. 28(3):213-27, 2017
4. Patil R et al: Endoscopic ultrasound-guided fine-needle aspiration in the diagnosis of adrenal lesions. Ann Gastroenterol. 29(3):307-11, 2016

Anisonucleosis With Smooth Contours

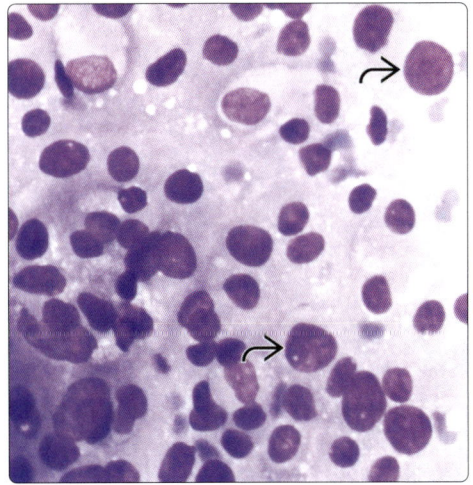

Stripped Nuclei

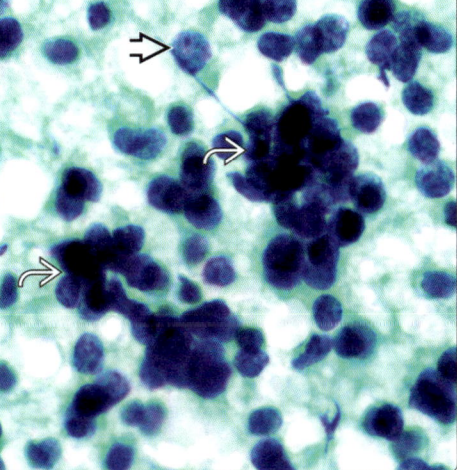

(Left) Anisonucleosis is common in ACA, but nuclear contours are smooth without nuclear pleomorphism or mitoses, as seen on this Diff-Quik stain. (Right) Pap-stained cluster of cells illustrates a common diagnostic pitfall: Misinterpretation of stripped nuclei in ACA as metastatic small cell carcinoma. Note that the surrounding cells have smooth nuclear contours with small nucleoli and lack mitoses or necrosis.

Adrenal Cortical Carcinoma

KEY FACTS

CLASSIFICATION
- Adrenal cortical carcinoma (ACC) is malignant epithelial tumor of adrenal cortical cells.

CLINICAL ISSUES
- Rare tumor (1-2 per million), more common in females
- Peak age: 60-70 years
- Most tumors are functional with excess hormones
- 40% with metastases at presentation
- Overall 5-year survival rate: 50-70%

CYTOPATHOLOGY
- Cellular smear with dyscohesive cells and often necrosis
- Vacuolated, eosinophilic, or granular cytoplasm
- Pleomorphic nuclei with irregular contours, coarse chromatin, prominent nucleoli, and active mitoses

MACROSCOPIC
- Large, red-brown, fleshy mass (often > 5 cm or 200 g)

ANCILLARY TESTS
- Positive: Inhibin, Melan-A, calretinin, synaptophysin
- Negative: AE1/AE3, PAX8

TOP DIFFERENTIAL DIAGNOSES
- Adrenal cortical adenoma
  - Slow-growing mass, usually smaller than ACC
  - More dispersal of cells with prominent naked nuclei
  - Lacks mitotic figures, necrosis, or diffuse atypia
- Clear cell renal cell carcinoma
  - Clear cells with intricate and branching blood vessels
  - PAX8(+), CD10(+), RCC(+), Melan-A (-), inhibin (-)
- Pheochromocytoma
  - Isolated large cells with marked anisonucleosis
  - Chromogranin (+), Melan-A (-), inhibin (-)
- Metastatic tumors
  - More likely to be bilateral and multiple
  - Correlation with history and immunohistochemistry

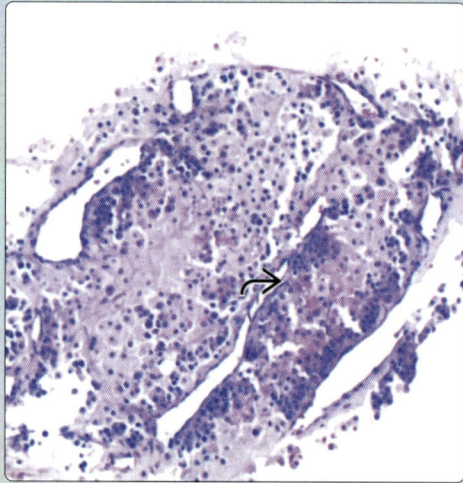
Core Needle Biopsy

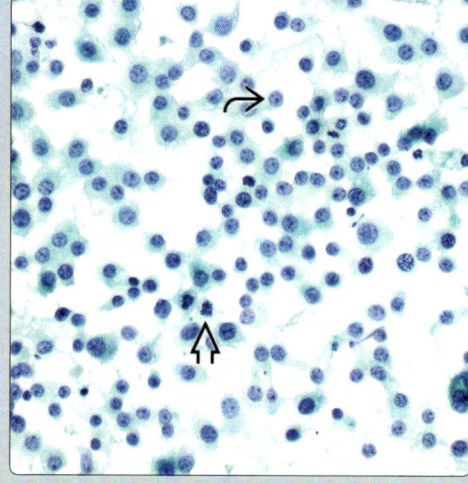
Active Mitosis and Prominent Nucleoli

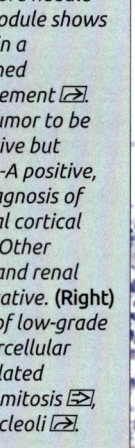

(Left) CT-guided core needle biopsy of a lung nodule shows a vascular tumor in a somewhat thickened trabecular arrangement ➡. IHC showed the tumor to be cytokeratin negative but inhibin and Melan-A positive, confirming the diagnosis of metastatic adrenal cortical carcinoma (ACC). Other pulmonary, liver, and renal markers were negative. (Right) Pap-stained FNA of low-grade ACC yields a hypercellular smear with vacuolated cytoplasm, active mitosis ➡, and prominent nucleoli ➡.

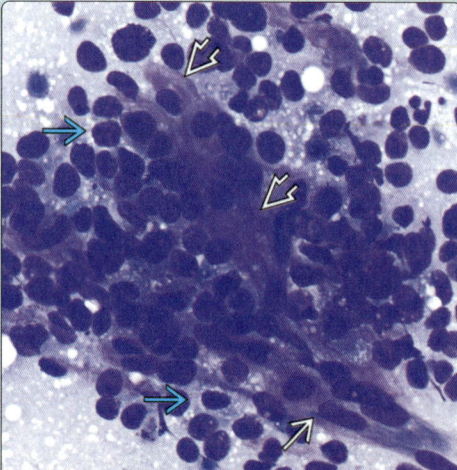
Spindle Cells With Eosinophilic Cytoplasm

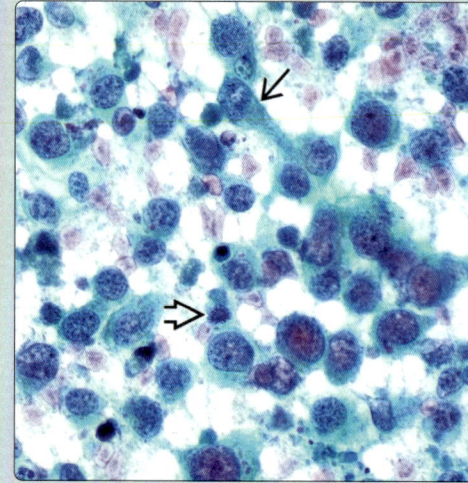
Granular Cytoplasm and Nuclear Atypia

(Left) Diff-Quik-stained FNA of high-grade ACC shows round to focal spindle cells ➡ with eosinophilic cytoplasm ➡ devoid of apparent fat vacuoles, most likely representing transgressing vessels. The background nonspindle cells show varying degrees of cytoplasmic vacuoles ➡. (Right) Pap-stained FNA of high-grade ACC demonstrates pleomorphic nuclei, irregular chromatin, prominent nucleoli, mitoses ➡, and granular cytoplasm without obvious fat vacuoles ➡.

Adrenal Cortical Carcinoma

CLINICAL ISSUES

Epidemiology
- Very rare; 1-2 per million
- Age: 60-70 years; minor peak < 2 years
- May be associated with Beckwith-Wiedemann syndrome, Li-Fraumeni syndrome, multiple endocrine neoplasia type 1, Carney complex, congenital adrenal hyperplasia

Presentation
- Most tumors are functional with excess glucocorticoid, mineralocorticoid, or sex hormones
- 40% with metastases at presentation

Treatment and Prognosis
- Complete radical surgical resection
- Overall 5-year survival rate: 50-70%

IMAGING

Radiographic Findings
- Inhomogeneous masses with low fat content, irregular borders, and necrosis

CYTOPATHOLOGY

Cellularity
- Hypercellular aspirate

Pattern
- Dyscohesive single cells or loose clusters

Background
- Many naked nuclei; necrosis often present

Cells
- Large, polygonal cells; may be bizarre or spindle in poorly differentiated tumor

Nuclear Details
- Pleomorphic nuclei, irregular nuclear membranes, coarse chromatin, and prominent nucleoli
- Mitosis can be brisk; occasional intranuclear inclusions

Cytoplasmic Details
- Vacuolated or clear in well-differentiated carcinomas
- Eosinophilic or granular in high-grade tumors
- Intracytoplasmic hyaline globules may be seen

ANCILLARY TESTS

Immunohistochemistry
- Positive: Inhibin, Melan-A, calretinin, synaptophysin
- Negative: AE1/AE3, PAX8

Genetic Testing
- Overexpression of *IGF2*, somatic mutations of *TP53* or *RB*, low expression of *P57*, *H19*, and *MYC*

DIFFERENTIAL DIAGNOSIS

Adrenal Cortical Adenoma
- Difficult to distinguish from low-grade adrenal cortical adenoma (ACA)
- ACA often smaller and slow-growing
- More dispersal of cells and prominent naked nuclei
- Lacks mitotic figures, necrosis, or diffuse atypia

Renal Cell Carcinoma
- Clear cells with intricate and branching blood vessels
- PAX8(+), CD10(+), RCC(+), Melan-A (-), inhibin (-)

Pheochromocytoma
- Isolated large cells with marked anisonucleosis
- Chromogranin (+), Melan-A (-), inhibin (-)

Metastatic Tumors
- More likely to be bilateral and multiple
- Correlation with history and immunohistochemistry

SELECTED REFERENCES

1. Point du Jour KS et al: Adrenal gland fine needle aspiration: a multi-institutional analysis of 139 cases. J Am Soc Cytopathol. 10(2):168-74, 2021
2. Torti JF et al: Adrenal cancer. StatPearls, 2021
3. Mete O et al: Immunohistochemical biomarkers of adrenal cortical neoplasms. Endocr Pathol. 29(2):137-49, 2018

Bizarre Tumor Cells

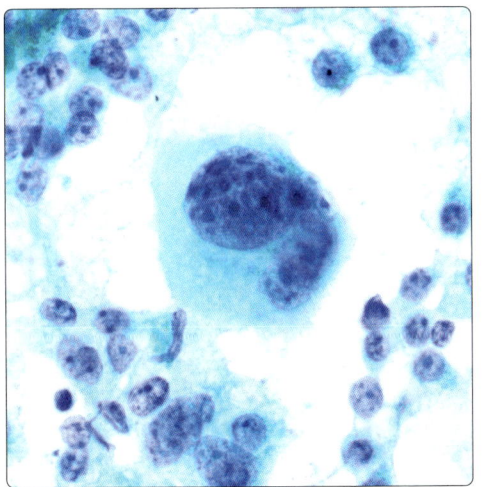

Histologic Features of ACC

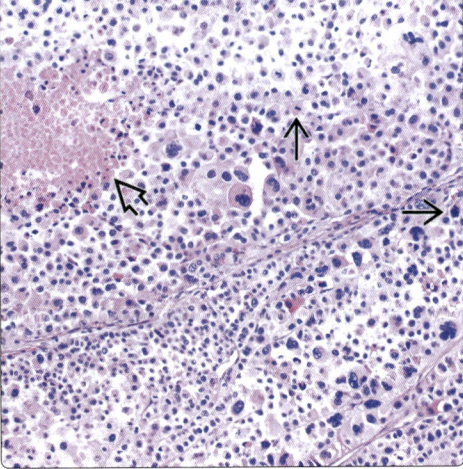

(Left) Pap stain shows a bizarre tumor cell with giant nucleus, marked irregularity of chromatin, and granular cytoplasm. *(Right)* On H&E, the tumor has prominent nuclear pleomorphism, eosinophilic cytoplasm, active mitosis ⇨, and tumor necrosis ⇨. Tumor necrosis is an important histologic criterion in all schemes for differentiation between benign and malignant adrenal cortical neoplasms.

Metastatic Tumors to Adrenal Gland

KEY FACTS

CLINICAL ISSUES
- Adrenal gland is 4th most common site for extranodal metastasis after lung, liver, and bone
- ~ 33-46% of adrenal FNA represent metastatic malignancies
- Lung is most common primary site (35-60%), followed by kidney, melanoma, stomach, esophagus, and liver
- ~ 50-60% of adrenal metastases are unilateral

CYTOPATHOLOGY
- Cytologic features dictated by primary tumor type
  - Metastatic adenocarcinoma is most common
- Background necrosis or mucin may be seen
- Cell block with IHC can be valuable in cytologic evaluation
  - Metastatic tumors often retain distinct morphologic and IHC features of primary tumors

TOP DIFFERENTIAL DIAGNOSES
- Clear cell renal cell carcinoma
  - Clear cells with intricate and branching blood vessels
  - PAX8, RCC, CD10 (+); inhibin, Melan-A (-)
- High-grade adenocarcinomas
  - AE1/AE3, CEA (+); inhibin, Melan-A (-)
- Small cell carcinoma
  - AE1/AE3, TTF-1 often (+); inhibin, Melan-A (-)

DIAGNOSTIC CHECKLIST
- Most malignant adrenal masses represent metastases
- Common metastatic tumors usually differ from primary adrenal tumors in morphology and immunohistochemistry
- Cytologic features unusual for distinctive adrenal tumors should alert one to consider possibility of metastasis
- Correlation with clinical history and radiologic findings are essential during cytologic evaluation
- Review of cytology and histology material of previous tumor (if available) can be helpful
- Cell block should be attempted for possible immunohistochemistry and molecular testing

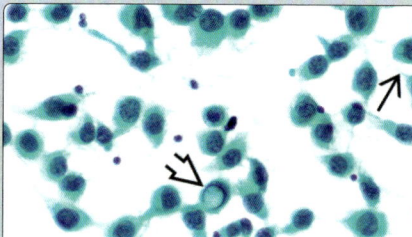

Metastatic Lung Adenocarcinoma

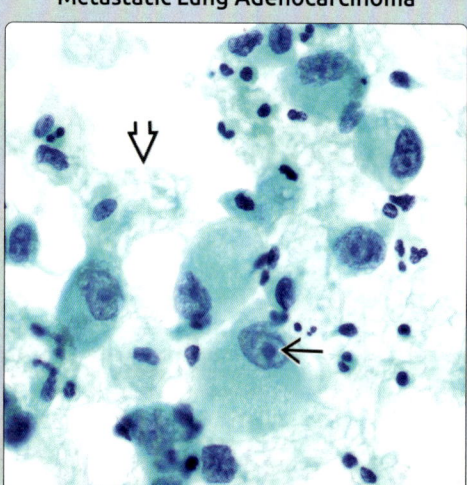

Metastatic Melanoma

(Left) *Metastatic lung adenocarcinoma on Pap stain shows abundant clear to vacuolated cytoplasm ➡ and prominent nucleoli ➡ that mimic adrenal cortical carcinoma (ACC) or clear cell renal cell carcinoma (RCC).* (Right) *Pap stain of a metastatic melanoma displays plasmacytoid cells, multiple cytoplasmic projections ➡, binucleation ➡, intranuclear inclusions ➡, and prominent nucleoli.*

Metastatic Hepatocellular Carcinoma

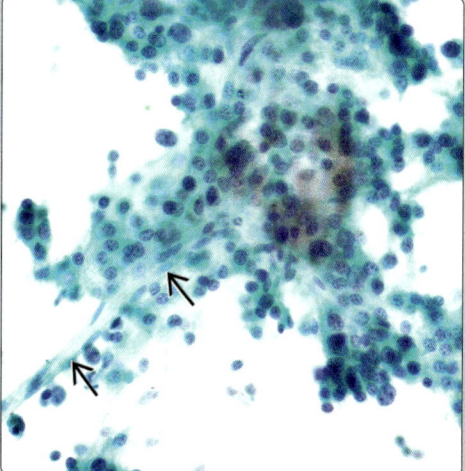

Metastatic Hepatocellular Carcinoma, Touch Preparation

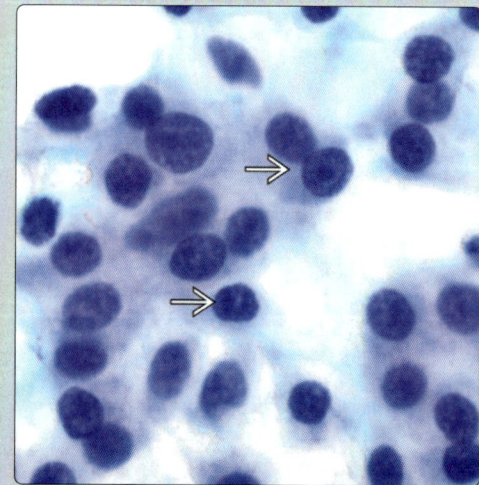

(Left) *Pap stain of an FNA from a metastatic hepatocellular carcinoma demonstrates thick trabeculae with transgressing blood vessels ➡, abundant granular cytoplasm, and pleomorphic nuclei.* (Right) *Pap-stained touch preparation of an adrenal mass core needle biopsy shows prominent nucleoli ➡. The typical features of hepatocellular carcinoma seen on FNA are not seen. Work-up of core is important, so the tissue has to be gently handled to retain the cells in the core.*

Metastatic Tumors to Adrenal Gland

CLINICAL ISSUES

Epidemiology
- Incidence
  - Adrenal gland is 4th most common site for extranodal metastasis after lung, liver, and bone
  - Adrenal metastasis has been documented in 9-20% cancer patients at autopsy
  - ~ 33-46% of adrenal FNA represent metastatic malignancies
  - Common primary sites: Lung (35-60%), kidney, melanoma, stomach, esophagus, and liver

Presentation
- Only 4% of adrenal lesions are symptomatic

CYTOPATHOLOGY

Background
- May have background mucin or necrosis

Cells
- Cytologic features dictated by primary tumors
- Adenocarcinoma is most common (~ 50%)
- Usually not challenging in differential diagnosis

Cell Block Findings
- Cell block can be very helpful for confirmatory immunohistochemistry

MACROSCOPIC

General Features
- ~ 50-60% of adrenal metastases are unilateral
- Mean size: 2.0 cm (SD = 1.9 cm)

ANCILLARY TESTS

Histochemistry
- Mucicarmine is negative in adrenal cells but often positive in metastatic adenocarcinomas

Immunohistochemistry
- Adrenal tissue (IHC profile)
  - Usually inhibin, Melan-A, calretinin, vimentin (+); cytokeratin (-)
- Metastatic carcinomas (IHC profile)
  - Usually cytokeratin, EMA (+); inhibin, Melan-A, vimentin, and calretinin (-)
- Other specific markers may also be useful depending on type of primary tumor

DIFFERENTIAL DIAGNOSIS

Clear Cell Renal Cell Carcinoma
- Cytologic features could readily be confused with adrenal cortical adenoma or adenocarcinoma
- Adrenal involvement by clear cell renal cell carcinoma is seen in 60% of radical nephrectomies and 90% of patients at autopsy
- Presence of renal mass is clue
- Clear cells with intricate and branching blood vessels
- PAX8, RCC, CD10 (+); inhibin, and Melan-A (-)

High-Grade Adenocarcinomas
- Often simulating adrenal cortical carcinoma
- AE1/AE3, CEA, mucicarmine (+); inhibin, Melan-A (-)

Small Cell Carcinoma
- May resemble clusters of naked nuclei of adrenal cortical cells
- Typically has active mitosis, apoptosis, necrosis, and lacks bubbly background
- AE1/AE3, TTF-1 often (+); inhibin, Melan-A (-)

Tumors With Clear or Oncocytic Cells
- May be seen in lung, breast, or salivary gland
- Usually inhibin, Melan-A (-)

SELECTED REFERENCES
1. Cingam SR et al: Adrenal metastasis. StatPearls, 2021
2. Satturwar S et al: An update on touch preparations of small biopsies. J Am Soc Cytopathol. 9(5):322-31, 2020

Core Needle Biopsy of Adrenal With Metastatic Small Cell Carcinoma

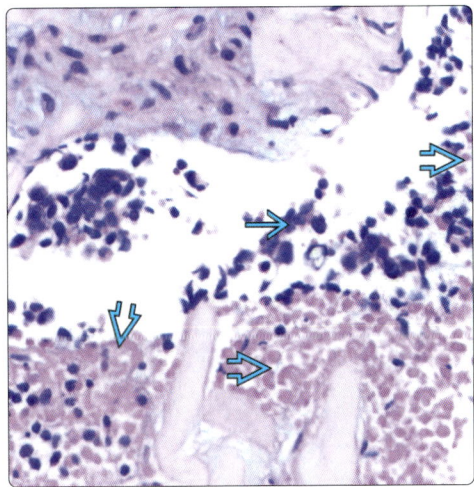

Metastatic Breast Lobular Carcinoma

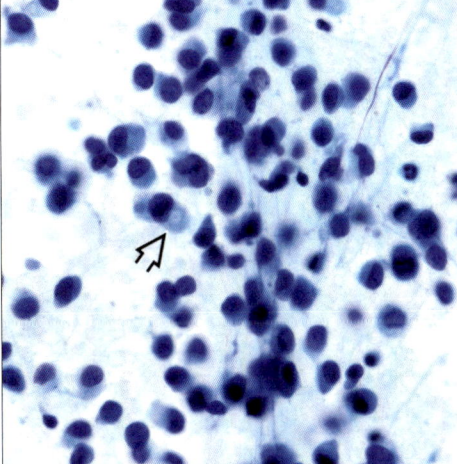

(Left) This H&E-stained core needle biopsy shows a small blue cell tumor ➡, which, on further work-up, was a metastasis of a small cell lung carcinoma. Note the extensive necrosis ➡, which can be problematic for accurate diagnosis if viable tumor is not present. *(Right)* Metastatic breast lobular carcinoma shows dyscohesive plasmacytoid cells with targetoid intracytoplasmic vacuoles ➡ on Pap stain.

Pheochromocytoma

KEY FACTS

CLASSIFICATION
- Neuroendocrine tumor of adrenal medulla; similar tumors in other locations are termed paraganglioma
- Adrenal pheochromocytomas (PCCs) account for 90% of sympathetic paragangliomas

ETIOLOGY/PATHOGENESIS
- 30-40% of PCCs are hereditary
- *SDH* mutations seen in 80% of familial PCCs

CLINICAL ISSUES
- Signs and symptoms of catecholamine excess
- Metastasis in 10-15%, associated with *SDHB* mutation, aberrant CAIX and MAX, and Ki-67 index > 3%

CYTOPATHOLOGY
- Hypercellular and bloody aspirate
- Dyscohesive or loose groups of cells with blood vessels
- Polygonal, spindle, or extremely anisocytotic
- Nuclei vary from bland to marked anisonucleosis
- Abundant fragile and granular cytoplasm

ANCILLARY TESTS
- Chromogranin (+), synaptophysin (+), CD56(+), AE1/AE3(-)
- *RET* (causes MEN2A and 2B), *VHL*, *NF1*, *SDH* mutations

TOP DIFFERENTIAL DIAGNOSES
- Adrenal cortical carcinoma
  - Nuclear pleomorphism, mitoses and necrosis often seen
  - Inhibin (+), synaptophysin (+), chromogranin (-)
- Metastatic high-grade malignancies
  - Nuclear pleomorphism and necrosis are often seen
  - Usually lack of neuroendocrine features

DIAGNOSTIC CHECKLIST
- Emergency treatment should be ready before performing FNA on possible PCCs
- PCCs should not be signed out as benign; all patients receive long-term follow-up

Bloody and Hypercellular Aspirate

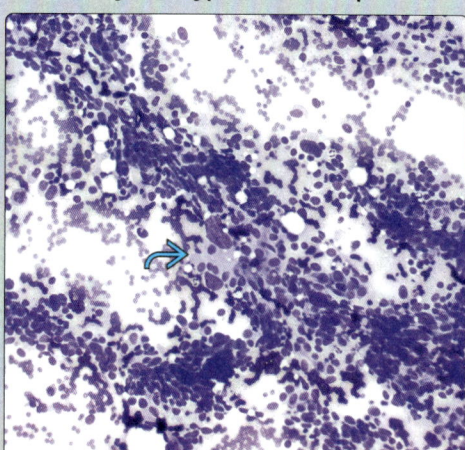

Granular Cytoplasm With Indistinct Borders

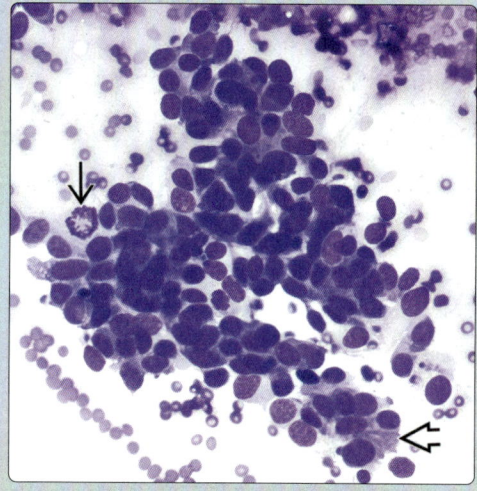

(Left) Diff-Quik-stained FNA of pheochromocytoma (PCC) yields a bloody and hypercellular smear with prominent anisocytosis ⊿. (Right) Higher magnification of a Diff-Quik stain shows polygonal cells with granular cytoplasm ⊿, indistinct cell borders, round to oval nuclei, smooth nuclear contours, and occasional mitoses ⊿.

Nuclear Pseudoinclusions

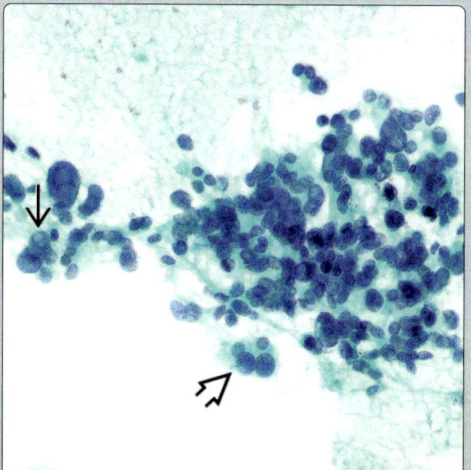

Marked Anisokaryosis

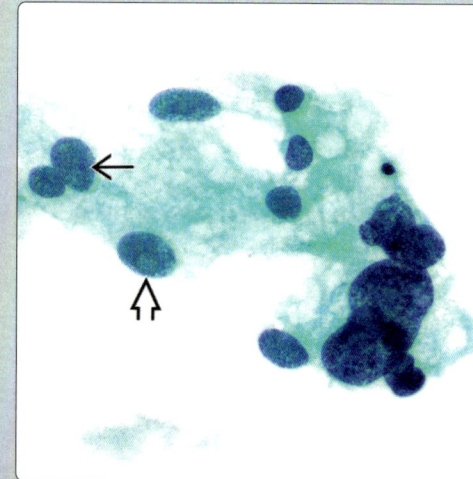

(Left) Pap stain demonstrates prominent anisokaryosis ⊿ with nuclear pseudoinclusions ⊿. (Right) High magnification of a Pap stain shows marked nuclear enlargement and anisokaryosis with fine, granular to coarse clumped chromatin, nuclear pseudoinclusion ⊿, and a prominent nucleolus ⊿. Note that marked irregularity of nuclear membranes is not seen.

Pheochromocytoma

CLINICAL ISSUES

Epidemiology
- 30-40% of pheochromocytomas (PCCs) are associated with hereditary genetic abnormalities involving > 20 genes, including *SDH* mutations (80%), *RET*, *VHL*, *NF1*, *TMEM127*, *MAX*, etc.

Site
- 90% of sympathetic paragangliomas are adrenal PCCs

Presentation
- Sympathoadrenal PCCs usually cause signs and symptoms of catecholamine excess

Treatment
- Complete surgical excision

Prognosis
- Patients with metastases often die from complications of excess catecholamines or destructive local growth

Malignancy
- Malignancy is defined by presence of metastases (10-15%)
- Metastasis is seen in 30% of patients with *SDHB* mutation

IMAGING

MR Findings
- Intense T2-weighted image (light bulb sign)

CYTOPATHOLOGY

Cellularity
- Hypercellular with bloody background

Pattern
- Dyscohesive or loose groups of cells, often with vessels

Cells
- Polygonal, spindle, or extremely anisocytotic
- Abundant fragile and granular cytoplasm with fine red granules

Nuclear Details
- Vary from bland with fine chromatin (carcinoidal) to marked anisonucleosis with hyperchromasia, pseudoinclusions, and prominent nucleoli
- Mitoses and necrosis are usually rare

MICROSCOPIC

Histologic Features
- Small nests of neuroendocrine cells (zellballen) with interspersed small blood vessels

ANCILLARY TESTS

Immunohistochemistry
- Chromogranin (+), synaptophysin (+), CD56(+), AE1/AE3(-)

Genetic Testing
- *RET* (causes MEN2A and 2B), *VHL*, *NF1*, *SDH* mutations

DIFFERENTIAL DIAGNOSIS

Adrenal Cortical Carcinoma
- Mitoses and necrosis often seen
- Inhibin (+), chromogranin (-), synaptophysin (+), calretinin (+), SF1(+)

Metastatic High-Grade Malignancies
- Nuclear pleomorphism and necrosis are often seen
- Usually lack neuroendocrine features
- Clinical history and immunohistochemistry are crucial

SELECTED REFERENCES

1. Garcia-Carbonero R et al: Multidisciplinary practice guidelines for the diagnosis, genetic counseling and treatment of pheochromocytomas and paragangliomas. Clin Transl Oncol. 23(10):1995-2019, 2021
2. Granberg D et al: Metastatic pheochromocytomas and abdominal paragangliomas. J Clin Endocrinol Metab. 106(5):e1937-52, 2021
3. Juhlin CC: Challenges in paragangliomas and pheochromocytomas: from histology to molecular immunohistochemistry. Endocr Pathol. 32(2):228-44, 2021
4. Papathomas TG et al: What have we learned from molecular biology of paragangliomas and pheochromocytomas? Endocr Pathol. 32(1):134-53, 2021

Anisocytosis and Anisokaryosis With Regular Nuclear Contours

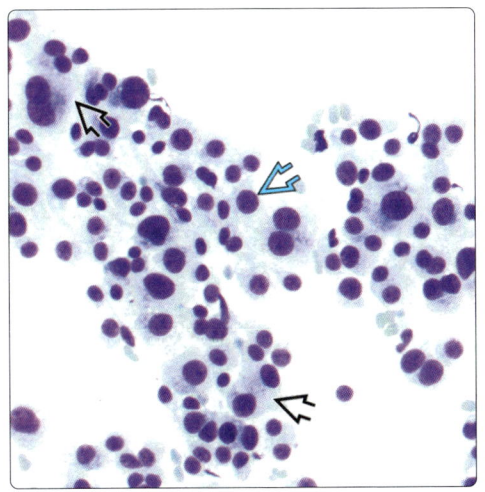

Focal Spindle Cell Morphology

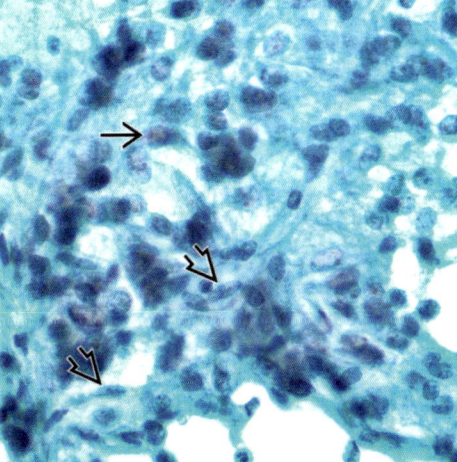

(Left) Diff-Quik stain of PCC shows prominent anisocytosis and anisokaryosis but mostly with regular nuclear contours ⮕. The cytoplasm is fragile with fine, red granules ⮕. *(Right)* Some tumor cells may have hyperchromasia, prominent nucleoli ⮕, or focal spindle cell morphology ⮕, as seen on this Pap stain.

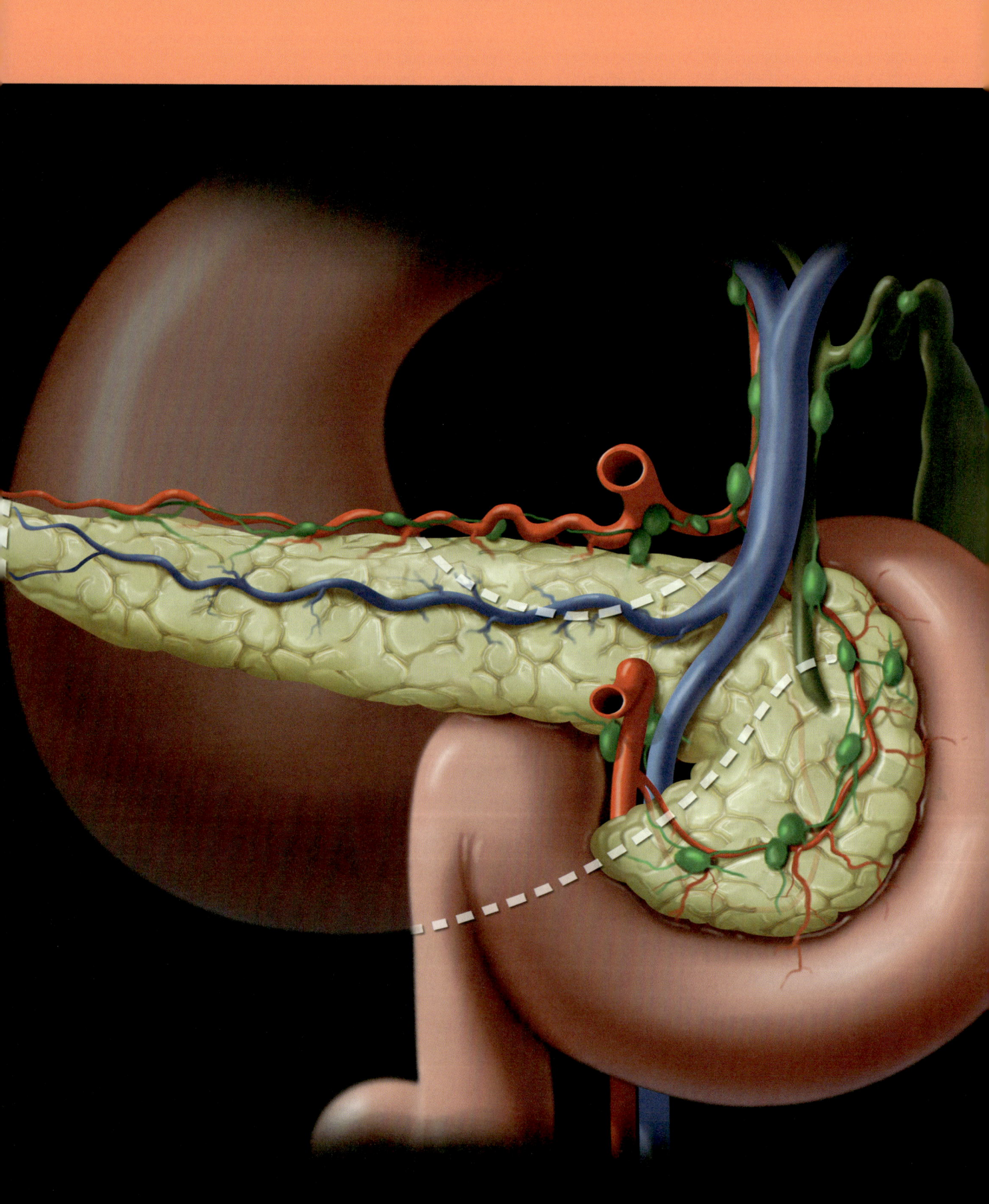

PART IV
SECTION 6
Pancreas

Overview

Cytology of Normal Pancreas	570
Pancreaticobiliary Cytology Reporting Terminology, Cyst Evaluation	572

Nonneoplastic Lesions

Pancreatitis	574
Lymphoepithelial Cyst of Pancreas	576
Intra- and Peripancreatic Splenules	577

Neoplasms

Serous Microcystic Adenoma	578
Mucinous Cystic Neoplasm	580
Intraductal Papillary Mucinous Neoplasm	582
Solid Pseudopapillary Neoplasm	584
Pancreatic Neuroendocrine Tumor	586
Pancreatic Ductal Adenocarcinoma	588
Unusual Variants of Ductal Carcinoma	590
Acinar Cell Carcinoma	594
Lymphoma and Secondary Tumors of Pancreas	596

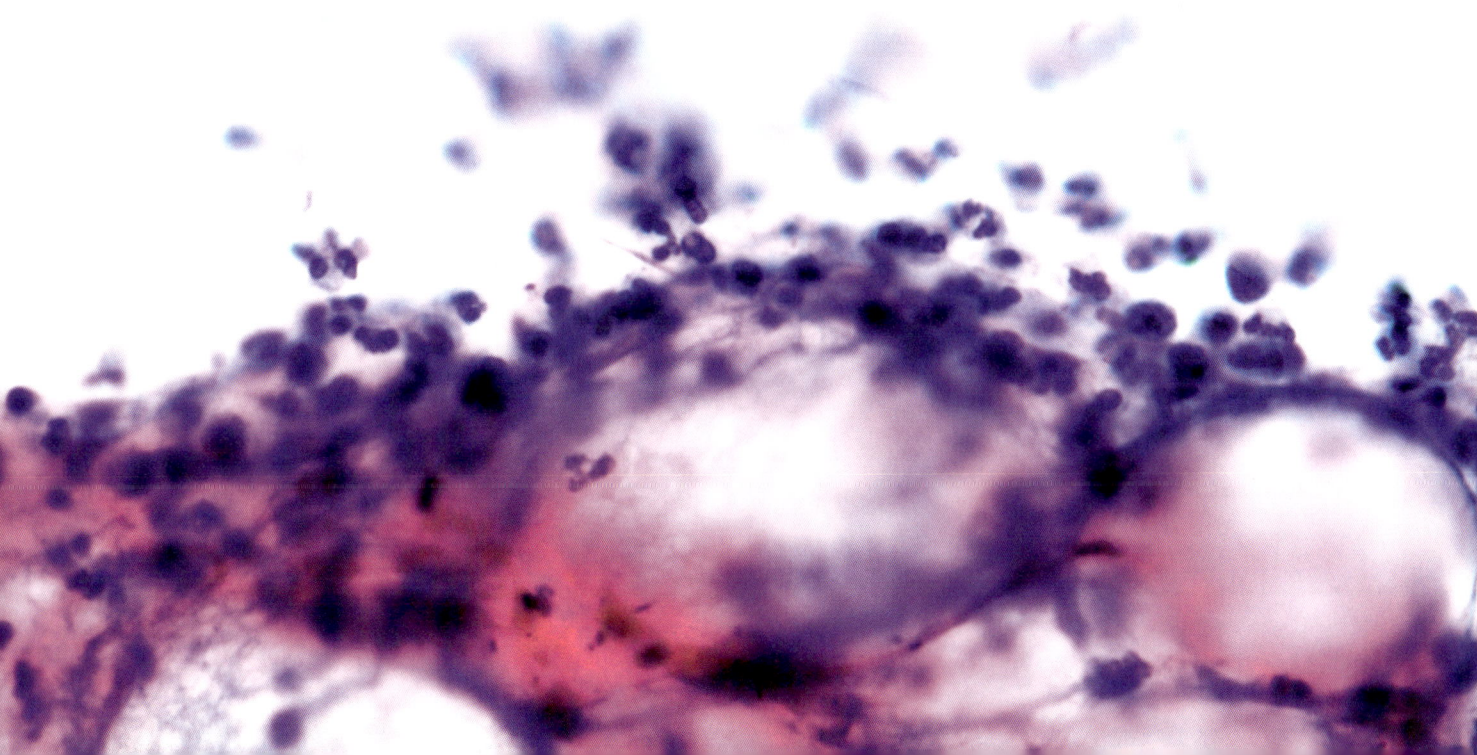

Cytology of Normal Pancreas

TERMINOLOGY

Anatomic Features
- Size and location
  - Retroperitoneal organ bordered by stomach anteriorly and aorta, splenic vein, and left kidney posteriorly
  - Divided into head (lies in C-shaped curve of duodenum), body (crosses midline of human body), and tail (extends to hilum of spleen)
  - Usually 60-140 g; average: 15 cm in length

Architectural Organization
- Exocrine pancreas
  - Acinar cells compose majority of pancreas; acini lead into duct system and main pancreatic duct
  - Zymogen granules contain digestive enzymes
- Endocrine pancreas
  - Islets of Langerhans

Clinical Utility of Pancreas FNA
- Indications for pancreas FNA
  - Image-guided FNA or core needle biopsies are effective and safe modality for sampling pancreatic lesions
  - Principal indication is for sampling radiologically detected lesion
    - Confirmation of solid primary pancreatic tumor (70% occur in head of pancreas): Pancreatic adenocarcinoma, pancreatic endocrine neoplasms, acinar cell carcinoma, solid-solid pseudopapillary tumor, lymphoma
    - Evaluation of cystic mass of pancreas (neoplastic cysts such as serous cystadenoma, mucinous cystic neoplasm, and intraductal papillary mucinous neoplasm vs. nonneoplastic cysts)
    - Cyst fluid analysis can aid in diagnosis of malignancy by measuring levels of amylase, CEA, CA125, CA15-3 and molecular profiling
    - Confirmation of metastatic disease to pancreas
- Diagnostic accuracy
  - Sensitivity: 86-98% for CT-guided FNA; 75-94% for EUS-guided FNA per current literature

Normal Pancreas: Posterior View

Normal Pancreatic Lobule

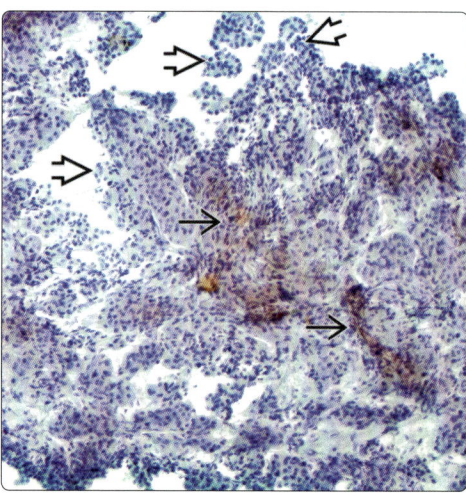

(Left) Based on the location of the pancreas and its relationship to the adjacent organs, lesions/masses in the body or tail of the pancreas are typically aspirated through the stomach ➡. Pancreatic head and uncinate process lesions are aspirated through the duodenum ➡. The location of the aspirate determines the type of contaminants inadvertently picked up at time of EUS FNA of pancreas. (Right) Pap-stained grape-like clusters ➡ of acini have a central duct ➡. The entire lobule was aspirated in this microbiopsy.

Normal Pancreatic Acinus

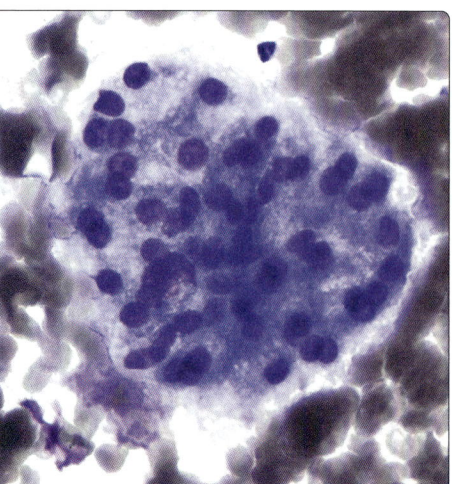

Normal Pancreas

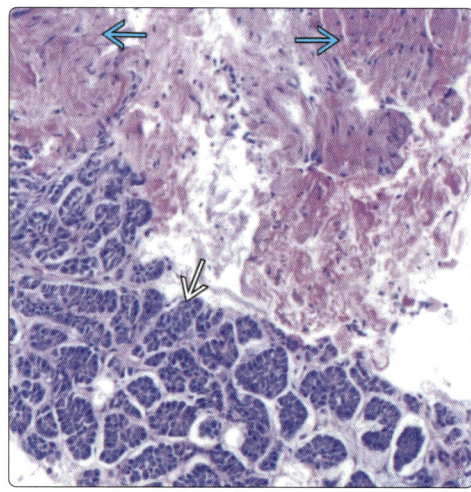

(Left) Diff-Quik-stained smear demonstrates a cluster of acinar cells with granular cytoplasm and round nuclei. (Right) Normal pancreatic acini ➡ and duodenal or gastric wall smooth muscle ➡ are often seen in EUS-guided CNBs of pancreatic masses. The epithelial component of the contaminant depends on whether the biopsy is through the duodenum (pancreatic head masses) or gastric (body/tail).

Cytology of Normal Pancreas

- Specificity for EUS-guided FNA is virtually 100%; EUS-guided CNB replacing FNA
- Greater sensitivity and specificity reported for institutions with greater experience with EUS
- Most common causes of false-negative diagnoses
  - Difficulty in distinguishing well-differentiated adenocarcinoma
  - Sampling error due to location of lesion or small size
  - Presence of chronic pancreatitis
- False-positive diagnoses
  - Less commonly encountered
  - Usually due to overinterpretation of reactive atypia for malignancy in setting of acute pancreatitis
  - Mistaking GI tract contaminants for neoplastic epithelium
- Contraindications and complications of EUS-guided pancreatic FNA
  - Upper gastrointestinal obstruction, bleeding disorders
  - Complications are rare
    - Most common major complication is acute pancreatitis; incidence: 1-3%
    - Other major complications include perforation, leaks, or major hemorrhage
    - Minor complication usually involves pain or minor hemorrhage; incidence: 1-5%
- Sample collection and preparation
  - Image-guided pancreas FNA performed by radiologists or gastrointestinal endoscopists ensures sampling of targeted lesion
  - Cytology preparation includes air-dried Diff-Quik slides or Carnoy fixed slides for rapid Pap stain or routine Pap stain
  - Diff-Quik- and Pap-stained slides are complementary in highlighting cytoplasmic and nuclear features for accurate diagnosis
  - Material for cell block sections should be collected when possible
  - Real-time and on-site adequacy checks by cytopathologists ensure quality and adequacy of material obtained for diagnosis and ancillary studies
  - Description of radiologic appearance of lesion (cystic, solid, solitary, multifocal) should be noted
  - Collection of designated passes for molecular testing may be indicated in certain situations
  - CNB directly collected in formalin and processed as surgical specimen; if fragmented, then best to process as cell block

Cytology

- Normal pancreas can be moderately cellular with combination of ductal and acinar elements
- Islet cells are rarely seen in FNAs
- Relatively clean background if there is no evidence of pancreatitis or neoplasm
- Acinar cells present as single cells or small clusters
  - Indistinct cell borders, abundant granular cytoplasm
  - Round eccentrically placed nuclei, fine chromatin pattern, small inconspicuous nucleoli
- Ductal cells are cohesive, in sheets, honeycomb pattern
  - Single cells are rare
  - Well-defined cell borders, moderate amount of cytoplasm
  - Round to oval nuclei, granular chromatin pattern, evenly distributed nuclei (no crowding or overlap)

Ancillary Studies

- Acinar cells: Positive for trypsin, chymotrypsin, PAS
- Ductal epithelial cells: Positive for CK19, CA19-9
  - Loss of SMAD4 expression in pancreatic ductal adenocarcinomas
- Islet cells: Synaptophysin, chromogranin, CD56

Differential Diagnosis

- Due to anatomic relationships, miscellaneous normal elements may be found in pancreatic FNA
  - Mesothelial cells may be mistaken for adenocarcinoma
  - Hepatocytes have granular cytoplasm and round nuclei, mistaken for acinar cells
  - Gastric or intestinal epithelium, wall or Brunner glands
    - Goblet cells or mucinous epithelium may be mistaken for mucinous neoplasm of pancreas

Duodenal Contaminant on EUS

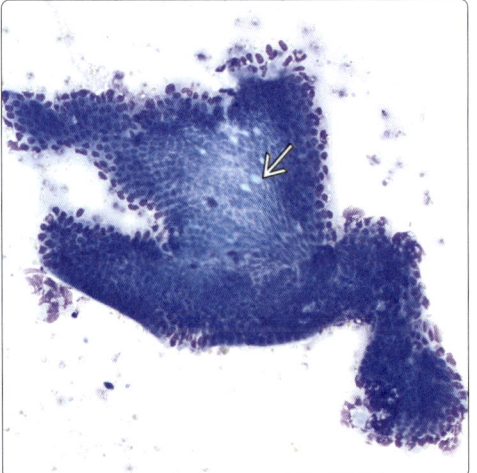

Normal Gastric Body Parietal and Chief Cells

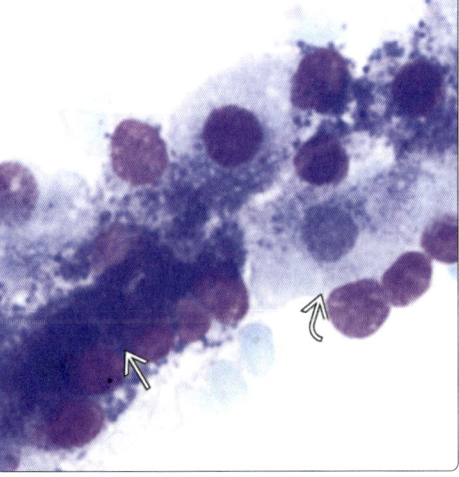

(Left) Diff-Quik-stained smear from EUS-guided FNA of a pancreatic head mass shows goblet cells ➡ that are indicative of duodenal contaminants and can be a pitfall. Knowing the site (stomach or duodenum) through which FNA was performed is key. **(Right)** Diff-Quik-stained example shows normal parietal ➡ cells with abundant granular cytoplasm. The chief cells have a clear, less granular cytoplasm ➡.

Pancreaticobiliary Cytology Reporting Terminology, Cyst Evaluation

REPORTING TERMINOLOGY

WHO International System for Reporting Pancreatic Cytopathology

- **Insufficient/inadequate/nondiagnostic**
  - Unable to make diagnosis of targeted lesion for qualitative or quantitative reason
  - Normal pancreatic tissue in presence of defined mass (may call it benign but explain)
  - Ancillary tests (cyst fluid testing, molecular testing) can help in defining lesion
  - Risk of malignancy (ROM) 5-25%; repeat sampling warranted
- **Negative for malignancy**
  - Includes autoimmune pancreatitis (AIP), acute and chronic pancreatitis, accessory/ectopic spleen, lymphoepithelial cyst, lymphangioma, pseudocyst, adrenal rests, serous cystadenoma, schwannoma, and other benign lesions
  - Unequivocally benign on cytology but may not be diagnostic of specific process or neoplasm
  - Benign neoplasms (serous cystadenoma) and nonneoplastic conditions
  - ROM for pancreatic FNA: 0-15%; conservative management with clinical correlation
- **Atypical**
  - Generally features of benign condition/lesions/neoplasms but with minimal changes concerning for malignant process
  - ROM for pancreatic FNA: 30-40%
- **Pancreatic neoplasm, low risk/grade (PaN-low)**
  - Intraductal papillary mucinous neoplasm (IPMN) and mucinous cystic neoplasm (MCN) with low- to intermediate-grade dysplasia
  - Ancillary studies, such as cyst fluid CEA, glucose, amylase, next-generation sequencing (NGS), helpful for diagnosis
  - ROM is 5-20%; usually conservative clinical management
- **Pancreatic neoplasm, high risk/grade (PaN-high)**
  - IPMN and MCN with high-grade dysplasia (used to be "neoplastic: other" in Papanicolaou Reporting system)
  - Includes high-grade dysplasia and high risk of disease progression

IPMN With Thick Mucin, Diff-Quik Stain
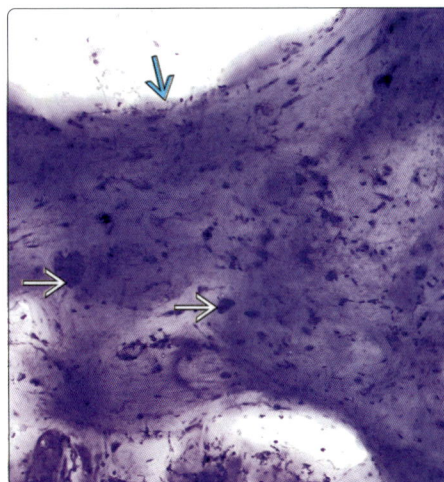

IPMN With Thick Mucin, Pap Stain
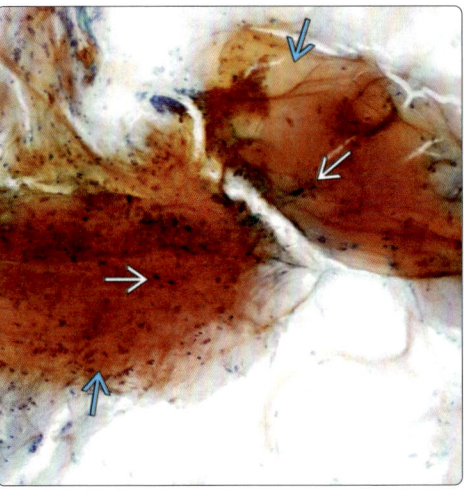

(Left) Diff-Quik-stained smear shows thick mucin ➡ with cellular debris ➡ from a case of intraductal papillary mucinous neoplasm (IPMN). The presence of histiocytes and debris is indicative of mucinous cyst/duct contents, in contrast to watery mucin without histiocytes or cellular debris from GI tract contaminants. *(Right)* Pap-stained smear shows thick mucin ➡ with entrapped cellular debris ➡ from a case of IPMN.

IPMN With Low-Grade Atypia
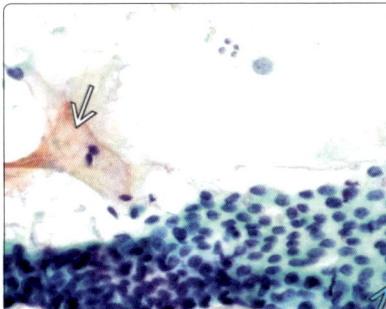

IPMN With High-Grade Atypia
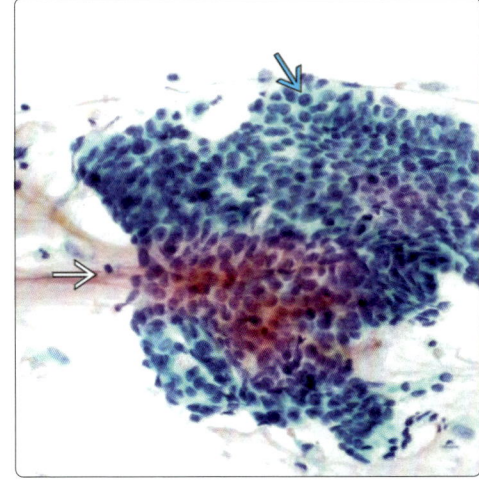

(Left) Pap-stained smear shows a large sheet of cells in a mucinous ➡ background showing low-grade atypia ➡. *(Right)* Pap-stained aspirate with thick mucin ➡ and a large sheet of cells with nuclear crowding and high-grade atypia ➡ is shown.

Pancreaticobiliary Cytology Reporting Terminology, Cyst Evaluation

Ancillary and Molecular Testing in Pancreatic Cysts/Cystic Neoplasms

Cyst Type	CEA	Glucose	Amylase	KRAS	GNAS	VHL	RNF43	CTNNB1	TP53	PIK3CA	PTEN	CDK2A	SMAD4 NOTCH1
Pseudocyst	-	↑	↑	-	-	-	-	-	-	-	-	-	-
IPMN	↑	↓	↑	+	+	-	+	-	+*	+*	+*	+*	+*
MCN	↑	↓	-	+**	-	-	-	-	-	+*	+*	+*	+*
Serous cystadenoma	-	↑	-	-	-	+	-	-	-	-	-	-	-
Solid pseudopapillary	-	↑	-	-	-	-	-	+	+†	+†	-	-	-
PanNET	-	↑	-	-	-	-	-	-	-	-	-	-	-
Nonneoplastic (other)	-	↑	-	-	-	-	-	-	-	-	-	-	-

*Seen in malignant/advanced disease; **up to 14% RAS positive, the rest negative; † seen in rare instances; IPMN = intraductal papillary mucinous neoplasm; MCN = mucinous cystic neoplasm; PanNET = pancreatic neuroendocrine tumor.

- Intraductal oncocytic papillary neoplasm and intraductal tubulopapillary neoplasm fall into this category
- ROM is 60-95%; usual management is surgical resection of lesion

- **Suspicious for malignancy**
  - Features are qualitatively or quantitatively short of unequivocal diagnosis of malignancy
  - ROM is 80-100%; management is repeat FNA for neoadjuvant therapy or surgical resection in appropriate clinical setting
- **Malignant**
  - Carcinoma, including pancreatic ductal, acinar, neuroendocrine and cholangiocarcinoma; pancreatic neuroendocrine tumor, including well-differentiated, pancreatoblastoma; metastatic malignancy; solid-pseudopapillary neoplasm
  - Unequivocal cytopathologic features of malignancy
  - ROM is 99-100%; management per clinical stage

Approach to Cytologic Analysis of Pancreatic Cysts

- **Is cyst mucinous or nonmucinous**
  - Mucin is thick, viscous, sticky, and colloid-like and described as such by gastroenterologist performing procedure
  - Cellular debris and histiocytes in cyst contents indicate origin from cyst and not gastrointestinal tract contamination
  - Elevated cyst fluid CEA, low cyst fluid glucose (≤ 50 mg/dl) or detection of KRAS/GNAS mutation may be necessary to support mucinous etiology
  - Presence of mucin, elevated CEA, low glucose, KRAS/GNAS mutation alone does not distinguish benign from malignant cyst
  - Negative mucin stain does not exclude mucinous cyst
- **Are cells high grade or not**
  - Atypia classified as low or high grade
  - High-grade criteria: Cell size < 12 μm (size of duodenal enterocyte), increased N:C ratio, abnormal chromatin pattern, and background necrosis

Proposed WHO International System for Reporting Biliary Cytopathology (BC)

- **Insufficient/inadequate, nondiagnostic**
- **Benign/negative for malignancy**
  - ROM: ~ 0-25%; conservative management with clinical correlation
- **Atypical**: ROM: ~ 25-50%; Rx repeat or consider FISH or NGS
- **Suspicious for malignancy**: ROM: 75-90%; repeat cytology, FISH/NGS, or surgical management if clinically appropriate
- **Malignant**: ROM: 96-100%

Role of Molecular Testing in Pancreatic Aspirates

- Provides information that may be helpful in cyst classification, risk stratification, and patient management
- Pancreatic cysts/neoplasms
  - Includes assessment of KRAS, GNAS, DNA quantity and quality, loss of heterozygosity, other markers
    - Absence of GNAS or KRAS mutations does not exclude intraductal papillary mucinous neoplasm (IPMN)
    - BRAF mutations and occasional MAP2K1 mutations found in subset of IPMNs, which are KRAS wild type
  - NGS allows evaluation of more mutations

SELECTED REFERENCES

1. Ardeshna DR et al: Recent advances in the diagnostic evaluation of pancreatic cystic lesions. World J Gastroenterol. 28(6):624-34, 2022
2. Hoda RS et al: Risk of malignancy associated with diagnostic categories of the proposed World Health Organization International System for Reporting Pancreaticobiliary Cytopathology. Cancer Cytopathol. 130(3):195-201, 2022
3. HooKim K et al: Atypical cells in fine needle aspiration biopsies of pancreas: causes, work-up, and recommendations for management. Diagn Cytopathol. 50(4):196-207, 2022
4. Nikas IP et al: Evaluating pancreatic and biliary neoplasms with small biopsy-based next generation sequencing (NGS): doing more with less. Cancers (Basel). 14(2), 2022

Pancreatitis

KEY FACTS

ETIOLOGY/PATHOGENESIS
- Gallstones, biliary sludge, periampullary diverticulum, neoplasms, duodenal stricture or obstruction, autoimmune pancreatitis (AIP)
- AIP divided into types I and II
  - Type I: Lobulocentric, older males, higher serum IgG4 levels, and extrapancreatic manifestations
  - Type II: Ductulocentric, younger individuals, and M = F; less stromal response and IgG4

CLINICAL ISSUES
- Abdominal pain, elevated serum amylase
- Elevated serum IgG4 in AIP

CYTOPATHOLOGY
- Acute inflammation, fat necrosis, calcifications in acute pancreatitis
- Mixed lymphohistiocytic infiltrate, fibrosis in chronic pancreatitis
- Fibroblastic stromal fragments with plasma cells and lymphocytes in AIP
- Nuclear features, such as prominent nucleoli, mild hyperchromasia, or minimal nuclear enlargement, are less worrisome for adenocarcinoma if background features of inflammation and repair are present
- Ductal epithelium with reactive atypia, especially in AIP
  - Cells are regularly spaced from each other
- In AIP, plasma cells express IgG4; lymphocytes are mostly CD4(+) with few CD8(+) T-lymphocytes and few B-lymphocytes

ANCILLARY TESTS
- Absence of *KRAS* mutation is supportive of diagnosis of AIP when differential involves carcinoma

TOP DIFFERENTIAL DIAGNOSES
- Pancreatic adenocarcinoma
  - Marked atypia

Reactive Ductal Epithelium
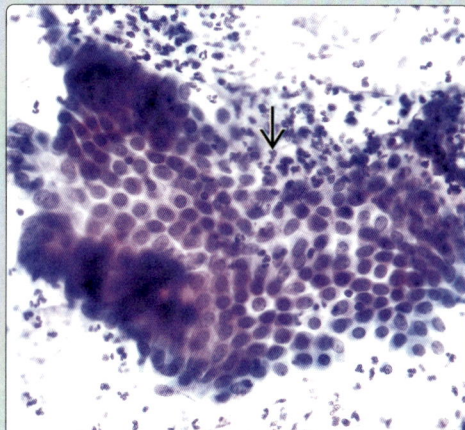

Calcifications
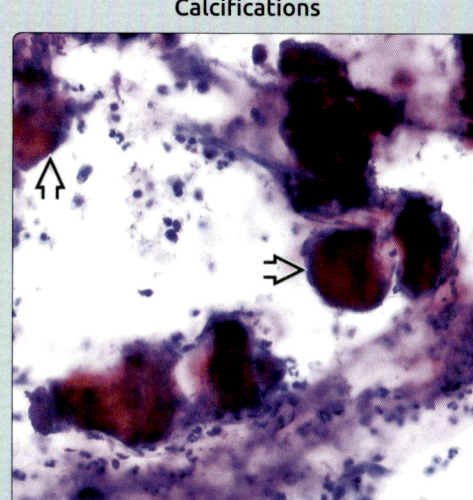

(Left) Pap-stained smear shows reactive pancreatic ductal epithelium with regularly spaced and slightly enlarged nuclei, relatively smooth nuclear borders, and infiltrating neutrophils ➡. (Right) Pap-stained smear shows numerous calcifications ➡. There is inflammation and debris in the background, supporting pancreatitis as the underlying cause of the calcium deposition.

Multinucleated Giant Cell
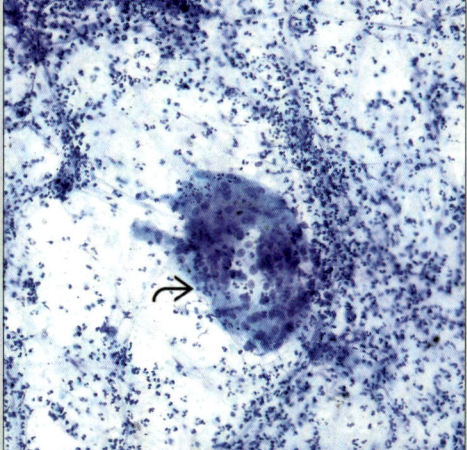

Core Biopsy of Autoimmune Pancreatitis
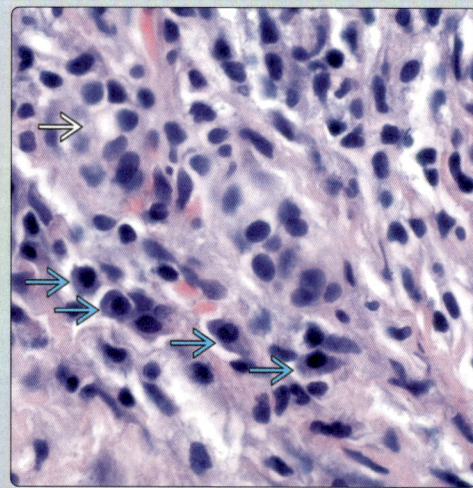

(Left) Pap-stained smear shows an intense neutrophilic infiltrate and a large multinucleated giant cell ➡. (Right) Core biopsy stained with H&E shows loss of acini with only rare, partially destroyed ducts ➡. The inflammatory infiltrate consists of lymphocytes and numerous plasma cells ➡. The plasma cells stained with IgG4 by immunohistochemistry.

Pancreatitis

TERMINOLOGY

Definitions
- Acute or chronic inflammatory process of pancreas

ETIOLOGY/PATHOGENESIS

Mechanical
- Gallstones, biliary sludge, periampullary diverticulum, neoplasms, duodenal stricture, or obstruction

Toxic
- Ethanol, scorpion venom, organophosphate poisoning

Trauma, Metabolic, Vascular, Drug Induced
- Blunt or penetrating abdominal injury, iatrogenic
- Hyperlipidemia type V and hypercalcemia
- Ischemia, hemorrhagic shock, atheroembolism, vasculitis

Drug Induced
- Numerous drugs implicated

Infectious Agents
- Virus: Mumps virus, coxsackievirus, cytomegalovirus, herpes simplex virus, HIV
- Bacteria: *Mycoplasma, Legionella, Leptospira, Salmonella*
- Parasites: *Toxoplasma, Cryptosporidium, Ascaris*

Idiopathic
- 10-25% of patients have no identifiable cause

Autoimmune Pancreatitis
- Types I and II, elevated serum IgG4, IgG4(+) plasma cells
- May be misdiagnosed as malignancy clinically and cytologically

CLINICAL ISSUES

Presentation
- Acute upper abdominal pain, nausea, vomiting
- Elevated serum amylase and lipase, IgG4 in autoimmune

CYTOPATHOLOGY

Cellularity
- Acute: Low cellularity
- Chronic: Early stages more cellular, later stages less cellular

Background
- Acute inflammation, fat necrosis, calcifications in acute pancreatitis
- Mixed lymphohistiocytic infiltrate, fibrosis in chronic pancreatitis
- Fibroblastic stromal fragments with plasma cells and lymphocytes in autoimmune pancreatitis (AIP)

Cells
- Ductal epithelium with reactive atypia, especially in AIP
- Cells are regularly spaced from each other
- In AIP, plasma cells express IgG4; lymphocytes are mostly CD4(+) with few CD8(+) T-lymphocytes and few B-lymphocytes

Nuclear Details
- Minimal nuclear enlargement, mild hyperchromasia, prominent nucleoli, smooth nuclear contours, occasional mitoses

ANCILLARY TESTS

Genetic Testing
- Absence of *KRAS* mutation is supportive of diagnosis of AIP when differential involves carcinoma

DIFFERENTIAL DIAGNOSIS

Pancreatic Adenocarcinoma
- Marked atypia

SELECTED REFERENCES

1. Okasha HH et al: Cystic pancreatic lesions, the endless dilemma. World J Gastroenterol. 27(21):2664-80, 2021

Fibrosis
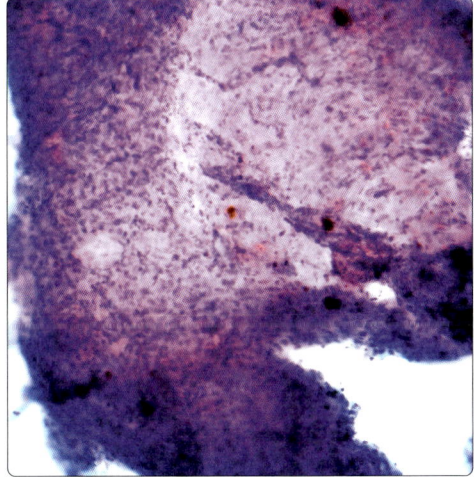

Fat Necrosis
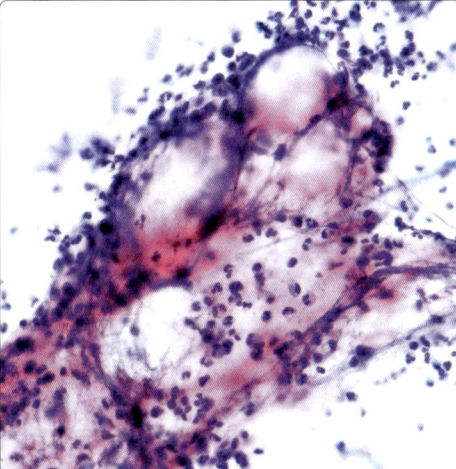

(Left) Pap-stained smear shows fibrosis in a case of chronic pancreatitis. Attention must be paid to the associated cells to rule out malignant desmoplastic fibrosis. **(Right)** Admixed acute inflammation and fat necrosis in acute pancreatitis are seen in a Pap-stained smear.

Lymphoepithelial Cyst of Pancreas

KEY FACTS

CLINICAL ISSUES

- Rare, nonneoplastic, cystic benign lesion consisting of squamous epithelial-lined cyst with surrounding benign lymphoid tissue
- Can be unilocular (40%) or multilocular (60%)
- Accounts for 0.5% of cystic lesions of pancreas
- M:F = 4:1; mean age: 56 years
- Size: 1.5-17 cm
- Presents with nonspecific symptoms
- No association with salivary gland lymphoepithelial cysts or underlying conditions associated with salivary cysts
- On gross examination, contents consist of cheesy keratinous debris
- Lymphoid tissue in wall has germinal centers with intervening T lymphocytes

MICROSCOPIC

- Variable cellularity consisting of nucleated and anucleated squames; may have keratinous debris
- Background has scattered lymphocytes
- Rarely, granulomatous reaction to squamous debris, cholesterol clefts, foamy histiocytes may be seen
- May have elevated cyst fluid CEA levels, potential pitfall

TOP DIFFERENTIAL DIAGNOSES

- Gastrointestinal tract contamination
  - Dismissing squamous cells as swallowed squames from GI tract contents in cases with paucity of lymphocytes may result in nondiagnostic interpretation
- Epidermoid cyst
  - Arising from intrapancreatic accessory spleen
  - Lacks lymphoid component with germinal centers
- Lymphangioma
  - Multiloculated with endothelial lining, lymphocytes, and lack of squamous component
- Pseudocyst
  - Contains debris, lacks epithelial lining

CT of Abdomen Showing 3.5-cm Mass
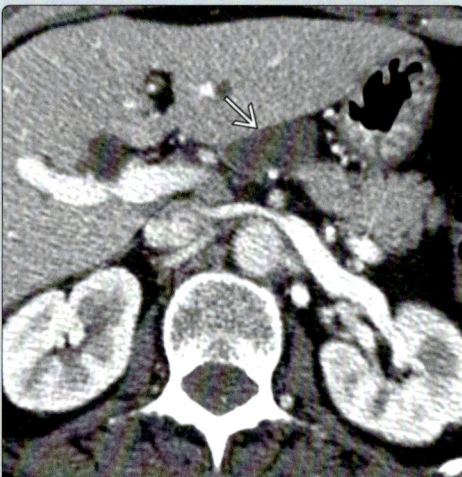

Lymphoepithelial Cyst Cytology
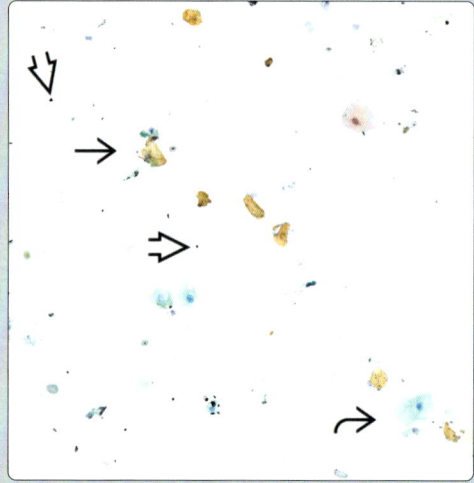

(Left) A 3.5 x 1.7-cm hypodense mass anterior to the pancreatic neck along the posterior surface of the lateral left lobe of the liver ➡ is shown. The enhancement is equivocal. The radiologist thought this may represent a mucinous neoplasm. Endoscopic biopsy/aspiration was recommended. The pancreas is otherwise unremarkable. **(Right)** Pap stain of an aspirate from a lymphoepithelial cyst of the pancreas shows mature anucleate ➡, nucleated squamous cells ➡, and rare lymphocytes ➡.

Histology of Lymphoepithelial Cyst
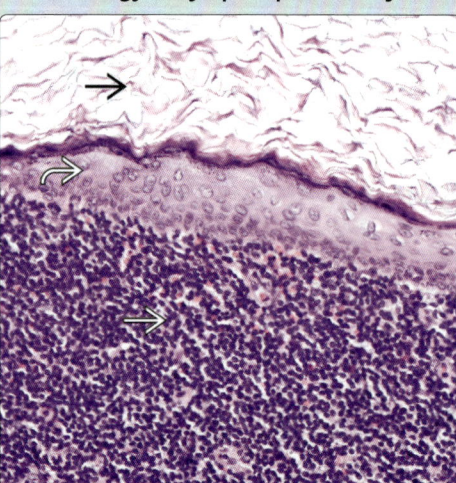

Lymphangioma With Lymphocytes Only
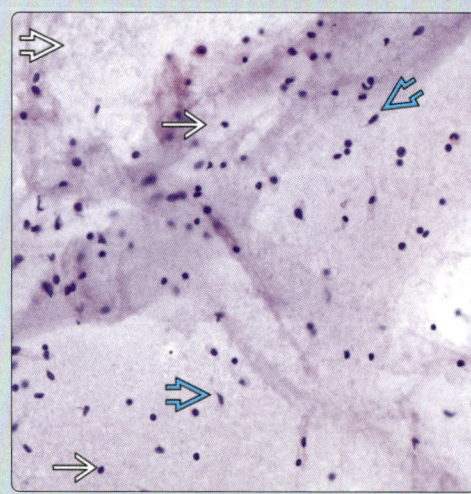

(Left) H&E-stained section of a lymphoepithelial cyst of the pancreas shows a basketweave pattern of anucleate squames ➡, squamous epithelium ➡, and underlying lymphocytes ➡. **(Right)** H&E-stained touch prep from a lymphangioma shows lymphocytes ➡ and a granular precipitate ➡ in the background derived from the lymph in a lymphocele. Note the conspicuous absence of squamous cells. A few bland spindled endothelial cells ➡ are noted.

Intra- and Peripancreatic Splenules

KEY FACTS

CLINICAL ISSUES
- Usually asymptomatic but identified radiographically by characteristic location and appearance, rarely aspirated
- Located in tail of pancreas and splenic hilum
- Other sites for accessory spleen/splenules include splenic vessels, gastrosplenic or splenorenal ligaments, wall of stomach or bowel, greater omentum or mesentery, pelvis, and scrotum
- Occasionally epidermal inclusion cysts may be seen in intrapancreatic accessory spleen
- Ultrasound-guided aspiration is important for accurate diagnosis and avoids unnecessary surgery if not radiologically recognized

CYTOPATHOLOGY
- Polymorphous population of predominantly lymphocytes as well as eosinophils, plasma cells, and endothelial cells
- Tissue fragments containing small vessels with adherent lymphocytes may be seen
- Numerous platelet aggregates in background is also clue
  - Platelets are smaller than lymphoglandular bodies

ANCILLARY TESTS
- Immunohistochemistry on cell block or core shows CD8 positivity in cells lining sinusoids/vessels, highlighting sinusoidal endothelial cells

TOP DIFFERENTIAL DIAGNOSES
- **Pancreatic neuroendocrine tumor or nodule (if < 5 mm)**
  - Occur in splenic hilum/tail of pancreas
  - Lacks hematopoietic elements and platelet aggregates or lymphoglandular bodies
  - Larger cells with more cytoplasm and eccentric nuclei characterized by neuroendocrine chromatin
  - Chromogranin, synaptophysin positive
- **Enlarged lymph node/lymphoma**
  - Many tingible body macrophages, flow cytometry helpful

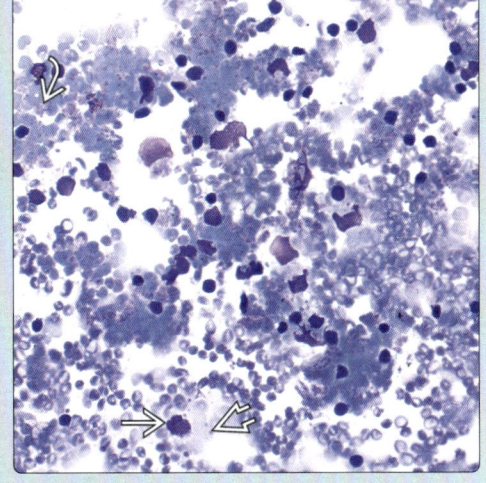

Polymorphous Population of Lymphocytes

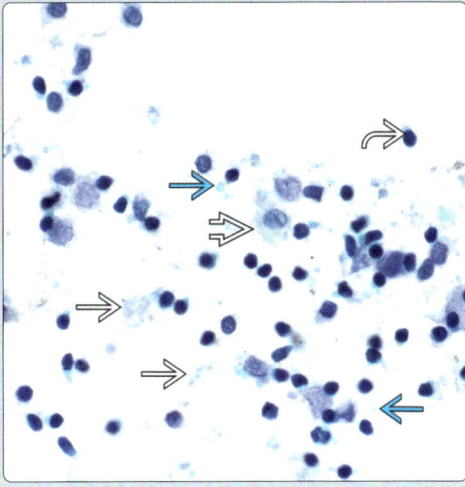

Platelet Aggregates, Histiocytes, and Lymphocytes

(Left) Diff-Quik-stained smear shows a hemorrhagic background with a polymorphous population of lymphocytes ➡, histiocytes, lymphoglandular bodies ➡, and aggregates of platelets ➡, which are smaller than lymphoglandular bodies. (Right) Pap-stained smear shows large aggregates of platelets ➡ between lymphocytes ➡ and histiocytes ➡. The lymphoglandular bodies ➡ are larger than individual platelets in the aggregates.

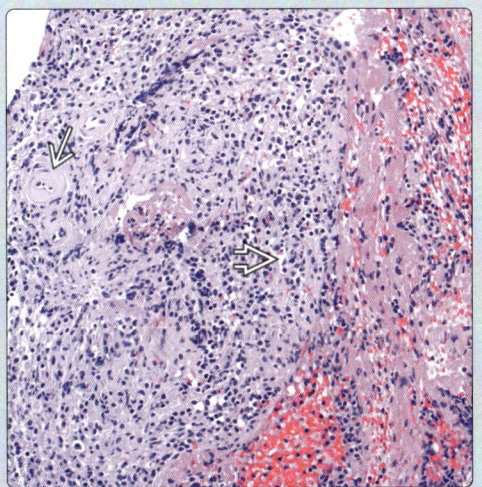

Cell Block With Microbiopsy Fragment

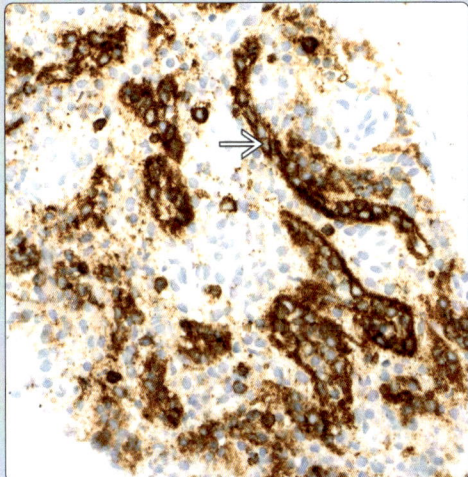

CD8 Stain of Sinusoidal Endothelial Cells

(Left) H&E-stained cell block containing a microbiopsy of the accessory spleen is shown. Note the arterioles ➡, sinusoids ➡, and hematolymphoid population of cells. (Right) Cell block of an intrapancreatic accessory spleen shows CD8-positive staining of the cytoplasm of sinusoidal endothelial cells ➡.

Serous Microcystic Adenoma

KEY FACTS

CLINICAL ISSUES
- Benign cystic epithelial neoplasm
- Accounts for 10% of surgically resected cystic pancreatic lesions
- Anywhere in pancreas
- Grayscale US and CECT are best imaging modalities
  - Central stellate scar with microlacunae separated by delicate septa

CYTOPATHOLOGY
- Microcystic, oligocystic, solid variants cytologically similar
  - No atypia, necrosis, or mitotic activity
- Generally paucicellular or acellular
- Clear, thin fluid; may be bloody
- Epithelial cells form small and flat sheets
  - May be mistaken for gastrointestinal epithelium
- Small and round nuclei
- Clear or vacuolated cytoplasm with distinct borders

ANCILLARY TESTS
- Immunohistochemistry
  - Positive for cytokeratin, α-inhibin, calponin, GLUT1, MUC6
  - Negative for vimentin, CEA, HMB-45, melan-A, MUC5, chromogranin, trypsin
- Granular cytoplasmic positivity for periodic acid-Schiff stain sensitive to diastase digestion
- von Hippel-Lindau (*VHL*) gene alteration detected even in sporadic cases

TOP DIFFERENTIAL DIAGNOSES
- von Hippel-Lindau-associated pancreatic cysts
- Pseudocyst
- Mucinous cystic neoplasm
- Lymphangioma
- Metastatic renal cell carcinoma
- Combined well-differentiated neuroendocrine neoplasm/serous microcystic adenoma

Gross Appearance

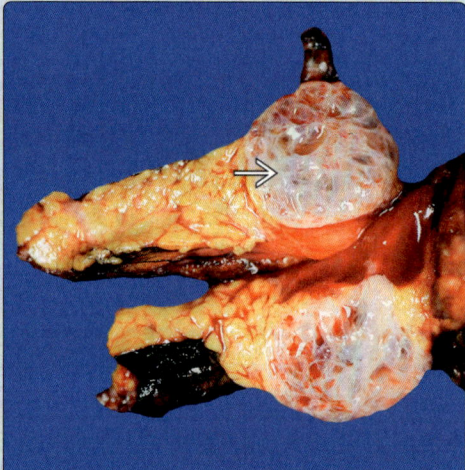

Epithelial Fragment

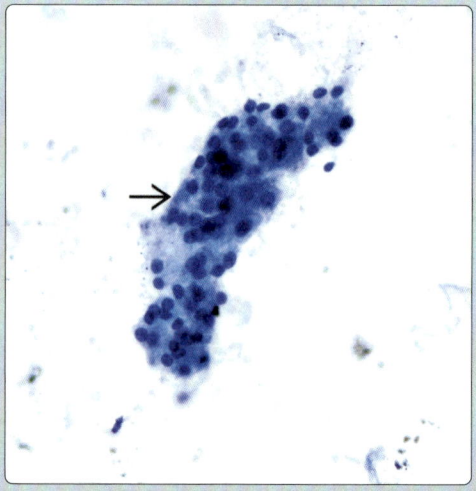

(Left) This well-circumscribed pancreatic mass ➡ has numerous smooth-walled microcysts containing clear serous fluid. (Courtesy G. Kim, MD.) (Right) Pap-stained FNA smear of serous microcystic adenoma shows a fragment of benign epithelial cells ➡ with a moderate amount of cytoplasm and round nuclei with smooth nuclear borders. This can easily be misinterpreted as gastrointestinal mucosal contaminant.

Serous Microcystic Adenoma

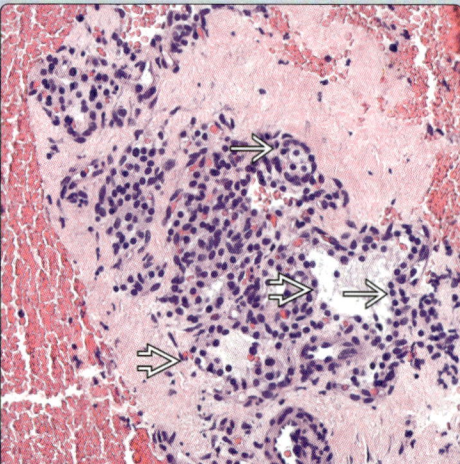

Round Nuclei and Delicate Cytoplasm

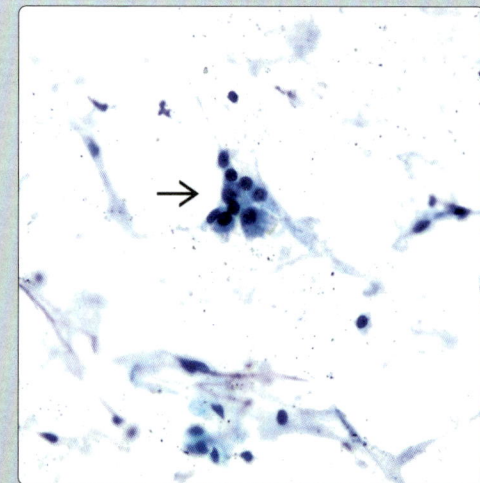

(Left) Endoscopic US-guided fine-needle biopsy of serous microcystic adenoma shows small cystic spaces ➡ lined by benign cuboidal epithelium ➡ with round nucleus and clear cytoplasm. (Right) Pap-stained FNA smear of serous microcystic adenoma shows a cluster of benign epithelial cells ➡ with round nuclei and moderate amount of delicate cytoplasm.

Serous Microcystic Adenoma

TERMINOLOGY

Synonyms
- Serous cystadenoma (SCA)
- Clear cell or glycogen-rich adenoma

Definitions
- Benign cystic epithelial neoplasm

CLINICAL ISSUES

Epidemiology
- Sex
  - Female predominance

Site
- Anywhere in pancreas

IMAGING

Radiographic Findings
- Grayscale US and CECT are best imaging modalities
  - Microlacunae separated by delicate septa
  - Central stellate scar

CYTOPATHOLOGY

Cellularity
- Generally paucicellular or acellular

Background
- Clear, thin fluid; may be bloody

Cells
- Microcystic, oligocystic, solid variants cytologically similar
- Epithelial cells form small and flat sheets

Nuclear Details
- Small and round nuclei

Cytoplasmic Details
- Clear or vacuolated cytoplasm with distinct borders

ANCILLARY TESTS

Histochemistry
- Granular cytoplasmic positivity for PAS stain sensitive to diastase digestion

Immunohistochemistry
- Positive for cytokeratin, α-inhibin, MUC6, MUC1, carbonic anhydrase 9 (CA9), HIF-1-α

DIFFERENTIAL DIAGNOSIS

von Hippel-Lindau-Associated Pancreatic Cysts
- Histologically identical to SCA, but distribution differs: Multifocal or diffuse cysts

Pseudocyst
- Unilocular cyst with thick fibrous wall

Mucinous Cystic Neoplasm
- Multilocular thick-walled cyst with mucoid material
- Ovarian-type stroma with overlying mucinous epithelium with variable degree of cytologic atypia

Lymphangioma
- Multilocular cyst lined by endothelial cells and lymphoid aggregates
- Immunoreactive for CD34, CD31, and D2-40

Metastatic Renal Cell Carcinoma
- Has glycogen-rich clear cells but is cytologically atypical

Combined Well-Differentiated Neuroendocrine Neoplasm/Serous Microcystic Adenoma
- Occurs in patients with von Hippel-Lindau syndrome

SELECTED REFERENCES

1. Jhala N et al: Role of ancillary testing on endoscopic US-guided fine needle aspiration samples from cystic pancreatic neoplasms. Acta Cytol. 64(1-2):124-35, 2020
2. Song SJ et al: Diagnosing pancreatic serous cystadenoma on ThinPrep. Diagn Cytopathol. 48(11):1134-6, 2020

CT Appearance
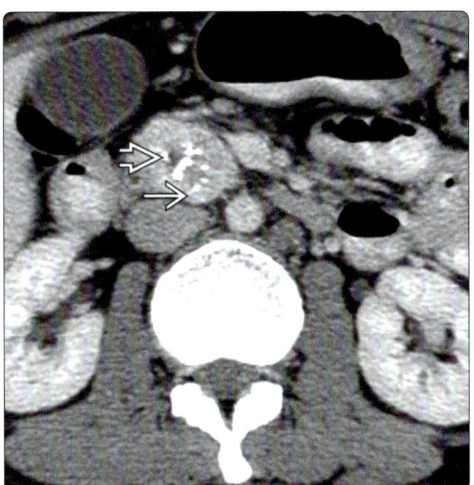

Background Thin Fluid and Histiocytes
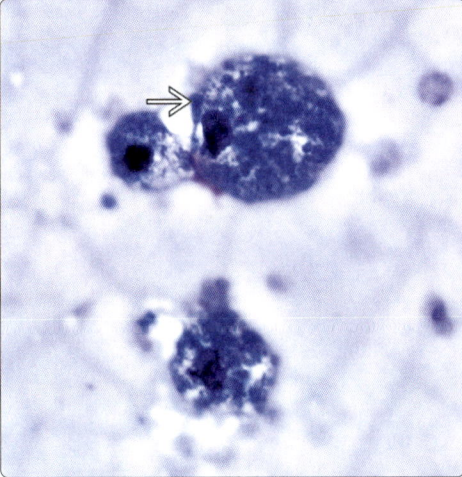

(Left) CT shows a well-defined mass within the pancreatic head with focal calcifications ➡ and a central stellate scar ➡. *(Courtesy G. Kim, MD.)* *(Right)* Diff-Quik-stained FNA smear of serous microcystic adenoma shows rare histiocytes ➡ in a background of thin proteinaceous fluid.

Mucinous Cystic Neoplasm

KEY FACTS

CLINICAL ISSUES
- Neoplasm composed of mucin-producing epithelial cells associated with ovarian-type stroma
- 10% of cystic lesions in pancreas
- Average age at diagnosis: 40-50 years; predominantly female (F:M = 20:1)
- 90% in body or tail of pancreas
- Usually well-demarcated, thick-walled multilocular cystic mass with peripheral calcification
- Main pancreatic duct/large interlobular ducts do not communicate with cysts in majority of cases

CYTOPATHOLOGY
- Columnar or cuboidal mucin-producing cells in sheets or clusters with varying grades of dysplasia
- Extracellular mucin and muciphages in background

ANCILLARY TESTS
- Increased CEA and low amylase levels in cyst fluid analysis

TOP DIFFERENTIAL DIAGNOSES
- Pseudocyst
  - Typically associated with history of pancreatitis and elevated serum amylase levels
  - More common in men than in women
- Intraductal papillary mucinous neoplasms (branch duct type)
  - More often seen in head of gland than in body/tail
  - More common in men than in women
  - Communicates with pancreatic duct system and lacks ovarian-type stroma
- Serous cystic neoplasm
  - Smaller cysts, central stellate scar, and glycogen-rich cuboidal lining cells
  - No mucin in background
- Normal gastrointestinal tract contaminants
  - Small intestine/gastric epithelium and scant mucin from contaminants can be confused with mucinous lesion

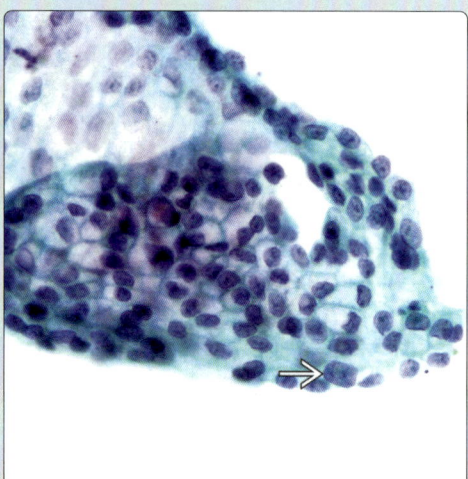

Moderately Atypical Cell Cluster

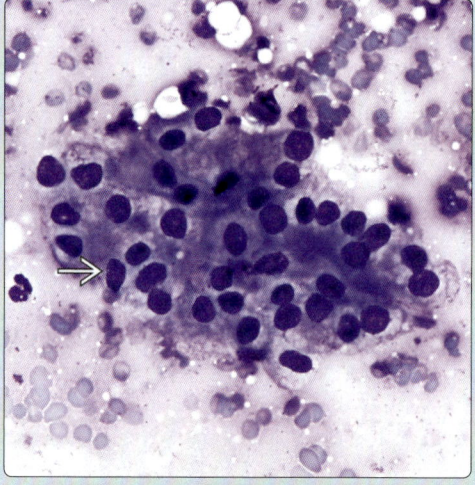

Bland Tumor Cells

(Left) Pap-stained FNA smear demonstrates a sheet of epithelial cells with well-defined cell borders, cytoplasmic mucin, and moderate nuclear atypia ➡. (Right) Diff-Quik-stained FNA smear of mucinous cystadenoma illustrates a small cluster of bland, mucin-containing epithelial cells ➡ with oval-round and regular nuclei and even chromatin pattern.

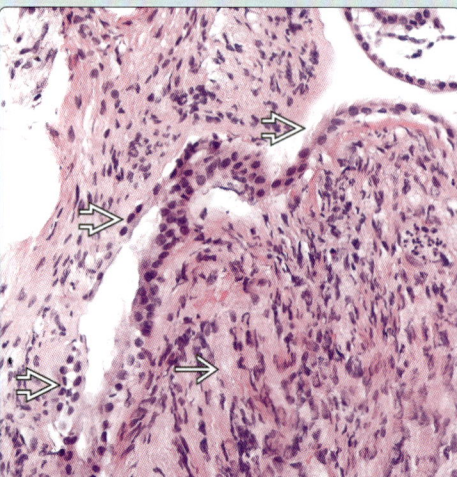

Mucinous Cystic Neoplasm Biopsy

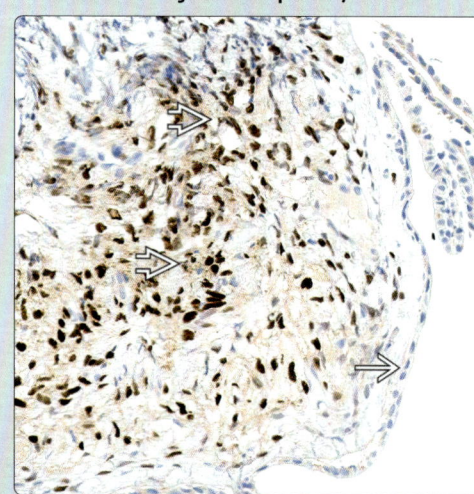

Mucinous Cystic Neoplasm, PR Stain

(Left) Endoscopic ultrasound-guided fine needle biopsy of a pancreatic mucinous cystic neoplasm shows cystic spaces lined by mucinous cuboidal epithelial cells ➡ and bordered by stroma that resembles ovarian stroma ➡. (Right) Endoscopic ultrasound-guided fine needle biopsy immunostained with PR shows positive staining in the ovarian-type stroma surrounding the cystic spaces ➡ that are lined by mucinous glandular epithelium ➡.

Mucinous Cystic Neoplasm

TERMINOLOGY

Definitions
- Neoplasm composed of mucin-producing epithelial cells associated with ovarian-type stroma

CLINICAL ISSUES

Epidemiology
- Incidence
  - 10% of cystic lesions in pancreas
- Age
  - Average age at diagnosis: 40-50 years
- Sex
  - Predominantly female (F:M = 20:1)

Prognosis
- Excellent for patients with benign mucinous cystic neoplasm (MCN) and MCN with noninvasive carcinoma

IMAGING

CT Findings
- Usually well-demarcated, thick-walled multilocular cystic mass with peripheral calcification

ERCP Findings
- Main pancreatic duct/large interlobular ducts do not communicate with cysts in majority of cases

CYTOPATHOLOGY

Pattern
- Columnar mucinous cells in honeycomb pattern, small clusters, or flat sheets in cystadenoma

Background
- Variable amounts of extracellular mucin, muciphages, or foamy histiocytes represent cyst contents

Cells
- Single columnar cells, small clusters, or flat sheets of mucinous epithelial cells

Nuclear Details
- Low grade: Basally located, round, regular nuclei
- High grade/carcinoma: Crowded irregular nuclei and prominent nucleoli

Cytoplasmic Details
- Cytoplasmic mucin can be seen in epithelial cells

MACROSCOPIC

General Features
- 90% in body or tail of pancreas
- Usually multiloculated with thick walls
  - Filled with thick, tenacious mucoid material

DIFFERENTIAL DIAGNOSIS

Pseudocyst
- Typically associated with history of pancreatitis and elevated serum amylase levels

Intraductal Papillary Mucinous Neoplasm (Branch Duct Type)
- Communicates with pancreatic duct system and lacks ovarian-type stroma

Serous Cystic Neoplasm
- Smaller cysts, central stellate scar, and glycogen-rich cuboidal lining cells

Normal Gastrointestinal Tract Mucosa
- Small intestine/gastric epithelium and scant mucin from gastric contamination can be confused for mucinous lesion

SELECTED REFERENCES
1. Wang H et al: The value of serum tumor markers and blood inflammation markers in differentiating pancreatic serous cystic neoplasms and pancreatic mucinous cystic neoplasms. Front Oncol. 12:831355, 2022
2. Sun LQ et al: Validation of serum tumor biomarkers in predicting advanced cystic mucinous neoplasm of the pancreas. World J Gastroenterol. 27(6):501-12, 2021
3. Abdelkader A et al: Cystic lesions of the pancreas: differential diagnosis and cytologic-histologic correlation. Arch Pathol Lab Med. 144(1):47-61, 2020

Cell Clusters and Mucin

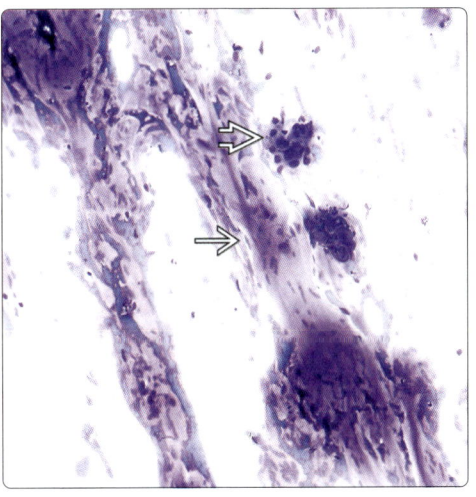

Muciphages Within Mucin

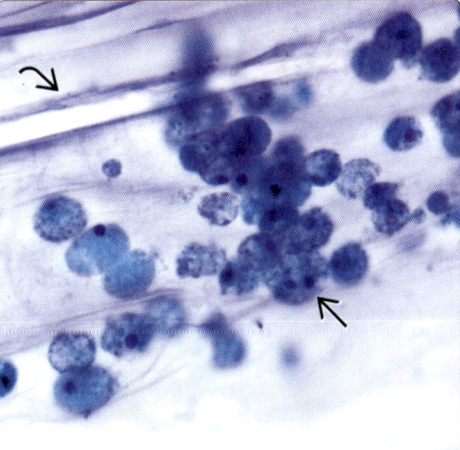

(Left) Diff-Quik-stained FNA smear of a mucinous cystic neoplasm shows thick background mucin ➡ and a small cluster of bland mucinous epithelial cells ➡. *(Right)* Diff-Quik-stained smear of a mucinous cystic neoplasm demonstrates muciphages ➡ in a background of thin extracellular mucin ➡.

Intraductal Papillary Mucinous Neoplasm

KEY FACTS

CLINICAL ISSUES
- Most common cystic tumor of pancreas
- Range: 25-94 years (average: 63 years)
- Slightly more common in men
- Grossly visible, mucin-producing epithelial neoplasm that primarily grows within main duct &/or its branches
- Classic endoscopic finding: Mucin extravasation from patulous ampulla of Vater

CYTOPATHOLOGY
- Small clusters, flat sheets, or papillary groups of glandular epithelial cells
  - ± intracytoplasmic mucin; dense oncocytic cytoplasm in oncocytic type
- Colloid-like, thick mucin in background
- Glandular epithelial cells can exhibit varying grades of atypia ranging from low-grade to high-grade dysplasia

ANCILLARY TESTS
- Mutations in *KRAS2* and *GNAS*
- High amylase, variable CEA levels in cyst fluid

TOP DIFFERENTIAL DIAGNOSES
- Mucinous cystic neoplasm
  - Usually involves body/tail of pancreas
  - Does not communicate with pancreatic ducts; has ovarian-like stroma
  - More common in younger women
- Pancreatic intraepithelial neoplasm
  - Smaller than IPMN (usually < 5 mm in diameter)
- Serous cystic neoplasm
  - Cysts lined by bland cuboidal epithelial cells with cytoplasmic glycogen; no mucin in background
  - Does not communicate with pancreatic ducts
- Retention cysts
  - Unilocular and lined by flat ductal epithelium without mucinous epithelium; no mucin in background

Gross Morphology
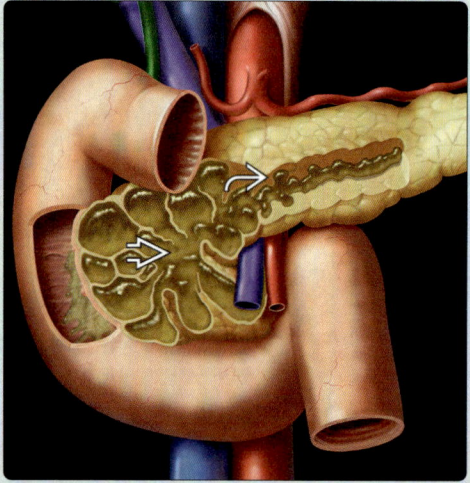

Branch-Duct Type
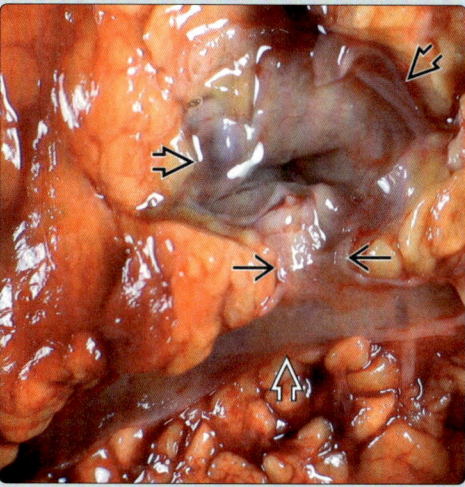

(Left) Graphic shows intraductal papillary mucinous neoplasm (IPMN) involving a dilated main pancreatic duct ➡ and mucin-filled cysts involving dilated branch ducts ➡. (Right) IPMN, branch-duct type, features a small cyst with a smooth lining ➡ connected to the main pancreatic duct ➡ through a dilated branch duct ➡.

Glandular Cells in Mucin
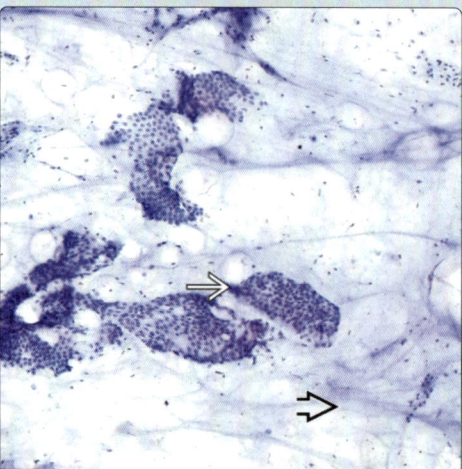

Low-Grade Histology
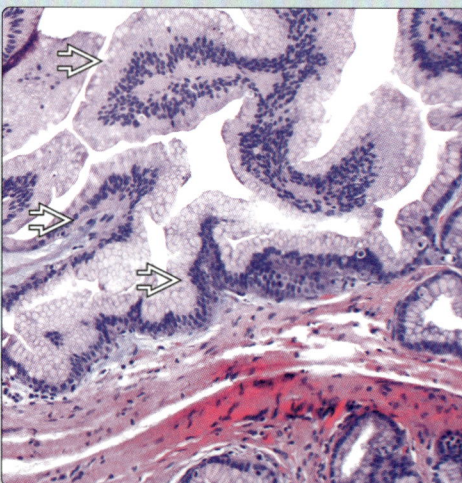

(Left) Pap-stained FNA smear of IPMN shows few clusters of glandular epithelial cells ➡ without atypia in a background of abundant extracellular mucin ➡. (Right) Low-grade IPMN shows mucinous glandular epithelial cells without atypia forming papillae ➡.

Intraductal Papillary Mucinous Neoplasm

TERMINOLOGY

Abbreviations
- Intraductal papillary mucinous neoplasm (IPMN)

Definitions
- Grossly visible, mucin-producing epithelial neoplasm that primarily grows within main duct &/or its branches
- Subclassification based on type of duct involvement
  - Main-duct, combined, or branch-duct type

CLINICAL ISSUES

Epidemiology
- Incidence
  - Most common cystic tumor of pancreas

IMAGING

ERCP Findings
- Dilated main pancreatic duct &/or branch ducts
- Filling defects

CYTOPATHOLOGY

Cellularity
- Variable quantity of cells

Pattern
- Flat sheets or honeycomb pattern, papillary clusters, or single columnar mucinous cells
  - ± intracytoplasmic mucin

Background
- Colloid-like, thick mucin

Cells
- Range from bland columnar mucinous cells to high-grade dysplasia/carcinoma in situ

Nuclear Details
- Low grade
  - Round, bland, basally located nuclei
- High grade
  - Irregular, crowded, hyperchromatic nuclei with loss of polarity

Cytoplasmic Details
- Dense oncocytic cytoplasm in oncocytic type

ANCILLARY TESTS

Genetic Testing
- Mutations in *KRAS2* and *GNAS*

Cyst Fluid Analysis
- High amylase, variable CEA levels

DIFFERENTIAL DIAGNOSIS

Mucinous Cystic Neoplasm
- Usually involves body/tail of pancreas
- Does not communicate with pancreatic ducts

Pancreatic Intraepithelial Neoplasm
- Smaller than IPMN (usually < 5 mm in diameter)

Serous Cystic Neoplasm
- Cysts lined by bland cuboidal epithelial cells with cytoplasmic glycogen; no mucin in background
- Does not communicate with pancreatic ducts

Retention Cysts
- Usually unilocular and lined by nonmucinous pancreatic duct epithelium; no mucin in background

Solid Pseudopapillary Neoplasm
- Composed of poorly cohesive, uniform neoplastic cells that form pseudopapillae

SELECTED REFERENCES

1. Gilani SM et al: Endoscopic ultrasound-guided fine needle aspiration cytologic evaluation of intraductal papillary mucinous neoplasm and mucinous cystic neoplasms of pancreas. Am J Clin Pathol. 154(4):559-70, 2020

High-Grade Dysplasia

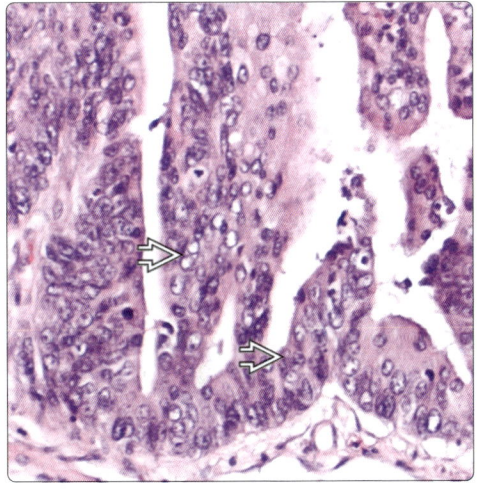

Papillary Fronds

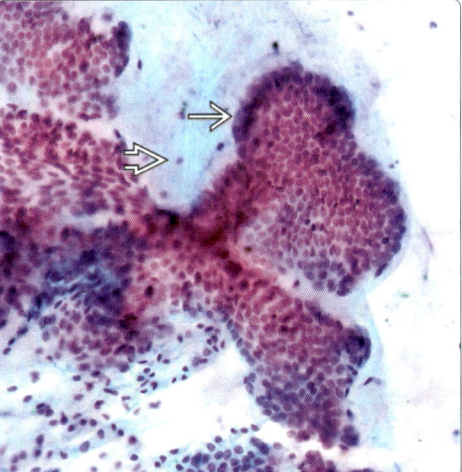

(Left) High-grade IPMN shows dysplasia of the glandular epithelium ➡ forming papillae. *(Right)* Pap-stained FNA smear of IPMN shows papillary fronds of mucinous epithelial cells ➡ with minimal atypia in a background of mucin ➡.

Solid Pseudopapillary Neoplasm

KEY FACTS

CLINICAL ISSUES
- Typically in young female patients, in body/tail of pancreas
- Most solid pseudopapillary neoplasms are indolent, slow growing, and nonaggressive
- Uncommon, 1-2% of pancreatic exocrine tumors
- > 80% cured with surgical resection
- 10-15% of cases have metastases or recurrence

CYTOPATHOLOGY
- Pseudopapillae with tumor cell layer(s) arranged around capillaries; nuclei oriented away from capillaries
- ± pericapillary metachromatic myxoid or hyaline stroma
- Bland nuclei ± longitudinal grooves
  - Finely dispersed chromatin, indistinct to small nucleoli, absent/rare mitoses
- Long, slender cytoplasmic processes (cercariform morphology)
- Intracytoplasmic hyaline globules

ANCILLARY TESTS
- PAS-D(+) hyaline globules
- Positive for β-catenin (nuclear and cytoplasmic), α-1-antitrypsin, CD10, vimentin, PR, CD56, CD99 (paranuclear dot-like pattern); ± synaptophysin &/or pancytokeratin, negative for E-cadherin (membranous)

TOP DIFFERENTIAL DIAGNOSES
- Pancreatic endocrine neoplasm
  - Finely stippled salt and pepper chromatin pattern
  - Strongly positive for synaptophysin, chromogranin, and pancytokeratin
  - Negative for β-catenin (nuclear), CD10, and vimentin
- Acinar cell carcinoma
  - More nuclear pleomorphism, prominent nucleoli, coarse chromatin, coarsely granular or clear cytoplasm
  - Negative for β-catenin (nuclear); positive pancytokeratin, trypsin, &/or chymotrypsin

Eccentric Nuclei
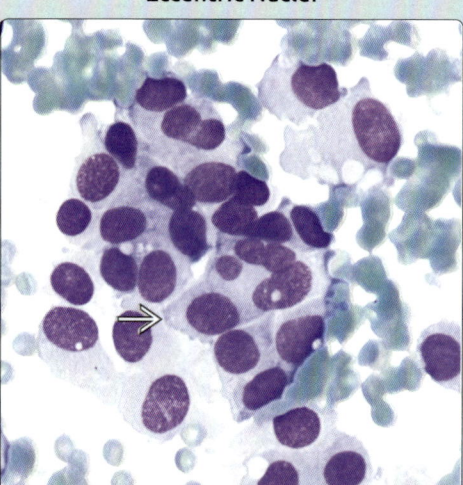

Tumor Cells Around Capillary
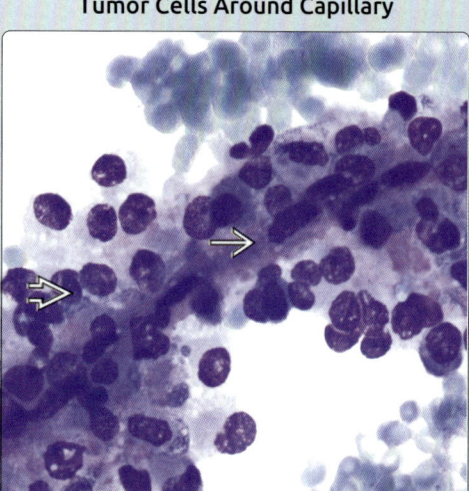

(Left) Diff-Quik-stained FNA smear of a solid pseudopapillary tumor shows tumor cells with round to oval, eccentrically placed nuclei ➡, condensed nuclear chromatin, and a moderate amount of delicate cytoplasm. (Right) Diff-Quik-stained FNA smear of a solid pseudopapillary tumor shows pseudopapillae composed of a capillary channel ➡ bordered by tumor cells ➡.

Capillaries and Cercariform Cells
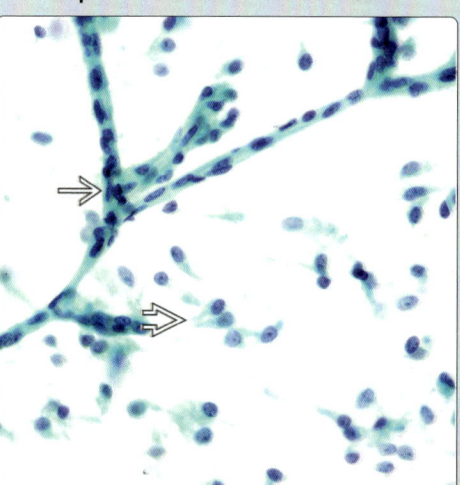

Bland Nuclear Features
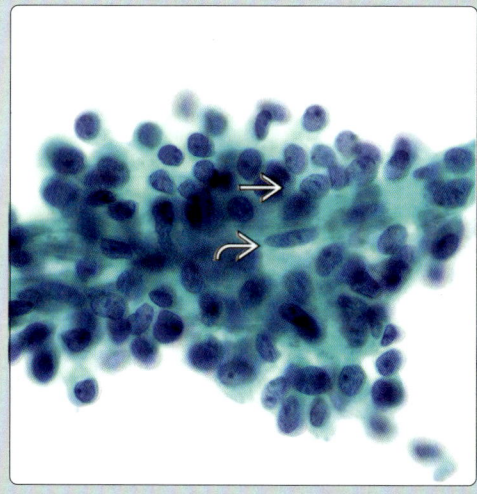

(Left) Pap-stained FNA smear of solid pseudopapillary tumor shows "naked" branched capillaries ➡ with a background of dispersed tumor cells that have slender cytoplasmic processes ➡. (Right) Pap-stained FNA smear of a solid pseudopapillary tumor shows a capillary ➡ surrounded by multiple layers of tumor cells ➡ with finely dispersed chromatin and small nucleoli.

Solid Pseudopapillary Neoplasm

TERMINOLOGY

Definitions
- Low-grade malignant neoplasm of uncertain cellular derivation

CLINICAL ISSUES

Epidemiology and Presentation
- Uncommon, 1-2% of pancreatic exocrine tumors
- Female predominance; rare in men

Treatment and Prognosis
- Surgical resection is treatment of choice for solid pseudopapillary neoplasm
- Excellent prognosis
  - > 80% cured with surgical resection
  - 10-15% of cases have metastases or recurrence

IMAGING

General Features
- Usually in pancreatic body or tail, large, solitary, well demarcated, variably cystic, ± calcified margins

CYTOPATHOLOGY

Cellularity
- Varies from paucicellular to highly cellular

Pattern
- Singly dispersed cells, loose fragments
- Characteristic pseudopapillae with tumor cell layer(s) arranged around capillaries
  - Tumor nuclei oriented away from capillaries, cytoplasmic zone oriented toward capillaries
  - ± pericapillary metachromatic myxoid or hyaline stroma

Cells
- Relatively bland and uniform

Nuclear Details
- Eccentric, round to oval, ± longitudinal grooves ("coffee bean" nuclei)
- Finely dispersed chromatin, indistinct to small nucleoli, absent/rare mitoses

Cytoplasmic Details
- Scant to moderate amount of eosinophilic cytoplasm, may be clear with vacuoles
  - Long, slender cytoplasmic processes are characteristic

ANCILLARY TESTS

Immunohistochemistry
- Positive for β-catenin (nuclear and cytoplasmic), α-1-antitrypsin, CD10, vimentin, PR, CD56, NSE, CD99 (paranuclear dot-like pattern), SOX11; negative for ER, E-cadherin (membranous), and chromogranin; may be focal and weakly positive for synaptophysin &/or pancytokeratin

Histochemistry
- Intracytoplasmic PAS-D(+) hyaline globules

DIFFERENTIAL DIAGNOSIS

Pancreatic Endocrine Neoplasm
- Finely stippled salt and pepper chromatin pattern
- Strongly positive for synaptophysin, chromogranin, and pancytokeratin
- Negative for β-catenin (nuclear), CD10, and vimentin

Acinar Cell Carcinoma
- More nuclear pleomorphism, prominent nucleoli, coarse chromatin, coarsely granular or clear cytoplasm
- Negative for β-catenin (nuclear); positive pancytokeratin, trypsin, &/or chymotrypsin

SELECTED REFERENCES

1. Dinarvand P et al: Utility of SOX11 for the diagnosis of solid pseudopapillary neoplasm of the pancreas on cytological preparations. Cytopathology. 33(2):216-21, 2022

Hyaline Globules

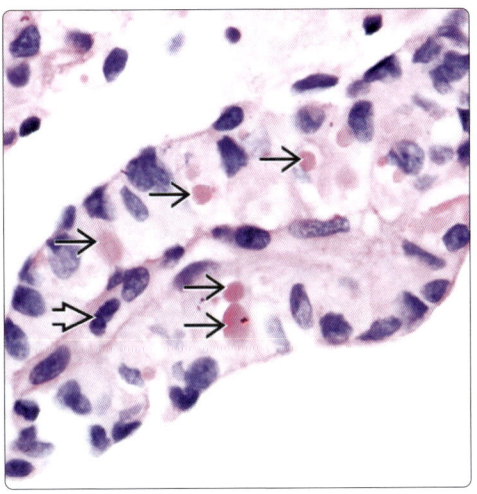

β-Catenin Positive

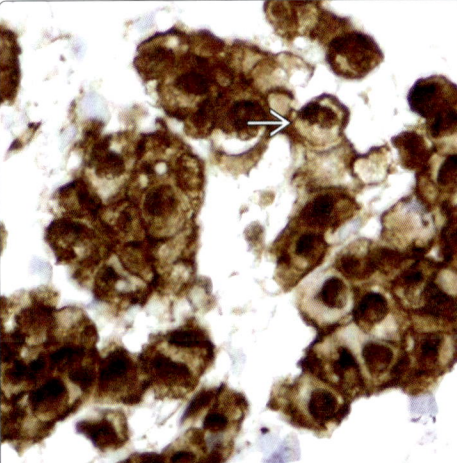

(Left) *H&E-stained cell block section of a solid pseudopapillary tumor shows pseudopapillae with a central capillary ➡ and hyaline globules ➡ within the tumor cell cytoplasm. The globules can be highlighted by PAS stain.* **(Right)** *β-catenin stain of a cell block section of a solid pseudopapillary tumor shows nuclear and cytoplasmic-positive staining of the tumor cells ➡.*

Pancreatic Neuroendocrine Tumor

KEY FACTS

CLINICAL ISSUES
- Typically in adults, in body or tail of pancreas
- Some associated with MEN1, VHL, TSC, or NF1
- Usually slow growing but all considered malignant
- Prognostic factors include mitotic count, Ki-67 staining, tumor size, extent of local invasion &/or metastases, functional status

CYTOPATHOLOGY
- Highly cellular, dispersed, and loosely cohesive sheets of monotonous cells ± endocrine atypia, often plasmacytoid
- Finely stippled salt and pepper chromatin texture
- Moderate amounts of finely granular cytoplasm

ANCILLARY TESTS
- Positive for neuroendocrine markers (synaptophysin, chromogranin, INSM1, NSE, CD56), CK (especially CK8/18/CAM5.2), E-cadherin
- Negative for β-catenin (nuclear), vimentin, pancreatic enzymes

TOP DIFFERENTIAL DIAGNOSES
- Acinar cell carcinoma
  - Positive for pancreatic enzymes; can be focally positive for neuroendocrine markers
- Solid pseudopapillary neoplasm
  - β-catenin (nuclear +), E-cadherin (-), can be focally positive for neuroendocrine markers
- Ductal adenocarcinoma
  - More nuclear atypia, pleomorphism, mitoses; negative for neuroendocrine markers
- Lymphoma/plasmacytoma
  - Lymphoglandular bodies, perinuclear hof, clock face chromatin pattern, monoclonal immunophenotype
- Metastatic tumors
  - Clinical history and immunohistochemistry useful

Salt and Pepper Chromatin

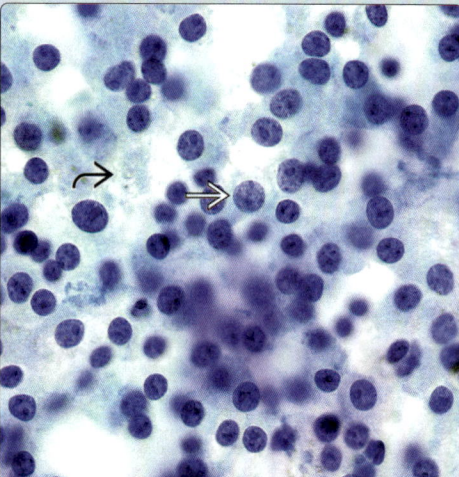

Plasmacytoid Tumor Cells

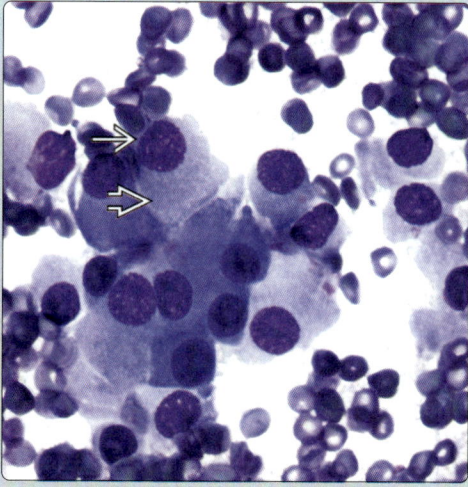

(Left) Pap-stained smear shows singly dispersed tumor cells with salt and pepper chromatin ➡ in a background of disrupted granular cytoplasmic material ➡. (Right) Diff-Quik-stained FNA smear of pancreatic neuroendocrine tumor shows plasmacytoid tumor cells with an eccentrically placed, round nucleus ➡ and abundant granular cytoplasm ➡.

Pancreatic Neuroendocrine Tumor

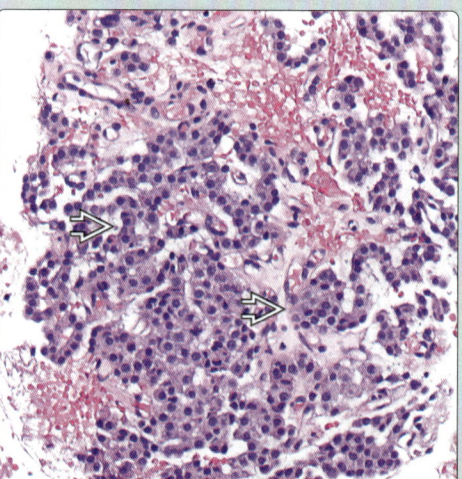

Pancreatic Neuroendocrine Tumor

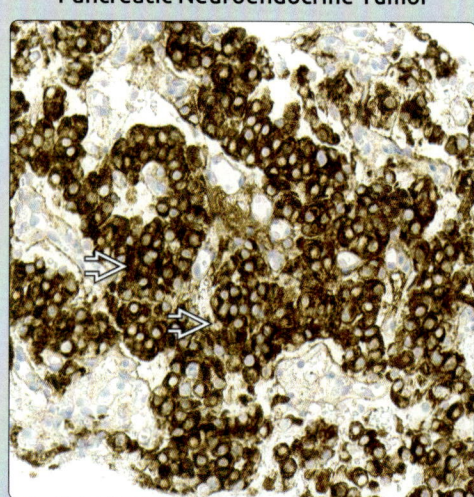

(Left) Core biopsy of pancreatic neuroendocrine tumor, well-differentiated and stained with H&E, shows cords and sheets of tumor cells ➡ with relatively uniform round nucleus and a moderate amount of granular cytoplasm. (Right) Core biopsy of pancreatic neuroendocrine tumor immunostained with synaptophysin shows diffuse and strong cytoplasmic staining in the tumor cells ➡.

Pancreatic Neuroendocrine Tumor

TERMINOLOGY

Definitions
- Pancreatic neoplasm composed of endocrine cells
- Limited to well-differentiated pancreatic endocrine tumors; if poorly differentiated, called neuroendocrine carcinoma
  - Well differentiated: Subdivided into low grade (G1) and intermediate grade (G2)
    - G1: < 2 mitoses per 10 HPF or < 3% Ki-67 index
    - G2: 2-20 mitoses per 10 HPF or 3-20% Ki-67 index

CLINICAL ISSUES

Epidemiology
- 1-2% of all pancreatic neoplasms

Prognosis
- Usually slow growing but all considered malignant

Image Findings
- Usually body or tail, well circumscribed, solid ± cystic area

CYTOPATHOLOGY

Cellularity
- Usually hypercellular smears

Pattern
- Single cells, ribbons, rosettes, loosely cohesive flat sheets
- Capillaries with attached tumor cells characteristic

Cells
- Relatively monotonous small cells, often plasmacytoid; round to oval (rarely spindle-shaped) nuclei; bi- and multinucleation common
  - ± scattered pleomorphic cells (endocrine atypia)

Background
- ± amyloid (especially with insulinomas), ± psammoma bodies (especially with somatostatinomas)

Nuclear Details
- Characteristic salt and pepper chromatin texture
- Variably inconspicuous to prominent nucleoli

Cytoplasmic Details
- Usually moderate amount of finely granular cytoplasm
  - Amphophilic to eosinophilic or clear
  - ± fine red granules on Romanowsky stains

ANCILLARY TESTS

Immunohistochemistry
- Positive for neuroendocrine markers (synaptophysin, chromogranin, NSE, CD56, INSM1, CK (especially CK8/18/CAM5.2), E-cadherin

DIFFERENTIAL DIAGNOSIS

Acinar Cell Carcinoma
- More abundant PAS-D(+) granular or foamy cytoplasm, prominent nucleoli, coarser chromatin
- Positive for pancreatic enzymes

Solid Pseudopapillary Neoplasm
- Pseudopapillae ± myxoid/hyalinized pericapillary layer
- β-catenin (nuclear +), E-cadherin (-), PAS-D(+) globules

Ductal Adenocarcinoma
- More nuclear atypia, pleomorphism, mitoses
- ± cytoplasmic mucin; lacks neuroendocrine markers

Lymphoma/Plasmacytoma
- Lymphoglandular bodies, perinuclear hof, clock face chromatin pattern, monoclonal immunophenotype

Metastatic Tumors to Pancreas
- Metastatic neuroendocrine carcinoma, melanoma
- Clinical history and immunohistochemistry useful

SELECTED REFERENCES
1. Crinò SF et al: Comparison between EUS-guided fine-needle aspiration cytology and EUS-guided fine-needle biopsy histology for the evaluation of pancreatic neuroendocrine tumors. Pancreatology. 21(2):443-50, 2021

Abundant Granular Cytoplasm

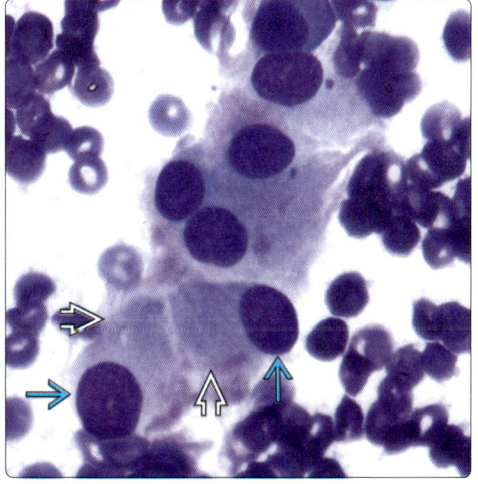

Loosely Cohesive Monotonous Cells

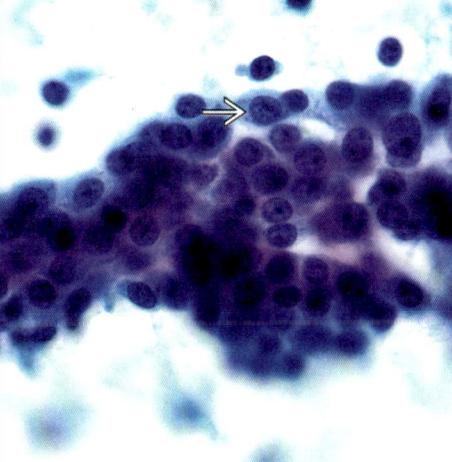

(Left) Diff-Quik-stained FNA smear of pancreatic endocrine tumor shows a tumor cell group with eccentrically located nuclei ➡ and abundant granular cytoplasm ➡. *(Right)* Pap-stained FNA smear of pancreatic neuroendocrine tumor shows a loosely cohesive group of monotonous tumor cells with round nuclei ➡.

Pancreatic Ductal Adenocarcinoma

KEY FACTS

CLINICAL ISSUES
- 2/3 located in pancreatic head
- May present with pain, weight loss, signs of biliary obstruction, ± migratory thrombophlebitis
- Overall 5-year survival rate: 2-4%

CYTOPATHOLOGY
- "Drunken honeycombs" with irregular spacing and overlap of nuclei
- "Tombstone" isolated malignant cells
- Nuclear enlargement with marked size variation (≥ 4:1 within same cell group)
- Nuclear contour irregularities and irregular chromatin distribution
- Cytoplasmic mucin

ANCILLARY TESTS
- Positive: CK7, CK8/18/CAM5.2, CK19, CK20 (33%), MUC5AC, mesothelin, S100P, pVHL, IMP-3, maspin
- Negative: MUC2, chromogranin/synaptophysin, trypsin/chymotrypsin
- Mutations in *KRAS* (~ 90%), *CDKN2A* (> 95%), *TP53* (~ 60%), *SMAD4* (deletion in ~ 50%)

TOP DIFFERENTIAL DIAGNOSES
- Acinar cell carcinoma
  - More uniform malignant cells
  - Trypsin/chymotrypsin (+)
- Pancreatic endocrine neoplasm
  - Synaptophysin/chromogranin (+)
  - Salt and pepper chromatin
- Metastatic carcinoma
  - Correlate with clinical &/or imaging information
  - Pertinent immunostains
- Nonneoplastic ductal epithelium with reactive changes (chronic pancreatitis, stent atypia, radiation)
  - Less cellular, less pronounced cytologic alterations
  - Correlate with clinical and imaging findings

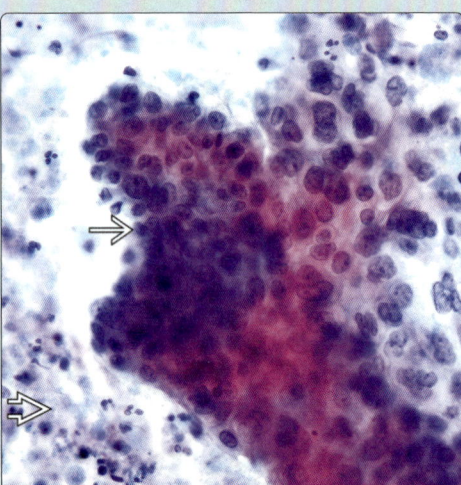
Sheet of Malignant Cells

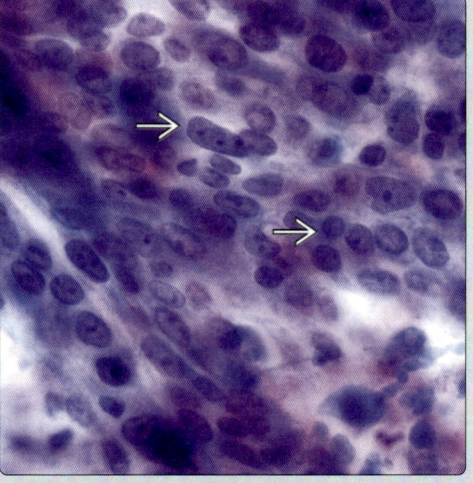
Marked Anisonucleosis

(Left) Pap-stained FNA smear of pancreatic ductal adenocarcinoma shows a sheet of crowded tumor cells ➔ in a background of necrotic debris ➔ and neutrophils. *(Right)* Pap-stained FNA smear of pancreatic ductal adenocarcinoma depicts marked anisonucleosis (≥ 4:1 size variation) of tumor cells ➔ within the same cell group.

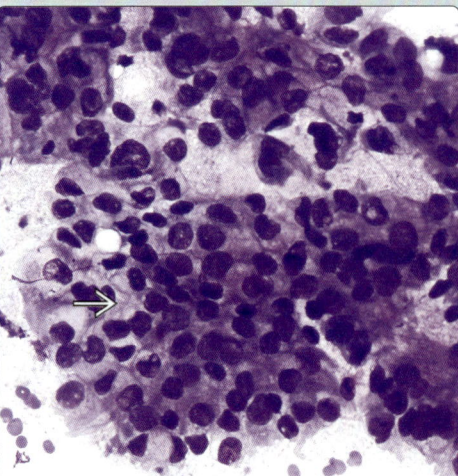
"Drunken Honeycomb"

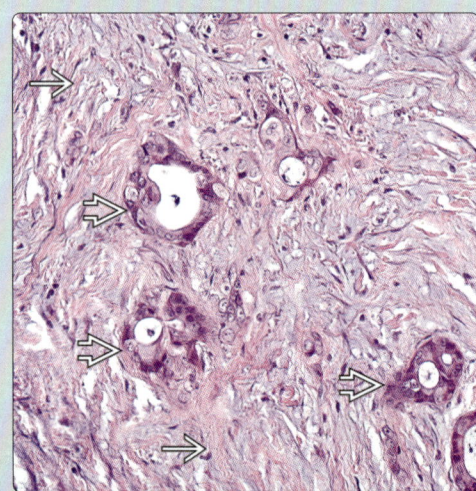
Pancreatic Ductal Adenocarcinoma

(Left) Diff-Quik-stained FNA smear of pancreatic ductal adenocarcinoma shows the irregularly spaced nuclei ➔ of a "drunken honeycomb." *(Right)* Tissue section of pancreatic surgical resection stained with H&E shows neoplastic glands ➔ lined by moderately pleomorphic tumor cells distributed in a desmoplastic stroma ➔.

Pancreatic Ductal Adenocarcinoma

TERMINOLOGY

Definitions
- Malignant epithelial neoplasm derived from pancreatic ductal system

ETIOLOGY/PATHOGENESIS

Precursor Lesions
- Pancreatic intraepithelial neoplasm, mucinous cystic neoplasm, intraductal papillary mucinous neoplasm

CLINICAL ISSUES

Epidemiology
- M:F = 1.3:1; typical age: 60-80 years

Presentation
- 90% of all pancreatic neoplasms; 2/3 are located in pancreatic head

CYTOPATHOLOGY

Cellularity
- Usually highly cellular, but less so if fibrotic

Pattern
- Sheets of disordered ductal cells ("drunken honeycombs"), 3D groups, isolated malignant cells (elongated "tombstones")

Cells
- Most are moderately differentiated but variable
- ± squamous differentiation, ± anaplastic/sarcomatoid features, ± signet-ring cells, ± osteoclast-type giant cells

Nuclear and Cytoplasmic Details
- Nuclear enlargement, size variation (≥ 4:1 within same cell group), contour irregularities, irregular chromatin distribution, hyperchromatic or pale nuclei, usually distinct nucleoli, ± mitoses
- Variably abundant cytoplasm, mucin (+)

ANCILLARY TESTS

Immunohistochemistry
- Positive: CK7, CK8/18/CAM5.2, CK19, CK20 (33%), MUC5AC, p53, mesothelin, S100P, pVHL, IMP-3, maspin
- Negative: MUC2, chromogranin/synaptophysin, trypsin/chymotrypsin
- Loss of expression: p16 (nuclear; > 90%), SMAD4/DPC4 (nuclear and cytoplasmic; 55%)

Genetic Testing
- Mutations in *KRAS* (~ 90%), *CDKN2A* (> 95%), *TP53* (~ 60%), *SMAD4* (deletion in ~ 50%)

DIFFERENTIAL DIAGNOSIS

Acinar Cell Carcinoma
- Trypsin/chymotrypsin (+)

Pancreatic Endocrine Neoplasm
- Synaptophysin/chromogranin (+)

Metastatic Carcinoma
- Immunohistochemistry is useful

High-Grade Pancreatic Intraepithelial Neoplasm
- Cytologically similar but low cellularity in FNA smears unlike ductal adenocarcinoma

Reactive Nonneoplastic Ductal Epithelium
- Less cellular, less pronounced cytologic alterations

SELECTED REFERENCES

1. Kandel P et al: Comparison of endoscopic ultrasound-guided fine-needle biopsy versus fine-needle aspiration for genomic profiling and DNA yield in pancreatic cancer: a randomized crossover trial. Endoscopy. 53(4):376-82, 2021
2. Levine I et al: Endoscopic ultrasound fine needle aspiration vs fine needle biopsy for pancreatic masses, subepithelial lesions, and lymph nodes. World J Gastroenterol. 27(26):4194-207, 2021
3. Visani M et al: Molecular alterations in pancreatic tumors. World J Gastroenterol. 27(21):2710-26, 2021
4. Hoda RS et al: Risk of malignancy in the categories of the Papanicolaou Society of Cytopathology system for reporting pancreaticobiliary cytology. J Am Soc Cytopathol. 8(3):120-7, 2019

Cytoplasmic Mucin

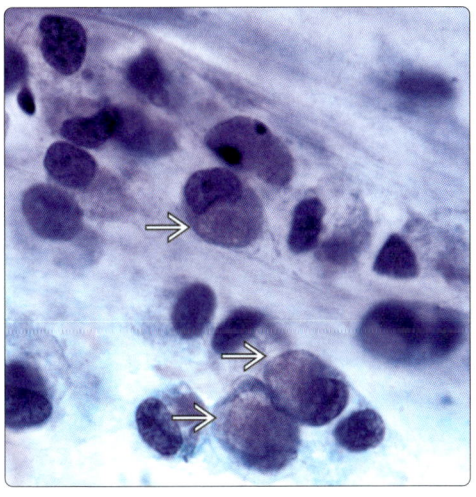

Irregular Nuclear Contours

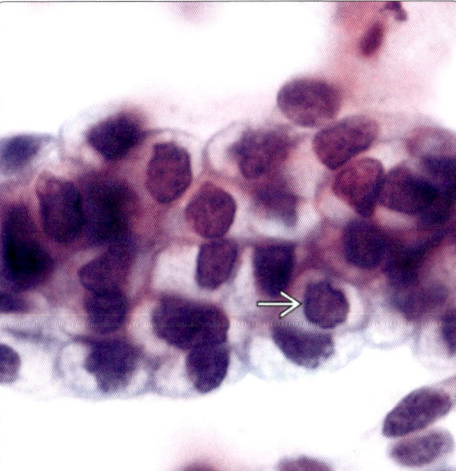

(Left) Pap-stained FNA smear of pancreatic ductal adenocarcinoma shows signet-ring cells ➡ with large cytoplasmic mucin accumulation indenting and displacing the nucleus to the side. **(Right)** Pap-stained FNA smear of pancreatic ductal adenocarcinoma shows a "drunken honeycomb" sheet of tumor cells with nuclear contour irregularities ➡.

Unusual Variants of Ductal Carcinoma

KEY FACTS

CLINICAL ISSUES

- Variants of pancreatic ductal carcinoma that have distinct clinical, morphological, or prognostic significance
- Several variants
  o Adenosquamous carcinoma
  o Colloid carcinoma
  o Medullary carcinoma
  o Signet-ring cell carcinoma
  o Hepatoid carcinoma
  o Undifferentiated carcinoma
  o Carcinoma with mixed differentiation, including variable combinations with neuroendocrine and acinar cells
- Prognosis is dismal for most variants
  o Colloid carcinoma and medullary carcinoma variants have better prognosis than conventional ductal carcinoma

CYTOPATHOLOGY

- Unusual cell morphologies can be seen depending on variant type
  o Squamous cells with keratinization
  o Signet-ring cells
  o Hepatocyte-like cells
  o Bizarre tumor giant cells
  o Acinar cells
  o Neuroendocrine cells
- Benign osteoclast-like giant cells and abundant extracellular mucin are noted in background of specific variants

TOP DIFFERENTIAL DIAGNOSES

- Melanoma
- Choriocarcinoma
- Metastatic anaplastic carcinoma from sites such as lung and thyroid gland
- Pancreatoblastoma
- Metastatic squamous carcinoma
- Metastatic hepatocellular carcinoma
- Metastatic gastric or breast carcinoma with signet-ring cells
- Giant cells associated with reactive processes

Undifferentiated Carcinoma Cytology

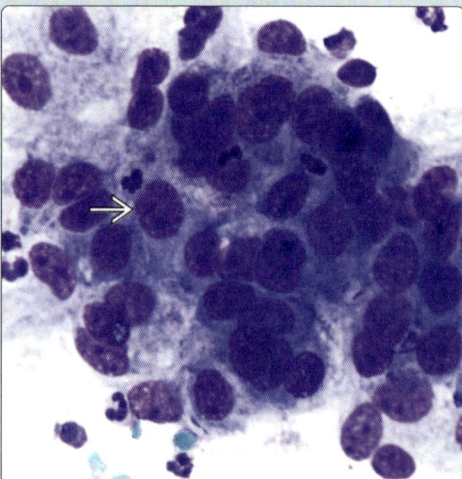

Undifferentiated Carcinoma Histology

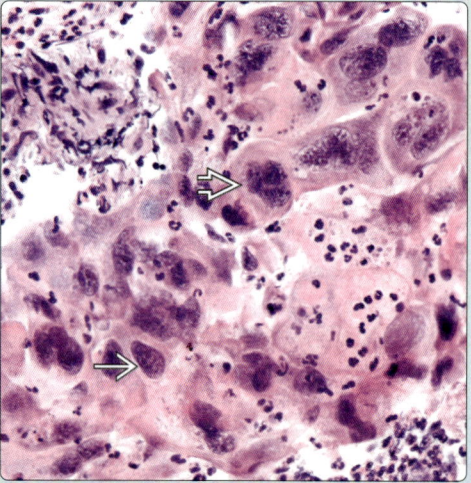

(Left) Diff-Quik-stained FNA smear of undifferentiated carcinoma of the pancreas shows a fragment of mononuclear tumor cells with large pleomorphic nuclei ➡ and a moderate amount of cytoplasm. (Right) H&E-stained cell block section of undifferentiated anaplastic carcinoma of the pancreas shows sheets of mononuclear large tumor cells ➡ and tumor giant cells with bizarre hyperchromatic nuclei ➡.

Adenosquamous Carcinoma Cytology

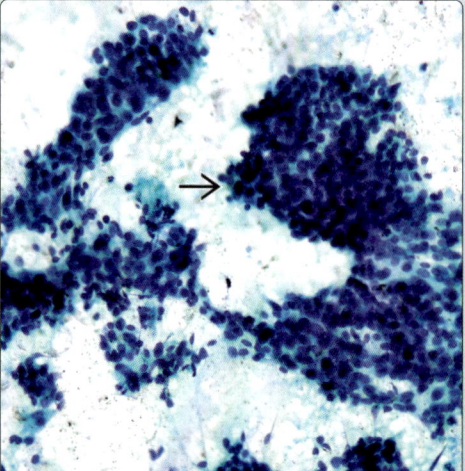

Adenosquamous Carcinoma Histology

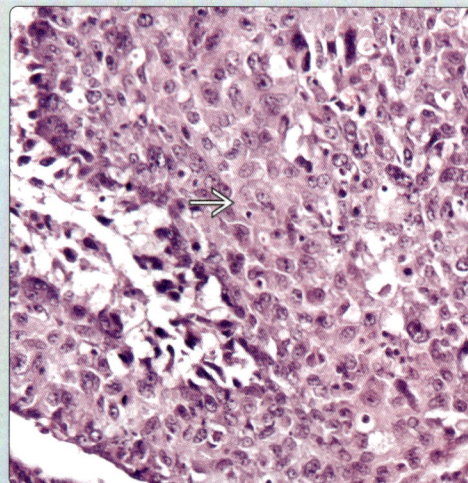

(Left) Pap-stained FNA smear of adenosquamous carcinoma of the pancreas shows large fragments of tumor cells with hyperchromatic nuclei associated with features suggestive of squamous differentiation ➡. (Right) H&E-stained section of adenosquamous carcinoma of the pancreas shows sheets of polygonal tumor cells ➡ with dense, eosinophilic cytoplasm and intercellular junctions, all of which support squamous differentiation of the tumor.

Unusual Variants of Ductal Carcinoma

TERMINOLOGY

Definitions

- Malignant epithelial neoplasms that include variants of ductal adenocarcinoma with distinct clinical, morphological, or prognostic significance
  - Adenosquamous carcinoma
    - Malignant epithelial neoplasm with ductal and squamous differentiation; at least 30% of neoplasm consists of squamous component
  - Colloid carcinoma
    - Infiltrating ductal epithelial neoplasm characterized by presence of large, extracellular stromal mucin pools in at least 80% of neoplasm
    - Arises in association with intestinal-type intraductal papillary mucinous neoplasm
  - Hepatoid carcinoma
    - Extremely rare malignant epithelial neoplasm with significant component of hepatocellular differentiation
    - Hepatoid differentiation involving entire tumor or as component of ductal adenocarcinoma, acinar cell carcinoma, or neuroendocrine neoplasm
  - Medullary carcinoma
    - Malignant epithelial neoplasm characterized by poor differentiation, limited gland formation, and prominent syncytial growth pattern
  - Signet-ring cell carcinoma
    - Adenocarcinoma composed almost entirely of signet-ring cells
  - Undifferentiated (anaplastic) carcinoma
    - Malignant epithelial neoplasm in which significant component of neoplasm does not show definitive direction of differentiation
    - 3 variants
      - Anaplastic giant cell carcinoma
      - Sarcomatoid carcinoma
      - Carcinosarcoma
  - Undifferentiated carcinoma with osteoclast-like giant cells
    - Rare malignant neoplasm composed of round to spindle-shaped, highly pleomorphic, neoplastic mononuclear cells associated with many nonneoplastic multinucleated histiocytic giant cells
    - In most cases there is associated in situ or invasive adenocarcinoma or associated mucinous cystic neoplasm
  - Carcinomas with mixed differentiation
    - Malignant epithelial neoplasms of pancreas with significant components of > 1 distinct direction of differentiation; each component should comprise at least 30% of entire tumor mass
      - Mixed acinar-ductal carcinoma
      - Mixed acinar-neuroendocrine-ductal carcinoma
      - Mixed ductal-neuroendocrine carcinoma
      - Mixed acinar-neuroendocrine carcinoma also occurs without ductal component

CLINICAL ISSUES

Epidemiology

- Incidence
  - Rare; < 1% of pancreatic neoplasms, occurring in older adult patients

Prognosis

- Majority of variants of ductal carcinoma have poorer prognosis than ductal adenocarcinoma with survival often < 1 year
- Colloid carcinoma and medullary carcinoma often have better prognosis than usual-type ductal adenocarcinoma

CYTOPATHOLOGY

Adenosquamous Carcinoma

- Highly cellular smears with malignant squamous and glandular elements
- Glandular component can show 3D clusters, sheets, loosely cohesive tumor cells, and single tumor cells similar to ductal adenocarcinoma
- Glandular component of tumor can be composed of tumor cells with delicate eosinophilic cytoplasm, clear cells, or signet-ring cells
- Intracellular mucin in tumor cells and extracellular mucin can be present
- Squamous cell carcinoma component is composed of nests and sheets of polygonal neoplastic cells with hard eosinophilic cytoplasm and varying degrees of keratinization
- Malignant squamous cells forming squamous pearls and individual cell keratinization with intercellular bridges can be seen

Colloid Carcinoma

- Clusters, strands, and sheets of malignant glandular epithelium exhibiting varying grades of atypia associated with abundant extracellular mucin

Hepatoid Carcinoma

- Large polygonal cells with abundant eosinophilic cytoplasm resembling hepatocytes

Medullary Carcinoma

- Syncytial sheets of high-grade, poorly differentiated tumor cells with high nuclear:cytoplasmic ratio, prominent nucleoli, and significant mitotic activity
- Often associated with marked lymphocytic infiltration

Signet-Ring Cell Carcinoma

- Very cellular smears composed predominantly of signet-ring cells with intracytoplasmic mucin pushing nucleus to periphery
- Variable amount of extracellular mucin

Undifferentiated Anaplastic Carcinoma

- Anaplastic giant cell carcinoma
  - Cellular smears with mononuclear tumor cells exhibiting significant pleomorphism, including bizarre tumor giant cells with eosinophilic cytoplasm
- Sarcomatoid carcinoma
  - Fragments, sheets, and single tumor cells of high nuclear grade with significant mitotic activity

Unusual Variants of Ductal Carcinoma

- Carcinosarcoma
  - Fragments, clusters, and sheets of high-grade spindle cells and epithelial tumor cells in varying proportions

Undifferentiated Carcinoma With Osteoclastic Giant Cells

- Malignant pleomorphic mononuclear epithelial tumor cells associated with benign reactive multinucleated osteoclastic giant cells and mononuclear histiocytoid cells

Carcinoma With Mixed Differentiation

- Variable combinations of tumor cells with ductal, neuroendocrine, and acinar cell differentiation
- Fragments of glandular epithelium of varying grades, including 3D clusters, sheets, and single tumor cells representing ductal component of tumor
- Acinar cell component: Loose clusters and abundant single tumor cells with large nucleus, prominent nucleolus, and moderate to abundant amounts of granular cytoplasm
- Neuroendocrine component: Loose clusters and single tumor cells often with eccentrically placed nucleus with stippled nuclear chromatin and moderate amount of granular cytoplasm

ANCILLARY TESTS

Immunohistochemistry

- Tumor cells of undifferentiated carcinoma are usually positive for cytokeratins, including CK7, CK8, CK18, and CK19, although staining may be very focal
- Majority also express CEA, CA19-9, and MUC1
- Squamous component of adenosquamous carcinoma will be positive for p63 and p40
- Osteoclast-like giant cells express CD68, CD45, and α-1-antitrypsin
- Colloid carcinoma shows strong expression of CDX2 and MUC2
- Hepatoid carcinoma shows expression of α-fetoprotein, Hep-Par1, glypican-3, arginase, and canalicular staining with polyclonal CEA and CD10
- Medullary carcinoma often shows loss of mismatch repair genes

Genetic Testing

- Most cases of adenosquamous carcinoma harbor *KRAS* mutations in codon 12
- Immunohistochemistry shows loss of CDKN2A, DPC4 protein, and strong nuclear staining for p53
- Medullary carcinoma can arise in patients with Lynch syndrome
  - Biallelic mutation of DNA mismatch repair genes
    - Most patients are microsatellite unstable and have wild-type *KRAS*
    - *BRAF* mutations can occur in these patients

DIFFERENTIAL DIAGNOSIS

Metastatic Melanoma

- Can mimic undifferentiated anaplastic carcinoma
- Clinical history and ancillary immunostaining are useful
  - Melanoma markers: S100, HMB-45, and Melan-A (+)

Choriocarcinoma

- Undifferentiated anaplastic carcinoma with bizarre tumor giant cells can mimic choriocarcinoma
- Affects younger patients; will be positive for β-HCG, unlike undifferentiated anaplastic carcinoma

Metastatic Anaplastic Carcinoma

- Giant cell anaplastic carcinoma from sites such as lung and thyroid may mimic undifferentiated anaplastic carcinoma of pancreas
- Clinical history and imaging findings may be useful for distinction

Multinucleated Giant Cells

- Benign multinucleated giant cells can be noted in several conditions, such as pseudocysts and infection
- Malignant neoplasms, such as lymphoma and sarcoma, can have tumor giant cells that can mimic giant cells seen in undifferentiated carcinoma
- Undifferentiated carcinoma of pancreas with osteoclast-like giant cells has mixed population of benign and malignant cells unlike other causes, which show either benign or malignant giant cells but not both

Pancreatoblastoma

- Squamous islands in pancreatoblastoma are associated with sheets and fragments of acinar cells, unlike adenosquamous carcinoma
- Occurs in younger individuals than adenosquamous carcinoma

Metastatic Squamous Carcinoma

- Shows features similar to primary pancreatic squamous carcinoma and cannot be distinguished based on cytologic features
- Clinical and imaging findings are useful for distinction

Metastatic Hepatocellular Carcinoma

- Primary hepatoid carcinoma cannot be distinguished from metastatic hepatocellular carcinoma
- Clinical history and imaging findings are useful for distinction

Metastatic Gastric or Breast Carcinoma With Signet-Ring Cells

- Primary pancreatic signet-ring cell carcinoma should be distinguished from metastatic carcinoma from stomach or breast
- Clinical history and ancillary immunostaining may be useful for distinction

SELECTED REFERENCES

1. Demetter P et al: Undifferentiated pancreatic carcinoma with osteoclast-like giant cells: what do we know so far? Front Oncol. 11:630086, 2021
2. Lenkiewicz E et al: Genomic and epigenomic landscaping defines new therapeutic targets for adenosquamous carcinoma of the pancreas. Cancer Res. 80(20):4324-34, 2020
3. Reid MD et al: Cytologic features and clinical implications of undifferentiated carcinoma with osteoclastic giant cells of the pancreas: An analysis of 15 cases. Cancer Cytopathol. 125(7):563-75, 2017
4. Muraki T et al: Undifferentiated carcinoma with osteoclastic giant cells of the pancreas: clinicopathologic analysis of 38 cases highlights a more protracted clinical course than currently appreciated. Am J Surg Pathol. 40(9):1203-16, 2016

Unusual Variants of Ductal Carcinoma

Adenosquamous Carcinoma With Vacuoles

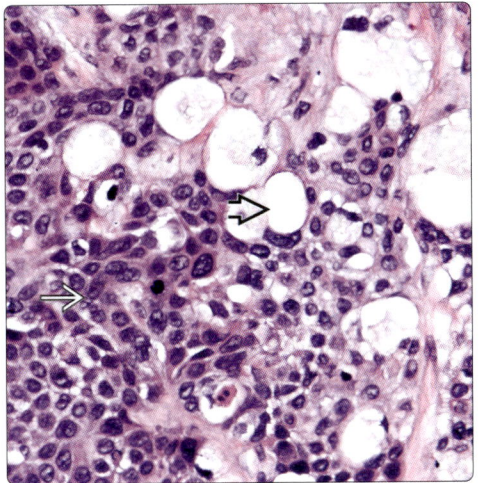

Adenosquamous Carcinoma p63 Positivity

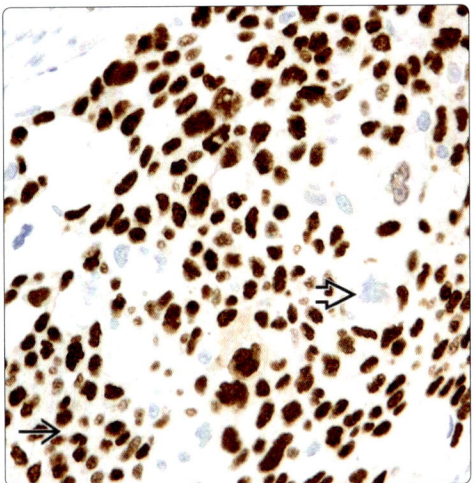

(Left) H&E-stained section of adenosquamous carcinoma of the pancreas shows sheets of polygonal tumor cells exhibiting features of squamous carcinoma ⇒ associated with tumor cells showing glandular differentiation with abundant, vacuolated cytoplasm ⇒. (Right) Immunohistochemical stain of adenosquamous carcinoma of the pancreas shows the squamous component of the tumor to be positive for p63 ⇒, whereas the glandular tumor cells are negative ⇒.

Colloid Carcinoma Histology

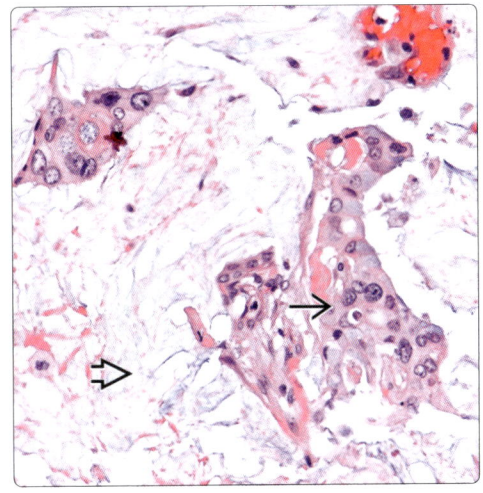

Osteoclastic Giant Cells in Carcinoma

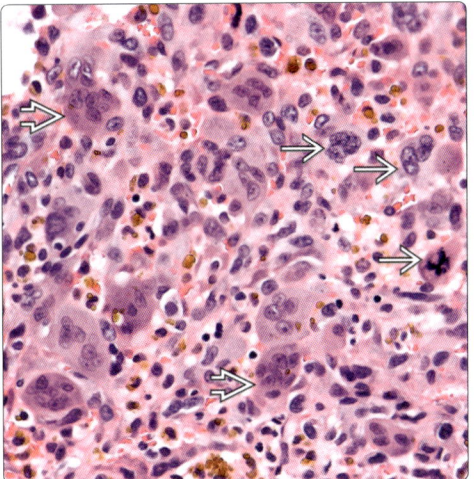

(Left) H&E-stained section of primary colloid carcinoma of the pancreas shows small sheets of high-grade tumor cells ⇒ associated with abundant extracellular mucin ⇒. (Right) H&E-stained section of undifferentiated tumor with osteoclastic giant cells of the pancreas shows high-grade mononuclear and giant tumor cells ⇒ associated with many benign osteoclastic giant cells ⇒ and histiocytes.

Dyscohesive Tumor Cells in Cytology

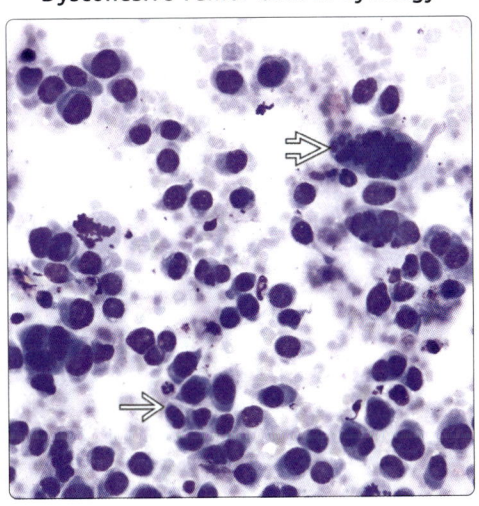

Dyscohesive Tumor in Cell Block

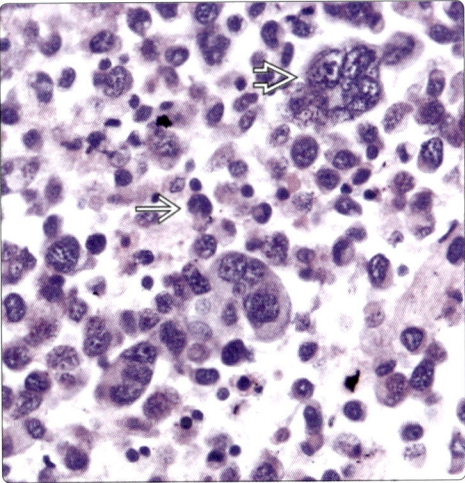

(Left) Diff-Quik-stained smear of undifferentiated carcinoma of pancreas shows dyscohesive tumor cells ⇒ and a multinucleated tumor giant cell ⇒. (Right) H&E-stained cell block of undifferentiated carcinoma shows dyscohesive tumor cells ⇒ and multinucleated tumor giant cells ⇒.

Acinar Cell Carcinoma

KEY FACTS

CLINICAL ISSUES
- Malignant epithelial neoplasm resembling pancreatic acinar cells with evidence of pancreatic exocrine enzyme production
- Outcome better than that of stage-matched infiltrating ductal carcinoma

CYTOPATHOLOGY
- Moderately to highly cellular smears with sheets, 3D, and acinar clusters; many single cells
- Tumor cells with eccentric nucleus with prominent nucleolus and abundant granular cytoplasm
- Mitotic activity is variable

ANCILLARY TESTS
- PAS(+), resistant to diastase digestion
- Immunopositive for trypsin, chymotrypsin, and lipase

TOP DIFFERENTIAL DIAGNOSES
- Normal pancreatic acinar tissue
  - Pancreatic acinar cells without atypia admixed with ductal cells forming acini and clusters without many single cells
- Pancreatic endocrine neoplasm/mixed endocrine/acinar neoplasm/pancreatoblastoma
  - Tumor cells with stippled "salt and pepper" chromatin with diffuse positivity for synaptophysin and chromogranin
    - Tumor cells including small round blue cells admixed with cells resembling acinar cells, spindle cells, and squamous pearls
- Solid pseudopapillary neoplasm
  - Commonly occurs in tail of pancreas of young women, unlike acinar cell carcinoma, which occurs in head of pancreas
    - Tumor cells show nuclear grooves and are CD10 and β-catenin (+)

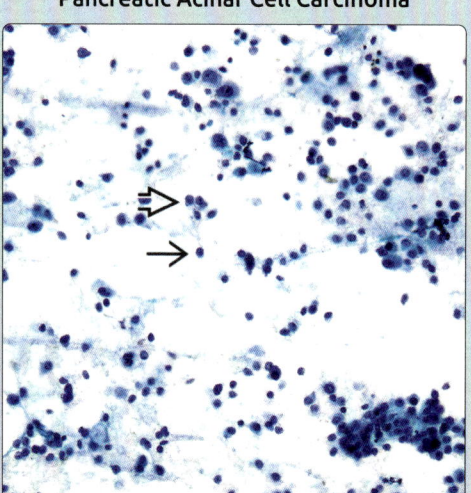

Pancreatic Acinar Cell Carcinoma

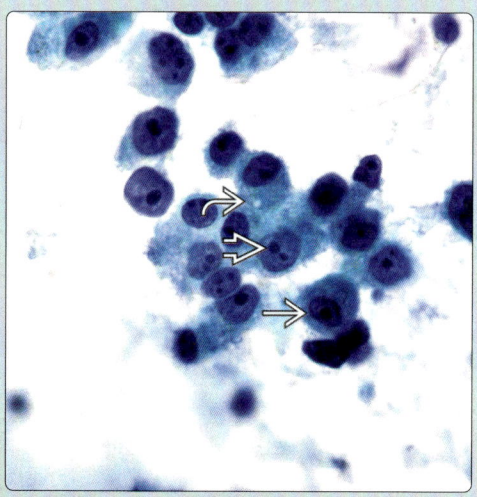

Pancreatic Acinar Cell Carcinoma, Eccentric Nucleus

(Left) Pap-stained FNA smear from a case of pancreatic acinar cell carcinoma (ACC) shows abundant cellularity with few loose clusters ➡ and many single tumor cells ➡. (Right) Pap-stained FNA smear of pancreatic ACC shows tumor cells with an eccentrically placed nucleus ➡, prominent nucleolus ➡, and a moderate amount of granular cytoplasm ➡.

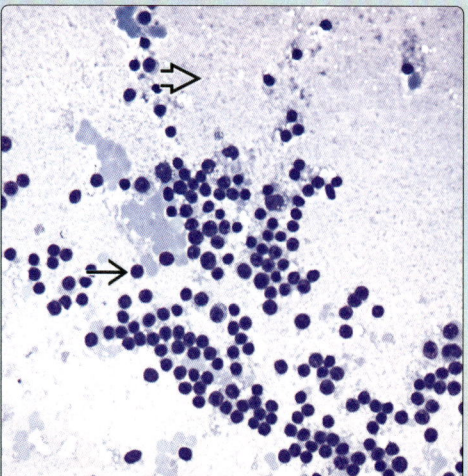

Pancreatic Acinar Cell Carcinoma, Naked Nuclei

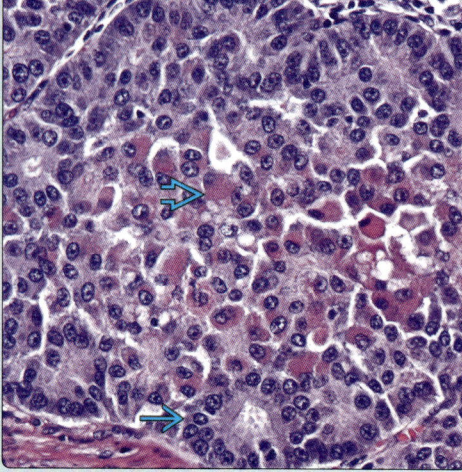

Pancreatic Acinar Cell Carcinoma, Acini Formation

(Left) Diff-Quik-stained FNA smear of pancreatic ACC shows granular material ➡ in the background and many naked tumor nuclei ➡. (Right) H&E-stained tissue section of pancreatic ACC shows tumor cells forming acini ➡ with a strikingly granular cytoplasm ➡.

Acinar Cell Carcinoma

TERMINOLOGY

Abbreviations
- Acinar cell carcinoma (ACC)

Definitions
- Malignant epithelial neoplasm composed of cells resembling pancreatic acinar cells with evidence of pancreatic exocrine enzyme production

CLINICAL ISSUES

Epidemiology
- Incidence: 1-2% of pancreatic exocrine neoplasms in adults
- Age: Average 58 years
- Sex: M > F

Prognosis
- Outcome better than that of stage-matched infiltrating ductal carcinoma
- Metastasis to sites such as liver and lymph nodes can be seen

IMAGING

General Features
- Large, circumscribed, homogeneously enhancing bulky mass, usually in head of pancreas, with average size of 11 cm

CYTOPATHOLOGY

Cellularity
- Moderately to highly cellular smears with sheets, crowded 3D clusters, microacinar clusters, and many single cells

Cells
- Tumor cells resemble benign pancreatic acinar cells with usually eccentrically placed round to oval nucleus with minimal pleomorphism
- Cytoplasm is moderate in amount, granular due to presence of zymogen granules, or clear due to granule disruption
- Disruption of cytoplasm results in presence of many naked tumor nuclei and granular material in background

Nuclear Details
- Nuclear chromatin can be fine, granular, or coarsely clumped with prominent nucleolus; mitotic activity is variable

ANCILLARY TESTS

Immunohistochemistry
- CK8(+) and CK18(+)
- Trypsin and chymotrypsin (+) in > 95%
- Lipase (+) in 70%
- CEA(+) in 50%
- Focally (+) for chromogranin and synaptophysin in 35-54%
- α-fetoprotein (+) in younger patients
- Usually CK7(-), CK19(-), and CK20(-)

Electron Microscopy
- Zymogen granules in cytoplasm of tumor cells
- PAS(+)
- Resistant to diastase digestion

DIFFERENTIAL DIAGNOSIS

Normal Pancreatic Acinar Tissue
- Pancreatic acinar cells without atypia admixed with ductal cells forming acini and clusters without many single cells

Pancreatic Endocrine Neoplasm
- Tumor cells with stippled "salt and pepper" chromatin with diffuse positivity for synaptophysin and chromogranin

Solid Pseudopapillary Neoplasm
- Commonly occurs in tail of pancreas of young women, unlike ACC; IHC shows CD10 and β-catenin (+)

SELECTED REFERENCES
1. Liu Y et al: Exome sequencing of pancreatic acinar carcinoma identified distinctive mutation patterns. Pancreas. 50(7):1007-13, 2021
2. Mustafa S et al: Acinar cell carcinoma of the pancreas: a clinicopathologic and cytomorphologic review. J Am Soc Cytopathol. 9(6):586-95, 2020

Pancreatic Acinar Cell Carcinoma, Cell Block

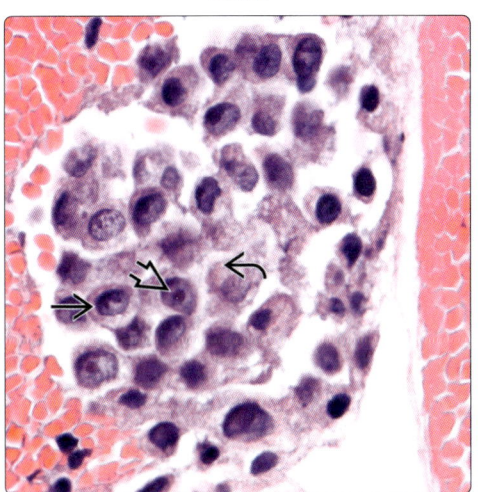

Pancreatic Acinar Cell Carcinoma, Positive for Trypsin

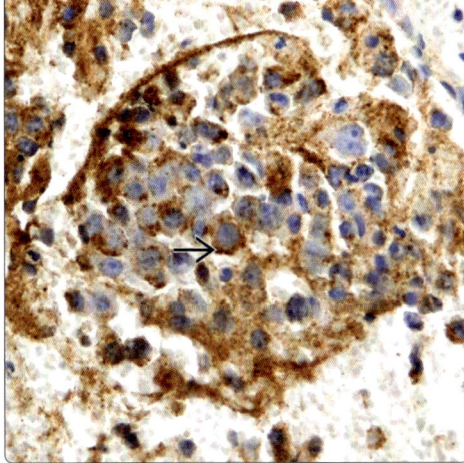

(Left) H&E-stained cell block section of pancreatic ACC shows a cluster of tumor cells with an eccentrically placed nucleus ➔, prominent nucleolus ➔, and moderate amounts of granular cytoplasm ➔. (Right) Immunostaining of a cell block section of pancreatic ACC for trypsin shows diffuse granular (+) staining ➔ in all the tumor cells.

Lymphoma and Secondary Tumors of Pancreas

KEY FACTS

CLINICAL ISSUES
- Lymphoma, usually B-cell type: Follicular lymphoma, mucosa-associated lymphoid tissue lymphoma, diffuse large B-cell lymphoma
- Secondary tumor: Renal cell carcinoma, melanoma, colorectal carcinoma, lung carcinoma, breast carcinoma, sarcoma

CYTOPATHOLOGY
- Lymphoma
  - Neoplastic lymphoid cells demonstrate cytomorphological features based on type of lymphoma and can show small lymphoid cells, mixed small and large cells, or large lymphoid cells
- Secondary tumor
  - Similar to primary tumor

ANCILLARY TESTS
- Flow cytometry and panel of immunomarkers

TOP DIFFERENTIAL DIAGNOSES
- Autoimmune pancreatitis
  - MALT lymphoma can mimic autoimmune pancreatitis
    - Immunophenotyping by flow cytometry will show clonal population of lymphoid cells in MALT lymphoma
      - ↑ levels of IgG4 in serum and IgG4-expressing plasma cells in autoimmune pancreatitis, unlike MALT lymphoma
- Accessory spleen
  - Aspiration smears may mimic low-grade primary lymphoma of pancreas; flow cytometry to exclude clonal population of lymphoid cells is useful
- Primary pancreatic tumor
  - Metastatic adenocarcinoma and melanoma can mimic primary pancreatic malignant epithelial tumors
    - Clinical history, imaging findings, and ancillary immunostaining may be useful for distinguishing from primary tumors

Primary Pancreatic Large Cell Lymphoma | **Metastatic Melanoma**

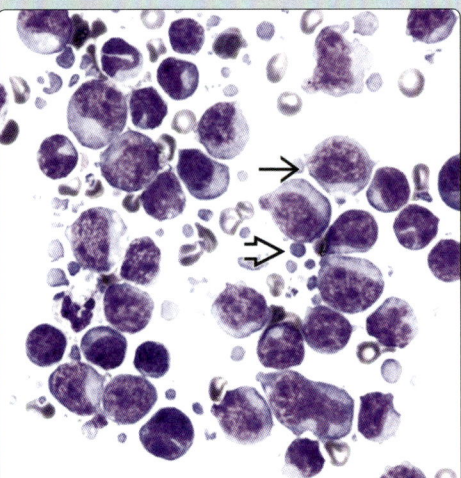 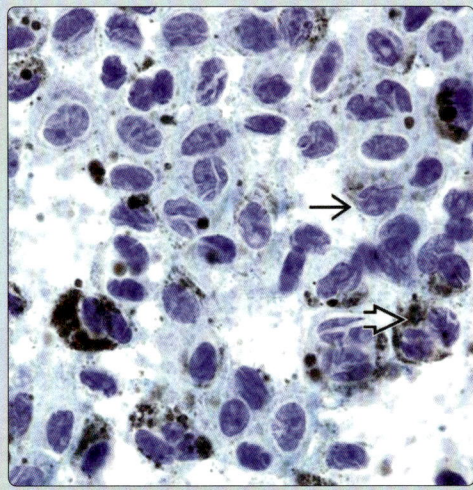

(Left) Diff-Quik-stained cytospin preparation of primary pancreatic lymphoma shows large and pleomorphic lymphoid cells ➡ associated with lymphoglandular bodies ➡ in the background. (Right) Pap-stained FNA smear of metastatic melanoma to pancreas shows dyscohesive tumor cells ➡ with nuclear grooves and dusty brown melanin pigment in the cytoplasm ➡.

Large Cell Lymphoma | **Diffuse Large Cell Lymphoma**

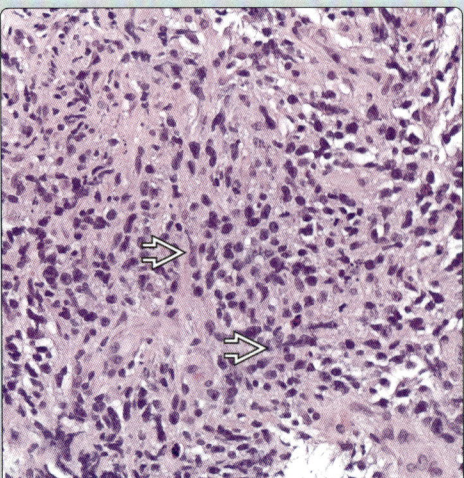 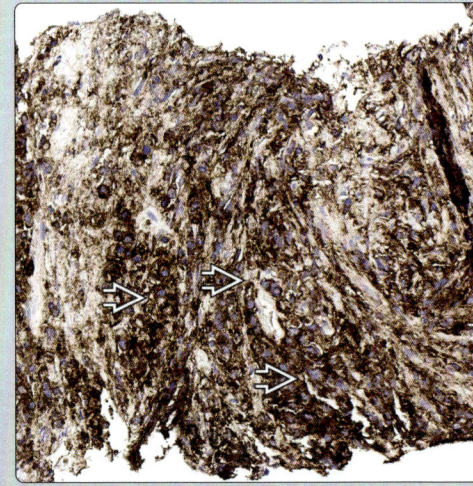

(Left) Core biopsy of large cell lymphoma in the pancreas shows large lymphoid cells ➡ with distortions in many cells associated with scant cytoplasm and fibrosis. The high-grade lymphoma mimics a poorly differentiated carcinoma. (Right) Core biopsy of large cell lymphoma immunostained for CD45 shows the large tumor cells to be positive ➡, which supports the diagnosis.

Lymphoma and Secondary Tumors of Pancreas

TERMINOLOGY

Definitions
- Lymphoma
  - Extranodal lymphoma arising in pancreas with bulk of disease localized to pancreas
  - Primary pancreatic lymphomas are usually of B-cell phenotype
    - Follicular lymphoma, lymphoma of mucosa-associated lymphoid tissue (MALT lymphoma), and diffuse large B-cell lymphoma can occur
- Secondary tumors
  - Direct extension or lymphatic and hematogenous spread of extrapancreatic primary malignant tumor
  - Common malignancies to metastasize to pancreas include renal cell carcinoma, melanoma, colorectal carcinoma, breast carcinoma, and sarcoma

CYTOPATHOLOGY

Cellularity
- Lymphoma: Usually cellular smears with individually distributed lymphoid cells
- Secondary tumors: Variably cellular

Background
- Lymphoma: Lymphoglandular bodies in background

Cells
- Lymphoma
  - Neoplastic lymphoid cells demonstrate cytomorphological features based on type of lymphoma and can show small lymphoid cells, mixed small and large cells, or large lymphoid cells
- Secondary tumors
  - Morphology similar to tumor in primary site

ANCILLARY TESTS

Flow Cytometry
- Immunophenotyping by flow cytometry to demonstrate clonality of lymphoid cells

Immunostaining
- Panel of immunomarkers to establish organ of origin of suspected metastatic tumors and their distinction from primary pancreatic tumors

DIFFERENTIAL DIAGNOSIS

Autoimmune Pancreatitis
- MALT lymphoma can mimic autoimmune pancreatitis
  - Immunophenotyping by flow cytometry will show clonal population of lymphoid cells in MALT lymphoma
- ↑ levels of IgG4 in serum and IgG4-expressing plasma cells in autoimmune pancreatitis, unlike MALT lymphoma

Accessory Spleen
- Aspiration smears may mimic low-grade primary lymphoma of pancreas; flow cytometry to exclude clonal population of lymphoid cells is useful

Primary Pancreatic Tumor
- Secondary tumors arising from other sites (such as bile duct, duodenum, gastric, lung, breast) can very closely mimic primary pancreatic ductal adenocarcinoma
- Metastatic melanoma with large tumor cells with prominent nucleolus and brisk mitotic activity can mimic acinar cell carcinoma or medullary carcinoma of pancreas
- Clinical history, imaging findings, and ancillary immunostaining may be useful for distinguishing from secondary tumors

SELECTED REFERENCES

1. Centeno BA: Metastases, secondary tumors, and lymphomas of the pancreas. Monogr Clin Cytol. 26:109-21, 2020
2. Facchinelli D et al: Primary pancreatic lymphoma: clinical presentation, diagnosis, treatment, and outcome. Eur J Haematol. 105(4):468-75, 2020
3. Kopel J et al: Primary B cell lymphoma of the pancreas. J Gastrointest Cancer. 51(3):1077-80, 2020
4. Hou Y et al: Endoscopic ultrasound-guided fine-needle aspiration diagnosis of secondary tumors involving pancreas: an institution's experience. J Am Soc Cytopathol. 7(5):261-7, 2018
5. Sadaf S et al: Role of endoscopic ultrasound-guided-fine needle aspiration biopsy in the diagnosis of lymphoma of the pancreas: a clinicopathological study of nine cases. Cytopathology. 28(6):536-41, 2017

Metastatic Renal Cell Carcinoma

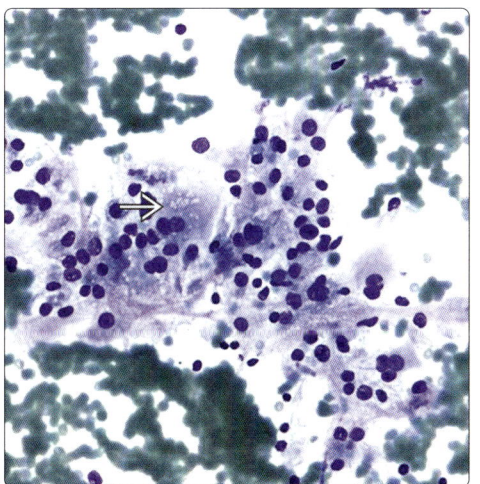

Metastatic Renal Cell Carcinoma

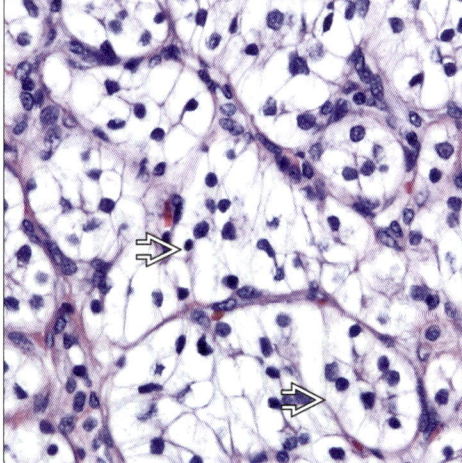

(Left) Diff-Quik-stained FNA smear of metastatic renal cell carcinoma to the pancreas shows a fragment of tumor cells with abundant vacuolated cytoplasm ➡. (Right) Core biopsy of metastatic renal cell carcinoma, conventional clear cell type to pancreas, shows tumor cells ➡ with abundant vacuolated clear cytoplasm.

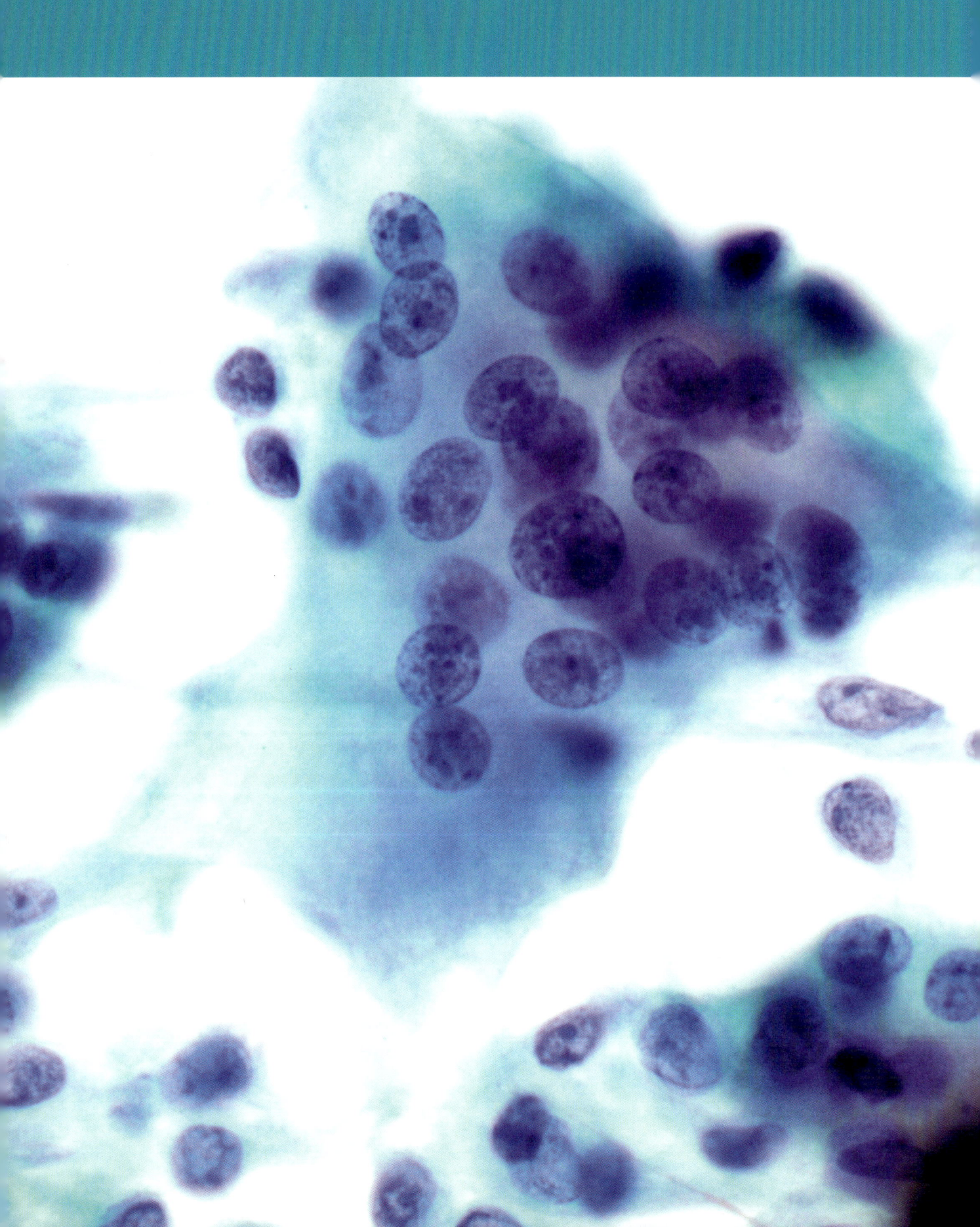

PART IV
SECTION 7
Bone

Overview
Approach to Cytologic/Small Biopsy Diagnosis of Primary Bone Tumors	600

Neoplasms
Chondromas of Bone and Soft Tissue	602
Chondroblastoma	604
Giant Cell Tumor	606
Osteoblastoma	608
Adamantinoma	610
Langerhans Cell Histiocytosis	612
Chordoma	614
Osteosarcoma	616
Chondrosarcoma	620
Ewing Sarcoma	624
Bone Lymphoma	628
Metastatic Tumors of Bone	630

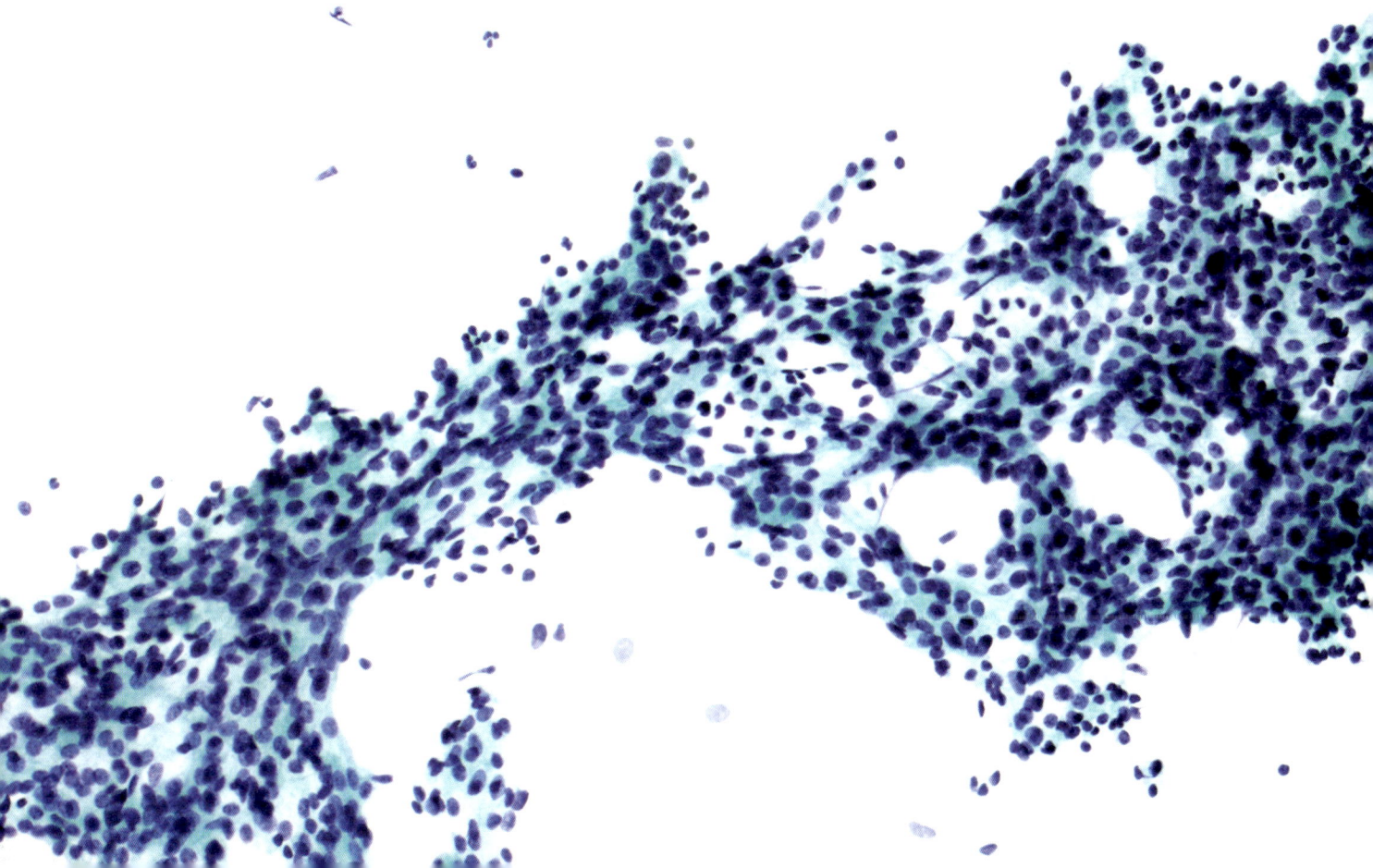

Approach to Cytologic/Small Biopsy Diagnosis of Primary Bone Tumors

EPIDEMIOLOGY

Age Range

- Primary bone tumors occur in all ages
  - Exclude metastasis 1st based on history and radiographs
  - Tend to be location-specific; most occur in tight age range
- Certain tumors are more prevalent in pediatric/adolescent patients, others in older adults
- 0-30 years of age
  - Benign: Chondroma, chondroblastoma, chondromyxoid fibroma, osteoblastoma
  - Malignant: Osteosarcoma, Ewing sarcoma, lymphoma/leukemia/Langerhans cell histiocytosis
- 20-40 years of age
  - Benign: Chondroma, chondroblastoma, chondromyxoid fibroma, osteoblastoma, giant cell tumor
  - Malignant: Ewing sarcoma, chondrosarcoma, osteosarcoma (in 20s), lymphoma/leukemia
- ≥ 40 years of age
  - Benign: Chondroma (tubular bones), giant cell tumors (epiphyseal/metaphyseal), osteoblastoma (all locations), chondroblastoma in small bones
  - Malignant: Chondrosarcoma, chordoma, lymphoma/leukemia/myeloma
- **Adequacy/rapid onsite evaluation and triage during biopsy/FNA of primary**
  - If small round blue cell tumor without osteoid or chondroid, look for lymphoglandular bodies (LBs), as they indicate lymphoma/leukemia in differential
    - If LBs are present, collect in RPMI/Hanks for flow cytometry as well as cell block
    - Collect for cultures if infectious
  - If no LBs, consider PNET/Ewing or related tumors
    - Collect enough for cell block/core biopsy
    - Collect fresh sample in appropriate medium if/as required by molecular lab
    - Most testing can be done from cell blocks, cores, smears, and cytospins, but exceptions exist
  - If spindle cells are present, look for osteoid and bland vs. pleomorphic spindle cells

Osteoid Matrix and Malignant Spindle Cells

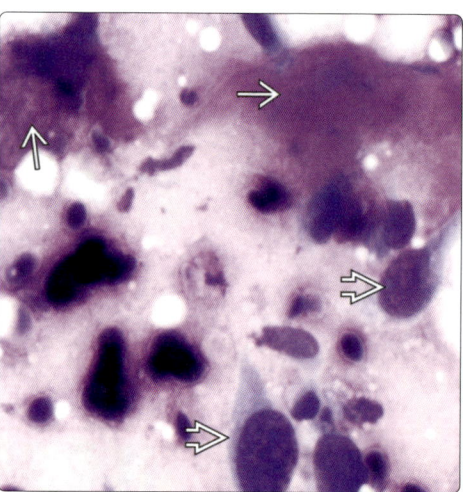

(Left) Diff-Quik stain shows magenta osteoid ➡ and pleomorphic malignant spindle cells ➡ in an osteosarcoma. In the absence of osteoid, such cells would be best interpreted as a high-grade spindle cell sarcoma without a specific diagnosis. (Right) Pap stain of low-grade chondrosarcoma shows chondroid matrix ➡ and binucleate chondrocytes ➡. The age, radiographic appearance, matrix, and cellular atypia, or lack of it, are important characteristics to consider.

Chondroid Matrix

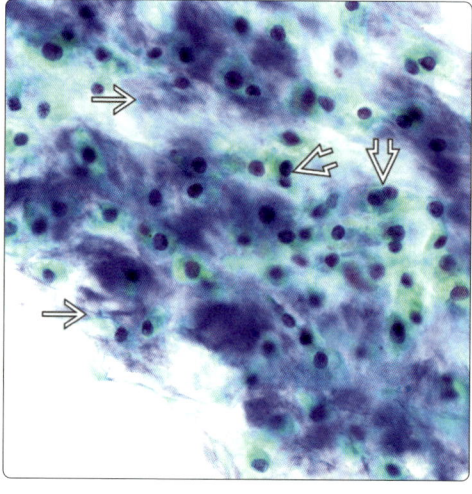

Core Needle Biopsy of Chordoma

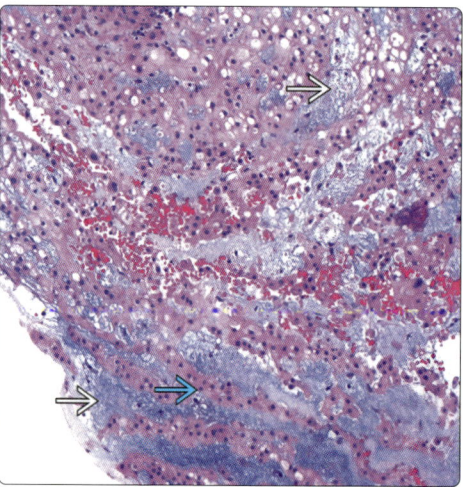

(Left) H&E-stained core needle biopsy of a sacral mass shows a mucoid/myxoid background ➡ with cords and nests ➡ of cells. These cells and background are easily shed on touch preparations, which are used for rapid onsite evaluation. (Right) Pap-stained smear shows an osteoclastic giant cell ➡ with > 40 bland vesicular nuclei. Several bone tumors are characterized by osteoclasts. The patient's age, location of the lesion, and radiographic appearance further narrow the differential diagnosis.

Osteoclastic Giant Cells

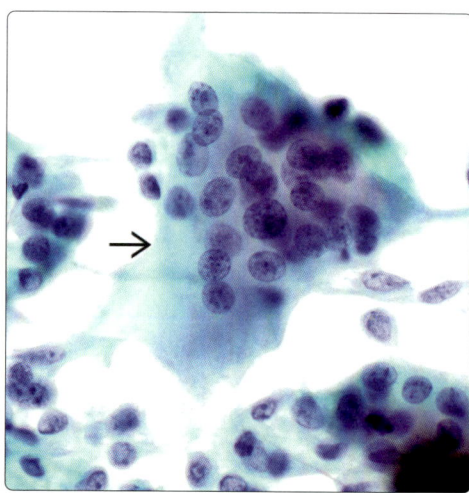

Approach to Cytologic/Small Biopsy Diagnosis of Primary Bone Tumors

Approach to Initial Evaluation of Primary Bone Tumors*

Osteoid Matrix	Chondroid Matrix	Mucoid/Myxoid Matrix	Small Round Blue Cell Tumor	Giant Cells
Benign with usual age range at presentation				
Fracture callus (all ages)	Fracture callus (all ages)	Benign notochordal tumor (location is key)	Chronic osteomyelitis (all ages)	Giant cell lesion of small bones (< 30; OGC)
Osteoid osteoma (5-25)	Chondromas (all ages)			Brown tumor of hyperparathyroidism (all ages; OGC)
Intermediate (includes locally aggressive and rarely metastasizing) with usual age range at presentation				
Osteoblastoma (10-30)	Chondromyxoid fibroma (10-30)		Langerhans cell histiocytosis (< 20)	Giant cell tumor (25-45; OGC)
	Chondroblastoma (10-25; open growth plates; also under tumors with OGC)			Chondroblastoma (10-25; OGC)
	Atypical cartilaginous tumor/grade I chondrosarcoma (30-80)			Aneurysmal bone cyst (< 20; OGC)
Malignant with usual age range at presentation				
Osteosarcoma (10-20, and > 50)	Chondrosarcoma (40-60 for grades II and III; 30-80 for dedifferentiated)	Chordoma (30-70; location is key)	Ewing sarcoma (< 17 in long bones)	Undifferentiated pleomorphic high-grade sarcoma (> 40; previously known as MFH; has pleomorphic giant cells)
	Chondroblastic osteosarcoma (10-20)		Lymphomas/hematopoietic malignancies/myeloma (all ages; type varies by age; lymphoglandular bodies)	Any primary malignant tumor with fracture can show some OGC
	Mesenchymal chondrosarcoma (10-30), also falls under SRBCT		Undifferentiated non-Ewing round cell sarcoma (6-62; CIC::DUX4)	

MFH = malignant fibrous histiocytoma; OGC = has osteoclastic giant cells; PNET = primitive neuroectodermal tumor; SRBCT = small round blue cell tumor.
*Limited list of lesions most likely to be aspirated.

- Bland: Consider fibrous dysplasia, adamantinoma, nonossifying fibroma
- Pleomorphic and malignant: Consider undifferentiated high-grade pleomorphic sarcoma

CLINICAL IMPLICATIONS

Clinical Presentation

- Most present with pain or fracture
- Aggressive tumors like Ewing sarcoma may have large soft tissue component and are warm to touch
- Tend to be location specific within bone (e.g., epiphyseal, metaphyseal, or diaphyseal)
  o Are also age range specific
  o Some carry specific mutations
    - Molecular testing is key
  o If unfamiliar with bone tumors, obtain consultation from expert, as misdiagnosis can be disastrous
- Plain radiographs depict sclerotic rims in benign/slow-growing tumors (e.g., chondroblastoma, osteoid osteoma)
- Lack of sclerotic rim in well-defined lytic lesion indicates faster growth (e.g., giant cell tumor)
- Malignant/aggressive tumors can have moth-eaten appearance or destructive bone lesion
- Periosteal reaction can be seen in benign and malignant bone tumors
- CT and MR give better idea of extension, edema, and other details
- Knowing age, location, and radiographic appearance can narrow differential diagnosis of primary tumors to 2-3 choices
- FNA/core needle biopsy can definitively confirm diagnosis in context of consonant radiographic and clinical findings

SELECTED REFERENCES

1. Hartmann W et al: Giant cell-rich tumors of bone. Surg Pathol Clin. 14(4):695-706, 2021
2. Köster J et al: Comparative cytological and histological assessment of 828 primary soft tissue and bone lesions, and proposal for a system for reporting soft tissue cytopathology. Cytopathology. 32(1):7-19, 2021
3. Agrawal T et al: Musculoskeletal small biopsies from small patients: current status in 2 academic hospitals. J Am Soc Cytopathol. 9(5):442-9, 2020
4. Chambers M et al: Fine-needle aspiration biopsy for the diagnosis of bone and soft tissue lesions: a systematic review and meta-analysis. J Am Soc Cytopathol. 9(5):429-41, 2020
5. Satturwar S et al: An update on touch preparations of small biopsies. J Am Soc Cytopathol. 9(5):322-31, 2020
6. Macagno N et al: [Benign and malignant giant-cell rich lesions of bone: pathological diagnosis with special emphasis on recent immunohistochemistry and molecular techniques.] Ann Pathol. 38(2):92-102, 2018

Chondromas of Bone and Soft Tissue

KEY FACTS

CLINICAL ISSUES
- Develops in all age groups
- Treatment is excision of mass/curettage
- Recurrences are uncommon

CYTOPATHOLOGY
- Cellularity is variable but can be high, especially in children and in enchondromas from short tubular bones
- Magenta chondroid matrix usually adherent to chondrocytes on Diff-Quik
- Mature chondrocytes seen in lacunar spaces
- Bland, round, small nuclei with occasional small nucleoli and condensed chromatin
- **Core biopsy and cell block**
  - Can be useful to evaluate atypical enchondromas in long tubular bones in older adults
  - Only aspirated or biopsied if there is clinical concern for chondrosarcoma

ANCILLARY TESTS
- *IDH1/IDH2* mutations identified in > 50% of enchondromas as well as in chondrosarcomas
- Cannot be used to differentiate chondromas from chondrosarcomas

TOP DIFFERENTIAL DIAGNOSES
- **Low-grade chondrosarcoma**
  - Can be difficult to distinguish from chondroma solely on cytologic basis
  - Correlation with radiologic and clinical findings is important
- **Osteosarcoma**
  - Demonstrates more cytologic atypia and contains neoplastic bone formation
- **Chordoma** (if spine based)
  - Sacrococcygeal, clivus, or thoracic spine location
  - Physaliferous cells present; brachyury, keratin, and EMA (+)

Enchondroma, Plain Radiograph
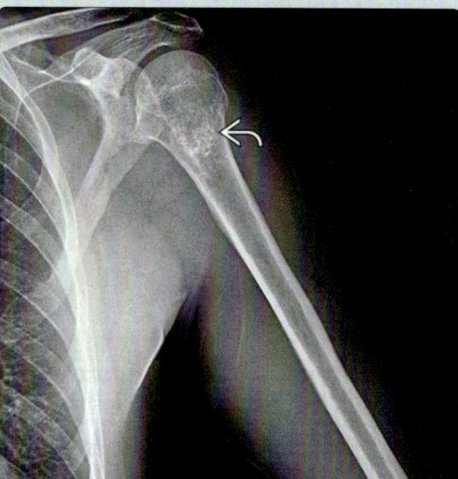

Enchondroma Cytology, Diff-Quik Stain
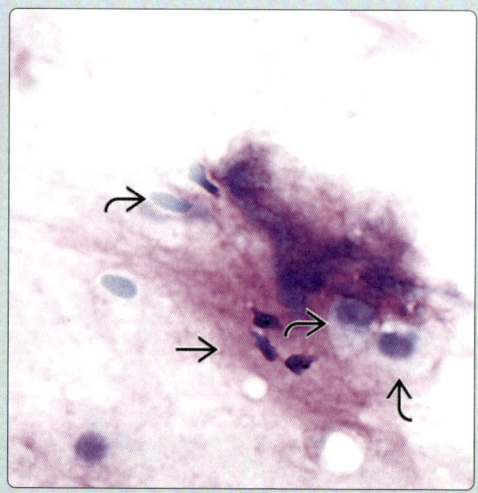

(Left) Radiograph shows a lesion at the upper end of the humerus with punctate calcifications ➡ that presented with pain. Atypical lesions are biopsied to rule out chondrosarcoma. **(Right)** Diff-Quik-stained touch prep shows fibrillar magenta matrix ➡ with bland uninucleate chondrocytes ➡ with abundant cytoplasm. There is lack of necrosis, mitosis, and atypia.

Enchondroma Cytology, Pap Stain
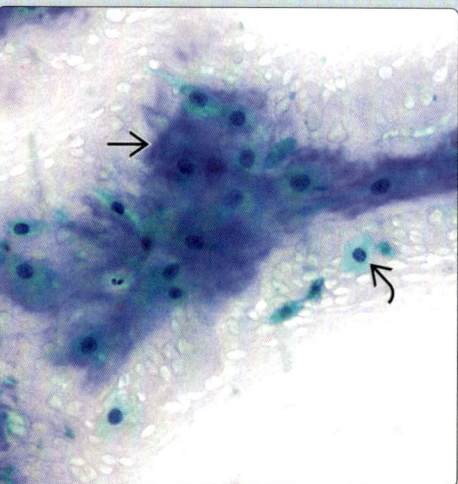

Chondroma Histology
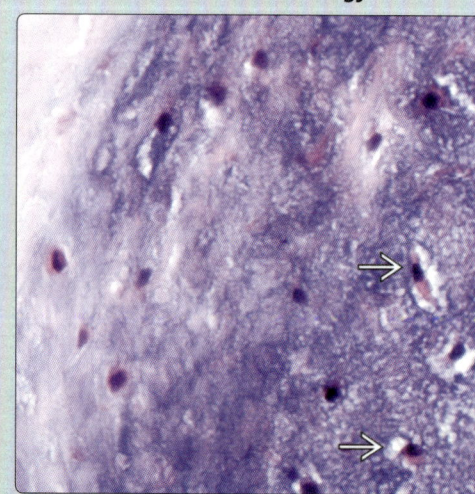

(Left) Pap stain shows a chondroma with chondroid matrix ➡, bland uninucleate chondrocytes, and abundant cytoplasm ➡. Note the lack of mitosis, necrosis, or atypia. **(Right)** H&E stain of a core needle biopsy shows a soft tissue chondroma with chondrocytes in lacunar spaces ➡.

Chondromas of Bone and Soft Tissue

TERMINOLOGY

Definitions
- Benign cartilage tumor that can arise in bone (enchondroma), on surface of cortex beneath periosteum (juxtacortical and periosteal chondromas), or in soft tissue [soft tissue chondroma (STC)]

CLINICAL ISSUES

Epidemiology
- Age
  - Develops in all age groups

Site
- Periosteal chondromas: Surfaces of tubular bones are characteristic sites of origin
  - Particularly metaphyseal or diaphyseal regions of humerus and femur and short tubular bones of hand and foot
- Enchondromas: Small bones of hands and feet followed by long tubular bones
- STCs: Fingers, toes, or soft tissue near tendons and joints

Prognosis
- Recurrences are uncommon
- Malignant transformation is extremely rare

IMAGING

Radiographic Findings
- Predominately radiolucent and lobulated
- May contain punctate calcifications
- Has well-defined margins
- Underlying cortex is superficially eroded (in enchondromas)

MR Findings
- Similar to other benign cartilage tumors
  - Bright on T2- and dark on T1-weighted images
- May show peripheral enhancement

CT Findings
- Shows size and round or oval shape
  - Clearly identifies extent of tumor involvement of medullary cavity
  - May show matrix calcifications and scalloping of underlying cortex in periosteal chondromas

CYTOPATHOLOGY

Cellularity
- Variable but can be high, especially in children and in enchondromas from short tubular bones
- Touch preps of cores have low cellularity (as cells do not easily shed) or may show thick groups
- High cellularity in patients with enchondromatosis

Background
- Magenta chondroid matrix usually adherent to chondrocytes on Diff-Quik
- More difficult to appreciate on Pap stain where it is pale and waxy
- Variably thick cartilaginous fragments with sharp edges

Cells
- Mature chondrocytes seen in lacunar spaces

Nuclear Details
- Bland, round, small nuclei with occasional small nucleoli and condensed chromatin
- No mitosis; very rare or no binucleation

Cytoplasmic Details
- Most cells in lacunae, but cytoplasm is abundant

Adequacy Criteria
- Adequate if it explains clinical and radiographic scenario

Core Biopsy and Cell Block Findings
- Can be useful to evaluate atypical enchondromas in long tubular bones in older adults
- Only aspirated or biopsied if there is clinical concern for chondrosarcoma

MICROSCOPIC

Histologic Features
- Neoplastic matrix is hypo- to moderately cellular
- Chondrocytes are bland
- May demonstrate mild to moderate atypia in form of nuclear enlargement, prominent nucleoli, and binucleation
- Matrix is composed of hyaline cartilage
  - May be focally myxoid

ANCILLARY TESTS

Molecular Testing
- *IDH1/IDH2* mutations identified in > 50% of enchondromas as well as in chondrosarcomas
- Cannot be used to differentiate chondromas from chondrosarcomas

DIFFERENTIAL DIAGNOSIS

Low-Grade Chondrosarcoma
- Can be difficult to distinguish from chondroma solely on cytologic basis
- Usually larger, more cellular, and demonstrates more cytologic atypia than chondroma
- Correlation with radiologic and clinical findings is important
- Permeative growth pattern
- In difficult cases, sign out as benign vs. low-grade hyaline cartilaginous neoplasm

Osteosarcoma
- Demonstrates more cytologic atypia and contains neoplastic bone formation

Chordoma
- Spine based (sacrococcygeal, clivus, or thoracic spine)
- Physaliferous cells present; brachyury, keratin, and EMA (+)

SELECTED REFERENCES

1. Engel H et al: Chondrogenic bone tumors: the importance of imaging characteristics. Rofo. 193(3):262-75, 2021
2. Suster D et al: Differential diagnosis of cartilaginous lesions of bone. Arch Pathol Lab Med. 144(1):71-82, 2020

Chondroblastoma

KEY FACTS

CLINICAL ISSUES
- Age range: 10-25 years, epiphysis-based tumor
- Skeletally immature individuals, usually treated by curettage

IMAGING
- Intramedullary, eccentric or central, well-defined tumor with sclerotic margins
- Predominately radiolucent but frequently contains scattered punctate calcifications
- May scallop cortex or result in its destruction

CYTOPATHOLOGY
- 2 populations of cells: Mononuclear and multinucleated giant cells
- Osteoclastic giant cells and smaller giant cells with nuclei similar to mononuclear cells
- Mononuclear cells have nuclear grooves and reniform or coffee bean-shaped nuclei
- Rare intranuclear cytoplasmic inclusions

ANCILLARY TESTS
- Clonal abnormalities, especially involving chromosomes 5 and 8, have been identified
- Chondroblasts on IHC express nuclear H3K36M, S100 protein, and SOX9

TOP DIFFERENTIAL DIAGNOSES
- Giant cell tumor of bone
  - Skeletally mature individuals, radiographically more aggressive
  - Mononuclear cells in giant cell tumor of bone are H3K36M, S100 negative but express H3G34W, p63
- Chondroblastoma-like osteosarcoma
  - Radiologically and cytologically aggressive
  - Does not contain chondroid matrix or chicken-wire calcifications

Plain Film of Chondroblastoma
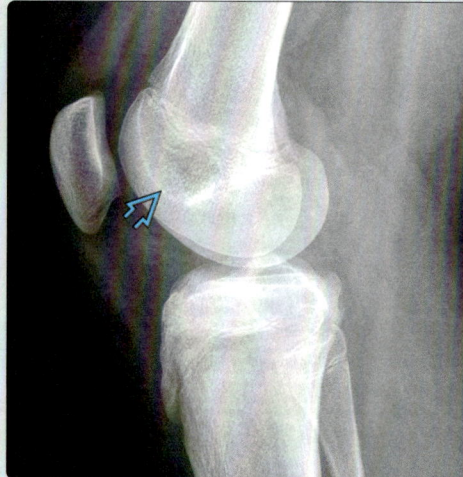

Chondroblastoma, Core Needle Biopsy
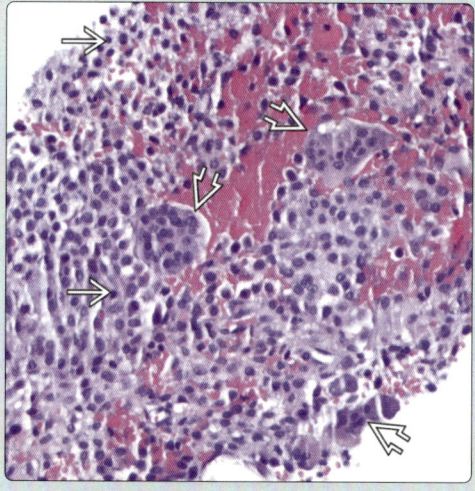

(Left) Plain film shows a lytic lesion of the epiphysis of the femur in a skeletally immature individual. The sclerotic rim ⇨ indicates a slow-growing benign lesion. **(Right)** Hematoxylin and eosin-stained core shows a bimorphic population of multinucleated osteoclastic-type giant cells ⇨ in a background of mononuclear chondroblasts ⇨.

Chondroblastoma Cellular Details
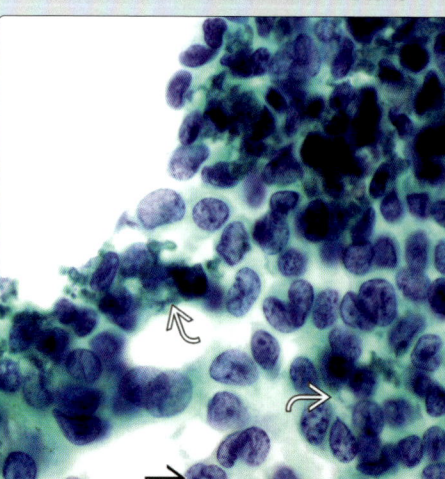

Chondroblastoma Cells and Stroma
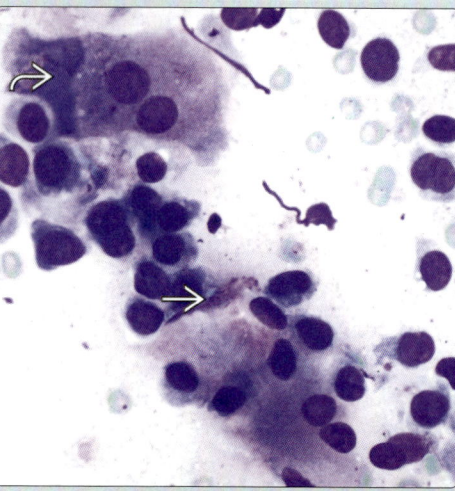

(Left) Pap stain shows mononuclear cells of chondroblastoma with nuclear grooves ⇨ and chicken-wire calcifications ⇨. **(Right)** Diff-Quik stain on adequacy evaluation demonstrates a dual population of cells. The multinucleated cells ⇨ alternate with mononuclear cells. There is a hint of magenta chondroid matrix ⇨.

Chondroblastoma

TERMINOLOGY

Definitions
- Benign, cartilage-producing neoplasm composed of chondroblasts

CLINICAL ISSUES

Epidemiology
- Incidence
  - Accounts for ~ 1% of primary bone tumors, < 3% of benign bone tumors, M:F = 2:1
  - Affected individuals are typically skeletally immature (i.e., with open growth plates), between ages 10-25 years

Site
- Typically develops in epiphysis of long tubular bones (66%)
- Other locations include talus, calcaneus, patella, acetabulum, iliac crest, temporal bone, and skull base

CYTOPATHOLOGY

Cellularity
- Specimens are usually cellular (can be operator dependent)

Pattern
- Dispersed population of uninucleate and multinucleated giant cells; uninucleate cells predominate and can form loose aggregates or cluster

Background
- None or bloody; may demonstrate chondroid matrix
- Romanowsky (Diff-Quik) stain: Brilliant, magenta-like stroma reminiscent of pleomorphic adenomas
- Pap stain: Waxy, green, and not very dramatic stroma

Cells
- 2 populations of cells: Mononuclear and multinucleated giant cells
- Giant cells can be osteoclastic type with numerous bland nuclei and inconspicuous nucleoli or can be smaller giant cells with nuclei similar to mononuclear cells
- Mononuclear cells are dispersed singly, in small aggregates, or entrapped in cartilaginous stroma
- Some mononuclear cells may be surrounded by characteristic chicken-wire calcification, which surrounds individual cells and results in necrosis
  - Best seen on lightly or nondecalcified cell blocks, core needle biopsy with H&E stains, or Pap-stained smears

Nuclear Details
- Mononuclear cells have characteristic nuclear grooves and reniform/bean-shaped nuclei
- Rare intranuclear cytoplasmic inclusions

Cell Block Findings
- Dual population of cells with mononuclear cells predominating; chicken-wire calcifications best seen on lightly decalcified H&E-stained cell block or small needle biopsy

ANCILLARY TESTS

Immunohistochemistry
- Chondroblasts express nuclear H3K36M, S100 protein, and SOX9

DIFFERENTIAL DIAGNOSIS

Giant Cell Tumor of Bone
- Large tumor that spans epiphysis and metaphysis in skeletally mature individuals
- Mononuclear cells in giant cell tumor of bone are H3K36M, S100 negative but express H3G34W, p63

Chondroblastoma-Like Osteosarcoma
- Tumor cells are similar to mononuclear cells in chondroblastoma and can express S100 protein but negative for H3K36M

SELECTED REFERENCES
1. Rekhi B et al: Immunohistochemical analysis of 36 cases of chondroblastomas: a single institutional experience. Ann Diagn Pathol. 44:151440, 2020

Nuclear Grooves in Chondroblastoma

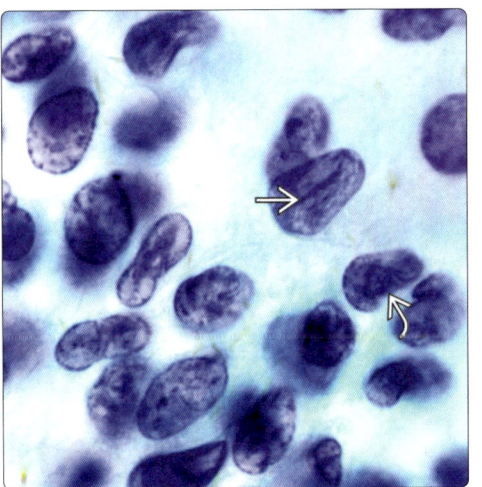

H3K36M Immunohistochemistry

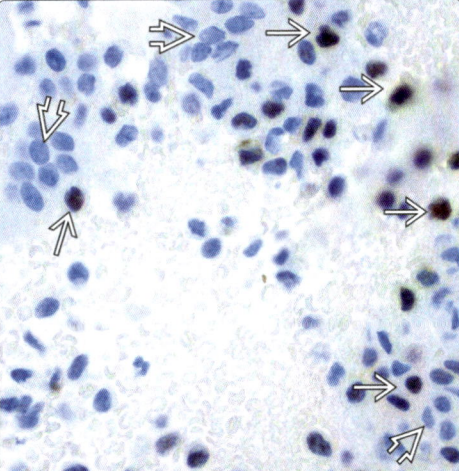

(Left) High magnification of a Pap-stained smear demonstrates nuclear grooves ➡ and coffee bean-shaped nuclei ➡. The chromatin is fine and dispersed without nucleoli. *(Right)* H3K36M IHC shows positive nuclear staining in the uninucleate chondroblasts ➡. The multinucleated giant cells are negative ➡.

Giant Cell Tumor

KEY FACTS

CLINICAL ISSUES
- Represents ~ 6% of primary bone tumors
- Pain and swelling
- Epiphyseal metaphyseal lytic lesion in distal long bone extending to subchondral area in adult patient is characteristic

CYTOPATHOLOGY
- Cellular aspirates that may be bloody
- Dispersed or checkerboard pattern of giant cells and uninucleate stromal cells, which may be spindle-shaped or round
- Giant cells may have up to 100 nuclei
- Nuclei of stromal and giant cells are similarly characterized by vesicular chromatin and nucleoli
- Uninucleate stromal cells can be mitotically active
- Giant cells have abundant cytoplasm; uninucleate cells have variable amounts of trailing cytoplasm
- Both can contain vacuoles and metachromatic granules on Diff-Quik stain
- Following receptor activator of nuclear factor-κ B (RANK) ligand inhibitor therapy (denosumab), giant cells disappear, mononuclear tumor cells decrease, and bone formation increases

ANCILLARY TESTS
- Molecular testing for H3F3A [in > 90% of giant cell tumors (GCTs)] and H3F3B helps differentiate between GCT and chondroblastoma
- IHC for H3G34W sensitive and specific for GCT; small percentage negative due to alternate mutations

TOP DIFFERENTIAL DIAGNOSES
- Nonossifying fibroma, chondroblastoma, giant cell reparative granuloma, aneurysmal bone cyst, giant cell-rich osteosarcoma

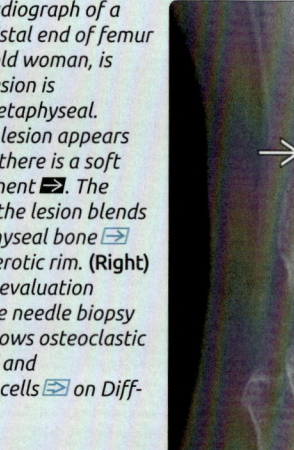

(Left) Plain radiograph of a lytic lesion, distal end of femur in a 23-year-old woman, is shown. The lesion is epiphyseal-metaphyseal. Although the lesion appears well defined, there is a soft tissue component ➡. The upper end of the lesion blends into the diaphyseal bone ➡ without a sclerotic rim. (Right) Rapid on-site evaluation (ROSE) of core needle biopsy touch prep shows osteoclastic giant cells ➡ and mononuclear cells ➡ on Diff-Quik stain.

Radiograph of Giant Cell Tumor
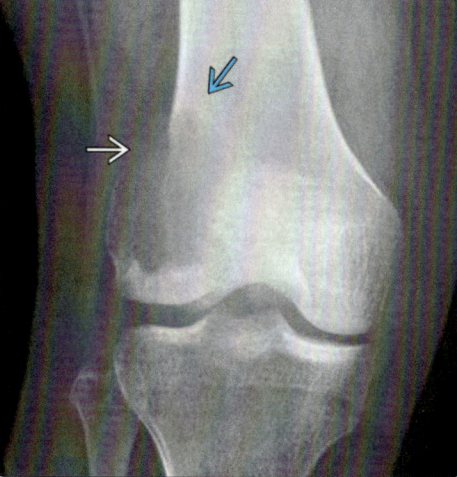

Touch Prep of Core Needle Biopsy Rapid On-Site Evaluation
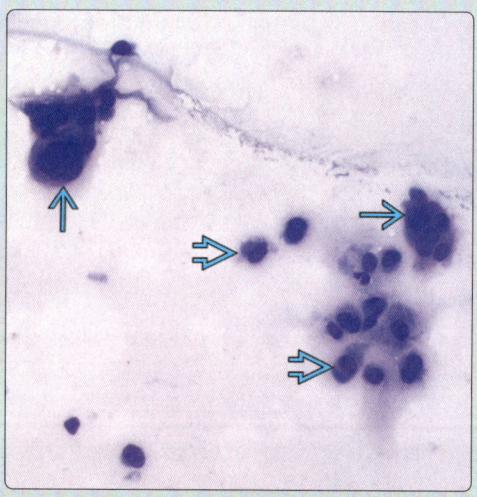

(Left) Low magnification of a Pap-stained FNA smear shows a checkerboard pattern caused by alternating giant cells ➡ and mononuclear stromal cells ➡. (Right) Pap stain shows osteoclastic giant cells with numerous nuclei. The nuclei of the stromal cells ➡ resemble those of the giant cells ➡.

Giant Cell Tumor Checkerboard Pattern
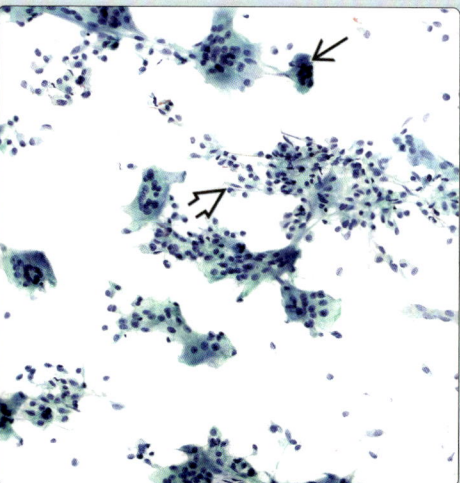

Osteoclastic Giant Cells
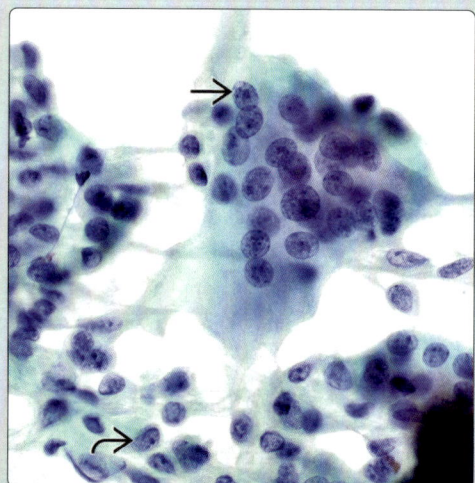

Giant Cell Tumor

CLINICAL ISSUES

Epidemiology
- Incidence
  - Represents ~ 6% of primary bone tumors
    - Represents ~ 20% of benign bone tumors
- Age
  - Skeletally mature individuals during 3rd-5th decades of life

Site
- Vast majority arise in epiphyseal-metaphyseal region of long tubular bones, especially around knees and distal radius, 5-15 cm
- Uncommon sites include vertebral bodies, short tubular bones of hands and feet, craniofacial bones, and patella

Prognosis
- Although giant cell tumor (GCT) of bone is classified as benign neoplasm, 1-2% eventually metastasize, primarily to lungs

IMAGING

Radiographic Findings
- Large, lytic, intramedullary, and frequently eccentric
- Usually from metaphysis to subchondral bone plate
  - Very large tumors may involve adjacent diaphysis, focally destroy cortex, and invade neighboring soft tissues
- Medullary margins are well defined, may have moth-eaten appearance, and are usually not sclerotic

CYTOPATHOLOGY

Cellularity
- Cellular with dispersed cells or checkerboard pattern
- Bloody if aneurysmal bone cyst component

Cells
- Osteoclastic giant cells with numerous nuclei and uninucleate spindle stromal cells

Nuclear Details
- Nuclei of stromal and giant cells are similarly characterized by vesicular chromatin and nucleoli
- Uninucleate stromal cells can be mitotically active

Cytoplasmic Details
- Giant cells have abundant cytoplasm; uninucleate cells have variable amounts of trailing cytoplasm
  - Both can contain vacuoles and metachromatic granules on Diff-Quik stain

ANCILLARY TESTS

Immunohistochemistry
- Molecular testing for H3F3A (in > 90% of GCTs) and H3F3B helps differentiate between GCT and chondroblastoma
- H3G34W-mutant-specific IHC is highly sensitive and specific surrogate marker for mutation; < 10% are negative due to alternate mutations

DIFFERENTIAL DIAGNOSIS

Nonossifying Fibroma/Benign Fibrous Histiocytoma
- Most GCTs have areas that resemble benign fibrous histiocytoma or nonossifying fibroma

Chondroblastoma
- Seen in skeletally immature individuals with open growth plate and centered in epiphysis; IHC for H3K36M positive

Giant Cell Reparative Granuloma/Brown Tumor
- IHC for H3G34W negative

Aneurysmal Bone Cyst
- FISH for t(16;17) present in primary aneurysmal bone cyst

Giant Cell-Rich Osteosarcoma
- Infiltrative pattern, cytologically malignant cells

SELECTED REFERENCES
1. Yamamoto H et al: Histone H3.3 mutation in giant cell tumor of bone: an update in pathology. Med Mol Morphol. 53(1):1-6, 2020

Giant Cell Tumor Cell Types

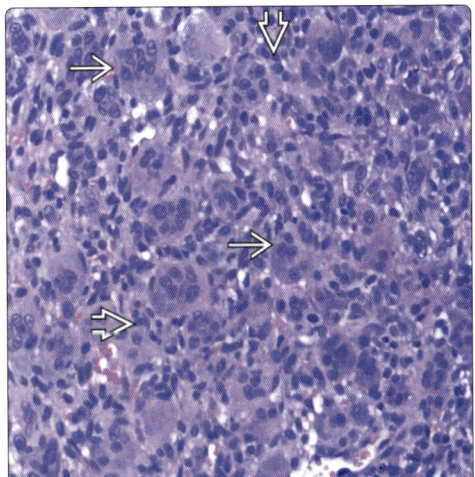

H3G34W Immunohistochemistry

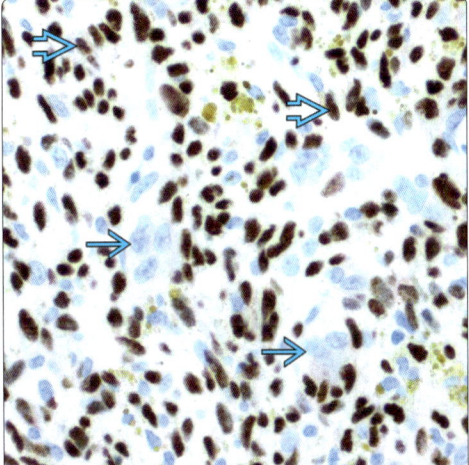

(Left) Core needle biopsy on an H&E stain shows giant cells ➡ alternating with mononuclear stromal cells ➡. (Right) The giant cells ➡ do not stain for H3G34W by immunohistochemistry, whereas the mononuclear cells are strongly positive ➡.

Osteoblastoma

KEY FACTS

TERMINOLOGY
- Benign, bone-forming neoplasm composed of woven bone trabeculae lined by osteoblasts
- Tumor > 2 cm in dimension by definition

CLINICAL ISSUES
- Diagnosed in adolescents and young adults, M:F = 2:1
- Uncommon; accounts for 1% of primary bone tumors
- Responsible for 3% of primary benign bone tumors
- Frequently involve metadiaphyseal region of tubular bones
- 30% arise in spinal column

CYTOPATHOLOGY
- Cellular specimen with plasmacytoid osteoblasts and osteoclastic giant cells
- Rare bland spindle cells and stromal fragments in background
- No atypia, necrosis, or mitotic activity
- Pink osteoid surrounded by osteoblasts may be seen

MICROSCOPIC
- Histology shows neoplastic woven bone trabeculae in haphazard, interconnecting, or sheet-like patterns
  - Bone rimmed by osteoblasts and scattered osteoclasts
  - Osteoblasts are ovoid or round with moderate amounts of eosinophilic or purple cytoplasm and eccentric nuclei with fine chromatin
  - Scattered mitoses with no atypical forms; necrosis usually absent or focal
  - Rarely cystic change mimicking aneurysmal bone cyst
  - Diagnosis is made based on clinical, radiologic, and microscopic findings
  - *FOS* IHC positivity in nuclei or FISH for rearrangement

TOP DIFFERENTIAL DIAGNOSES
- Osteoid osteoma
  - < 2 cm; characteristic clinical symptoms
- Aneurysmal bone cyst
- Osteoblastoma-like osteosarcoma

Osteoblastoma of Spine
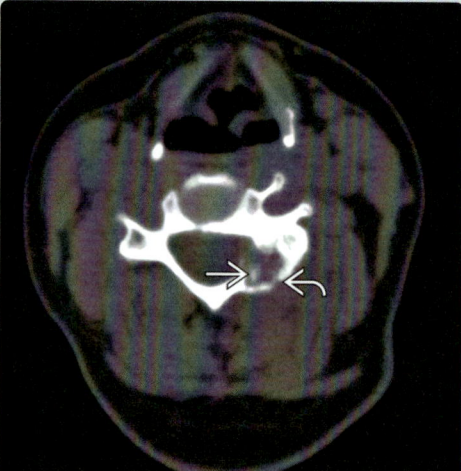

Osteoblastoma Touch Prep of Core
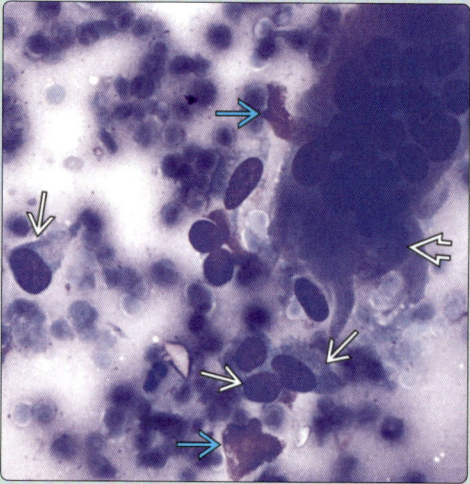

(Left) Axial CT of the C5 cervical spine without contrast in bone windows demonstrates a lytic, expansile lesion of the posterior elements of the spine ➡ with internal matrix ➡. (Courtesy A. Ayala, MD.) (Right) Diff-Quik-stained touch preparation of a core needle biopsy at time of rapid on-site evaluation shows uninucleate osteoblasts ➡ with an occasional multinucleated osteoclastic giant cell ➡. Magenta-staining stromal/osteoid fragments ➡ are also seen in a bloody background.

Osteoblasts and Giant Cell
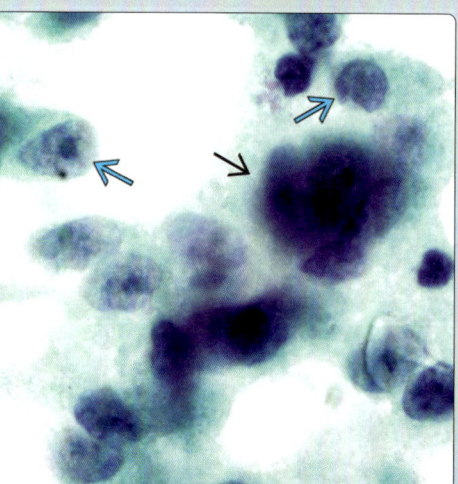

Osteoblastoma Core Needle Biopsy
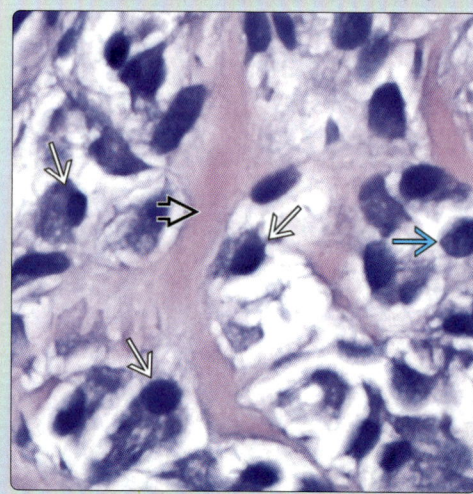

(Left) Pap-stained smear shows uninucleate osteoblasts with ➡ plasmacytoid features, nuclei protruding from cytoplasm, and prominent nucleoli. An osteoclastic giant cell ➡ is also present. (Right) Hematoxylin and eosin stain shows osteoblasts ➡ rimming the osteoid ➡. The osteoblasts have nuclei, which appear to protrude out of the cell and have nucleoli ➡.

Osteoblastoma

TERMINOLOGY

Definitions
- Benign, bone-forming neoplasm composed of woven bone trabeculae lined by osteoblasts, > 2 cm in dimension

CLINICAL ISSUES

Epidemiology
- Incidence
  - Uncommon; accounts for 1% of primary bone tumors
    - Responsible for 3% of primary benign bone tumors
- Age
  - Diagnosed in adolescents and young adults (2nd-4th decades)
- Sex
  - M:F = 2:1

Site
- Most commonly arises in tubular bones
  - ~ 60% develop in appendicular skeleton
    - Often involve metadiaphyseal region of tubular bones
- Axial skeleton is also frequently affected
  - 30% arise in spinal column
    - Originate in posterior elements (lamina and pedicles)
- Craniofacial bones involved in 10% of cases

IMAGING

Radiographic Findings
- Expansile, well-defined, oval, mixed lytic and blastic mass
  - Peripheral lucent halo surrounds central area of mineralization
  - Poorly defined margins in small minority

CYTOPATHOLOGY

Cellularity
- Usually cellular specimen with dispersed cells in bloody background (FNA and Touch preparations of core needle biopsies for ROSE)

Cells
- Combination of uninucleate plasmacytoid osteoblasts and osteoclastic giant cells
- Rare bland spindle cells and stromal fragments
- No atypia, necrosis, or mitotic activity
- Pink osteoid surrounded by osteoblasts may be seen

Nuclear Details
- Osteoblasts resemble plasma cells but lack chunky, spoke-wheel chromatin pattern
  - Uninucleate with eccentrically placed nucleus, which almost protrudes out of cell; nucleolus present
- Osteoclasts have many nuclei with nucleoli

Cytoplasmic Details
- Fine granular cytoplasm without perinuclear hof in osteoblasts

ANCILLARY TESTS

In Situ Hybridization
- Rearrangement of FOS in osteoblastoma and osteoid osteoma by FISH in ~90% or nuclear staining of osteoblasts by IHC; FOSB rearrangement in ~3%

DIFFERENTIAL DIAGNOSIS

Osteoid Osteoma
- < 2 cm; characteristic clinical symptoms

Aneurysmal Bone Cyst
- No haphazardly joining trabeculae of woven bone

Osteoblastoma-Like Osteosarcoma
- Grows with infiltrative pattern
- Absence of FOS by FISH or immunohistochemistry

SELECTED REFERENCES
1. Lam SW et al: Utility of FOS as diagnostic marker for osteoid osteoma and osteoblastoma. Virchows Arch. 476(3):455-63, 2020
2. Amary F et al: FOS expression in osteoid osteoma and osteoblastoma: a valuable ancillary diagnostic tool. Am J Surg Pathol. 43(12):1661-7, 2019

Osteoblasts on Diff-Quik Stain

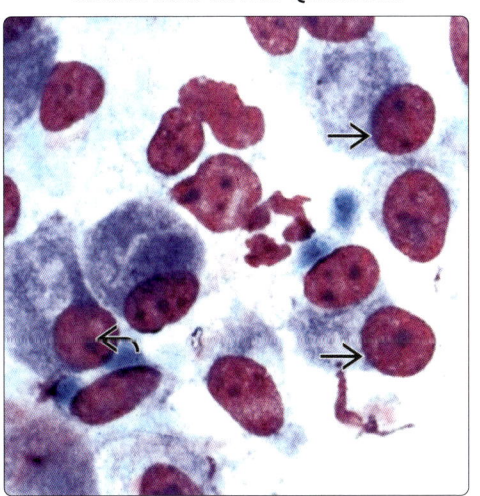

Osteoblasts on Pap Stain

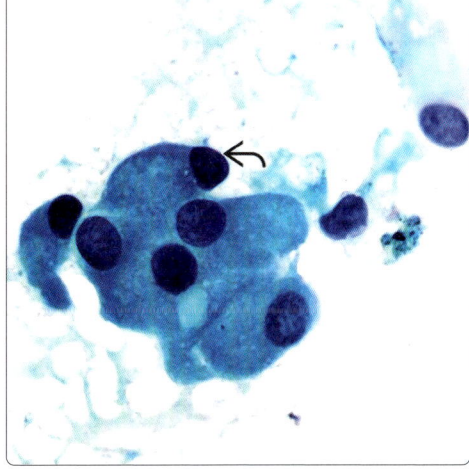

(Left) Diff-Quik shows many osteoblasts characterized by eccentrically placed nuclei ➡ that protrude out of the cytoplasm. Nucleoli ➡ are seen. The chromatin differs from plasma cells by lack of spoke-wheel pattern. **(Right)** Pap stain shows osteoblasts with nuclei ➡ protruding out of the cytoplasm. Any process where there is aggressive bony remodeling, such as a fracture, Paget disease of bone, or certain osteoblastic metastasis as well as osteoblastomas, will show osteoblasts.

Adamantinoma

KEY FACTS

CLINICAL ISSUES
- Almost exclusively in tibia ± involvement of fibula
- Wide surgical excision with reconstructive surgery

IMAGING
- Diaphyseal, well-circumscribed intracortical lytic foci showing characteristic soap bubble appearance
- Adjacent cortex is irregularly thickened and sclerotic

CYTOPATHOLOGY
- Usually low cellularity but can vary depending upon amount of epithelial component compared with fibrous elements
- Clean background, but rarely debris in squamoid variant
- Biphasic pattern with islands of bland spindle and epithelioid cells; more epithelioid cells in classic type
- No atypia, necrosis, or mitosis
- Cell block or core needle biopsy helpful for cytokeratin stain

- Dedifferentiated variants are high-grade tumors and can only be diagnosed on resected specimens and need background of classic ADA

ANCILLARY TESTS
- Epithelial cells are positive for keratin, EMA, p63, and podoplanin and have profile similar to basal layer cells of epidermis
- Keratins expressed are usually types 14 and 19
- In contrast, other mesenchymal tumors with epithelial features like synovial sarcoma, chordoma, and epithelioid sarcoma express keratins 8 and 18

TOP DIFFERENTIAL DIAGNOSES
- Osteofibrous dysplasia
  - Lacks epithelial cell aggregates
- Adamantinoma (ADA)-like Ewing sarcoma
  - Demonstrates t(11;22)
- Intraosseous synovial sarcoma
  - Genetic/FISH profile of synovial sarcoma

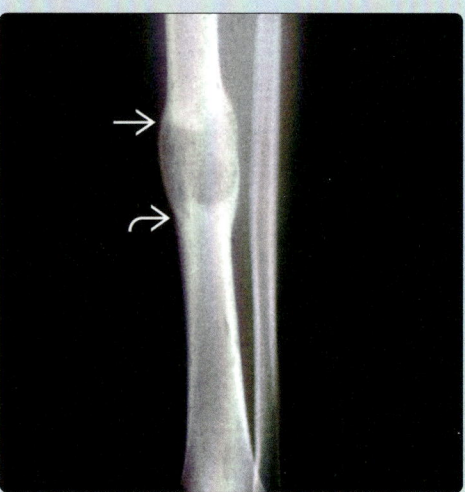

Adamantinoma Plain Film

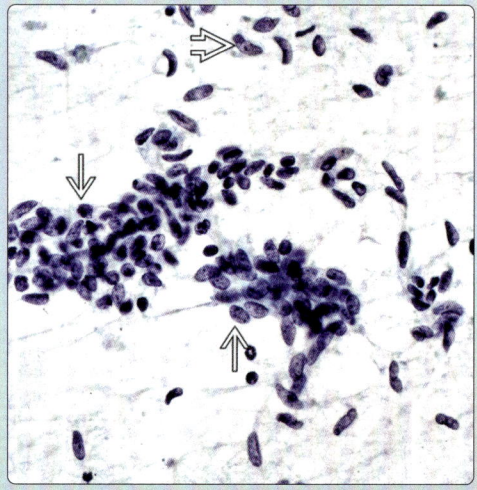

Adamantinoma Epithelial Islands

(Left) Plain film shows a middiaphyseal lesion with a soap bubble appearance. There is a sclerotic rim at the top ➡ and bottom ➡, indicating a slowly growing lesion. The cortex is mostly replaced. (Right) Pap stain of tibial adamantinoma shows a background of spindle cells ➡, scattered in which are epithelial islands ➡ of varying sizes and shapes. Some of the nuclei in the islands may resemble those in the background, possibly resulting in an underdiagnosis of fibrous dysplasia by cytology.

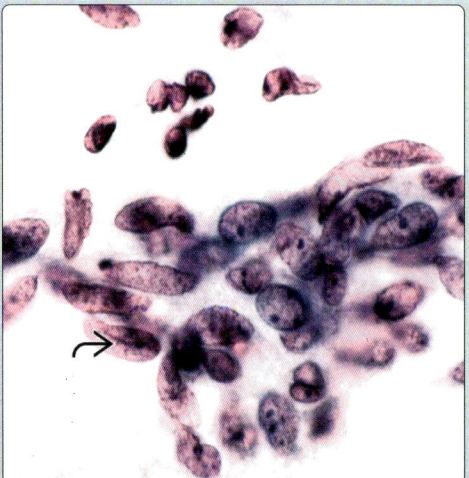

Adamantinoma Epithelial Islands

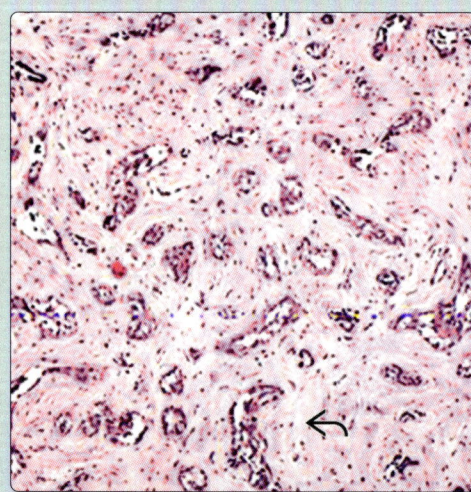

Well-Differentiated Adamantinoma

(Left) Pap stain shows epithelioid aggregates of spindle to oval cells with scant cytoplasm and nuclear grooves ➡. Note the absence of atypia, mitosis, or necrosis. (Right) Well-differentiated adamantinoma with fibrous dysplasia-like stroma ➡ is shown.

Adamantinoma

TERMINOLOGY

Abbreviations
- Adamantinoma (ADA)

Definitions
- Low-grade biphasic malignant neoplasm of bone, composed of epithelial and mesenchymal elements

CLINICAL ISSUES

Epidemiology
- Incidence
  - Uncommon; < 1% of primary malignant bone tumors
- Age
  - Classic ADA affects patients > 20 years
  - Well-differentiated ADA affects patients < 20 years

Site
- Almost exclusively in tibia, ± involvement of fibula

Treatment
- Surgery with wide excision and reconstruction

Prognosis
- Tendency for local recurrence, particularly with close surgical margins
- Metastases usually develop after long clinical course and occur in ~ 12-29% of patients
  - All metastatic lesions are classic ADA or dedifferentiated

IMAGING

Radiographic Findings
- Diaphyseal, well-circumscribed intracortical lytic foci showing characteristic soap bubble appearance
- Adjacent cortex is irregularly thickened and sclerotic
- Dedifferentiated ADA has aggressive radiologic appearance and soft tissue extension

CYTOPATHOLOGY

Cellularity
- Usually low cellularity but can vary depending upon amount of epithelial component compared with fibrous elements
- Greater in classic ADA and dedifferentiated variants

Pattern
- Dispersed bland spindle nuclei and clumps of epithelial cells
- Metachromatic material may be seen on Diff-Quik stain

Background
- Usually clean but rarely there is debris in squamoid variant

Cells
- Biphasic pattern with spindle, ovoid, and epithelioid cells
  - More epithelioid cells in classic type
- Spindle bipolar bland nuclei without mitosis or atypia
- Epithelial islands show benign rounded or spindled nuclei
- Scant to absent cytoplasm in spindle and clustered epithelioid cells
- No atypia, necrosis, or mitosis (unless dedifferentiated)

MICROSCOPIC

Histologic Features
- Groups or sheets of epithelial cells
- Variable amount of osteofibrous dysplasia-like tissue
- Classic ADA
  - Epithelial component is prominent, whereas osteofibrous dysplasia-like areas are inconspicuous
- Well-differentiated ADA
  - Predominance of osteofibrous dysplasia-like areas
- Dedifferentiated ADA
  - Highly malignant component in background of classic ADA

ANCILLARY TESTS

Immunohistochemistry
- Epithelial cells are keratin positive with profile similar to basal layer cells of epidermis
- Keratins expressed are usually CK14 and CK19

DIFFERENTIAL DIAGNOSIS

Osteofibrous Dysplasia
- Lacks aggregates of epithelial cells

Adamantinoma-Like Ewing Sarcoma
- Demonstrates t(11;22)

Intraosseous Synovial Sarcoma
- Genetic/FISH profile of synovial sarcoma

SELECTED REFERENCES

1. Ali NM et al: Comprehensive molecular characterization of adamantinoma and OFD-like adamantinoma bone tumors. Am J Surg Pathol. 43(7):965-74, 2019

Characteristic Features of Classic and Well-Differentiated Adamantinoma

Features	Classic	Well Differentiated	Dedifferentiated
Age	Typically > 20 years	Typically < 20 years	Middle-aged to older adults
Location	Intracortical ± medullary or extraosseous spread	Purely intracortical	Aggressive with extracortical extension and metastasis
Osteofibrous dysplasia-like component	Minority, epithelial predominant	Dominant with rare epithelial cells	Pleomorphic/sarcomatoid cells
Metastasis	~ 20%	Extremely rare	Frequent, aggressive, high grade

Langerhans Cell Histiocytosis

KEY FACTS

CLINICAL ISSUES
- Usually diagnosed during first 3 decades of life
- Can develop in any bone but is most common in skull and jaw; monostotic and polyostotic types
- Patients with monostotic skeletal involvement have excellent prognosis
- Commonly involves skeleton
- Other common sites of involvement include skin, lungs, and lymph nodes
- Associated with variety of clinical syndromes that vary due to symptoms and number, site, and size of tumors
- Localized pain
- Large tumors may undergo pathologic fracture

CYTOPATHOLOGY
- Usually cellular with scattered eosinophils, inflammatory cells, and larger histiocytic cells
- Langerhans cells are mononuclear or multinucleated histiocyte-like cells
- Nuclei are vesicular and kidney-shaped with mitosis, including atypical forms
- Some have longitudinal groove running through nucleus ("coffee bean" nuclei)
- Cytoplasm is abundant and may contain phagocytized debris
- CD1a, CD207 (langerin), S100 positive; Birbeck granules on electron microscopy
- MAPK pathway gene mutations in > 85%; *BRAF* V600 most common

TOP DIFFERENTIAL DIAGNOSES
- Acute or chronic osteomyelitis with increased eosinophils
  - Acute osteomyelitis has prominent neutrophilic and fibrinous exudate and bone necrosis
- Fungal and parasitic infections
- Foreign body giant cell reactions
- Hodgkin and non-Hodgkin lymphoma
- Rosai-Dorfman disease

Langerhans Cell Histiocytosis
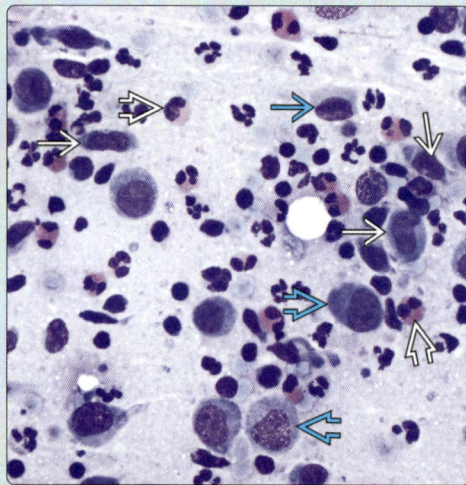

Pap Stain of Langerhans Cell Histiocytosis
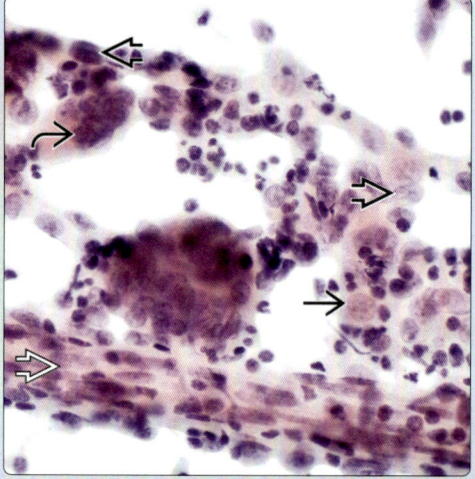

(Left) Diff-Quik-stained smear/touch preparation at time of rapid on-site evaluation shows a mixed population of cells, some with reniform nuclei ⟶ or nuclear grooves ⟶ in a background of eosinophils ⟶, histiocytic cells ⟶, and other inflammatory cells. **(Right)** Pap stain shows histiocytic cells ⟶, giant cells ⟶, blood vessels ⟶, and inflammatory cells in the background. The chromatin of the Langerhans cells is open and vesicular with linear nuclear grooves ⟶.

Core Needle Biopsy of Langerhans Cell Histiocytosis
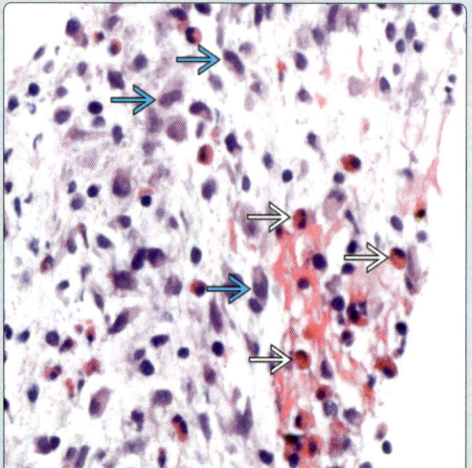

CD1a Stain in Langerhans Cell Histiocytosis
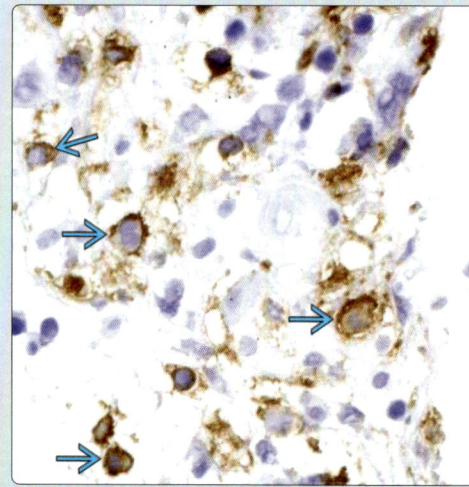

(Left) H&E-stained core needle biopsy shows Langerhans cells with bean-shaped nuclei and nuclear grooves ⟶. These were Cd1a positive. A collection of eosinophils ⟶ is also present. **(Right)** CD1a-positive Langerhans cells ⟶ show cytoplasmic staining in a core needle biopsy, aiding in confirmation of the diagnosis of Langerhans cell histiocytosis.

Langerhans Cell Histiocytosis

TERMINOLOGY

Abbreviations
- Langerhans cell histiocytosis (LCH)
  - Histiocytosis X, eosinophilic granuloma (for solitary lesions) is not recommended
    - Multifocal and multisystem terminology, such as Hand-Schuller-Christian disease or Letterer-Siwe disease, are not recommended

Definitions
- Clonal neoplastic proliferation of myeloid dendritic cells with Langerhans cell phenotype, driven by MAPK pathway activation mutation (*BRAF* V600E in most)

CLINICAL ISSUES

Epidemiology
- Incidence
  - Rare: Accounts for < 1% of all bone tumors
- Age
  - Usually diagnosed during first 3 decades of life
  - Disseminated disease with extraosseous lesions typically occurs in first 2 years of life

Site
- LCH commonly involves skeleton
  - Monostotic more common than polyostotic
- Other common sites of involvement include skin, lungs, and lymph nodes
- Can develop in any bone but most commonly occurs in craniofacial bones

Prognosis
- Patients with monostotic skeletal involvement have excellent prognosis
  - Usually remain disease-free after adequate therapy
- Multifocal systemic disease has guarded prognosis

IMAGING

Radiographic Findings
- Well-defined lytic lesion
  - Minority of cases have ill-defined and permeative margins, resembling osteomyelitis
  - Sequestrum may be seen
- Discretely punched-out lesions may involve tables of skull unevenly, resulting in beveled edge appearance
- Cortical involvement may elicit periosteal reaction that may be more extensive than would be expected from degree of cortical destruction

CYTOPATHOLOGY

Cellularity
- Usually cellular with scattered eosinophils, inflammatory cells, and larger histiocytic cells

Pattern
- Dispersed cell pattern with occasional blood vessels
- Cells may adhere to blood vessels

Cells
- Mononuclear or multinucleated histiocyte-like cells
- Nuclei are vesicular and kidney-shaped with usual mitosis but no atypical forms
- Some have longitudinal groove running through nucleus ("coffee bean" nuclei)
- Cytoplasm is abundant and may contain phagocytized debris
- Cell borders are distinct; no atypia
- Rare osteoclast-like giant cells may be seen

MICROSCOPIC

Histologic Features
- Proliferating Langerhans cells are ovoid or round, histiocytic cells, 10-15 μm in diameter, and arranged in aggregates, sheets, or individually
- Cells have eosinophilic cytoplasm and contain central ovoid/coffee bean-shaped or deeply indented nuclei that have pale chromatin and inconspicuous nucleoli
  - Coffee bean appearance produced by linear grooves that traverse length of nuclei
- Most Langerhans cells are mononuclear
  - Some cells contain multiple nuclei
- Mitotic figures are commonplace; atypical forms are absent
- Eosinophils, present in varying numbers, are distributed evenly or arranged in clusters
- Other types of inflammatory cells and osteoclast-type giant cells
- Necrosis may be seen in minority of cases

ANCILLARY TESTS

Immunohistochemistry
- Langerhans cells express CD1a, S100, CD207 (langerin), CD68
- *BRAF* V600 mutation detected by specific antibody or molecular testing

Electron Microscopy
- Birbeck granules (tubular pentilaminar membrane-bound cytoplasmic organelles) resembling tennis racket or lollipop

DIFFERENTIAL DIAGNOSIS

Acute and Chronic Osteomyelitis
- Acute osteomyelitis has prominent neutrophilic and fibrinous exudate and bone necrosis
- Chronic osteomyelitis exhibits mixed inflammatory infiltrate ± histiocytes, not Langerhans cells

Granuloma-Inducing Processes
- Fungal and parasitic infections, foreign body reactions, Hodgkin and non-Hodgkin lymphoma, Rosai-Dorfman

Chondroblastoma
- Chondroblasts CD1a and CD207 negative, H3K36M positive

SELECTED REFERENCES
1. Rodriguez-Galindo C et al: Langerhans cell histiocytosis. Blood. 135(16):1319-31, 2020

Chordoma

KEY FACTS

CLINICAL ISSUES

- Accounts for ~ 5% of primary malignant bone tumors
- Usually diagnosed during 4th-8th decades; M > F
- Only 5% of tumors develop in patients < 20 years
- Virtually restricted to axial skeleton
- Most (~ 50%) arise in sacrum, 35% in skull base
- Mobile spine is site of origin in 15%
- Tumors in children usually arise in skull base

IMAGING

- Destructive &/or lytic with soft tissue extension ± calcifications
- In sacrum, soft tissue component is anterior

CYTOPATHOLOGY

- Cellular specimens with magenta background stroma on Romanowsky stains
- Combination of large vacuolated cells and smaller cells with granular cytoplasm
- Large physaliferous/spider cells with multiple vacuoles and cytoplasmic processes that stretch from nucleus to periphery of cell separated by vacuoles may be seen
- Correlation of radiologic, clinical, and cytologic findings is key to diagnosis

ANCILLARY TESTS

- Keratin, S100, T-Brachyury (nuclear) positive

TOP DIFFERENTIAL DIAGNOSES

- Metastatic adenocarcinoma
  - S100 and T-Brachyury negative in adenocarcinomas
- Chondrosarcoma
  - Negative for keratin, EMA, and T-Brachyury
- Metastatic renal cell carcinoma
  - T-Brachyury negative, PAX8 positive
- Benign notochordal cell tumor
  - Confined to bone and lack extracellular myxoid matrix histologically

Core Needle Biopsy of Chordoma

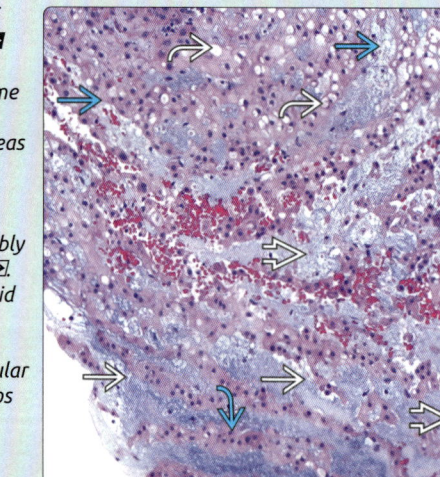

Chordoma Cells and Background

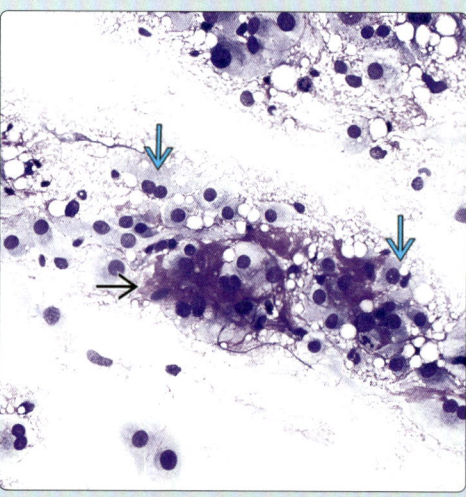

(Left) Core needle biopsy of chordoma shows ribbons ⇨ and cords ⇨ of cells in a mucoid ⇨ background. Some cells have vacuolated and bubbly cytoplasm ⇨, whereas others have a pink granular cytoplasm ⇨. (Right) Diff-Quik stain for adequacy evaluation shows large bubbly cells in a magenta matrix ⇨. The large cells are epithelioid with cytoplasmic vacuoles. The majority of cells are nonvacuolated with a granular cytoplasm and low N:C ratios ⇨.

Chordoma Touch Prep for ROSE

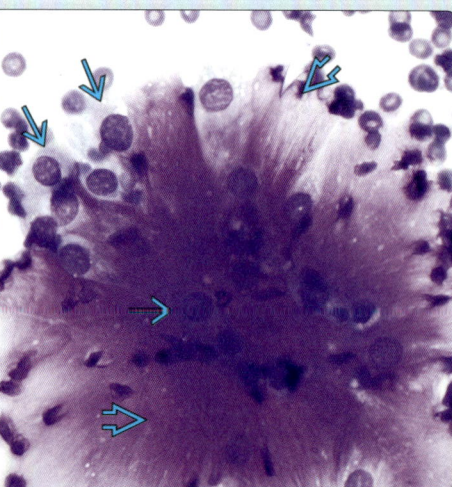

Chordoma Cell Types

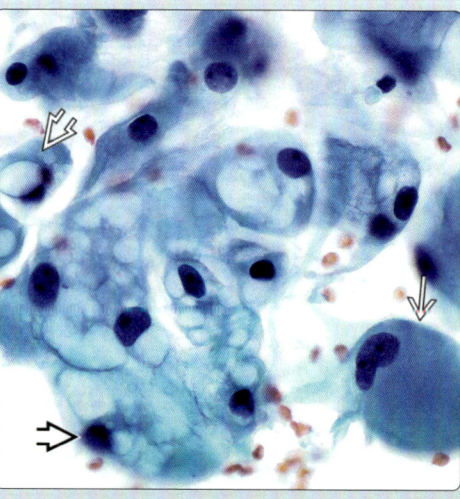

(Left) Diff-Quik-stained touch preparation for rapid on-site evaluation (ROSE) shows uninucleate cells with low N:C ratios and regular nuclear contours ⇨ embedded in a brilliant magenta stroma ⇨. Differential includes chordoma, chondrosarcoma, and other matrix-producing tumors. (Right) Pap stain shows cells with abundant cytoplasm and low N:C ratios ± vacuolated cytoplasm ⇨. Some cells have a signet-ring appearance ⇨. Note the presence of a physaliferous cell ⇨.

Chordoma

TERMINOLOGY

Definitions
- Primary malignant tumor of bone with phenotype that recapitulates notochord and usually arises within bones of axial skeleton
- Chondroid chordoma: Tumor with areas of conventional chordoma and regions resembling low-grade, hyaline-type chondrosarcoma
- Dedifferentiated chordoma contains chordoma juxtaposed to high-grade sarcoma

CLINICAL ISSUES

Site
- Virtually restricted to axial skeleton
- Most (~ 50%) arise in sacrum, 35% in skull base
- Mobile spine is site of origin in 15%
- Chondroid chordoma usually arises in skull base
  - Much less frequently in mobile spine and sacrococcygeal region

Prognosis
- Affected by tumor subtype, location, size, and resectability
- Dedifferentiated chordomas that have high-grade sarcomatous areas and poorly differentiated chordomas, which are SMARCB1 (INI1) negative, have worst prognosis
- Sacral chordomas have best prognosis and longest overall survival, as they can be resected with negative margins

IMAGING

Radiographic Findings
- Destructive &/or lytic with soft tissue extension ± calcifications

MR Findings
- Extremely bright on T2-weighted images
- May show lobulated pattern

CYTOPATHOLOGY

Background
- Abundant mucoid background that stains magenta on Romanowsky stains (Diff-Quik) at time of adequacy evaluation; rarely fibrillary

Cells
- 2 populations
  - Large cells with signet-ring appearance due to cytoplasmic vacuoles
    - Or large physaliferous/spider cells with multiple vacuoles and cytoplasmic processes that stretch from nucleus to periphery of cell separated by vacuoles
  - Smaller cells with granular cytoplasm; nuclei are small and bland with dispersed to vesicular chromatin and occasional nucleoli or chromocenters

ANCILLARY TESTS

Immunohistochemistry
- Conventional chordoma typically expresses epithelial markers, keratin and EMA
- Vast majority stain for nuclear transcription factor T-Brachyury and for S100
- Variable numbers may also stain with antibodies to carcinoembryonic antigen and glial fibrillary acidic protein

DIFFERENTIAL DIAGNOSIS

Metastatic Adenocarcinoma
- Mucinous adenocarcinoma can mimic chordoma on small biopsy sample
- S100 and T-Brachyury negative in adenocarcinomas

Chondrosarcoma, Especially Myxoid Type
- Negative for keratin, EMA, and T-Brachyury

SELECTED REFERENCES
1. Layfield LJ et al: Myxoid neoplasms of bone and soft tissue: a pattern-based approach. J Am Soc Cytopathol. 10(3):278-92, 2021

Chordoma Physaliferous Cell

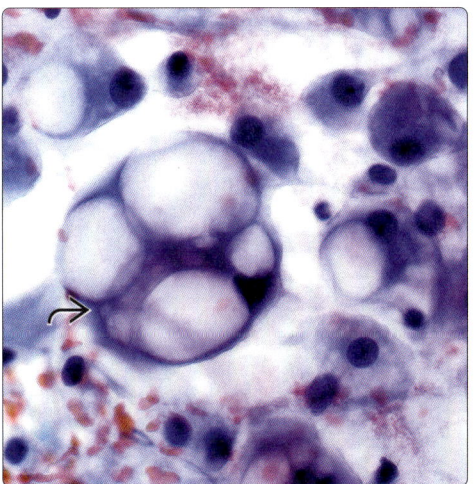

Brachyury Nuclear Positivity in Chordoma

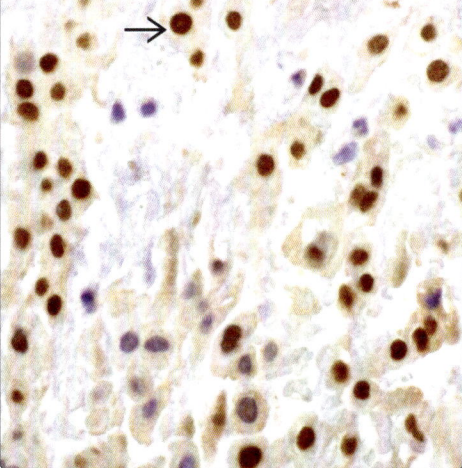

(Left) Pap-stained smear, higher power, shows a multivacuolated physaliferous cell with vacuoles indenting the nucleus and strands of cytoplasm extending from the nucleus to the periphery of the cell ➡. These characteristic cells are typically rare. Most cells resemble the cells in the background. *(Right)* Immunohistochemical staining for T-Brachyury on a cell block shows nuclear positivity in chordoma ➡. Chondroblastomas, chondrosarcomas, and other similar-appearing tumors are negative for Brachyury.

Osteosarcoma

KEY FACTS

CLINICAL ISSUES

- Most common primary malignant tumor of bone, exclusive of hematopoietic malignancies
  - Accounts for ~ 20% of primary bone sarcomas
- Commonly occurs at 10-20 years of age
- Most commonly arises in long tubular bones
  - Distal femur > proximal tibia > proximal humerus
  - 50% of cases occur in knee region
- In older individuals, pelvis and axial skeleton are most common locations
- Primary osteosarcoma is most common type; arises de novo
  - Secondary osteosarcoma arises in diseased bones in patients with history of Paget disease, radiation exposure, chemotherapy, trauma, foreign body (orthopedic implants), and certain genetic abnormalities
- Permeative and destructive lesion centered around metaphysis of long bones

CYTOPATHOLOGY

- Usually high cellularity with fragments, loose clusters, and single cells
- Malignant spindle and epithelioid tumor cells with significant pleomorphism and increased mitotic activity; tumor giant cells are commonly present
- Osteoid production by tumor cells is characteristic feature
- Chondroblasts with cartilaginous matrix, small round blue cells, and osteoclastic giant cells can be noted in variants

TOP DIFFERENTIAL DIAGNOSES

- Undifferentiated pleomorphic sarcoma
- Chondrosarcoma/dedifferentiated chondrosarcoma
- Giant cell tumor
- Ewing sarcoma/primitive neuroectodermal tumor
- Metastatic carcinoma
- Aneurysmal bone cyst
- Osteoblastoma

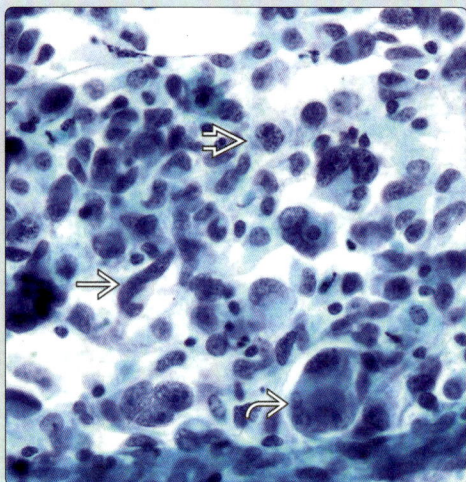

Spindled and Epithelioid Tumor Cells

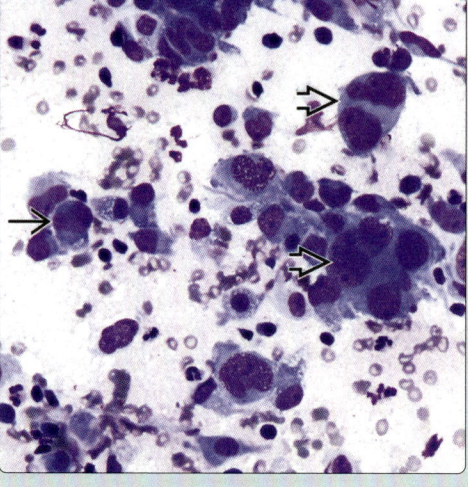

Epithelioid Tumor Cells

(Left) Pap-stained FNA smear of osteosarcoma shows spindled ➡ and epithelioid ➡ individual tumor cells and tumor giant cells ➡. (Right) Diff-Quik-stained FNA smear from a case of osteosarcoma shows malignant epithelioid tumor cells ➡ and tumor giant cells ➡.

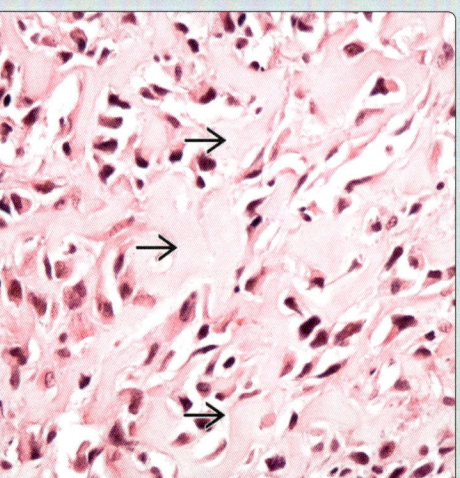

Osteoid Production

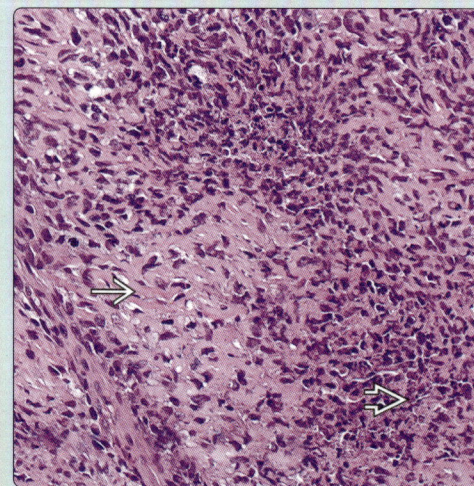

Osteosarcoma

(Left) H&E-stained cell block section shows abundant lace-like osteoid ➡ production by the tumor cells, thereby supporting the diagnosis of osteosarcoma. (Right) Core biopsy of a bone tumor stained with H&E shows high-grade spindle cells ➡ with osteoid production ➡. The overall features are consistent with osteosarcoma, high grade.

Osteosarcoma

TERMINOLOGY

Abbreviations
- Osteosarcoma (OSA)

Definitions
- High-grade malignant tumor in which neoplastic cells produce bone

ETIOLOGY/PATHOGENESIS

Neoplastic Process
- Primary OSA is most common type; arises de novo without known predisposing condition
- Secondary OSA arises within diseased bone in patients with history of Paget disease, radiation exposure, chemotherapy, trauma, foreign body (orthopedic implants), and certain genetic abnormalities

CLINICAL ISSUES

Epidemiology
- Incidence
  - Most common primary malignant tumor of bone, exclusive of hematopoietic malignancies
    - Account for ~ 20% of primary bone sarcomas
- Age
  - Most patients are young (10-20 years)
  - 2nd peak occurs in patients > 50 years
- Sex
  - M:F = 1.3:1

Site
- Most commonly arises in long tubular bones: Distal femur > proximal tibia > proximal humerus
  - 50% of cases occur in knee region
- In older individuals, pelvis and axial skeleton are most common locations
  - < 10% of cases occur in mandible and craniofacial bones

Prognosis
- Relapse-free survival rates: 50-80% (median: ~ 70%)

IMAGING

Radiographic Findings
- Permeative and destructive lesion centered around metaphysis of long bones
  - < 10% of lesions are diaphyseal in location
  - Rarely, OSA can occur in epiphysis
- Poorly defined mixed lytic and blastic mass transgressing cortex and forming large soft tissue component with cloud-like pattern of radiodensity with lack of sclerotic rim
  - Periosteal reaction: Reactive woven bone is deposited between cortex and periosteum elevated by tumor; appears as multiple layers (onion skin) or has radiating (sunburst) appearance
  - Codman triangle: Term used to describe periosteal reaction at diaphyseal end of tumor at angle created by cortex and elevated periosteum
- Entirely lytic appearance is characteristic of telangiectatic variant
  - Lower grade tumors tend to be more mineralized

CYTOPATHOLOGY

Cellularity
- Highly cellular smears in majority of cases
- Some variants of OSA may yield smears of low cellularity

Pattern
- Variably sized fragments, loose clusters, and single tumor cells

Cells
- Spindle and epithelioid tumor cells exhibiting significant pleomorphism
  - Tumor giant cells are commonly present
- Malignant epithelioid cells often have oval or plasmacytoid appearance resembling osteoblasts
- Osteoid or unmineralized bone matrix production by tumor cells is characteristic feature of OSA
- Osteoid is hyaline or finely fibrillar in Pap stain, metachromatic in Romanowsky stains, and faintly birefringent; osteoid can be difficult to distinguish from dense collagen
- Osteoid can also be present as dense irregular clumps without associated tumor cells
- Variants of conventional OSA
  - Osteoblastic: Predominant population of malignant cells includes singly distributed plasmacytoid cells with eccentrically placed nucleus resembling osteoblasts
    - Malignant spindle cells and pleomorphic tumor giant cells will also be present
    - Osteoid production by tumor cells will also be noted
  - Chondroblastic: Spindle and epithelioid tumor cells with significant pleomorphism associated with cartilaginous matrix and abundant osteoid production
    - Fragments of hyaline cartilage with malignant cells residing in lacunar spaces are commonly encountered
- Other types of OSA
  - Telangiectatic: Pleomorphic spindle and epithelioid cells, including tumor giant cells associated with minimal osteoid matrix
    - Aspiration smears are very bloody
  - Fibroblastic: High-grade spindle cell tumor with varying range of atypia associated with very focal areas of osteoid production
  - Small cell: Small round blue cell tumor mimicking Ewing sarcoma (EWS)/primitive neuroectodermal tumor (PNET) except for presence of osteoid in association with tumor cells
    - Tumor cell demonstrates round to oval nucleus with fine chromatin, inconspicuous nucleolus, and scant cytoplasm
  - Low-grade central OSA arising from medullary cavity: Mild to moderately atypical spindle cells with variable amounts of osteoid production
  - Periosteal OSA arising on surface of bone: Features similar to chondroblastic OSA, usually of intermediate grade
  - Parosteal OSA arising on surface of bone: Low-grade tumor with spindle cells showing minimal atypia associated with areas of cartilaginous differentiation
    - Fragments of bone ± osteoblastic rimming

Osteosarcoma

   o High-grade surface OSA (high-grade bone-forming tumor arising from surface of bone) and secondary OSA arising in Paget disease, post radiation, or in course of bone diseases show features similar to conventional OSA

Nuclear Details
- Spindle and epithelioid tumor cells in conventional OSA have round to oval and spindle-shaped nucleus with coarse chromatin, significant pleomorphism, prominent nucleolus, and increased mitotic activity
- Tumor giant cells in conventional OSA can demonstrate very large bizarre multilobated nucleus or can be multinucleated with coarse nuclear chromatin and irregular nuclear membrane

Cell Block Findings
- Osteoid is more easily appreciated in cell blocks

ANCILLARY TESTS

Immunohistochemistry
- Immunoprofile is nonspecific and of minimal help in diagnosis
   o Cartilaginous areas in chondroblastic OSA will be positive for S100
   o CD99 is frequently positive in small cell OSA
- May be focally positive for keratin and EMA

DIFFERENTIAL DIAGNOSIS

Undifferentiated Pleomorphic Sarcoma
- Cytologic findings are similar to those of OSA except for presence of osteoid in association with tumor cells in OSA and not in undifferentiated pleomorphic sarcoma
- Usually occurs in older individuals and presents as lytic lesion in bone on imaging (unlike OSA)
- Distinction between intraosseous undifferentiated pleomorphic sarcoma and OSA is academic one
   o Clinical management is similar

Chondrosarcoma
- In chondroblastic type of OSA and some gnathic OSAs, tumor cells are associated with abundant cartilaginous matrix mimicking chondrosarcoma
- Presence of osteoid in focal areas in OSA is only distinguishing factor
- Cartilaginous tumor with marked atypia, particularly in 2nd and 3rd decades of life, is highly suspicious for OSA
- Presence of *IDH1* or *IDH2* mutations supports diagnosis of chondrosarcoma

Dedifferentiated Chondrosarcoma
- Fragments of high-grade sarcoma in dedifferentiated chondrosarcoma can show osteoid, thereby mimicking OSA
- Presence of fragments is suggestive of low-grade cartilaginous neoplasm admixed with high-grade sarcoma (*dedifferentiated* component) noted in this type of tumor (unlike OSA)

Giant Cell Tumor
- Reactive woven bone frequently found at periphery of giant cell tumor may mimic osteoid produced by tumor cells of OSA
- Unlike OSA, osteoid in giant cell tumor is not lined by atypical tumor cells but by osteoblasts without any evidence of cytologic atypia
- Location of tumor in metaphysis and imaging findings may be useful for distinction

Ewing Sarcoma/Primitive Neuroectodermal Tumor
- Small cell variant of OSA may mimic EWS
   o Presence of osteoid amidst tumor cells will be useful
- While both small cell OSA and EWS/PNET can be positive for CD99, EWS/PNET alone will be positive for FLI-1 and show characteristic cytogenetic alteration t(11;22)(q24;q12)

Metastatic Carcinoma
- Metastatic breast or prostate carcinoma may evoke robust osteoblastic reaction with reactive bone formation that can mimic OSA
   o Appropriate immunohistochemical studies assist in making this distinction

Osteoblastoma
- Fragments of bone lined by plump osteoblasts may mimic osteoblastoma-like OSA
- OSA is usually larger than osteoblastoma and demonstrates significantly more atypia than benign-appearing osteoblasts in osteoblastoma
- Features supporting diagnosis of OSA include infiltration of preexisting bony trabeculae on imaging, large size (> 5 cm), atypical mitotic figures, and abundant lace-like osteoid

Aneurysmal Bone Cyst
- May mimic telangiectatic OSA based on imaging findings
- Cells in cyst wall are not severely atypical (unlike in OSA)

SELECTED REFERENCES

1. Gupta P et al: Cytological diagnosis of osteosarcoma with emphasis on diagnostic pitfalls. Cytopathology. 32(2):243-9, 2021
2. Vangala N et al: Fine-needle aspiration cytology in preoperative diagnosis of bone lesions: a three-year study in a tertiary care hospital. Acta Cytol. 65(1):75-87, 2021
3. Corre I et al: The osteosarcoma microenvironment: a complex but targetable ecosystem. Cells. 9(4):976, 2020
4. Osasan S et al: Osteogenic sarcoma: a 21st century review. Anticancer Res. 36(9):4391-8, 2016
5. VandenBussche CJ et al: Chondroblastic osteosarcoma: cytomorphologic characteristics and differential diagnosis on FNA. Cancer Cytopathol. 124(7):493-500, 2016
6. Kansara M et al: Translational biology of osteosarcoma. Nat Rev Cancer. 14(11):722-35, 2014
7. Sathiyamoorthy S et al: Osteoblastic osteosarcoma: cytomorphologic characteristics and differential diagnosis on fine-needle aspiration. Acta Cytol. 56(5):481-6, 2012
8. Akerman M et al: Cytological features of bone tumours in FNA smears I: osteogenic tumours. Monogr Clin Cytol. 19:18-30, 2010
9. Bishop JA et al: Small cell osteosarcoma: cytopathologic characteristics and differential diagnosis. Am J Clin Pathol. 133(5):756-61, 2010
10. Layfield LJ: Cytologic diagnosis of osseous lesions: a review with emphasis on the diagnosis of primary neoplasms of bone. Diagn Cytopathol. 37(4):299-310, 2009
11. Fleshman R et al: Fine-needle aspiration biopsy of high-grade sarcoma: a report of 107 cases. Cancer. 111(6):491-8, 2007
12. Klijanienko J et al: Cyto-histological correlations in primary, recurrent, and metastatic bone and soft tissue osteosarcoma. Institut Curie's experience. Diagn Cytopathol. 35(5):270-5, 2007
13. Domanski HA et al: Fine-needle aspiration of primary osteosarcoma: a cytological-histological study. Diagn Cytopathol. 32(5):269-75, 2005
14. Handa U et al: Fine needle aspiration cytology in the diagnosis of bone lesions. Cytopathology. 16(2):59-64, 2005

Osteosarcoma

Osteoid Matrix
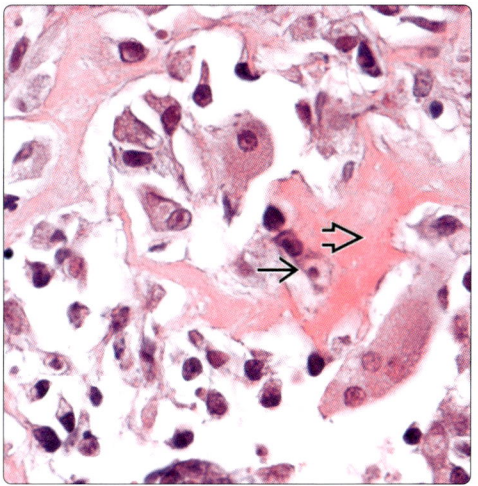

Osteoblast-Like Tumor Cells
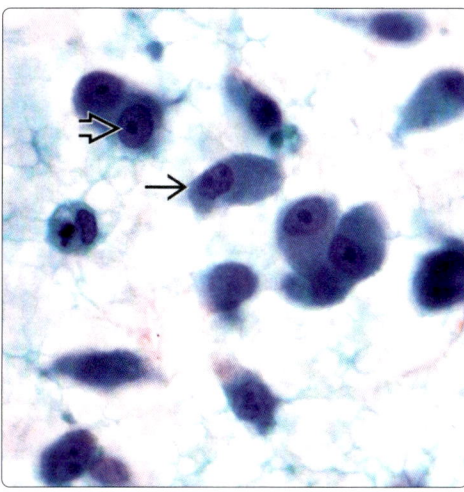

(Left) H&E-stained cell block section of osteosarcoma shows epithelioid tumor cells ⇨ intimately associated with osteoid matrix ⇨, which is present between the tumor cells. (Right) Pap-stained FNA smear of a case of osteoblastic osteosarcoma shows malignant epithelioid tumor cells ⇨ with an eccentrically placed nucleus with prominent nucleolus ⇨, resembling osteoblasts.

Osteosarcoma, Chondroblastic Type
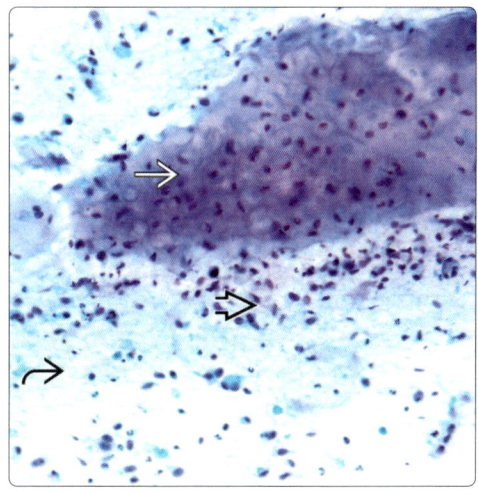

Chondroid and Osteoid Production
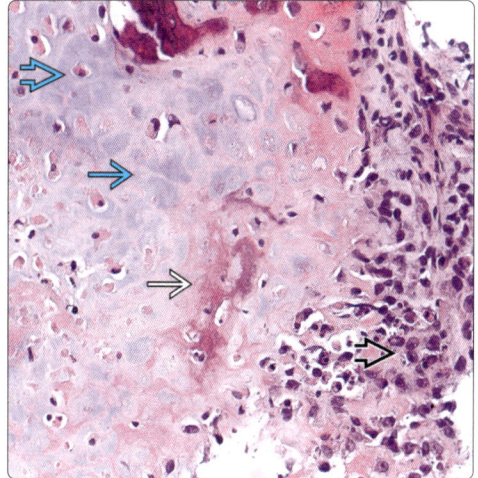

(Left) Pap-stained FNA smear of chondroblastic osteosarcoma shows a fragment of hyaline cartilage ⇨ with malignant tumor cells in lacunar spaces associated with many individual tumor cells ⇨ in a background myxoid matrix ⇨. (Right) Core needle biopsy stained with H&E shows high-grade epithelioid tumor cells ⇨ with osteoid production ⇨ and chondroid matrix ⇨, including tumor cells in lacunar spaces ⇨.

Osteosarcoma Cell Block
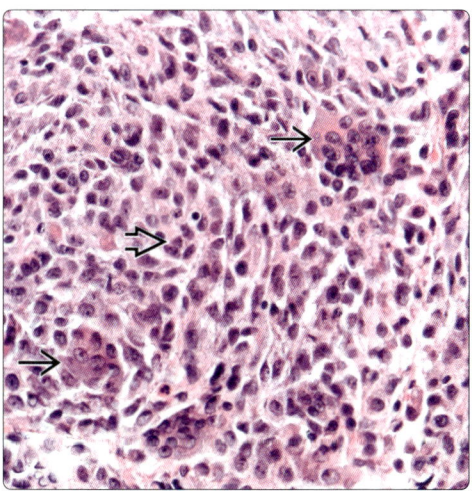

High-Grade Nuclear Features and Mitoses
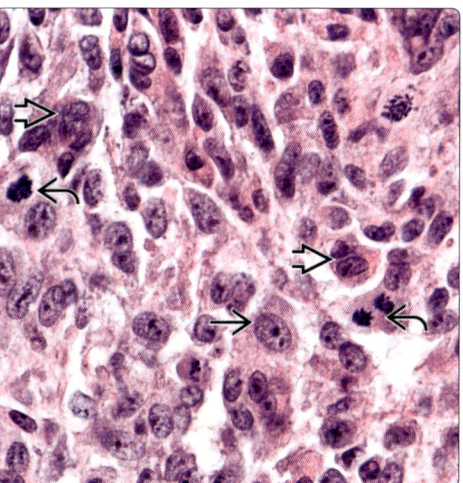

(Left) H&E-stained cell block section of a case of osteosarcoma shows high-grade spindle and epithelioid tumor cells ⇨ associated with many osteoclast-like multinucleated giant cells ⇨. (Right) H&E-stained cell block section shows high-grade epithelioid tumor cells ⇨ with large nucleus and prominent nucleolus, tumor giant cells ⇨, and significantly increased mitotic activity ⇨ of the tumor cells.

Chondrosarcoma

KEY FACTS

CLINICAL ISSUES

- Conventional intramedullary chondrosarcoma (CSA) accounts for > 90% of all CSAs
- Primary CSA usually develops in adults in 5th-7th decades of life
- Most tumors originate in pelvis and femur
- Patients usually present with pain or enlarging mass
- Primary CSA; arises in normal bone
- Secondary CSA; arises in association with
  - Preexisting benign tumor: Enchondroma/enchondromatosis, osteochondroma, fibrous dysplasia
    - Diseased bone: Radiation, Paget disease

CYTOPATHOLOGY

- Variable cellularity and atypia that increase with increasing grade of tumor
- Fragments of hyaline cartilage and cartilaginous matrix in background
- Graded on scale of 1-3 based on cellularity and nuclear atypia
- Dedifferentiated CSA shows features of enchondroma or low-grade CSA with abrupt transition to high-grade sarcoma
- Mesenchymal CSA shows small round blue cell tumor admixed with fragments of hyaline cartilage
- Clear cell CSA shows chondrocytes with centrally located nucleus with minimal atypia associated with abundant clear/vacuolated cytoplasm

TOP DIFFERENTIAL DIAGNOSES

- Enchondroma
- Fracture callus
- Chondromyxoid fibroma
- Chordoma
- Chondroblastic osteosarcoma

Chondrosarcoma: Low Grade

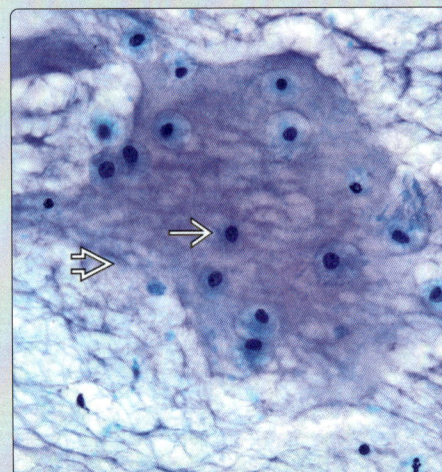

Chondrosarcoma: Low Grade

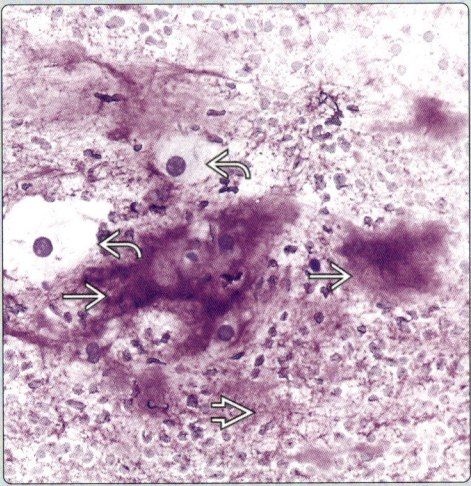

(Left) Pap-stained FNA smear of low-grade chondrosarcoma (CSA) shows a fragment of hyaline cartilage ➡ with mildly increased cellularity. Chondrocytes ➡ are uniform in size with minimal atypia. (Right) Diff-Quik-stained FNA smear of low-grade CSA shows intensely metachromatic fragments of cartilage ➡ and myxoid matrix in the background ➡. The chondrocytes show small round nuclei and abundant cytoplasm ➡.

Chondrosarcoma: Atypical Chondrocytes

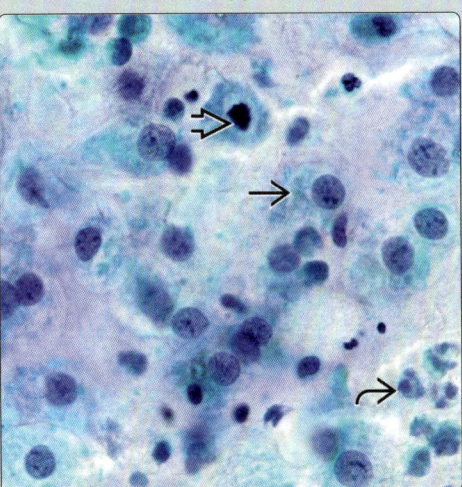

Chondrosarcoma, Intermediate Grade

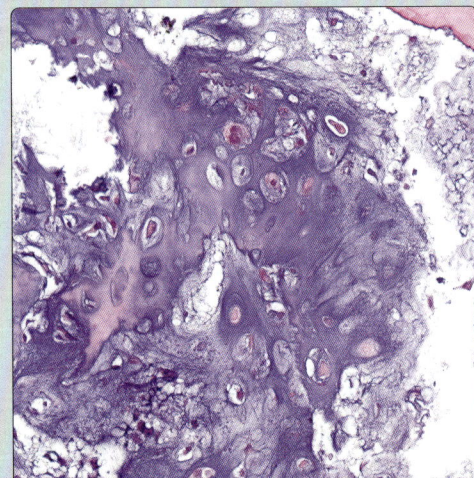

(Left) Pap-stained FNA smear of grade 2 CSA shows increased cellularity with chondrocytes ➡ exhibiting large nuclei with coarse nuclear chromatin. There is a mitotic figure in 1 of the tumor cells ➡ as well as evidence of necrosis ➡ of the tumor. (Right) Core biopsy of CSA, intermediate grade shows increased cellularity, including atypical chondrocytes with moderate nuclear pleomorphism.

Chondrosarcoma

TERMINOLOGY

Abbreviations
- Chondrosarcoma (CSA)

Definitions
- Malignant tumor producing cartilaginous matrix

Types
- Primary CSA
  - Arises in normal bone
- Secondary CSA
  - Arises in association with
    - Preexisting benign tumor
      - Enchondroma/enchondromatosis, osteochondroma, fibrous dysplasia
    - Diseased bone
      - Radiation, Paget disease
- Periosteal CSA (a.k.a. juxtacortical CSA)
  - Arises on surface of bone
- Dedifferentiated CSA
  - Distinct variant of CSA containing well-differentiated cartilage tumor, either enchondroma or low-grade CSA, with abrupt transition to high-grade noncartilaginous tumor
- Mesenchymal CSA
  - Rare malignant tumor with bimorphic pattern composed of highly undifferentiated small round cells and islands of well-differentiated hyaline cartilage
- Clear cell CSA
  - Rare low-grade variant of CSA with distinct histology

ETIOLOGY/PATHOGENESIS

Neoplastic
- Etiology for most CSAs is unknown
- Malignant transformation of sporadic enchondroma
  - Risk is very low (< 1%)
- Patients with enchondromatosis (e.g., Ollier disease or Maffucci syndrome) have increased risk of developing CSA
  - Risk of malignant transformation is 35-40%
- Malignant transformation of sporadic osteochondroma
  - Estimated incidence is 0.4-2.0%
- Patients with osteochondromatosis have 5-25% chance of developing CSA

CLINICAL ISSUES

Epidemiology
- Incidence
  - Primary CSA is 2nd most common primary malignant bone tumor after osteosarcoma, accounting for 20% of malignant bone tumors
  - Conventional intramedullary CSA accounts for > 90% of all CSAs
- Age
  - Primary CSA usually develops in adults in 5th-7th decades of life
  - Dedifferentiated CSA occurs usually at 50-60 years
  - Mesenchymal CSA can occur at any age
  - Clear cell CSA age range: 12-84 years
- Sex
  - Males are affected slightly more frequently than females

Site
- Most originate in pelvis, especially in ilium, followed by proximal femur, proximal humerus, distal femur, and ribs
  - Infrequently develop in small bones of hand and feet (1% of CSA)
  - In long bones, usually involve metaphysis or diaphysis
- Most CSAs arising in osteochondroma originate in pelvis or femur
- CSA of cranium usually involves skull base
- Periosteal CSA most commonly involves distal femur
- Dedifferentiated CSA usually involves pelvis, femur, or humerus
- Mesenchymal CSA can involve sites, such as craniofacial bones, jawbones, ribs, ilium, and vertebra
- Clear cell CSA involves epiphyseal ends of long bones

Presentation
- Patients present with pain, enlarging mass, and (infrequently) fracture of bone
- Skull base tumors frequently cause headache, diplopia, and cranial nerve palsies
- In patients with osteochondroma/enchondromatosis, any change in clinical symptoms or increase in size after puberty should raise suspicion of malignant transformation

Prognosis
- Histologic grade is single most important prognostic factor
- Grade 1 CSAs behave in locally aggressive manner
  - 5-year survival rate: ~ 85%
  - Deaths usually result from local recurrence
  - Metastases are rare
- Grades 2 and 3 CSAs have much worse prognosis
  - 5-year survival rate: ~ 50%
- Prognosis of CSA arising in osteochondroma is excellent unless there is dedifferentiation
- Periosteal CSA tends to recur locally
- Dedifferentiated CSA has dismal prognosis
- Mesenchymal CSA has strong tendency for local recurrence and distant metastasis that can occur several years after initial diagnosis
- Surgical excision with clear margins usually results in cure of clear cell CSA

IMAGING

Radiographic Findings
- Lytic with scattered radiodensities that take form of rings, arcs caused by endochondral ossification and reactive bone formation, and irregular spiculations caused by irregular calcification of matrix

CYTOPATHOLOGY

Cellularity
- Cellularity is low in low-grade CSAs and increases with increasing grade of tumor

Pattern
- Fragments of hyaline cartilage of variable cellularity associated with cartilaginous matrix

Chondrosarcoma

Background
- Myxoid matrix resulting from chondroid matrix liquefaction with clusters and single chondrocytes
- Cartilaginous matrix can be thick and dense to watery and fibrillar
- Intensely metachromatic in Romanowsky stains

Cells
- Chondrocytes located in lacunar spaces in fragments of hyaline cartilage or in cartilaginous matrix in background show varying grades of cytologic atypia depending on tumor grade
- Dedifferentiated CSA shows features of low-grade conventional CSA with abrupt transition to high-grade sarcoma
- Mesenchymal CSA shows biphasic pattern with undifferentiated small round cells admixed with islands of hyaline cartilage
- Clear cell CSA shows features of low-grade CSA with chondrocytes exhibiting centrally located nucleus with minimal atypia, abundant clear cytoplasm, and distinct cytoplasmic membrane
    - Multinucleated osteoclastic giant cells are commonly present

Nuclear Details
- Nuclei are round or oval
    - Low-grade CSA: Fine nuclear chromatin with inconspicuous nucleolus
    - High-grade CSA: Coarse nuclear chromatin, often with prominent nucleolus and significant mitotic activity
- Nuclear atypia, binucleation, multinucleation, and mitotic activity increase with increasing grade of tumor
- Conventional CSA is graded on scale of 1-3 based on cellularity, nuclear size, and nuclear hyperchromasia
    - Grading of CSA can be useful in predicting behavior
- Grade 1: Moderate cellularity; small and dark or slightly enlarged nuclei with fine chromatin of uniform size; occasional binucleated cells are present; cytology is similar to enchondroma
- Grade 2: Higher cellularity; larger hyperchromatic nuclei, often with irregular nuclear membrane with coarse nuclear chromatin; infrequent mitoses
- Grade 3: Higher cellularity; significant nuclear atypia; nuclear pleomorphism and mitoses are easily detected

Cytoplasmic Details
- Moderate to abundant cytoplasm
- Vacuoles are often noted on Romanowsky stains

ANCILLARY TESTS

Genetic Testing
- Isocitrate dehydrogenase genes *IDH1* and *IDH2* are mutated in many CSAs
    - Primary CSA: 38-70%
    - Secondary CSA: 86%
    - Periosteal CSA: 100%
- Mutation analysis can be used in difficult cases to distinguish CSA from chondroblastic osteosarcoma in small specimens

DIFFERENTIAL DIAGNOSIS

Enchondroma
- Enchondromas yield few fragments of hyaline cartilage; chondrocytes lack atypia
    - Cytologic features overlap with those of CSA
- Relatively well-circumscribed tumor without infiltrative pattern by imaging studies
- Permeation of bony trabeculae can be appreciated on histology specimens alone

Fracture Callus
- Fragments of hyaline cartilage with minimal atypia in fracture callus can mimic low-grade CSA
    - Correlation with clinical history and imaging findings will be useful for distinction

Chondromyxoid Fibroma
- Contains spindle and stellate tumor cells, chondrocytes, and giant cells associated with chondromyxoid matrix (unlike CSA)
- Well-circumscribed, expansile, lytic tumor by imaging studies

Chordoma
- Chondroid chordomas can be difficult to differentiate from low-grade CSA
- Chondroid chordomas usually arise in skull base (unlike CSA)
- Whereas both types of tumors can be positive for S100, chordomas alone stain with keratin and brachyury

Chondroblastic Osteosarcoma
- Fragments of cartilage with high-grade nuclei associated with cartilaginous matrix in background can mimic high-grade CSA
    - Presence of osteoid in cartilaginous tumor is useful to support diagnosis of chondroblastic osteosarcoma
- Different imaging findings from high-grade CSA

SELECTED REFERENCES
1. Wakely PE Jr: Extraskeletal myxoid chondrosarcoma: combining cytopathology with molecular testing to achieve diagnostic accuracy. J Am Soc Cytopathol. 10(3):293-9, 2021
2. Wangsiricharoen S et al: Cytopathology of chondromyxoid fibroma: a case series and review of the literature. J Am Soc Cytopathol. 10(4):366-81, 2021
3. Amer KM et al: Survival and prognosis of chondrosarcoma subtypes: SEER Database Analysis. J Orthop Res. 38(2):311-9, 2020
4. Mohammad N et al: Characterisation of isocitrate dehydrogenase 1/isocitrate dehydrogenase 2 gene mutation and the d-2-hydroxyglutarate oncometabolite level in dedifferentiated chondrosarcoma. Histopathology. 76(5):722-30, 2020
5. Huang R et al: Identifying the prognosis factors and predicting the survival probability in patients with non-metastatic chondrosarcoma from the SEER Database. Orthop Surg. 11(5):801-10, 2019
6. Chow WA: Chondrosarcoma: biology, genetics, and epigenetics. F1000Res. 7, 2018
7. McHugh KE et al: Fine needle aspiration biopsy diagnosis of primary clear cell chondrosarcoma: a case report. Diagn Cytopathol. 46(2):165-9, 2018
8. Speetjens FM et al: Molecular oncogenesis of chondrosarcoma: impact for targeted treatment. Curr Opin Oncol. 28(4):314-22, 2016
9. Chhabra S et al: Cytomorphologic features of chondroid neoplasms: a comparative study. Acta Cytol. 54(6):1101-10, 2010
10. Cabay RJ et al: Cytologic features of primary chondroid tumors of bone in crush preparations. Diagn Cytopathol. 36(10):758-61, 2008
11. Dodd LG: Fine-needle aspiration of chondrosarcoma. Diagn Cytopathol. 34(6):413-8, 2006
12. Trembath DG et al: Cytopathology of mesenchymal chondrosarcomas: a report and comparison of four patients. Cancer. 99(4):211-6, 2003

Chondrosarcoma

Chondrosarcoma: High Grade
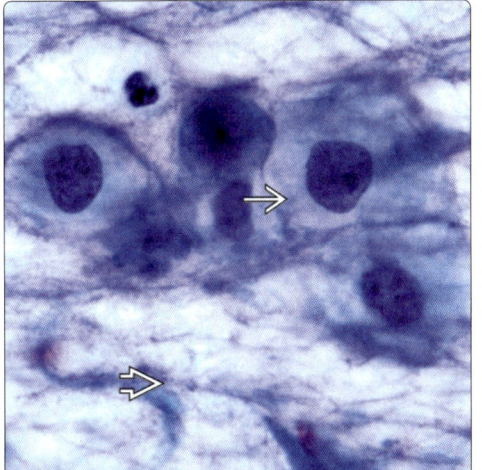

Chondrosarcoma: High Grade
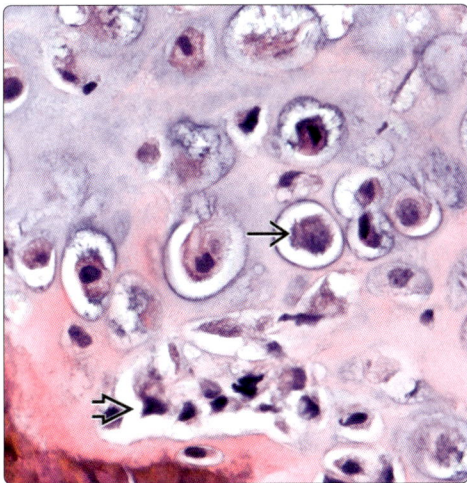

(Left) Pap-stained FNA smear of a case of high-grade CSA shows very large chondrocytes ➡ distributed in a myxoid matrix ➡. (Right) H&E-stained cell block section of a high-grade CSA shows large, atypical chondrocytes ➡ in lacunae. Some of the tumor cells are dying with shrunken hyperchromatic nuclei ➡.

Chondrosarcoma: Low Grade
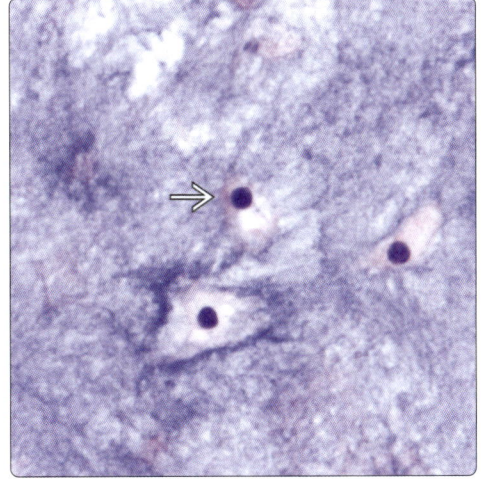

Chondrosarcoma: Low Grade
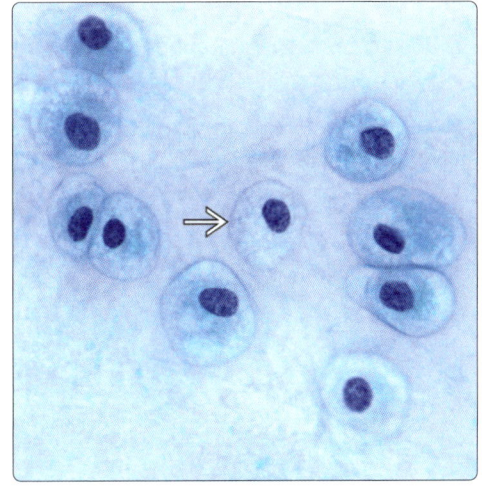

(Left) Pap-stained FNA smear of CSA, low grade, shows few chondrocytes with minimal atypia ➡. (Right) Pap-stained smear of CSA, low grade, shows chondrocytes with a low nuclear:cytoplasmic ratio exhibiting a single nucleus with clumped chromatin and regular nuclear membrane ➡.

Chondrosarcoma: Dedifferentiated
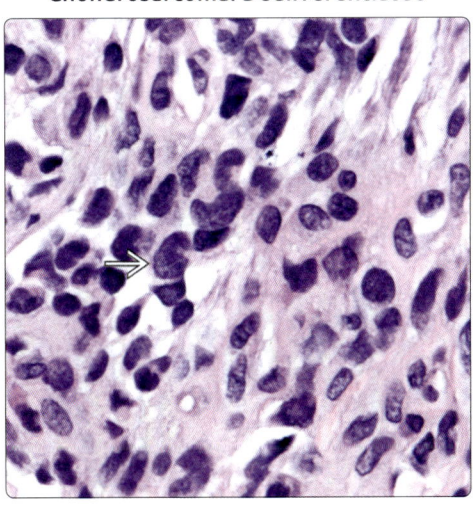

Mesenchymal Chondrosarcoma
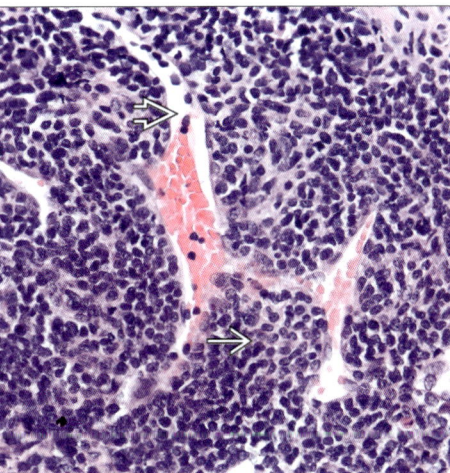

(Left) H&E-stained tissue section of dedifferentiated CSA shows 1 of the components of the tumor with features of a high-grade spindle cell ➡ sarcoma. (Right) H&E-stained tissue section of mesenchymal CSA shows sheets of small round blue tumor cells ➡ with blood vessels demonstrating a hemangiopericytoma-like pattern ➡.

Ewing Sarcoma

KEY FACTS

CLINICAL ISSUES
- Accounts for ~ 6-10% of primary malignant bone tumors
- Usually arises in diaphysis or metadiaphysis of long tubular bones and flat bones of pelvis

CYTOPATHOLOGY
- High cellularity with single tumor cells 1-2x size of lymphocytes
- Tumor cells have round to oval nucleus with fine chromatin, inconspicuous nucleolus, and scant, often vacuolated cytoplasm
- Tumor cell cytoplasm is rich in glycogen
  - Disruption of tumor cells results in naked nuclei with vacuolated background
- Common variant: Large cell Ewing sarcoma with larger tumor cells with prominent nucleolus, irregular nuclear membrane, and more cytoplasm

ANCILLARY TESTS
- Cells express vimentin, CD99 (90%), and FLI-1 (90%)
  - CD99 is also expressed by many other malignant small round cell tumors, including lymphoblastic lymphoma, small cell osteosarcoma, mesenchymal chondrosarcoma, and small cell carcinoma
  - Small cell osteosarcoma, lymphoblastic lymphoma, and mesenchymal chondrosarcoma are negative for FLI-1, unlike Ewing sarcoma
- Molecular testing: ~ 85% harbor t(11;22)(q24;q12)

TOP DIFFERENTIAL DIAGNOSES
- Malignant lymphoma
- Neuroblastoma
- Small cell osteosarcoma
- Mesenchymal chondrosarcoma

Ewing Sarcoma: Small Round Blue Tumor Cells

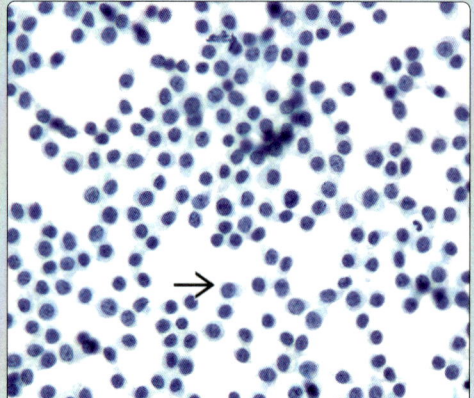

Ewing Sarcoma: Tigroid Background

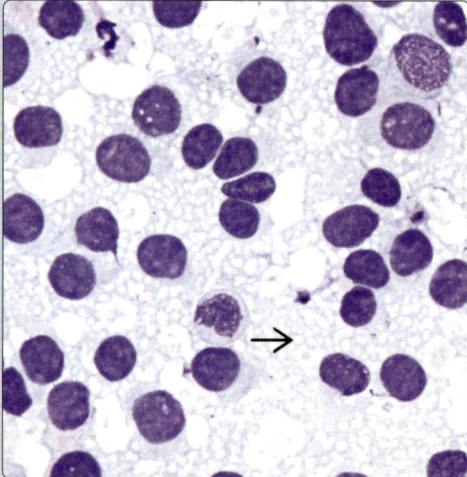

(Left) Pap-stained FNA smear of Ewing sarcoma shows individually distributed monotonous small round blue tumor cells ➡. (Right) Diff-Quik-stained smear of Ewing sarcoma shows a vacuolated tigroid background ➡ caused by glycogen derived from a disrupted cytoplasm of tumor cells.

Ewing Sarcoma

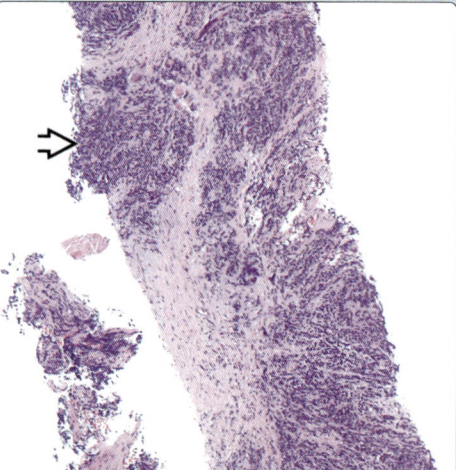

Ewing Sarcoma

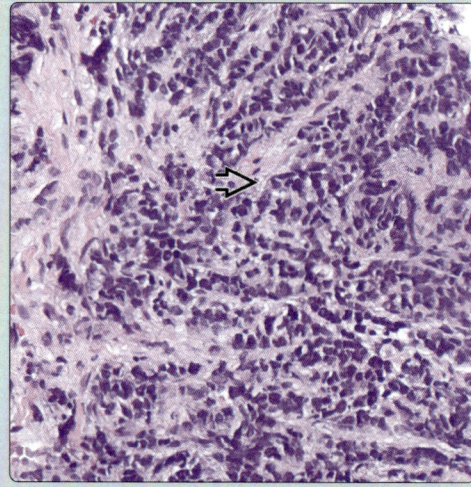

(Left) Core needle biopsy stained with H&E shows sheets of tumor cells ➡ with no particular arrangement. (Right) Core biopsy stained with H&E shows tumor cells with moderate nuclear pleomorphism, inconspicuous nucleolus, and scant cytoplasm ➡. The tumor demonstrates characteristic EWS::FLI1 fusion by molecular testing as a result of t(11;22)(q24;q12) translocation. Morphological features in conjunction with genomic changes are consistent with Ewing sarcoma.

Ewing Sarcoma

TERMINOLOGY

Abbreviations
- Ewing sarcoma (EWS)

Synonyms
- Peripheral neuroepithelioma; Askin tumor

Definitions
- Round cell sarcoma showing variable degree of neuroectodermal differentiation

ETIOLOGY/PATHOGENESIS

Neoplasm
- Evidence suggests stem cell origin

CLINICAL ISSUES

Epidemiology
- Incidence
  - Accounts for 6-10% of primary malignant bone tumors
  - Follows osteosarcoma and chondrosarcoma in frequency in adults
  - Follows osteosarcoma in frequency in children and adolescents
- Age
  - Most patients are 10-15 years old
    - ~ 80% of patients are < 20 years old
- Sex
  - M:F = 1.3-1.4:1
- Ethnicity
  - Striking predilection for White patients (3 per 1 million)
  - Africans, Asians, and Native American patients are rarely affected (0.2 per 1 million)

Site
- Can arise in any portion of skeleton
- Usually develops in diaphysis or metadiaphysis of long tubular bones and flat pelvic bones
- ~ 22% arise in femur, followed by ilium, tibia, humerus, fibula, and ribs
- Tumor that originates in chest wall is called Askin tumor

Presentation
- Painful enlarging mass; affected site is frequently tender, warm, and swollen
- Some patients present with systemic findings that mimic infection with fever, elevated sedimentation rate, anemia, and leukocytosis
- Pathologic fracture is uncommon presentation

Treatment
- Usually treated with neoadjuvant chemotherapy followed by surgery

Prognosis
- Effective chemotherapy has improved 5-year survival rate from 5-15% to 75%
  - At least 50% are long-term cures
  - Important factors influencing prognosis are stage of disease at time of diagnosis and site of tumor
  - Other prognostic factors: Type of translocation, percentage of chemotherapy-related tumor necrosis, presence of chimeric transcripts in peripheral blood or bone marrow cells after treatment, and local recurrence of tumor

IMAGING

Radiographic Findings
- Intraosseous destructive and lytic tumor with poorly defined margins
- Permeation of cortex usually results in concentric soft tissue mass that can be very large
  - Extraosseous tumor frequently erodes outer cortex, producing "saucerization" of bone
- Displaced periosteum deposit layers of reactive bone in onion skin-like or sunburst-like fashion

CT Findings
- Large, destructive intraosseous mass with extension into soft tissues

CYTOPATHOLOGY

Cellularity
- High cellularity

Pattern
- Tumor cells are predominantly singly distributed with few small sheets and loose clusters
- Homer Wright rosettes with central neuropil suggesting neural differentiation can be seen with primitive neuroectodermal tumor (PNET) but not with EWS

Background
- Vacuolated tigroid background due to disruption of tumor cells with high glycogen content in cytoplasm
- Necrosis is variable

Cells
- Tumor cells are 1-2x size of lymphocytes
- Dimorphic or 2-cell population of light and dark cells is often noted, particularly on Romanowsky stains
- Light and dark cells reflect viable and dying tumor cells
- Variants of EWS
  - Large cell variant: Large tumor cells with prominent nucleolus, irregular nuclear membrane, and more cytoplasm
  - Adamantinoma-like variant: Clusters of moderately pleomorphic tumor cells with peripheral palisading and desmoplasia
  - Spindle cell sarcoma-like variant: Spindle tumor cells mimicking other spindle cell sarcomas
  - Sclerosing variant: Tumor cells associated with hyalinized matrix

Nuclear Details
- Viable (light) cells show round to oval nuclei, fine nuclear chromatin, and inconspicuous nucleolus
- 1-3 small nucleoli can be seen in tumor cells
- Dying (dark) cells resemble lymphocytes with dense nuclear chromatin and thin rim of scant cytoplasm
- Binucleation and multinucleation are usually absent
- Mitotic activity is variable

Ewing Sarcoma

Cytoplasmic Details
- Cytoplasm can be vacuolated or clear due to glycogen content
- Cytoplasmic vacuoles can be coarse and punched-out in Romanowsky stain or delicately vacuolated and clear in Pap stain

Variants
- Large cell EWS: Larger tumor cells with prominent nucleolus, irregular nuclear membrane, and more cytoplasm
- Adamantinoma-like variant: Clusters of moderately pleomorphic cells with peripheral palisading and desmoplasia
- Spindle cell sarcoma-like variant: Spindle tumor cells resembling synovial sarcoma
- Sclerosing variant: Tumor cells associated with hyalinized matrix

ANCILLARY TESTS

Immunohistochemistry
- Cells express vimentin, CD99 (90%), and FLI-1 (90%)
  - Other tumors, such as small cell osteosarcoma, mesenchymal chondrosarcoma, and lymphoblastic lymphoma, can also be positive for CD99 but are negative for FLI-1
  - Tumors with neuroectodermal differentiation express 1 or more neural markers, including NSE, CD57, and S100
- Neurofilament and keratin positivity can be seen in ~ 20% of cases

Molecular Pathology
- ~ 85% harbor t(11;22)(q24;q12)
- 5-10% have t(21;22)(q22;q12)
- < 1% of tumors show *EWSR1* fusion with *ETV4* (7p220), *E1AF* (17q12), or *FEV* (2q33)
- Some EWS-negative tumors have been shown to harbor *FUS::ERG* fusion t(16;21)
  - Tumors negative for *FUS/ERG* may show *CIC::DUX4* fusion

DIFFERENTIAL DIAGNOSIS

Malignant Lymphoma
- Cells in large cell lymphoma are frequently larger and exhibit more cytoplasm; their nuclei are often irregular, cleaved, and hyperlobated, unlike EWS
- Lymphoblastic lymphoma is composed of uniform round cells that can be similar to EWS
  - Presence of lymphoglandular bodies in background of smears will be useful
- Lymphomas express lymphoid antigens
- Lymphomas can also express CD99 but are FLI-1 negative and TdT positive, unlike EWS
- Ultrastructurally, tumor cells of lymphoma have marginated chromatin, lack intercellular junctions, and do not contain glycogen
- Chromosomal translocations associated with malignant lymphoma do not include those identified in EWS

Neuroblastoma
- Cytologic features of metastatic undifferentiated neuroblastoma are similar to those of EWS
  - Presence of neuropils and ganglion cells in neuroblastoma may be useful for distinction
- Negative for CD99 and FLI-1, unlike EWS
- Shows *MYCN* amplification and loss of 1p, whereas EWS::PNET shows characteristic t(11;22)(q24;q12)

Small Cell Osteosarcoma
- Tumor cells of small cell osteosarcoma and EWS may be similar
  - Presence of neoplastic osteoid in small cell osteosarcoma may be useful for distinction
  - EWS may contain reactive woven bone that can cause confusion with osteosarcoma
    - Osteoblastic rimming of woven bone may be useful
  - Ancillary immunostain for FLI-1 and cytogenetic analysis are useful

Mesenchymal Chondrosarcoma
- Tumor cells may mimic those of EWS
- Areas of chondroid differentiation admixed with tumor cells
  - This characteristic is useful in differentiating from EWS
- Can be positive for CD99 but negative for FLI-1 and does not show characteristic cytogenetic alteration of EWS

SELECTED REFERENCES

1. Flucke U et al: EWSR1-the most common rearranged gene in soft tissue lesions, which also occurs in different bone lesions: an updated review. Diagnostics (Basel). 11(6), 2021
2. Riggi N et al: Ewing's sarcoma. N Engl J Med. 384(2):154-64, 2021
3. Lott-Limbach AA et al: Mediastinal sarcomas: experience using fine needle aspiration cytopathology. Mediastinum. 4:14, 2020
4. Salguero-Aranda C et al: Breakthrough technologies reshape the Ewing sarcoma molecular landscape. Cells. 9(4), 2020
5. Sbaraglia M et al: Ewing sarcoma and Ewing-like tumors. Virchows Arch. 476(1):109-19, 2020
6. Kao YC et al: BCOR-CCNB3 fusion positive sarcomas: a clinicopathologic and molecular analysis of 36 cases with comparison to morphologic spectrum and clinical behavior of other round cell sarcomas. Am J Surg Pathol. 42(5):604-15, 2018
7. Kilpatrick SE et al: Ewing sarcoma and the history of similar and possibly related small round cell tumors: from whence have we come and where are we going? Adv Anat Pathol. 25(5):314-26, 2018
8. Machado I et al: Review with novel markers facilitates precise categorization of 41 cases of diagnostically challenging, "undifferentiated small round cell tumors". A clinicopathologic, immunophenotypic and molecular analysis. Ann Diagn Pathol. 34:1-12, 2018
9. Russell-Goldman E et al: NKX2.2 immunohistochemistry in the distinction of Ewing sarcoma from cytomorphologic mimics: diagnostic utility and pitfalls. Cancer Cytopathol. 126(11):942-9, 2018
10. Schaefer IM et al: Diagnostic immunohistochemistry for soft tissue and bone tumors: an update. Adv Anat Pathol. 25(6):400-12, 2018
11. Wong KS et al: Cytologic diagnosis of round cell sarcomas in the era of ancillary testing: an updated review. J Am Soc Cytopathol. 7(3):119-32, 2018
12. Antonescu CR et al: Sarcomas with CIC-rearrangements are a distinct pathologic entity with aggressive outcome: a clinicopathologic and molecular study of 115 cases. Am J Surg Pathol. (7):941-9, 2017
13. Chebib I et al: Round cell sarcoma with CIC-DUX4 gene fusion: discussion of the distinctive cytomorphologic, immunohistochemical, and molecular features in the differential diagnosis of round cell tumors. Cancer Cytopathol. 124(5):350-61, 2016
14. Kovar H et al: The second European interdisciplinary Ewing sarcoma research summit–a joint effort to deconstructing the multiple layers of a complex disease. Oncotarget. 7(8):8613-24, 2016
15. Machado I et al: Ewing sarcoma and the new emerging Ewing-like sarcomas: (CIC and BCOR-rearranged-sarcomas). A systematic review. Histol Histopathol. 31(11):1169-81, 2016

Ewing Sarcoma

Ewing Sarcoma

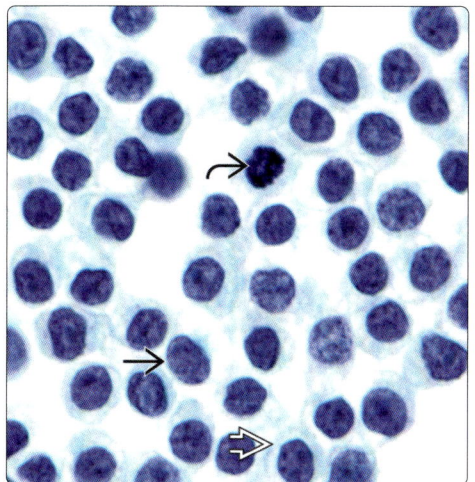

Ewing Sarcoma: Dark and Light Tumor Cells

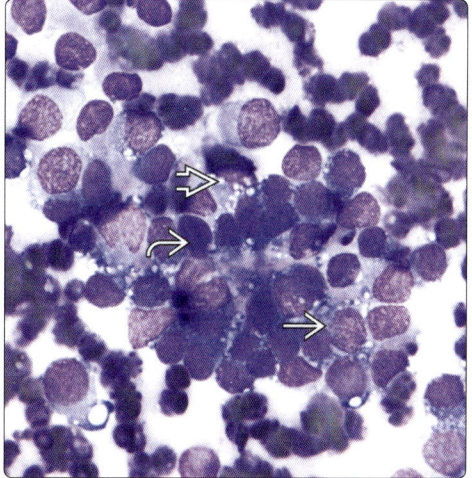

(Left) Pap-stained FNA smear of Ewing sarcoma shows tumor cells with a round nucleus, fine nuclear chromatin, inconspicuous nucleolus ⇨, rare mitosis ⇨, and a moderate amount of clear cytoplasm ⇨. (Right) Diff-Quik-stained FNA smear of Ewing sarcoma shows a loose cluster of tumor cells with dark (dying) ⇨ and light (viable) ⇨ tumor cells with coarse vacuoles ⇨ in many of the tumor cells.

Ewing Sarcoma: Variant

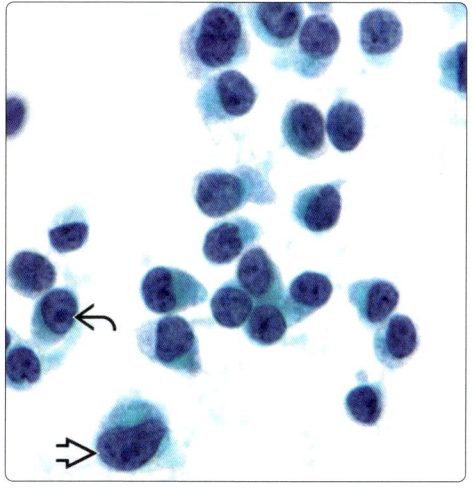

Ewing Sarcoma: Cytoplasmic Vacuoles

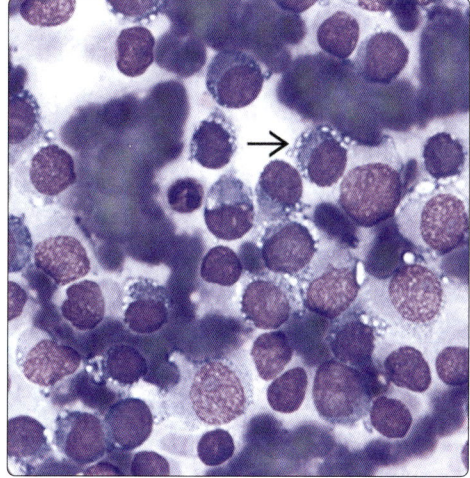

(Left) Pap-stained FNA smear shows a variant Ewing sarcoma with larger tumor cells ⇨ with more cytoplasm ⇨ than classic Ewing sarcoma and prominent nucleolus in some of the tumor cells. (Right) Diff-Quik-stained FNA smear of Ewing sarcoma shows tumor cells with a moderate amount of cytoplasm, some with punched-out vacuoles ⇨.

Ewing Sarcoma: Cell Block

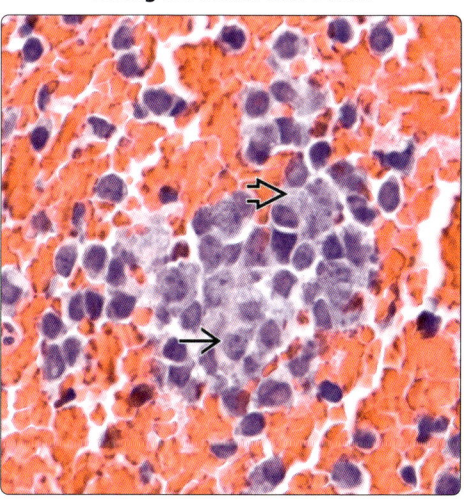

Ewing Sarcoma: CD99-Positive Tumor Cells

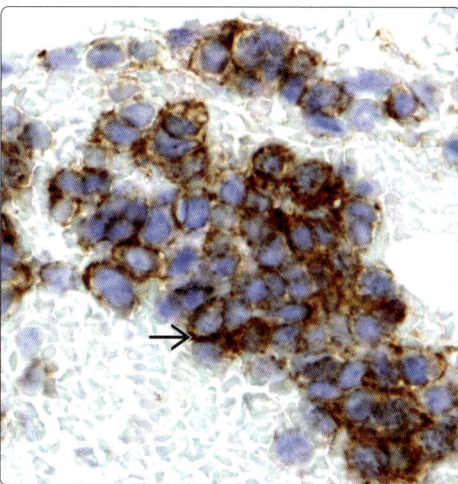

(Left) H&E-stained cell block section of Ewing sarcoma shows a loose cluster of tumor cells with fine nuclear chromatin, small nucleolus ⇨ in some of the tumor cells associated with moderate amounts of cytoplasm ⇨. (Right) Cell block section of Ewing sarcoma immunostained for CD99 (MIC2) shows positive staining of tumor cells with a membranous pattern of staining ⇨.

Bone Lymphoma

KEY FACTS

TERMINOLOGY
- Primary lymphoma originating in bone ± soft tissue extension

CLINICAL ISSUES
- Usually adults
  - ~ 50% are > 40 years
- Femur is most common location, followed by pelvis, vertebrae, and humerus
- ~ 10-40% of cases of lymphoma are multifocal/polyostotic
- Several lesions in 1 bone or multiple bones involved concurrently
- Produces pain, erythema, swelling
- Treatment with radiation and chemotherapy of large B-cell lymphoma has 75% 10-year survival

CYTOPATHOLOGY
- Dispersed population of round or cleaved blue cells
- Round blue cells with morphology that varies depending upon type of lymphoma
- Diffuse large B-cell lymphoma is most common in all ages
- Lymphoblastic lymphoma is 2nd most common type to arise in children (40% of cases)
- Anaplastic large cell lymphoma is rare but most common primary T-cell lymphoma of bone
- At time of adequacy evaluation, it is of paramount importance to collect adequate material in appropriate medium for immunophenotyping by flow cytometry and molecular studies
- Cell block is helpful for immunohistochemistry and molecular studies

ANCILLARY TESTS
- Immunoprofile varies according to type

TOP DIFFERENTIAL DIAGNOSES
- Small round blue cell lesions

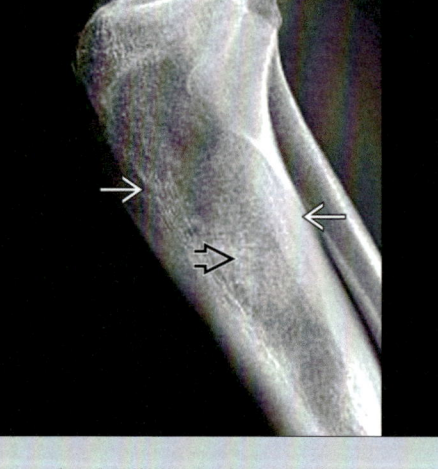

Plain Film: Bone Lymphoma

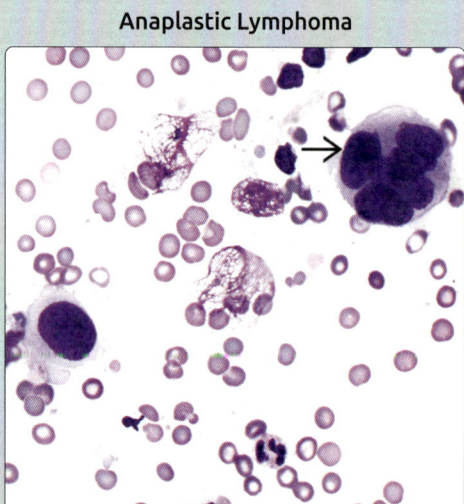

Coronal MR: Tibia

(Left) Radiograph of the proximal tibial metaphysis shows a lytic lesion with endosteal resorption anteriorly and posteriorly ➡. The distal component is indistinct with an area of sclerosis ➡. (Courtesy A. Rosenberg, MD.) (Right) Fluid-sensitive coronal MR with fat saturation shows small, hyperintense soft tissue component with intact-appearing cortex, which indicates the permeative nature of the lesion ➡. (Courtesy A. Rosenberg, MD.)

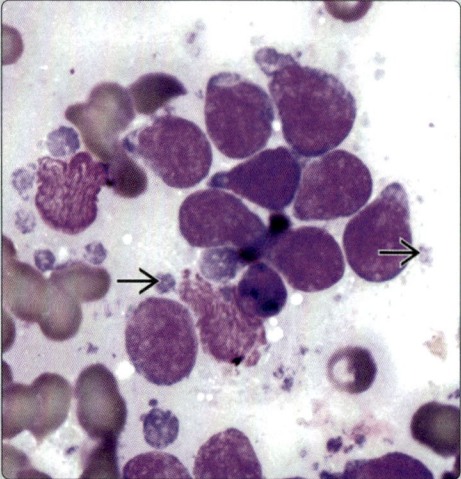

Lymphoglandular Bodies in Primary Bone Lymphoma

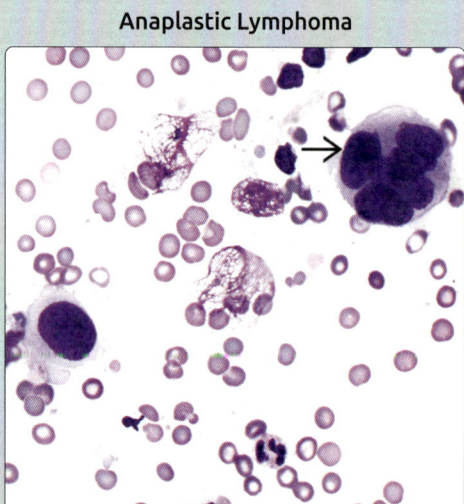

Anaplastic Lymphoma

(Left) Diff-Quik stain of bone aspirate shows dispersed round blue cells with lymphoglandular bodies ➡ in the background, indicating the lymphoid nature of the cells. (Right) Diff-Quik stain shows unilobated and multilobated nuclei ➡ in a bloody background from an anaplastic lymphoma of the bone. Note the low cellularity and absence of lymphoglandular bodies.

Bone Lymphoma

TERMINOLOGY

Definitions
- Primary lymphoma originating in bone ± soft tissue extension
  - Lymphoma should not be identified elsewhere; however, some studies include patients with regional lymph node involvement
  - No extraosseous distant disease should be identified within 4-6 months of initial diagnosis
- Does not include leukemia involving bone

ETIOLOGY/PATHOGENESIS

Etiology
- Most primary bone lymphomas are sporadic and of unknown etiology
- Rarely reported in patients with HIV, longstanding osteomyelitis, or Paget disease of bone

CLINICAL ISSUES

Epidemiology
- Incidence
  - Rare and accounts for ~ 5% of primary malignant bone tumors and ~ 5% of all extranodal lymphomas
    - < 1% of all lymphomas arise in bone with slightly higher incidence in children
- Age
  - Usually adults; ~ 50% are > 40 years
  - Minority arise in children and adolescents

Site
- Femur is most common location, followed by pelvis, vertebrae, and humerus
- Usually arises in metadiaphyseal region
- ~ 10-40% of cases are multifocal (polyostotic), producing several lesions in 1 bone or involving multiple bones concurrently

IMAGING

Radiographic Findings
- Large, lytic, and destructive
- May erode cortex and form soft tissue mass
- Bone margins are "moth eaten" or permeative
- "Onion skin" periosteal reaction may be present
- Because of highly infiltrating growth pattern, soft tissue mass tends to be concentrically distributed around affected bone
- In some cases, tumor may elicit extensive medullary sclerosis
- Occasionally, findings on plain radiography are minimal with abnormalities only recognized on bone scan, CT, or MR

MR Findings
- Provides important information regarding extent of bone and soft tissue involvement

CYTOPATHOLOGY

Cellularity
- Usually cellular unless very bloody

Pattern
- Dispersed population of round or cleaved blue cells

Background
- Lymphoglandular bodies and blood

Cells
- Round blue cells with morphology that varies depending on type of lymphoma
- Diffuse large B-cell lymphoma is most common type in adults and children
- Lymphoblastic lymphoma is 2nd most common type to arise in children (40% of cases)
- Anaplastic large cell lymphoma is rare but most common primary T-cell lymphoma of bone
- Primary Hodgkin lymphoma in bone is very rare

Adequacy Criteria
- At time of adequacy evaluation, it is of paramount importance to collect adequate material in appropriate medium for immunophenotyping by flow cytometry and molecular studies

Cell Block Findings
- Can be helpful for immunohistochemistry and molecular studies

ANCILLARY TESTS

Immunohistochemistry
- Immunoprofile varies according to type
- Large B-cell lymphomas express leukocyte common antigen (LCA) and B-cell markers
- Anaplastic large cell lymphoma may be positive or negative for ALK
  - ALK(+) tumors affect mainly children
  - ALK(-) tumors affect adults
- Lymphoblastic lymphoma may not express LCA and can be CD99(+)

DIFFERENTIAL DIAGNOSIS

Round Cell Lesions
- Osteomyelitis
- Langerhans cell histiocytosis
- Ewing sarcoma/primitive neuroectodermal tumor
- Metastatic small cell carcinoma
- Neuroblastoma
- Rhabdomyosarcoma
- Other round cell malignancies
- Immunohistochemistry, electron microscopy, and cytogenetic analysis may be necessary to distinguish between these possibilities

DIAGNOSTIC CHECKLIST

Pathologic Interpretation Pearls
- Think lymphoma if malignant round cell tumor with extensive necrosis or crush artifact

SELECTED REFERENCES
1. Tazi I et al: [Adult non-Hodgkin bone lymphomas.] Bull Cancer. 108(4):424-34, 2021

Metastatic Tumors of Bone

KEY FACTS

CLINICAL ISSUES
- Metastases far more common than primary bone tumors (25:1)
- Most common primary sites: Lung, breast, prostate, kidney, and thyroid
- Predilection for regions containing red marrow
- Commonly involved bones include skull, spine, ribs, pelvis, humerus, and femur
- Pain typical presenting symptom of skeletal metastases

CYTOPATHOLOGY
- Usually cellular, however, can be bloody and hypocellular
- Epithelial, cohesive cells in carcinomas
- Crush effect and chromatin streaking: Think small cell carcinoma/lymphoma
- Clear cells: Consider renal cell, lung
- In general, metastases try to imitate primary

ANCILLARY TESTS
- Real-time PCR assay may assist in identifying primary site
- Decalcification may degrade DNA and RNA, making molecular tests difficult to apply on bone biopsy material
- Renal cell carcinoma: RCC, PAX8, CD10 (+)
- Lung adenocarcinoma: Most are CK7, TTF-1, napsin A (+); CK20(-)
- Thyroid: PAX8, TTF-1, thyroglobulin, and calcitonin (medullary)
- Prostate: PSA, PSAP, NKX3.1
- Breast: ER, PR, BRST-2, GCDFP-15, and GATA3 (especially triple-negative tumors)
- Cervix: HPV and p16 (+) for HPV-driven tumors
- Müllerian (ovary, endometrium, tubes): PAX8, ER, PR, WT1, p53, vimentin depending upon site
- Epithelioid vascular tumors, osteosarcoma, and adamantinoma are keratin (+) primary bone tumors

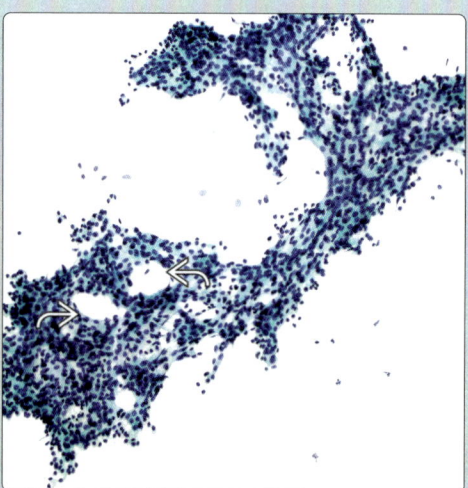

Metastatic Prostate Carcinoma

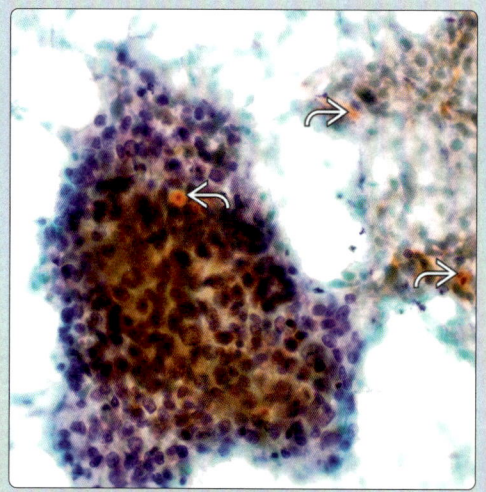

Metastatic Squamous Cell Carcinoma

(Left) Pap stain of metastatic prostate carcinoma shows cribriform pattern characterized by punched-out intrasheet lumina ⇨. The cells are cohesive and in sheets and clearly do not belong in the bone. (Right) Pap stain shows a large, syncytial cluster of malignant cells with abrupt keratinization ⇨ that indicates the squamous nature of this poorly differentiated carcinoma.

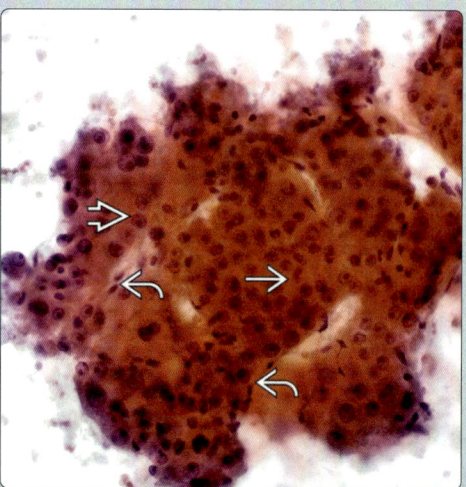

Metastatic Hepatocellular Carcinoma

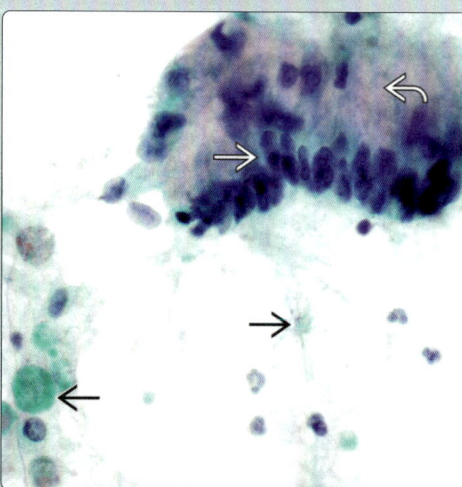

Metastatic Colon Carcinoma

(Left) Pap stain shows metastatic hepatocellular carcinoma with thickened trabeculae ⇨ and endothelial wrapping ⇨. The trabeculae are 4-8 cells thick, and the nuclei have prominent nucleoli ⇨. (Right) Pap stain of metastatic colon carcinoma shows a strip of mucin-producing columnar cells ⇨ that contain cigar-shaped, vertically oriented nuclei ⇨ in a necrotic background ⇨.

Metastatic Tumors of Bone

CLINICAL ISSUES

Epidemiology
- Incidence
  - Far more common than primary bone tumors (25:1)
  - Most common primary sites: Lung, breast, prostate, kidney, and thyroid
    - Other tumors include lymphoma, melanoma, neuroendocrine carcinoma (NEC), and hepatocellular carcinoma
    - Rarely, osteosarcoma shows bone-to-bone metastasis
  - After lungs and liver, skeleton 3rd most frequent site of metastatic disease
  - ~ 40-90% of patients with advanced carcinoma have skeletal metastases during course of disease
- Age
  - More common in older adult population

Site
- Predilection for regions containing red marrow
- Commonly involved bones include skull, spine, ribs, pelvis, humerus, and femur
- Metastases distal to knee are rare
  - Distal metastases typically from lung
- In long bones, metastatic deposits tend to involve metaphysis
  - Solitary metastasis in long bones may mimic primary sarcoma

Presentation
- Pain typical presenting symptom of skeletal metastases
- Pathologic fracture
- Neurologic symptoms with spinal metastasis

IMAGING

Radiographic Findings
- Single or multiple lesions
- Lesions may be entirely sclerotic or lytic or combination of both
- Typically lytic metastases: Renal, thyroid
- Typically sclerotic metastases: Prostate, breast, neuroendocrine

CT Findings
- Bone scan and PET/CT very sensitive for detection of bone metastasis
- Sensitivity: 80-90%
  - Bone scan more sensitive than plain film or CT

CYTOPATHOLOGY

Cellularity
- Usually cellular, however, can be bloody and hypocellular
- Fine-needle aspiration or touch preparations from core needle biopsies of pathologic fracture sites can be bloody, fibrotic, and show few malignant cells with hemosiderin

Pattern
- Depends upon primary tumor
  - Dispersed for lymphomas, melanomas
  - Cohesive for carcinoma

Background
- Varies from bloody to necrotic to clean

Cells
- Epithelial, cohesive cells in carcinomas
- Arrangements can be in gland forms (adenocarcinomas), cribriform (prostate), or dispersed with high nuclear:cytoplasmic ratios (lymphomas, melanomas, NECs)
- Crush effect and chromatin streaking usually indicate small cell carcinoma or lymphoma
- Clear cells
  - Consider renal cell, lung
- In general, metastases try to imitate primary

Cell Block Findings
- Helpful in tumor with unknown primary to work-up using IHC or molecular testing
- Note decalcification can affect molecular testing and rarely some IHC markers

Cytology-Histology Correlation
- Compare with primary when available
  - Should show some morphologic similarity
- If morphologically or immunohistochemically different, consider 2nd primary

ANCILLARY TESTS

Immunohistochemistry
- Renal cell carcinoma: RCC, PAX8, CD10
- Lung adenocarcinoma: Most are CK7, TTF-1, napsin A (+); CK20(-)
- Thyroid: PAX8, TTF-1, thyroglobulin, and calcitonin (medullary)
- Prostate: PSA, PSAP, NKX3.1 (+)
- Breast: ER, PR, BRST-2, GCDFP-15, and GATA3 (especially triple-negative tumors)
- Epithelioid vascular tumors, osteosarcoma, and adamantinoma are keratin (+) primary bone tumors
- Cervix: HPV and p16 (+) for HPV-driven tumors
- Müllerian (ovary, endometrium, tubes): PAX8, ER, PR, WT1, p53, vimentin depending upon site

DIFFERENTIAL DIAGNOSIS

Osteosarcoma
- Osteoblastic metastasis, such as prostatic metastasis, may mimic osteosarcoma
  - Osteosarcoma may be focally keratin (+)
  - Osteosarcoma cells are PSA ,PSAP, NKX3.1 (-)

Epithelioid Vascular Tumors
- Epithelioid hemangioma, epithelioid hemangioendothelioma, and angiosarcoma may all be diffusely keratin (+)
- All 3 vascular tumors (+) for endothelial cell markers
  - CD31, CD34, FVIIIRAg, ERG

SELECTED REFERENCES
1. Huang X et al: Mutational characteristics of bone metastasis of lung cancer. Ann Palliat Med. 10(8):8818-26, 2021

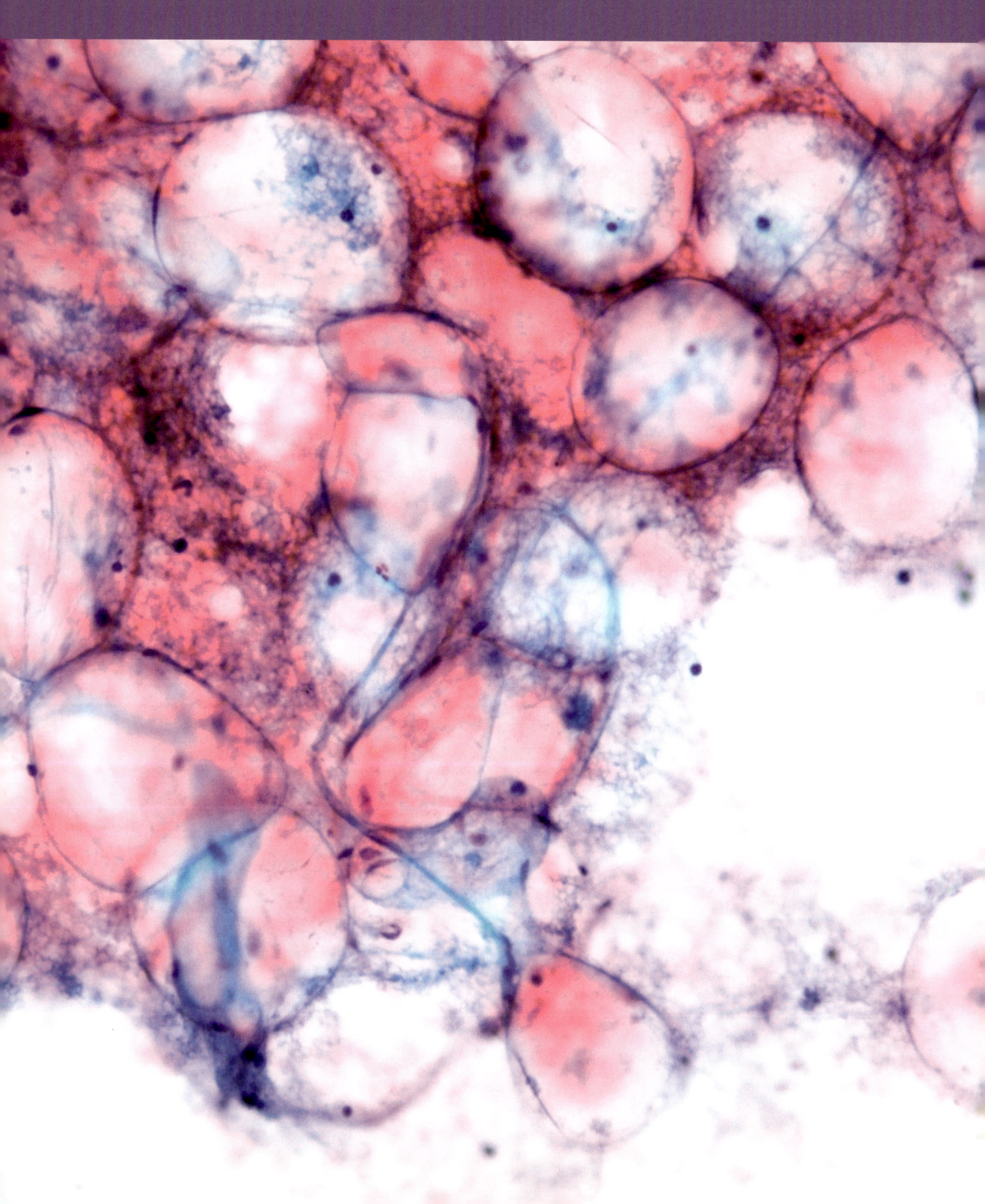

PART IV
SECTION 8
Soft Tissue

Overview
Approach to Cytologic/Small Biopsy Diagnosis of Primary Soft Tissue Lesions	634

Adipocytic Tumors
Benign Adipose Tissue Tumors	636
Liposarcoma	638

Fibroblastic/Myofibroblastic Lesions
Fibrosarcoma	642
Myofibroblastoma	644
Low-Grade Myofibroblastic Sarcoma	646

Fibrohistiocytic Tumors
Giant Cell Tumor of Tendon Sheath	648
Undifferentiated Pleomorphic Sarcoma	650

Tumors of Muscle Origin
Smooth Muscle Tumors	652
Skeletal Muscle Tumors	654

Vascular Tumors
Hemangioma, Soft Tissue	658
Epithelioid Hemangioendothelioma	660
Angiosarcoma	662

Other Tumors
Other Reactive and Neoplastic Soft Tissue Entities	664
Mesenchymal Chondrosarcoma	666
Solitary Fibrous Tumor	667
Intramuscular Myxoma	668
Synovial Sarcoma	670
Epithelioid Sarcoma	672
Alveolar Soft Part Sarcoma	674
Clear Cell Sarcoma of Soft Tissue	676
Desmoplastic Small Round Cell Tumor	678

Approach to Cytologic/Small Biopsy Diagnosis of Primary Soft Tissue Lesions

EPIDEMIOLOGY

Age Range
- Primary soft tissue neoplasms tend to be age range specific

Subcutaneous/Soft Tissue Tumors: Questions
- Is it reactive or neoplastic?
- If neoplastic, is it benign or malignant?
- If malignant, is it metastasis (more common) or primary (rare)?
  - If primary, is it SRBCT or other tumor?
  - If SRBCT, is it hematopoietic or nonhematopoietic?
  - If not SRBCT, is it spindled, epithelioid, biphasic, or other, and is it low or high grade?
    - Can ancillary techniques be utilized to specify exact type?
    - Collect specimen accordingly for flow cytometry (if hematopoietic), molecular (nonheme SRBCT), cell block and cores for immunohistochemistry, cytospins/smears or cell blocks for FISH, etc.

Mesenchymal Lesions: Helpful Cytologic Features
- Cellularity, presence or absence of tissue fragments
- Presence or absence of matrix, tissue culture-like appearance
- Types of cells
  - If spindle, are they plump spindle cells or pleomorphic?
- Fibrillar ground substance between cells
- Necrosis and mitosis, especially atypical ones

Important Clinical Findings
- Age, location, size, presentation, type, and grade
- Pathologists interpreting these rare FNAs/small biopsies should be familiar with soft tissue tumors/pathology
- Recommend low threshold to send out for consultation

General Criteria for Cytologic Grading (Non-SRBCT)
- Cellularity: 1 point for low, 3 for high
- Nuclear atypias: 1 point for minimal, 3 for marked
- Number of mitoses/200 cells: 1 point if 0-2, 3 points if > 5
- Tumor necrosis: 1 point if absent, 3 if present
- Grade 1 if scores 4-6, grade 3 if scores 10-12

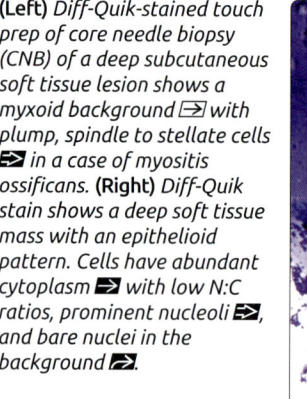

(Left) Diff-Quik-stained touch prep of core needle biopsy (CNB) of a deep subcutaneous soft tissue lesion shows a myxoid background ⇨ with plump, spindle to stellate cells ⇨ in a case of myositis ossificans. (Right) Diff-Quik stain shows a deep soft tissue mass with an epithelioid pattern. Cells have abundant cytoplasm ⇨ with low N:C ratios, prominent nucleoli ⇨, and bare nuclei in the background ⇨.

Low Cellularity With Myxoid Background

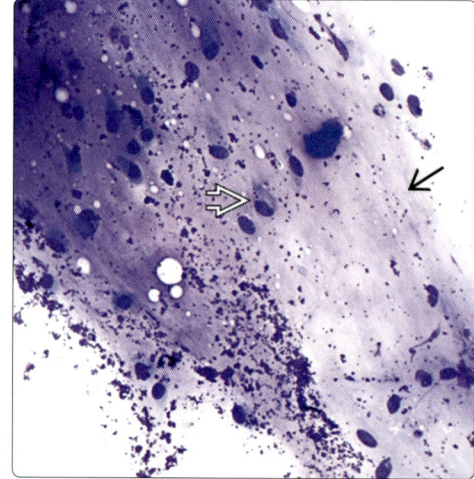

Epithelioid Pattern With Abundant Cytoplasm

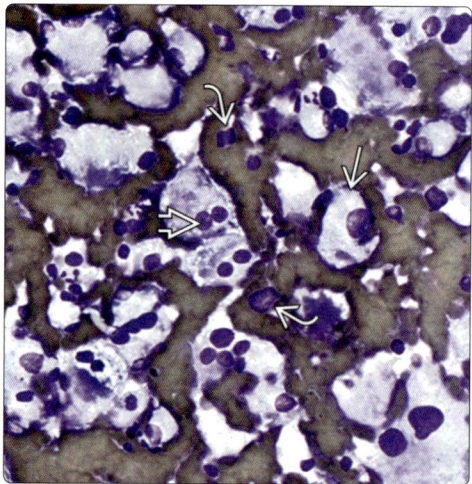

(Left) Diff-Quik stain shows a small round blue cell tumor with lymphoglandular bodies ⇨, indicative of hematopoietic origin. Immunophenotyping by flow cytometry is preferred in most cases. (Right) Diff-Quik-stained touch prep of low-grade fibromyxoid sarcoma shows spindle cells ⇨ and fibrillar stroma ⇨ but no atypia, necrosis, or mitosis.

Hematopoietic Malignancy With Lymphoglandular Bodies

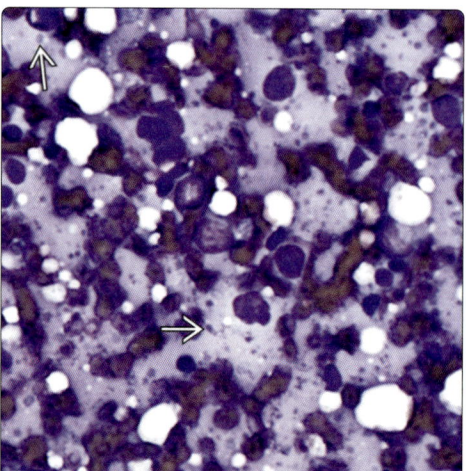

Spindle Cell Pattern, Benign vs. Low Grade

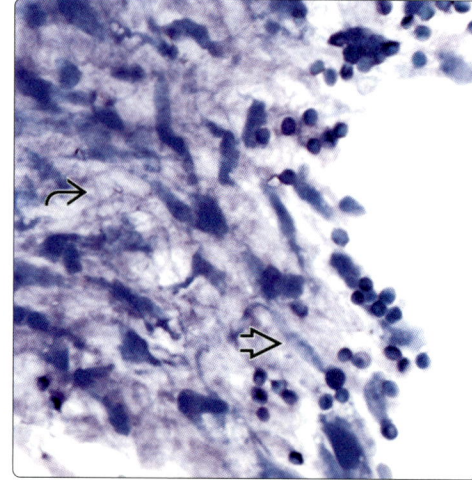

Approach to Cytologic/Small Biopsy Diagnosis of Primary Soft Tissue Lesions

Cytologic/Small Biopsy Categorization of Primary Soft Tissue Tumors by Cell Types

Lipogenic Tumors	Myxoid/Mucoid Background	Small Round Blue Cell Tumors	Epithelioid Tumors	Pleomorphic Cells	Spindle Cells	Biphasic Tumors
Benign						
Lipomas	Intramuscular myxoma, NF, MO	Myelolipoma	Granular cell tumor	Not applicable	NF, proliferative myositis, MO, AGM, schwannoma, ganglioneuroma, myofibroblastoma	Not applicable
Locally Aggressive						
Well-differentiated liposarcoma	AGM, LGFMS, myxoinflammatory fibroblastic sarcoma	Not applicable	Not applicable	Atypical fibroxanthoma	AGM, solitary fibrous tumor, DFSP, LGFMS	Not applicable
Malignant						
Myxoid liposarcoma, round cell, pleomorphic types	Chordoma, myxoid liposarcoma, pleomorphic myxoid liposarcoma, mesenchymal chondrosarcoma, myxoid chondrosarcoma, myxofibrosarcoma, extraskeletal myxoid chondrosarcoma	Ewing, round cell sarcoma with *EWSR1*::non-ETS fusions embryonal RMS, mesenchymal chondrosarcoma, hematopoietic, DSRCT, BCOR and CIC-rearranged sarcoma	ASPS, CCS, EHE, AS, epithelioid sarcoma, rhabdoid tumor epithelioid GIST; always consider metastatic carcinoma or melanoma	PUS, pleomorphic liposarcoma, pleomorphic RMS, pleomorphic undifferentiated carcinoma, or melanoma	Leiomyosarcoma, monophasic SS, AS, GIST, neurofibrosarcoma	SS, AS, mesothelioma

Depending on age of patient, malignant melanomas and sarcomatoid carcinomas should be added to differential. AGM = aggressive angiomyxoma; AS = angiosarcoma; ASPS = alveolar soft part sarcoma; CCS = clear cell sarcoma; DFSP = dermatofibrosarcoma protuberans; DSRCTL = desmoplastic small round cell tumor; EHE = epithelioid hemangioendothelioma; GIST = gastrointestinal stromal tumor; LGFMS = low-grade fibromyxoid sarcoma; MO = myositis ossificans; NF = nodular fasciitis; PNET = primitive neuroectodermal tumor; PUS = pleomorphic undifferentiated sarcoma; RMS = rhabdomyosarcoma; SS = synovial sarcoma.

- In practice, low vs. high is what matters
- In reality, distinction between benign and low-grade malignant spindle cell tumors most difficult area of soft tissue interpretation
  o In difficult cases, best to sign out as benign vs. low-grade malignant spindle cell tumor/neoplasm

Soft Tissue Sarcomas (Non-SRBCT): Prognostic Factors

- Size: Smaller (< 5 cm) is better
- Location: Extremity is better
- Grade: Low is better
- Differentiation
- Mitosis, necrosis

Ancillary Testing

- For SRBCT with lymphoglandular bodies, can do immunophenotyping by flow cytometry
- For other soft tissue neoplasms, immunohistochemistry if cell block or core needle biopsy (CNB) is available
- FISH on cytospins, smears, cell block, or CNB
- RT-PCR from fresh smears or cell block/CNB
- Electron microscopy is rarely performed

Proposed IAC-IARC-WHO Reporting System for Soft Tissue Cytopathology/Small Biopsies

- Insufficient/inadequate/nondiagnostic
  o Specimen is qualitatively or quantitatively insufficient to render diagnosis
  o No consistent cellular definition of adequacy; any atypia excludes this diagnosis
  o Incidence 2-30% (4% if cores included)
  o Reported risk of malignancy (ROM) ~ 40%
- Benign
  o Unequivocal benign cytopathologic/small biopsy features; includes mass-forming inflammatory processes, benign neoplasms, spindle and multinucleated giant cell processes/masses
- Atypical
  o Morphologic abnormalities that preclude diagnosis of negative but insufficient for suspicious classification
- Soft tissue neoplasm of uncertain malignant potential
  o Neoplasms that cannot be unequivocally diagnosed as benign or malignant by morphology &/or ancillary testing; incidence: ~ 10%; ROM: ~ 27%
  o Specific tumor types include DFSP, SFT, inflammatory myofibroblastic tumor, angiomatoid MFH, GIST, PEComa
- Suspicious for malignancy
  o Features suggest malignancy but qualitatively or quantitatively fall short of unequivocal malignancy
- Malignant
  o Incidence: ~ 25%; ROM: ~ 97%

SELECTED REFERENCES

1. Choi JH et al: The 2020 WHO Classification of Tumors of Soft Tissue: selected changes and new entities. Adv Anat Pathol. 28(1):44-58, 2021

Benign Adipose Tissue Tumors

KEY FACTS

ETIOLOGY/PATHOGENESIS
- Benign tumor of mature adipocytes

CLINICAL ISSUES
- Painless mass; large lesions can be painful
- Recurrence in < 5% cases; higher recurrence rate in intramuscular lipoma
- Surgical excision is curative

CYTOPATHOLOGY
- Variable cellularity, uniform size of adipocytes
- Adipocytes with peripheral flattened nucleus without atypia and univacuolated cytoplasm
- Atypical stromal nuclei (floret-like cell nuclei) may be seen in pleomorphic lipoma
- Myxoid background may be present (myxolipoma)
- Additional mesenchymal component may be present
  - Spindle cell lipoma, chondrolipoma, osteolipoma, myolipoma

- Other variants that can be encountered
  - Myelolipoma, intramuscular lipoma, pleomorphic lipoma, hibernoma

TOP DIFFERENTIAL DIAGNOSES
- Atypical lipomatous tumor
  - Deep-seated intramuscular lipoma may be mistaken for atypical lipomatous tumor
    - Intramuscular lipomas show no nuclear atypia
- Myxoid liposarcoma
  - Myxolipoma may be mistaken for myxoid liposarcoma
    - Myxolipoma does not contain lipoblasts or plexiform vasculature
- Normal fibroadipose tissue
  - Does not form distinct mass
    - Not circumscribed or encapsulated

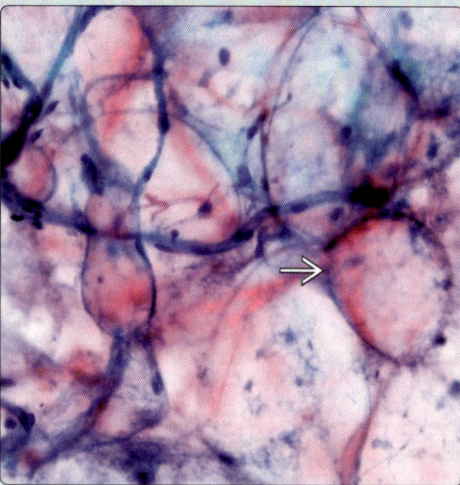

Usual Appearance of Lipoma

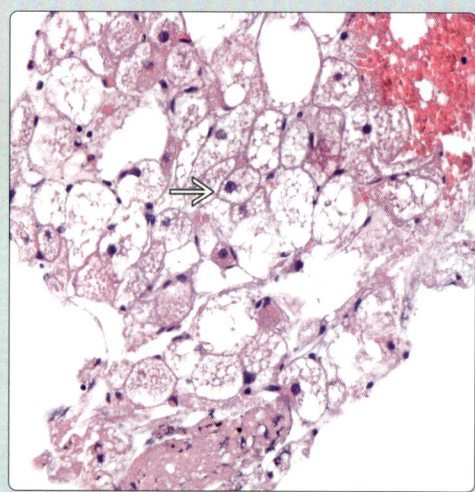

Hibernoma in Cell Block

(Left) Pap-stained FNA smear of lipoma shows a fragment of mature adipose tissue comprised of adipocytes ➡ without any atypia. (Right) H&E-stained cell block section of hibernoma shows the tumor cells ➡ with distinct cytoplasmic borders, multivacuolated cytoplasm, and central round nuclei without atypia.

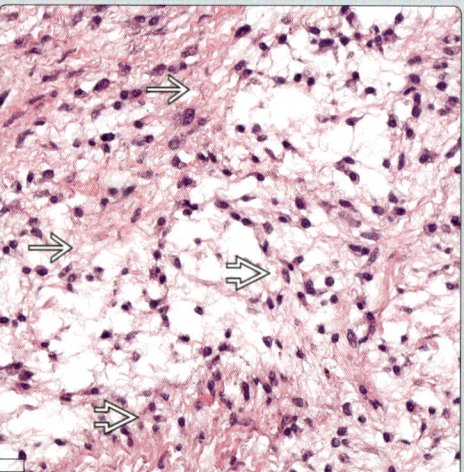

Spindle Cell Lipoma

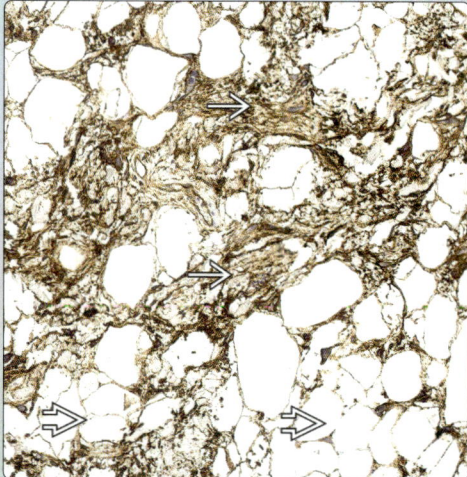

CD34 in Spindle Cell Lipoma

(Left) Core biopsy of spindle cell lipoma stained with H&E shows plump spindle cells ➡ without atypia associated with ropy collagen fibers ➡ in the stroma. (Right) Core biopsy of spindle cell lipoma immunostained for CD34 shows diffuse positivity in the spindle cells ➡ and associated adipose tissue ➡.

Benign Adipose Tissue Tumors

TERMINOLOGY

Definitions
- Benign tumor of mature adipocytes

ETIOLOGY/PATHOGENESIS

Unknown
- Lipomas tend to occur more commonly in obese individuals

CLINICAL ISSUES

Epidemiology
- Most common between 40-60 years of age

CYTOPATHOLOGY

Cellularity and Pattern
- Variable cellularity, uniform size of adipocytes

Background and Cells
- May see myxoid background in myxolipoma
- Adipocytes with peripheral flattened nuclei
- Variants
  - Prominent spindle cells in spindle cell lipoma
  - Myxoid background in myxolipoma
  - Chondroid matrix in chondrolipoma
  - Bone marrow elements in myelolipoma
  - Floret-like cells in pleomorphic lipoma

Nuclear:Cytoplasmic Ratio Details
- Small, bland nuclei with no nuclear atypia
  - Atypical stromal nuclei (floret-like cell nuclei) may be seen in pleomorphic lipoma
- Usually large univacuolated cytoplasm; multivacuolated cytoplasm in hibernoma

MICROSCOPIC

Variants
- Additional mesenchymal component may be present in some lipomas
  - Abundant fibrous tissue: Fibrolipoma
  - Cartilage: Chondrolipoma
    - Mature hyaline cartilage admixed with adipose tissue
  - Bone: Osteolipoma
  - Myxoid stromal change: Myxolipoma
    - Some may have prominent vascular component (e.g., angiomyolipoma)
  - Smooth muscle: Myolipoma
  - Spindle cell lipoma
    - Plump spindle cells without atypia associated with mature adipose tissue and ropy collagen in stroma
    - Loss of *RB1* locus demonstration helpful in selected cases
- Intramuscular lipoma
  - Entrapped skeletal muscle at periphery
- Hibernoma
  - Derived from brown fat; express brown fat marker gene *UCP1*

ANCILLARY TESTS

Immunohistochemistry
- S100(+), CD34(+) and RB1(-) in spindle cell lipoma

DIFFERENTIAL DIAGNOSIS

Atypical Lipomatous Tumor
- Intramuscular lipomas show no nuclear atypia

Myxoid Liposarcoma
- Has lipoblasts and plexiform vasculature

Normal Fibroadipose Tissue
- Does not form distinct mass

SELECTED REFERENCES

1. Bala N Jr et al: A diagnostic dilemma in fine-needle aspiration cytology: spindle cell/pleomorphic lipoma. Cureus. 14(1):e20919, 2022
2. Van Treeck BJ et al: Updates in spindle cell/pleomorphic lipomas. Semin Diagn Pathol. 36(2):105-11, 2019
3. Magro G: Differential diagnosis of benign spindle cell lesions. Surg Pathol Clin. 11(1):91-121, 2018

Myelolipoma

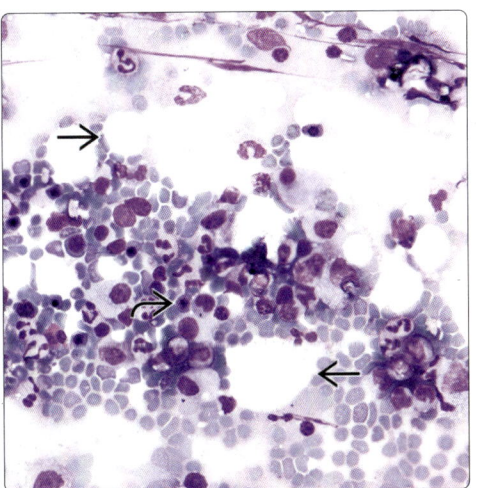

Pleomorphic Lipoma, Floret-Like Giant Cell

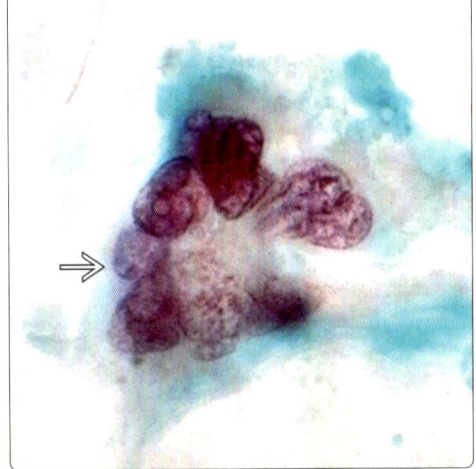

(Left) Diff-Quik-stained FNA smear shows ghost outlines of adipocytes ➔ with hematopoietic elements ➔ in an adrenal gland myelolipoma. *(Right)* Pap-stained smear demonstrates a floret-like giant cell ➔ from a case of pleomorphic lipoma. The nuclear pleomorphism may raise concern for malignancy.

Liposarcoma

KEY FACTS

CLINICAL ISSUES
- Age: Older adult patients, children, and young adults
- Sites of occurrence: Extremities, retroperitoneum, intraabdominal, mediastinum

CYTOPATHOLOGY
- Atypical lipomatous tumor/well-differentiated liposarcoma (ALT/WD): Mature adipose tissue, variably sized adipocytes, atypical cells within stroma, and (rarely) lipoblasts
- Myxoid liposarcoma (ML): Round/oval cells, myxoid background, and chicken-wire vessels
- Round cell liposarcoma (RL): Small round cells, scattered lipoblasts, and intracytoplasmic vacuoles
- Pleomorphic liposarcoma (PL): Bizarre nuclei
- Dedifferentiated liposarcoma (DL): Nonlipogenic sarcoma in background of ALT/WD
- Myxoid pleomorphic liposarcoma (MPL): Round/oval cells, myxoid background, chicken-wire vessels, bizarre pleomorphic nuclei

ANCILLARY TESTS
- ALT/WD: Aberrations of 12q14-15, supernumerary ring chromosomes
  - MDM2(+) &/or CDK4(+) by immunohistochemistry
  - MDM2 amplification by FISH
- ML/RL: t(12;16)(q13;p11) or rarely t(12;22)(q13;p11)
- PL: Complex cytogenetic aberrations
- DL: Supernumerary ring chromosomes, aberrations of 12q13-21
- MPL: MDM2(-), CDK4(-), inactivation of RB1

TOP DIFFERENTIAL DIAGNOSES
- ALT/WD: Normal fat, fat necrosis, and lipoma
- ML: Low-grade fibromyxoid sarcoma
- PL: Undifferentiated pleomorphic sarcoma or other pleomorphic sarcomas and carcinomas
- DL: Undifferentiated pleomorphic sarcoma
  - May be indistinguishable from other sarcomas
- RL: Other small round cell tumors

(Left) H&E-stained cell block section shows cells with atypical nuclei ➡ within fibrous septa in a case of atypical lipomatous tumor/well-differentiated liposarcoma. (Right) Pap-stained FNA smear of myxoid liposarcoma shows round to oval cells, delicate branching vessels ➡, and a myxoid background.

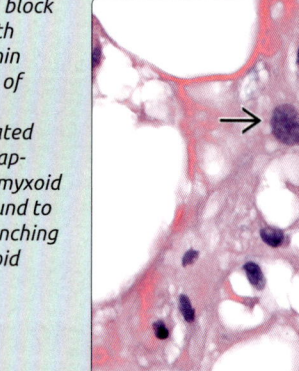
Atypical Lipomatous Tumor Cell Block Appearance

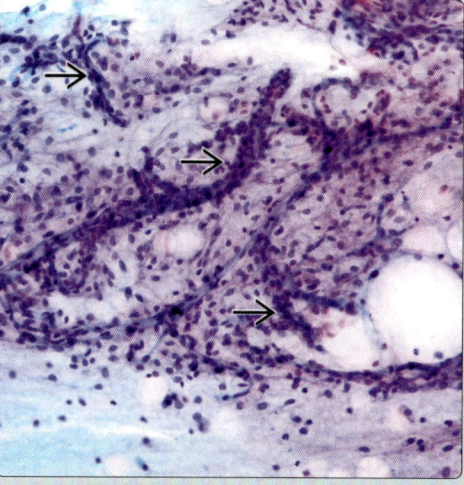
Myxoid Liposarcoma With Branching Vessel

(Left) Core biopsy of atypical lipomatous tumor/well-differentiated liposarcoma stained with H&E shows atypical cells ➡ distributed in fibromyxoid tissue associated with adipocytes. (Right) Core biopsy of dedifferentiated liposarcoma shows malignant spindle tumor cells ➡ exhibiting significant nuclear pleomorphism, including the presence of bizarre tumor giant cells ➡.

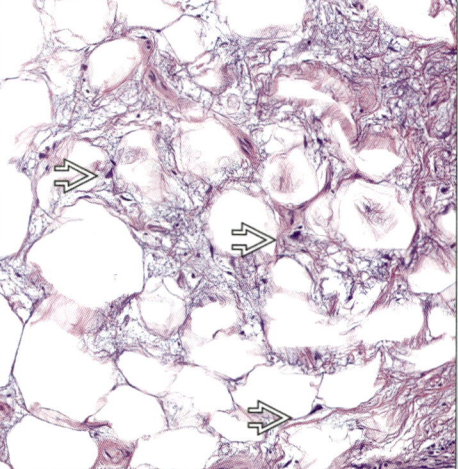
Atypical Lipomatous Tumor/Well-Differentiated Liposarcoma

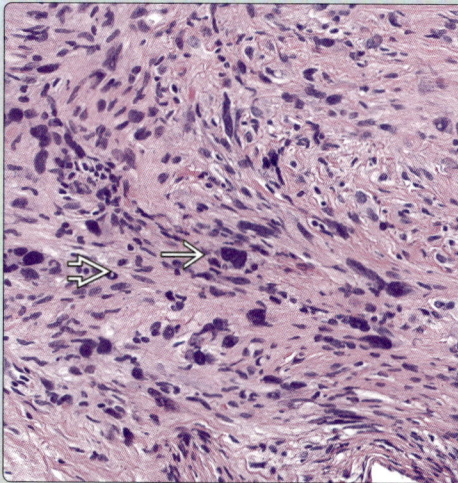
Dedifferentiated Liposarcoma

Liposarcoma

TERMINOLOGY

Abbreviations
- Atypical lipomatous tumor/well-differentiated liposarcoma (ALT/WD)
- Myxoid/round cell liposarcoma (ML/RL)
- Pleomorphic liposarcoma (PL)
- Dedifferentiated liposarcoma (DL)
- Myxoid pleomorphic liposarcoma (MPL)

Definitions
- Malignant tumor of adipose tissue origin

CLINICAL ISSUES

Epidemiology
- Incidence
  - Extremely rare
- Age
  - Older adult patients
  - MPL occurs in children and young adults
- MPL: Some cases associated with Li-Fraumeni syndrome

Site
- Extremities, retroperitoneum, mediastinum, intraabdominal

Presentation
- Painless, slow-growing mass

CYTOPATHOLOGY

Cellularity
- ALT/WD: Variable cellularity; PL: High cellularity

Background
- ML and MPL: Myxoid matrix is present; branching capillary network may be seen

Cells
- ALT/WD: Resembles mature adipose tissue and fibrous septa with atypical cells and (rarely) lipoblasts
- ML: Uniform round/oval cells and delicate capillary network
- RL: Small round cells with minimal cytoplasm
- PL: Pleomorphic tumor cells
- DL: Sheets of spindle to pleomorphic cells without intervening adipose tissue; high grade
- MPL: Admixture of bland zones with features similar to ML and cellular areas resembling PL

Nuclear Details
- ML: Uniform round/oval nuclei
- RL: Round, enlarged nuclei
  - May see background naked nuclei
- PL and DL: Bizarre pleomorphic tumor nuclei
- MPL: Features similar to ML and PL

Cytoplasmic Details
- Lipoblasts are multivacuolated; signet-ring in ML

MACROSCOPIC

General Features
- Large, often multinodular neoplasms
- May contain cystic and solid tumor areas

MICROSCOPIC

Histologic Features
- ALT/WD: Mature adipose tissue with variably sized adipocytes; fibromyxoid stroma with atypical cells
- ML: Monomorphic cells without atypia, myxoid background, chicken-wire vessels
- RL: Small round cells; areas of necrosis and increased mitotic activity
- PL: Enlarged round to bizarre nuclei
- DL: Component of nonlipogenic sarcoma
- Grading of mixed-type liposarcoma is related to different tumor components
- MPL: Admixture of areas with features of ML and PL

ANCILLARY TESTS

Immunohistochemistry
- S100(+) in all types
- MDM2(+) &/or CDK4(+) in ALT/WD and DL; MDM2(-) in MPL

Genetic Testing
- ALT/WD: Aberrations of 12q14-15, supernumerary ring chromosomes
  - MDM2 amplification can be demonstrated by FISH
    - Amplification of *CDK4*, *HMGA2*, *YEATS4*, *CPM*, *FRS2*
- ML/RL: t(12;16)(q13;p11); *FUS::DDIT3* gene fusion in 95%
  - t(12;22)(q13;p11); *DDIT3::EWSR1* gene fusion
- PL: Complex cytogenetic aberrations
- DL: Supernumerary ring chromosomes, aberrations of 12q13-21
- MPL: *FUS::EWSR1::DDIT3* fusions are absent

DIFFERENTIAL DIAGNOSIS

Atypical Lipomatous Tumor/Well-Differentiated Liposarcoma
- Nonneoplastic adipose tissue, fat necrosis, lipoma

Myxoid Liposarcoma
- Low-grade fibromyxoid sarcoma
- Extraskeletal myxoid chondrosarcoma

Pleomorphic Liposarcoma
- Undifferentiated pleomorphic sarcoma

Dedifferentiated Liposarcoma
- Difficult to distinguish from other sarcomas
  - History of ALT/WD may be required

Round Cell Liposarcoma
- Other small round cell tumors (lymphoma, melanoma, Ewing sarcoma/primitive neuroectodermal tumor)

Myxoid Pleomorphic Liposarcoma
- Bland zones may mimic ML, low-grade fibromyxoid sarcoma; cellular zones may mimic PL and other pleomorphic sarcomas or carcinomas

SELECTED REFERENCES

1. Choi JH et al: The 2020 WHO Classification of Tumors of Soft Tissue: selected changes and new entities. Adv Anat Pathol. 28(1):44-58, 2021

Liposarcoma

Atypical Lipomatous Tumor: Diff-Quik

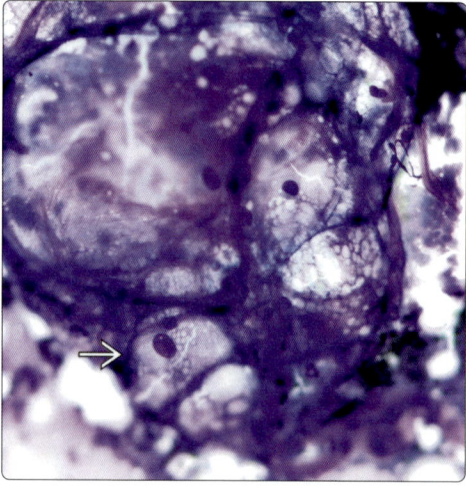

Atypical Lipomatous Tumor: Pap Stain

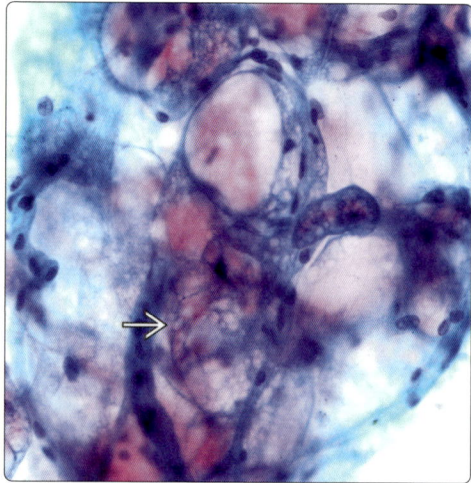

(Left) *Diff-Quik-stained FNA smear of atypical lipomatous tumor/well-differentiated liposarcoma shows adipocytes ➡ with vacuolated cytoplasm that resemble normal adipose tissue.* **(Right)** *Pap-stained FNA smear of atypical lipomatous tumor/well-differentiated liposarcoma shows adipocytes with a vacuolated cytoplasm ➡.*

Myxoid Liposarcoma With Monotonous Cells

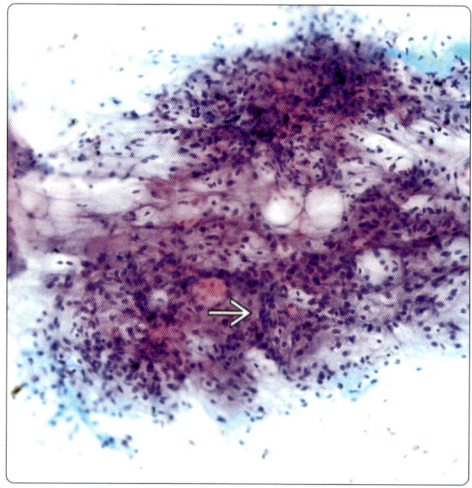

Myxoid Liposarcoma With Myxoid Background

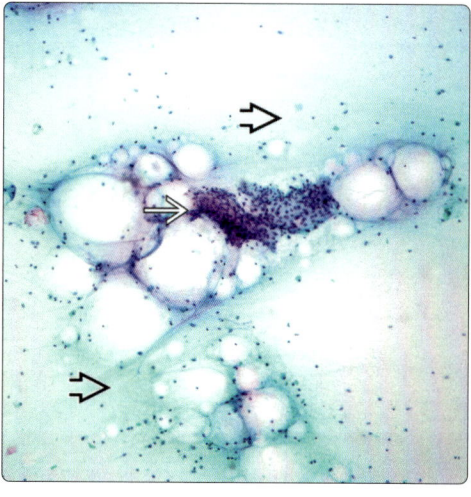

(Left) *Pap-stained FNA smear of myxoid liposarcoma demonstrates numerous monotonous round to oval cells ➡ in a myxoid background.* **(Right)** *Pap-stained FNA smear of myxoid liposarcoma shows a fragment of round/oval cells ➡ in a prominent myxoid background ➡.*

Myxoid Liposarcoma With Vascular Network

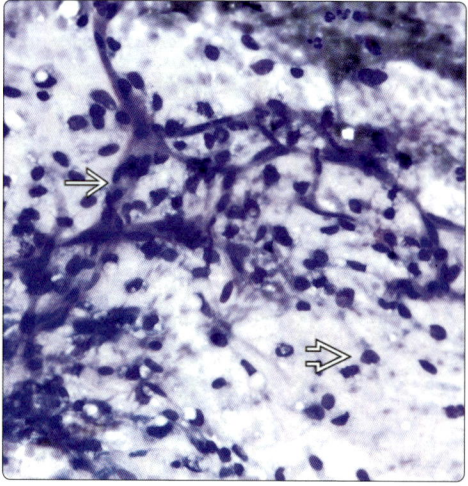

Myxoid Liposarcoma With Tumor Cells in Myxoid Background

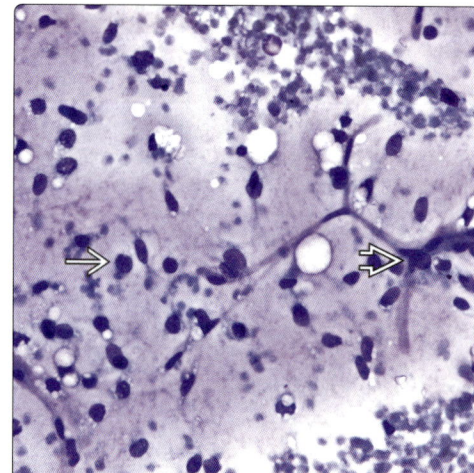

(Left) *Diff-Quik-stained FNA smear of myxoid liposarcoma shows a network of capillary channels ➡ associated with round/oval tumor cells ➡.* **(Right)** *Diff-Quik stained FNA smear of myxoid liposarcoma shows round and oval tumor cells ➡ distributed in a myxoid background. Note thin-walled capillary vessels ➡ in the background.*

Liposarcoma

Myxoid Liposarcoma With Chicken-Wire Vessels

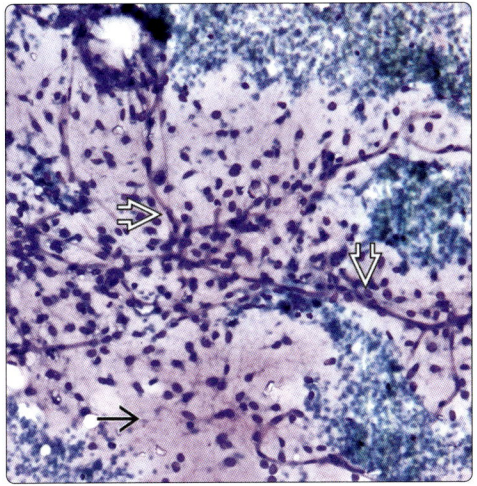

Myxoid Liposarcoma Cell Block Appearance

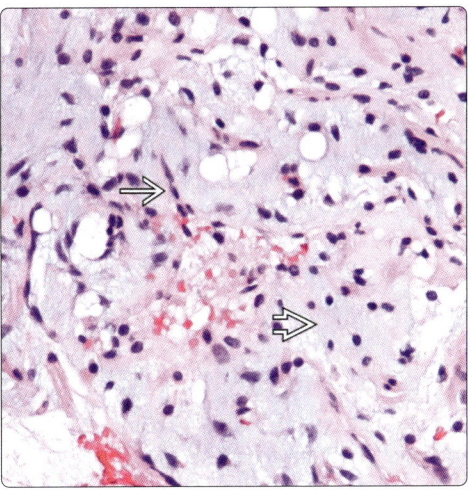

(Left) Diff-Quik-stained FNA smear of myxoid liposarcoma shows delicate branching capillaries ➡, commonly referred to as the chicken-wire pattern, within a myxoid matrix ➡. *(Right)* H&E-stained cell block section of myxoid liposarcoma demonstrates round/oval mononuclear cells, a network of delicate branching capillaries referred to as chicken-wire pattern ➡, and a myxoid background ➡.

Pleomorphic Liposarcoma Lipoblasts

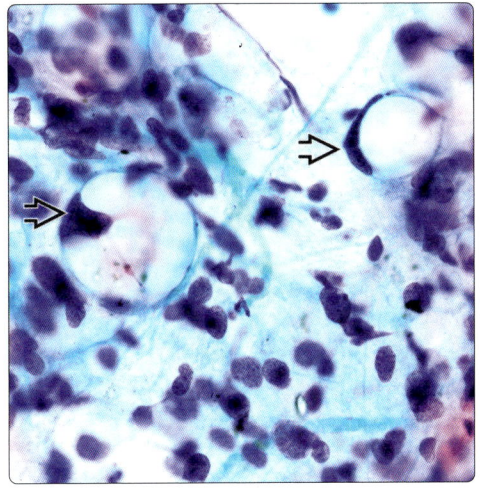

Pleomorphic Liposarcoma Giant Cells

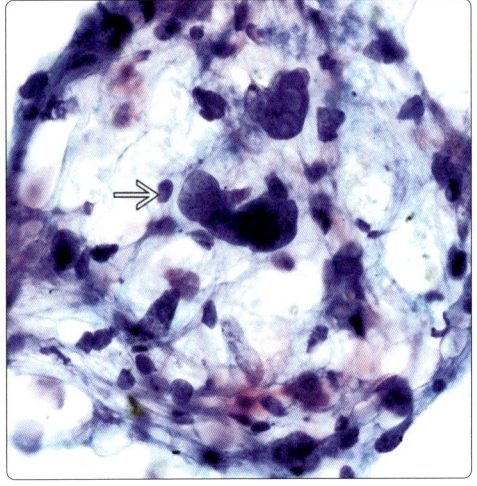

(Left) Pap-stained FNA smear of pleomorphic liposarcoma demonstrates lipoblasts ➡ with pleomorphic nuclei. *(Right)* Pap-stained FNA smear of pleomorphic liposarcoma shows large pleomorphic giant tumor cells ➡.

Dedifferentiated Liposarcoma With Prominent Nucleoli

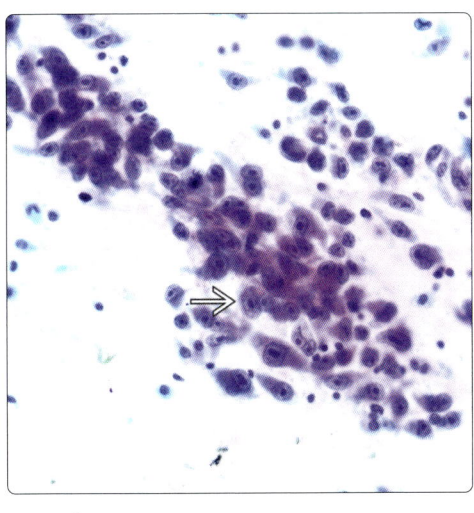

Dedifferentiated Liposarcoma Cell Block Appearance

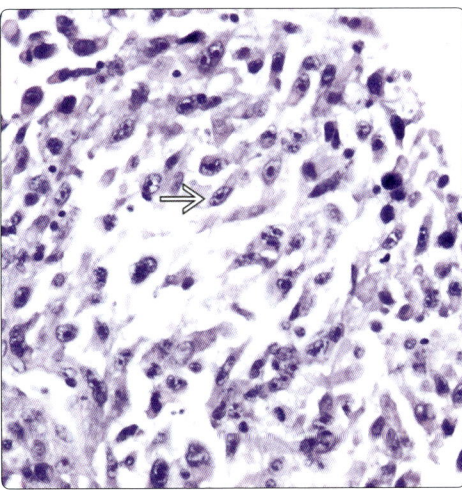

(Left) Pap-stained FNA smear of dedifferentiated liposarcoma shows spindled and epithelioid tumor cells with prominent nucleoli ➡. *(Right)* H&E-stained cell block section of dedifferentiated liposarcoma shows spindle cells ➡ with prominent nucleoli and a moderate amount of cytoplasm.

Fibrosarcoma

KEY FACTS

CLINICAL ISSUES
- Soft tissue sarcoma composed of fibroblasts
- Now very rare; mostly diagnosis of exclusion
- Etiology/pathogenesis
  - De novo: Very rare
  - Arising in course of other tumor
    - Dermatofibrosarcoma, solitary fibrous tumor
  - Post irradiation
- Occurs in deep soft tissues of extremities, trunk, and head and neck

CYTOPATHOLOGY
- Spindle cells with slender, wavy, and tapered nuclei
- Variable hyperchromasia, pleomorphism, mitotic activity

ANCILLARY TESTS
- Most cases are negative for all immunohistochemical markers except vimentin
  - Some express CD34 focally or diffusely
- Some superficial examples have *COL1A1::PDGFB* fusion transcripts like dermatofibrosarcoma

TOP DIFFERENTIAL DIAGNOSES
- Low-grade fibromyxoid sarcoma
  - Myxoid and fibrous areas with whorling
  - Specific translocation t(7;16)(q34;p11)
- Low-grade myofibrosarcoma
  - Cells have more cytoplasm
  - Multifocal positivity for SMA
- Synovial sarcoma
  - Biphasic pattern with gland formation in 1/3
  - Specific translocation t(X;18)(p11;q11)
- Malignant peripheral nerve sheath tumor
  - Spindle cells with wavy or bullet-shaped nuclei
  - S100 protein (+) in 2/3 of cases
- Fibromatosis
  - Less cellular, cells evenly dispersed in mature collagen
  - Nuclear immunoreactivity for β-catenin

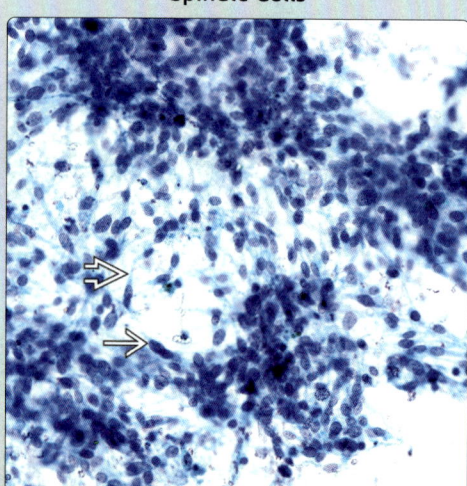
Spindle Cells

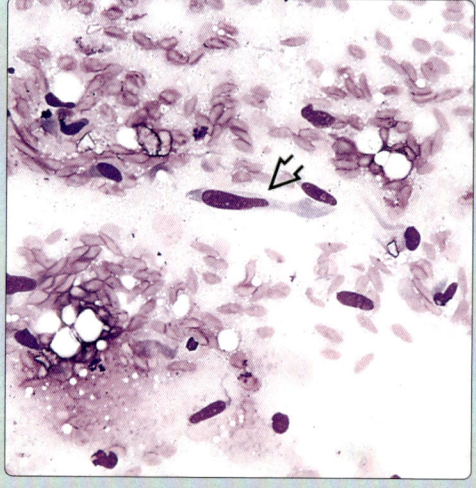
Tapered Nuclei

(Left) Pap-stained FNA smear shows numerous spindle cells ➡ with elongated cytoplasmic processes ➡. Note the lack of collagen or myxoid material in the background. (Right) Diff-Quik-stained FNA smear of fibrosarcoma demonstrates slender, wavy, and tapered nuclei ➡. These features are not specific to fibrosarcoma.

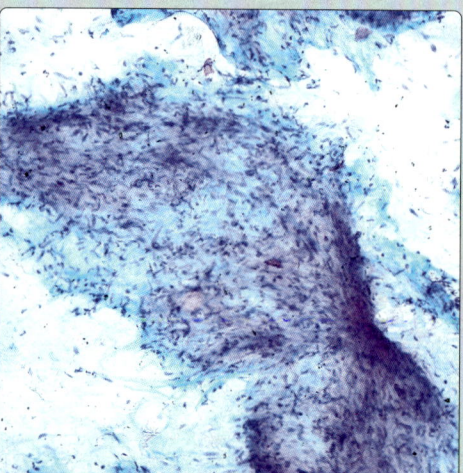
Low-Power Appearance

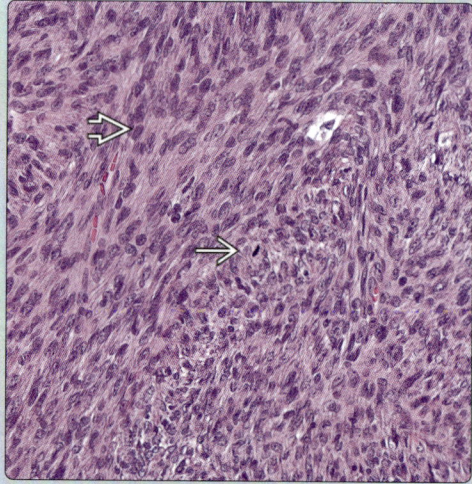
Fibrosarcoma

(Left) Pap-stained FNA smear of fibrosarcoma shows a large bundle of spindled cells on low power. The spindled nuclei are for the most part aligned but do not form any distinctive pattern. (Right) Core biopsy of fibrosarcoma shows spindled tumor cells ➡ arranged in fascicles with minimal nuclear pleomorphism and scattered mitotic figures ➡.

Fibrosarcoma

TERMINOLOGY

Definitions
- Soft tissue sarcoma composed of fibroblasts
  - Lacks features of named fibrosarcoma subtypes
  - Now very rare; mostly diagnosis of exclusion
  - Pleomorphic variants are currently classified as undifferentiated pleomorphic sarcoma

ETIOLOGY/PATHOGENESIS

De Novo
- Exceptionally rare if strictly defined

Arising in Course of Other Tumor
- Fibrosarcoma in dermatofibrosarcoma
  - Probable origin of many superficial adult fibrosarcomas
- Malignant solitary fibrous tumor
- Component of other fibrosarcoma subtypes (e.g., sclerosing epithelioid fibrosarcoma)

CYTOPATHOLOGY

Background
- May have focal myxoid change or stromal collagen

Cells
- Elongated spindle cells with slender, tapered, and wavy nuclei and scant, delicate cytoplasm

Nuclear Details
- Variable hyperchromasia, pleomorphism, mitotic activity

Cell Block Findings
- May show herringbone or chevron pattern

ANCILLARY TESTS

Immunohistochemistry
- Most cases are negative for mesenchymal markers except for vimentin and very focal SMA
- Some cases arising in dermatofibrosarcoma protuberans or solitary fibrous tumor express CD34 focally or diffusely

Genetic Testing
- Some superficial examples have *COL1A1::PDGFB* fusion transcripts like dermatofibrosarcoma
- Recent report of *STRN3::NTRK3* fusion suggests link to other *NTRK*-rearranged mesenchymal neoplasms

DIFFERENTIAL DIAGNOSIS

Low-Grade Fibromyxoid Sarcoma
- Less cellular
- Myxoid and fibrous areas with whorling
- Specific translocation t(7;16)(q34;p11)

Low-Grade Myofibrosarcoma
- Cells have more cytoplasm
- Multifocal positivity for SMA

Synovial Sarcoma
- Biphasic pattern with gland formation in 1/3
- Shorter, ovoid uniform cells, overlapping nuclei
- Specific translocation t(X;18)(p11;q11)

Malignant Peripheral Nerve Sheath Tumor
- Spindle cells with wavy or bullet-shaped nuclei
- S100 protein (+) in 2/3 of cases

Fibromatosis
- Less cellular, cells evenly dispersed in mature collagen
- Myofibroblasts, punctate nucleoli
- Nuclear immunoreactivity for β-catenin

SELECTED REFERENCES

1. Chen Y et al: Novel TNC-PDGFD fusion in fibrosarcomatous dermatofibrosarcoma protuberans: a case report. Diagn Pathol. 16(1):63, 2021
2. Wakely PE Jr: Cytopathology of myxofibrosarcoma: a study of 66 cases and literature review. J Am Soc Cytopathol. 10(3):300-9, 2021
3. Folpe AL: "Hey! Whatever happened to hemangiopericytoma and fibrosarcoma?" An update on selected conceptual advances in soft tissue pathology which have occurred over the past 50 years. Hum Pathol. 95:113-36, 2020
4. Lopez LV et al: Dermatofibrosarcoma protuberans with fibrosarcomatous transformation: our experience, molecular evaluation of selected cases, and short literature review. Int J Dermatol. 58(11):1246-52, 2019

Elongated Cytoplasm

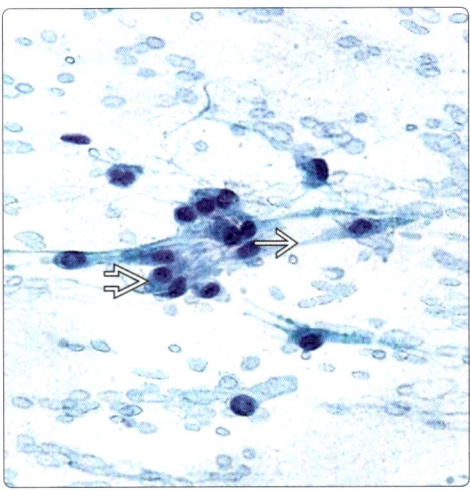

Wavy Nuclei

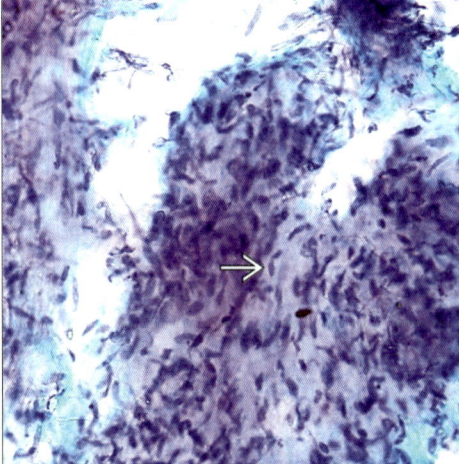

(Left) Pap-stained FNA smear shows cells with delicate elongated cytoplasm ➡ and round to oval nuclei ➡ in a case of fibrosarcoma. *(Right)* Pap-stained FNA smear of fibrosarcoma shows spindle cells ➡ with slender, wavy nuclei.

Myofibroblastoma

KEY FACTS

CLINICAL ISSUES
- Well-circumscribed, solitary, slow-growing nodule
- Locations: Head and neck, back, buttocks, anterior abdominal wall
- May be related to spindle cell lipoma &/or solitary fibrous tumor
- Excellent prognosis following surgical excision

CYTOPATHOLOGY
- Single spindle cells and cohesive clusters of spindle cells
- Round to oval nuclei with fine chromatin pattern, minimal cytoplasm
- Cells may be embedded within extracellular matrix material
- No necrosis, rare/no mitotic activity

ANCILLARY TESTS
- Immunostains: Positive for CD34, desmin, BCL2, ER, PR; negative for S100

- Molecular: Deletions similar to spindle cell lipoma: 13q-, 16q-

TOP DIFFERENTIAL DIAGNOSES
- Fibromatosis
  - Not well circumscribed
  - Long fascicular arrangement of spindle cells without thick collagen bands
  - Spindle cells generally parallel to each other
- Low-grade myofibroblastic sarcoma
  - Increased cellular atypia, infiltrating borders, increased mitotic activity
  - Fusiform nuclei with evenly distributed chromatin
- Nodular fasciitis
  - Infiltrative borders and mucoid stroma
  - Storiform or fascicular pattern
  - Inflammatory cells and myxoid stroma can be present

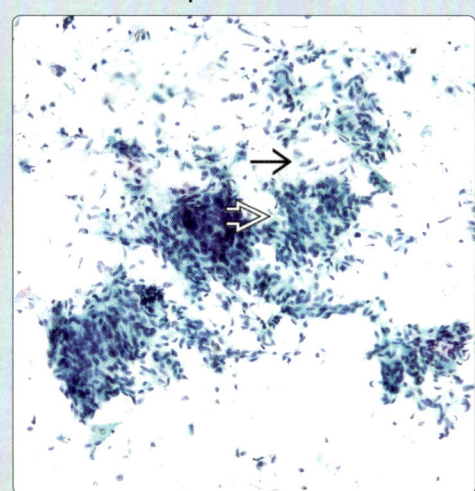

Spindle Cells

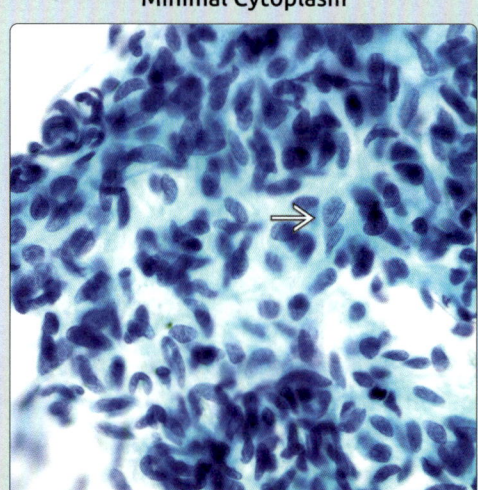

Minimal Cytoplasm

(Left) Pap-stained smear shows single dispersed spindle cells ➡ along with cohesive clusters of spindle cells ➡. (Right) Pap-stained smear of myofibroblastoma demonstrates spindle cells ➡ with minimal cytoplasm and round to oval nuclei with fine nuclear chromatin and without atypia.

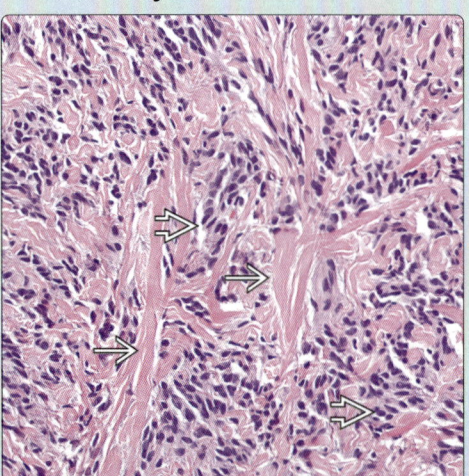

Myofibroblastoma

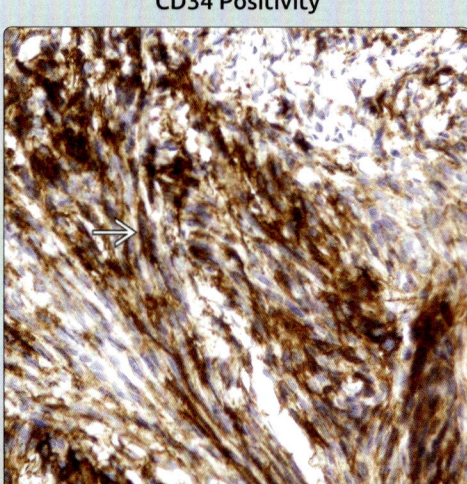

CD34 Positivity

(Left) Core biopsy of myofibroblastoma stained with H&E shows plump spindle cell proliferation with uniform nuclear chromatin ➡ without atypia associated with thick hyalinized collagen bundles ➡ amidst them. (Right) Immunohistochemical stain for CD34 shows strong and diffuse positivity of the spindle cells ➡ in myofibroblastoma.

Myofibroblastoma

TERMINOLOGY

Definitions
- Benign soft tissue spindle cell tumor composed of myofibroblasts

CLINICAL ISSUES

Site
- Head and neck, back, buttocks, anterior abdominal wall

Presentation
- Usually well-circumscribed, solitary, slow-growing nodule

Treatment
- Surgical excision

Prognosis
- Excellent

CYTOPATHOLOGY

Cellularity
- Variable

Background
- Spindle cells may be embedded within extracellular matrix

Cells
- Single bland spindle cells or cohesive groups of spindle cells without atypia associated with extracellular matrix
  - Occasional mast cells can be seen

Nuclear Details
- Oval nuclei with fine chromatin pattern, rare nuclear grooves, or nucleoli may be seen

Cytoplasmic Details
- Minimal cytoplasm

MICROSCOPIC

Histologic Features
- Uniform spindle cells arranged in fascicles with pushing borders
- Hyalinized collagen bands may separate spindle cells
- No necrosis and rare/no mitotic activity

ANCILLARY TESTS

Immunohistochemistry
- Positive for ER, PR, desmin, BCL2, CD34, vimentin; negative for S100

Genetic Testing
- Aberrations similar to spindle cell lipoma: 13q-, 16q-

DIFFERENTIAL DIAGNOSIS

Nodular Fasciitis
- Infiltrative borders and mucoid stroma; inflammatory cells may be present
- Storiform or fascicular pattern
- May have increased mitotic figures but no atypical forms

Low-Grade Myofibroblastic Sarcoma
- Increased cellular atypia, infiltrating borders, increased mitotic activity
- Fusiform nuclei with evenly distributed chromatin

Fibromatosis
- Not well circumscribed
  - Absence of thick collagen bands
- Long fascicular arrangement of spindle cells

SELECTED REFERENCES

1. Tajiri R et al: Potential pathogenetic link between angiomyofibroblastoma and superficial myofibroblastoma in the female lower genital tract based on a novel MTG1-CYP2E1 fusion. Mod Pathol. 34(12):2222-8, 2021
2. Wickre M et al: Mammary and extramammary myofibroblastoma: multimodality imaging features with clinicopathologic correlation, management and outcomes in a series of 23 patients. Br J Radiol. 94(1120):20201019, 2021

Extracellular Matrix

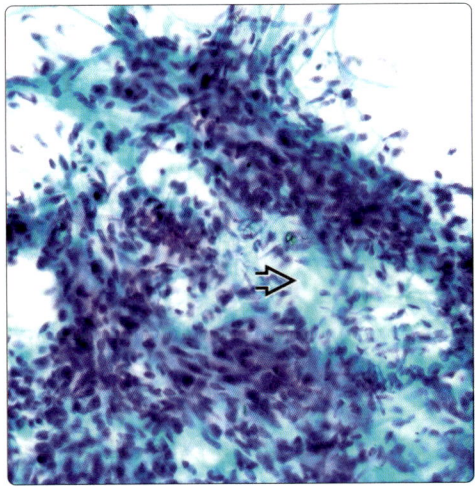

Fine Nuclear Chromatin

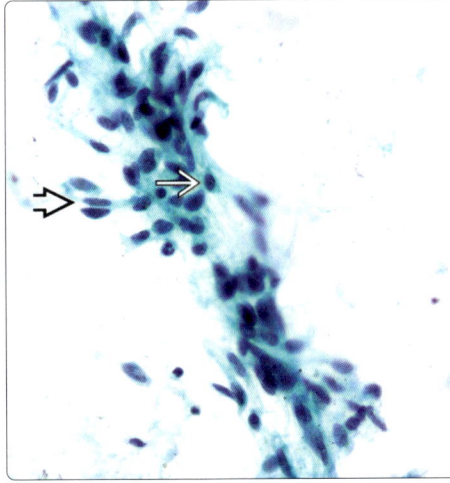

(Left) Pap-stained smear shows cohesive clusters of bland spindle cells within an extracellular matrix ➡. (Right) Pap-stained smear of myofibroblastoma demonstrates spindle cells with oval ➡ and elongated nuclei ➡ with fine nuclear chromatin and without atypia.

Low-Grade Myofibroblastic Sarcoma

KEY FACTS

CLINICAL ISSUES
- Predominantly in adult patients
  - Rarely in children
- Occurs frequently in head and neck region and extremities
  - Tongue and oral cavity preferred locations
- Subcutaneous and deep soft tissue
- Increased rate of local recurrences
- Metastases occur only rarely and often after prolonged time interval

CYTOPATHOLOGY
- Spindle-shaped tumor cells with fusiform nuclei
- Nuclei elongated with evenly distributed chromatin
- Nuclei vesicular with indentations and small nucleoli
- Moderate nuclear atypia with enlarged, hyperchromatic, and irregular nuclei
- Ill-defined, pale eosinophilic cytoplasm
- Associated with numerous thin-walled capillaries

ANCILLARY TESTS
- SMA(+/-), vimentin (+), desmin (+/-), calponin (+/-)
- S100, EMA, CD34, h-caldesmon, nuclear β-catenin (-)

TOP DIFFERENTIAL DIAGNOSES
- Desmoid fibromatosis
  - No cytologic atypia; β-catenin (+)
- Leiomyosarcoma
  - Spindled tumor cells with deep eosinophilic, fibrillar cytoplasm; h-caldesmon (+)
- Inflammatory myofibroblastic tumor
  - Prominent inflammatory infiltrate; ALK(+)
- Solitary fibrous tumor
  - Well-circumscribed, nodular neoplasms; CD34(+)
- Low-grade fibromyxoid sarcoma
  - Bland, elongated, spindle-shaped cells; often EMA(+)

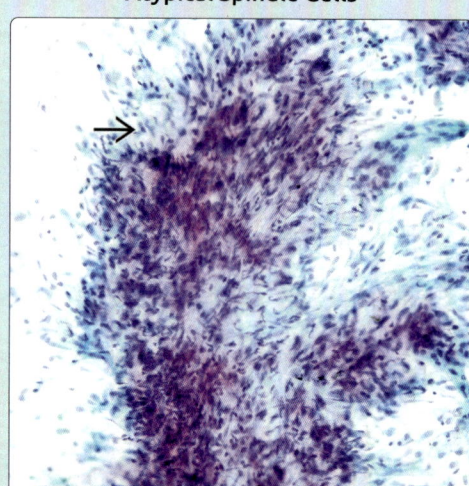
Atypical Spindle Cells

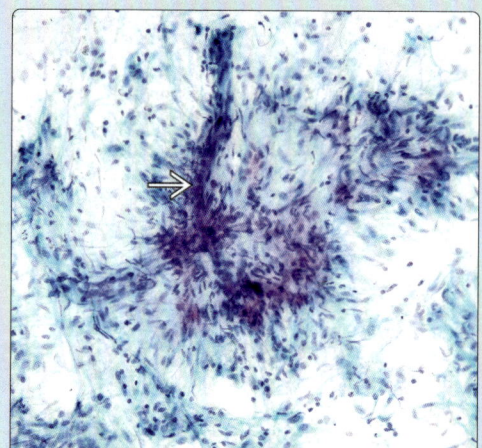
Traversing Capillaries

(Left) Pap-stained FNA smear of low-grade myofibroblastic sarcoma demonstrates proliferation of atypical spindle cells ➡. *(Right)* Pap-stained FNA smear of low-grade myofibroblastic sarcoma shows thin-walled capillaries ➡ traversing clusters of atypical spindle cells.

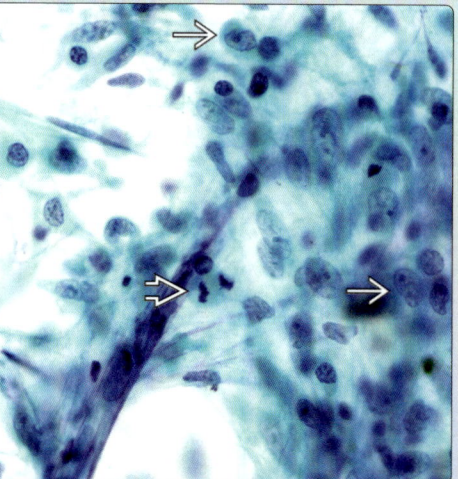
Prominent Nucleoli and Mitosis

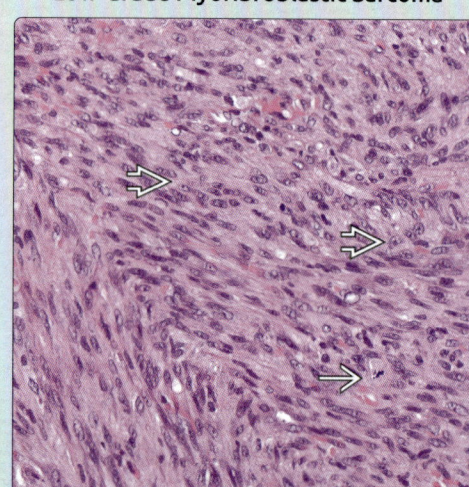
Low-Grade Myofibroblastic Sarcoma

(Left) Pap-stained FNA smear of low-grade myofibroblastic sarcoma demonstrates atypical spindle cells with nuclear membrane indentations and prominent nucleoli ➡. A mitotic figure ➡ is also present. *(Right)* Core biopsy of low-grade myofibroblastic sarcoma shows myofibroblastic proliferation, including spindle cells ➡ with elongated vesicular nucleus, mild nuclear pleomorphism, and scattered mitotic figures ➡.

Low-Grade Myofibroblastic Sarcoma

TERMINOLOGY

Definitions
- Distinct atypical myofibroblastic neoplasm with fibromatosis-like morphologic features

CLINICAL ISSUES

Site
- Wide anatomic distribution
- Occurs frequently in head and neck region
  - Tongue and oral cavity preferred locations
- Occurs frequently in extremities

Prognosis
- Locally aggressive behavior

CYTOPATHOLOGY

Cells
- Spindle-shaped tumor cells

Nuclear Details
- Moderate nuclear atypia; enlargement and hyperchromasia
- Elongated vesicular nuclei with indentations/clefts and small nucleoli

Cytoplasmic Details
- Ill-defined, pale eosinophilic cytoplasm

ANCILLARY TESTS

Immunohistochemistry
- SMA(+/-), vimentin (+), desmin (+/-), calponin (+/-)
- S100, EMA, CD34, h-caldesmon, nuclear β-catenin (-)

DIFFERENTIAL DIAGNOSIS

Desmoid Fibromatosis
- Infiltrative growth but no diffuse "growing through preexisting structures"
- No cytologic atypia
- β-catenin (+)

Leiomyosarcoma
- Spindled tumor cells with deep eosinophilic, fibrillar cytoplasm
- H-caldesmon (+)

Inflammatory Myofibroblastic Tumor
- Prominent inflammatory infiltrate
- ALK(+)

Infantile Fibrosarcoma
- Children and adolescents affected
- Plump, spindle, round tumor cells with enlarged nuclei

Myofibroma/Myofibromatosis
- Biphasic growth
  - Primitive mesenchymal tumor cells associated with hemangiopericytoma-like growing capillaries
  - Mature myofibroblastic tumor cells set in collagenous/myxohyaline stroma
- No desmin expression

Solitary Fibrous Tumor
- Well-circumscribed, nodular neoplasms
- CD34(+)

Low-Grade Fibromyxoid Sarcoma
- Bland, elongated, spindle-shaped tumor cells
- EMA expression in many cases

SELECTED REFERENCES

1. Kim JH et al: Surgical treatment and long-term outcomes of low-grade myofibroblastic sarcoma: a single-center case series of 15 patients. World J Surg Oncol. 19(1):339, 2021
2. Xu Y et al: Is there a role for chemotherapy and radiation in the treatment of patients with low-grade myofibroblastic sarcoma? Clin Transl Oncol. 23(2):344-52, 2021
3. Taweevisit M et al: Distinctive features of low-grade myofibroblastic sarcoma on aspiration cytology: a case report. Cytopathology. 29(6):578-81, 2018

Enlarged Indented Nuclei

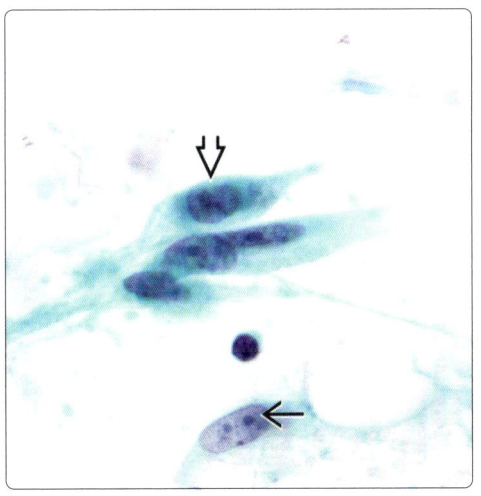

Intranuclear Inclusion

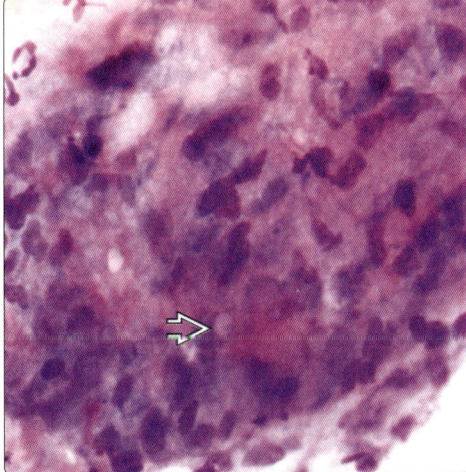

(Left) Few spindle cells with wispy cytoplasm and nuclear atypia are seen in this Pap-stained smear of low-grade myofibroblastic sarcoma. The nuclei are enlarged with indentations ⇨ and prominent nucleoli ⇨. (Right) Diff-Quik stain of low-grade myofibroblastic sarcoma demonstrates a cluster of atypical spindle cells. A rare intranuclear inclusion ⇨ is also present.

Giant Cell Tumor of Tendon Sheath

KEY FACTS

CLINICAL ISSUES
- Benign soft tissue tumor of synovial origin
- Any age; peak: 3rd-4th decades; F:M = 2:1
- Most commonly found in digits of hand (85%)
- Also seen in large joints (10%)
  - Intraarticular tumors are referred to as localized pigmented villonodular synovitis
- Benign but recurs locally (~ 20%)

CYTOPATHOLOGY
- Polymorphous population
  - Stromal cells with pale cytoplasm and round, spindle-shaped, or reniform nuclei
  - Large, epithelioid macrophages with eosinophilic cytoplasm and vesicular nuclei
  - Osteoclast-like giant cells
  - Xanthoma cells and siderophages
- Intracellular hemosiderin pigment
- Extracellular hemosiderin pigment in background

ANCILLARY TESTS
- Stromal cells: CD68(+), few cells SMA(+), desmin (+) in 50% of tumors
- Giant cells: CD68(+), TRAP(+)

TOP DIFFERENTIAL DIAGNOSES
- Diffuse-type tenosynovial giant cell tumor/pigmented villonodular synovitis
  - Diffuse intraarticular tumors form villonodular masses
  - Large joints; knee most common site
- Giant cell tumor of soft tissue
  - More uniform, less polymorphous mononuclear stromal cell population
- Hemosiderotic synovitis
  - Deposition of hemosiderin pigment in synovial membrane secondary to intraarticular hemorrhage
  - Presence of hemosiderin-laden macrophages and hemosiderin pigment deposition

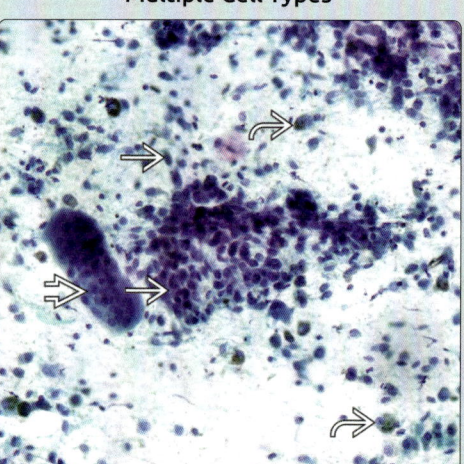

Multiple Cell Types

(Left) Pap-stained FNA smear of a giant cell tumor of the tendon sheath shows loose clusters and individually distributed stromal cells ⇨, osteoclastic giant cells ⇨, and few hemosiderin-laden histiocytoid cells ⇨.

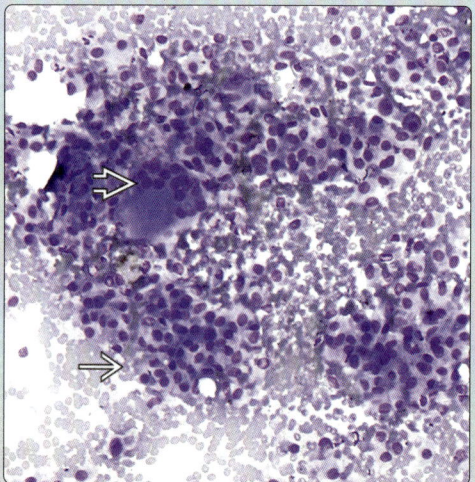

Multinucleated Giant Cell Among Mononuclear Cells

(Right) Diff-Quik-stained FNA smear shows clusters of mononuclear stromal cells ⇨ and a multinucleated osteoclastic giant cell ⇨.

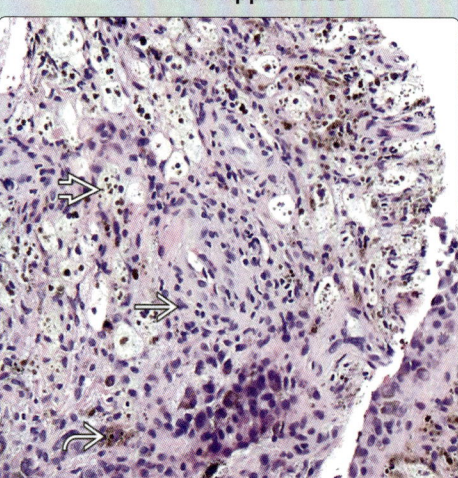

Cell Block Appearance

(Left) H&E-stained cell block of a giant cell tumor of the tendon sheath shows many stromal cells ⇨, hemosiderin-laden histiocytoid cells ⇨, and extracellular hemosiderin pigment deposition ⇨.

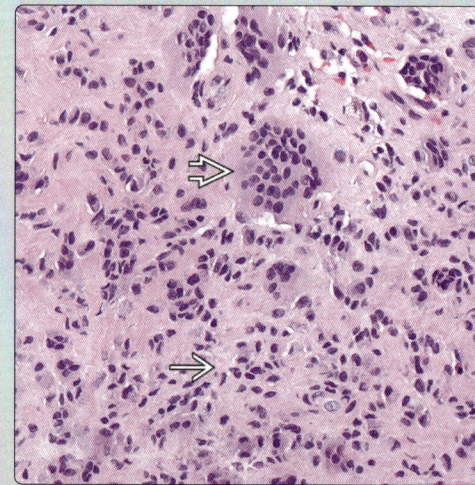

Giant Cell Tumor of Tendon Sheath

(Right) Core biopsy stained by H&E shows mononuclear stromal cells ⇨ without significant atypia and multinucleated osteoclastic giant cells ⇨.

Giant Cell Tumor of Tendon Sheath

TERMINOLOGY

Synonyms
- Localized tenosynovial giant cell tumor
- Localized pigmented villonodular synovitis
- Nodular tenosynovitis

Definitions
- Benign soft tissue tumor of synovial origin
  o Polymorphous population of neoplastic stromal cells, macrophages, and osteoclast-like giant cells
  o Well circumscribed, noninvasive

ETIOLOGY/PATHOGENESIS

Histogenesis
- Neoplastic growth
  o Balanced translocation involving 1p13 (*CSF1* gene) in many tumors

CLINICAL ISSUES

Epidemiology
- Age
  o Any age; peak: 3rd-4th decades
- Sex
  o F:M = 2:1

Site
- Digits (85%)
- Large joints (10%)

Prognosis
- Benign but recurs locally (~ 20%)

CYTOPATHOLOGY

Background
- Extracellular hemosiderin pigment

Cells
- Polymorphous population
  o Stromal cells with pale cytoplasm and round, spindle-shaped, or reniform nuclei
  o Large, epithelioid macrophages with eosinophilic cytoplasm and vesicular nuclei
  o Osteoclast-like giant cells
    – Giant cells can be sparse in some tumors
  o Xanthoma cells and siderophages
- Intracellular hemosiderin pigment

Nuclear Details
- Round nuclei, vesicular chromatin pattern, pinpoint nucleoli
- Mitotic figures can be noted, sometimes abundant

ANCILLARY TESTS

Immunohistochemistry
- Stromal cells: CD68(+), few cells SMA(+), desmin (+) in 50% of tumors
- Giant cells: CD68(+), TRAP(+)

DIFFERENTIAL DIAGNOSIS

Diffuse-Type Tenosynovial Giant Cell Tumor/Pigmented Villonodular Synovitis
- Similar microscopically to giant cell tumor of tendon sheath

Giant Cell Tumor of Soft Tissue
- More uniform, less polymorphous mononuclear stromal cell population

Hemosiderotic Synovitis
- Deposition of hemosiderin pigment in synovial membrane secondary to intraarticular hemorrhage

SELECTED REFERENCES

1. Ota T et al: Tumor location and type affect local recurrence and joint damage in tenosynovial giant cell tumor: a multi-center study. Sci Rep. 11(1):17384, 2021
2. Mastboom MJL et al: Surgical outcomes of patients with diffuse-type tenosynovial giant-cell tumours: an international, retrospective, cohort study. Lancet Oncol. 20(6):877-86, 2019
3. Ozben H et al: Giant cell tumor of tendon sheath in the hand: analysis of risk factors for recurrence in 50 cases. BMC Musculoskelet Disord. 20(1):457, 2019

Mononuclear Stromal Cells and Hemosiderin-Laden Histiocytoid Cells

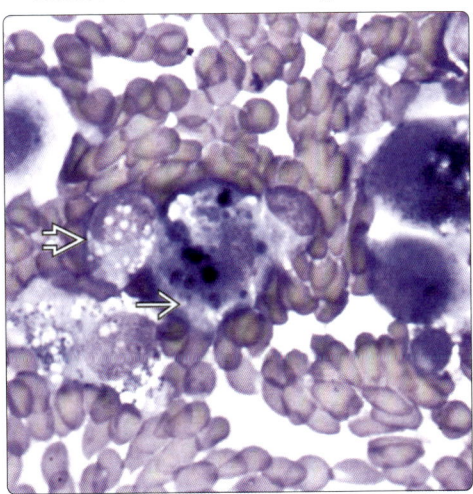

Prominent Hemosiderin

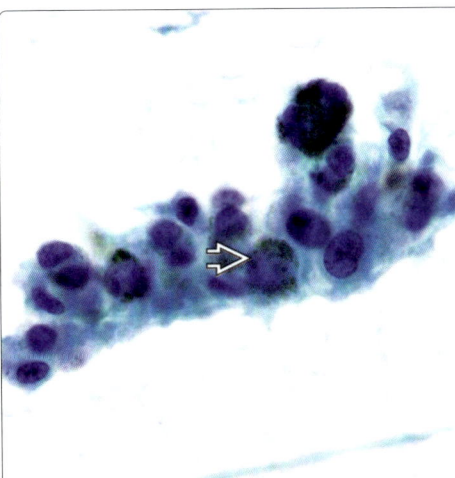

(Left) Diff-Quik-stained FNA smear of a giant cell tumor of the tendon sheath shows hemosiderin-laden histiocytoid cells ➡ and mononuclear stromal cells ➡. (Right) Pap-stained FNA smear of a giant cell tumor of the tendon sheath shows intracellular, coarse, golden-brown pigment ➡ consistent with hemosiderin.

Undifferentiated Pleomorphic Sarcoma

KEY FACTS

TERMINOLOGY
- High-grade malignant neoplasm characterized by spindle and histiocytoid tumor cells with diffuse pleomorphism in absence of specific line of differentiation

CLINICAL ISSUES
- Tumor of late adult life: 50-70 years
- M > F; > 2/3 of cases occur in men
- Most commonly arises in lower extremities, particularly thigh, followed by upper extremities
- Local recurrence in 19-31%
- Metastasis to sites, such as lung, bone, liver in 31-35%

CYTOPATHOLOGY
- Plump, spindle, and histiocyte-like cells with significant nuclear atypia
- Pleomorphic cells with single or multiple nuclei
- Osteoclast-like giant cells with high-grade nuclei
- Many typical and atypical mitotic figures

ANCILLARY TESTS
- Positive for vimentin, SMA (focal), CD34 (variable)
- Desmin (-), caldesmon (-)
- Rare cytokeratin (+) cells
- Complex and nonspecific cytogenetic abnormalities

TOP DIFFERENTIAL DIAGNOSES
- Pleomorphic nonmesenchymal neoplasms
  - Sarcomatoid carcinoma
  - Melanoma
  - Anaplastic lymphoma
- Pleomorphic leiomyosarcoma
- Pleomorphic rhabdomyosarcoma
- Pleomorphic malignant peripheral nerve sheath tumor
- Pleomorphic liposarcoma
- Dedifferentiated pleomorphic sarcoma
  - Features of low-grade sarcoma along with undifferentiated pleomorphic sarcoma

(Left) Pap-stained FNA smear of undifferentiated pleomorphic sarcoma shows plump spindled cells with significant nuclear atypia ➡. (Right) Pap-stained FNA smear of undifferentiated pleomorphic sarcoma shows pleomorphic giant tumor cells ➡ and atypical spindle cells ➡.

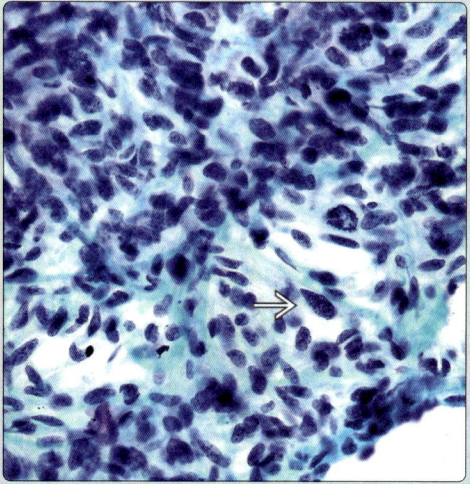
Plump Spindle Cells With Marked Atypia

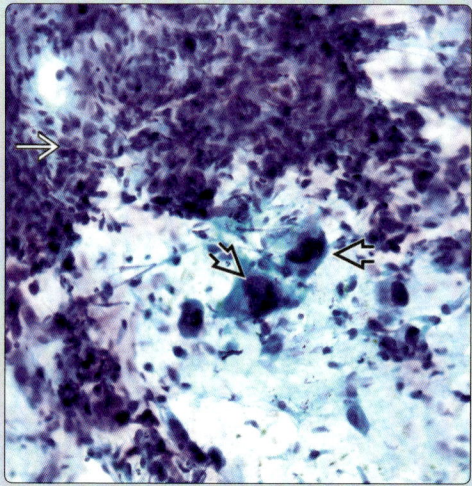
Pleomorphic Giant Cells

(Left) Diff-Quik-stained FNA smear of undifferentiated pleomorphic sarcoma demonstrates atypical pleomorphic spindle and epithelioid tumor cells ➡. (Right) Core biopsy of undifferentiated pleomorphic sarcoma stained with H&E shows plump spindle and epithelioid tumor cells ➡ with significant pleomorphism, including tumor giant cells ➡.

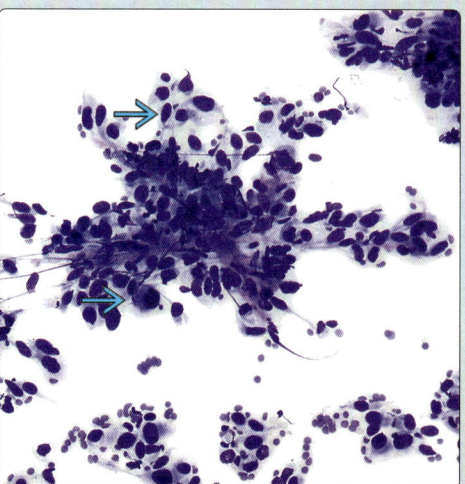
Diff-Quik Appearance

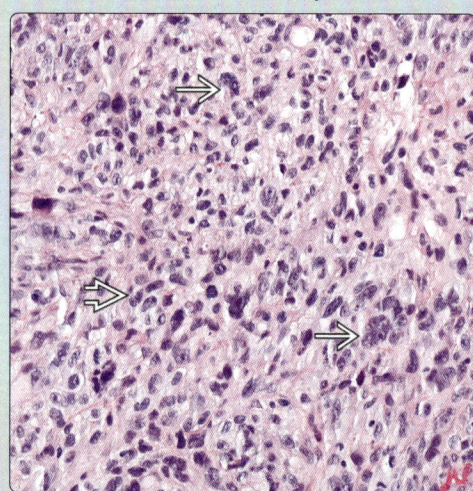
Undifferentiated Pleomorphic Sarcoma

Undifferentiated Pleomorphic Sarcoma

TERMINOLOGY

Abbreviations
- Undifferentiated pleomorphic sarcoma (UPS)
  - Previously termed malignant fibrous histiocytoma (MFH)

Definitions
- High-grade malignant neoplasm characterized by spindle and histiocytoid tumor cells with diffuse pleomorphism and absence of specific line of differentiation

CLINICAL ISSUES

Epidemiology
- Incidence
  - MFH accounts for significant proportion of sarcomas
- Age
  - Tumor of late adult life: 50-70 years
    - Rare in children
- Sex
  - M > F; > 2/3 of cases occur in men

Site
- Lower extremities, particularly thigh, followed by upper extremity

Presentation
- Painless, slowly enlarging mass

Natural History
- Local recurrence in 19-31%
- Metastasis in 31-35%
  - Metastatic sites: Lung (90%), bone (8%), liver (1%)
- Local recurrence and distant metastasis often develop within 12-24 months after diagnosis

Prognosis
- 5-year survival rate: 65-70%
- Factors correlating with metastasis and survival
  - Tumor size, grade, necrosis, depth, and local recurrence

CYTOPATHOLOGY

Cellularity
- Usually very high

Background
- Chronic inflammatory cells, xanthoma cells
- Fragments of fibrocollagenous tissue, rarely osteoid or chondroid material

Cells
- Plump spindle cells arranged in short fascicles
- Histiocyte-like cells admixed with spindle cells
- Pleomorphic cells with single or multiple nuclei
- Osteoclast-type giant cells with high-grade nuclei
- Giant cells can show ingested lipid material or hemosiderin pigment in cytoplasm

Nuclear Details
- Significant nuclear atypia and pleomorphism in spindle and histiocyte-like cells
- Many typical and atypical mitotic figures

ANCILLARY TESTS

Immunohistochemistry
- Positive for vimentin, SMA (focal), CD34 (variable)
- Negative for desmin, caldesmon
- Rare cytokeratin (+) cells
- Diagnosis of exclusion if no specific line of differentiation

Genetic Testing
- Complex and nonspecific cytogenetic abnormalities
- MFH demonstrates striking similarities with pleomorphic leiomyosarcoma by comparative genomic hybridization

DIFFERENTIAL DIAGNOSIS

Pleomorphic Nonmesenchymal Neoplasms
- Sarcomatoid carcinoma
  - Location in skin, mucosal surface, or parenchymal organ
  - High and low molecular weight cytokeratin (+), p63(+)
- Melanoma
  - S100(+), panmelanoma marker (+), SOX10(+)
- Anaplastic lymphoma
  - CD30(+), ALK1(+)

Pleomorphic Leiomyosarcoma
- Tumor cells with blunt-ended nuclei with perinuclear vacuole and deeply eosinophilic cytoplasm
- SMA(+), desmin (+), caldesmon (+)

Pleomorphic Rhabdomyosarcoma
- Tumor cells with eosinophilic cytoplasm and cross striations
- Desmin (+), myogenin (+), MyoD1(+)

Pleomorphic Malignant Peripheral Nerve Sheath Tumor
- History of neurofibromatosis type 1
- S100(+), SOX10(+)

Pleomorphic Liposarcoma
- Multivacuolated pleomorphic lipoblasts
- S100(+)

Dedifferentiated Pleomorphic Sarcoma
- Transformation of low-grade sarcoma, such as well-differentiated liposarcoma/atypical lipomatous tumor
  - Features of low-grade sarcoma along with UPS

SELECTED REFERENCES

1. Thway K et al: Undifferentiated and dedifferentiated soft tissue neoplasms: immunohistochemical surrogates for differential diagnosis. Semin Diagn Pathol. 38(6):170-86, 2021
2. Carvalho SD et al: Pleomorphic sarcomas: the state of the art. Surg Pathol Clin. 12(1):63-105, 2019
3. Hornick JL: Subclassification of pleomorphic sarcomas: how and why should we care? Ann Diagn Pathol. 37:118-24, 2018
4. Domansk HA et al: Undifferentiated/unclassified sarcomas. Monogr Clin Cytol. 22:122-4, 2017
5. Goldblum JR: An approach to pleomorphic sarcomas: can we subclassify, and does it matter? Mod Pathol. 27 Suppl 1:S39-46, 2014
6. Le Guellec S et al: Are peripheral purely undifferentiated pleomorphic sarcomas with MDM2 amplification dedifferentiated liposarcomas? Am J Surg Pathol. 38(3):293-304, 2014
7. Schaefer IM et al: Myxoid variant of so-called angiomatoid "malignant fibrous histiocytoma": clinicopathologic characterization in a series of 21 cases. Am J Surg Pathol. 38(6):816-23, 2014

Smooth Muscle Tumors

KEY FACTS

CLINICAL ISSUES
- Most common overall sarcoma type if uterine/other visceral leiomyosarcoma (LMS) included
- Primary sites: Pelvic, retroperitoneal, intraabdominal, extremities
- Usually middle-aged to older adults
- Retroperitoneal and inferior vena cava lesions more common in female patients
- Associated with radiation and with Epstein-Barr virus (EBV) in immunosuppressed patients

CYTOPATHOLOGY
- Low-grade LMS: Plump spindle cells with cigar-shaped nuclei and fibrillar/finely granular cytoplasm with indistinct cytoplasmic borders
- High-grade LMS: ↑ atypia, mitoses, necrosis, pleomorphism
- Features that may be seen: Perinuclear vacuoles, nuclear indentations, cytoplasmic nuclear inclusions, palisading, myxoid stroma

ANCILLARY TESTS
- Positive: Desmin, SMA, MSA, calponin, caldesmon, vimentin
  - Positive: EBER by in situ hybridization in EBV-associated smooth muscle tumor
- Variably positive: Keratin, EMA, CD99
- Usually negative: S100, β-catenin (nuclear), CD34, C-kit, DOG1, TLE1, ALK, MyoD1, myogenin, p63, cyclin-D1

TOP DIFFERENTIAL DIAGNOSES
- Benign entities: Leiomyoma, nerve sheath tumors, desmoid fibromatosis, solitary fibrous tumor
- Malignant entities: Gastrointestinal stromal tumor, rhabdomyosarcoma, malignant peripheral nerve sheath tumor, sarcomatoid carcinoma, melanoma, fibrosarcoma, myofibrosarcoma, synovial sarcoma, pleomorphic sarcomas, desmoplastic mesothelioma
- Immunostains, tests for genetic alterations, and clinical information useful to narrow differential

Fascicular Group of Cells

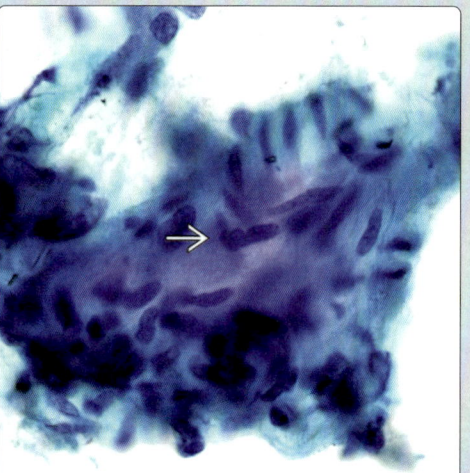

Diff-Quik Appearance

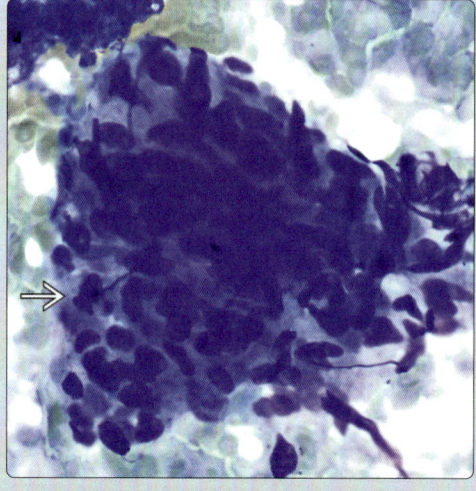

(Left) Pap-stained FNA smear of leiomyosarcoma shows a fascicular fragment of spindle cells with moderate nuclear atypia ➡. (Right) Diff-Quik-stained FNA smear of leiomyosarcoma shows crowded, ovoid, and elongated nuclei in a tumor fragment ➡.

Leiomyosarcoma

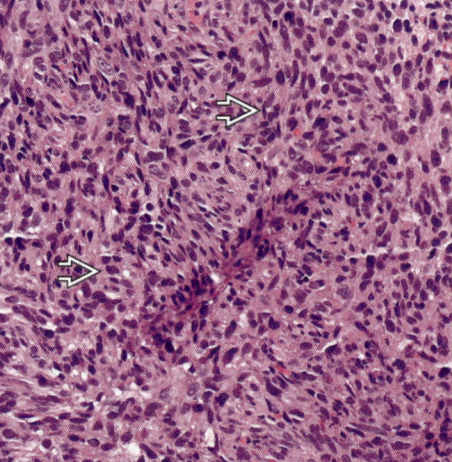

Leiomyosarcoma

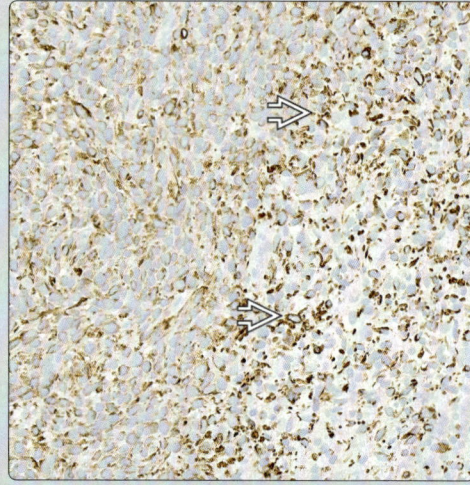

(Left) Core biopsy of leiomyosarcoma stained with H&E shows malignant spindle cells ➡ exhibiting hyperchromatic nucleus and significant nuclear pleomorphism. (Right) Core biopsy immunostained with desmin shows positive staining ➡ in malignant spindle cells, which supports the diagnosis of leiomyosarcoma.

Smooth Muscle Tumors

TERMINOLOGY

Definitions
- Leiomyosarcoma (LMS): Malignant neoplasm with smooth muscle differentiation
  - Epstein-Barr virus (EBV)-associated smooth muscle tumor
    - Inflammatory leiomyosarcoma

CLINICAL ISSUES

Epidemiology
- Incidence
  - Most common overall sarcoma type if uterine/other visceral LMS included
- Age
  - Usually middle-aged to older adults
- Sex
  - Excluding uterine LMS, no sex preference overall
    - Retroperitoneal and inferior vena cava lesions more common in female patients
- Associated factors: EBV in immunosuppressed patients, radiation, primary immunodeficiency, posttransplant immunosuppression

Presentation
- Pelvic, retroperitoneal, intraabdominal, extremities
  - EBV-associated smooth muscle tumors commonly arise in visceral organs
    - Inflammatory LMSs arise in deep soft tissue, most commonly in lower limb, trunk, and retroperitoneum

CYTOPATHOLOGY

Pattern
- Fascicular fragments, naked nuclei, ± intact single cells

Background
- ± myxoid stroma, ± necrosis
  - Inflammatory infiltration, including small lymphocytes, plasma cells, and histiocytes often as aggregates of foam cells

Cells
- Spindle cells with indistinct borders, ± rounded/polygonal cells, ↑ pleomorphism with tumor grade

Nuclear Details
- Cigar-shaped, elongated nuclei with blunt ends, ± indentations, ± cytoplasmic nuclear inclusions, ± palisading
- Atypia and mitoses ↑ with tumor grade
- Granular chromatin, ± striated appearance, usually inconspicuous nucleoli

Cytoplasmic Details
- Abundant, finely granular/fibrillar, ± perinuclear vacuoles

ANCILLARY TESTS

Immunohistochemistry
- Positive: Desmin, SMA, MSA, calponin, caldesmon
- Variably positive: Keratin, EMA, CD99
- Usually negative: S100, β-catenin (nuclear), CD34, C-kit, DOG1, TLE1, ALK, MyoD1, myogenin, p63, cyclin-D1

DIFFERENTIAL DIAGNOSIS

Benign Entities
- Leiomyoma, benign nerve sheath tumors, solitary fibrous tumor, desmoid fibromatosis

Malignant Entities
- Gastrointestinal stromal tumor, rhabdomyosarcoma, malignant peripheral nerve sheath tumor, sarcomatoid carcinoma, melanoma, fibrosarcoma, myofibrosarcoma, synovial sarcoma, pleomorphic sarcomas, mesothelioma

SELECTED REFERENCES

1. Stubbins RJ et al: Epstein-Barr virus associated smooth muscle tumors in solid organ transplant recipients: incidence over 31 years at a single institution and review of the literature. Transpl Infect Dis. 21(1):e13010, 2019

Nuclear and Cytoplasmic Features

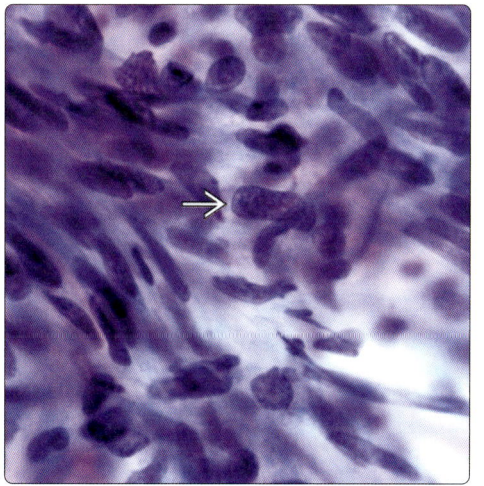

Histologic Appearance

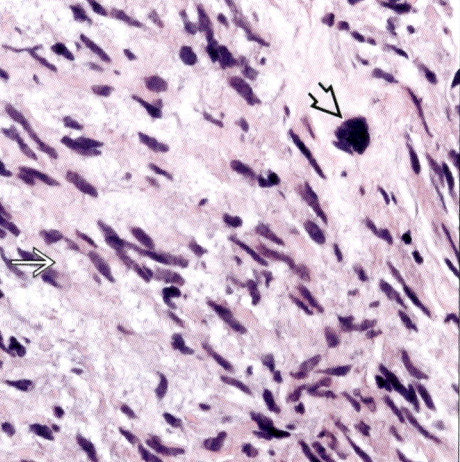

(Left) Pap-stained FNA smear of leiomyosarcoma shows mostly blunt-ended ➡, elongated nuclei with granular chromatin and indistinct nucleoli. (Right) Core needle biopsy of leiomyosarcoma shows the fascicular arrangement ➡ of spindle cells. Note the occasional pleomorphic tumor cell ➡.

Skeletal Muscle Tumors

KEY FACTS

CLINICAL ISSUES
- Rhabdomyoma (RMO): Rare benign tumor
- Embryonal and alveolar rhabdomyosarcoma (ERMS and ARMS): Most common pediatric soft tissue sarcomas

CYTOPATHOLOGY
- RMO: No atypia, necrosis, or mitotic activity; most common type [adult-type (ARMO)] resembles skeletal muscle
- ERMS: Myxoid stroma, no alveoli, spindle rhabdomyoblasts >> small round blue cells, giant cells rare, uniform nuclei with fine chromatin, indistinct nucleoli
- ARMS: Fibrotic stroma, small round blue cells predominate, giant/floret cells, more variable nuclei, coarser chromatin, prominent nucleoli
- Pleomorphic RMS (PMRS): Large pleomorphic/bizarre cells, abundant eosinophilic cytoplasm rarely with cross striations
- Spindle cell/sclerosing RMS (SRMS): Spindle cells with ovoid or elongated nuclei, vesicular chromatin, inconspicuous nucleoli, scant eosinophilic cytoplasm

ANCILLARY TESTS
- Immunochemistry: (+) for vimentin, desmin, MSA, MyoD1, myogenin; +/- PAX3, PAX7; +/- aberrant S100, cytokeratin, GFAP, neuroendocrine, B-cell markers
- ARMS has translocations: t(2;13)(q35;q14) in > 50% and t(1;13)(p36;q14) in ~ 20%
- ERMS: Complex karyotype, hallmark loss of heterozygosity at 11p15.5
- SRMS: Molecular testing for *VGLL2/NCOA2/CITED2*, *TFCP2/NCOA2* rearrangements, and *MYOD1* mutation

TOP DIFFERENTIAL DIAGNOSES
- ARMO: Normal striated muscle, granular cell tumor
- ERMS: RMO, sarcomas with myxoid stroma, other small round blue cell tumors
- ARMS: Other small round blue cell tumors, small cell/neuroendocrine carcinoma
- PRMS: Other pleomorphic malignancies
- SRMS: Other spindle cell malignancies

Rhabdomyoma: Pap Stain

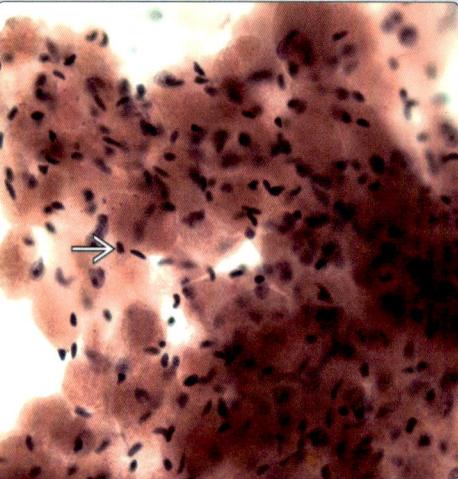

Rhabdomyoma: Cell Block

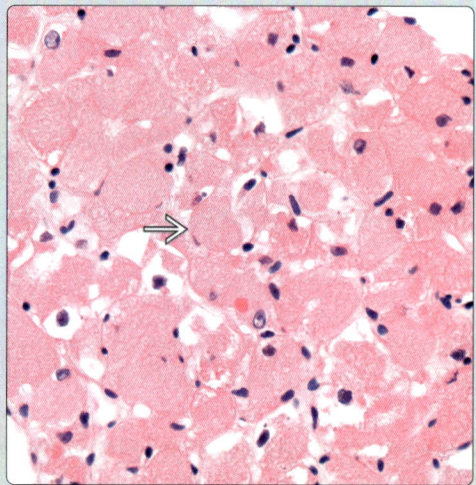

(Left) Pap-stained FNA smear of adult-type rhabdomyoma shows tumor cells with peripherally placed nuclei ➡, abundant cytoplasm, and a resemblance to skeletal muscle. (Courtesy A. Limbach, MD.) (Right) H&E-stained section of cell block preparation from an FNA rinse of adult-type rhabdomyoma shows large polygonal cells with abundant eosinophilic cytoplasm ➡. (Courtesy A. Limbach, MD.)

Alveolar Rhabdomyosarcoma

Pleomorphic Rhabdomyosarcoma

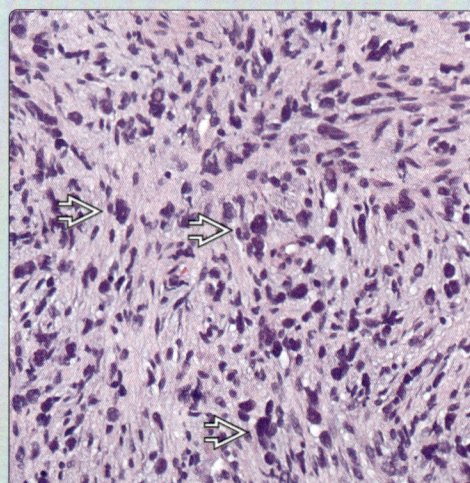

(Left) Core biopsy of alveolar rhabdomyosarcoma (ARMS) stained with H&E shows malignant cells with polygonal nucleus, variation in nuclear size, fine nuclear chromatin with inconspicuous nucleolus, and a scant to moderate amount of cytoplasm ➡. (Right) Core biopsy of pleomorphic rhabdomyosarcoma (PRMS) stained with H&E shows pleomorphic tumor cells, including many bizarre tumor giant cells ➡.

Skeletal Muscle Tumors

TERMINOLOGY

Definitions
- Rhabdomyoma (RMO): Benign neoplasm of cells with skeletal muscle differentiation
  - Cardiac RMO is considered to be hamartoma and often associated with tuberous sclerosis
- Rhabdomyosarcoma (RMS): Malignant neoplasm of cells with skeletal muscle differentiation

RMO Types
- Fetal type (FRMO), adult type (ARMO), genital type (GRMO)

RMS Types
- Embryonal type (ERMS), alveolar type (ARMS), pleomorphic type (PRMS), spindle cell/sclerosing (SRMS)

CLINICAL ISSUES

Epidemiology
- Incidence
  - RMO: Extremely rare (< 2% of skeletal muscle tumors)
  - RMS: Most common pediatric sarcoma (ERMS most common subtype)
- Age and sex
  - RMO: ARMO: M:F = 3:1, mean age: 50 years; FRMO: M > F, classic subtype in young children, intermediate subtype in adults; GRMO: F > M, mean age: 42 years
  - RMS: ERMS: Mean age 6.5 years; ARMS: Mean age: 12 years; PRMS occurs in adults; ERMS and PRMS: M > F; ARMS: M = F; SRMS: M > F

Site
- RMO
  - ARMO and FRMO: > 90% in head and neck region
  - GRMO: Genital tract
- RMS
  - ERMS: Head and neck, urogenital tract
  - ARMS: Trunk, extremities, head and neck
  - PRMS: Extremities (especially thigh)
  - SRMS: Head and neck, extremities, paratesticular region (pediatric population)

CYTOPATHOLOGY

Cells and Background
- ARMO
  - Large round to polygonal cells with abundant eosinophilic cytoplasm
  - Round peripherally or centrally located nuclei (± multiple), vesicular chromatin, conspicuous nucleoli
  - ± intranuclear cytoplasmic inclusions, characteristic cytoplasmic cross striations, cytoplasmic vacuoles (glycogen or lipid) with spider cells in cell block, cytoplasmic crystalloids of Z-band material
  - No atypia/mitoses/necrosis
- FRMO
  - Myocytes with range of maturation
  - No atypia/mitoses/necrosis
- ERMS
  - Small round blue cells, hyperchromatic nuclei, fine chromatin, inconspicuous nucleoli, mitoses, necrosis, myxoid matrix
  - ± spindle cells, strap cells, anaplasia, cytoplasmic glycogen vacuoles, cytoplasmic inclusion-like condensations, tigroid background
- ARMS
  - Small round blue cells, bi-/multinucleation common, mitoses, necrosis, floret or giant cells with eosinophilic &/or clear cytoplasm
  - ± variation in nuclear size/shape, coarser chromatin, prominent nucleoli, alveolar structures, fibrotic stroma
- PRMS
  - Large pleomorphic/bizarre cells, abundant eosinophilic cytoplasm rarely with cross striations, mitoses, ± necrosis
- SRMS
  - Spindle cells with ovoid or elongated nuclei, vesicular chromatin, inconspicuous nucleoli, scant eosinophilic cytoplasm

ANCILLARY TESTS

Immunohistochemistry
- Positive: Vimentin, desmin, MSA, MyoD1, myogenin; +/- aberrant staining for nonmuscle markers

Genetics
- ARMS: t(2;13)(q35;q14) in > 50%, t(1;13)(p36;q14) in ~ 20%
  - *FOXO1* on chromosome 13
  - *PAX3* and *PAX7* on chromosomes 2 and 1, respectively
- ERMS: Complex karyotype, hallmark loss of heterozygosity at 11p15.5
- PRMS: Complex karyotype
- SRMS: Aneuploidy with whole chromosome gains and nonrecurrent structural changes
  - *VGLL2*/*NCOA2*/*CITED2* rearrangements in congenital spindle cell SRMS
  - *MYOD1* mutation in *MYOD1*-mutant SRMS
  - *TFCP2*/*NCOA2* rearrangements in intraosseous spindle cell SRMS

DIFFERENTIAL DIAGNOSIS

Adult-Type Rhabdomyoma
- Nonneoplastic: Normal striated muscle
- Neoplasms: Granular cell tumor, hibernoma, paraganglioma, salivary gland oncocytoma, Hürthle cell neoplasm, lymphoplasmacytic lymphoma with immunoglobulin inclusions, alveolar soft part sarcoma

Embryonal-Type Rhabdomyosarcoma
- FRMO, GRMO, sarcomas with myxoid stroma, other small round blue cell tumors

Alveolar-Type Rhabdomyosarcoma
- Other small round blue cell tumors

Pleomorphic-Type Rhabdomyosarcoma
- Other pleomorphic malignancies

Spindle Cell/Sclerosing Rhabdomyosarcoma
- Other spindle cell malignancies

SELECTED REFERENCES
1. Giannikopoulos P et al: Rhabdomyosarcoma: how advanced molecular methods are shaping the diagnostic and therapeutic paradigm. Pediatr Dev Pathol. 24(5):395-404, 2021

Skeletal Muscle Tumors

Embryonal Rhabdomyosarcoma: Pap Stain

Embryonal Rhabdomyosarcoma: Diff-Quik

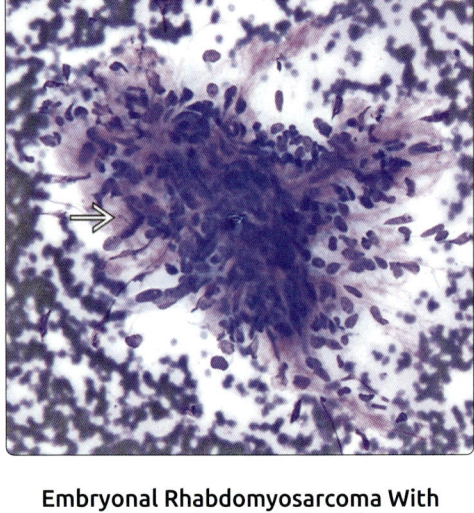

(Left) *Pap-stained FNA smear of embryonal rhabdomyosarcoma (ERMS) shows a fragment ⇒ of tumor cells with hyperchromatic round to ovoid nuclei. Faintly cyanophilic matrix ⇒ is seen in the center of the tumor fragment.* (Right) *Diff-Quik-stained FNA smear of ERMS shows spindle tumor cell nuclei enmeshed in a metachromatic myxoid matrix ⇒.*

Embryonal Rhabdomyosarcoma: High-Power Features

Embryonal Rhabdomyosarcoma With Hyperchromatic Nuclei

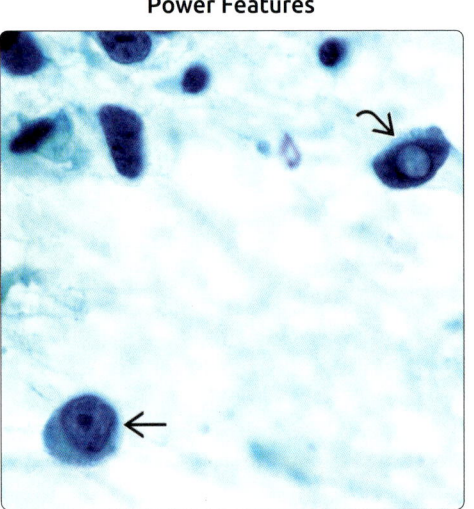

(Left) *Pap-stained FNA smear of ERMS shows 1 tumor cell with a nuclear cytoplasmic inclusion ("hole") ⇒ and another tumor cell ⇒ with an eccentrically placed nucleus, distinct nucleolus, and moderately abundant cyanophilic cytoplasm.* (Right) *Pap-stained FNA smear of ERMS shows hyperchromatic, ovoid tumor nuclei ⇒ with indistinct nucleoli.*

Myogenin (+)

Desmin (+)

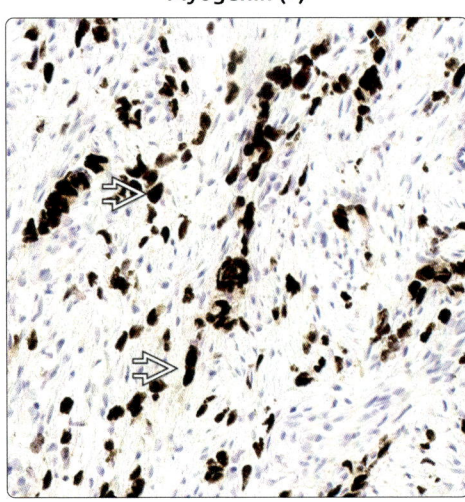 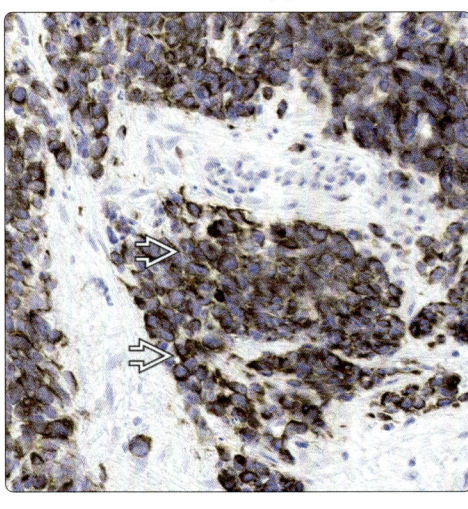

(Left) *Core biopsy of ARMS immunostained for myogenin shows positive nuclear staining ⇒.* (Right) *Core biopsy of ARMS immunostained for desmin shows positive cytoplasmic staining ⇒.*

Skeletal Muscle Tumors

Alveolar Rhabdomyosarcoma With Fibrocollagenous Alveolar Structure

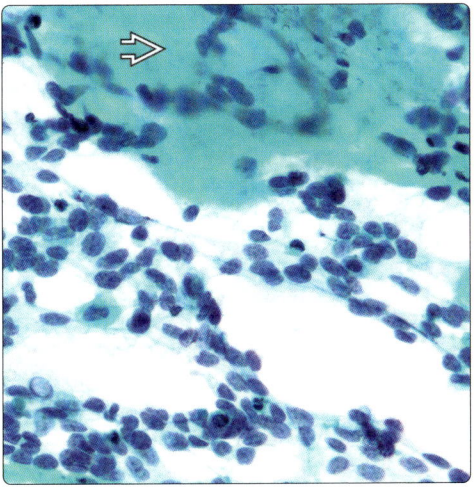

Alveolar Rhabdomyosarcoma Rhabdomyoblast: Pap Stain

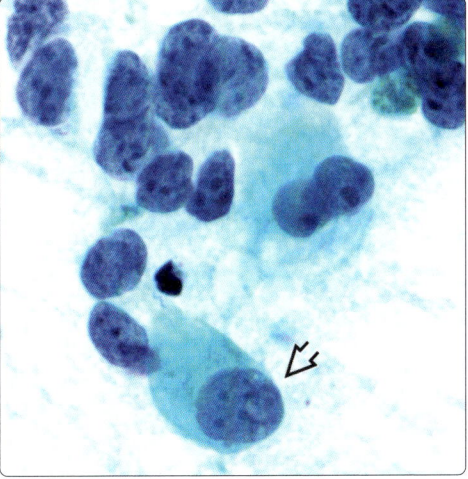

(Left) Pap-stained FNA smear of ARMS shows dyscohesive small round blue cells and cyanophilic stroma ➡ corresponding to fibrocollagenous alveolar structure. *(Right)* Pap-stained FNA smear of ARMS shows small round blue cells and a rhabdomyoblast ➡ with eccentrically placed nucleus and abundant cytoplasm, suggesting skeletal muscle differentiation.

Alveolar Rhabdomyosarcoma With Floret Cell

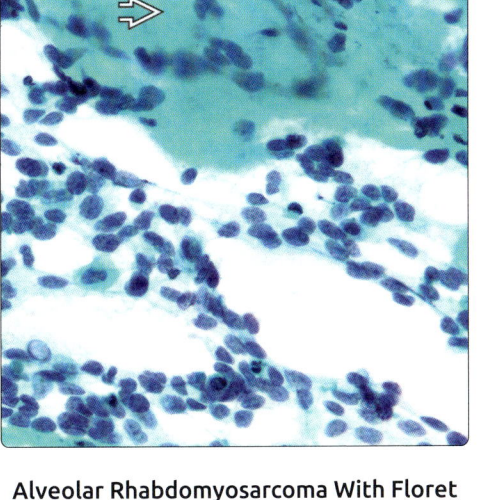

Alveolar Rhabdomyosarcoma With Small Round Cells and Giant Cell

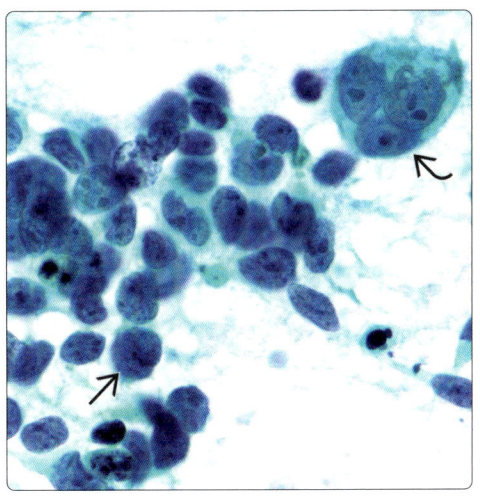

(Left) Pap-stained FNA smear of ARMS shows a characteristic floret type of giant tumor cell ➡ with wreath-like, peripherally arranged nuclei. *(Right)* Pap-stained FNA smear of ARMS shows small round tumor cells ➡ and a multinucleated giant tumor cell ➡.

Alveolar Rhabdomyosarcoma Rhabdomyoblast: Diff-Quik

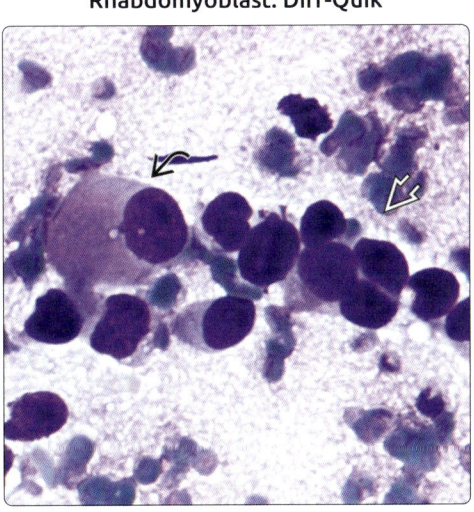

Alveolar Rhabdomyosarcoma: MyoD1 (+)

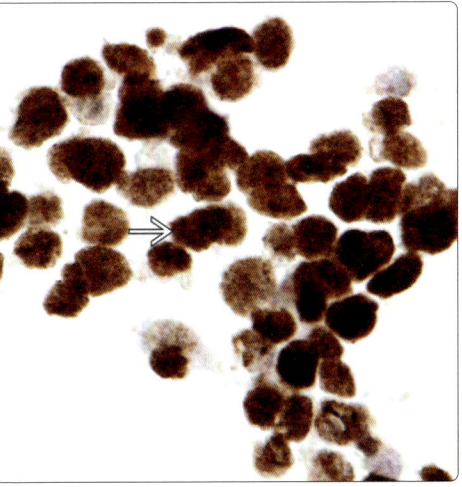

(Left) Diff-Quik-stained FNA smear of ARMS shows a large rhabdomyoblast ➡ with eccentrically located nucleus and abundant cytoplasm adjacent to a group of small round blue cells ➡. *(Right)* MyoD1 immunoperoxidase stain of ARMS FNA smear shows strong nuclear staining ➡ in tumor cells.

Hemangioma, Soft Tissue

KEY FACTS

CLINICAL ISSUES
- In skin/subcutaneous tissue, liver, and other sites; single or multiple
- Most are clinically obvious and not aspirated
  - FNA to exclude malignancy if not clinically obvious

CYTOPATHOLOGY
- Scanty to acellular FNA
- Rare, single spindle &/or polygonal cells with moderate cytoplasm
  - ± cell tangles/swirls
- Oval nuclei ± longitudinal groove
  - Fine chromatin with indistinct nucleoli
  - ± minimal atypia

ANCILLARY TESTS
- Positive for immunohistochemistry endothelial markers: CD31, CD34, FLI-1, ERG

- Cell block preparation of FNA can be diagnostic if tissue fragments show benign vascular channels

TOP DIFFERENTIAL DIAGNOSES
- Epithelioid hemangioendothelioma
  - More cellular
  - Greater nuclear pleomorphism and atypia
  - May have intracytoplasmic lumina
  - May have myxohyaline stroma
- Angiosarcoma
  - More cellular
  - Obvious malignant features
- Kaposi sarcoma
  - More cellular
  - May have hyaline globules within or outside spindle cells
  - Associated with immunosuppression and HHV-8
- Organizing thrombus/hematoma
  - History and imaging are helpful

Bland Ovoid Nuclei

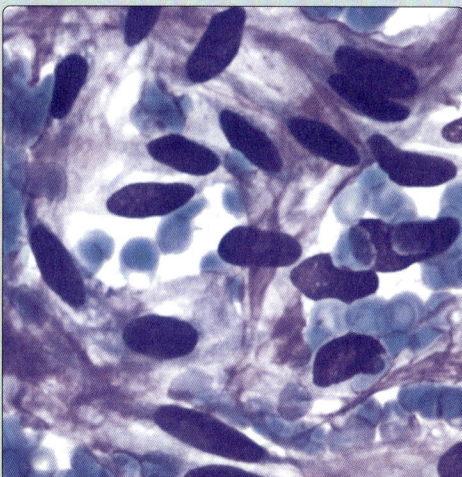

Fragment With Spindle Cells and Stroma

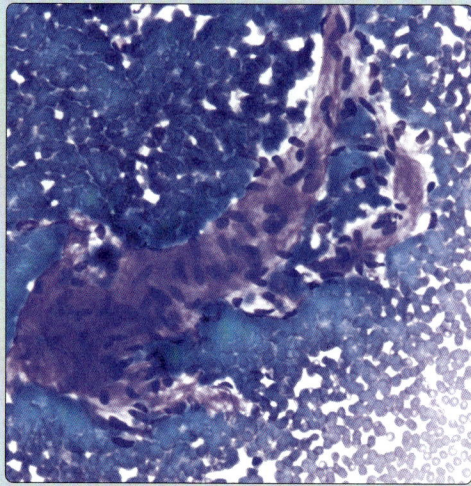

(Left) Diff-Quik-stained FNA high-power view shows uniform, bland, ovoid hemangioma nuclei. The cells have moderate cytoplasm with a spindled morphology. (Right) Diff-Quik-stained FNA shows a fragment of cavernous hemangioma with spindle cells associated with stroma in a background of red blood cells.

Spindle Cells Within Stroma

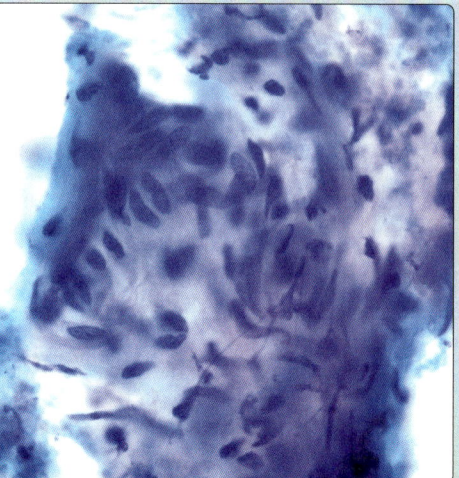

Fibrous Walls With Spindle Cells

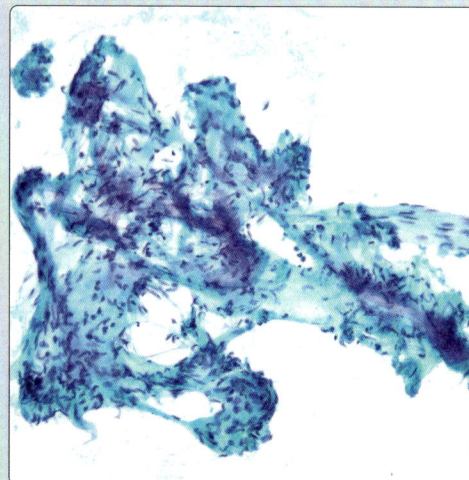

(Left) Pap-stained FNA of hemangioma shows bland, elongated/spindle-shaped nuclei and associated stroma. (Right) Pap-stained FNA shows cyanophilic stroma of fibrous walls associated with bland spindle cells.

Hemangioma, Soft Tissue

TERMINOLOGY

Definitions
- Benign tumor of blood vessels

CLINICAL ISSUES

Presentation
- Common soft tissue tumor at any age
- Most often in skin/subcutaneous tissue but also in liver and other sites
- Single or multiple
- Most are clinically obvious and not aspirated
  - Some deep sites receive FNA to exclude malignancy if diagnosis is not obvious

CYTOPATHOLOGY

Cellularity
- Scanty to acellular; often nondiagnostic

Pattern
- Rare tissue fragments or isolated spindle cells; rarely polygonal cells ± tangles/swirls of cells

Background
- Very bloody ± fibrous stromal fragments

Cells
- Bland, uniform spindle cells; rarely polygonal cells ± minimal pleomorphism

Nuclear Details
- Elongate/oval nuclei ± longitudinal groove/fold in nuclear membrane, fine chromatin, indistinct nucleoli

Cytoplasmic Details
- Moderate amount, varies from pale to dense

Cell Block Findings
- Can be diagnostic if obtained tissue shows vascular channels lined by benign endothelium

ANCILLARY TESTS

Immunohistochemistry
- Endothelial markers: Factor VIII, CD31, CD34, FLI-1, ERG, ± D2-40 (podoplanin) ± *Ulex europaeus*

DIFFERENTIAL DIAGNOSIS

Other Vascular Lesions
- Epithelioid hemangioendothelioma
  - Usually more cellular
  - Myxohyaline stroma
  - Epithelioid cells with abundant cytoplasm ± intracytoplasmic lumina ("neolumina")
  - ± moderate nuclear pleomorphism/atypia
- Angiosarcoma
  - Usually more cellular
  - More cytologic atypia
  - Mitoses generally identified
  - ± necrosis and apoptosis
- Kaposi sarcoma
  - Usually more cellular
  - HHV-8(+)
  - ± hyaline globules inside &/or outside spindle cells
  - Patients usually immunosuppressed, African children/middle-aged adults, or older men of Mediterranean/Eastern European extraction
- Organizing thrombus/hematoma
  - Patient history and clinical/imaging information are usually helpful

SELECTED REFERENCES

1. Flucke U et al: Soft tissue special issue: perivascular and vascular tumors of the head and neck. Head Neck Pathol. 14(1):21-32, 2020
2. Shon W et al: Epithelioid vascular tumors: a review. Adv Anat Pathol. 26(3):186-97, 2019
3. Sharma S et al: Cytological diagnosis of deep-seated cellular hemangioma of the parotid gland by using cell button technique. J Cytol. 33(3):174-6, 2016

Fibrous Walls With Bland Endothelial Cells

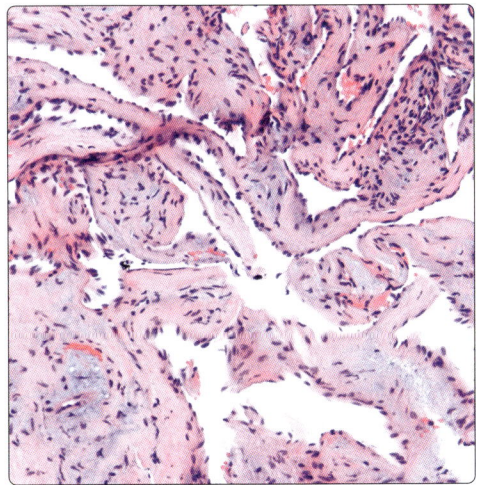

Endothelium-Lined Spaces Containing Red Blood Cells

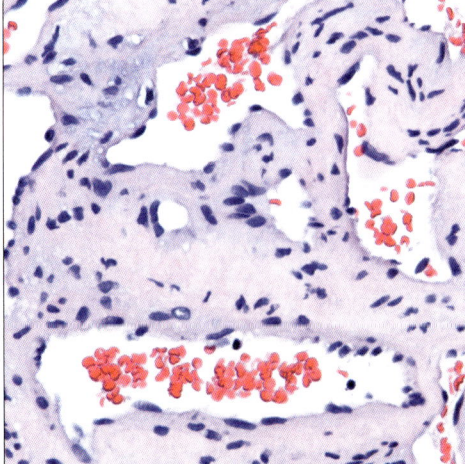

(Left) H&E-stained section of a core needle biopsy of a hepatic cavernous hemangioma shows bland fibrous walls lined by flattened endothelial cells. (Right) Higher power view of an H&E-stained core needle biopsy shows bland endothelial cell nuclei lining spaces containing red blood cells.

Epithelioid Hemangioendothelioma

KEY FACTS

CLINICAL ISSUES
- Low-grade malignant vascular neoplasm
- Rare tumor arising in soft tissues, bone, lung, liver, and other organs
- Behavior intermediate between hemangioma and angiosarcoma
- Wide age range but rare in children
- Solitary or multicentric, especially in viscera

CYTOPATHOLOGY
- Epithelioid (polygonal) vacuolated blister cells, plasmacytoid cells, spindle cells, ± moderate pleomorphism/atypia
- Large, irregular/lobulated/folded nuclear shapes, vesicular chromatin, prominent nucleoli, ± bi-/multinucleation, ± cytoplasmic intranuclear inclusions
- Abundant cytoplasm with vacuoles (neolumina) ± intact or fragmented RBC contents

ANCILLARY TESTS
- Positive immunostains: CD31, CD34, ERG, factor VIII, FLI-1, vimentin
  - ± D2-40, cytokeratin, SMA, and CD10
- Negative immunostains: Mucin, EMA, CEA, AFP, S100, CD117, glypican-3
- Translocation t(1;3)(p36.3;q25); *WWTR1::CAMTA1* fusion in 90% cases
- *YAP1::TFE3* fusion in < 5%

TOP DIFFERENTIAL DIAGNOSES
- Adenocarcinoma
- Epithelioid vascular tumors
  - Epithelioid hemangioma
  - Epithelioid angiosarcoma
  - Pseudomyogenic hemangioendothelioma
- Epithelioid sarcoma
- Melanoma

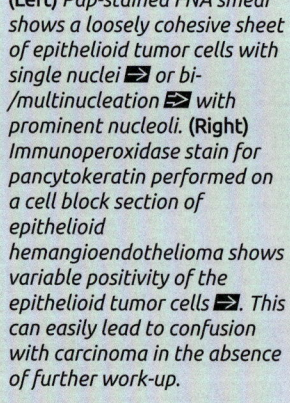

(Left) Pap-stained FNA smear shows a loosely cohesive sheet of epithelioid tumor cells with single nuclei ➡ or bi-/multinucleation ➡ with prominent nucleoli. (Right) Immunoperoxidase stain for pancytokeratin performed on a cell block section of epithelioid hemangioendothelioma shows variable positivity of the epithelioid tumor cells ➡. This can easily lead to confusion with carcinoma in the absence of further work-up.

Cells With Single or Multiple Nuclei

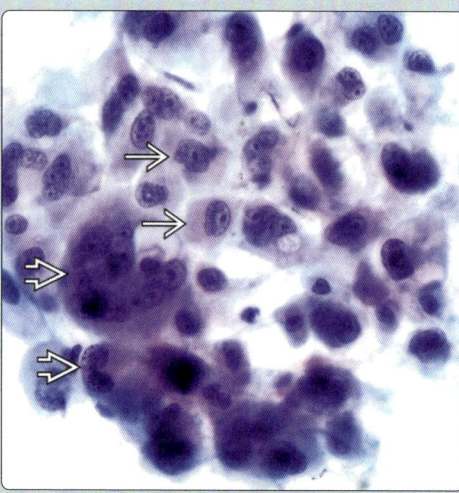

Variable Positivity for Pancytokeratin

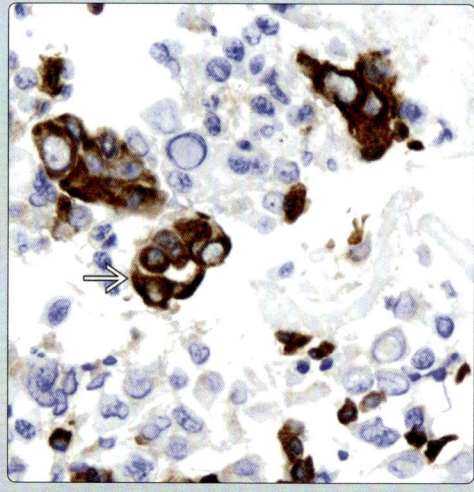

(Left) Pap-stained FNA smear of epithelioid hemangioendothelioma shows large cytoplasmic intranuclear inclusions in some of the tumor cells ➡. (Right) Diff-Quik-stained FNA smear of epithelioid hemangioendothelioma shows epithelioid tumor cells with eccentrically located nuclei ➡.

Intranuclear Inclusions

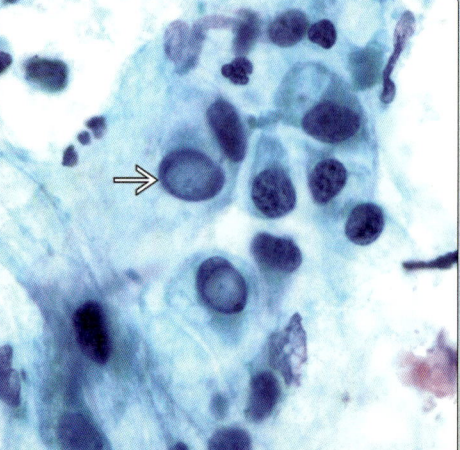

Diff-Quik Appearance

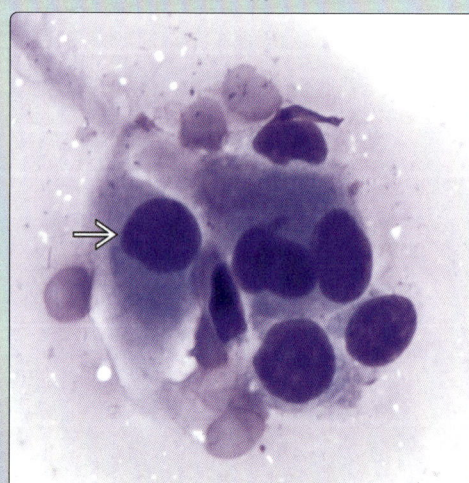

Epithelioid Hemangioendothelioma

TERMINOLOGY

Definitions
- Low-grade malignant vascular neoplasm

CLINICAL ISSUES

Epidemiology
- Rare tumor arising in soft tissues, bone, lung, liver, and other organs
- Wide age range but rare in children
- Solitary or multicentric, especially in viscera

Treatment and Prognosis
- Intermediate behavior between hemangioma and angiosarcoma

CYTOPATHOLOGY

Pattern
- Loosely cohesive sheets, cell clusters, whorls, single cells

Cells
- Epithelioid (polygonal) vacuolated blister cells, plasmacytoid cells, spindle cells, ± moderate pleomorphism/atypia

Nuclear Details
- Large, irregular/lobulated/folded nuclear shapes, vesicular chromatin, prominent nucleoli, ± bi-/multinucleation, ± cytoplasmic intranuclear inclusions

Cytoplasmic Details
- Abundant with vacuoles (neolumina)
- May have intact or fragmented RBCs in vacuoles

ANCILLARY TESTS

Genetic Testing
- t(1;3)(p36.3;q5) translocation, *WWTR1::CAMTA1* fusion in 90%; *YAP1::TFE3* fusion in < 5%

Immunohistochemistry and Histochemistry
- Positive: CD31, CD34, ERG, factor VIII, FLI-1, vimentin, D2-40 (podoplanin) ±, cytokeratin ±, SMA ±, CD10 ±, CAMTA1 ± (90%), TFE3 ± (< 5%)
- Negative: Mucin, EMA, CEA, AFP, S100, CD117, glypican-3

DIFFERENTIAL DIAGNOSIS

Adenocarcinoma
- Negative for vascular markers, positive for pancytokeratin and EMA
- Vacuoles in adenocarcinoma are mucin positive and lack RBC contents

Epithelioid Hemangioma
- Less cellular, lacks myxohyaline stroma and intracytoplasmic lumina, ± RBCs

Epithelioid Sarcoma
- Pancytokeratin and EMA positive, CD31 positive, loss of INI1 expression

Epithelioid Angiosarcoma
- More atypia, mitotic activity, tumor necrosis, and apoptosis
  - Lacks genomic findings, including t(1;3)(p36.3;q25), *WWTR1::CAMTA1* fusion

Melanoma
- Positive for melanocytic markers

Pseudomyogenic Hemangioendothelioma
- Plump spindled and epithelioid cells with abundant eosinophilic cytoplasm, coexpression of keratin and endothelial markers; *SERPINE1::FOSB* fusion

SELECTED REFERENCES

1. Abd El Hafez A: Primary diagnosis of epithelioid hemangioendothelioma in pleural effusion based on cytologic features and vascular marker immunocytochemical staining. J Cytol. 38(2):101-3, 2021
2. Jebastin Thangaiah J et al: Cytologic features and immunohistochemical findings of epithelioid hemangioendothelioma (EHE) in effusion: a case series. Diagn Cytopathol. 49(1):E24-30, 2021

Blister Cells
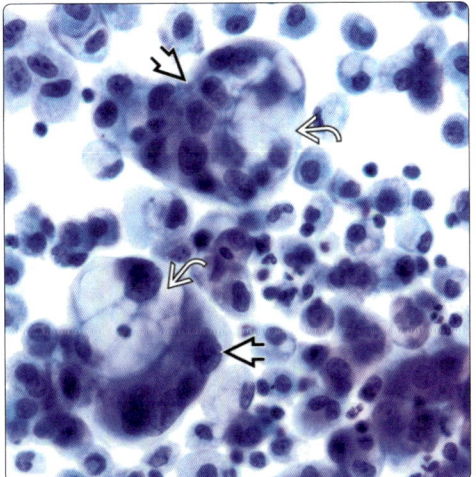

Cell Block
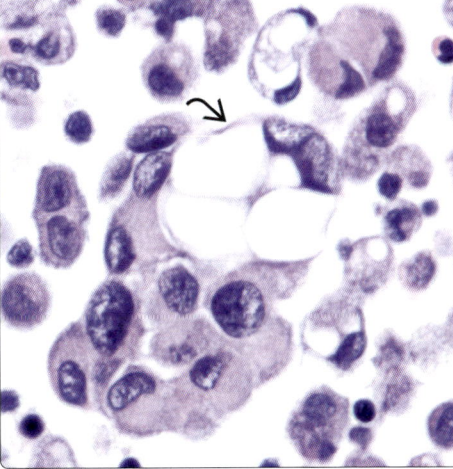

(Left) Pap-stained cytocentrifuge preparation of pleural effusion from a patient with epithelioid hemangioendothelioma involving the right lung and pleura shows large clusters ➡ of tumor cells with enlarged nuclei and abundant, focally vacuolated cytoplasm. Note the blister cells ➡. (Right) H&E-stained cell block preparation of the effusion shows another blister cell ➡ amidst the loose cluster of epithelioid tumor cells.

Angiosarcoma

KEY FACTS

CLINICAL ISSUES
- Most occur in older adults, rarely in children
- Widely distributed with most occurring in cutaneous soft tissue and visceral sites
  - Epithelioid subtype most often in deep soft tissues
- Risk factors/associations: Lymphedema, radiation, sun exposure, Thorotrast, arsenicals, polyvinyl chloride, cirrhosis, foreign bodies
- Treatment: Aggressive surgical resection with wide tumor-free margins if possible &/or XRT &/or chemotherapy

CYTOPATHOLOGY
- Epithelioid, spindle, or mixed tumor cell morphology
- Variable cytologic atypia, ranging from moderate to marked
- May show evidence of vasoformation (neolumens ± RBCs, anastomosing sieve-like vascular channels, endothelial multilayering, and papillary formation)
- Isolated cells and cells in groups (syncytia, clusters, whorls, rosette-like structures, pseudoacini)

ANCILLARY TESTS
- Endothelial markers [CD31, FLI-1, ERG, factor VIII (+/-), CD34(+/-), D2-40(+/-)] can be used to support diagnosis
- Other lineage markers to be used to exclude other entities in differential diagnosis
- Epithelioid angiosarcoma may be (+) for pancytokeratin &/or EMA
- MYC amplifications in some, secondary to radiation/chronic lymphedema
- Neolumens are mucin (-)

TOP DIFFERENTIAL DIAGNOSES
- Wide differential includes many benign and malignant spindle cell &/or epithelioid proliferations
- Melanoma, carcinoma, other sarcomas, mesothelioma, gastrointestinal stromal tumor, hemangioma, atypical vascular lesion, epithelioid hemangioendothelioma

Spindle Cells
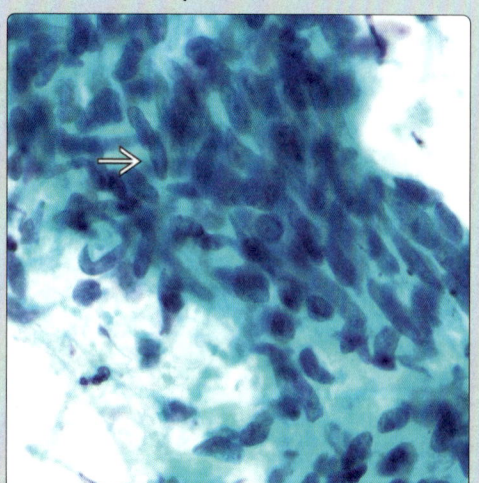

Vascular Channels
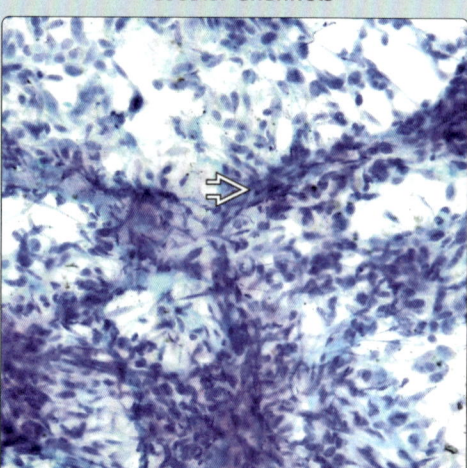

(Left) Pap-stained FNA smear of high-grade angiosarcoma shows a densely cellular fragment of proliferating spindle cells ➡. (Right) Pap-stained FNA smear of high-grade angiosarcoma shows spindled tumor cells forming vascular channels ➡.

Angiosarcoma
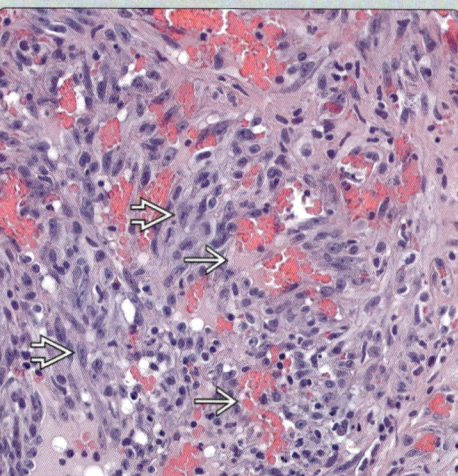

CD31 immunostain
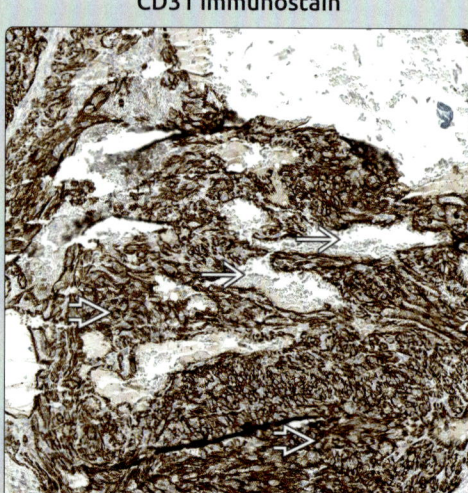

(Left) Skin excision stained with H&E shows malignant spindle cells with elongated nucleus, prominent nucleolus, and scant cytoplasm ➡. There are vascular spaces containing red blood cells ➡ amidst the tumor cells. The overall features are consistent with angiosarcoma. (Right) Skin excision specimen immunostained with CD31 shows the malignant spindle cells forming vascular spaces ➡ to be positive ➡, which supports the diagnosis of angiosarcoma.

Angiosarcoma

CLINICAL ISSUES

Site
- Can arise anywhere in body

Presentation
- May present with purple plaques/patches/nodules on skin, symptomatic or asymptomatic mass in soft tissue, bone, or viscera, coagulation dysfunction

Prognosis
- Poor prognosis with 5-year survival rate of ~ 30%

CYTOPATHOLOGY

Cellularity
- Variable: Very well-differentiated tumors tend to be hypocellular and bloody; more poorly differentiated tumors are usually more cellular

Pattern
- Isolated cells, cells in groups (syncytia, clusters, whorls, rosette-like structures, pseudoacini ± luminal RBCs), tumor fragments

Cells
- Bland to mildly atypical to markedly anaplastic, depending on tumor differentiation
- Variable morphology: Spindled, epithelioid, signet ring cell-like, rhabdoid, pleomorphic, bi-/multinucleated

Cytoplasmic Details
- Finely to coarsely vacuolated, ± intracytoplasmic lumina (neolumens), ± RBC content, ± hemosiderin

Cell Block Findings
- ± features suggestive of vasoformation (neolumens, anastomosing sieve-like vascular channels, endothelial multilayering, and papillary formation)

ANCILLARY TESTS

Immunohistochemistry
- CD31, FLI-1, and ERG (+); epithelioid variants ± pancytokeratin &/or EMA

Genetic Testing
- *MYC* amplifications in some secondary to radiation/chronic lymphedema

DIFFERENTIAL DIAGNOSIS

Hemangioma and Atypical Vascular Lesion
- Hypocellular and bloody
- Has well-formed vascular structures, no prominent cytologic atypia, no/few mitoses of endothelial cells, no endothelial multilayering/papillary formation, no *MYC* amplifications

Epithelioid Hemangioendothelioma
- May show neolumens ± RBCs, no vessel formation; moderate cytologic atypia; mitotic activity not high
- IHC for endothelial markers (+) but EMA(-)

Melanoma
- Immunohistochemistry (IHC) for endothelial markers (-), melanocytic markers (+)

Poorly Differentiated Carcinoma
- IHC for endothelial markers (-), epithelial markers (+)

Other Sarcomas
- IHC for endothelial markers (-) except for CD34(+/-)
- Epithelioid sarcoma: Loss of nuclear *INI1* expression, CD34 (+) but (-) for more specific endothelial markers (CD31, FLI-1, ERG)

SELECTED REFERENCES

1. Khandakar B et al: Ultrasound-guided fine needle aspiration cytology of angiosarcoma of head and neck: a review of cytomorphologic features and discussion of diagnostic pitfall of aspiration cytology of vascular lesions. Diagn Cytopathol. 49(7):902-6, 2021

Epithelioid-Type Cell Block Findings

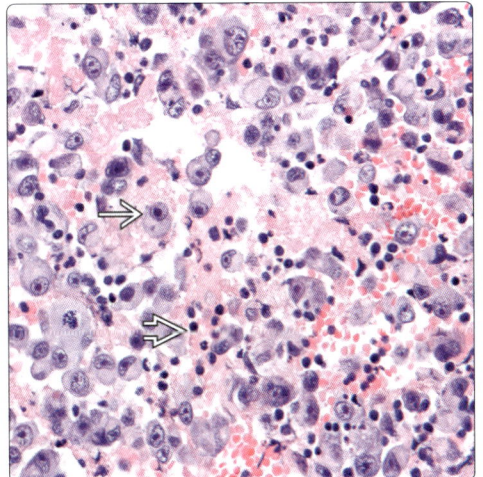

Angiosarcoma, CD31(+)

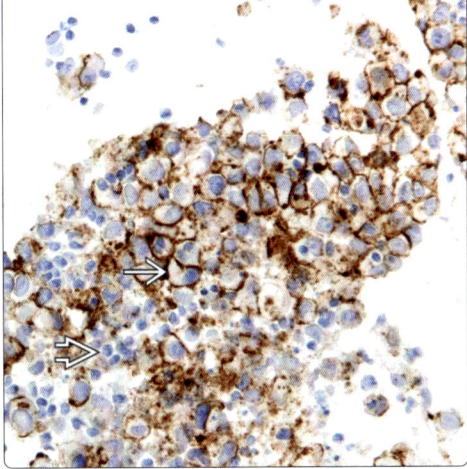

(Left) H&E-stained cell block preparation of epithelioid angiosarcoma shows numerous epithelioid tumor cells ➡ with admixed small lymphocytes ➡. *(Right)* Immunoperoxidase-stained cell block preparation of epithelioid angiosarcoma shows tumor cells to be strongly positive for CD31 ➡, while surrounding small lymphocytes are negative for CD31 ➡.

Other Reactive and Neoplastic Soft Tissue Entities

NODULAR FASCIITIS

General Features

- Benign, self-limited but rapidly growing myofibroblastic mass that produces cellular proliferation and is mitotically active in its early stages
- Head and neck areas, upper trunk, and upper extremities; superficial location; patients usually in 3rd-4th decades
- Histologically, loose storiform feathery pattern with tissue culture-like appearance and loose myxoid stroma ± cystic spaces and dense keloid-like collagen
- Osteoclast-like giant cells, histiocytes, lymphocytes, and extravasated erythrocytes can be seen
- 3 forms correlating with duration of lesion: Myxoid [earliest (within days)], cellular, and fibrous
- **Molecular**: Majority (> 90%) overexpress *USP6* gene rearrangement (located on 17p13) with most common partner (in 60%) being *MYH9*, (located on 22q12.3-q13); FISH testing available and helpful on cytology specimens and in difficult cases
- **IHC**: Cytokeratin, CD34, muscle markers, and nuclear β-catenin negative

Cytology

- Aspirates can be cellular depending on phase of lesion
- Background can be myxoid with scattered lymphocytes, macrophages, and (rarely) osteoclastic giant cells
- Mitosis may be seen but is not atypical
- Loosely arranged plump to stellate spindle cells
- May be misdiagnosed as sarcoma
    - Superficial location and age are important

PROLIFERATIVE MYOSITIS/FASCIITIS

General Features

- Tumefactive intramuscular or subcutaneous proliferation featuring ganglion-like fibroblasts in background of myofibroblasts and fibroblasts, similar to nodular fasciitis
- Presents in middle age and older adults with painless, poorly circumscribed mass, growing rapidly along connective tissue septa

Nodular Fasciitis Touch Prep

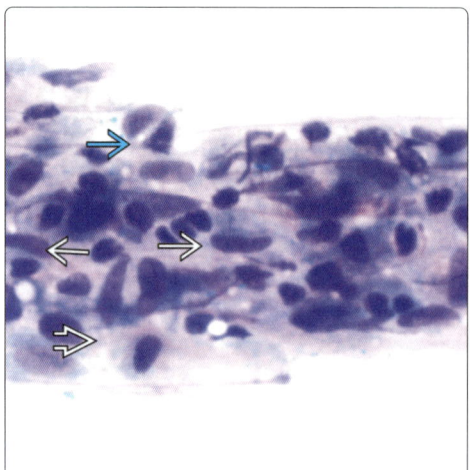

Proliferative Myositis

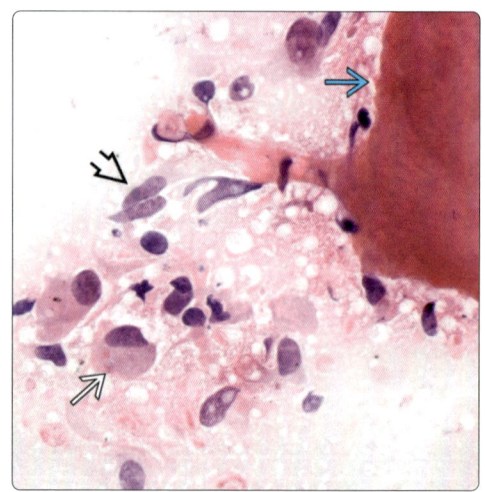

(Left) Diff-Quik-stained touch prep shows bipolar spindle cells ➡ and plump to stellate cells ➡ in a loose myxoid stromal background ➡. *(Right)* H&E-stained touch prep shows large ganglion-like cells ➡, spindle cells ➡, and degenerating skeletal muscle ➡. The background can be myxoid or have a precipitate.

Myositis Ossificans

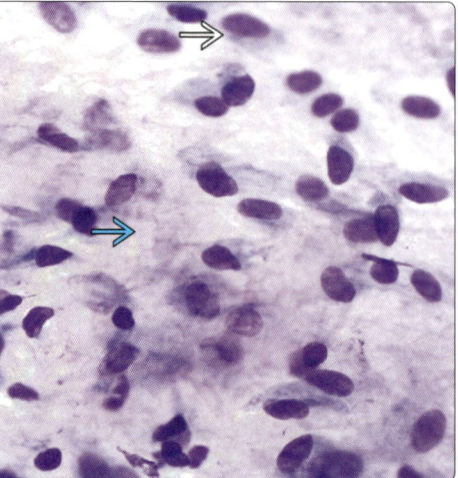

Ganglioneuroma

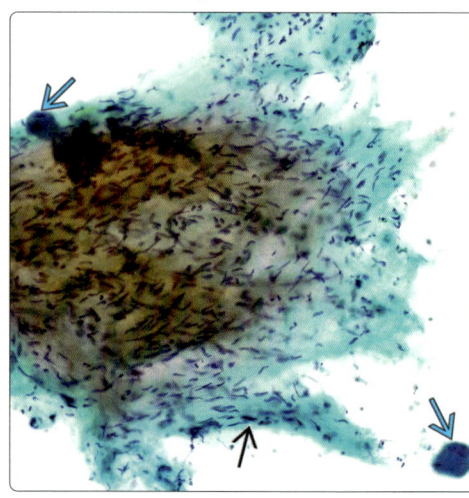

(Left) Diff-Quik-stained touch prep of a core needle biopsy for rapid on-site evaluation of a calcified mass in a zonal pattern shows plump spindle cells ➡ in a repair-like pattern with a loose myxoid ➡ background. *(Right)* Pap-stained smear of a retroperitoneal ganglioneuroma shows spindle cells with elongated nuclei ➡ and fibrillary ill-defined cytoplasm. The large ganglion cells ➡ are easily visible in this smear and may contain cytoplasmic pigment.

Other Reactive and Neoplastic Soft Tissue Entities

- Histologically characterized by plump stellate to spindle-shaped myofibroblasts and fibroblasts with background lymphocytes and extravasated erythrocytes
- Large ganglion-like cells with macronucleoli and abundant cytoplasm
- Brisk mitotic activity may result in misinterpretation as sarcoma; *USP6* gene rearrangement demonstrated by FISH

Cytology
- Variably cellular aspirates with large ganglion-like cells with prominent nucleoli
- Background stellate cells, myxoid stroma, lymphocytes, and erythrocytes
- Degenerating skeletal muscle fibers with striations may be seen
- **Differential diagnosis**: Pleomorphic undifferentiated sarcoma, rhabdomyosarcoma

MYOSITIS OSSIFICANS
General Features
- Localized, self-limited, benign, fibroosseous pseudotumor of digits or soft tissues; wide age range, mean: ~ 30 years
- Radiologically and histologically classic zonation with cellular central area and peripheral ossification
- Central portion with myofibroblastic proliferation with active mitosis reminiscent of nodular fasciitis

Cytology
- Plump stellate fibroblasts
- Loose myxoid stroma with scattered lymphocytes and histiocytes; *USP6* gene rearrangement demonstrated by FISH
- **Differential diagnosis**: Extraskeletal osteosarcoma, which lacks zonation and is markedly atypical

GANGLIONEUROMA
General Features
- Benign, well-differentiated neoplasm containing ganglion cells and arising from sympathetic or peripheral nerves
- Usually solitary, painless mass in posterior mediastinum or retroperitoneum, rarely adrenal and other locations
- Age: 10-30 years

Cytology
- Uniform tight bundles of spindle, nerve-like/Schwann cells with scattered large ganglion cells
- Ganglion cells may contain fine cytoplasmic granular pigment
- **IHC**: S100(+) in Schwann cells; synaptophysin (+) in ganglion cells
- **Differential diagnosis**: Ganglioneuroblastoma: Younger age and contains immature neuroblasts; neurofibroma and schwannoma, which lack ganglion cells

ABDOMINAL FAT PAD ASPIRATION FOR AMYLOID
General Features
- Performed for diagnosis of systemic amyloidosis
- Sensitivity: Low (19-70%); specificity: Close to 100%
- If positive, then speciation by immunohistochemistry or mass spectrometry is crucial for management

Cytology
- Fat pad aspiration between umbilicus and symphysis pubis is performed using 21-gauge needle
- Smears on frosted slides and cell block should be prepared
- Alkaline Congo red stain on smears and cell block
- Congophilia with apple-green birefringence is diagnostic
- Alternatively, electron microscopy can be performed for diagnosis and is thought by some to be more sensitive
- Congophilia should follow contours of adipocytes or around blood vessels
- Apple-green birefringence should be fine and in same pattern as congophilia

SELECTED REFERENCES
1. Hasegawa K et al: Abdominal fat pad fine-needle aspiration for diagnosis of cardiac amyloidosis in patients with non-ischemic cardiomyopathy. Int Heart J. 63(1):49-55, 2022

Congo Red (+) Fat Pad Aspiration

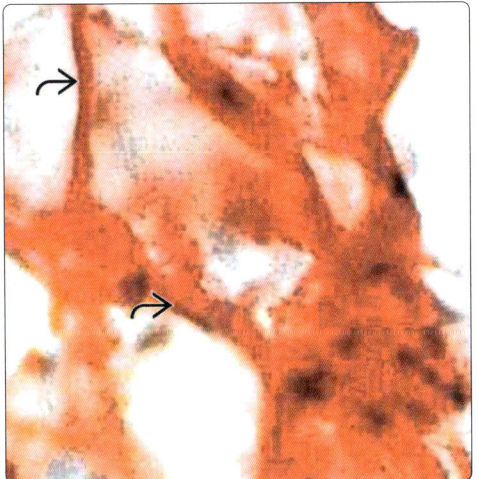

Apple Green Birefringence

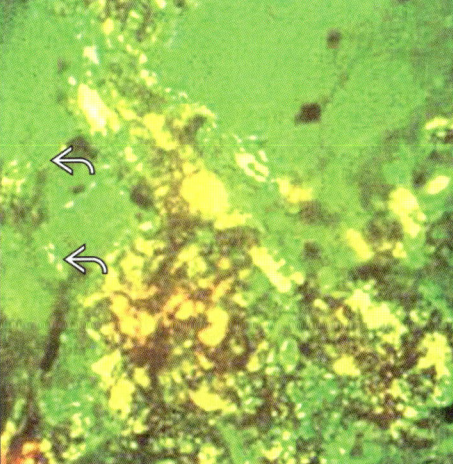

(Left) Congo red stain of an abdominal fat pad aspirate shows congophilia following the contours of the adipocytes ➔. *(Right)* Polarization shows apple green birefringence of the congophilic fibers following the adipocyte contours in a fine fibrillar pattern ➔, characteristic of amyloid.

Mesenchymal Chondrosarcoma

KEY FACTS

CLINICAL ISSUES
- Primary can be in skeleton (2/3) or extraskeletal
- Wide age range: 2-75 years; most between 10-40 years
- Any bone or soft tissue site can be involved; in long bone, arises in diaphyses
- Symptoms and presentation depend on site of origin
- Radiographically destructive tumor with stippled calcifications in bone
- Soft tissue masses can be large depending on location and may appear well circumscribed
- 5-year survival: 55%; 10-year survival: 28%

MICROSCOPIC
- Bimorphic pattern of small round or spindle cells with hyaline cartilaginous islands
- Cellular specimen on FNA or touch preps of cores
- Small, round blue cells or spindle cells with hyperchromasia and scant cytoplasm
- Cartilaginous stroma can be hyaline or fibrillary (similar to pleomorphic adenoma)
- Coarse nuclear chromatin; may show small nucleoli
- Pericytomatous vessels seen on histology but rare on cytology/small biopsy

ANCILLARY TESTS
- CD99 and SOX9 (+), NKX2.2(+) in up to 75%, desmin (+) in 50%, EMA(+) in 35%
- S100 and ERG (+) in cartilage only
- FLI1, STAT6, CD45, SMA, GFAP, keratin, and myogenin (-); MyoD1 [very rare focal (+)]
- Recurrent *HEY1::NCOA2* fusion (in 90%) detectable by RT-PCR (or FISH)

TOP DIFFERENTIAL DIAGNOSES
- Other primitive small round blue or spindle cell tumors, such as Ewing sarcoma, synovial sarcoma, rhabdomyosarcoma, osteosarcoma, malignant solitary fibrous tumor, extraskeletal myxoid chondrosarcoma

Fibrillary Stroma and Small Blue Cells

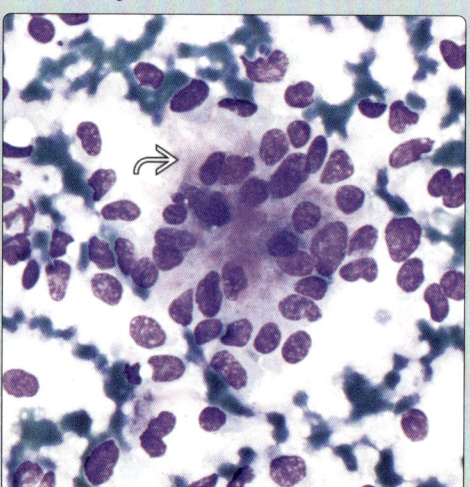

Nuclear Details on Pap Stain

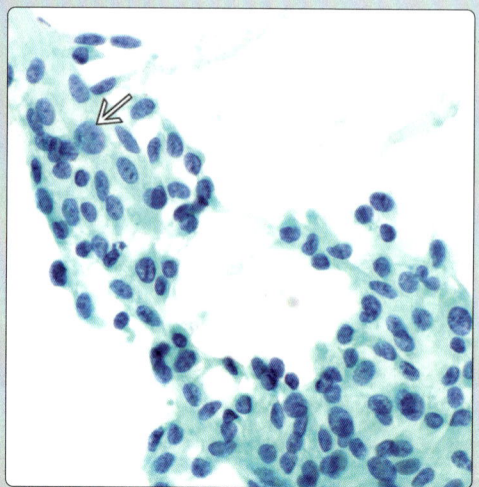

(Left) Diff-Quik stain of a mesenchymal chondrosarcoma shows a monotonous population of small blue cells with fibrillary magenta stroma ⇨ and lack of lymphoglandular bodies in the background. (Right) Cells show round to oval nuclei with smooth contours and occasional small nucleoli/chromocenters ➔. There is a uniform heterogeneity to the nuclear sizes and shapes.

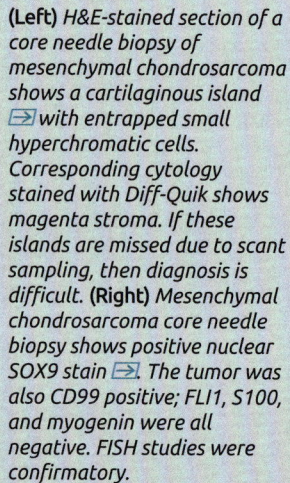

Core Biopsy With Cartilaginous Island

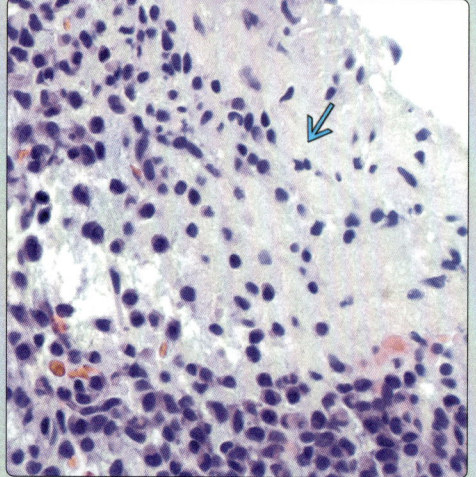

Nuclear SOX9 in Core Needle Biopsy

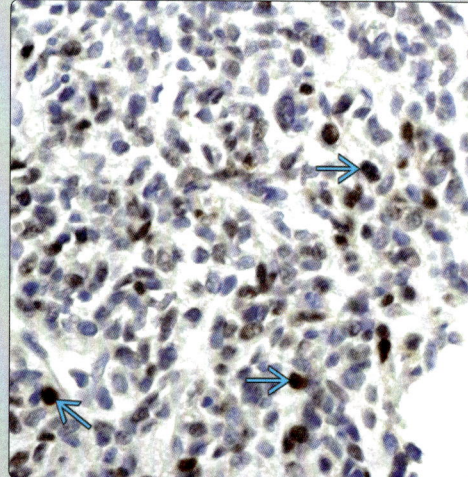

(Left) H&E-stained section of a core needle biopsy of mesenchymal chondrosarcoma shows a cartilaginous island ➔ with entrapped small hyperchromatic cells. Corresponding cytology stained with Diff-Quik shows magenta stroma. If these islands are missed due to scant sampling, then diagnosis is difficult. (Right) Mesenchymal chondrosarcoma core needle biopsy shows positive nuclear SOX9 stain ➔. The tumor was also CD99 positive; FLI1, S100, and myogenin were all negative. FISH studies were confirmatory.

Solitary Fibrous Tumor

KEY FACTS

TERMINOLOGY
- Solitary fibrous tumor (SFT)
- Tumors previously known as hemangiopericytomas now classified as SFT
- Fibroblastic mesenchymal tumor, characteristically featuring prominent branching staghorn vascular pattern (hemangiopericytomatous vessels)

CLINICAL ISSUES
- Usually adults 20-70 years; M > F; lobulated, circumscribed; 1-20 cm
- Can occur in any body site, including pleura, where it has characteristic radiologic appearance
- Can be benign or malignant; risk stratification model based on patient age, tumor size, mitosis/mm², and necrosis

MICROSCOPIC
- Falls in differential diagnosis of spindle cell soft tissue neoplasms
- Plump spindle cells with bland nuclei, either dispersed or embedded in metachromatically staining ropy collagen
- Malignant SFTs are pleomorphic and mitotically active (> 4/10 HPF)
- Mast cells common, occasional multinucleated giant stromal cells
- Lipomatous and giant cell rich types recently described

ANCILLARY TESTS
- Strong and diffuse nuclear STAT6(+) is diagnostic; CD34(+), often diffuse, can be patchy but not specific
- Nuclear β-catenin, BCL2, CD99, EMA can also be (+) in subset
- Keratin, S100 protein, desmin, CD117, DOG1, CD31 (-)

TOP DIFFERENTIAL DIAGNOSES
- Other benign and low-grade spindle cell neoplasms
  - Schwannoma, low-grade malignant nerve sheath tumors, GIST, monophasic synovial sarcoma, leiomyosarcoma

Ropy Collagen and Spindle Cells
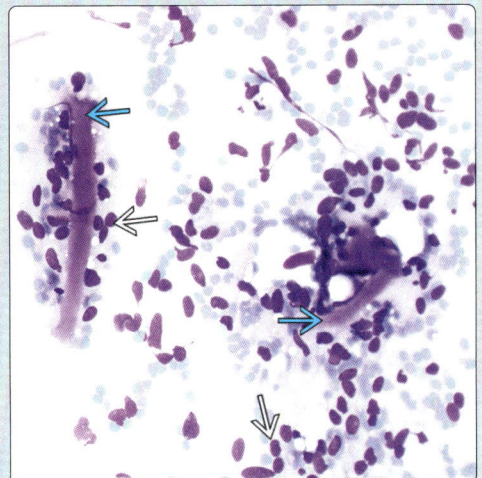

Dense Stroma and Spindle Cells
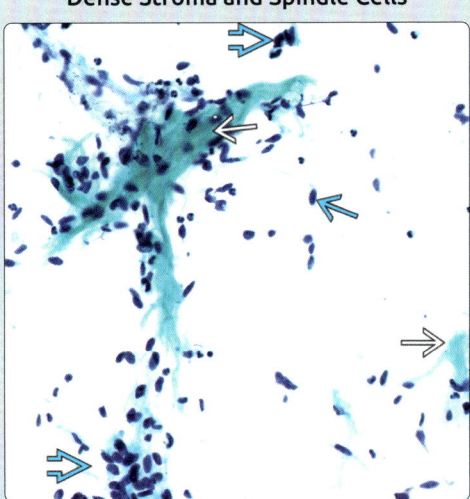

(Left) Diff-Quik stain of a touch prep of a core needle biopsy for rapid onsite evaluation is shown. The magenta-staining ropy collagen ➡ is easily visible. The plump spindle cells ➡ are either attached to the collagen or dispersed singly. *(Right)* Pap-stained smear of a solitary fibrous tumor (SFT) shows dense, ropy collagenous stroma ➡. The spindle cells are adherent to the stroma as well as seen singly ➡ or in small groups ➡ in the background away from the collagen.

Cellular and Collagenous Areas
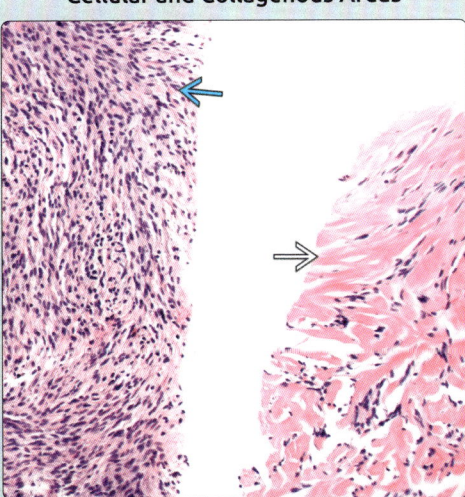

Nuclear Positive STAT6
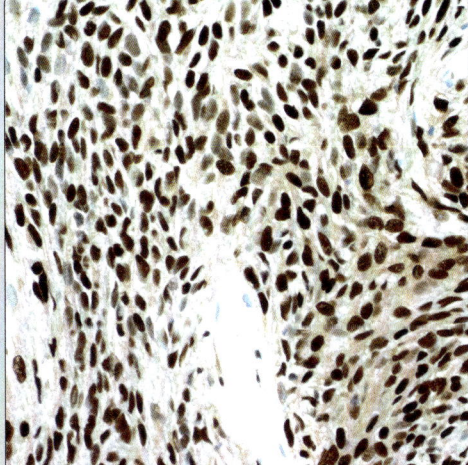

(Left) H&E-stained small biopsy of SFT shows 2 cores, one of which is cellular ➡, and the other is hypocellular with dense, ropy collagen ➡ that is also seen on cytology. Note the lack of mitosis or necrosis in this benign SFT. *(Right)* Immunohistochemistry for STAT6 in this biopsy specimen shows strong nuclear positivity, diagnostic for SFT. CD34 was also positive.

Intramuscular Myxoma

KEY FACTS

CLINICAL ISSUES
- Benign neoplasm of mesenchymal cells that produces hyaluronic acid-rich stroma
- Most in ages 40-70; slight female predominance
- Usually slow-growing, painless mass in large muscles of thighs, shoulders, buttocks, upper arms
- Cured by complete local excision; nonmetastasizing

CYTOPATHOLOGY
- Low cellularity but may be mildly increased in cellular myxoma variant
- Scattered single spindle/stellate cells with long slender cytoplasmic processes
  - ± mild atypia in spindle cells
  - ± "school of fish" cell groups "swimming" in myxoid background
- Myxoid material in background
  - Basophilic and fibrillar on Pap, metachromatic and granular on Romanowsky
- Sparse to absent background nonarborizing, thin-walled blood vessels, ± mast cells, ± macrophages, ± fibrosis, ± skeletal muscle cells

ANCILLARY TESTS
- Positive for actin, desmin, CD34; negative for S100, *GNAS* mutations

TOP DIFFERENTIAL DIAGNOSES
- Nonneoplastic lesions
  - Nodular fasciitis, intramuscular ganglion, focal mucinosis, localized myxoid edema
- Benign neoplasms
  - Myxoid nerve sheath tumors, myxoid leiomyoma, angiomyxoma
- Malignant neoplasms
  - Malignant peripheral nerve sheath tumor, low-grade fibromyxoid sarcoma (Evans tumor), myxoid chondrosarcoma, myxoid liposarcoma, low-grade myxofibrosarcoma, embryonal rhabdomyosarcoma

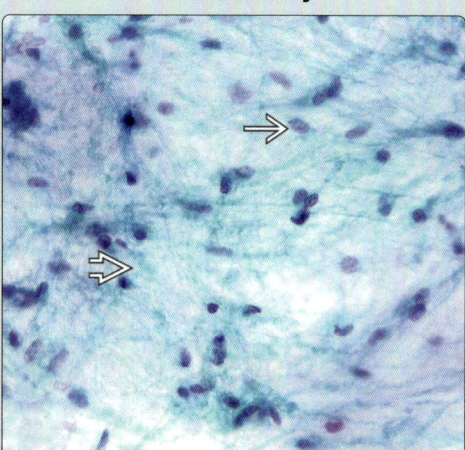

Paucicellularity

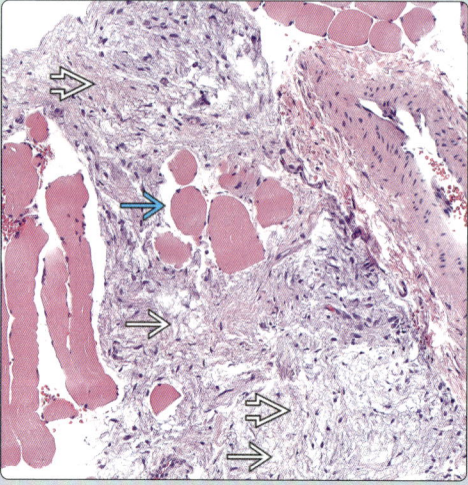

Intramuscular Myxoma

(Left) Pap-stained FNA smear shows a paucicellular spindle cell proliferation ➡ with finely fibrillar material in the background ➡. (Right) Core biopsy of intramuscular myxoma stained with H&E shows spindle cells ➡ without atypia associated with a fibrillary stroma ➡, including skeletal muscle fibers ➡ in the background.

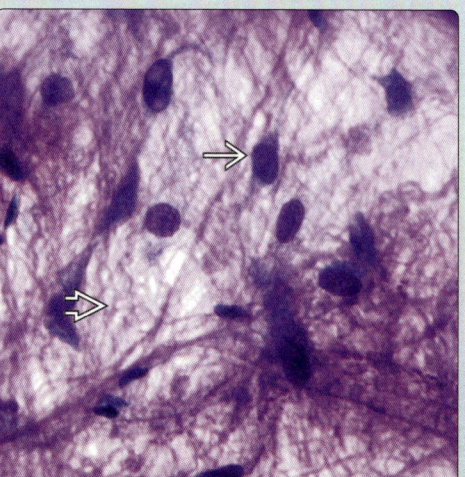

Metachromatic Fibrillary Background

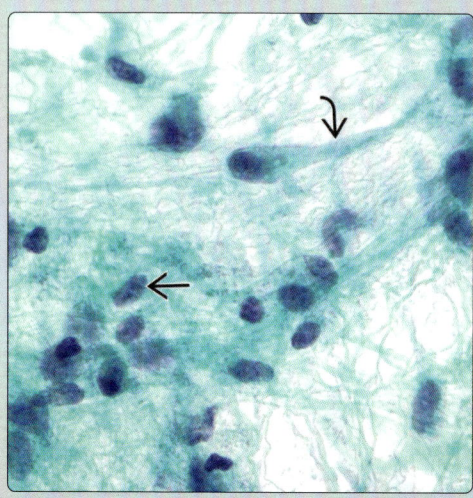

Long Cytoplasmic Process

(Left) Diff-Quik-stained FNA smear of intramuscular myxoma shows tumor cells with a round/ovoid nucleus ➡ without atypia with fibrillary material in the background ➡. (Right) Pap-stained FNA smear of intramuscular myxoma shows tumor cells with an ovoid nucleus ➡. Note the characteristic long, slender, cytoplasmic process ➡ exhibited by one of the tumor cells.

Intramuscular Myxoma

TERMINOLOGY

Definitions
- Benign neoplasm of mesenchymal cells that produces hyaluronic acid-rich stroma

CLINICAL ISSUES

Presentation
- Most in ages 40-70; slight female predominance
- Sporadic or in Mazabraud syndrome (patients have fibrous dysplasia of same extremity bone)
- Usually slow-growing, painless mass in large muscles of thighs, shoulders, buttocks, upper arms

Treatment and Prognosis
- Cured by complete local excision; nonmetastasizing

CYTOPATHOLOGY

Cellularity
- Low but may be increased in cellular myxoma variant

Pattern
- Usually single spindle cells, ± "school of fish" cell groups "swimming" in myxoid background

Background
- Myxoid material: Basophilic and fibrillar on Pap, metachromatic and granular on Romanowsky
- Sparse to absent, nonarborizing, thin-walled blood vessels
- ± mast cells, ± macrophages, ± fibrosis, ± muscle cells

Cells
- Bland spindle/stellate cells, ± mild atypia

Nuclear and Cytoplasmic Details
- Nuclear: Elongate/ovoid, smooth (nonindented) nuclear outlines; fine chromatin; usually indistinct nucleoli
- Cytoplasmic: Characteristic long, slender processes, ± cytoplasmic vacuoles

Cytology-Histology Correlation
- Biopsy is frequently done due to difficulty in making definitive diagnosis on FNA alone
- Histology mirrors FNA with scarce, bland, spindle-shaped, or small stellate cells in paucivascular hyaluronidase-sensitive myxoid matrix

ANCILLARY TESTS

Immunohistochemistry
- Positive for actin, desmin, CD34
- Negative for S100

Genetic Testing
- *GNAS* mutations found in some cases

DIFFERENTIAL DIAGNOSIS

Nonneoplastic Lesions
- Nodular fasciitis, intramuscular ganglion, focal mucinosis, localized myxoid edema

Benign Neoplasms
- Myxoid nerve sheath tumors, myxoid leiomyoma, angiomyxoma

Malignant Neoplasms
- Malignant peripheral nerve sheath tumor, low-grade fibromyxoid sarcoma (Evans tumor), myxoid chondrosarcoma, myxoid liposarcoma, low-grade myxofibrosarcoma, embryonal rhabdomyosarcoma

SELECTED REFERENCES

1. Al Awadhi A et al: A case of intramuscular lumbar myxoma: uncertainty in the preoperative diagnosis of a spinal soft tissue tumour. Neurochirurgie. ePub, 2021
2. Layfield LJ et al: Myxoid neoplasms of bone and soft tissue: a pattern-based approach. J Am Soc Cytopathol. 10(3):278-92, 2021
3. Libbrecht L et al: Next generation sequencing for GNAS uncovers CD34 as a sensitive marker for intramuscular myxoma. Ann Diagn Pathol. 43:151409, 2019
4. Wakely Jr PE et al: The cytopathology of soft tissue mxyomas: ganglia, juxta-articular myxoid lesions, and intramuscular myxoma. Am J Clin Pathol. 123(6):858-65, 2005

Diff-Quik Appearance
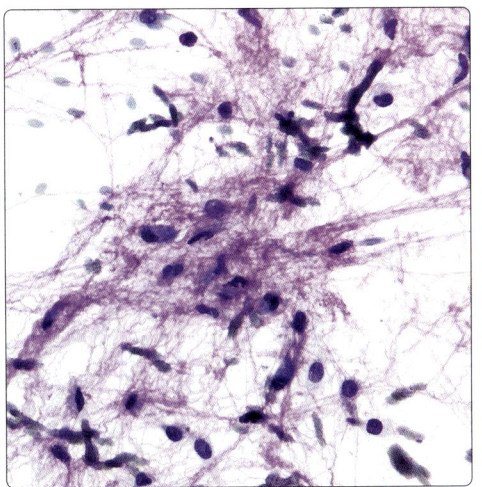

Intramuscular myxoma
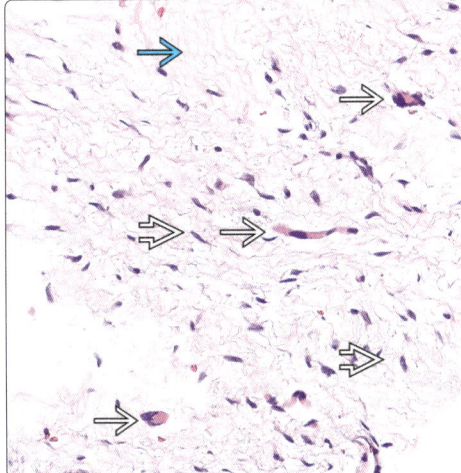

(Left) *Romanowsky-stained FNA shows a paucicellular spindle cell proliferation in a metachromatic, finely fibrillar background.* (Right) *Core biopsy of intramuscular myxoma shows spindle cell proliferation ➡ distributed in a fibrillary background ➡ that includes scattered atrophic skeletal muscle fibers ➡.*

Synovial Sarcoma

KEY FACTS

CLINICAL ISSUES
- 5-10% of soft tissue sarcomas
- Most patients are 15-35 years old, rarely > 50 years, M > F
- In almost any anatomic site, most near large extremity joint, especially knee
- Slow-growing mass, often painful; most deep seated
- Local recurrences are common
- Metastases (often late) most often in lung, bone, lymph nodes

CYTOPATHOLOGY
- Monophasic synovial sarcoma: Small- to medium-sized bland spindle cells, no significant atypia, ovoid nuclei, scant tapered cytoplasm
- Biphasic synovial sarcoma: Spindle and epithelial cells, ± clusters, acini, &/or papillary fragments
- Pleomorphic synovial sarcoma: Variants may have small round cells, larger pleomorphic cells, &/or rhabdoid cells
- Spindle cells: Scant, finely fibrillar, tapering cytoplasm with ill-defined borders
- Background ± mast cells, calcification, myxoid/fibrous matrix, siderophages, cholesterol crystals, and hyaline globules

ANCILLARY TESTS
- IHC and genetic analysis essential for diagnosis
- EMA/pancytokeratin (focally +), vimentin (+), TLE1(+), BCL2(+), CD56(+), CD99(+/-), S100(+/-), FLI-1(+/-), SMARCB1/INI1/BAF47 [(+), reduced expression]
- TLE1 highly specific for synovial sarcoma
- If CD34(+), consider other diagnoses
- Identification of t(X;18)(p11.q11) and corresponding fusion transcripts are diagnostic

TOP DIFFERENTIAL DIAGNOSES
- Malignant peripheral nerve sheath tumor, spindle cell carcinoma, leiomyosarcoma, solitary fibrous tumor, rhabdomyosarcoma, Ewing sarcoma/PNET

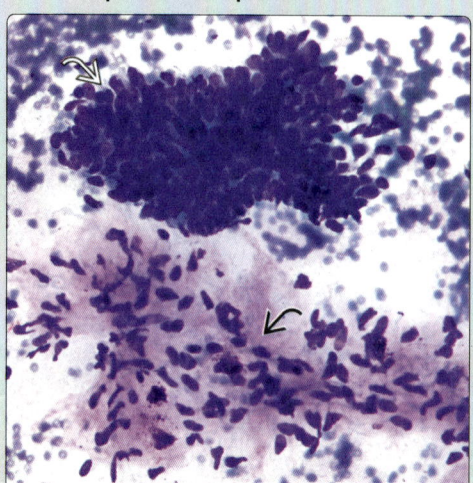

Spindle and Epithelial Cells

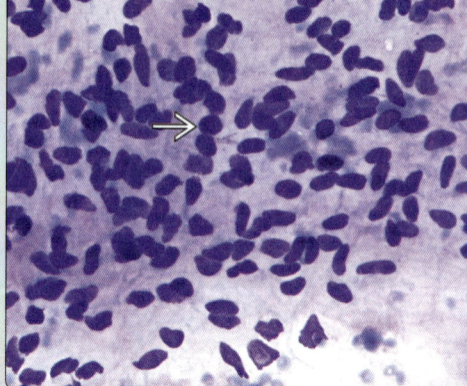

Bland Spindle Cells

(Left) Diff-Quik-stained FNA of biphasic synovial sarcoma shows both epithelial cell ⇨ and spindle cell ⇨ components. (Right) Diff-Quik-stained FNA smear of monophasic synovial sarcoma shows spindle tumor cells with ovoid nuclei ⇨ without significant atypia.

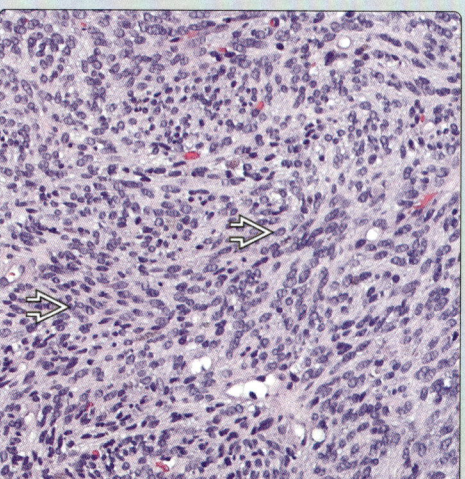

Synovial Sarcoma, Monophasic

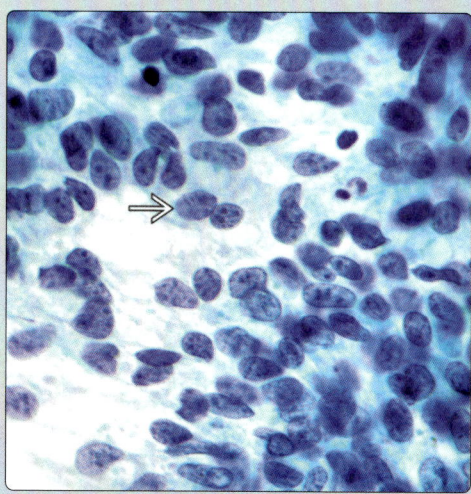

Nuclear Features

(Left) Core biopsy stained with H&E shows monophasic synovial sarcoma composed of intersecting fascicles of spindle cells ⇨ with hyperchromatic nucleus and scant cytoplasm. The tumor showed SS18 (SYT) gene rearrangement by fluorescence in situ hybridization. (Right) Pap-stained FNA smear of monophasic synovial sarcoma shows spindle cells with small, ovoid nuclei with granular chromatin and indistinct nucleoli ⇨.

Synovial Sarcoma

TERMINOLOGY

Definitions
- Malignant mesenchymal spindle cell tumor with variable epithelial differentiation
  - > 90% have chromosomal translocation t(X;18)(p11;q11)

Subtypes
- Biphasic synovial sarcoma (BSS), monophasic spindle synovial sarcoma (MSS), poorly differentiated synovial sarcoma (PSS)

CLINICAL ISSUES

Epidemiology
- 5-10% of soft tissue sarcomas
- Majority in 15-35 years of age, rare > 50 years, M > F

Presentation
- Slow-growing mass, often painful, most deep seated
- In almost any anatomic site, most commonly near large extremity joint, especially knee

CYTOPATHOLOGY

Pattern
- MSS: Singly dispersed cells
- BSS: May have alternating areas of singly dispersed and cohesive cells in clusters ± acini and fragments ± papillary features

Background
- ± mast cells, calcification, myxoid/fibrous matrix, siderophages, cholesterol crystals, and hyaline globules

Cells
- Small- to medium-sized uniform spindle cells with no significant atypia (unless PSS)
- BSS: Epithelial cells in addition to spindle cells
- PSS: Variants may have small round cells, larger pleomorphic cells, &/or rhabdoid cells

Nuclear Details
- Spindle cells: Nuclei bland, ovoid to elongate, hyperchromatic, finely granular chromatin, usually indistinct nucleoli, ± longitudinal fold, mitoses
- Epithelial cells: Nuclei round to ovoid, finely granular chromatin, usually distinct nucleoli, mitoses

Cytoplasmic Details
- Spindle cells: Scant, finely fibrillar, tapering, ill-defined borders

ANCILLARY TESTS

Immunohistochemistry
- EMA/pancytokeratin [(focally)+)], vimentin (+), TLE1(+), BCL2(+), CD56(+)
  - TLE1 is highly specific for SS
- Almost always negative for CD34, desmin, WT1

Cytogenetics/Molecular Genetics
- > 90% have tumor-specific translocation t(X;18)(p11;q11)

DIFFERENTIAL DIAGNOSIS

Malignant Peripheral Nerve Sheath Tumor
- Epithelial markers usually absent (unless glandular differentiation is present), S100/SOX10 (+/-)

Spindle Cell Carcinoma
- Cytokeratin positivity usually more diffuse, TLE1(-)

Leiomyosarcoma
- Desmin/SMA/muscle-specific actin/myosin (+), almost always pancytokeratin/EMA (-)

Solitary Fibrous Tumor
- CD34(+) but cytokeratin/EMA(-)

SELECTED REFERENCES
1. Gazendam AM et al: Synovial sarcoma: a clinical review. Curr Oncol. 28(3):1909-20, 2021

Cohesive Epithelial Cells
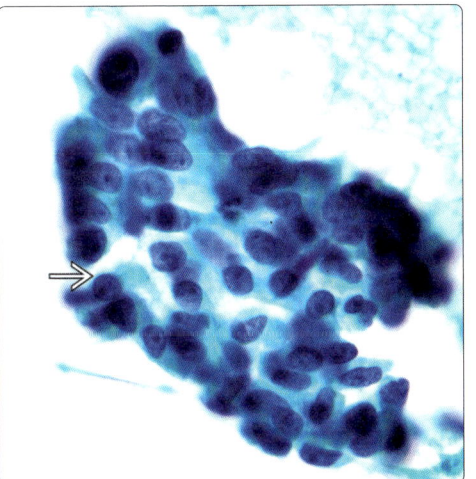

Epithelial Cells With Abundant Cytoplasm
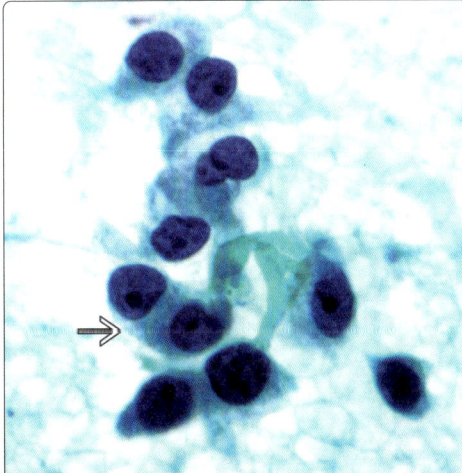

(Left) Pap-stained FNA smear of a biphasic synovial sarcoma shows a cohesive epithelial cell group ➡. (Right) Pap-stained FNA smear of a biphasic synovial sarcoma shows epithelial cells with round nuclei, distinct single, small nucleoli, and more abundant cytoplasm ➡.

Epithelioid Sarcoma

KEY FACTS

CLINICAL ISSUES
- Rare malignant mesenchymal tumor resembling carcinoma or granuloma
  - Shows epithelial and mesenchymal differentiation
- Classic epithelioid sarcoma (CES) occurs commonly in cutis/subcutis of distal extremities (especially hand and forearm) of adolescents and young adults
- Proximal-type ES (PES) occurs commonly in deep/superficial soft tissue of pelvis, perineum, inguinal areas in adults (median age: 40 years)
  - Can grow more rapidly than CES; metastasizes earlier than CES
- Multiple recurrences and relatively late metastases
- Metastases to regional lymph nodes, lungs, bone, brain, and soft tissue

CYTOPATHOLOGY
- Epithelioid &/or spindled, rhabdoid, or polygonal cell morphology
- May be binucleated or multinucleated
- CES bland/less atypical than PES
- May have rhabdoid inclusions of intermediate filaments
- Necrotic debris may be present

ANCILLARY TESTS
- Immunohistochemistry findings
  - Characteristic loss of INI1 expression
  - CK(+), EMA(+), vimentin (+)
  - CD34(+) in 50% of cases; rarely ERG(+) or desmin (+)
  - CD31(-), FLI-1(-), S100(-), HMB-45/MART-1(-), GFAP(-), myogenin/MYOD1(-)
- Chromosome 22q11.2 mutations/deletions in many

TOP DIFFERENTIAL DIAGNOSES
- Carcinoma: Usually more pleomorphism, history of primary
- Melanoma: Usually more pleomorphism, history, distinctive immunohistochemistry
- Epithelioid or rhabdoid sarcomas: Ancillary studies useful

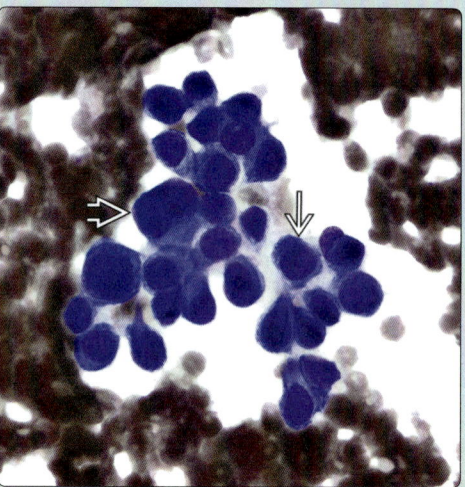

Single and Multiple Nuclei

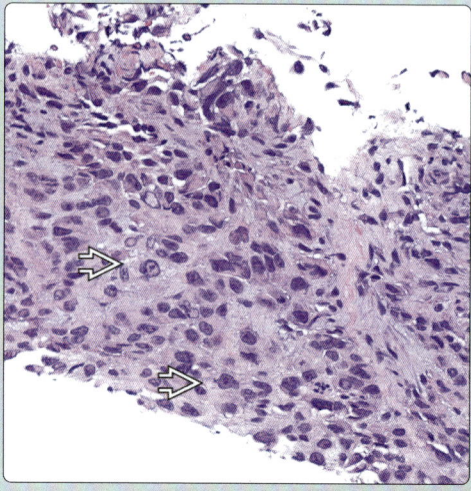

Epithelioid Sarcoma

(Left) Diff-Quik-stained FNA smear shows epithelioid tumor cells with a single nucleus ➡ in the majority of the tumor cells; rare tumor cells are multinucleated ➡. (Right) Core needle biopsy stained with H&E shows sheets of epithelioid tumor cells ➡ with a large polygonal nucleus, prominent nucleolus in many tumor cells, and a scant to moderate amount of cytoplasm. The histopathologic features very closely mimic poorly differentiated carcinoma.

Large Nuclei

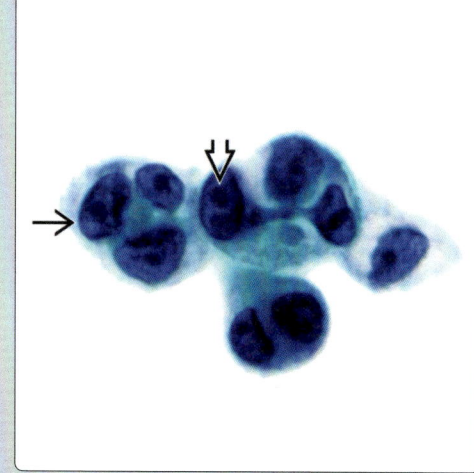

Prominent Nucleoli

(Left) Pap-stained FNA smear shows epithelioid tumor cells ➡ with a large nuclei, which may be central or eccentric, containing prominent nucleoli ➡. (Right) Pap-stained FNA smear of epithelioid sarcoma shows multinucleated epithelioid tumor cells ➡ with prominent nucleoli ➡ and a moderate amount of cytoplasm.

Epithelioid Sarcoma

TERMINOLOGY

Abbreviations
- Epithelioid sarcoma (ES)
  - Proximal-type ES (PES)
  - Classic ES (CES)

Definitions
- Malignant mesenchymal tumor, resembling carcinoma or granuloma, of unknown histogenesis that shows epithelial and mesenchymal differentiation

CLINICAL ISSUES

Epidemiology and Presentation
- Rare (< 1% of all soft tissue sarcomas); M > F
- CES: Slow-growing dermal or subcutaneous nodule, nonhealing ulcer in distal extremities (especially hand and forearm) of adolescents and young adults
- PES: Subcutaneous or deep soft tissue mass in perineal, pelvic, inguinal areas
  - Slightly older age group than CES (median age: 40 years); can grow more rapidly than CES

Behavior, Treatment, and Prognosis
- Multiple local recurrences and late metastatic disease; PES metastasizes earlier than CES
  - Metastases to regional lymph nodes, lungs, bone, brain, and soft tissue
- Optimal treatment: Wide local excision ± chemoradiotherapy
- 5-year survival rate: ~ 70% for CES, 35-65% for PES

CYTOPATHOLOGY

Background
- Necrotic debris may be present

Cells
- Epithelioid &/or spindled, rhabdoid, or polygonal
- Cells may be bi- or multinucleated
- Varying degrees of atypia, greater in PES than CES

Nuclear Details
- Central or eccentric location, vesicular chromatin, ± prominent nucleoli

Cytoplasmic Details
- May have rhabdoid inclusions of intermediate filaments

ANCILLARY TESTS

Immunohistochemistry
- CK(+), EMA(+), vimentin (+), CD34(+) in 50% of cases; rarely ERG(+) or desmin (+)
- Loss of nuclear INI1/BAF47/SMARCB1/hSNF5 expression
- CD31(-), FLI-1(-), S100(-), HMB-45/MART-1(-), GFAP(-), myogenin/MYOD1(-)

Genetic Testing
- Chromosome 22q11.2 mutations/deletions in many

DIFFERENTIAL DIAGNOSIS

Carcinoma
- Usually more pleomorphism, history of primary tumor, but may be very difficult to rule out

Melanoma
- Usually more pleomorphism, distinct immunohistochemistry

Epithelioid and Rhabdoid Sarcomas
- May be difficult by cytology alone; immunohistochemistry and genetic studies helpful

SELECTED REFERENCES
1. Simeone N et al: Tazemetostat for advanced epithelioid sarcoma: current status and future perspectives. Future Oncol. 17(10):1253-63, 2021
2. Gounder M et al: Tazemetostat in advanced epithelioid sarcoma with loss of INI1/SMARCB1: an international, open-label, phase 2 basket study. Lancet Oncol.21(11):1423-32, 2020
3. Li Y et al: Clinicopathologic features of epithelioid sarcoma: report of seventeen cases and review of literature. Int J Clin Exp Pathol. 12(8):3042-8, 2019

Nuclear INI1 Loss
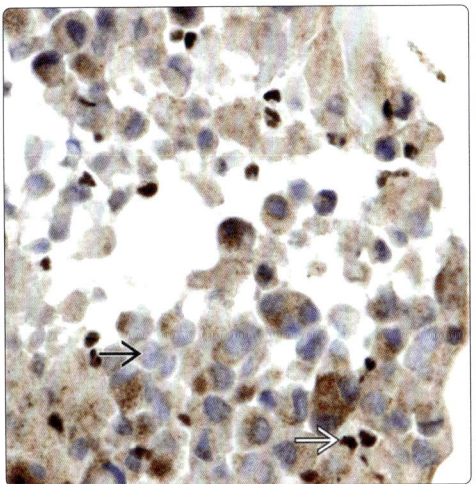

Pancytokeratin Positive
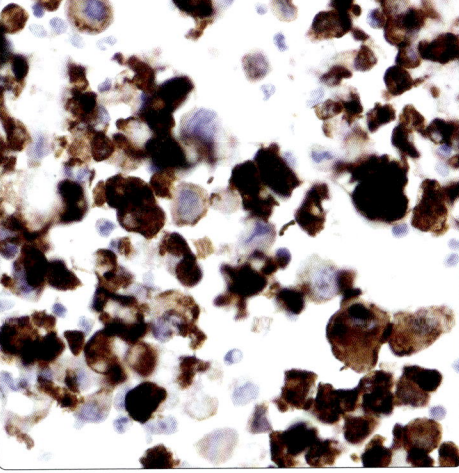

(Left) Immunoperoxidase stain of cell block preparation shows loss of nuclear INI1 expression ➔ in tumor cells with preservation of nuclear staining ➔ in admixed white blood cells. (Right) Immunoperoxidase stain of cell block preparation of epithelioid sarcoma shows tumor cells that are strongly positive for pancytokeratin. This finding may lead to confusion with carcinoma.

Alveolar Soft Part Sarcoma

KEY FACTS

CLINICAL ISSUES
- Malignant soft tissue tumor that mainly affects young adults and children
- Presents as painless, intramuscular, hemorrhagic mass
- Lymphatic invasion almost always present
- Deceptively indolent course
- Late recurrence and metastasis common
- Distant metastasis to lung, bone, and brain in 25%
- 5-year survival rate: 65%

CYTOPATHOLOGY
- Low to moderate cellularity; hemorrhagic background
- Epithelioid-type cells with abundant cytoplasm
- Eccentrically placed nuclei, vesicular chromatin pattern, prominent nucleoli, occasional intranuclear pseudoinclusions
- Finely granular cytoplasm, intracytoplasmic crystalline inclusions
- Granular background and bare nuclei due to cell disruption on smears
- Single cells or 3D alveolar-like clusters lined by endothelial cells

ANCILLARY TESTS
- TFE3(+) by immunohistochemistry, unbalanced translocation (X;17) by cytogenetics
- PAS(+), diastase-resistant granular to crystalline cytoplasmic material, varies from few to all cells
- Desmin focally positive
- Negative: Vimentin, MYOD1, HMB-45, S100, CD34, keratin

TOP DIFFERENTIAL DIAGNOSES
- Myomelanocytic tumor
- Paraganglioma
- Rhabdomyoma
- Granular cell tumor
- Renal cell carcinoma in children

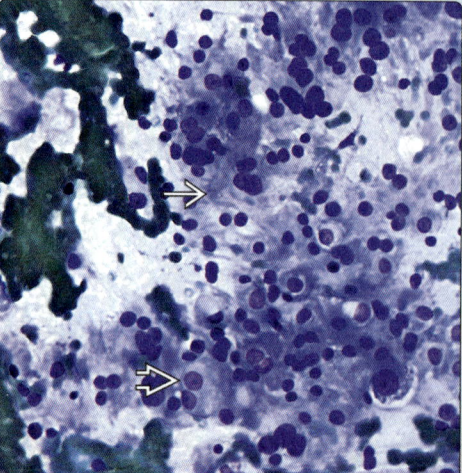

Appearance on Diff-Quik

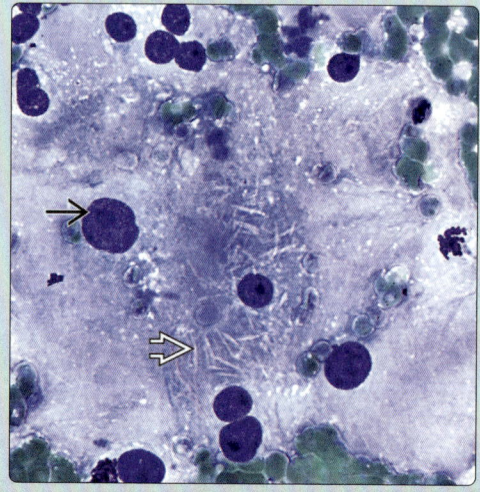

Crystalline Material in Cytoplasm

(Left) Diff-Quik-stained smear shows a sheet of neoplastic cells with finely granular and vacuolated cytoplasm ➡, round nuclei, and prominent nucleoli ➡. *(Right)* Diff-Quik stain demonstrates disrupted cytoplasm appearing as a granular background and nuclei with prominent nucleoli ➡. Intracytoplasmic crystalline structures ➡ are also seen.

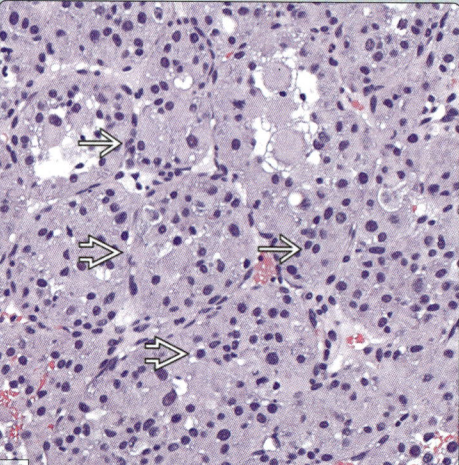

Alveolar Soft Part Sarcoma

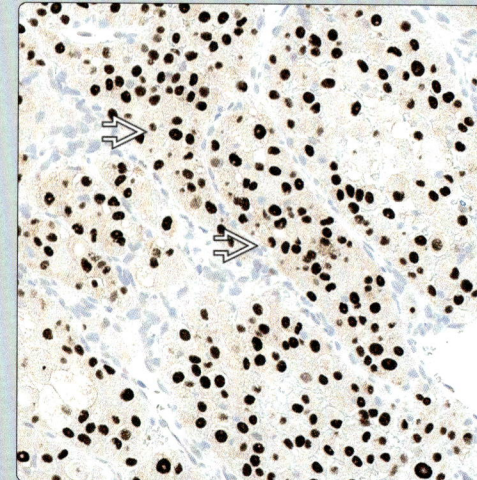

Alveolar Soft Part Sarcoma, TFE3 Positive

(Left) Core biopsy of alveolar soft part sarcoma stained with H&E shows an alveolar pattern of arrangement of tumor cells ➡ that demonstrate a round nucleus with moderate nuclear pleomorphism and abundant, finely granular, eosinophilic cytoplasm ➡. *(Right)* Core biopsy of alveolar soft part sarcoma immunostained for TFE3 shows positive nuclear staining in the tumor cells ➡.

Alveolar Soft Part Sarcoma

TERMINOLOGY

Definitions
- Malignant soft tissue tumor of uncertain phenotype that mainly affects young adults and children
- Clustering alveolar-like growth pattern separated by fibrous septa

CLINICAL ISSUES

Prognosis
- Distant metastasis to lung, bone, and brain present in 25%
- 5-year survival rate: 65%

CYTOPATHOLOGY

Cellularity
- Low to moderate cellularity; hemorrhagic background

Pattern
- Single cells or 3D alveolar clusters lined by endothelial cells

Background
- Granular background and bare nuclei due to cell disruption on smears

Cells
- Cells have abundant cytoplasm (when intact)

Nuclear Details
- Eccentrically placed nuclei, vesicular chromatin pattern, prominent nucleoli, occasional intranuclear pseudoinclusions

Cytoplasmic Details
- Fine granular cytoplasm, intracytoplasmic crystalline inclusions

ANCILLARY TESTS

Histochemistry
- PAS(+), diastase-resistant granular to crystalline cytoplasmic material, varies from few to all cells

Immunohistochemistry
- TFE3(+) by immunohistochemistry
- Desmin focally (+)
- Vimentin, MYOD1, HMB-45, S100, CD34, keratin (-)

Genetic Testing
- Unbalanced translocation (X;17) by cytogenetics
- Demonstration of *TFE3* rearrangement or *ASPSCR1*::*TFE3* fusion transcripts.
  - Same can be seen in Xp11 translocation renal cell carcinoma; PAX8(+) in renal cell carcinoma

DIFFERENTIAL DIAGNOSIS

Myomelanocytic Tumor
- Similar cell clustering; lymphatic invasion not present
- Positive for HMB-45 and desmin; negative for TFE3

Paraganglioma
- Similar zellballen pattern
- S100 protein (+) in sustentacular cells and chromogranin (+)

Rhabdomyoma
- Large polygonal and spider cells, no atypia; desmin and myoregulatory protein (+)

Granular Cell Tumor
- More granularity of cytoplasm
- Strongly (+) for S100 protein, unlike alveolar soft part sarcoma

Renal Cell Carcinoma in Children
- Xp11.2 translocation tumors have abundant clear/granular eosinophilic cytoplasm
  - TFE3 immunohistochemistry is (+) in both
- Absence of renal mass and PAX8(-) IHC would favor alveolar soft part sarcoma

SELECTED REFERENCES
1. Rekhi B et al: Revisiting cytomorphology, including unusual features and clinical scenarios of 8 cases of alveolar soft part sarcoma with TFE3 immunohistochemical staining in 7 cases. Cytopathology. 32(1):20-8, 2021

Large Tumor Cells With Abundant Cytoplasm

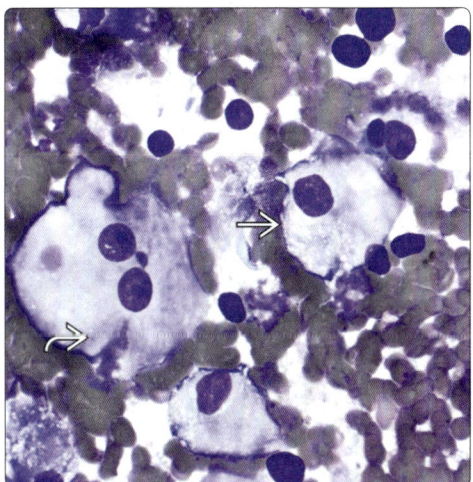

Pap Stain Appearance

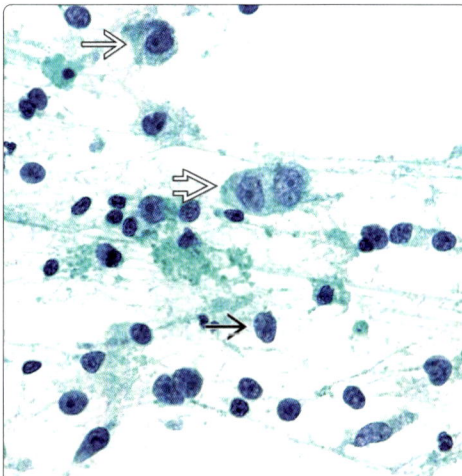

(Left) Diff-Quik-stained smear demonstrates large tumor cells ➡ with abundant granular cytoplasm, round to oval nuclei, and occasional binucleated cells ➡. (Right) Pap-stained smear of alveolar soft part sarcoma shows uni- ➡ and binucleated ➡ tumor cells with prominent nucleoli and abundant granular cytoplasm. Note the disrupted tumor cells resulting in many naked nuclei ➡ in the background.

Clear Cell Sarcoma of Soft Tissue

KEY FACTS

CLINICAL ISSUES

- Seen in young adults (3rd or 4th decades)
- Usually affects extremities (> 90%)
  - Foot most common site
- Behaves as high-grade sarcoma
- Metastasizes to lymph nodes and lung
- Often attached to tendon or aponeurosis
- Occasional visceral examples
  - Ileum most common gastrointestinal site

CYTOPATHOLOGY

- Moderate to high cellularity
- Round to oval nuclei with prominent macronucleoli
- Granular cytoplasm
  - May show melanin pigment
- Occasional pleomorphic cells may be seen
- Mitoses present

ANCILLARY TESTS

- Immunohistochemical profile similar to melanoma in most cases (positive for S100, HMB-45, MART-1)
- Most common cytogenetic abnormality
  - t(12;22)(q13;q12)
  - *EWS::ATF1* fusion
- *EWS::CREB1* fusion: Often in gastrointestinal clear cell sarcoma (lacks melanocytic differentiation)
  - Cases express S100 but not melanocytic markers

TOP DIFFERENTIAL DIAGNOSES

- Melanoma
- Epithelioid sarcoma
- Tenosynovial giant cell tumor
- Schwannoma
- Malignant peripheral nerve sheath tumor
- Perivascular epithelioid cell tumor

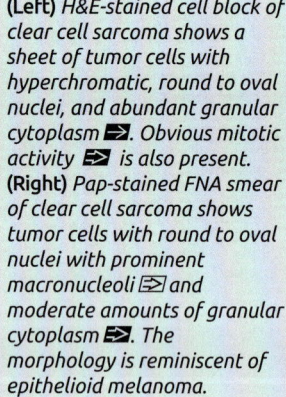

(Left) H&E-stained cell block of clear cell sarcoma shows a sheet of tumor cells with hyperchromatic, round to oval nuclei, and abundant granular cytoplasm ➡. Obvious mitotic activity ➡ is also present. **(Right)** Pap-stained FNA smear of clear cell sarcoma shows tumor cells with round to oval nuclei with prominent macronucleoli ➡ and moderate amounts of granular cytoplasm ➡. The morphology is reminiscent of epithelioid melanoma.

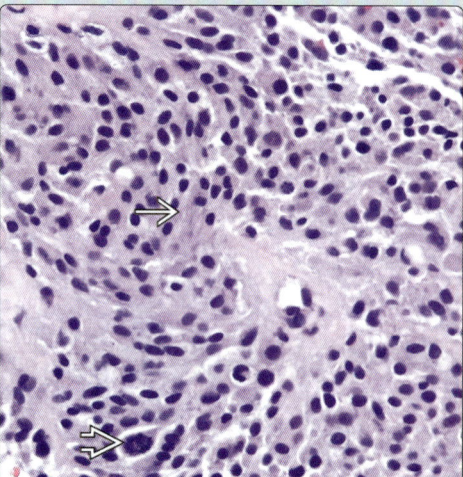

Clear Cell Sarcoma in Cell Block

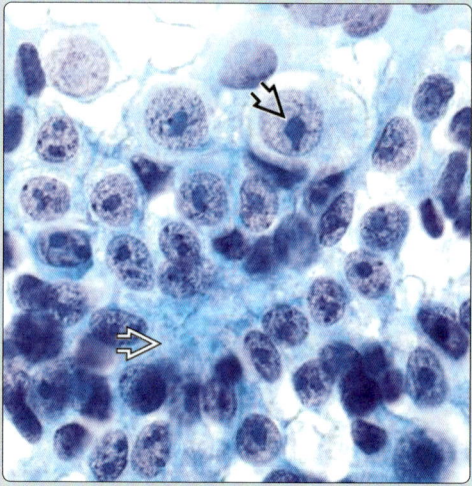

Granular Cytoplasm and Prominent Nucleoli

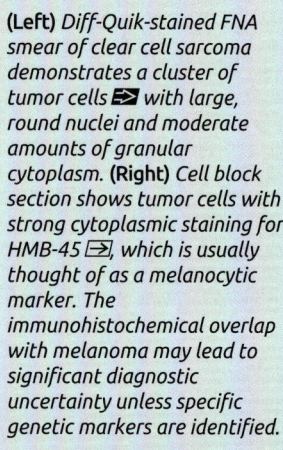

(Left) Diff-Quik-stained FNA smear of clear cell sarcoma demonstrates a cluster of tumor cells ➡ with large, round nuclei and moderate amounts of granular cytoplasm. **(Right)** Cell block section shows tumor cells with strong cytoplasmic staining for HMB-45 ➡, which is usually thought of as a melanocytic marker. The immunohistochemical overlap with melanoma may lead to significant diagnostic uncertainty unless specific genetic markers are identified.

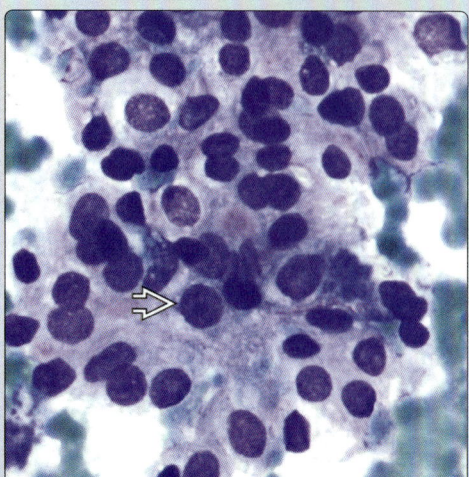

Clear Cell Sarcoma Stained by Diff-Quik

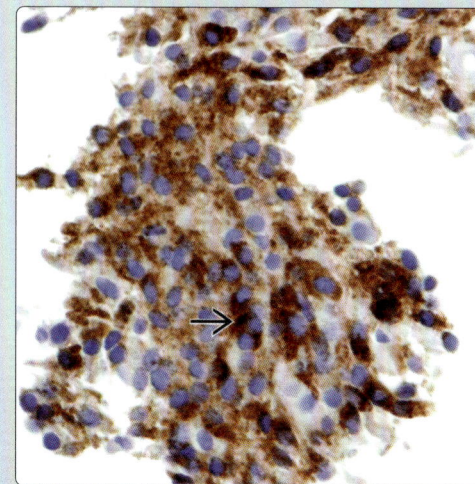

HMB-45(+) Stain in Clear Cell Sarcoma

Clear Cell Sarcoma of Soft Tissue

TERMINOLOGY

Synonyms
- Malignant melanoma of soft parts

Definitions
- Sarcoma showing melanocytic differentiation

CLINICAL ISSUES

Epidemiology
- Age
  - Young adults (3rd or 4th decades)

Prognosis
- Behaves as high-grade sarcoma
- Differs from behavior of melanoma despite overlapping features

CYTOPATHOLOGY

Cellularity
- Moderate to high cellularity, cohesive and dyscohesive cells, ± necrosis

Nuclear Details
- Round to oval nuclei with prominent macronucleoli
  - Intranuclear cytoplasmic pseudoinclusions

Cytoplasmic Details
- Granular to clear cytoplasm, rarely melanin pigment

ANCILLARY TESTS

Immunohistochemistry
- Profile similar to melanoma in most cases

Genetic Testing
- Hallmark is reciprocal translocation t(12;22)(q13;q12), which fuses *EWSR1* with *ATF*, seen in 70-90% of soft tissue cases
- t(2;22)(q13;q12)
  - Often in gastrointestinal cases
- Alternate *EWS::CREB1* fusion

DIFFERENTIAL DIAGNOSIS

Melanoma
- Associated with skin lesions
- Epithelioid melanomas express S100 and melanocytic markers
- Most have complex karyotypes unlike the characteristic translocation and fusion
- Some have *BRAF* mutations

Epithelioid Sarcoma
- Distal extremities (similar to clear cell sarcoma)
- Express CAM5.2 and AE1/AE3, often CD34(+)

Tenosynovial Giant Cell Tumor
- Usually in fingers, female predominance, CD68(+)

Schwannoma
- Common in head and neck, deep soft tissue, retroperitoneum, and posterior mediastinum; S100(+), melanocytic markers (-), keratin (-), variable CD34

Malignant Peripheral Nerve Sheath Tumor
- Deep large soft tissue lesions, usually of proximal extremities
- Usually only focal S100 expression, no melanocytic differentiation

Perivascular Epithelioid Cell Neoplasm
- Encompass angiomyolipoma, clear cell "sugar" tumor of lung, lymphangiomyomatosis, clear cell myelomelanocytic tumor of falciform ligament
- Expresses smooth muscle and melanocytic markers
  - But not keratins or S100

SELECTED REFERENCES
1. Li J et al: Whole-exome sequencing in clear cell sarcoma of soft tissue uncovers novel prognostic categorization and drug targets. Clin Transl Med. 11(12):e640, 2021
2. Huang X et al: Metastatic clear-cell sarcoma. N Engl J Med. 383(4):379, 2020

Nested Sheet of Tumor Cells in Cell Block

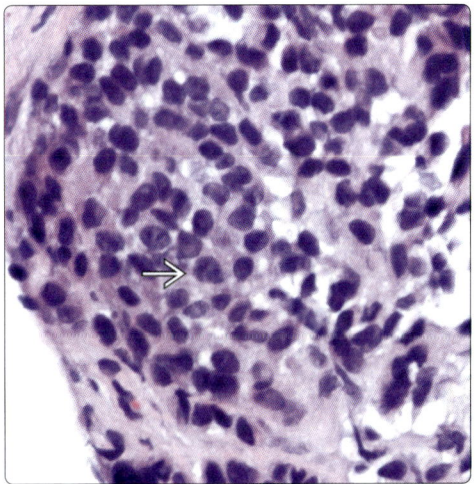

PEComa

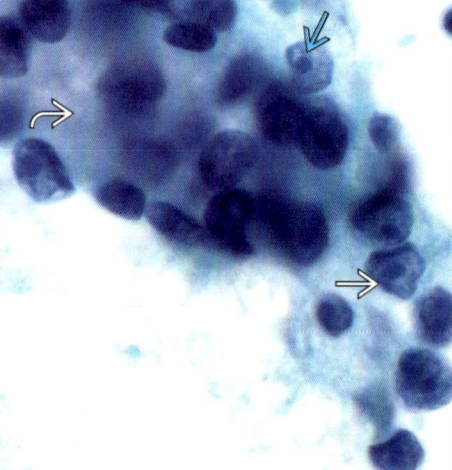

(Left) Cell block section of clear cell sarcoma stained by H&E shows a nested sheet of tumor cells ➡ with round/oval nuclei and moderate amounts of granular cytoplasm. (Right) Pap-stained cluster of cells shows abundant finely vacuolated cytoplasm ➡, nuclear contour irregularities ➡, and prominent nucleoli ➡ in this case of metastatic PEComa. The cells can be morphologically similar to clear cell sarcoma, melanoma, and other entities in the differential of clear cell sarcoma.

Desmoplastic Small Round Cell Tumor

KEY FACTS

CLINICAL ISSUES
- Most common in children and young adults
  - Median age: 20 years; male predilection
- Sites of occurrence: Peritoneal cavity, paratesticular region, ovary, lung, central nervous system, head and neck
- Poor prognosis; median survival: 24 months

CYTOPATHOLOGY
- Small- to intermediate-sized, round to oval cells with scant cytoplasm distributed as single cells, rosette-like groups, and 3D clusters
- Round to oval, hyperchromatic nuclei, finely granular chromatin pattern, small nucleoli, nuclear molding; high mitotic rate
- Collagenous or desmoplastic stroma

ANCILLARY TESTS
- Vimentin, cytokeratin, desmin, EMA, and WT1 consistently stain tumor cells in ~ 90% of cases
- Staining pattern for desmin and vimentin characteristically dot-like and paranuclear
- May also show focal positivity for CD56, NSE, chromogranin, synaptophysin, and S100
- Shows t(11;22)(p13;q12), similar to Ewing sarcoma
  - Unlike Ewing sarcoma, site on chromosome 11 is *WT1* gene rather than *FLI1* gene

TOP DIFFERENTIAL DIAGNOSES
- Ewing sarcoma
  - Lacks strong expression of polyphenotypic markers, such as desmin, cytokeratin, and WT1
- Metastatic neuroendocrine carcinoma
  - Positive for neuroendocrine markers (chromogranin, CD56, and synaptophysin)
- Lymphoma
  - Expresses CD45 and other lymphoid markers
- Alveolar rhabdomyosarcoma
  - Diffuse positivity for desmin and myogenin

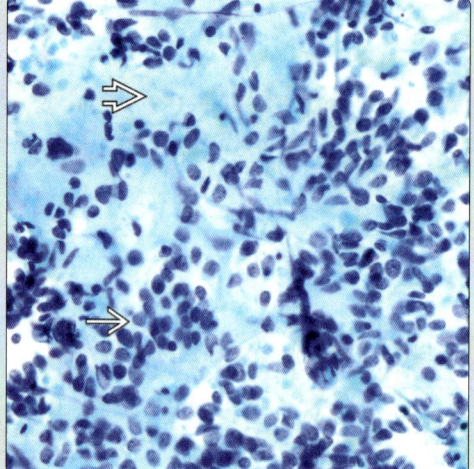
Small Round Cells in Stroma

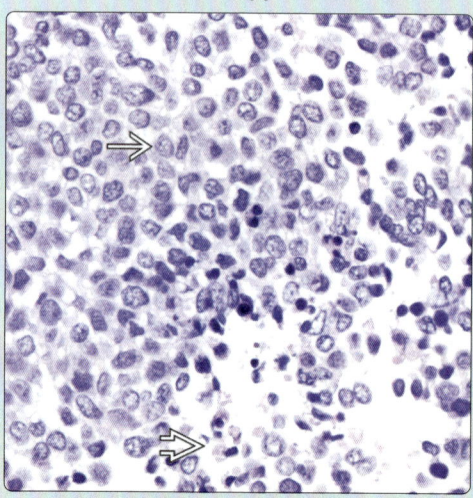
Cell Block Appearance

(Left) Pap-stained FNA smear shows small round cells ➡ distributed in a desmoplastic stroma ➡. **(Right)** Cell block section stained with H&E illustrates relatively uniform small round cells with hyperchromatic nuclei ➡ associated with necrosis ➡.

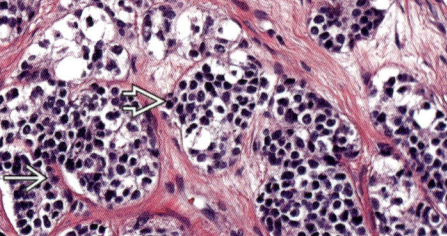
Desmoplastic Small Round Cell Tumor

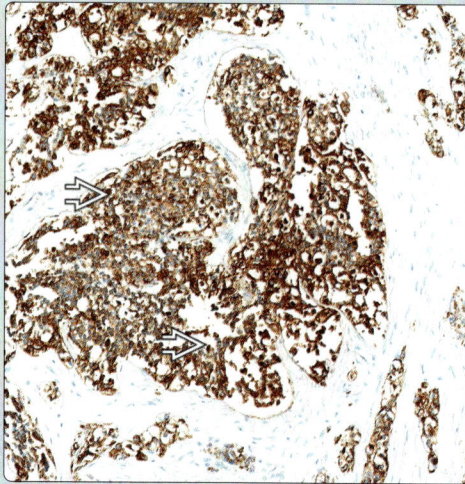
Desmoplastic Small Round Cell Tumor, Cytokeratin Positive

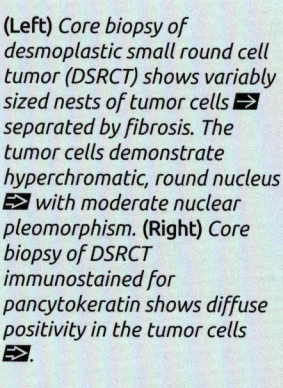

(Left) Core biopsy of desmoplastic small round cell tumor (DSRCT) shows variably sized nests of tumor cells ➡ separated by fibrosis. The tumor cells demonstrate hyperchromatic, round nucleus ➡ with moderate nuclear pleomorphism. **(Right)** Core biopsy of DSRCT immunostained for pancytokeratin shows diffuse positivity in the tumor cells ➡.

Desmoplastic Small Round Cell Tumor

TERMINOLOGY

Definitions
- Primitive malignant neoplasm arising in serosal surfaces with distinctive histology composed of primitive small round blue cells embedded in abundant desmoplastic stroma

CLINICAL ISSUES

Presentation
- Male predilection
- Median age: 20 years
- Peritoneal cavity, paratesticular region, ovary, lung, central nervous system, head and neck

CYTOPATHOLOGY

Pattern
- Single cells or rosette-like appearance and 3D clusters

Background
- Collagenous or desmoplastic stroma appears pink on Diff-Quik or pale blue on Pap-stained smears

Cells
- Small- to intermediate-sized, round to oval cells with scant cytoplasm

Nuclear Details
- Fine granular chromatin pattern; may show nuclear molding
- Hyperchromatic nuclei, small nucleoli
- High mitotic rate with typical mitoses

Cytoplasmic Details
- May have vacuolated cytoplasm

ANCILLARY TESTS

Immunohistochemistry
- Vimentin, cytokeratin, desmin, EMA, and WT1 consistently stain tumor cells in ~ 90% of cases
- Staining pattern for desmin and vimentin characteristically dot-like and paranuclear
- May also show focal positivity for CD56, NSE, chromogranin, synaptophysin, and S100

Genetic Testing
- Shows t(11;22)(p13;q12), similar to Ewing sarcoma/peripheral neuroectodermal tumor
- Unlike Ewing sarcoma, site on chromosome 11 is *WT1* gene rather than *FLI1* gene

DIFFERENTIAL DIAGNOSIS

Ewing Sarcoma
- Lacks strong expression of polyphenotypic markers, such as desmin, cytokeratin, and WT1
- Strongly positive for CD99 in most cases
- t(11;22)(p24;q12)

Metastatic Neuroendocrine Carcinoma
- Positive for neuroendocrine markers (chromogranin, CD56, and synaptophysin)
- Does not express EMA, desmin, or WT1

Lymphoma
- Expresses CD45 and other lymphoid markers

Alveolar Rhabdomyosarcoma
- Diffuse positivity for desmin and myogenin

SELECTED REFERENCES

1. Jayakrishnan T et al: Desmoplastic small round-cell tumor: retrospective review of institutional data and literature review. Anticancer Res. 41(8):3859-66, 2021
2. Lozano MD et al: A comprehensive diagnosis of a desmoplastic small round cell tumor of unusual location based on fine-needle aspiration cytology: report of a case arising in the parotid gland and review of the literature. Diagn Cytopathol. 48(9):827-32, 2020
3. Mohamed M et al: Desmoplastic small round cell tumor: evaluation of reverse transcription-polymerase chain reaction and fluorescence in situ hybridization as ancillary molecular diagnostic techniques. Virchows Arch. 471(5):631-40, 2017
4. Leça LB et al: Desmoplastic small round cell tumor: diagnosis by fine-needle aspiration cytology. Acta Cytol. 56(5):576-80, 2012

Desmoplastic Small Round Cell Tumor, Desmin Positive

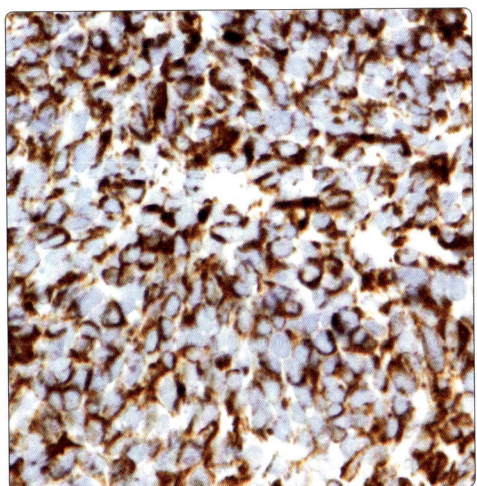

Small Round Tumor Cells

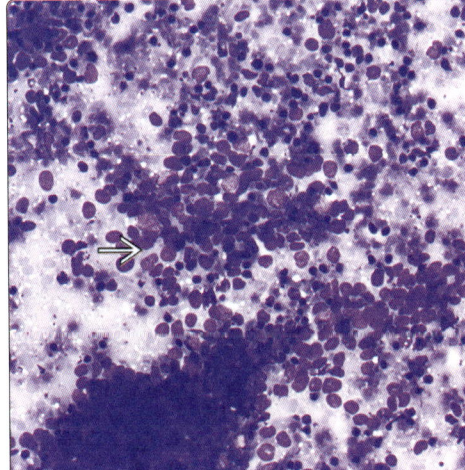

(Left) Immunostain for desmin performed on cell block section of DSRCT shows the characteristic perinuclear dot-like pattern of positivity. *(Right)* Diff-Quik-stained FNA smear demonstrates small round tumor cells ➡ with minimal cytoplasm and nuclear molding in a background of necrosis.

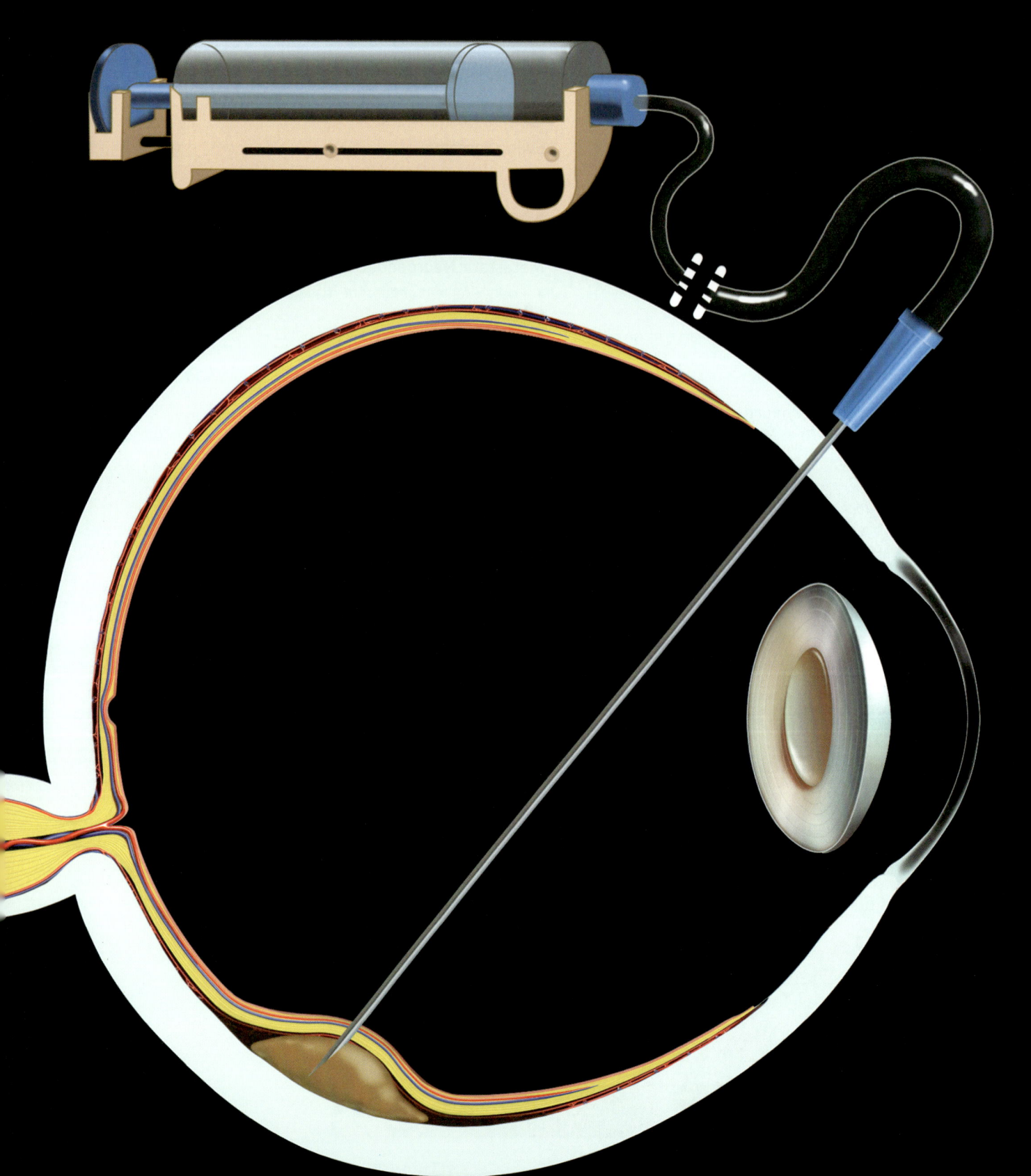

PART IV
SECTION 9
Ophthalmic and Neuropathology

Approach to Ophthalmic Cytology	682
Ophthalmic Cytopathology, Infectious	686
Ophthalmic Cytopathology, Neoplastic	690
Neuropathology Squash Preparations, Infectious	696
Neuropathology Squash Preparations, Glial Neoplasms	700
Neuropathology Squash Preparations, Nonglial Neoplasms	704

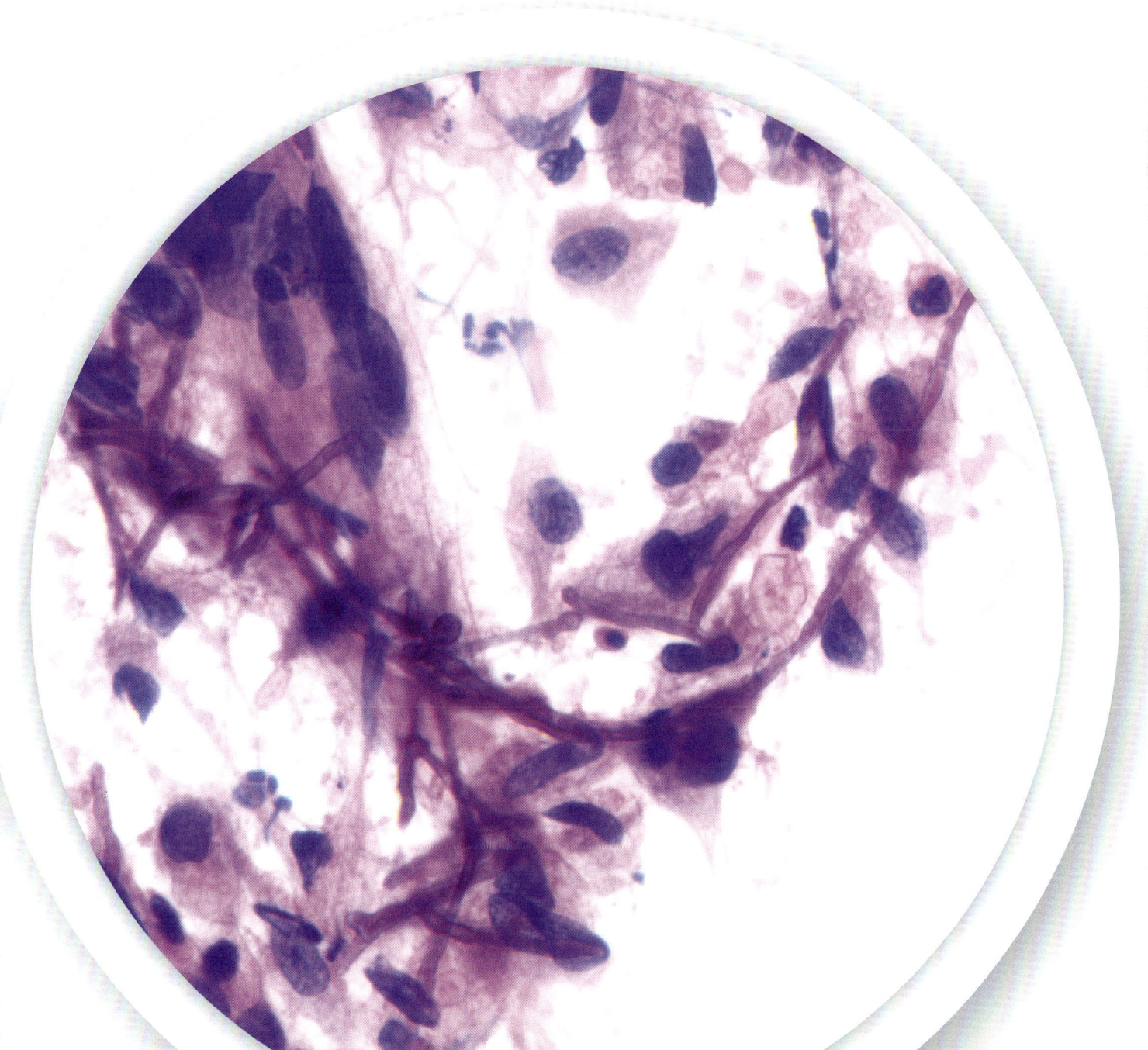

Approach to Ophthalmic Cytology

OPHTHALMIC CYTOLOGY

Types of Samples

- Vitreous biopsy or undiluted vitreous in syringe (~ 0.5 mL), obtained at beginning of procedure
  - Usually obtained specifically for diagnosis
- Vitrectomy specimen or diluted vitreous (in bag or cassette from vitrectomy machine)
  - Obtained during procedure, diluted with balanced salt solution, varies in amount
    - Sample is obtained as part of treatment to remove opacities &/or reattach retina &/or for diagnosis
- Anterior chamber sample is always received as undiluted sample (~ 0.05 to 0.2 mL) in syringe
  - Easiest to obtain for diagnosis in work-up of anterior uveitis &/or glaucoma
    - Most common ancillary tests performed in specimen are viral and parasitic PCRs
- FNA biopsy of intraocular lesions
  - If adequacy check is performed during procedure, cytology slides and material for cell block will be available
  - If adequacy check is not performed, only material for liquid-based cytology and cell block would be available
- Exfoliation cytology from cornea/conjunctiva is used to exclude organisms or to follow-up after local chemotherapy of ocular surface neoplasia
  - Slides are usually prepared by ophthalmologist as smears, rarely in CytoLyt or other fixative

CYTOLOGIC PREPARATION AND INTERPRETATION

Challenges

- For ophthalmologist, opacities in clear media of eye may appear similar, regardless of etiology
  - Cytology and other testing are necessary for diagnosis
- Diagnostic/therapeutic procedures should maintain clear media to preserve vision
  - Consequently, scant specimen is usually obtained
- Intraocular tumors may need genetic/molecular testing
  - Sharing of specimen for diagnosis and prognostic molecular testing is often necessary

Vitreous Opacities and Retinal Lesions

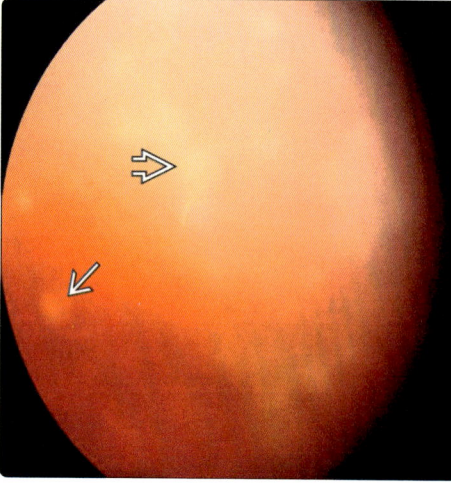

Transscleral Approach of Choroidal Tumor Biopsy: Transillumination

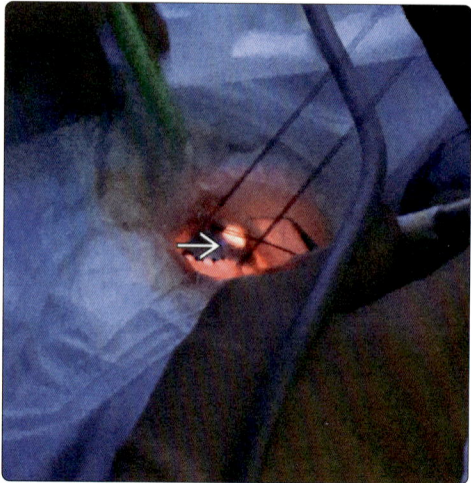

(Left) Fundus photograph shows an eye with vitreous opacities ⇨, haziness, and retinal lesions ⇨. Differential diagnosis includes inflammation, infectious and noninfectious, and lymphoma. (Right) Peripheral tumor located near the ciliary body may be approached through the sclera. Transillumination with marking of the borders of the opaque tumor is shown. The bright light shines through the pupil (left) ⇨ and the unaffected choroid/sclera. A smear is prepared (27-gauge needle) to assess adequacy.

Transvitreal Approach of Choroidal Tumor Biopsy: Operating Microscope

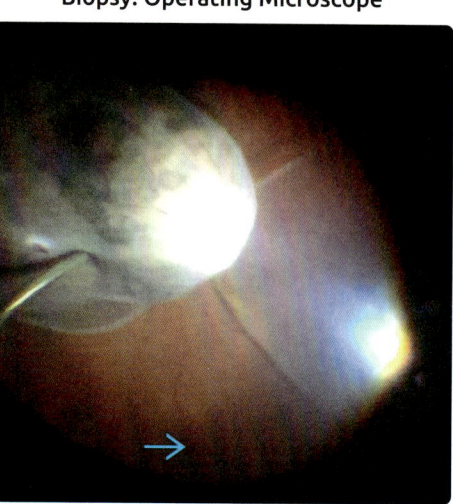

Vitreous Aspirate Appearance

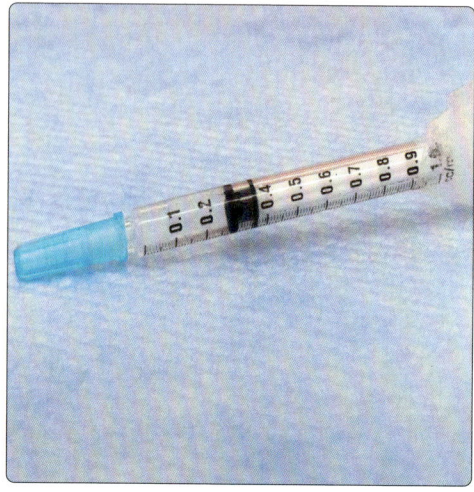

(Left) Equatorial or posterior choroidal tumors are approached through the vitreous with visualization using an operating microscope. The needle pierces the tumor and the biopsy is obtained. Note the previous biopsy site ⇨ inferior to the needle. A smear is prepared from the 27-gauge needle sample to assess adequacy. (Right) Undiluted vitreous aspirate in a syringe is shown. The usual amount received varies between 0.1-0.5 cc.

Approach to Ophthalmic Cytology

- Adequacy check in operating room may be necessary for adequate sampling and better yield for distribution into various tests
- Enclosed intraocular environment is conducive to rapid and often permanent damage by infectious organisms
  - Triaging of vitreous and anterior chamber samples is essential for timely and accurate diagnosis and treatment
- Communication between ophthalmologist and cytopathologist before procedure is desirable
  - Discussion of clinical suspicion and differential diagnosis facilitates guiding triage of specimen
  - Prompt report of unexpected results to referring physician is recommended, especially for
    - Acute inflammation
    - PCR detection of infectious organism
    - Organisms identified in cytologic preparation
    - Growth of organisms in cultures
    - Lymphoma is diagnosed
    - Other malignancy is diagnosed
- Communication between cytopathologist and other laboratory personnel (hematopathologist, molecular diagnostics, flow cytometry, etc.) is desirable if case is expected to need special &/or multiple different tests

TRIAGING OF VITREOUS AND AQUEOUS HUMOR

Evaluate Cellularity

- From undiluted sample, obtain liquid-based cytology to evaluate cellularity
- Use only 1 drop to spare sample for other tests
- If there are neutrophils, submit for cultures (aerobic, anaerobic, fungus, mycobacteria)
  - If only undiluted sample, submit all for cultures
  - If both undiluted and diluted samples, submit undiluted for cultures and diluted for cell block and special stains and keep small amount frozen for possible molecular testing
- If specimen shows scant small lymphocytes, few macrophages, and condensed vitreous with clinical suspicion of virus vs. lymphoma
  - Submit undiluted sample for PCR
    - Herpes zoster virus (HZV), herpes simplex virus 1 (HSV1), and HSV2, CMV, *Toxoplasma*, or other specific for clinical suspicion (EBV, etc.)
  - If diluted specimen is available, send 1/3 to cultures and 2/3 to cell block
    - Cell block for special stains and immunohistochemistry (CD3, CD20, CD68)
- If there are atypical large lymphocytes in background of necrotic debris, macrophages, and small lymphocytes
  - Submit undiluted sample for molecular viral (EBV) PCR, save frozen for molecular gene rearrangement; if sample cellular submit to flow cytometry (best yield for diagnosis is cell block if needing to choose)
  - Submit diluted sample for cell block for immunohistochemistry
    - CD3, CD20, CD68, and others (CD10, MUM1, BCL2, etc.) as needed to confirm diagnosis of lymphoma
  - From cell block, sample can be submitted for molecular gene rearrangement test if necessary
- From only diluted sample, also obtain liquid-based cytology to evaluate cellularity
  - Proceed similarly as with undiluted samples based on cytologic findings

INTRAOCULAR SOLID TUMORS

Uveal vs. Metastatic vs. Other Melanomas

- Melanoma of choroid may be biopsied before radiation plaque is placed, mostly for prognostic molecular testing
  - Adequacy check at time of biopsy may be necessary to assure sufficient sample for diagnosis and molecular
  - Desirable to obtain enough material for cell block
    - Cell block may be used for immunohistochemistry for diagnosis of melanoma when coexpression of HMB-45 and Ki-67 is present in melanocytic cells
    - Cell block may be used for molecular testing if not enough fresh sample was obtained during FNA
    - Typically, cytologic smears may have scant cellularity
    - > 2 passes may be needed to obtain enough material; average number of passes is 3
- Pitfall: Choroidal tissue contains melanocytes with abundant melanin and retina has pigmented epithelium
  - Therefore, presence of melanin pigment does not assure adequate sampling of suspicious lesion that clinically appears as choroidal melanoma
    - Spindle cells or epithelioid cells with occasional nucleoli are necessary for diagnosis of melanocytic tumor
- Other tumors: Treat similar to melanoma to confirm adequate cellularity for cell block and ancillary studies
  - Immunohistochemistry in cell block should be guided by patient history and cytomorphology

ACELLULAR SAMPLES

Opacities Secondary to Deposits

- Asteroid hyalosis is made of deposits of calcium and lipids
  - If sample is not diagnostic on Pap stain and polarization, specimen should be submitted for cytologic preparations to stain with oil red O &/or alcian blue
    - Deposits are birefringent under polarization
- Amyloidosis
  - Entire specimen should be submitted for cell block for special stains and possible immunohistochemistry
- Synchesis scintillans (cholesterol)
  - Fresh cytologic preparations are indicated to show crystals under polarization
- Retained lens fragments
  - Cell block is indicated if there is enough specimen to demonstrate lens material
- Spherulosis
  - Remote vitreous hemorrhage may form yellow-orange deposits reminiscent of lymphoma infiltrates
  - Composed of partially degenerated erythrocytes with round, spherical shapes and different sizes

SELECTED REFERENCES

1. Sehgal A et al: Diagnosing vitreoretinal lymphomas-an analysis of the sensitivity of existing tools. Cancers (Basel). 14(3):598, 2022
2. Shumilov E et al: Comprehensive laboratory diagnostic workup for patients with suspected intraocular lymphoma including flow cytometry, molecular genetics and cytopathology. Curr Oncol. 29(2):766-76, 2022

Approach to Ophthalmic Cytology

Inflammatory Sample

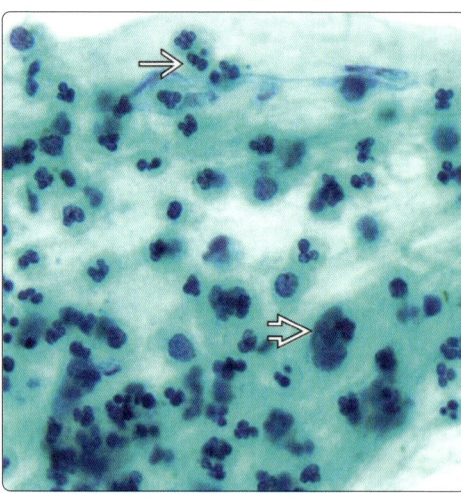

(Left) Pap stain on ThinPrep shows a drop of undiluted sample of mostly neutrophils ➡ and few macrophages ➡. **(Right)** Triaging for samples with acute and granulomatous infiltrate is shown. Securing a sample for cultures is essential, and if enough samples are available, cell block with ancillary studies is also recommended.

Triage Strategy for Acute Inflammatory and Granulomatous Vitreous Aspirates

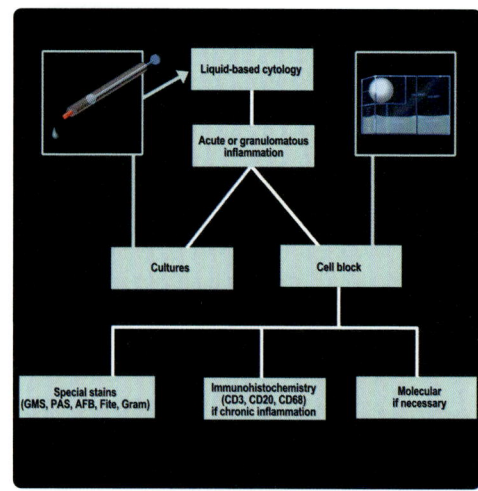

Small Scattered Lymphocytes in Suspected Viral Infection

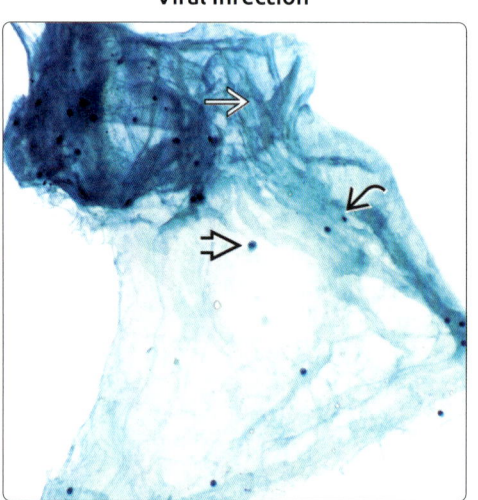

(Left) Pap stain shows condensed vitreous ➡ and rare small lymphocytes ➡ and macrophages ➡ in a patient with clinical suspicion of viral infection. Apoptotic cells may be seen. **(Right)** Triaging of samples with clinical suspicion of viral disease where the specimen shows scant cellularity of small lymphocytes, condensed vitreous, and rare macrophages is shown. Order PCR for viral organisms, and, if enough sample is available, submit for cultures and cell block.

Vitreous Triage Strategy in Suspected Viral Infection

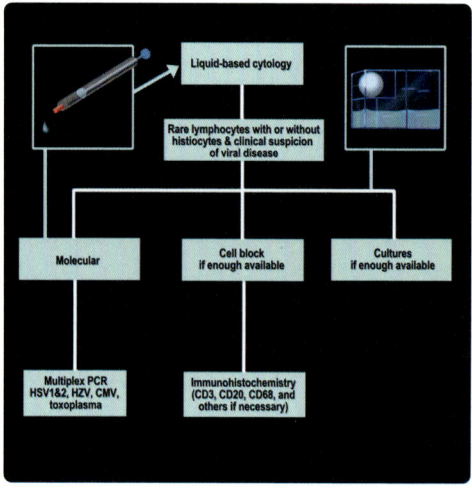

Large Atypical Lymphocytes in Suspected Lymphoma

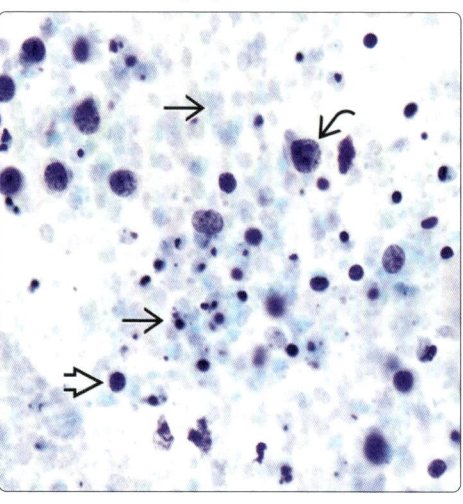

(Left) Pap-stained large atypical lymphocytes with prominent nucleoli ➡, lymphoglandular bodies, cellular debris ➡, small lymphocytes ➡, and macrophages are shown. Immunophenotyping the cells is essential for diagnosis. **(Right)** Triaging of specimens with large atypical lymphocytes and suspicion of lymphoma is shown. If available, flow cytometry should be ordered; otherwise, molecular testing of undiluted sample is indicated. Cell block and immunohistochemistry are useful.

Vitreous Aspirate Triage Strategy in Suspected Lymphoma

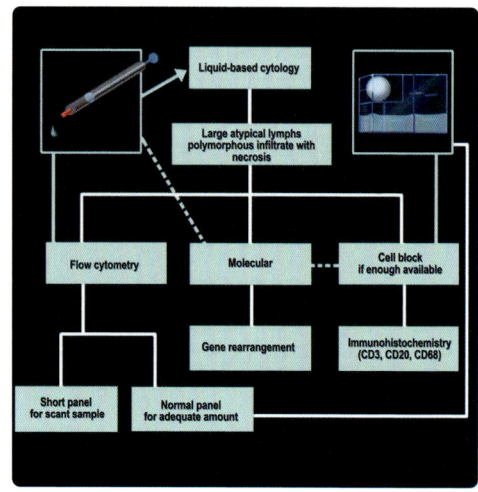

Approach to Ophthalmic Cytology

Granulomatous Chorioretinitis

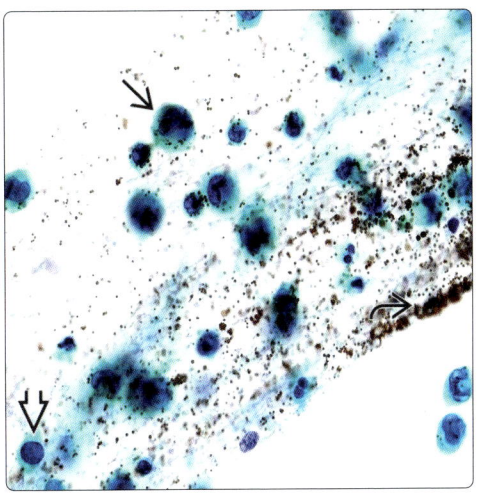

Candida Yeast and Pigment Granules

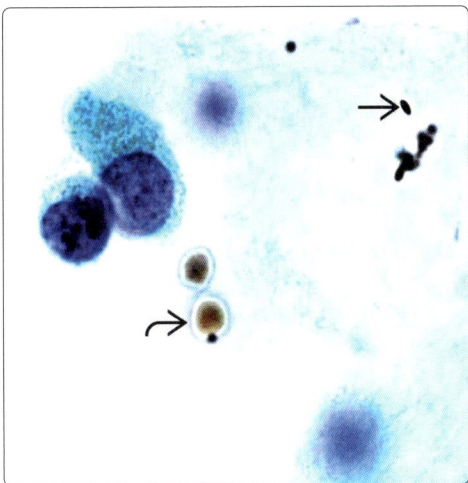

(Left) Undiluted sample of granulomatous chorioretinitis on Pap stain shows granulomatous inflammation, abundant melanin pigment ⇒, histiocytes ⇒, and rare retinal pigmented epithelium cells ⇒. PCR for infectious organisms and cell block with immunohistochemistry showed HZV. (Right) Pap stain of aqueous humor (0.2 cc) from a 2-week-old baby with anterior chamber infiltrate shows yeast forms ⇒ and football-shaped pigment granules (pigmented epithelium) ⇒. Cultures grew Candida species.

Sarcoid Granuloma in Vitreous Aspirate

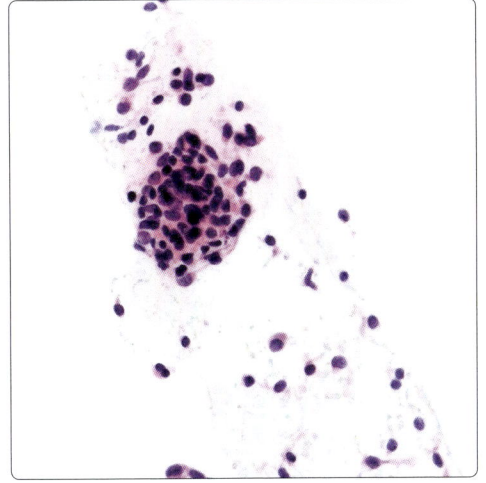

Polyclonal Plasma Cells and Granuloma

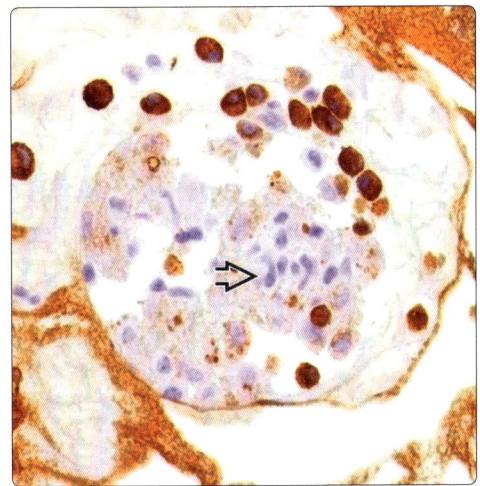

(Left) H&E stain shows a well-formed granuloma with epithelioid histiocytes in condensed vitreous. Cultures, PCRs for infectious organisms, and cell block for special stains were negative for organisms. Patient presentation was clinically consistent with sarcoidosis. (Right) Cell block with immunohistochemistry in the same case of sarcoidosis demonstrates a polyclonal plasma cell component surrounding an epithelioid granuloma ⇒.

Condensed Vitreous and Round Deposits

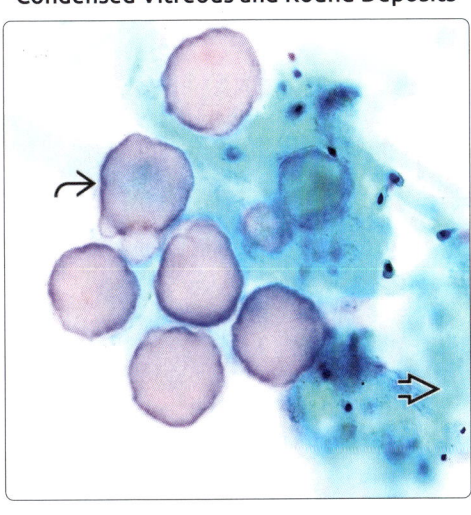

Asteroid Hyalosis on Polarization

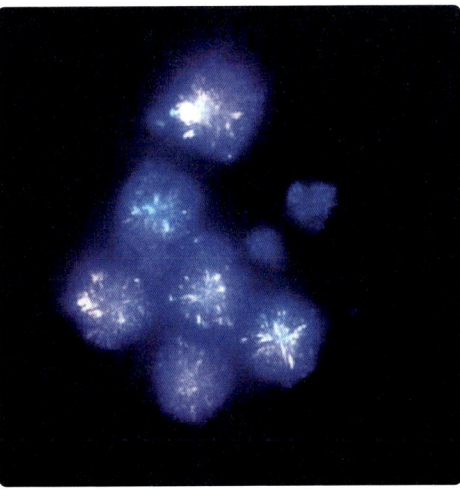

(Left) Pap stain shows a mostly acellular vitreous specimen with condensed vitreous ⇒ and round deposits ⇒ from a case of asteroid hyalosis. Cytologic preparation or cell block with special stains (alcian blue, oil red O) is used to highlight the calcium and phosphates or phospholipids in the deposits. (Right) Cytologic preparation from a case of asteroid hyalosis, upon polarization, shows the birefringent crystals of hydroxylapatite deposits.

Ophthalmic Cytopathology, Infectious

TERMINOLOGY

Ocular Infectious Diseases
- Acute and chronic keratitis, keratoconjunctivitis, and conjunctivitis
- Intraocular infections encompass anterior, intermediate, and posterior uveitis, vitreitis, and retinitis
- Infection of entire intraocular compartment is endophthalmitis, and involvement of entire eye is panophthalmitis
  - These may be endogenous or exogenous

EPIDEMIOLOGY

Worldwide Infectious Ocular Diseases
- In past, trachoma and onchocerciasis were main cause of blindness worldwide
- In last 20 years, incidence of these diseases has dropped significantly through international efforts coordinated by WHO
- Currently, corneal infections are most sight-threatening complications of contact lens use and refractive corneal surgery
- Early diagnosis and treatment are key to minimizing any sight-threatening sequelae
- Up to 20% of cases of fungal keratitis (particularly candidiasis) are complicated by bacterial coinfection
- Immunocompromised (primary, acquired, or secondary to treatments) and septicemic patients have higher risk of endophthalmitis
- Children and adolescents may develop parasitic endophthalmitis as they come in contact with cats and dogs (including puppies)
- Syphilis is rising cause of uveitis

ETIOLOGY/PATHOGENESIS

Ocular Infectious Diseases With Impact on Vision
- Most frequently caused by
  - Bacteria: *Streptococcus*, *Pseudomonas*, Enterobacteriaceae (including *Klebsiella*, *Enterobacter*, *Serratia*, and *Proteus*), and *Staphylococcus* species

Ring-Shaped Corneal Infiltrate
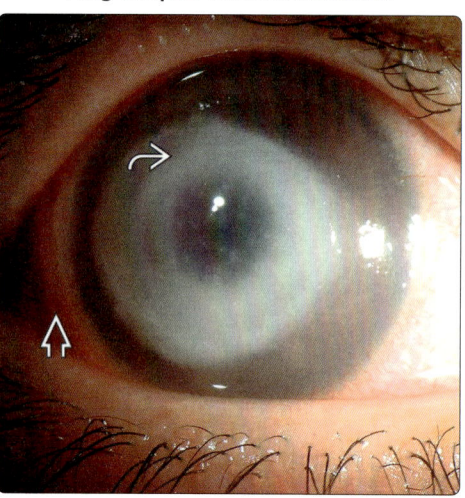

Anterior Segment of Eye, Normal and Endophthalmitis
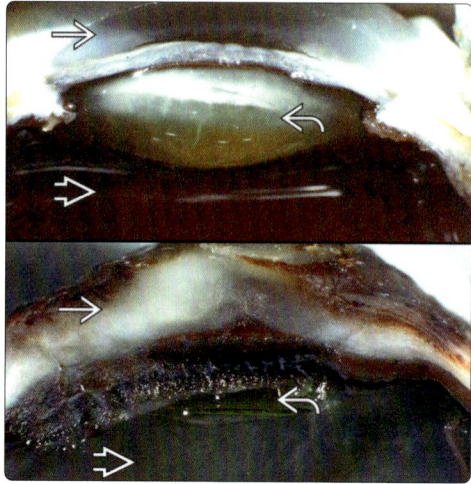

(Left) Clinical photograph shows an eye with a corneal infiltrate in a ring shape ➔, typical of Acanthamoeba keratitis. Notice the hyperemic conjunctiva ➔. (Right) Gross photograph shows the anterior segment of a normal eye (top) compared with an eye with endophthalmitis and corneal ulcer (bottom). Cornea ➔, lens ➔, and vitreous ➔ can all be seen.

Corneal Smear of Acanthamoeba: PAS
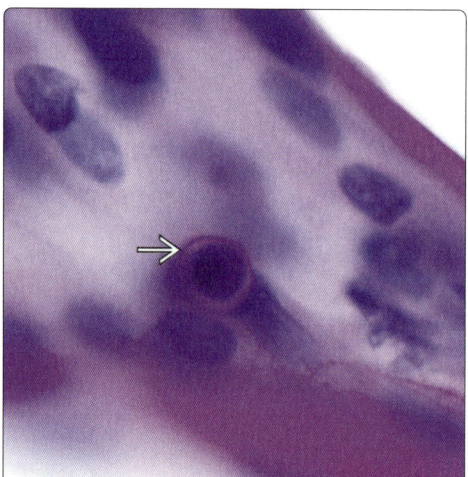

Cyst Wall and Nucleus of Acanthamoeba
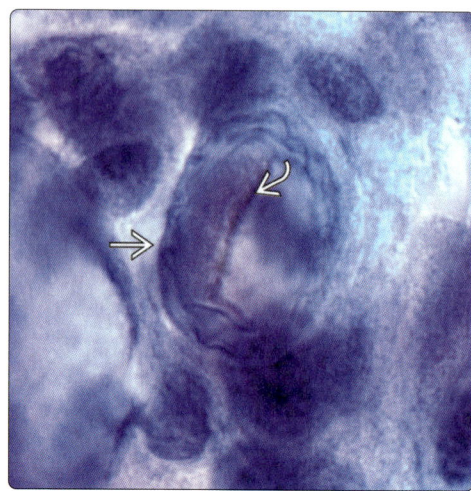

(Left) PAS stain highlights the outer wall ➔ of the cyst of acanthamoeba and shows the polygonal shape of the inner wall. Notice the prominent nucleosome typical of these parasites. (Right) A higher power image shows details of the nucleus ➔ and the wall of the cyst ➔, visible with Pap stain in a ThinPrep.

Ophthalmic Cytopathology, Infectious

- Atypical mycobacteria in cornea and *Mycobacterium tuberculosis* intraocular
o Viruses: Herpes simplex virus 1 (HSV1), HSV2, varicella-zoster virus, EBV, CMV
o Fungi: *Candida, Fusarium, Aspergillus*, Dematiaceae
o Parasites
  - Cornea and conjunctiva: *Acanthamoeba, Microsporidia*, microfilaria
  - Intraocular: *Toxoplasma, Toxocara, Cystericus*

CLINICAL IMPLICATIONS

Risk of Vision Loss Through Several Mechanisms
- Perforation of corneal ulcer with secondary endophthalmitis and large corneal opacities
- Most corneal and conjunctival infections are diagnosed clinically, and most respond to treatment without need of scraping, biopsy, or keratectomy

Clinical Risk Factors
- Contact lens wear
- Trauma (including previous surgery)
- Use of contaminated ocular medications
- Decreased immunologic defenses
- Aqueous tear deficiencies
- Recent corneal disease (e.g., herpetic keratitis, neurotrophic keratopathy)
- Structural alteration or malposition of eyelids
- Systemic infection (e.g., bacteremia or fungemia) or metastasis due to localized infection (e.g., fungal from lung, bacterial from colon carcinoma)

MACROSCOPIC

Specimen Handling
- Biopsy
  o Corneal scrapes: Ophthalmologists provide unstained slide(s) of scraping of surface of cornea &/or conjunctiva
    - If only 1 slide is available, Gram stain followed by destain and stain with periodic acid-Schiff (PAS) stain is recommended
    - PAS allows for interpretation of cellular component, presence of goblet cells, and identification of *Acanthamoeba* cysts and fungal elements
    - If other slides are available, they should be stained after evaluation of PAS-stained slide
    - Gram stain: Bacteria, *Microsporidia* (gram positive)
    - Modified trichrome stain: *Microsporidia*
    - Fite: Atypical mycobacteria, *Microsporidia* (variable)
    - Gomori methenamine silver (GMS): *Acanthamoeba*, fungus, *Microsporidia*
  o Vitreous or aqueous humor: From undiluted samples, obtain cytospin or preferably liquid-based preparation with Pap stain to evaluate type of cellularity
    - Acute inflammation: Submit for cultures, cell block, and special stains
    - Granulomatous inflammation: Submit for cultures, cell block, and special stains
    - Eosinophils in children: Submit vitreous for ELISA for *Toxocara canis*
    - Condensed vitreous with scant inflammation and necrosis: Submit for viral PCR and cell block

MICROSCOPIC

Bacterial Infections
- Acute inflammatory cells and necrotic debris; 16S (bacterial) rDNA sequencing is useful if available for scant specimens
- Corneal scrapes usually show bacteria in background
- Vitreous may have organisms at center of microabscesses
  o Some organisms are only diagnostic in cytology samples, as they are heavily pretreated and will not grow in cultures

Fungal Infections
- Acute inflammation in corneal scrapes with associated fungal elements; 18S (fungal) rDNA sequencing is useful if available for scant specimens
- Vitreous and aqueous samples may have granulomatous inflammation associated with milder acute inflammation
- Vitreous condensation and organisms at center of granulomata

Viral Infections
- Herpetic keratitis shows viral effect (Cowdry type A nuclear inclusions) and multinucleation in smears
- Vitreous samples show scant amount of lymphocytes and rare plasma cells in background of condensed focally necrotic vitreous (acute retinal necrosis syndrome)
- PCR for most common viruses is recommended (HSV1, HSV2, herpes zoster virus, CMV); cell block may be use to do immunohistochemistry

Parasitic Infections
- Acanthamoeba keratitis shows polygonal PAS-/GMS-positive cysts (10 μm to > 20 μm)
  o Trophozoites (25-50 μm) are difficult to distinguish from macrophages; trophozoites are larger and have single nucleus, dense nucleolus, and acanthopodia
- Microsporidial keratitis: Spores may be associated to epithelium or present in background
  o *Encephalitozoon* spp., *Vittaforma corneae, Anncaliia algerae*, and *Nosema* spp. with spores measuring 1.5-4 μm are most common
  o For identification, gold standard is transmission electron microscopy
  o Immunofluorescence assays and molecular methods are currently only used in research laboratories
- Intraocular: In children, toxocariasis is most frequent parasitosis, and main cytologic finding is presence of eosinophils
- *Toxoplasma gondii* is most common cause of infectious uveitis worldwide
  o Reactivations may present diagnostic challenge with mostly macrophages and chronic inflammation
  o PCR is preferred diagnostic tool for toxoplasma

SELECTED REFERENCES

1. Sharma K et al: Detection of viable Mycobacterium tuberculosis in ocular fluids using mRNA-based multiplex polymerase chain reaction. Indian J Med Microbiol. 40(2):254-7, 2022
2. Matoba A et al: Microsporidial stromal keratitis: epidemiological features, slit-lamp biomicroscopic characteristics, and therapy. Cornea. 40(12):1532-40, 2021
3. Chidambaram JD et al: In vivo confocal microscopy cellular features of host and organism in bacterial, fungal, and acanthamoeba keratitis. Am J Ophthalmol. 190:24-33, 2018

Ophthalmic Cytopathology, Infectious

Fungal Keratitis: Gram Stain

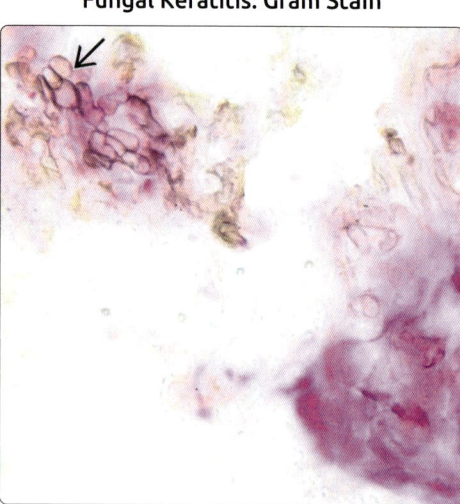

Fungal Keratitis: PAS

(Left) Gram stain shows abundant focally pigmented septate fungal organisms with wide, oval, and round conidia ➡, better seen on PAS stain. Cultures grew Curvularia species. **(Right)** PAS stain highlights the many hyphae with wide, oval, and round conidia ➡ (cultures grew Curvularia species) in a background of proteinaceous exudate and cellular debris.

Microsporidial Spores on Trichrome Stain

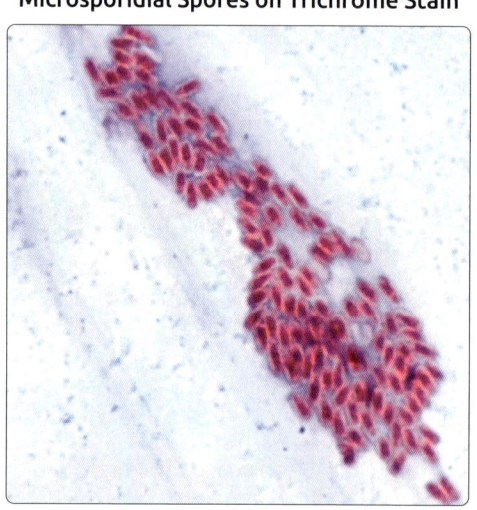

Gram-Positive Microsporidial Spores

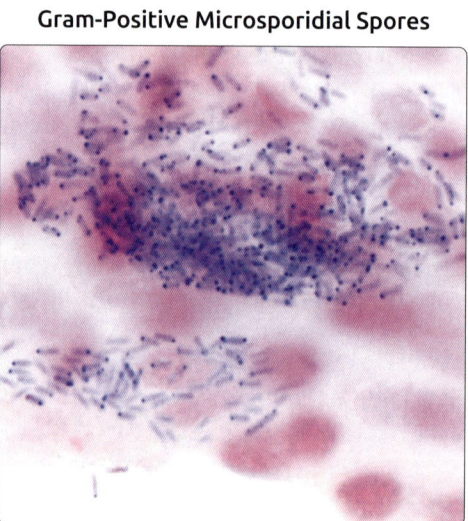

(Left) Modified trichrome stains the microsporidial spores pinkish-red in this scrape specimen. **(Right)** Scraping of cornea and conjunctiva shows background epithelium with many gram-positive microsporidial spores. Note the darker dot corresponding to the polar tube end in this case of microsporidial keratoconjunctivitis.

Herpetic Keratitis

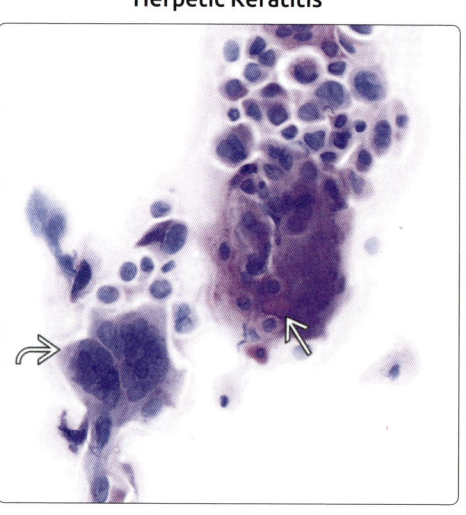

Acute Vitreous Inflammation

(Left) PAS stain highlights the viral herpetic (HSV-1) cytopathic changes in a corneal epithelium scraping. Note abundant cytoplasm and multinucleation of the cells with central nuclear clearing ➡ and intranuclear inclusions ➡. **(Right)** Undiluted vitreous shows acute inflammation and a few cocci ➡ (Pap stain; top). Cell block of the washings shows many neutrophils (H&E; bottom left) with cocci that are gram positive ➡ (Gram stain; bottom right). Cultures grew Staphylococcus aureus in this case of acute bacterial endophthalmitis.

Ophthalmic Cytopathology, Infectious

Lymphocytes Due to HZV Infection

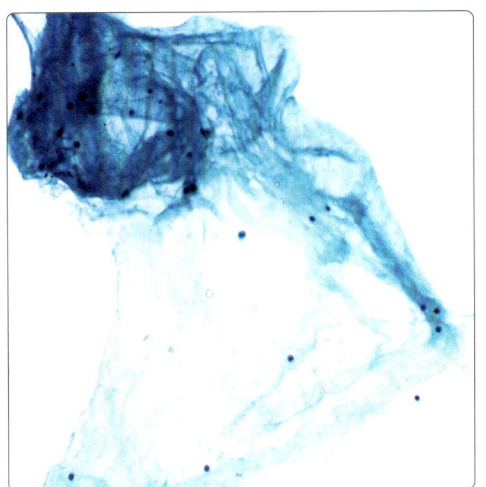

Granulomas and Mixed Inflammation

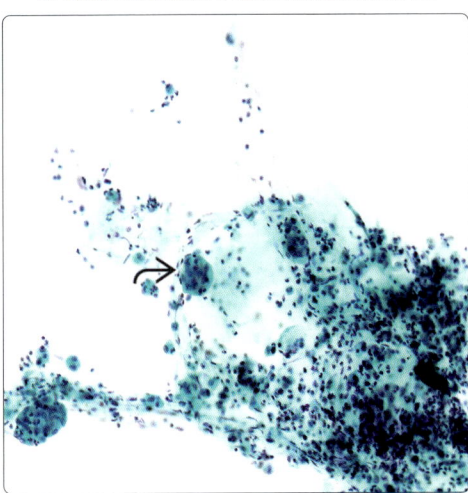

(Left) Pap-stained undiluted vitreous specimen on liquid-based cytology shows condensation of vitreous with rare lymphocytes and plasma cells. Immunohistochemistry in a cell block and PCR in an undiluted vitreous were positive for HZV in this case of acute retinal necrosis syndrome. **(Right)** Pap stain of an undiluted vitreous sample on liquid-based cytology shows condensation of vitreous and mixed inflammation with granulomas ⇨ in Candida endophthalmitis.

Candida Yeast Forms

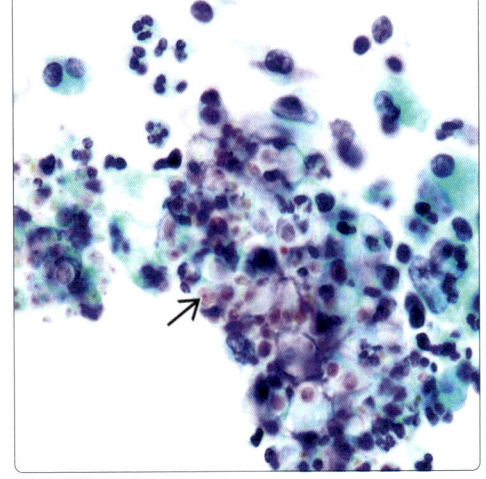

Yeast on PAS Stain

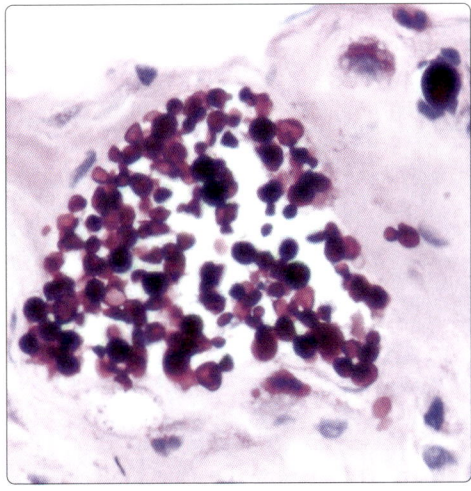

(Left) Higher magnification of the granulomatous inflammation shows many yeast forms ⇨ surrounded by neutrophils and macrophages on this Pap-stained ThinPrep. **(Right)** Cell block of the same case shows the granulomatous and acute vitreoretinitis stained with PAS to show the budding yeast forms, consistent with Candida species.

Eosinophils in *Toxocara canis* Infection

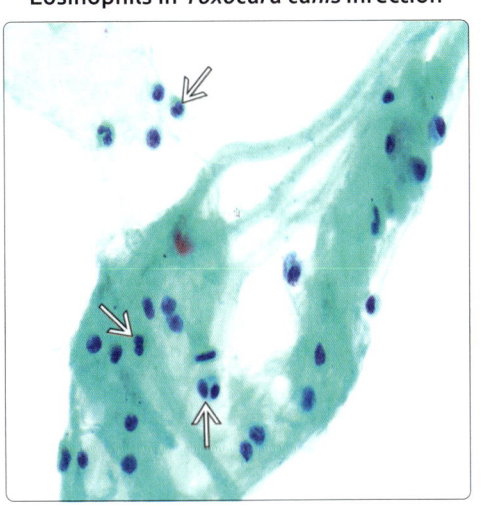

Eosinophil on Pap Stain

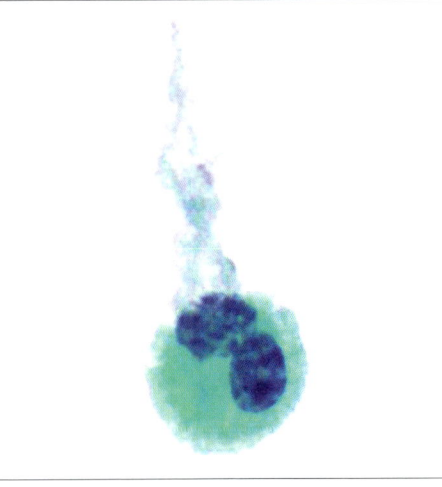

(Left) Liquid-based cytology Pap stain of a vitreous tap in a 9-year-old girl shows condensed vitreous containing lymphocytes, plasma cells, and eosinophils ⇨. ELISA in vitreous and serum showed high Toxocara canis titers. Note that the granules in eosinophils are better seen on Diff-Quik stain. **(Right)** High-power view shows an eosinophil in this case of Toxocariasis. Note that on Pap stain, eosinophils show bilobed nuclei and greenish cytoplasm with granules.

Ophthalmic Cytopathology, Neoplastic

TYPES OF CYTOLOGY

Aspiration Cytology
- Intraocular biopsies of anterior chamber fluid, iris lesions, vitreous, retina, and uvea (choroid and ciliary body) are most common
  - Orbital FNA may rarely be performed
  - Liquid biopsy for retinoblastoma (RB) using aqueous humor and analysis of cfDNA is possibility

Touch Imprint Cytology
- Frequently used to evaluate adequacy of sampling during intraoperative consultation of orbital tumors

Exfoliative Cytology
- May be used rarely on ocular surface neoplasia (cornea or conjunctiva) for diagnosis but more often for follow-up

NEOPLASIA IN CHILDREN

Orbital Neoplasia
- Most often performed to evaluate adequacy intraoperatively and for triaging for genetic/molecular testing
  - Touch imprints of orbital malignant tumors show cellular specimens with medium size, high nuclear:cytoplasmic (N:C) ratio, and hyperchromatic cells
- Metastatic neuroblastoma to orbit, typically in children 3-5 years old
  - Shows neuroendocrine salt and pepper nucleus with scant cytoplasm
- Rhabdomyosarcoma of orbit, typically in children 7-9 years old, is rapidly growing lesion, often located in superior nasal orbit
  - Shows strap cells with rare striations and abundant cytoplasm in embryonal type

FNA of Choroidal Tumor

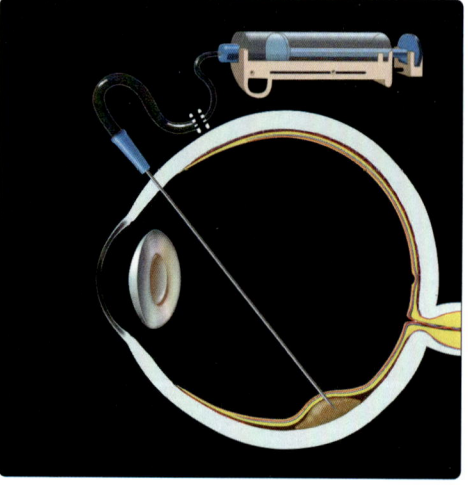

Diff-Quik Adequacy, Uveal Melanoma Smear

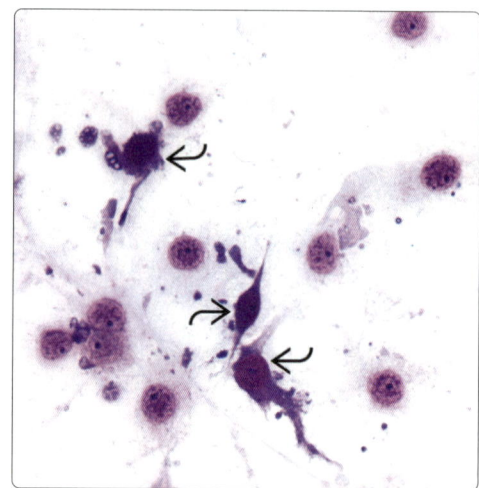

(Left) Graphic illustrates an FNA of choroidal tumor with a 27- or 30-gauge needle. *(Right)* Diagnostic cells are focally present in a predominantly paucicellular smear. Three spindled melanoma cells ⇒ with prominent nucleoli and scant melanin are seen in a background of naked nuclei.

Spindled Uveal Melanoma Cell, Liquid-Based Cytology

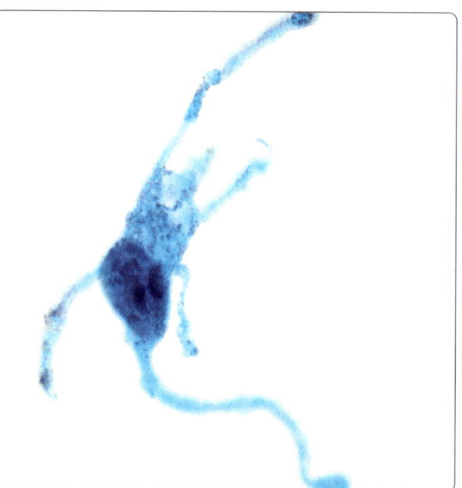

Choroidal Melanoma

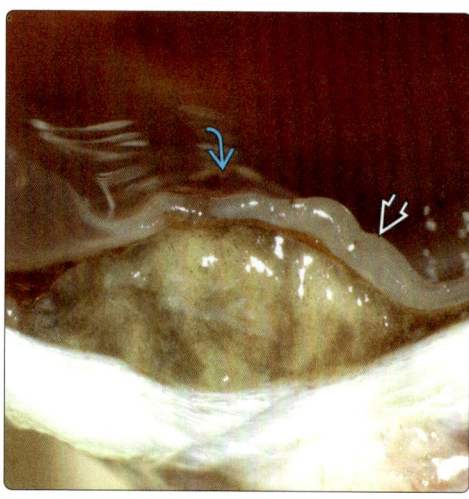

(Left) A spindled cell diagnostic of uveal melanoma in a ThinPrep shows the delicate cytoplasmic (jellyfish-like) prolongations and the oval nuclei with prominent nucleoli. *(Right)* Gross photograph shows a choroidal melanoma (8.0 x 5.0 mm) under the retina ⇒. Note the site of needle entrance and focal hemorrhage ⇒.

Ophthalmic Cytopathology, Neoplastic

Intraocular Retinoblastoma
- RB: Most frequent malignant intraocular tumor in children and most frequent intraocular malignancy worldwide
  - Not usually biopsied before radical treatment (to avoid needle tract seeding and metastasis)
- Cytology of FNA in RB may be cellular or scant with medium to large cells with scant cytoplasm and rosettes
  - Mitosis and apoptosis should be found before rendering diagnosis of RB
  - Pitfall: FNA of normal retina may show medium to large cells with high N:C ratio that are neurons
    - These features may be present in Coats disease or hyperplastic persistent primary vitreous (frequent differential diagnoses of RB)
  - During fresh tumor retrieval, touch imprint of tumor is used to evaluate adequacy of sampling and to serve as comparison to touch imprint of optic nerve (ON) cut margin to rule out margin involvement
    - Normal ON imprint shows blood and rare meningothelial cells that are bland cohesive cells with abundant cytoplasm

NEOPLASIA IN ADULTS
Orbital Neoplasia
- Adult orbital neoplasia is evaluated intraoperatively by touch imprint for triaging
  - Lymphoproliferative lesions should be submitted for flow cytometry/molecular testing to exclude clonality
  - Touch imprints are obtained instead of frozen sections to spare scant tissue available
  - Most lesions are reactive and represent idiopathic orbital inflammation with polymorphous infiltrate: Eosinophils, plasma cells, lymphocytes, tingible body macrophages
  - Lymphoma is usually of low-grade B-cell type
    - Most frequent is extranodal marginal zone lymphoma [mucosa-associated lymphoid tissue (MALT) type] with monomorphous infiltrate and occasional plasmacytoid cells; followed by follicular lymphoma
    - Pitfall: Mantle cell lymphoma should be excluded in seemingly low-grade lymphomas if positive for cyclin-D1 immunostain
  - Other hematopoietic lesions include diffuse large B-cell lymphomas or plasmacytoma/multiple myeloma
- Orbital FNA is seldom performed due to possible complications
  - Retrobulbar hemorrhage, perforation of globe, and unintended entry into cranial cavity
  - Vascular lesions and cystic lesions are not usually aspirated, and they represent large portion of orbital pathologies

Intraocular Neoplasia
- Not biopsied before treatment because clinical and ancillary studies are highly accurate to reach diagnosis and to avoid potential hemorrhage, retinal detachment, and tumor seeding
- FNA of vitreous is most frequent specimen received to exclude primary intraocular lymphoma (PIOL)
- PIOL (large B-cell lymphoma) involves retina, ON, and vitreous, often masquerades as chronic uveitis, and requires adequate triaging of vitreous samples
  - Cytologic findings include cellular specimen with necrotic background, condensed vitreous, macrophages, and small lymphocytes admixed with large, highly atypical lymphocytes with occasional nucleoli
  - Pitfall: Presence of numerous reactive cells may mislead to benign diagnosis
  - Pitfall: Flow cytometry may not be diagnostic due to scant material, large size, and necrosis of cells
    - Cell block should be attempted to confirm diagnosis by immunohistochemistry/molecular gene rearrangement
  - Main differential diagnosis is granulomatous vitritis (condensed vitreous, hypocellularity, or moderate cellularity of macrophages, and small lymphocytes)
- Choroidal lymphomas are low-grade B-cell lymphomas, usually secondary to systemic lymphoma, not often sampled
- Rarely, large T-cell lymphomas may also involve vitreous, retina, and ON, and carry poor prognosis
- FNA of intraocular solid tumors, if performed, is obtained to access adequacy for molecular testing and occasionally for diagnosis
  - Metastases to choroid are most frequent malignant intraocular tumors in adults, may mimic amelanotic melanoma; cytomorphology and immunohistochemistry are essential for accurate diagnosis
  - Melanoma of uveal tract is most common primary malignant intraocular tumor in adults and has high incidence (50%) of metastasis and death
- Melanoma of uveal tract is biopsied before plaque radiation treatment for molecular prognosis and rarely to exclude metastasis
  - Genetic/molecular prognostication tests stratify patients into high- or low-risk groups for metastasis
  - Melanoma cytology is often hypocellular: Epithelioid cells (worse prognosis), spindle B cells (plump with nucleoli), and spindle A cells (slender nuclei with central groove)
  - Cell block using double immunohistochemistry HMB-45 and Ki-67 (MIB-1) highlights melanoma cells with > 3% double-stained cells

SELECTED REFERENCES
1. Lin V et al: Biopsy for molecular risk stratification in uveal melanoma: yields and molecular characteristics in 119 patients. Clin Exp Ophthalmol. 50(1):50-61, 2022
2. Amer HZM et al: Intraocular metastases of lung origin: case reports and cytology correlates. Cytopathology. 32(5):677-83, 2021
3. Ozawa H et al: Iris metastasis as the initial presentation of metastatic esophageal cancer diagnosed by fine needle aspiration biopsy: a case report. Medicine (Baltimore). 100(22):e26232, 2021
4. Xu L et al: Establishing the clinical utility of ctDNA analysis for diagnosis, prognosis, and treatment monitoring of retinoblastoma: the aqueous humor liquid biopsy. Cancers (Basel). 13(6):1282, 2021
5. Han LM et al: The diagnostic utility of next-generation sequencing on FNA biopsies of melanocytic uveal lesions. Cancer Cytopathol. 128(7):499-505, 2020
6. Corrêa ZM et al: Indications for fine needle aspiration biopsy of posterior segment intraocular tumors. Am J Ophthalmol. 207:45-61, 2019
7. Kim RS et al: Histopathologic analysis of transvitreal fine needle aspiration biopsy needle tracts for uveal melanoma. Am J Ophthalmol. 174:9-16, 2017

Ophthalmic Cytopathology, Neoplastic

Touch Imprint of Tumor

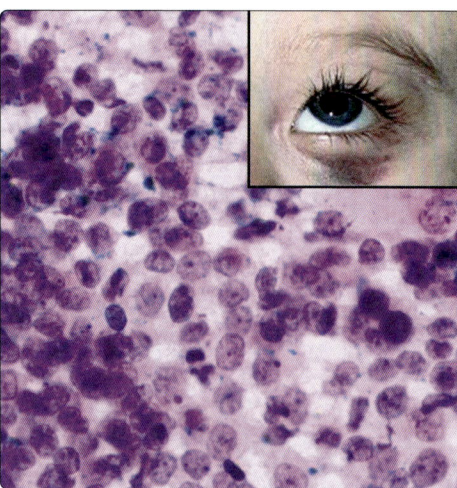

MR of Superotemporal Lesion

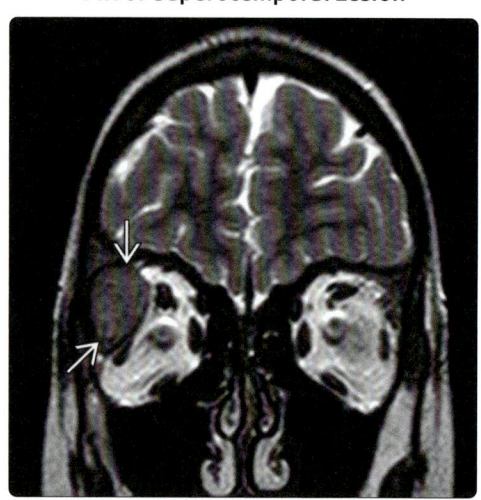

(Left) Inset shows a photograph of a 3-year-old girl with sudden proptosis with hematoma. Touch imprint of the biopsy shows large cells with scant cytoplasm and hyperchromatic nuclei. (Right) MR shows a superotemporal lesion expanding the lacrimal gland ➡ in a 14-year-old girl with a history of lymphoblastic B-cell leukemia.

Chorioretinal Lesions, FNAB

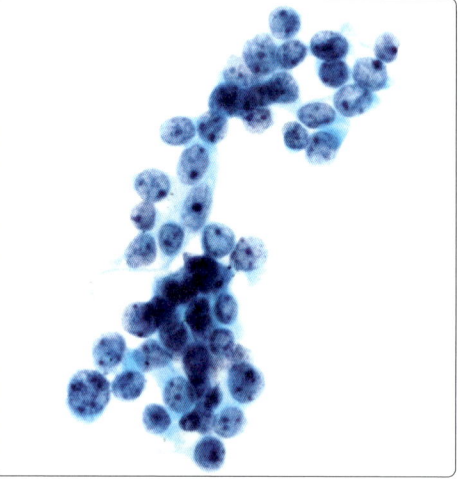

CK7 Immunohistochemistry

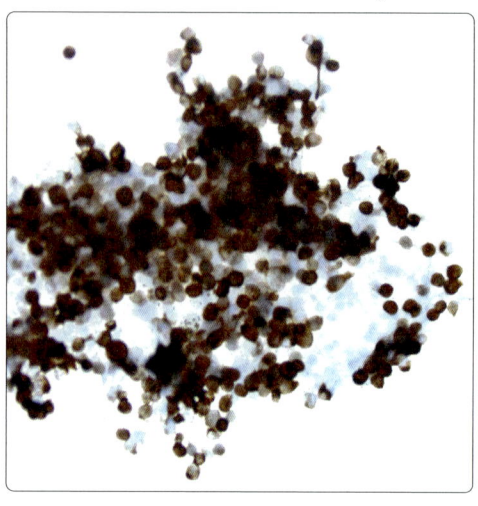

(Left) Predominantly choroid lesions with some extending into the retina are present in a 37-year-old man. The high nuclear:cytoplasmic ratio with prominent nucleoli and salt and pepper chromatin with cohesive groups raise suspicion for a metastatic neuroendocrine carcinoma in this Pap stain. (Right) Immunostains for TTF-1 and CK7 (seen here) are positive in the same case, consistent with a metastatic small cell carcinoma, neuroendocrine type.

Touch Imprint of Liver Core Biopsy in Metastatic Uveal Melanoma

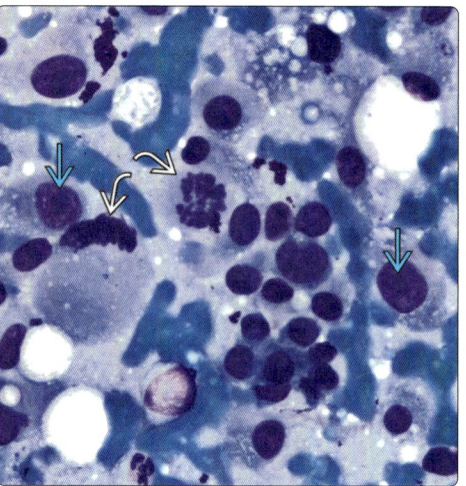

Core Biopsy of Metastatic Uveal Melanoma to Liver

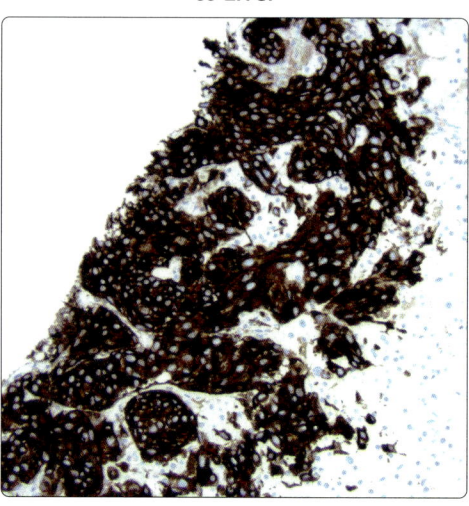

(Left) This liver core biopsy touch imprint stained with Diff-Quik, in a patient with known uveal melanoma, has large epithelioid amelanotic cells with mitoses ➡ and prominent nucleoli ➡. (Right) Notice the groups and single malignant cells mostly replacing and expanding the sinusoids of the liver, highlighted by the strongly positive melanoma marker HMB-45.

Ophthalmic Cytopathology, Neoplastic

Mantle Cell Lymphoma

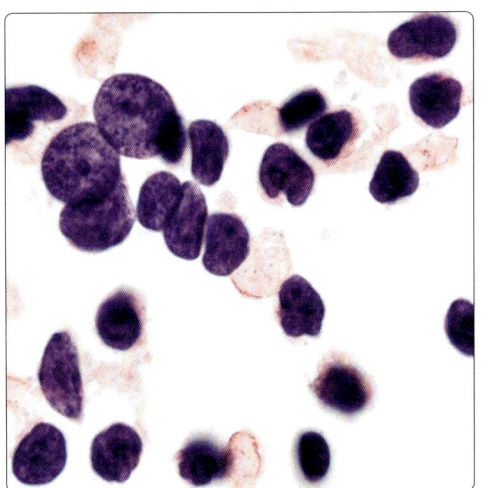

Plasmacytoma

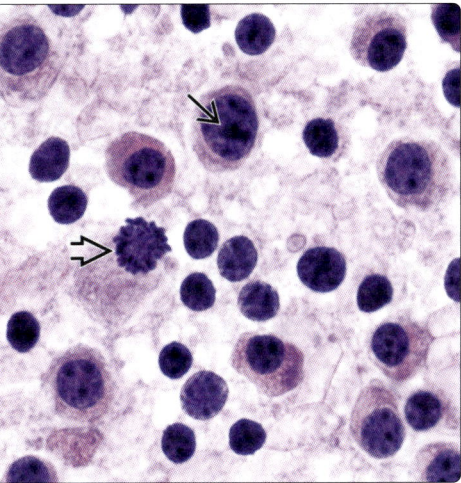

(Left) H&E touch imprint of a superotemporal orbital mass in a 60-year-old man shows small lymphocytes with irregular nuclear contours. Flow cytometry and permanent sections of the biopsy were diagnostic of mantle cell lymphoma. (Right) H&E touch imprint in a 75-year-old woman with a superior orbital mass shows many plasma cells that are atypical and large with occasional nucleoli ➡ and mitosis ➡. Plasma cells were κ-light chain restricted, which is consistent with plasmacytoma.

Primary Intraocular Lymphoma

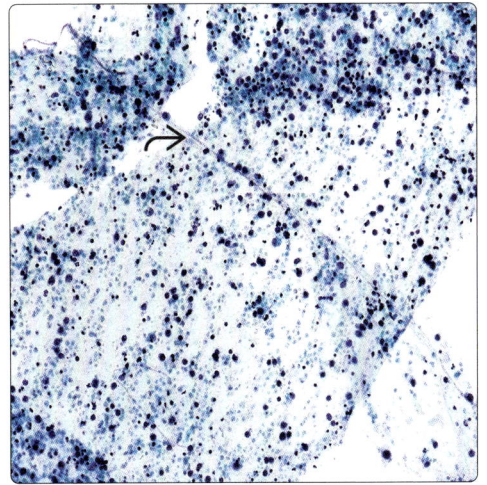

Large B-Cell Lymphoma

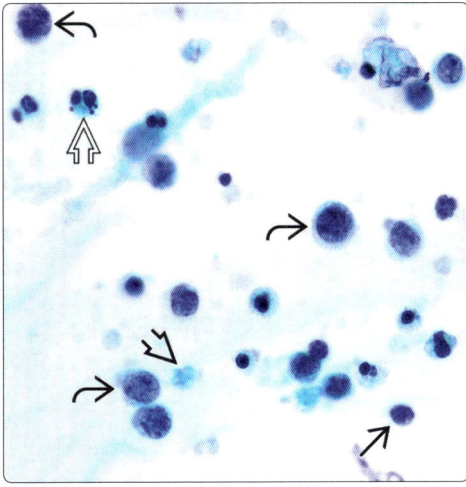

(Left) Vitreous biopsy was taken from a 70-year-old woman with floaters and visual loss. Pap stain of primary intraocular lymphoma (PIOL), large B-cell lymphoma, shows cellular, polymorphous infiltrate and background debris with condensed vitreous ➡ on liquid-based cytology. (Right) Liquid-based cytology of PIOL (large B-cell lymphoma diagnosed on flow cytometry) shows large, atypical lymphocytes ➡, small lymphocytes ➡, apoptotic cells ➡, and lymphoglandular bodies ➡.

Cell Block With CD20 Stain

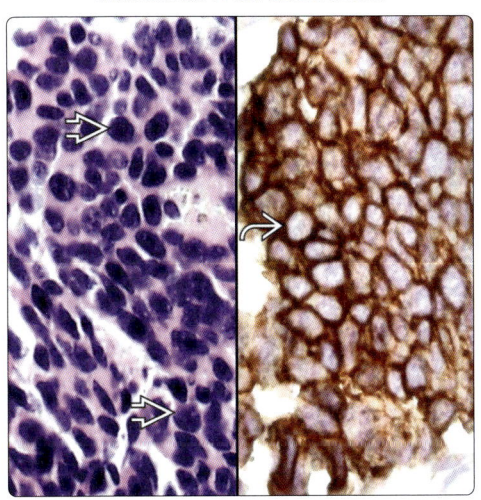

Large T-Cell Lymphoma

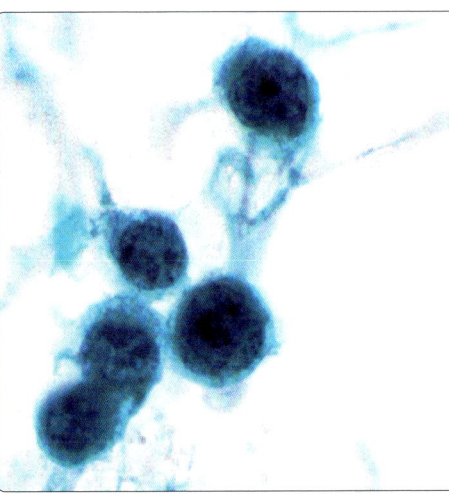

(Left) Cell block of the same case of PIOL shows large, atypical hyperchromatic cells on H&E ➡. Uniform CD20 cytoplasmic staining by immunochemistry ➡ is seen. (Right) Bedside FNA of a 72-year-old woman with rapid progression of vitreous opacity and altered mental status shows large lymphocytes on Pap stain. Short-panel flow cytometry was consistent with large T-cell lymphoma. The patient had CNS involvement and died 3 weeks later.

Ophthalmic Cytopathology, Neoplastic

(Left) Pigment from the retinal pigment epithelium (RPE) is oval (football-shaped), mildly refractile, and slightly orange in this H&E-stained touch imprint. Epithelioid and spindle melanoma cells are in the background. A lymphocyte ⇒ is associated with higher likelihood of metastasis and poor prognosis. **(Right)** Spindled melanoma cells show dusty, powder-like pigment in their cytoplasm in H&E-stained touch imprints, different from RPE pigment as seen in the previous image.

Touch Imprint of Uveal Melanoma With Other Cells
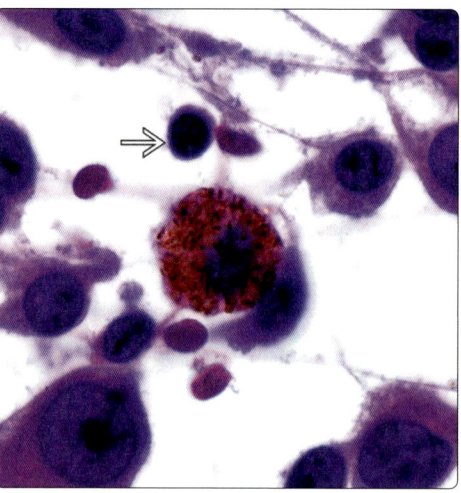

Touch Imprint of Uveal Melanoma
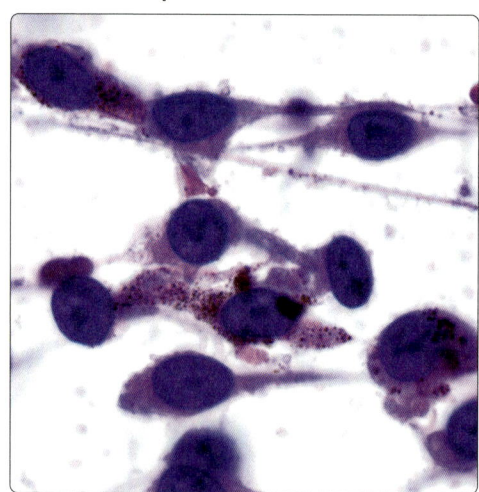

(Left) H&E stain of an amelanotic choroidal mass shows delicate cytoplasm and the tadpole shape ⇒ typically seen in melanoma spindle cells. Spindle A cells have a groove in the nucleus ⇒ and spindle B cells have nucleoli ⇒. Note the bland appearance of the cells. **(Right)** H&E stain of an amelanotic choroidal mass shows an epithelioid-type melanoma cell with abundant cytoplasm and prominent nucleoli ⇒ admixed with spindle B-type cells. Occasional intracytoplasmic melanin ⇒ is seen.

Amelanotic Melanoma
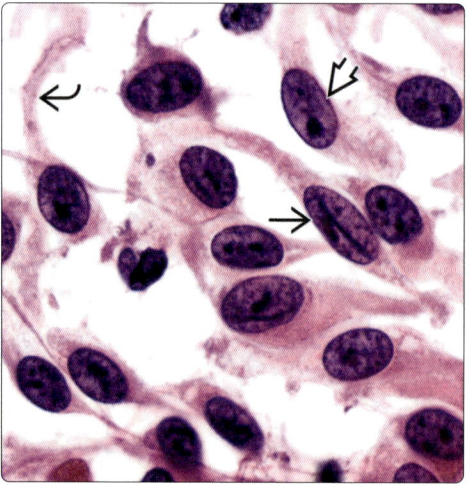

Epithelioid Melanoma of Choroid
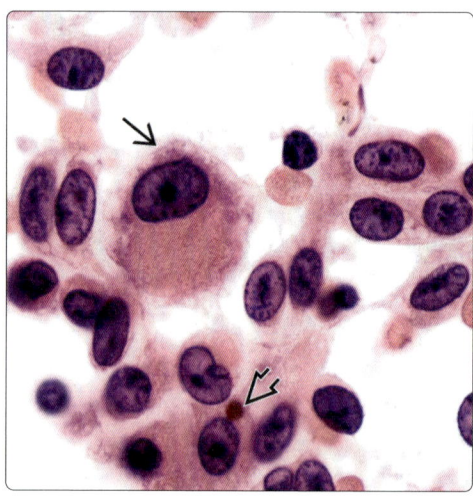

(Left) Cell block of FNA of a choroidal melanoma shows the clusters of slightly pigmented epithelioid and spindle B cells. Inset shows intense cytoplasmic positivity with Melan-A immunostain. **(Right)** Cell block of the FNA from choroidal melanoma double stained with HMB-45 (red-cytoplasmic) and Ki-67 (DAB brown-nuclear) shows proliferation of melanoma cells.

Pigmented Epithelioid and Spindle Cells
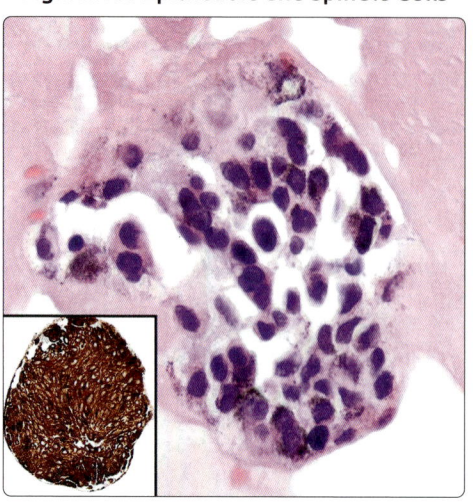

HMB-45 and Ki-67 Dual Stain
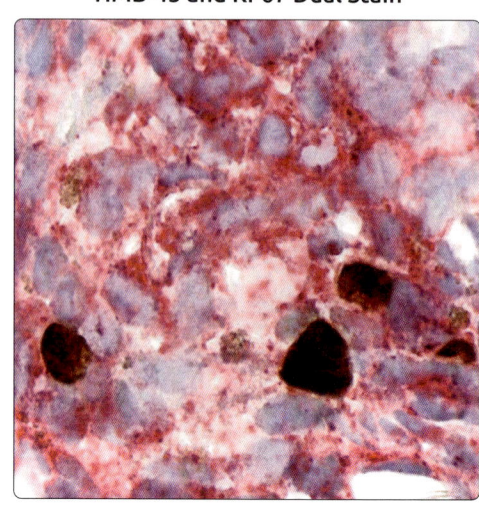

Ophthalmic Cytopathology, Neoplastic

Metastatic Lung Carcinoma to Iris

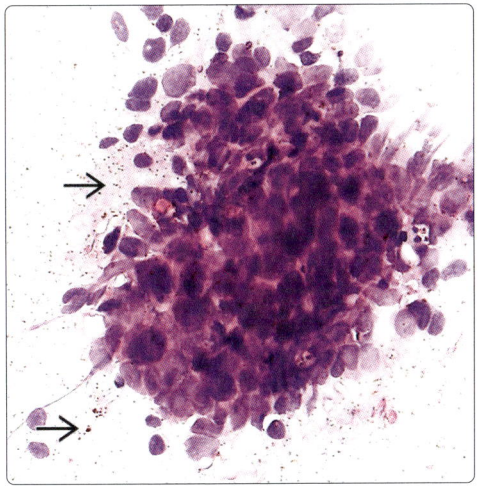

Retinoblastoma Rosettes, Mitoses, Necrosis

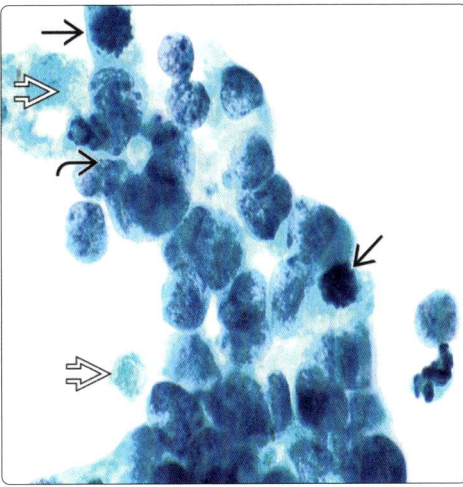

(Left) FNA in a patient with known lung carcinoma and a recently developed iris mass shows a crowded group of pleomorphic cells with a moderate amount of cytoplasm and background uveal pigment ➡. Immunohistochemistry on cell block showed CK7 and p63 positivity, consistent with pulmonary squamous cell carcinoma metastatic to iris. *(Right)* FNA in a 6-year-old child with anterior diffuse retinoblastoma shows large hyperchromatic cells with rosettes ➡, mitoses ➡, and necrosis ➡.

Retinoblastoma With Retinal Detachment

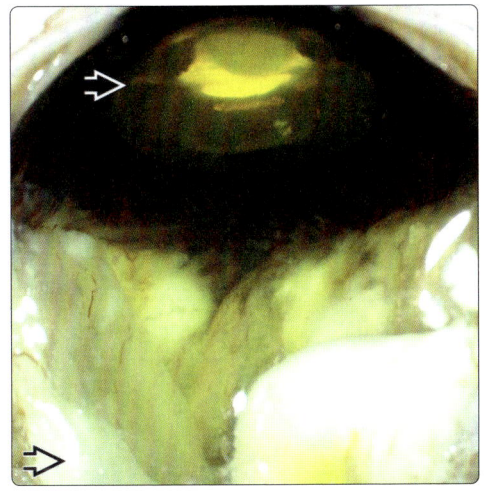

Liquid-Based Cytology of Retinoblastoma

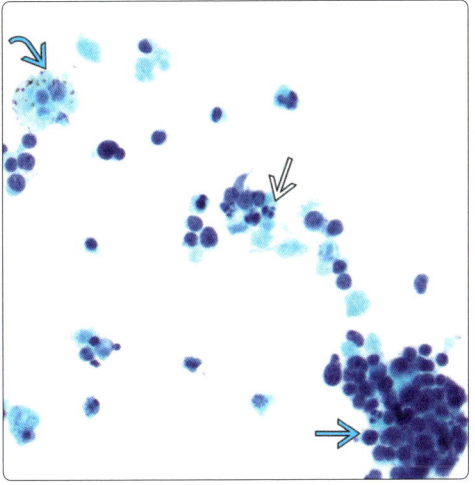

(Left) Gross photograph shows a retinoblastoma expanding and detaching the retina ➡ and filling most of the posterior portion of the eye. The lens ➡ is unremarkable. *(Right)* Notice the cohesive groups of neuroendocrine-type cells ➡ with some apoptosis ➡. The background contains cellular debris and some retinal pigment epithelial cells ➡.

Bone Marrow Metastasis of Retinoblastoma

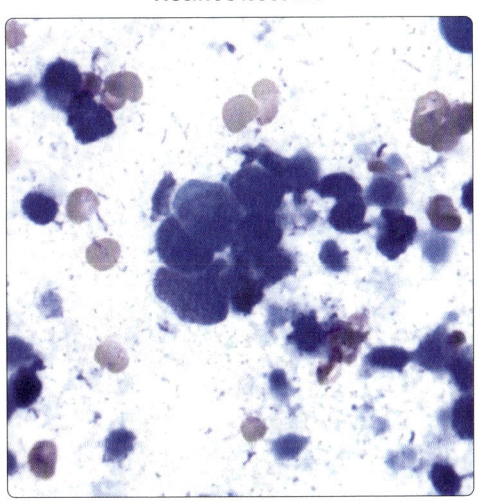

Bone Marrow Biopsy With Metastatic Retinoblastoma

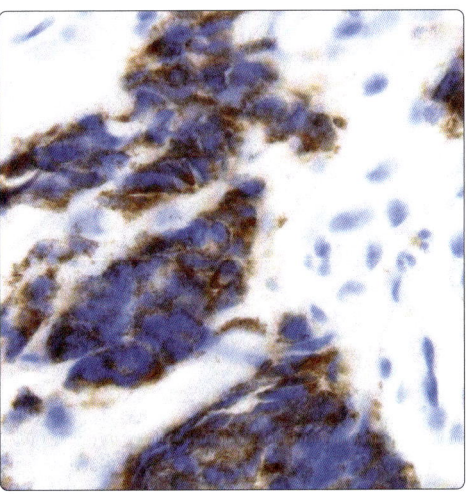

(Left) 3-year-old boy with massive choroidal invasion in enucleated eye presents 16 months later with bone marrow metastasis. Note the cohesive groups of large cells with high nuclear:cytoplasmic ratio in this Giemsa stain. *(Right)* Immunohistochemistry using synaptophysin highlights the cytoplasm of the cohesive neuroendocrine-type retinoblastoma cells in the bone marrow biopsy of the same case.

Neuropathology Squash Preparations, Infectious

TERMINOLOGY

Definitions

- Infection
  - Invasion of body or tissue by pathogenic microorganism (e.g., bacterium, virus, fungus, or protozoa) that subsequently produces tissue injury through cellular or toxic mechanisms
- Squash preparation
  - Performed at time of intraoperative consultation by "squashing" small portion of tissue between 2 glass slides for cytologic evaluation
  - Can be helpful in triaging of specimens, particularly those that may be infectious
    - PCR-based testing available for identification of many organisms

EPIDEMIOLOGY

Natural History

- Hematogenous dissemination from separate source in body: Lung, gastrointestinal tract, skin
- Direct extension from sinuses, dental work, trauma, surgery

ETIOLOGY/PATHOGENESIS

Bacterial

- Infection acquired hematogenously or through direct spread
- Increased risk of bacterial meningitis following head and neck or neurosurgical procedures
- Causes meningeal and parenchymal infection; can present as single mass, multiple masses, or diffuse disease

Tuberculosis

- Infection with *Mycobacterium tuberculosis*
- Up to 15% of cases involve nervous system
  - Children and immunocompromised patients are at increased risk
- Can be diffuse (meningitis) or localized (tuberculoma)

Fungal

- Infection acquired through inhalation of organism with nervous system involvement via hematogenous or direct spread from sinuses
- Can present as parenchymal mass, multiple masses, or diffuse disease
- Can be seen in immunocompromised and immunocompetent patients
- Large group of organisms with variable appearance
- Only relatively few organisms commonly infect nervous system

Toxoplasmosis

- Infection with *Toxoplasma gondii* (intracellular protozoan parasite)
  - Acquired through exposure to cat feces
- Seen most often in immunocompromised patients
- Can present as diffuse or mass-forming lesions

Cysticercosis

- Infection with *Taenia solium* (pork tapeworm)
  - Acquired through ingestion of contaminated food or water
- Most common nervous system parasitic infection worldwide
- Can occur in immunocompetent or immunocompromised individuals
- Can present as single or multiple small parenchymal cysts or large multiloculated cysts typically without organism (racemose form)

Viral

- Herpes simplex virus (HSV)
  - Type 1 is most common and typically causes encephalitis (affecting frontal and temporal lobes)
  - Type 2 is associated with Mollaret meningitis and neonatal infection
  - Can occur in immunocompetent or immunocompromised individuals
  - Rarely biopsied, only if cerebral spinal fluid (CSF) testing by polymerase chain reaction (PCR) is negative or presentation is atypical
- Progressive multifocal leukoencephalopathy (PML)
  - Caused by John Cunningham (JC) virus (polyomavirus)
  - Opportunistic infection in immunocompromised patients by reactivation of latent virus
    - Multiple sclerosis patients on immune modulators (e.g., natalizumab) are at increased risk
    - Also seen in patients with hematologic malignancies and on immunosuppressants post transplantation or for collagen vascular diseases
  - Multifocal, white matter lesions with little to no mass effect

MACROSCOPIC

Mass-Forming Lesions

- Abscess
  - Thick hyperemic capsule with purulent/necrotic center
- Tuberculoma

Diffuse Processes

- Meningitis
  - Purulent material overlying meninges
  - May have subarachnoid hemorrhages
- Cerebritis/encephalitis
  - Diffuse inflammation of brain parenchyma
  - Can be initial stage of abscess

MICROSCOPIC

Bacterial

- Necrosis, macrophages, neutrophils, and necroinflammatory debris on cytology
- May see fibroblasts from abscess wall and reactive gliosis from adjacent brain tissue
- Organisms can be difficult to see on hematoxylin and eosin (H&E) stain
- Filamentous bacterium can sometimes be identified on cytology
- Fite stain can help to distinguish *Nocardia* [Fite (+)] from *Actinomyces* [Fite (-)]

Neuropathology Squash Preparations, Infectious

Tuberculosis
- Epithelioid histiocytes, lymphocytes, plasma cells, multinucleated giant cells, and necrosis on cytology
- May see well-formed granulomas with central necrosis
- Bacilli are not easily identified on H&E and may also be difficult to identify on acid-fast bacillus (AFB) stain

Fungal
- Histiocytes, multinucleated giant cells, and lymphocytes on cytology
- Fungal organisms can occasionally be identified on squash preparation
- *Cryptococcus neoformans*
  - Commonly involves nervous system
  - Round yeast forms
    - Varying size (4-7 μm)
    - Thick capsule
- *Aspergillus*
  - Septate hyphal forms with acute angle branching
- Zygomycetes (*Rhizopus*, *Mucor*)
  - Opportunistic
  - Nonseptate or minimally septate hyphal forms with irregular branching
- *Blastomyces dermatitidis*
  - Nervous system involvement is uncommon but can occur, typically in immunocompetent patients
  - Dimorphic fungus
  - Yeast form with broad-based budding at body temperature
  - Thin capsule
- *Histoplasma capsulatum*
  - Nervous system involvement is uncommon
  - Small yeast forms
    - 2-4 μm in size
    - No capsule
  - Intracellular organisms seen in macrophages
- *Coccidioides immitis*
  - Seen in both immunocompetent and compromised individuals
  - Large (30- to 60-μm) sporangia with multiple endospores within
  - Large multinucleated giant cells are often present
- Dematiaceous fungi
  - Group of pigmented (melanized) fungi often found in soil
  - Seen in both immunocompetent and compromised individuals
  - Can have variable morphology from filamentous to yeast-like
    - Common feature is heavily pigmented (melanized) appearance

Toxoplasmosis
- Necrotic debris
- Mixed acute and chronic inflammation
- Typically seen in tachyzoite form in human tissues
- Can be seen as encysted bradyzoites (clustered tachyzoites) or as individual tachyzoites

Cysticercosis
- Organism is best identified on histology
- On cytologic preparation, findings are nonspecific
  - Normal to mildly gliotic neural tissue and mild chronic inflammation in viable larval stage
  - Mixed acute and chronic inflammation and eosinophils in degenerating larval stage
  - Necrosis, gliosis, fibrosis, and calcified nodules in remote infection
- No organism is present in racemose forms

Viral
- HSV1: Herpes simplex encephalitis
  - Necrosis, hemorrhage, and mixed inflammation on cytology
  - May see intranuclear Cowdry A inclusion in some infected cells (neurons, astrocytes, oligodendrocytes)
- JC virus: PML
  - Macrophages, bizarre astrocytes
    - May see multinucleated (Creutzfeldt) astrocytes
  - Oligodendrocytes may have enlarged nuclei with ground-glass viral inclusions

DIFFERENTIAL DIAGNOSIS

On Cytologic Preparation
- Presence of microorganisms on squash preparation aids in diagnosis
  - Unfortunately, many times no organism will be seen on preparations
- Differential diagnosis of cytologic preparations can be reached based on observed features
  - Acute inflammation, necrosis, and fibroblasts
    - Acute inflammation is suggestive of abscess; however, presence of fibroblasts and gliotic neuropil can mimic high-grade glioma
    - In glioma, look for pleomorphic glial cells and mitoses
    - Although acute inflammation can be seen in glioma, it is usually minimal
  - Macrophages
    - Presence of numerous macrophages on squash preparation is unusual in context of tumor but does play role in differential inflammatory and infectious processes
    - Stroke: Numerous macrophages, necrotic debris, hemosiderin
    - Demyelinating plaque: Foamy macrophages, Creutzfeldt astrocytes, granular mitoses
    - PML: Foamy macrophages, bizarre astrocytes, ground-glass intranuclear inclusions in oligodendrocytes
    - Tuberculosis: Epithelioid histiocytes, reactive lymphocytes, necrotic debris
    - Fungal infection: Epithelioid histiocytes, mixed inflammation
    - Sarcoidosis: Epithelioid histiocytes (may be multinucleated), reactive lymphocytes
    - Langerhans cell histiocytosis: Histiocytes, eosinophils
    - Rosai-Dorfman disease: Histiocytes, lymphocytes, plasma cells, emperipolesis

SELECTED REFERENCES
1. Stebner A et al: Molecular diagnosis of polymicrobial brain abscesses with 16S-rDNA-based next-generation sequencing. Clin Microbiol Infect. 27(1):76-82, 2021

Neuropathology Squash Preparations, Infectious

Acute Bacterial Cerebritis

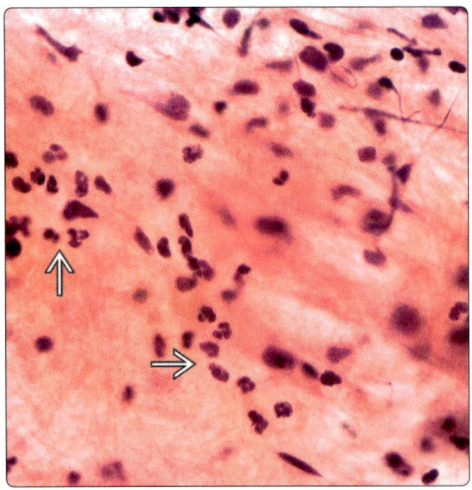

Viral Meningoencephalitis

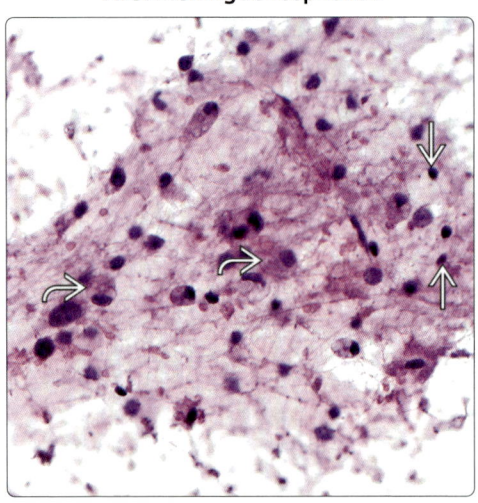

(Left) Bacterial and fungal infections can have varying degrees of acute inflammation ➡. On this image of an H&E-stained smear, the inflammation is within the reactive neuropil and was from a case of bacterial cerebritis. (Right) Squash preparation stained with H&E shows scattered macrophages ➡ and lymphocytes ➡ in a background of reactive neuropil and necrosis. The patient was found to have a viral meningoencephalitis.

Granulomatous Fungal Meningitis

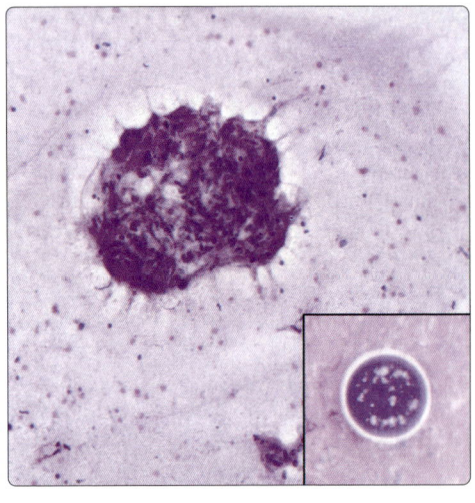

Nocardia in Neuropil

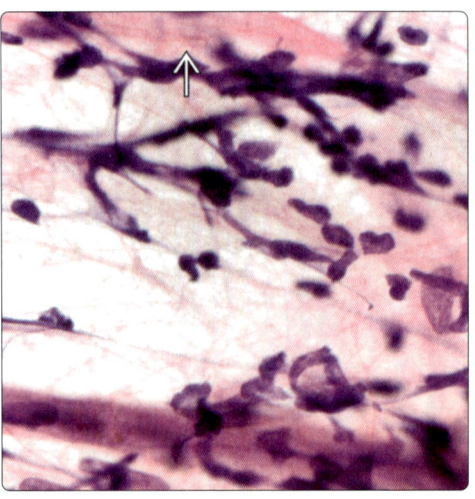

(Left) Granulomas like the one demonstrated by H&E in this fungal meningitis can be encountered not only in infectious processes but also in noninfectious entities, such as neurosarcoidosis. Identification of organisms is helpful to distinguish the 2. In this case, Coccidioides (inset) was identified on PAS stain. (Right) Identification of bacterial microorganisms can be exceedingly difficult on H&E-stained cytology. The reactive neuropil and mixed inflammation in this preparation helps to mask the filamentous bacterium ➡.

Nocardia With GMS and Gram Stain

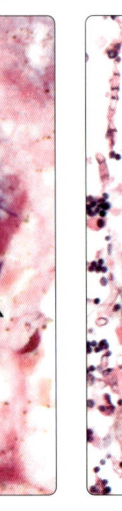

Mucormycosis

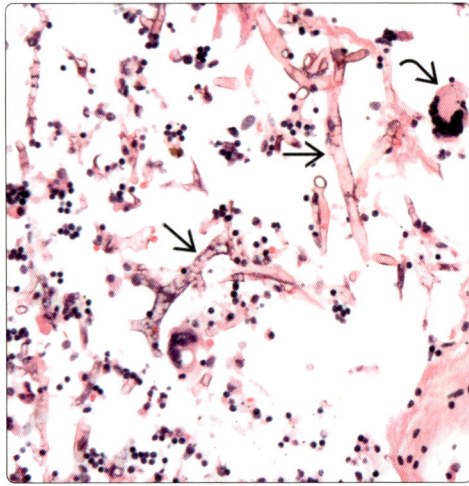

(Left) Most bacteria are better identified on special stains. The left panel shows a GMS stain highlighting numerous filamentous bacteria ➡. The right shows the same bacteria on Gram stain ➡. This organism was also Fite (+), consistent with Nocardia species. (Right) Many fungal organisms are often large enough to identify on H&E-stained squash preparation. This fungus ➡ shows the classic ribbon-like, aseptate forms of mucormycosis. Multinucleated giant cells ➡ can often be seen in fungal infections.

Neuropathology Squash Preparations, Infectious

Histoplasma in Macrophages

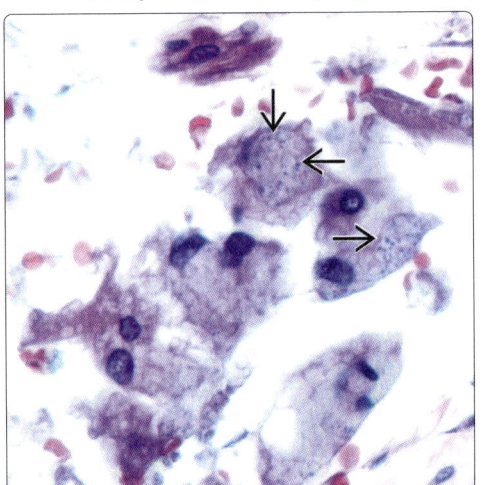

Dematiaceous Fungus

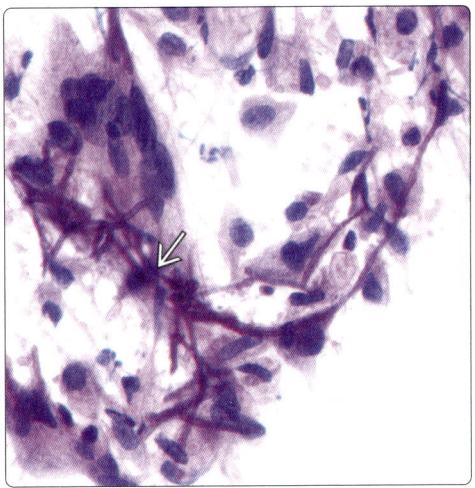

(Left) Other fungal forms can be more subtle in their appearance. This H&E shows macrophages with intracellular collections of Histoplasma ➡. (Right) H&E shows a squash preparation from a brain abscess. The slide is stained with H&E; a brown pigmented Cladophialophora organism ➡ is shown.

Toxoplasma

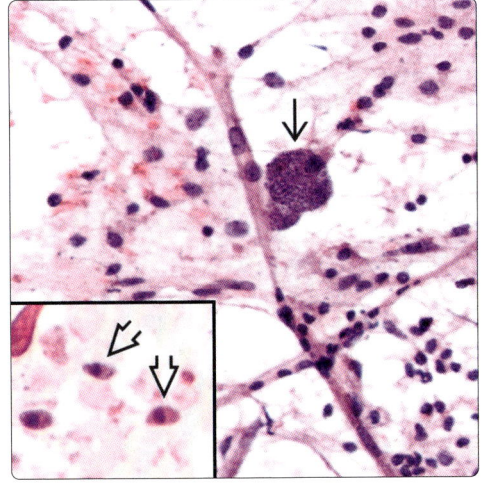

Neurocysticercosis Racemose Form

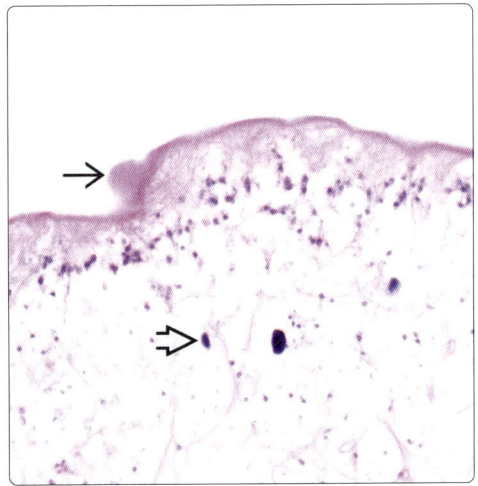

(Left) Some organisms can be concurrently present in multiple forms. Squash preparation stained with H&E shows an intact bradyzoite ➡, consistent with Toxoplasma infection. The organism is easier to identify when encysted vs. when in the individual tachyzoite form ➡. (Right) Cysticercosis can be encountered in the brain in a multiloculated cyst composed of the helminth cuticle layer ➡ and underlying reticular layer usually with calcifications ➡. No scolex is present in these forms.

Herpes Cowdry A Inclusion

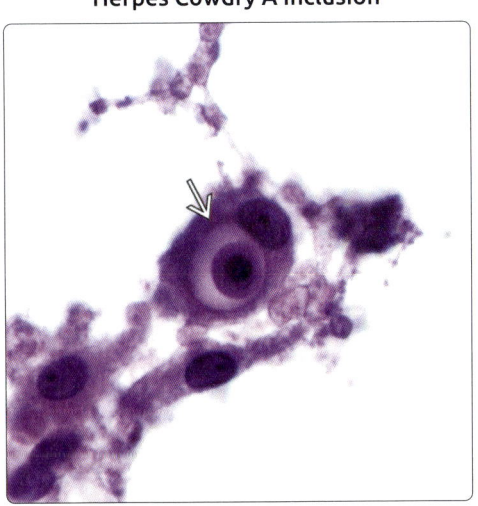

Oligodendrocyte With Ground-Glass Viral Inclusion

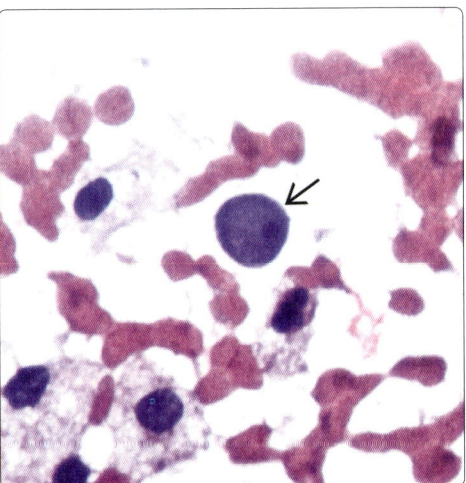

(Left) Viral cytopathic changes can also be seen on squash preparations. The image shows the Cowdry A inclusion ➡ of herpesvirus seen in a patient with encephalitis in an H&E-stained smear. (Right) The image of a smear stained with H&E shows an oligodendrocyte with ground-glass inclusions ➡, suggestive of progressive multifocal encephalopathy.

Neuropathology Squash Preparations, Glial Neoplasms

TERMINOLOGY

Abbreviations
- Glioblastoma (GBM), ganglioglioma (GG), pilocytic astrocytoma (PA), pleomorphic xanthoastrocytoma (PXA), adult-type diffuse astrocytoma (DA), subependymal giant cell astrocytoma (SEGA)

WHO CNS 2021
- Integrated diagnoses now include molecular results where possible
- Low grade
  ○ Grade 1: PA, SEGA, subependymoma, myxopapillary ependymoma
  ○ Grade 2: PXA, DA IDH mutant, oligodendroglioma IDH mutant and 1p19q codeleted, supratentorial ependymoma, supratentorial ependymoma ZFTA fusion positive, supratentorial ependymoma, YAP1 fusion positive, posterior fossa group A (PFA) and posterior fossa group B (PFB) ependymoma, spinal ependymoma
- High grade
  ○ Grade 3: DA, IDH mutant, oligodendroglioma IDH mutant and 1p19q codeleted, PXA, GG
  ○ Grade 4: GBM IDH-wildtype, diffuse midline glioma H3K27M mutant, DA, IDH mutant
  ○ **Integrated diagnoses (should be rendered if possible)**
    – DA IDH mutant, grade 2, grade 3, or grade 4
    – GBM, IDH-wildtype, grade 4
    – Diffuse midline glioma, H3K27M mutant, grade 4
    – Oligodendroglioma, IDH mutant and 1p/19q codeleted, grade 2 or grade 3
  ○ **Other astrocytic tumors, including "relatively" circumscribed types**
    – PA, SEGA, and PXA
  ○ **Ependymal tumors**
    – Subependymoma, grade 1
    – Myxopapillary ependymoma, grade 2
    – Ependymoma, grade 2
    – Supratentorial ependymoma, ZFTA fusion positive, and supratentorial ependymoma, YAP-1 fusion positive
    – PFA and PFB
    – Spinal ependymoma and spinal ependymoma MYCN amplified

ETIOLOGY/PATHOGENESIS

Molecular Alterations
- PA: Tandem duplication at chromosome 7q34 with resultant novel BRAF fusion gene (KIAA1549::BRAF fusion); rarely, BRAF V600E mutation
- Identification of isocitrate dehydrogenase I (IDH1) mutation (R132H) or, less commonly, other IDH1/IDH2 mutations are prognostically significant in gliomas and are **required** for integrated diagnosis
- Mutant IDH can separate DA from reactive process (gliosis) and differentiates between DA IDH mutant, grade 4 and GBM IDH-wildtype, grade 4
- 1p19q loss of heterozygosity (LOH) (FISH testing is gold standard) is molecularly characteristic coupled with IDH-mutant status for **required** integrated diagnosis of oligodendroglioma

CLINICAL IMPLICATIONS

Therapeutics
- 2021 CNS WHO grade is based on integrated diagnosis that includes not only histologic features as to cell type but immunohistochemical stain results for IDH1 R132H for DA coupled with 1p19q for O
- Other immunohistochemical stains, such as p53, ATRX, and proliferation rate assessment using Ki-67, are often performed in addition to molecular studies
- Results of these tests affect prognosis and clinical outcome; radiology features (i.e., location), patient's performance status (Karnofsky score), and extent of resection are also critical to patient prognosis
- Treatment for high-grade gliomas, whether of astrocytic or oligodendroglial lineage, includes both radiation and chemotherapy

(Left) H&E touch imprint highlights corkscrew-like, densely eosinophilic Rosenthal fibers ⇒ seen in pilocytic astrocytoma, which may also be seen in nonneoplastic conditions. A very fibrillary background is present. (Right) H&E touch imprint of pilocytic astrocytoma reveals an eosinophilic granular body (EGB) ⇒, characteristic of some neoplastic processes. EGB is composed of multiple proteinaceous globules of varying size.

Rosenthal Fibers

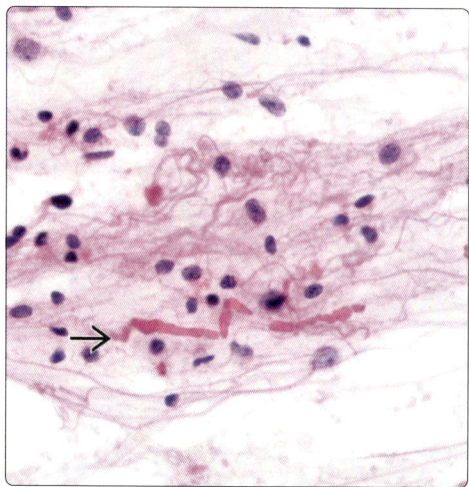

Eosinophilic Granular Body

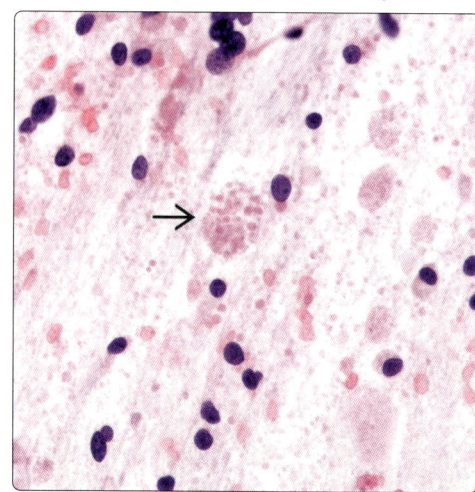

Neuropathology Squash Preparations, Glial Neoplasms

- *IDH1* R132H immunoreactivity (positive staining) in patients < 55 years should be confirmed with molecular studies (sequencing)
- Presence of LOH for 1p and 19q with *IDH1* mutation is diagnostic of oligodendroglioma and may spare patients radiation therapy (especially AO)
- *IDH1/IDH2* mutations, *BRAF* V600E mutations, and *KIAA1549::BRAF* fusion proteins are characteristic of low-grade glioma and also may impact therapeutic choices

MACROSCOPIC

Specimen Handling

- Most laboratories use both frozen tissue section and touch &/or squash cytologic preparation for intraoperative consultation
- H&E and Pap stains can be used for cytologic preparation with comparative quality for evaluation
- Squash preparations of glial tissue "spread" easily in comparison with those of nonglial (epithelial or mesenchymal) tissues
- Touch imprint preparations and squash preparations will identify fibrillar cytoplasmic processes in glial tumors (especially astrocytic neoplasms)
  - These must be distinguished from "stretch" artifact in meningothelial processes
- Even when very small amounts of tissue are present at time of frozen section, squash &/or touch preparations may provide more information than poorly prepared frozen section

MICROSCOPIC

General Features

- Oligodendrogliomas characteristically demonstrate perinuclear halos (fried egg appearance) in formalin-fixed tissue sections
  - Oligodendrogliomas have little cytoplasm with exception of minigemistocytes that may be present in grade 3 tumors
- Round-to-oval nuclei with generally darker chromatin (as compared with astrocyte nuclei) are characteristic of oligodendroglial and ependymal tumors
- Mild-to-moderate nuclear pleomorphism and hypercellularity in astrocytic tumors, particularly with escalation in grade
- Nuclear pleomorphism is less prominent in both oligodendroglial and ependymal neoplasms as compared with astrocytomas, even with escalation in grade
- Rosette formation (true ependymal rosettes and perivascular pseudorosettes) is characteristic of ependymomas
- Mitotic activity and necrosis may be identified in any of these tumors and increases with grade

Specific Cytologic Findings

- Oligodendroglioma: Monomorphic tumor cells with limited cytoplasm
  - Delicate, thin-walled blood vessels may be seen on squash preparation
  - Grade 3: Minigemistocytic tumor cells may be seen
- Ependymoma: Hypercellular on touch preparation
  - Round-to-oval nuclei with vesicular chromatin
  - Perivascular acellular zones (corresponding to perivascular pseudorosettes) may be found on squash preparation
- Myxopapillary ependymoma: "Blue balls" of myxoid material may be identified in fibrillary (glial) background
  - Secondary changes (e.g., hemorrhage) are common
- PA: Bland nuclear features and very long, delicate (hair-like) cytoplasmic processes
- Chronic processes: Indicated by Rosenthal fibers and eosinophilic granular bodies (EGBs)
  - Gliomas (e.g., PA, PXA, GG)
  - Gliotic tissue with Rosenthal fibers may surround cystic lesions; beware of overinterpretation of this finding as tumor
- Grade 4 astrocytoma: Necrotic background and microvascular proliferation (MVP)

DIFFERENTIAL DIAGNOSIS

Reactive vs. Neoplastic Glial Process

- Differentiation often difficult, even on histologic sections
- Cells with angulated hyperchromatic nuclei and mitotic activity favor neoplasm
- Multiple clumps of tissue on squash preparation favor reactive gliosis
- IDH1 immunoreactivity is consistent with neoplasm
- Diffuse strong p53 immunoreactivity is highly suggestive of neoplasm
  - Negativity of these immunostains does not exclude neoplasm

Astrocytic vs. Oligodendroglial Neoplasms

- Astrocytoma: Glial processes or large cells with generous eosinophilic cytoplasm; nuclear pleomorphism
- Oligodendroglioma: Round to oval bare nuclei; nuclear monomorphism
- MVP and necrosis do **not** distinguish high-grade astrocytoma from high-grade oligodendroglioma

Glioblastoma vs. Metastatic Malignancies (Carcinomas and Melanomas)

- Radiologically, both lesions show ring-enhancing mass
- Cytologically, both lesions show dirty background (due to necrosis and hemorrhage)
  - GBM: Dyscohesive or loosely cohesive atypical cells with glial processes
  - Metastatic carcinomas: Cohesive clusters of atypical cells
    - Intracytoplasmic mucin or keratinization can be seen
  - Metastatic melanoma: Dyscohesive, or loosely cohesive, atypical plasmacytoid tumor cells with prominent nucleoli
    - Identification of melanin pigments in tumor cells is almost diagnostic
    - ~ 50% of melanomas in brain are amelanotic

SELECTED REFERENCES

1. Perez A et al: The evolving classification of diffuse gliomas: World Health Organization updates for 2021. Curr Neurol Neurosci Rep. 21(12):67, 2021
2. WHO Classification of Tumours Editorial Board: Gliomas, glioneuronal tumours, and neuronal tumours. In Central Nervous System Tumours. 5th ed. 15-187, 2021

Neuropathology Squash Preparations, Glial Neoplasms

IDH1 R132H Immunohistochemical Stain

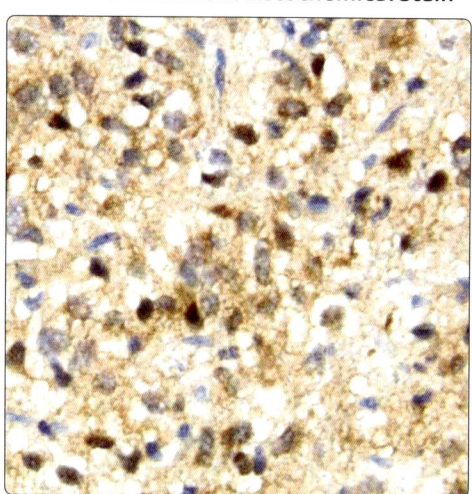

Astrocytoma With Atypical Mitosis

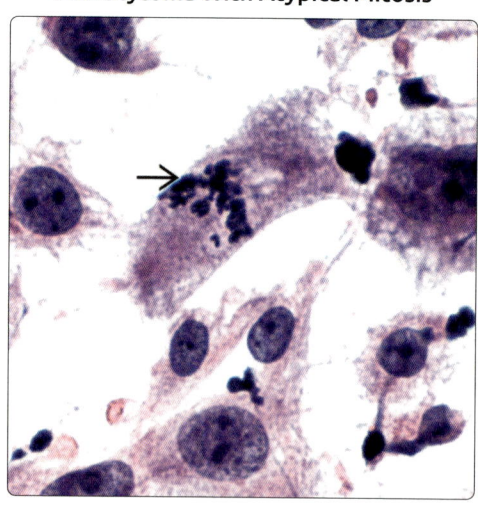

(Left) *IDH1-mutant glioma with nuclear and cytoplasmic immunoreactivity is shown.* (Right) *H&E-stained touch imprint of an astrocytoma with marked nuclear pleomorphism and fibrillary cytoplasmic processes reveals the presence of an atypical mitosis ➡.*

Vascular Proliferation in Glioblastoma

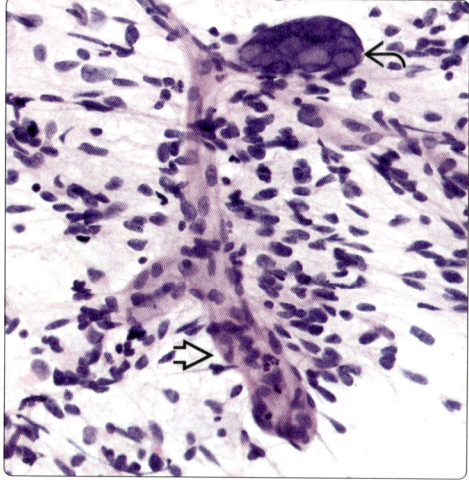

Nuclear Pleomorphism and Atypia in Glioblastoma

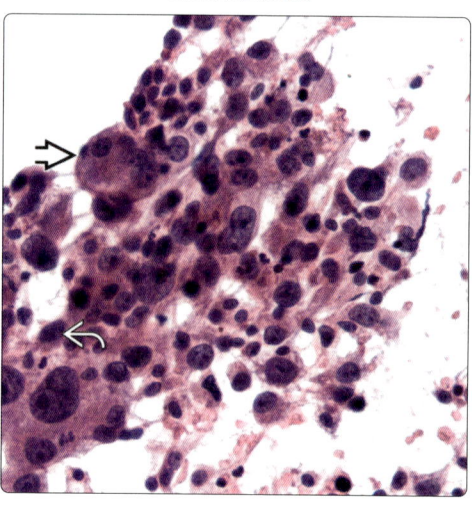

(Left) *H&E-stained smear preparation of a glioblastoma (GBM) shows a cellular glial neoplasm with pleomorphism and a prominent vessel with endothelial proliferation ➡. A bizarre nucleus ➡ is present. The background is fibrillary.* (Right) *H&E-stained touch imprint preparation of GBM highlights a cellular astrocytic neoplasm with several extremely large and pleomorphic cells with prominent nucleoli ➡ admixed with small cells with dense chromatin ➡. The background is necrotic.*

"Blue Balls" of Myxopapillary Ependymoma

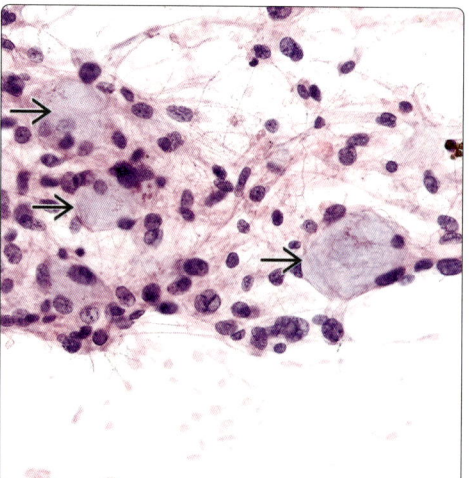

Eosinophilic Granular Body and Pilocytic Astrocytoma

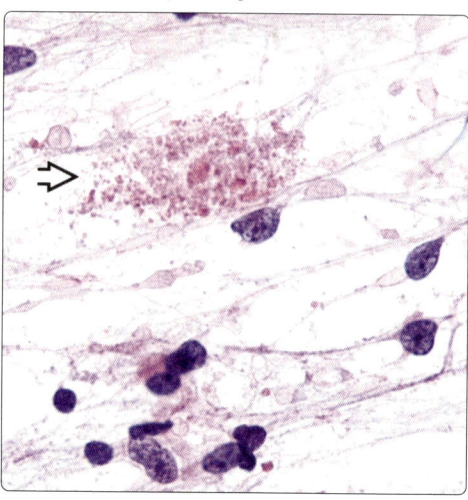

(Left) *H&E-stained touch imprint of a circumscribed mass of the filum terminale shows a neoplasm with a fibrillar glial background and "blue balls" of myxoid material ➡, characteristic of a myxopapillary ependymoma.* (Right) *EGB ➡ and piloid cells with fibrillar background in pilocytic astrocytoma are shown in this H&E-stained touch imprint. The EGB is somewhat distorted due to the preparation.*

Neuropathology Squash Preparations, Glial Neoplasms

Oligodendroglioma

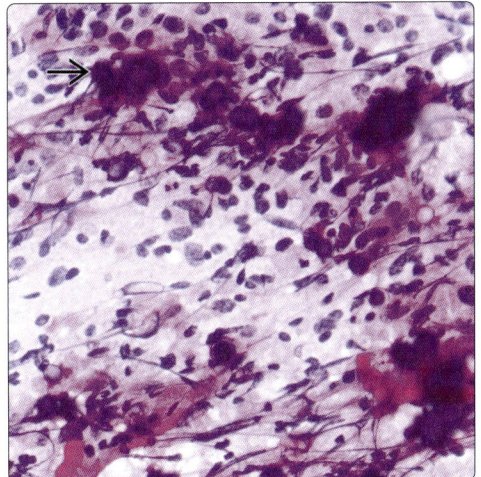

High-Power Touch Prep of Oligodendroglioma

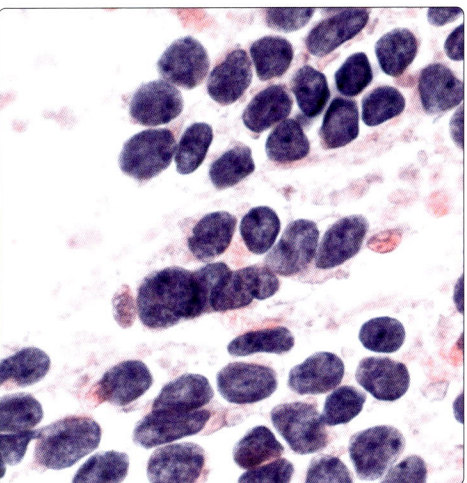

(Left) Touch imprint shows an oligodendroglioma with bland oval to round nuclei and calcifications ➡. (Right) H&E-stained touch imprint/smear shows round to oval cells with minimal cytoplasm and scattered chromocenters. Minimal nuclear pleomorphism without obvious glial processes is noted. These are nuclear features of an oligodendroglioma.

Oligodendroglioma

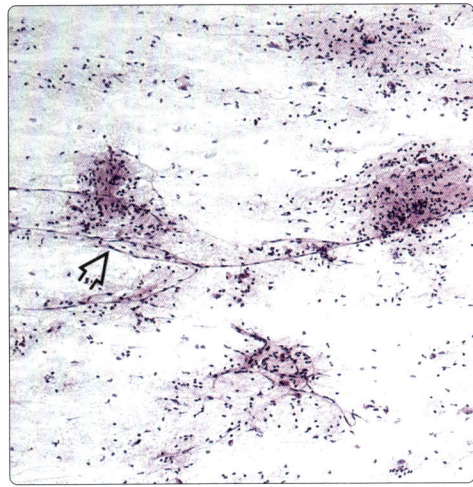

Minigemistocytes of Oligodendroglioma

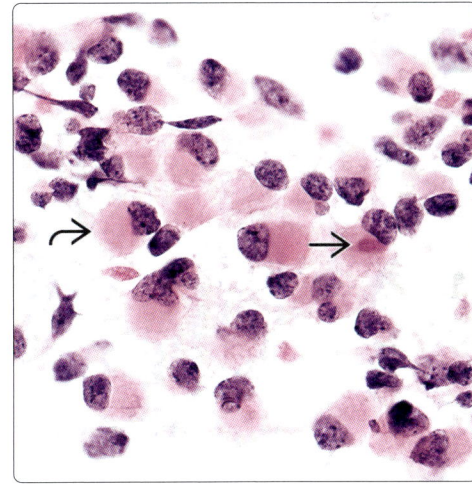

(Left) Cytologic squash preparation shows the delicate and thin vascular pattern characteristic of oligodendroglioma ➡. (Right) H&E smear of an anaplastic oligodendroglioma shows globular eosinophilic cytoplasm ➡ diagnostic of a minigemistocyte. Dense, eosinophilic inclusion ➡ (a.k.a. red crunchie) is another feature of oligodendroglioma. (Courtesy P. Burger, MD.)

Ependymoma

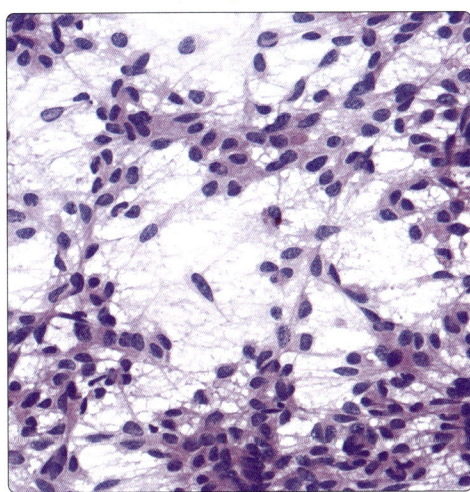

Subependymoma

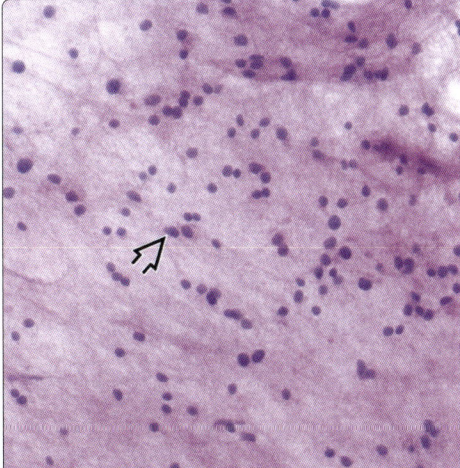

(Left) Cytologic squash preparation of a recurrent ependymoma stained with H&E is shown. Note hypercellularity and oval to spindled nuclei with process formation. (Right) H&E-stained cytologic squash preparation of a subependymoma with scattered bland, round cells in a myxoid matrix ➡ is shown.

Neuropathology Squash Preparations, Nonglial Neoplasms

TERMINOLOGY

Definitions

- Cytologic preparations
  - Squash preparations are performed by "squashing" small piece of tissue between glass slides for purpose of cytologic examination; this method can be used on most neuropathology specimens
  - Other methods of cytologic preparations include touch imprints, scraping, and dragging
  - Typically done at time of intraoperative consultation to aid frozen section interpretation
- Nonglial neoplasms
  - Tumors arising from tissues or cell types other than glial (astrocyte, oligodendroglia, ependyma) within nervous system or its surrounding structures

EPIDEMIOLOGY

Location

- Meningioma: Most commonly seen in convexities and sphenoid ridge; less commonly seen in posterior fossa, spinal, intraventricular, nerve sheath, and ectopic
- Solitary fibrous tumor (SFT): Dural based, often supratentorial, less commonly spinal (10%)
- Schwannoma: Involves peripheral nerves; often seen in cerebellopontine angle and spine
  - When bilateral cerebellopontine angle tumors, most likely associated with neurofibromatosis (NF) type 2
- Pituitary adenoma: Sella, suprasellar region; can extend into carotid sinus and invade bone
- Primary central nervous system lymphoma: Can often be multifocal; most commonly involves cerebral hemispheres
  - Secondary lymphoma can occur at any site, most often involve leptomeninges
- Metastatic tumors: Can occur anywhere along neuraxis involving brain, spinal cord, dura, and bone
- Chordoma: Most often associated with skull base, clival region, and sacral spine but can occur at any location along spine and, rarely, extraaxial bones and soft tissues

ETIOLOGY/PATHOGENESIS

Cell of Origin

- Meningioma: Neoplasm arising from meningothelial (arachnoid) cells, usually dural based
- SFT: Neoplasm thought to arise from fibroblasts; molecular hallmark *NAB2*::*STAT6* fusion
- Schwannoma: Neoplasm arising from Schwann cells of peripheral nerves
- Pituitary adenoma: Neoplasm arising from cells of anterior pituitary (adenohypophysis)
- Lymphoma: Malignant neoplasm arising from neoplastic lymphocytes
- Metastatic neoplasms: Neoplasms originating outside nervous system and spreading (typically via hematogenous routes) to nervous system
  - Cancers with higher incidence of brain metastasis include lung (particularly adenocarcinoma), breast, melanoma, renal cell, and colorectal
- Chordoma: Neoplasms arising from notochordal cells

MACROSCOPIC

General Features

- Meningioma: Typically solid, firm, well circumscribed, sometimes with attached dura
- SFT: Firm, fibrous tissue; may have attached dura
- Schwannoma: Firm tan-white tissue; cystic degeneration can be seen in larger specimens
- Pituitary adenoma: Often received as small gelatinous fragments; has very "sticky" quality, and tissue will easily adhere to most surfaces
  - Exception to squash preparation technique: Suspected pituitary adenomas should be lightly touched (touch preparation) to glass slide, not squashed, to assess cytologic appearance
- Lymphoma: Soft, tan-gray glistening appearance; can be hemorrhagic or necrotic
- Metastatic tumors: Variegated appearance; can be hemorrhagic, necrotic, or pigmented

Meningothelial Features on Smear

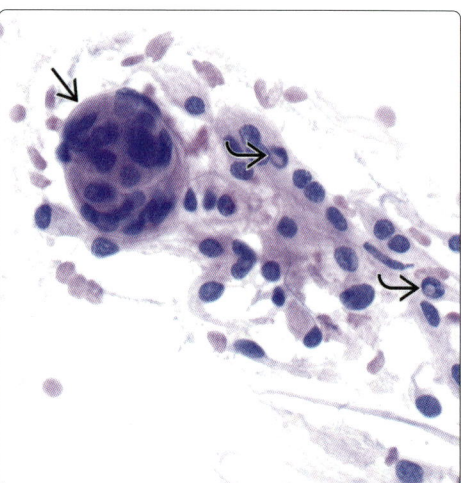

Psammoma Bodies

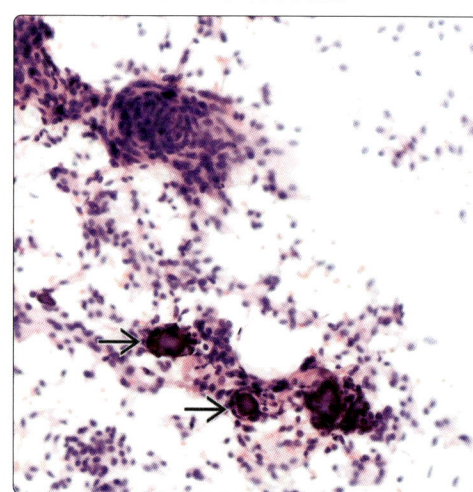

(Left) Meningothelial whorls ➡ are a classic feature of meningioma. Intranuclear pseudoinclusions ➡ are a common finding in both benign and neoplastic meningothelial cells. On H&E, the bland nuclei and abundant delicate cytoplasm can be easily appreciated. (Right) Psammoma bodies ➡, or psammomatous calcifications, are often seen in meningiomas, as in this H&E stain.

Neuropathology Squash Preparations, Nonglial Neoplasms

- Chordoma: Lobulated blue-gray appearance; can have gelatinous or more solid texture

MICROSCOPIC

Cytologic Features

- Meningioma
  - Cohesive clusters and sheets of monomorphic cells
  - Typically bland ovoid nuclei with delicate chromatin; may have intranuclear pseudoinclusions
  - Abundant wispy or feathery cytoplasm with indistinct cell borders
  - Meningothelial whorls and psammoma bodies are classic finding
  - 13 histologic subtypes of meningioma add to variable cytologic appearance
    - Secretory meningioma: Intracytoplasmic pseudopsammoma bodies, sometimes multiple
    - Rhabdoid meningioma: Rhabdoid cells
    - Microcystic and angiomatous meningioma: Can have marked nuclear pleomorphism
- SFT
  - Cellularity can vary based on grade; in central nervous system, high-grade SFTs have historically been referred to as hemangiopericytoma
  - Low-grade SFTs can have little to no shedding on touch preparations and will often show dense collagen on squash preparations
  - High-grade SFTs can show dyshesive round to ovoid cells with little to no cytoplasm
- Schwannoma
  - Difficult to squash, often forms cohesive fragments of spindle cells with blood vessels
  - Bland spindle cells with elongated nuclei with blunt ends and eosinophilic cytoplasm
  - Degenerative atypia can be present
- Pituitary adenoma
  - Sheets of individual bland monomorphic cells with little cytoplasm on touch preparation
  - Small round nuclei with small prominent nucleoli
  - Little to no mitotic activity
  - Necrosis can be seen in association with pituitary apoplexy/infarction
- Lymphoma
  - Dyshesive sheets of tumor cells with overall monomorphic appearance with variation in cell size
  - Irregular nuclear contours, coarse chromatin, and prominent nucleoli
  - Conspicuous mitotic figures are common
  - There may be extensive necrosis in patients previously treated with corticosteroids
  - Lymphoma on cytology can be complicated by gliotic neuropil background
- Metastatic tumors
  - Cytologic appearance varies with tumor type
  - Carcinoma
    - Most commonly exhibits cohesive clusters of cells
    - Large nuclei with mild to marked pleomorphism and abundant cytoplasm with distinct cell borders
    - Conspicuous mitotic activity
    - Often have necrotic background
  - Melanoma
    - Dyshesive tumor cells with moderate to marked nuclear pleomorphism, prominent nucleoli, ± intranuclear inclusions
    - Cytoplasmic melanin pigment is helpful but not always present
    - Mitotic activity present
- Chordoma
  - Clusters of cells with small typically bland rounded nuclei and abundant vacuolated "bubbly" cytoplasm (physaliphorous cells)
  - Can have myxoid or chondroid-appearing background

DIFFERENTIAL DIAGNOSIS

Meningioma, Fibrous Subtype

- SFT: Spindled to ovoid appearance on cytologic preparation; look for smaller, denser nuclei and little to no cytoplasm
- Schwannoma: Found in similar anatomic locations; has more elongated nucleus
  - Presence of hyalinized blood vessels, focal nuclear pleomorphism, and hemosiderin is suggestive

Meningioma, Microcystic/Angiomatous Subtype

- Hemangioblastoma: Cystic appearance and nuclear pleomorphism are seen in both; look for vacuolated stromal cells and lack of whorls and psammoma bodies

Schwannoma

- Fibrous meningioma: Spindled appearance on squash preparation; look for meningothelial whorls and psammoma bodies

Pituitary Adenoma

- Normal pituitary gland: Normal pituitary gland sheds very few cells on touch preparation; look for lack of monotony with variable cytoplasmic appearance
- Metastatic carcinoma: Pituitary adenomas can have epithelioid appearance; look for increased mitotic activity, nuclear pleomorphism, and gland formation
- Sellar region cysts: Rathke cleft cysts are common and can mimic cystic adenomas on imaging; look for ciliated respiratory-type epithelial cells

Lymphoma

- Melanoma: Due to dyshesive appearance and prominent nucleoli; look for presence of cytoplasm and melanin pigment to help differentiate on cytologic preparation
- Inflammatory process: Can be cytologically concerning
  - Lesions should have small, round reactive lymphocytes without atypia, and mitotic activity should be minimal

Chordoma

- Chondrosarcoma: Look for increased mitotic activity and nuclear atypia; physaliphorous cells are not typical in chondrosarcomas

SELECTED REFERENCES

1. Altshuler DB et al: Imaging errors in distinguishing pituitary adenomas from other sellar lesions. J Neuroophthalmol. 41(4):512-18, 2021
2. WHO Classification of Tumours Editorial Board: Central Nervous System Tumours. WHO Classification of Tumours Series. 5th ed, vol 6. International Agency for Research on Cancer, 2021

Neuropathology Squash Preparations, Nonglial Neoplasms

Pleomorphic Nuclei in Microcystic Meningioma

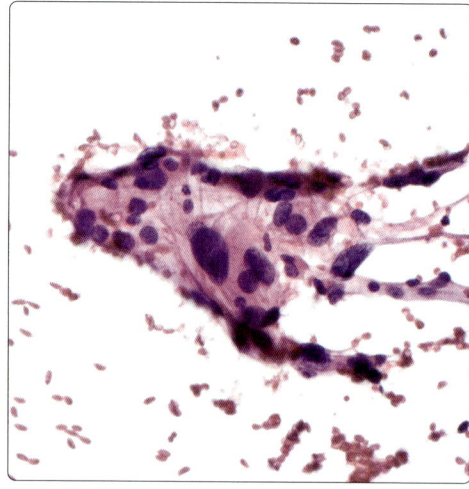

Rhabdoid Meningioma

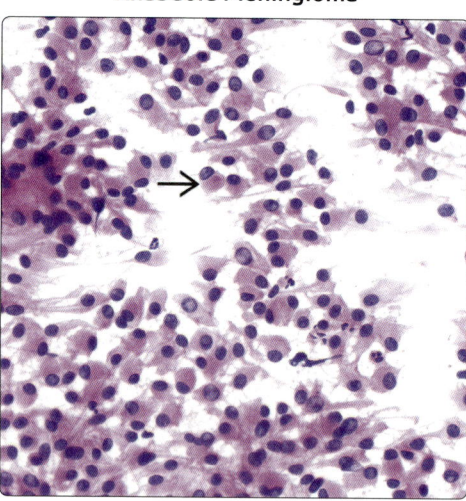

(Left) Microcystic meningiomas can have remarkable nuclear pleomorphism and even vacuolation, as seen in this H&E stain; however, this bears no impact on grade. (Right) Rhabdoid cells ⇨ like the ones seen in this H&E preparation are found in the eponymous WHO grade 3 rhabdoid meningioma; however, they can also represent a subset of cells in an otherwise lower grade meningioma. Tissue sections will help to confirm extent of rhabdoid morphology.

Solitary Fibrous Tumor

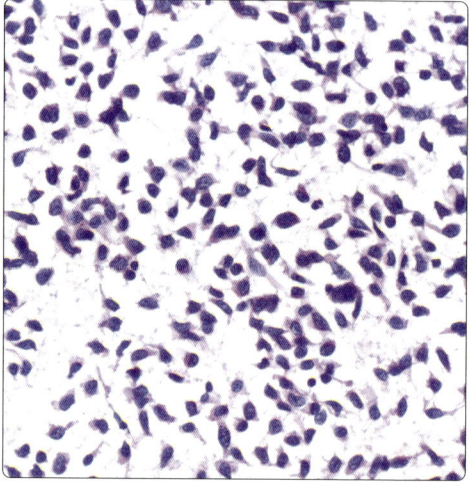

Hemangioblastoma

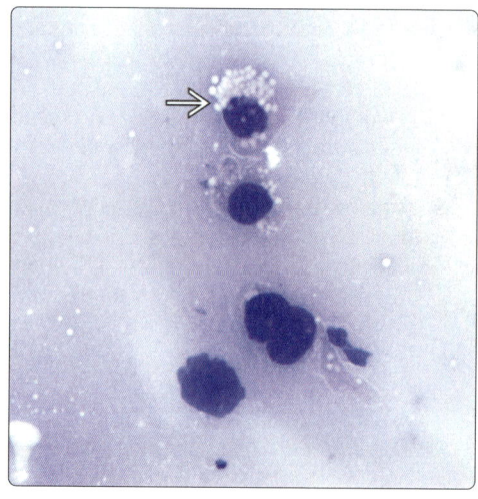

(Left) Solitary fibrous tumors (SFTs), like meningiomas, are dural-based lesions. The SFT cells seen here show round to ovoid cells with little to no cytoplasm. These cells lack the typical nuclear features (delicate chromatin, intranuclear pseudoinclusions) and abundant cytoplasm seen in meningothelial cells. (Right) Hemangioblastoma is a highly vascular tumor characterized by stromal cells with vacuolated cytoplasm ⇨ like the cell seen here on H&E. These tumors are often inhibin positive.

Schwannoma Nuclear Features

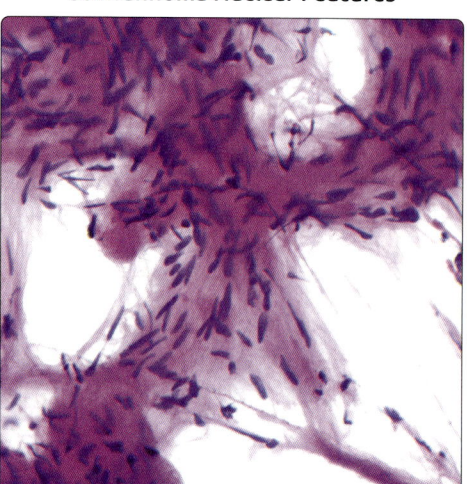

Verocay Bodies in Schwannoma

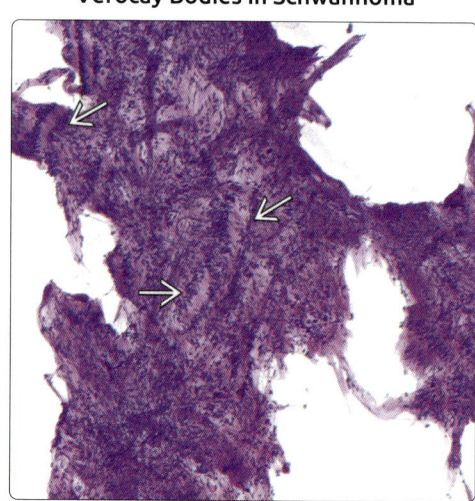

(Left) Schwannomas, compared with meningiomas, have darker, denser nuclei with more blunted ends, as seen on this H&E-stained squash preparation. (Right) Palisading nuclear structures classic for schwannoma, Verocay bodies ⇨, can sometimes be seen on cytologic preparations, such as this H&E-stained example.

Neuropathology Squash Preparations, Nonglial Neoplasms

Pituitary Adenoma Nuclear Features

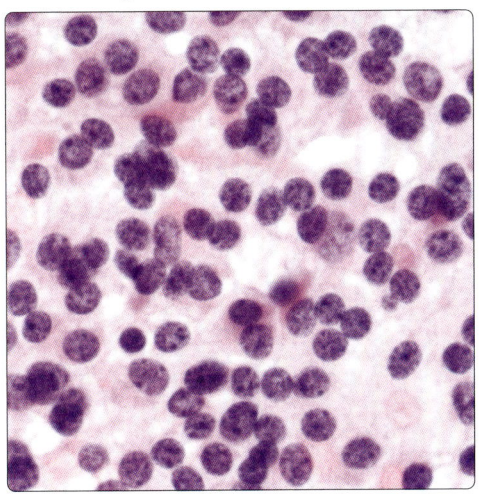

Rathke Cleft Cyst

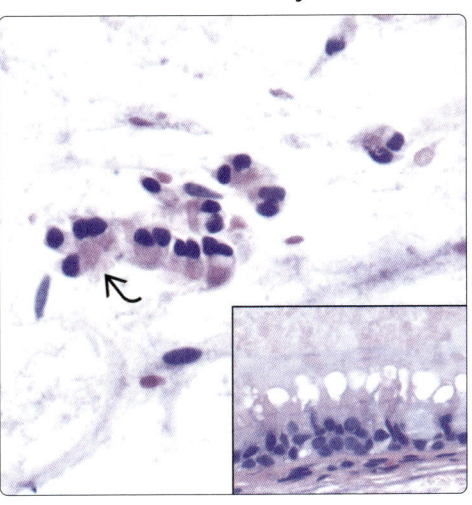

(Left) Pituitary adenoma cells have classic neuroendocrine appearance with small round nuclei and multiple nucleoli well-visualized on H&E stain. Moderate nuclear pleomorphism can be seen. There is an overall monomorphous appearance. (Right) Rathke, colloid, and neuroenteric cysts all have similar respiratory-type epithelium, as seen in the inset. Rare bland ciliated cells ⇨ in a background of proteinaceous debris seen on H&E touch preparations may be the only finding.

Lymphoma

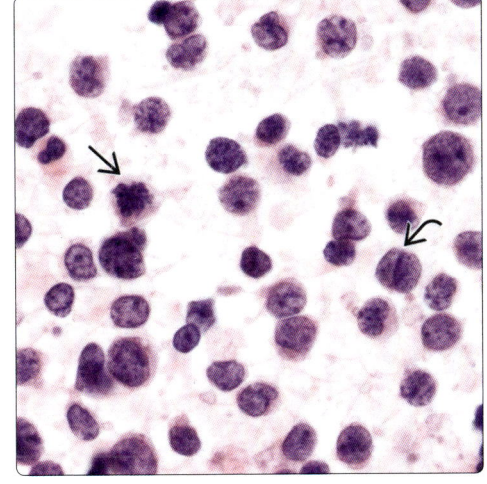

Melanoma

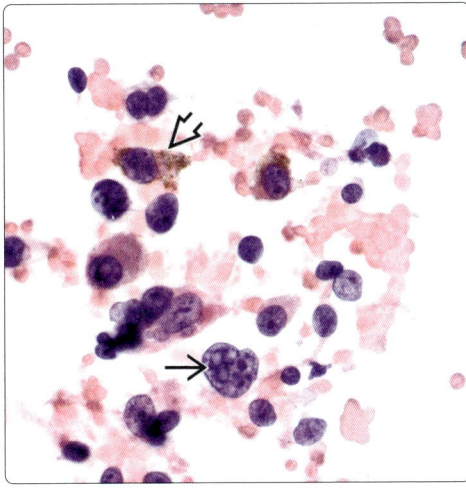

(Left) Lymphomas involving the nervous system are most often diffuse large B-cell tumors with cytologic preparations showing sheets of individual cells with irregular nuclear borders, prominent nucleoli, nuclear clefting ⇨, and little cytoplasm, seen by H&E stain. Mitoses ⇨ are often present. (Right) Melanomas often have marked nuclear pleomorphism with large nucleoli and nuclear vacuolation ⇨, seen here on H&E stain. Melanin pigment ⇨ is diagnostically helpful; however, it is not always present.

Metastatic Adenocarcinoma

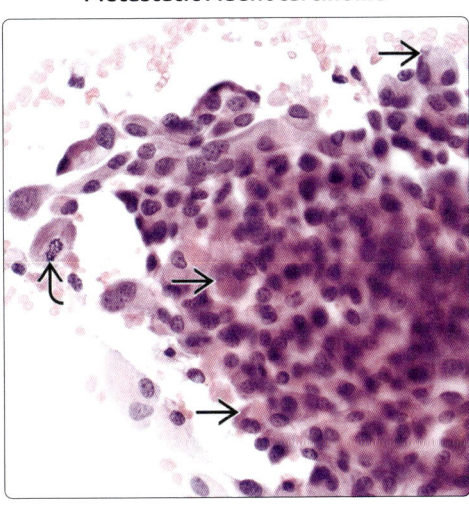

Physaliferous Cells of Chordoma

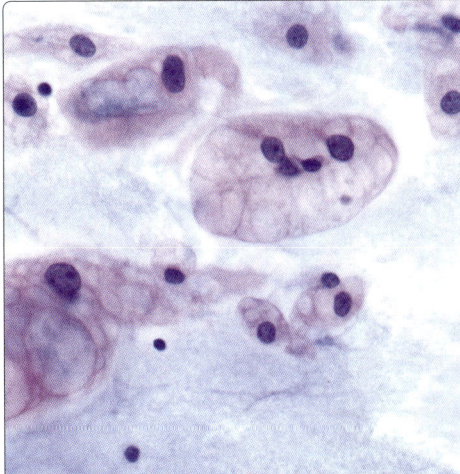

(Left) H&E-stained metastatic ductal breast carcinoma shows features of an adenocarcinoma: Large nuclei with conspicuous nucleoli, intracytoplasmic vacuoles ⇨, and defined cell borders. Mitoses ⇨ are easily identified. (Right) The classic hallmark of chordoma on cytologic preparations is the presence of vacuolated "physaliferous" cells in a myxoid background, seen here in this H&E-stained squash preparation.

PART V
Management and Ancillary Testing

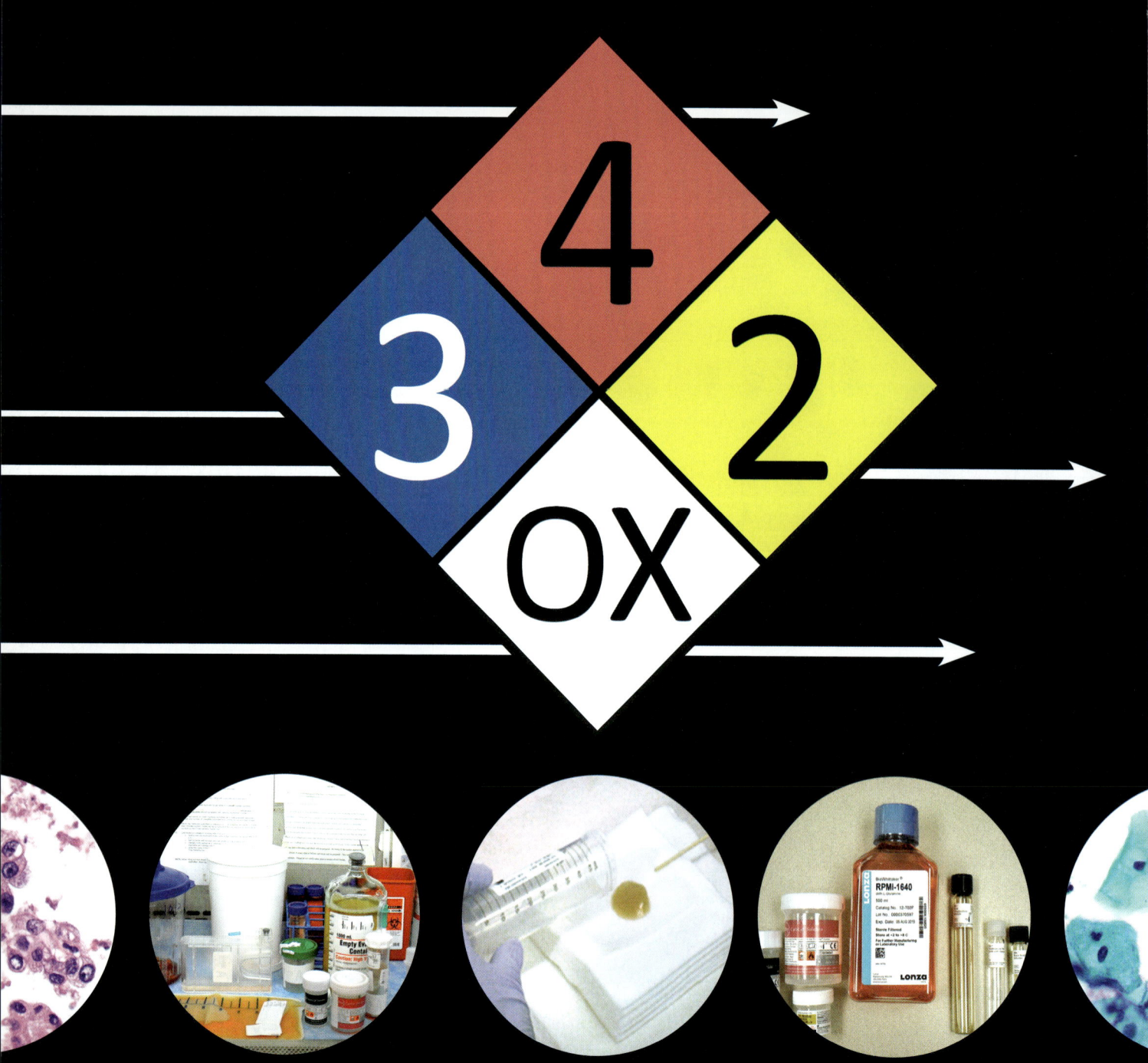

PART V
SECTION 1
Cytopreparatory and Quality Management

Cytopreparatory Techniques and Instrumentation in
   Nongynecologic Cytology   710
Quality Improvement and Laboratory Management for Cytopathology   716

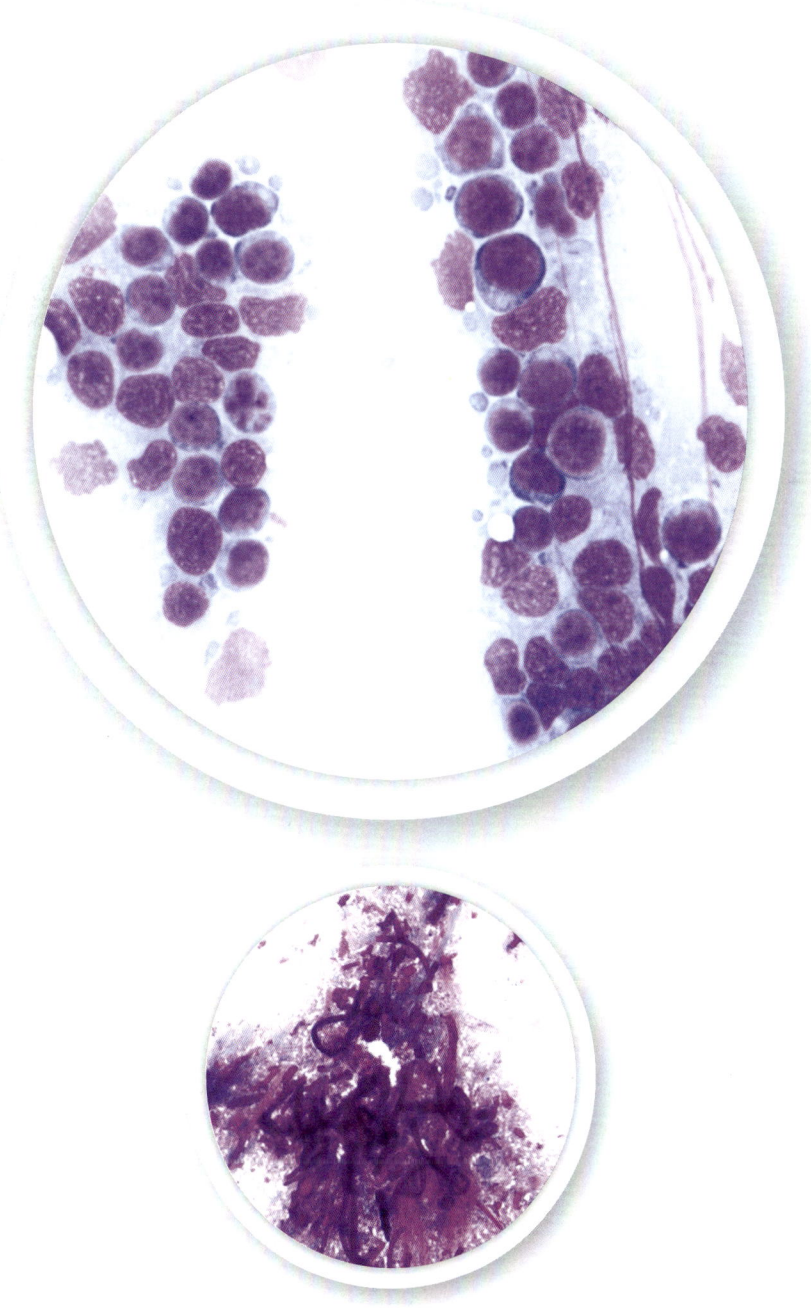

Cytopreparatory Techniques and Instrumentation in Nongynecologic Cytology

MAJOR STEPS IN CYTOLOGY PROCESSING

Specimen Receipt
- Document specimen was received in laboratory
  - Essential for calculating turnaround time
- Confirm order for cytology and scan requisition for ancillary test off cytology specimen (e.g., GMS, flow cytometry, FISH)
- Gross examination of color, turbidity, and volume of cytology specimen should be documented

Specimen Preparation Techniques
- **Cytocentrifugation**
  - Assessment of specimen: Macroscopic examination of specimen is used to select processing protocol (e.g., bloody, thick, watery, etc.)
  - Initial centrifugation: 5 minutes at 2,200 RPM; pour off supernatant
  - Critical resuspension of cell button: Depends on size of cell button
    - Resuspend in balanced electrolyte solution (RPMI) until slightly hazy suspension
  - Loading cytospin chambers: Sample chambers hold maximum of 0.5 mL (~ 20 drops) and ≥ 0.1 mL (~ 5-6 drops) should be used
    - Load enough drops so cells will not dry out during spin; filter will absorb excess liquid
    - Good cytospin preparation has monolayer of cells in tight cytospin circle
  - Cellular assessment slide: Diff-Quik stain can be done on cytospin to check thickness of preparation
    - Number of drops can be adjusted to increase or decrease cell distribution
- **ThinPrep nongynecologic processing**
  - Initial spin in CytoLyt: 5 minutes at 2,200 RPM
  - Evaluate cell pellet appearance: If cell pellet is not free of blood, mucus, or protein, add 30 mL of CytoLyt and recentrifuge
  - Determine amount of specimen to be transferred to PreservCyt: If pellet is not visible, transfer entire sample into PreservCyt; if pellet is > 1 mL, transfer 1 drop of specimen into PreservCyt
- **SurePath nongynecologic processing**
  - Transfer 50-mL aliquot (or entire amount for small specimens) and centrifuge for 10 minutes at 600 g (program 3)
  - Add 30 mL of BD CytoRich red preservative for all specimens except urine (add 30-mL SurePath preservative fluid for urine)
  - Centrifuge for 10 minutes at 600 g, then decant supernatant and vortex tubes
    - Use BD PrepStain instrument according to guidelines
- **ThinPrep and SurePath gynecologic processing**
  - Follow exact manufacturer-recommended protocol

Staining Methods
- **Regressive staining (Pap stain)**
  - Alcohol- or spray-fixed slides must be hydrated in preparation for aqueous hematoxylin stain (10 dips or 30 seconds)
  - Nucleus is overstained in Harris hematoxylin for 2 minutes and then rinsed in running water
  - To remove excess hematoxylin, slides are immersed in diluted HCl (1%) for 1-2 quick dips and then rinsed with water
    - Mild hydrochloric acid dip causes lysis of red blood cells; this is advantageous for bloody FNA slides and other bloody preps
  - Slides are dehydrated in 95% alcohol to prepare for cytoplasmic staining
    - 2 minutes in OG stain and 5 minutes in mixture of EA 50/65 with alcohol rinses in between
    - Final dehydration in 100% alcohol
  - Clearing with xylene will prepare slides for mounting medium
- **Progressive staining (Pap)**
  - Alcohol- or spray-fixed slides must be hydrated with water in preparation for aqueous hematoxylin stain (10 dips or 30 seconds)
  - Nucleus is stained in hematoxylin to desired intensity (~ 2 minutes) and rinsed with tap water
  - Bluing agent is used to set nuclear dye

Collection Devices

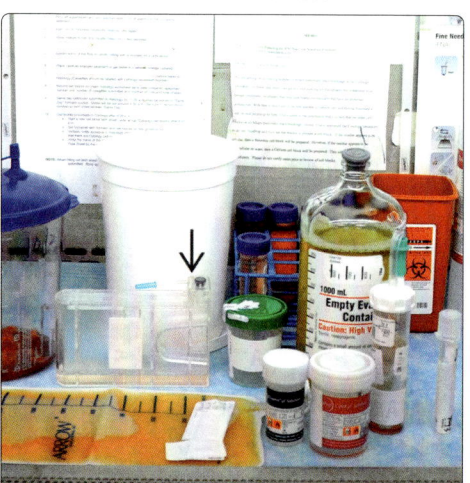

Slides and Blocks

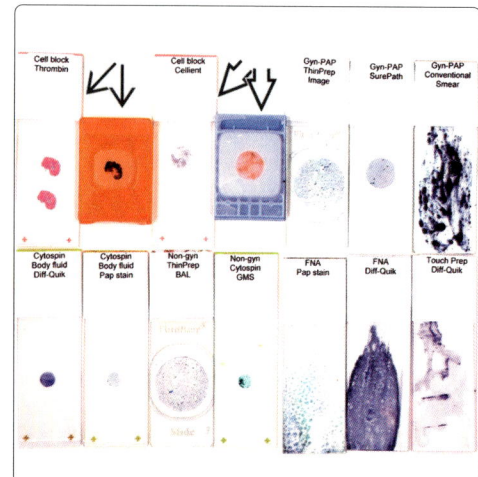

(Left) Clinical photograph shows various bottles and collecting devices in which nongynecologic cytology specimens are received in the laboratory, including a cassette for vitreous specimens ➡. *(Right)* Image depicts various preparations, including thrombin ➡ and Cellient ➡ cell blocks, smears, cytospins, ThinPrep, and SurePath stained with Pap, Diff-Quik, and H&E stains.

Cytopreparatory Techniques and Instrumentation in Nongynecologic Cytology

- – Scott's tap water substitute or tap water can be used if pH > 8
- o Follow steps for cytoplasmic staining, dehydration, and clearing with xylene
- **Diff-Quik stain**: Rapid differential stain that gives results similar to those of Wright-Giemsa stain within seconds
  - o Allow slides to air dry completely
  - o Follow with 10 dips in solution #1 (fixative), 10 dips in solution #2 (xanthene dye), and 10-20 dips in solution #3 (thiazine dye)
  - o Rinse in tap water
- **Rapid Pap**: Used in some laboratories for immediate evaluation and final diagnosis
  - o Slower than Diff-Quik but faster than complete Pap
    - – Total staining time: 90-130 seconds
  - o Several commercial kits are available with prepackaged solutions ready for use
  - o Modified ultrafast Pap (MUFP) stain can be used with reagents and solutions common in cytopathology laboratory
  - o Suggested MUFP method; air-dried smears placed in normal saline for 30 seconds
    - – Tap water (6 dips), Harris hematoxylin (30 seconds), tap water (6 dips), 95% isopropyl alcohol (6 dips), EA-36 (15 dips), 95% alcohol (6 dips), 100% isopropyl alcohol (6 dips), and xylene (10 slow dips)
- **Destaining**: Removes Pap stain from preparations to allow for restaining with same method or other stains
  - o Soak slides in xylene until coverslip comes off
    - – Place slide in xylene bath for 1-2 hours to remove residual mounting media
  - o Dip slides in Pap staining set-up in reverse order, skipping actual stains
    - – If using regressive staining method, allow slides to sit in 1% hydrochloric acid until slide is destaining
    - – Microscopically check progress of destaining
  - o Rinse slides in running water for 5 minutes to remove acid
  - o Check slide microscopically for decoloration
    - – Destain further if necessary
  - o Dehydrate by using 95% and 100% alcohol and clear in xylene before coverslipping

Coverslipping

- **Manual**
  - o Clearing, which is final step in staining process, is also important prior to coverslipping
    - – Clearing agent (typically xylene) should have refractive index of slide = 1.515
  - o Mounting media is substance that acts as permanent bond between glass slide and coverslip
    - – Mounting media should have refractive index similar to those of clearing agent and glass slide
  - o Coverslip must cover entire cellular area
    - – 24 x 55 mm is used for FNA slides, and 24 x 50 mm can be used for cytospin ThinPrep, SurePath, or preparations that cover ≤ 1/2 of slide
    - – No.1 coverslip is recommended for cytologic use
  - o Coverslipping should be done in well-ventilated space, preferably under fume hood
  - o 2 basic methods are used in coverslipping
    - – One method is to place 1 drop of mounting media on coverslip and place slide at 45° angle to allow mounting media to flow up slide, thereby attaching coverslip to slide
    - – Another method is to place 1 drop of mounting media on slide and drop coverslip on top of slide; care must be taken not to contaminate pipette used to drop media onto specimen
- **Automated**
  - o Many automated coverslippers are available, belonging to 2 types: Ones that use glass coverslips and ones that use coverslipper film
    - – Glass is preferred for cytology
  - o Automated coverslipper film is adhesive-backed film activated by xylene

FNA

- FNA procedures can be performed by trained cytopathologist, clinician, or radiologist
- Supplies needed to set up FNA clinic or traveling cart
  - o Alcohol preps, iodine swabs, sterile gauze, glass slides, sharps containers, cytology spray fixative, cytology/procedural forms, microscope
  - o FNA guns (e.g., INRAD, Cameco, Aspir-gun, Tao Aspirator, etc.)
  - o Syringes (10 cc or 20 cc), sterile needles (20-25 gauge)
  - o Solutions for needle rinses (CytoLyt or RPMI)
  - o Type of stain for immediate adequacy (Diff-Quik or Rapid Pap)
  - o Gloves (sterile and boxed)
- Simultaneous use of both wet-fixed and air-dried smears is recommended
  - o 2 slides complement each other and add to interpretation of case
- Most common way to prepare smears used in cytology
  - o Place bevel of needle directly on glass slide near frosted end, then use 2nd or spreader slide to make smears
  - o Spreader slide is gently lowered over droplet, which spreads out due to capillary action
  - o Spreader slide is gently pulled straight back in 1 smooth motion down length of slide
    - – If expressed material is scant, drop 2nd slide on top of specimen and pull up gently
- Material that remains in needle hub can be expressed in cytology preservative/solution (CytoLyt, RPMI, CytoRich Red, Saccomanno, etc.)

Real-Time Telecytology

- Can be time-efficient technique in busy cytopathology laboratories
  - o With training and equipment, this technique can be made available at remote locations
    - – Documentation of training on equipment required
    - – For CAP accreditation, items from telepathology section of Laboratory General Checklist apply
  - o Set-up requires use of high-resolution digital camera, video software, secure intranet, and validation
    - – Digital camera should transmit 20-30 frames per second and have fast, reliable network
    - – Laptop computer/tablet device that resides on cart is attached to camera through USB or FireWire

Cytopreparatory Techniques and Instrumentation in Nongynecologic Cytology

- □ Cellular phone with camera directly aligned with eyepiece may be sufficient for some applications
- Any variety of screen-sharing program can be used to share laptop/tablet screen with attached camera to view computer monitor in office/laboratory
  - □ Screen-sharing software can be purchased or downloaded as freeware, though confidentiality of information may be issue with some applications
- Case information is communicated between 2 stations via phones and used to pinpoint fields of interest or to maneuver microscope
  - □ Experienced microscope operator (such as cytotechnologist) is needed on-site to achieve optimal results
- Manufacturers offer all-encompassing telepathology solutions as alternative to self-assembled technologies

Examples of Commonly Used Cell Block Techniques

- **Thrombin**: Can be used on any specimen but works best with cellular specimens
  - Fluid is centrifuged for 5 minutes at 2,200 RPM
  - Supernatant is decanted, and 1 mL of plasma is added to cell button and vortexed to mix cells and plasma together
  - 1 mL of thrombin is added to mixture, and tube is slowly moved side-to-side until mixture clots
  - Clot is placed on piece of lens paper, then reduced in size by carefully and gently rolling it with wooden stick until it reaches pea size
  - Fold clot in lens paper and place in cassette
  - Submit cassette to histology laboratory for processing
- **HistoGel (propriety gel)**
  - Centrifugation of cell suspensions followed by adding HistoGel to pellet
- **Formalin**: Works on cellular specimens
  - Fluid is centrifuged for 5 minutes at 2,200 RPM
  - Pour off supernatant, resuspend pellet in 10 mL of 95% ethanol, and layer on 5 cc of 10% formalin
  - Centrifuge for additional 5 minutes at 2,200 RPM
  - Pour supernatant and drain tube well
  - Carefully remove packed sediment from centrifuge tube and wrap it in lens paper
  - Place lens paper in cassette and submit for processing
- **Collodion bag**: Can be used for enhanced cell collection
  - Cells can be effectively concentrated by sedimenting cell pellet into small collodion bag
    - Place 15-mL conical tube under vented fume hood
    - Slowly pour collodion to top of conical tube
    - Let stand for 10 minutes, then pour collodion solution back into bottle; conical tube is left with hardened collodion "bag"
    - Place tubes in rack upside down so that excess collodion can drain and tubes can dry
    - Place specimen in centrifuge tube and spin for 6 minutes at 1,500 RPM
    - After initial centrifugation, decant all but 10 mL, then remix specimen
    - Pour remixed specimen in collodion bag and centrifuge tube for 8 minutes at 1,500 RPM
    - Using disposable pipet, remove as much supernatant as possible
    - Carefully remove collodion sac, using scissors to cut off excess collodion bag
    - Fold collodion sac as close to cell button as possible
    - Wrap bag in 1 piece of tissue paper and place in tissue cassette
- **Blood clots as cell blocks**
  - Allow (bloody) sample to clot in syringe followed by aspiration of 10% formalin and transfer into formalin container
    - Small clots can be filtered, large clots can be sliced and submitted for processing as cell block
- **Cellient**: Can be used on any specimen; works well with specimens that are not very cellular
  - Cellient automated cell block system creates paraffin block using controlled vacuum to deposit layer of cells on filter and infiltrate cells with reagents and paraffin
  - System consists of
    - Cellient processor that processes sample
    - Cassette/filter assembly that captures sample and guides infusion of reagents and paraffin
    - Finishing station that is used to embed cell block in paraffin in preparation for cutting and slide preparation
    - Instrument then processes sample, dispensing stain (optional), dehydrating reagent, clearing reagent, and then infusing paraffin
  - Follow Cellient operator's manual for detailed operation
- **Nano cell block**
  - Proprietary preformed disks with wells and built-in markers to precisely indicate level of cells (Nano NextGen CelBloking, Micro NextGen CelBloking kits)

Ancillary Testing

- Most common ancillary tests using liquid-based Pap vials
  - Human papillomavirus
  - *Chlamydia trachomatis*/*Neisseria gonorrhoeae*
  - Herpes simplex virus types 1 and 2, *Trichomonas*, vaginosis panel
- Due to ability to acquire tissue with minimally invasive procedure, use of cytology nongynecologic specimens for molecular analysis has become common
  - Can be used to determine prognosis, response to therapy, and further classify diagnosis
  - Most common ancillary tests using nongynecologic/FNA specimens
    - UroVysion (FISH assay for detection of recurrent urothelial carcinoma): Probe set contains probes to centromeres of chromosomes 3, 7, and 17, and locus-specific probe to 9p21 band
    - FISH for biliary tract mutational analysis
    - EGFR: Can detect wild-type sequence and 29 known mutations, deletions, and insertions found in exons 18-21 of *EGFR* tyrosine kinase domain
    - ALK: Detects rearrangements of *ALK* gene
    - Afirma (thyroid FNA analysis): Measures expression of 142 genes and applies multidimensional algorithm to classify whether nodule with cytopathology diagnosis of indeterminate is benign or malignant

Cytopreparatory Techniques and Instrumentation in Nongynecologic Cytology

- ThyroSeq 3 and other commercially available tests for indeterminate thyroid FNAs performed from needle rinses in manufacturer-provided media
- Next-generation sequencing can be performed on any cytology specimen (smears, cell blocks, or CytoLyt fixed-needle rinses)

TROUBLESHOOTING COMMON PROBLEMS

Cell Button Assessment Slide
- Useful for determining make-up of fluid (e.g., bloody, inflammatory, mucinous, etc.)
  - After initial centrifugation, centrifuge for 5 minutes at 2,200 RPM
  - Pour off supernatant
  - Take wooden applicator stick and dip in cell button to obtain small amount of specimen
  - Smear on glass slide and stain with Diff-Quik
  - Use knowledge of what is on slide to help prepare specimen

Large-Volume Fluids (Vacutainer Bottles)
- Large-volume fluids present problem for laboratories that do not have enough room to store large Vacutainer bottles
- Alternative is to store some of fluid in 100-cc specimen containers and use it for cell blocks, flow cytometry, or repeating specimen
- Shake up bottle so cells become dispersed throughout fluid
  - Cells tend to settle to bottom of container
- Draw out 50 mL in centrifuge tube to make original specimen, and place 100 mL in specimen container to use for further processing and studies
- Large bottle can be kept for few days or discarded after dividing specimen as described

Bloody Specimens
- Ammonium chloride lyse is recommended for cases in which flow cytometry may be ordered
  - Grossly bloody specimens should be lysed
    - Lyse red blood cells by resuspending bloody cell button in ammonium chloride solution and allowing it to stand for 3-5 minutes
    - Centrifuge suspension at 2,200 RPM for 5 minutes
  - Ammonium chloride lyse 10x stock solution recipe
    - Weigh out 41.3 g of ammonium chloride, 5.0 g of potassium bicarbonate, and 0.19 g of EDTA
    - Dilute with 500 mL of deionized water and mix until completely dissolved (stable at 2-8 °C for 3 months)
    - To make working solution, add 100 mL of stock solution to 900 mL of deionized water (stable at 2-8 °C for 3 months)
- Use of regressive staining method can also lyse slightly bloody specimens

INSTRUMENTATION

Most Common Instrumentation in Cytology Laboratory
- **Biologic safety cabinet**: Class II-A2 is best suited and recommended for diagnostic cytology laboratory
  - Class I cabinet is similar to chemical fume hood and is usually hard ducted to exhaust system of building
  - Class II cabinet can be used as specimen-processing station
    - Air is recirculated back into room through high-efficiency particulate air (HEPA) filters with little risk to outside environment if cabinet is maintained properly and certified annually
    - Class II-A1 has positively pressurized contaminated air bordering air outside cabinet and is therefore less safe than class II-A2
    - Class II-A2 has negative pressure surrounding positively pressurized contaminated air; negative pressure ensures that contaminated air will not be pulled out of cabinet
  - Class III cabinet is designed for highly infectious agents that are not usually encountered in cytology specimens
- **Centrifuges**
  - Centrifugation is used to separate cells from fluid
  - Cell fractionation studies have shown that cells sediment best at 600x gravity in 10 minutes
    - This depends on actual centrifuge used and on rotating radius of centrifuge
  - Most commonly used centrifuge speed and time for cytology specimens are 1,200-1,500 RPM for 10 minutes or faster variation of 2,200 RPM for 5 minutes
- **Cytocentrifuges**
  - Cytospin is special instrument designed to deposit cells on glass slide to be stained for cytologic examination
  - Primary requirements are that specimen be cell suspension of single cells or cell groups and that cells are fresh and intact
- **Thin layer preparations**
  - **ThinPrep**: Can be used for gynecologic and nongynecologic specimens; sample preparation process involves
    - Dispersion to separate debris and disperse mucus
    - Cell collection for which cells are collected on exterior surface of filter membrane by gentle vacuum
    - Cell transfer in which cells are collected on membrane of filter and deposited on ThinPrep microscopic slide
  - **SurePath**: Can be used for gynecologic and nongynecologic specimens
    - There are different protocols for gynecologic and nongynecologic processing on PrepStain workstation
    - Refer to PrepStain slide processor operator's manual for procedures
- **Automatic stainers and automatic coverslippers**
  - Free up technologist time; consistent staining
- **Automatic cell block (Cellient)**
  - Advantages offered by automated cell block system
    - Shorter processing time to embed sample into block
    - Excellent structural detail and preservation of nucleic acid integrity

SELECTED REFERENCES

1. Shidham VB: Cell-blocks and other ancillary studies (including molecular genetic tests and proteomics). Cytojournal. 18:4, 2021
2. Shidham VB et al: CytoJournal monographs: first CMAS (CytoJournal Monograph/Atlas Series) on science of cell-block making, titled "CellBlockistry 101 (text book of cell-blocking science)". Cytojournal. 18:10, 2021
3. Tommola E et al: The contributory role of cell blocks in salivary gland neoplasms fine needle aspirations classified by the Milan system for reporting salivary gland cytology. Diagnostics (Basel). 11(10):1778, 2021

Cytopreparatory Techniques and Instrumentation in Nongynecologic Cytology

Collection Media

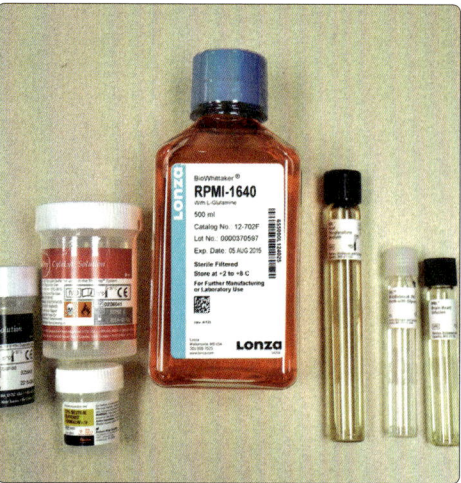

(Left) *Image depicts various collecting media: RPMI for flow cytometry, formalin for microbiopsies and rinses, CytoLyt for FNA needle rinses, and brushes and culture tubes for bacterial, fungal, or acid-fast cultures.* **(Right)** *Clinical photograph shows a class II biohazard cabinet under which nongynecologic specimens are processed. Sharps ➡ and biohazard disposal ➡ containers are also in the immediate vicinity.*

Class II Biohazard Cabinet

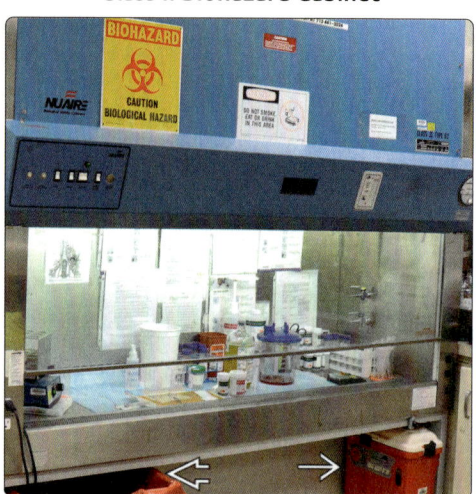

Cytospin Machine

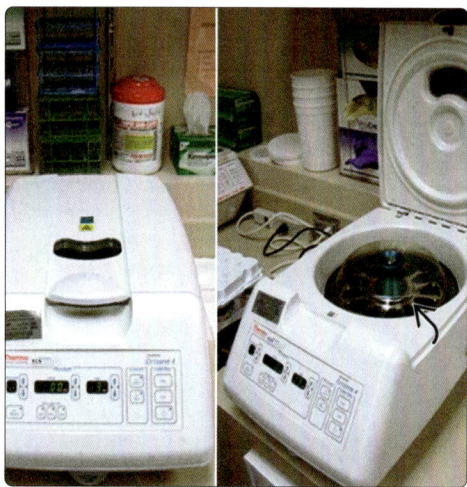

(Left) *Closed (left) and open (right) views of a Cytospin machine are shown. Note the chambers ➡.* **(Right)** *Endoscopic ultrasound-guided FNA can yield bloody specimens and long, worm-like blood clots ➡. Collecting them in a proprietary fixative that also contains a lysing agent can alleviate the problem of numerous bloody smears. A single liquid-based slide can be prepared, and the clotted "worm" along with the cell button can be made into a cell block.*

Processing Clots and Bloody Specimens

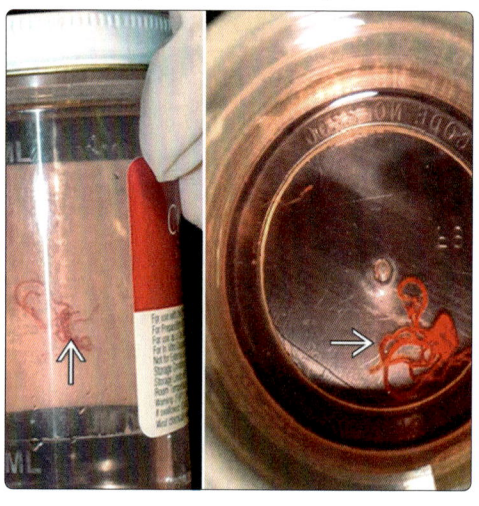

Thrombin Cell Block Preparation

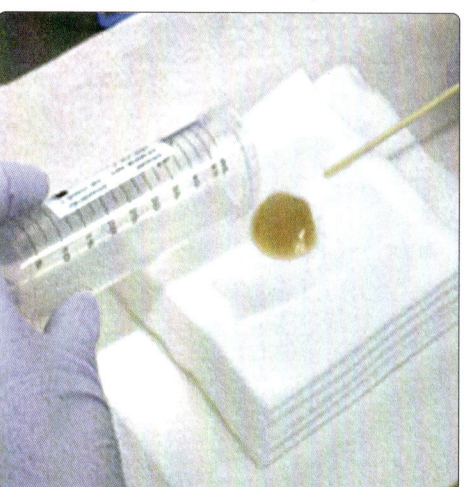

(Left) *Photograph shows thrombin cell block in the clot stage being poured from tube to a lens paper perched on gauze pads for absorption of excess fluid. The wooden stick is used to facilitate rolling of the clot to squeeze out excess fluid before wrapping in lens paper for formalin fixation.* **(Right)** *Paraffin block and H&E-stained section prepared with Nano NextGen CelBloking kit with a marker ➡. The cells are in the other wells ➡. The marker helps with cutting and locating the diagnostic cells, especially in IHC-stained sections.*

Propriety Nano Gel Disk With Wells

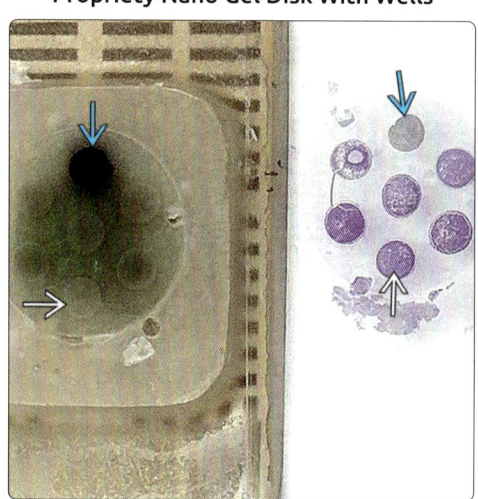

Cytopreparatory Techniques and Instrumentation in Nongynecologic Cytology

Cellient Cell Block Machine
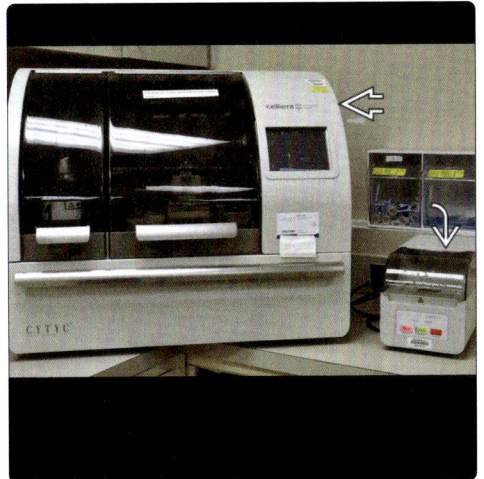

Cellient Cell Block Section
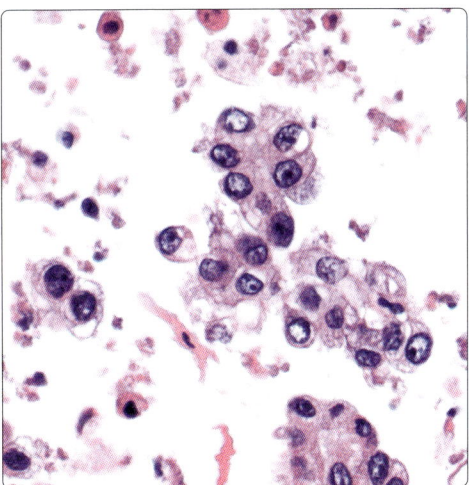

(Left) Cellient system by Cytyc Corporation consists of the Cellient processor ➡, which processes the sample, and the finishing station ➡, which is used to embed the cell block in paraffin to allow for cutting the block and preparing the slide. **(Right)** H&E-stained section from a Cellient cell block preparation of a sputum sample shows adenocarcinoma. The Cellient technique is designed to create a thin layer without the use of thrombin or HistoGel.

Cart With Microscope and Camera Set-Up
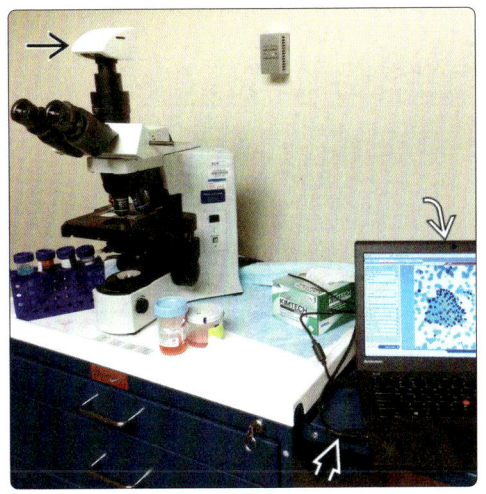

ThinPrep 2000 Processor
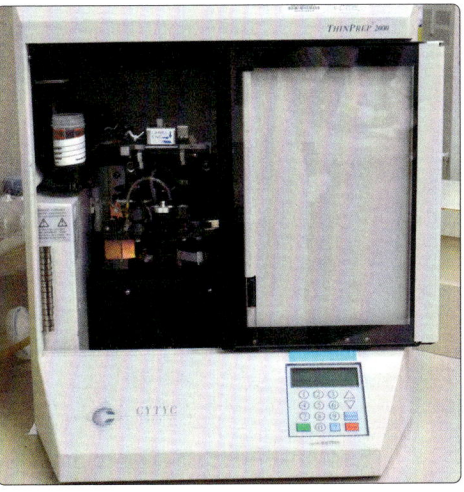

(Left) FNA and rapid on-site evaluation cart with microscope and camera ➡ are shown. The camera is connected to the laptop, which resides on a retractable table ➡. The laptop has secure access, and the live image ➡ is shared with the computer screen in the cytology laboratory. A trainee or cytologist is in the EUS suite moving the slide with a pathologist in the laboratory viewing. **(Right)** Nongynecologic specimens, both exfoliative and FNA rinses, can be processed in a ThinPrep 2000 processor.

Automatic Coverslipper
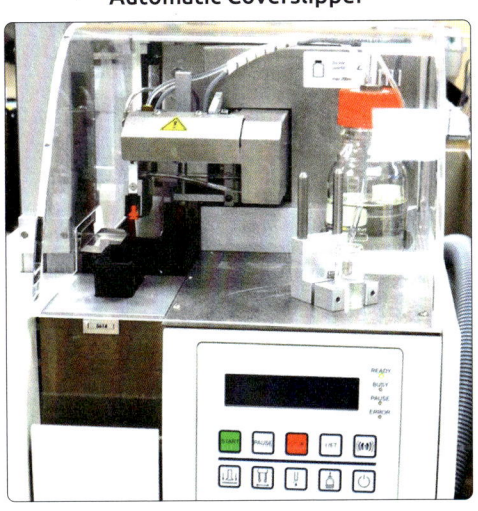

Superficial FNA Clinic
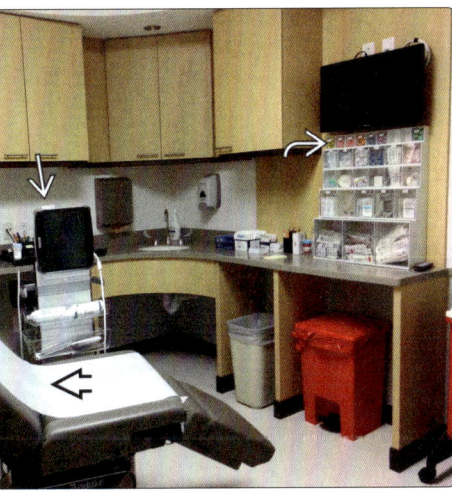

(Left) Photograph shows the Leica CV5030 robotic glass coverslipper for cytology specimens. **(Right)** FNA clinic room is shown with multifunctional chair/bed ➡, supplies ➡, and an ultrasound machine ➡.

Quality Improvement and Laboratory Management for Cytopathology

TOTAL QUALITY MANAGEMENT

Definition

- Integrative philosophy of management for continuously improving quality of products and processes
  - Quality of cytopathology services came under scrutiny with publication of series of articles in Wall Street Journal in 1987
    - Articles prompted United States Congress to pass Clinical Laboratory Improvement Amendments of 1988 (CLIA '88), which are center of any cytology laboratory quality management plan
- Laboratory must have clearly defined, documented quality management program that includes active surveillance of laboratory activities
  - College of American Pathologists Laboratory Accreditation Program checklist
- Quality management surveillance must be
  - Preanalytic: Specimen collection and processing
  - Analytic: Screening and interpretation
  - Postanalytic: Receipt of results, analysis of results, statistics, benchmarking
- Records must be kept to show conformance to and results of program
- Most cytology quality management functions in United States are driven by **CLIA '88 mandates**

QUALITY IMPROVEMENT

Definition

- Quantitative and qualitative methods to improve effectiveness, quality, efficiency, and safety of processes and systems
  - Annual quality improvement plan should provide means of monitoring accuracy and completeness of diagnostic reporting and identify potential areas for improvement
  - Examples include monthly quality assurance (QA) indicators, such as
    - Cytology-histology correlations [gynecologic (GYN) and nongynecologic (NGYN)] and fine-needle aspiration biopsies (FNAB)
    - Cytopathologist-to-cytotechnologist correlations (GYN and NGYN)
    - Turnaround time (NGYN and FNAB)
  - Quarterly monitoring of QA indicators
    - Cytopathologist peer review (prospective &/or retrospective)
    - Intradepartmental and extradepartmental consultations
    - HPV positivity rates for cases of atypical squamous cells of undetermined significance (ASC-US) in lab and individuals
    - Comparison of ASC:SIL ratio with HPV positivity rates for ASC-US can be used to monitor individuals (cytotechnologists and pathologists) for over- or undercalling
  - Site-specific review of processes or specimen categories to identify trends and areas for improvement
    - Pick organ (e.g., liver, lung) or procedure (e.g., endobronchial ultrasound), and look at everything in detail (preanalytic, analytic, and postanalytic), including cytology, histology, and clinical correlation
  - Cytotechnologist evaluation and workload limits
    - Every 6 months, CLIA '88 mandate
  - Continuous mechanisms of quality improvement
    - High-grade squamous intraepithelial lesion/carcinoma (HSIL/Ca) look-back of previous negative Paps
    - Incomplete requisitions, reasons, and locations
    - Final report review for completeness
  - External audit mechanisms, such as proficiency testing and interlaboratory comparison programs
  - Annual statistics summary of GYN, NGYN, and FNAB
- Accomplished by using results of quality control (QC) and QA monitoring to identify trends and target areas for improvement

QUALITY CONTROL

Definition

- System for monitoring level of quality as specimen moves through laboratory

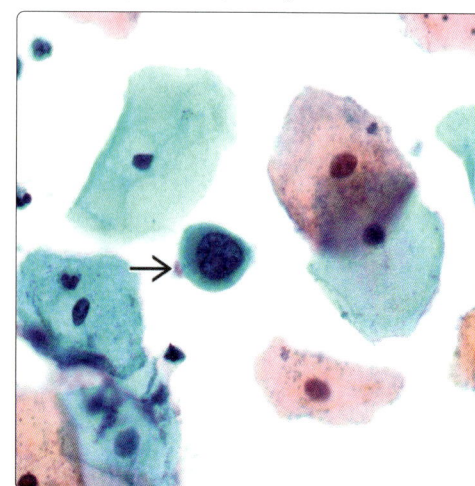

Wall Street Journal Article, Nov. 2, 1987

Rare, Isolated, Easily Missed Cell

(Left) Headline from one article in a series that led to the Clinical Laboratory Improvement Amendments of 1988 is shown. (Reprinted with permission of Wall Street Journal, Dow Jones & Company, Inc. License number 3318251347115.) (Right) Pap stain shows a rare, high-grade "litigation" cell ➔, which can easily be missed on screening.

Quality Improvement and Laboratory Management for Cytopathology

- Specimen is monitored from moment it arrives in lab until clinician receives report

Preanalytical Quality Control
- Specimen receipt
  - Documented criteria for rejection of specimens
  - Physician notification when unacceptable specimens are received (document in log)
  - All specimens must be labeled at time of collection to provide unique identification
    - 2 unique identifiers are required in USA
- Specimen preparation
  - Technical quality of preparations should be checked and documented daily by pathologist or supervisory-level cytotechnologist
    - If problem is found, documentation of solution can help if problem presents itself in future
- Specimen staining
  - Slides must be stained using Papanicolaou or modified Papanicolaou staining method
  - Effective measures to prevent cross-contamination between GYN and NGYN specimens during staining is required
  - NGYN specimens that have high potential for cross-contamination must be stained separately from other NGYN specimens
- Instruments and equipment
  - All equipment must be on routine maintenance schedule and documented in accordance with written procedures
  - Instrument maintenance, service, and repair records must be kept and available to technical staff operating machine
  - Refrigerators that store reagents &/or patient samples must have daily documented acceptable range of temperature
- Reagents
  - Should be labeled with date of receipt; expiration date should also be noted
  - Should be stored as per manufacturer's specifications and recommended temperature
  - Upon placement into use, all chemicals and reagents will be labeled with "date opened"
- Air quality checks should be performed in accordance with local, state, &/or federal guidelines
- Hand-off communications
  - Pending specimens processed between shifts
  - Documented communication within laboratory as to changes in procedures, processes, and personnel issues

QUALITY ASSURANCE

Definition
- Systematic monitoring of results and processes to detect, control, and prevent occurrence of errors
  - Assures that all QC functioned as intended
  - Used as learning tool if errors occurred
  - All QA processes must be described and documented in laboratory QA program

Cytology-Histology Correlations (GYN, NGYN, FNA)
- Lab must provide at least annual statistics on number of cases of HSIL or Ca (GYN) for which histology results are available for comparison and cases in which cytology and histology results are discrepant
- For gynecological specimens of HSIL or Ca (GYN), laboratory must send follow-up letters at certain laboratory-determined intervals (usually 3 and 6 months) to obtain patient follow-up information
  - Annual statistics should include this information
- There must be effort to correlate NGYN and FNAB cytopathology findings with histological and clinical findings

Retrospective Reviews (GYN)
- For each patient with current/new HSIL or Ca, laboratory must review all normal or negative GYN specimens received within previous 5 years
- If significant discrepancies are found that would affect current patient care, laboratory must notify patient's physician and issue revised report
- For NGYN and FNAB, certain percentage of cases can be retrospectively reviewed for interpretation and other variances (to be defined by laboratory)

Measures of Screening Performance
- Rescreening of ≥ 10% of each cytotechnologist's GYN cases that have been interpreted as negative
  - Required for laboratories subjected to CLIA '88 regulations
  - Should be performed by cytotechnologist supervisor with ≥ 3 years of full-time experience within preceding 10 years or designee who meets requirements
  - Must include some cases from high-risk patients based on criteria established by laboratory director
  - Certain percentage of prospective should include random non-high-risk cases as well
  - Results of cases selected for rescreening must not be reported until rescreen is completed
  - Slides processed by imaging instruments must be rescreened in their entirety
- Comparison between individual performance and overall laboratory performance
- Cytotechnologist-to-pathologist correlation
- Screening limits
  - CLIA '88 limit of maximum number of slides that can be screened (USA specific)
    - 100 slides/24 hours prorated to 12.5 slides/1 hour in 8-hour screening day
      - Note some states like NY, CA have lower limits
  - Slide counts must include new routine slides, 10% rescreen slides, 5-year look-back negative slides, proficiency testing slides, and other slides subject to full-screening techniques
  - GYN preparations
    - Liquid-based preparations (ThinPrep and SurePath): 1-slide count
    - Image-guided liquid-based preparations (ThinPrep and SurePath): 0.5-slide count (or 1.5-slide count if full manual review is done)
    - Conventional smear: 1-slide count
  - NGYN preparations

Quality Improvement and Laboratory Management for Cytopathology

- Cytospins or liquid-based preparations: 0.5-slide count
- FNAB slides or smears: 1-slide count
  - Pathologists who screen previously unscreened GYN and NGYN slides must document and adhere to maximum workload set by CLIA '88
    - Primary screening pathologists must also take GYN proficiency test in primary screener mode

Turnaround Time

- Laboratory needs to determine timeframes for reporting test results; no CLIA '88 mandate
  - Suggested turnaround time for NGYN tests: 48 hours
  - Turnaround time for GYN tests: 48-72 hours (large commercial labs) to 6-8 workdays (hospital labs)
- If unable to report patient test results in established timeframe, laboratory must determine and address delay

Examination of Unknown Slides (Peer Comparison Survey Programs)

- Interlaboratory comparison programs provide valuable educational opportunities for peer comparisons in both technical and diagnostic areas
- Also allows benchmarking with peers within lab as well as nationally
- Policy should be in place on remedial action if significant variance if found

Diagnostic Statistics

- Each laboratory should produce statistical summary of various aspects of diagnoses at regular intervals and develop thresholds for acceptable deviation from these statics
  - Diagnostic category (including unsatisfactory) by preparation type
  - Significant GYN and NGYN cytologic/histologic discrepancies (as defined by laboratory policy)
  - Total number of negative cases rescreened before sign-out (to include but not limited to 10% rescreen)
  - Cases for which rescreen resulted in reclassification as premalignant or malignant
  - Cases for which histopathology results are available to compare with malignant or HSIL

Proficiency Testing

- All screening personnel (cytotechnologist, secondary screening pathologist, and primary screening pathologist) must successfully complete annual proficiency test approved by Centers for Medicare and Medicaid Services
  - Required for USA laboratories and other laboratories subject to CLIA '88 regulations
- Written policies and records of proficiency testing results, failures, remedial training, and retesting must be kept for 2 years

RISK REDUCTION

Record Keeping per CLIA '88

- Requisitions &/or authorizations for tests should be retained for 2 years
- Proficiency test records should be retained for 2 years
- Quality system assessment records should be retained for 2 years
- Pathology test reports are to be retained for at least 10 years from date of reporting
- Records of intra- and extradepartmental consultations are retained for 10 years

Slide Handling and Retention

- All slides must be retrievable upon request
  - Receipt of slides loaned out for proficiency testing or for other purposes must be documented
- Cytology GYN and NGYN (non-FNAB) slides must be retained for 5 years
  - FNAB slides are retained for 10 years
- Cell block are to be retained for same duration as corresponding cytology slides
- It is important to remember that retention guidelines may vary from one regulatory agency to another and by countries

Amended Reports From Retrospective Reviews

- Laboratory should have written policy that defines term "significant discrepancy" and reporting protocols
- Amended reports issued only if it makes difference in **current clinical management**
- In absence of "significant discrepancy," this review should be for internal use only and used as teaching/learning tool

Solid Policies and Procedures

- Having well-written standard operating procedures (SOP) and updating them frequently will help ensure that personnel are knowledgeable about their jobs
- Annual review of procedures should be documented by medical director or designee

Documentation of Knowledge of Changes

- Laboratory must have procedure to document that employees have knowledge of any changes affecting their scope of work

Workload Limits

- Laboratory directors must assign individual screener workload limits based on competency assessments, and these must be reassessed every 6 months
  - Workload limits must be based on capability/documented performance evaluation
  - Performance can be evaluated on (but not limited to) following
    - Negative rescreen evaluation and 5-year HSIL/Ca lookbacks (GYN)
    - Comparison between cytotechnologist's interpretation of GYN specimens and final cytologic diagnosis
    - Comparison between cytotechnologist's interpretation of NGYN specimens and final cytologic diagnosis
    - Performance with respect to retrospective reviews
    - Comparison between individual's statistics and overall lab statistics
    - Competency assessment
- Documentation
  - Cytotechnologist must keep daily accurate workload records
  - Cytotechnologist must be in compliance with federally mandated workload limits

Quality Improvement and Laboratory Management for Cytopathology

- Best way to reduce risk to patient and laboratory is through evidence of accreditation, compliance with good policies and procedures, and good documentation
- Pap test false-negative notification: Policy should exist to educate providers of cervicovaginal specimens that Pap test is screening test for cervical cancer with inherent false-negative results
  - Preferred mechanism: Educational note on all negative Pap test reports
  - Other choices: Sending periodic educational information to providers, conferences, or presentations

Laboratory Safety

- Laboratory can be hazardous work environment
  - Employees can be exposed to many potential hazards, e.g., chemical, biological, and physical stresses
- Laboratory safety is governed by local, state, and federal regulations
- Employers must evaluate laboratory and develop plan for protecting their workers that includes immediate actions and long-term solutions
- Occupational Safety and Health Administration (OSHA) suggests framework of "hierarchy of controls" to select ways of addressing workplace hazards
  - Engineering controls that reduce workplace hazards
    - Chemical fume hoods
    - Biological safety cabinets
    - Processing equipment that has sealed chambers (cytospin), fume filters (automatic stainers), and other environmental controls
  - Administrative controls that minimize workers' exposure
    - Biological and chemical hygiene plan
    - SOP for biological and chemical handling
  - Procedures for safe and proper work practices that can reduce duration, frequency, or intensity of exposure
    - Disposal of infectious specimens and contaminated material
    - Universal precautions as all body substances may carry infectious agents
    - Proper disposal of chemicals
    - Storage of volatile reagents in safety storage cabinet for flammable liquids
    - Availability of material safety data sheets for all employees dealing with chemicals
    - Hand washing facilities, antiseptic hand cleansers, paper towels, eye wash stations
    - Formaldehyde and xylene vapor monitoring (8 hours and 15 minutes)
    - Housekeeping: All environmental surfaces should be cleaned daily with approved disinfectant
    - Employee ergonomic evaluation: Recommended approach is to achieve "neutral body" positioning, i.e., comfortable working posture in which joints are naturally aligned
  - Personal protective equipment (PPE): Protective gear to keep workers safe while performing jobs
    - OSHA defines PPE as appropriate if it does not permit blood or other potentially infectious materials to pass through or reach employee's clothes, undergarments, skin, mouth, eyes, or other mucous membranes
    - Laboratory coat: Impervious coat, gown, or uniform to prevent contamination of personal clothing
    - Hand protection: Disposable gloves in various sizes with appropriate glove types for employees who have skin sensitivity
    - Eye and face protection: Goggles, mask, face shield, or other splatter guard when working outside biological safety hood

Quality Assurance/Quality Control Specific to FNA Service

- **Preanalytic**: Informed consent form, to include patient name, physician performing FNA, site, patient assent, statement of satisfaction with information, anesthesia options, complications, accuracy of procedure, disclaimer, and patient and witness signatures
- **Analytic**: Procedure, to include "time out" and patient identification (2 identifiers, such as, name, date of birth), equipment in room, patient comfort and safety, adequacy/rapid on-site evaluation, postprocedure patient instructions, and interpretation
- **Postanalytic**: Result reporting, documentation of oral communication, cytology-histology-clinical correlation and reason for noncorrelates, (sampling vs. interpretation), turnaround times, statistics, amended reports and reasons

Telecytopathology for Rapid On-Site Evaluation

- Validation requirements, security and integrity requirements similar to other computer-based laboratory systems, including interface integrity, downtime procedures, and competency assessment of those operating system

Significant and Unexpected Findings

- Any significant and unexpected findings (as determined by cytopathology department) must be communicated to treating physician in timely or urgent manner
- Date and time of these communications has to be documented (either in report or separate binder, which should be made available if requested by inspector)

Dashboards for Performance Improvement

- Develop personalized dashboards for cytotechnologists and pathologists
- ASCUS:SIL ratios, HPV(+) ASCUS rates (%), thyroid AUS rates (%) and others
- Available on demand (confidentially) to individuals for benchmarking and performance improvement

SELECTED REFERENCES

1. Geisler DL et al: Accuracy of definitive rapid onsite evaluation cytopathology diagnoses: Assessment of potentially critical diagnoses as a quality assurance measure. J Am Soc Cytopathol. 11(3):133-141, 2022
2. Roberson J et al: Cross-contamination in cytology processing: a review of current practice. J Am Soc Cytopathol. 11(4):194-200, 2022
3. Trabzonlu L et al: Telecytology validation: is there a recipe for everybody? J Am Soc Cytopathol. 11(4):218-25, 2022
4. VanderLaan PA et al: Molecular testing results as a quality metric for evaluating cytopathologists' utilization of the atypia of undetermined significance category for thyroid nodule fine-needle aspirations. J Am Soc Cytopathol. 11(2):67-73, 2022
5. Weiss VL et al: All in for patient safety: a team approach to quality improvement in our laboratories. J Am Soc Cytopathol. 11(2):87-93, 2022
6. Compton ML et al: Targeted education as a method for reinforcing Paris System criteria and reducing urine cytology atypia rates. J Am Soc Cytopathol. 10(1):9-13, 2021
7. Green DM et al: Implementation and assessment of a telecytology quality assurance program. J Am Soc Cytopathol. 10(2):239-45, 2021

Quality Improvement and Laboratory Management for Cytopathology

Cytology-Specific Mandates Under Clinical Laboratory Improvement Amendments of 1988 (USA Specific)

Mandate	Applies to	Requirements	Details
Personnel standards	CT	Graduated from CAAHEP accredited school of cytotechnology and passed ASCP board of registry exam	Screen and sign-out negative GYN (Paps) (except reactive/repair); screen NGYN, assist in FNA and ROSE
	GS	As above + 3 years full-time experience as CT; (if no CT, then TS can also serve as GS)	Prospective rescreen (GYN) and 5-year retrospective rescreen for HSIL/Ca
	TS/medical director	MD or DO with board certification in anatomic pathology by American Board of Pathology	Sign-out abnormal GYN + reactive/repair, all NGYN cases, set workload limits, other medical director duties
Workload limits	CTs and primary screening pathologists (includes GYN and NGYN)	100 slides/8-hour day, prorated/hour (12.5/hour max); for GYN, conventional, and liquid-based slide count as 1; imaged slide = 0.5, with manual review = 1.5	Primary screener to maintain records and not exceed workload limits, which are evaluated and assigned 6 monthly
	GS	Same as CT	Keep own records and review other CTs
	TS	Only if primary screener	Responsible for CTs, GS, and other screeners (primary screening pathologists)
Hierarchical review of slides	Abnormal and reactive/repair Paps, all NGYN cases	Reviewed and signed out by pathologists	Mechanism for resolving major discrepancies between pathologist and CT diagnosis
Prospective rescreen (prior to case sign out)	Negative Pap slides	Minimum 10% rescreen by GS or TS or designee	Certain percentage of this 10% should include random negatives, others can be high risk; document results or rescreens and remedial actions (if needed)
Retrospective rescreen (look-backs)	Negative Paps only in past 5 years, if in lab file	Every time new high-grade squamous intraepithelial lesion/carcinoma (HSIL/Ca) is diagnosed on cytology	**Amended report issued by TS/pathologist only if it makes difference in current clinical management**
Performance evaluations	CTs for GYN and NGYN	Every 6 months by TS in consultation with GS and workload limits issued/evaluated	Use individual stats, rescreen misses, benchmarks, HPV(+) atypical squamous cells of undetermined significance rates, performance on proficiency testing (PT), and peer comparison
Lab statistics	GYN and NGYN cytology cases	At minimum, maintain by different types of specimens and diagnostic categories; can do so by individuals	For GYN, specimen reporting categories; for NGYN, specimen types and reporting categories
Proficiency testing	CTs and pathologists involved in GYN cytology	Annual testing; 4 failures (totaling 80 slides) is considered fail for year and reported to CMS	PT to be taken under normal work setting; different grading schemes for CTs and pathologists
Cytology-histology correlations	GYN and NGYN high-grade and malignant cases	Cytology has to be correlated with histology and clinical information	Correlation is mandated; timelines and details depend on lab and resources
Staining	GYN and NGYN	Permanent stain like Pap is used	Stains that fade should not be used
Slide retention	GYN and NGYN	5 years for exfoliative, 10 for FNAs	5 years due to HSIL/Ca look-back
Lab inspections	Laboratory	2 years or STAT if complaint or compliance issue is reported	CMS, ASCT, CAP, TJC, others with deemed status by CMS

ASCP = American Society for Clinical Pathology; ASCT = American Society of Cytotechnology; CA = carcinoma; CAAHEP = Commission on Accreditation of Allied Health Education Programs; CAP = College of American Pathologists; CMS = Center for Medicare and Medicaid Services; CT = cytotechnologists; GS = general supervisor; GYN = gynecologic; HSL = high-grade squamous intraepithelial lesion; NGYN = nongynecologic; ROSE = rapid on-site evaluations; TJC = The Joint Commission; TS = technical supervisor.

Quality Improvement and Laboratory Management for Cytopathology

Biohazard and Sharps Disposal

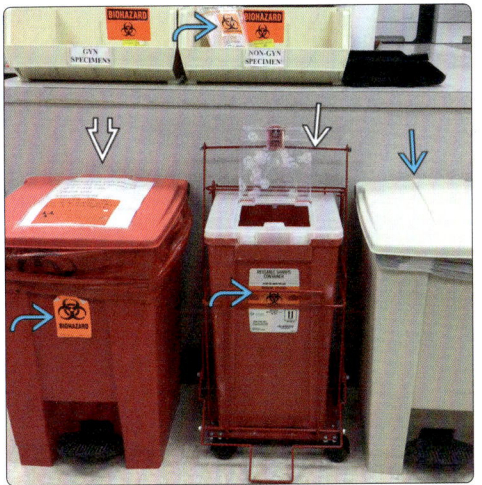

Fire Safety and Evacuation Route

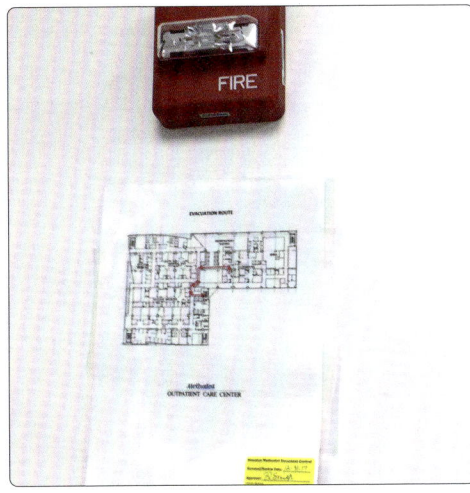

(Left) A biohazard waste disposal plan must address infectious waste and sharps that are capable of transmitting disease. The sharps container should be solid and upright ➡ with the appropriate signage ➡. Nonsharps are disposed in marked biohazard bags, which are held in red marked containers ➡. Regular trash is noted ➡. Specimens are received in marked, impervious bags. **(Right)** Fire safety plans must include the use of alarms and evacuation routes out of the laboratory in case of fire.

Signage on Cabinet or Room

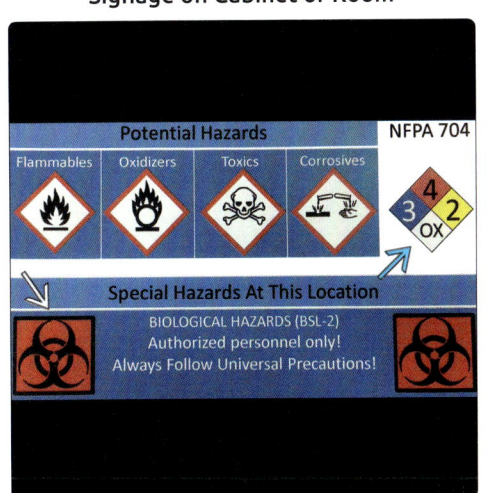

National Fire Protection Association Placard

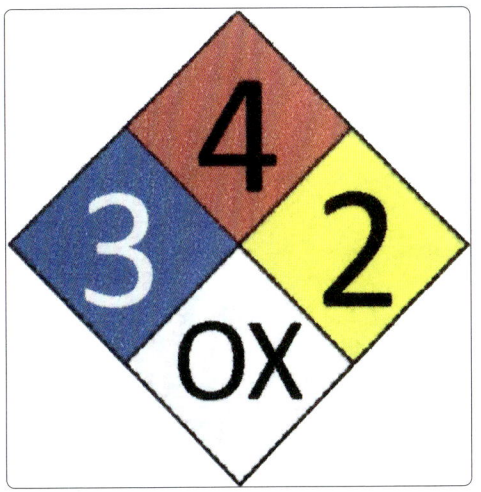

(Left) Signage for the storage unit of xylene, formalin, and alcohol is shown. The various symbols for flammables, oxidizers, toxins, and corrosives are depicted along with the biohazard symbol ➡ and the NFPA 704 diamond ➡. **(Right)** NFPA standards for health care facilities are: Red for flammability, yellow for instability and reactivity, white for special hazards, and blue for health hazard on a scale of 0 (indicating minimal to no hazard) to 4 (severe hazard). OX stands for oxidizable, under special hazard.

Biological Safety Hoods

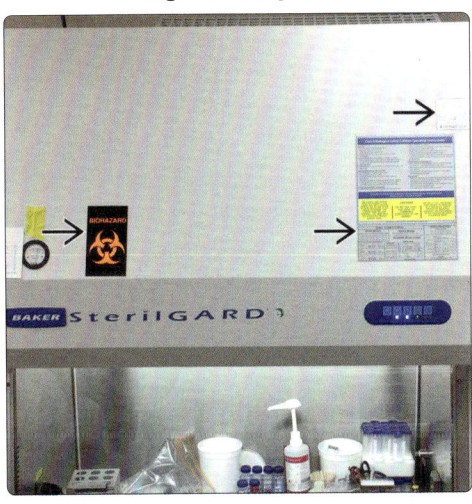

Ergonomically Proper Neutral Body Positioning

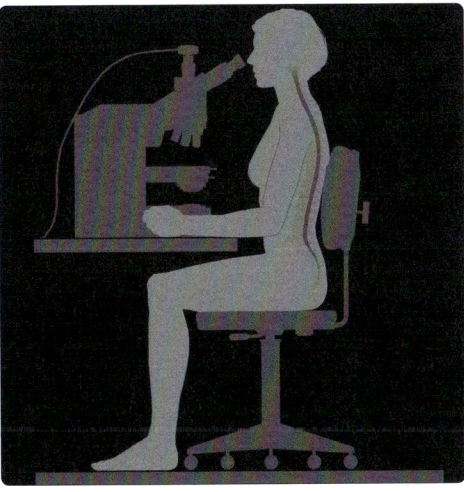

(Left) Certain procedures in which aerosols or splashes may occur are conducted in biologic safety hoods, which are periodically checked for proper working conditions with appropriate documentation/labels and inspection stickers ➡. **(Right)** Head, neck, and trunk face forward and are perpendicular to floor. Shoulders and upper arms are close to the body, in line with the torso. Forearms, wrist, and hands are straight. Thighs are parallel to floor with lower legs perpendicular. Feet are flat on floor or are supported by stable foot rest.

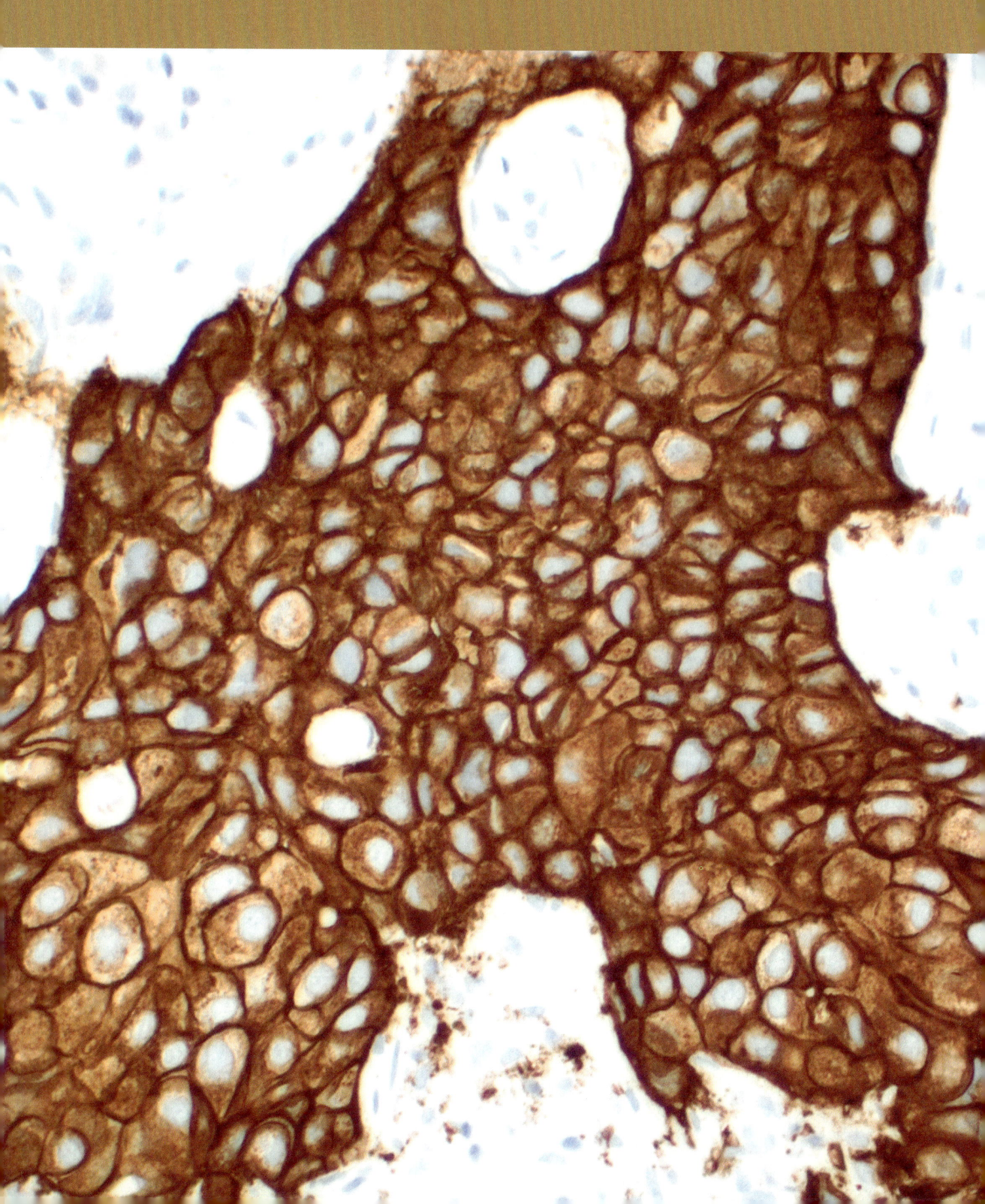

PART V
SECTION 2
Ancillary Testing

Immunocytochemistry	724
Molecular Techniques	728

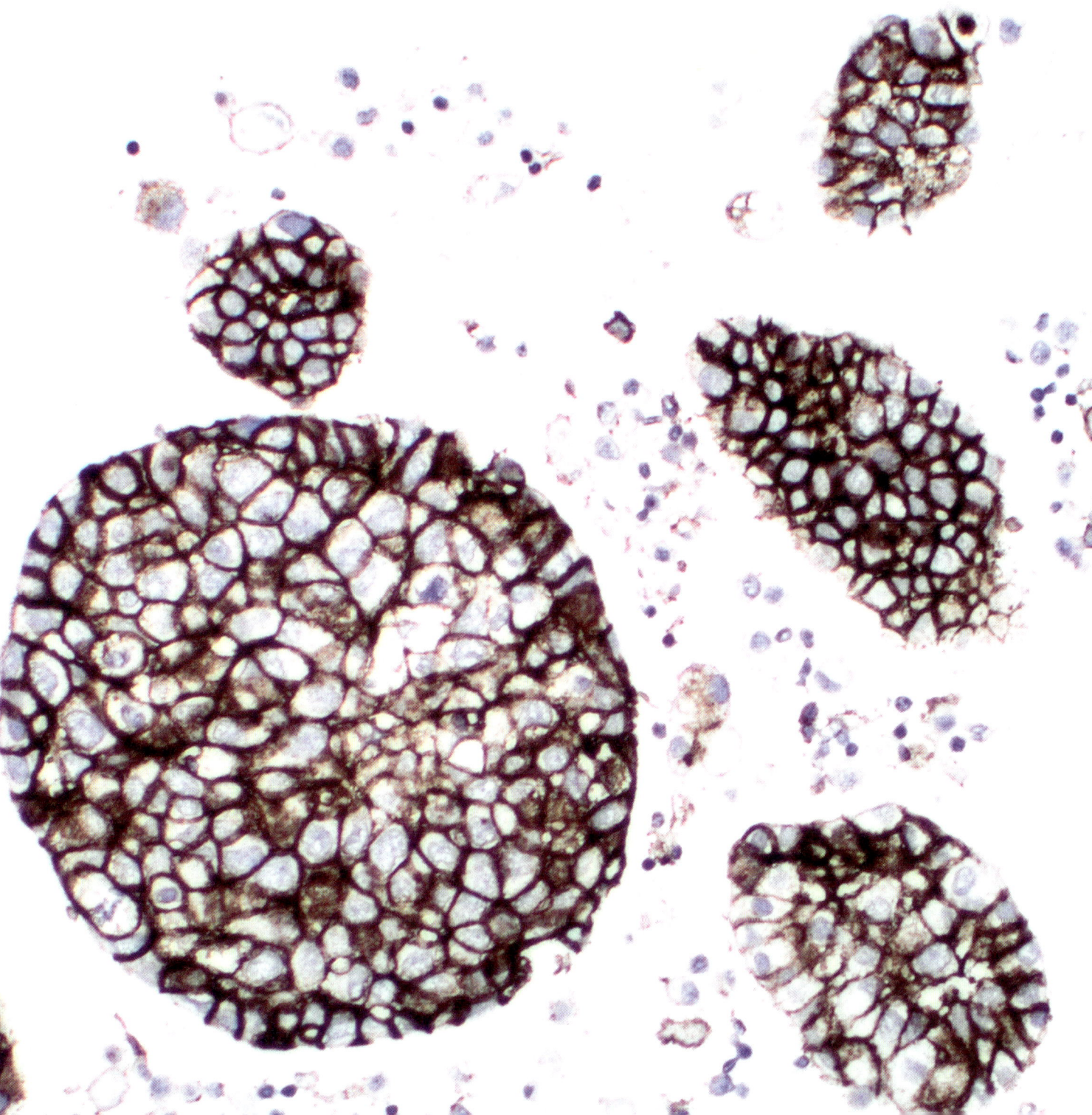

Immunocytochemistry

IMMUNOSTAINING USING CYTOLOGY AND CORE BIOPSY SPECIMENS

Special Issues
- Often limited quantity of specimen for testing
- Availability of different types of cytology specimen preparations for immunostaining
- Probability of nonspecific staining generally higher in cytology specimens in comparison to core biopsy due to presence of blood &/or necrosis
- Difficulty in using positive and negative cytology controls for immunostaining of cytology specimens
- Standardization and validation of antibodies usually uses formalin-fixed and paraffin-embedded tissue controls, necessitating validation of cytology specimens for immunomarkers using tissue control

Specimen Types
- Cell block, monolayer preparations/cytospins, FNA smears
- Core biopsy, cell-transferred preparations

Utility of Different Specimen Preparations
- Unstained tissue sections of core biopsy is optimal material for immunostaining
- Cell block is optimal cytology specimen preparation for immunostaining
- Limited material precluding preparation of cell blocks for immunostaining may necessitate use of alternatives
  - Often only stained smears prepared for conventional cytologic examination are available
  - Certain low cellularity cytology specimens, such as cerebrospinal fluid, usually do not permit preparation of cell block
- Previously stained materials can be reused
  - Diff-Quik-stained preparations can be fixed in formal saline prior to immunostaining
  - Pap-stained preparations can be used for immunostaining as such
  - Cells from Pap-stained preparations can be transferred to multiple slides to test multiple immunomarkers
  - Cell transfer of smears: Decoverslipped smears covered with thick mountant that can be floated in water and then cut into multiple pieces to be mounted on independent slides for testing
- Unstained smears, cytospins, and monolayer preparations can be fixed in different fixatives and used for immunostaining

Basic Principles of Interpretation
- Interpretation should always be made in context of morphology
- Immunostaining to be considered positive only if signal localization is correct for antibody
- Immunomarkers with nuclear staining are generally more valuable than those associated with cytoplasmic staining for cytology specimens
- Know immunoreactivity spectrum, cross reactivity, and pattern of immunostaining of utilized antibodies
- Recommend use of at least 1 antibody that would be positive for each differential diagnosis
- Immunomarkers with nuclear positivity are more useful than cytoplasmic markers when cytology smears are used for immunostaining

APPLICATIONS

Categorization and Typing of Epithelial Tumors
- Basic panel of immunomarkers for work-up of poorly differentiated malignant neoplasm
  - Pancytokeratin contains combination of high and low molecular weight cytokeratins
    - Positive in carcinoma
  - LCA in hematopoietic neoplasms
  - Melanoma cocktail usually contains tyrosinase, HMB-45, and MART-1 (+) in melanoma
- Cytokeratin profiles of carcinoma from different organ sites
  - CK7(+)/CK20(-) tumors: Lung (adenocarcinoma), breast, müllerian tract, thyroid, salivary gland, mesothelial
  - CK7(-)/CK20(+) tumors: Colorectal, Merkel cell carcinoma
  - CK7(+)/CK20(+) tumors: Pancreatic carcinoma, cholangiocarcinoma, urothelial carcinoma

Pan-Melanoma Marker

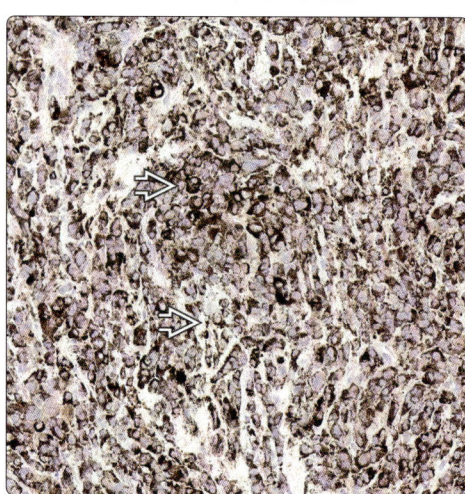

TRPS1

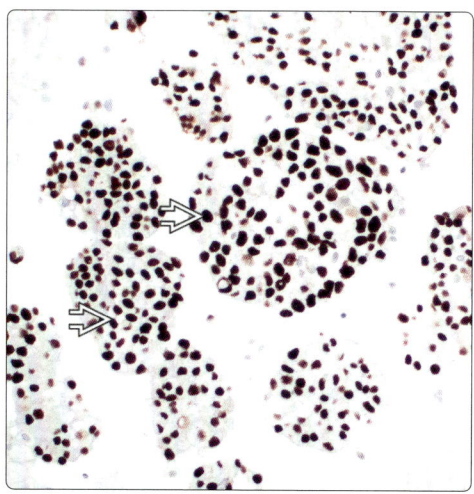

(Left) Core biopsy of metastatic melanoma immunostained for pan-melanoma marker shows cytoplasmic staining in the tumor cells ➡. (Right) Cell block section of metastatic breast carcinoma in pleural fluid immunostained for TRPS1 shows diffuse and strong nuclear staining in all the tumor cells ➡.

Immunocytochemistry

- CK7(-)/CK20(-) tumors: Adrenocortical, prostate, thymomas, renal cell carcinoma, carcinoids of lung and gastrointestinal tract, hepatocellular carcinoma, lung small cell carcinoma, lung and head and neck squamous cell carcinoma

Determine Organ of Origin of Malignant Tumors

- Sensitivity and specificity of marker for each site is variable
- Panel approach using > 1 marker may be necessary
- Lung: TTF-1, napsin A
- Breast: GATA3, ER, GCDFP-15, mammaglobin, TRPS1
- Müllerian tract: WT1, PAX8, CA 125, ER
- Mesothelium: Calretinin, D2-40, mesothelin, CK5/6, WT1
- Hepatocellular: HepPar1, glypican-3, arginase-1
- Gastrointestinal tract: CDX2, villin, SATB2, CDH17
- Thyroid gland: Thyroglobulin, TTF-1, PAX8
- Parathyroid gland: PTH, PAX8
- Adrenal gland: Calretinin, A103, inhibin, SF1
- Kidney: RCC marker, CD10, PAX2, PAX8
- Urinary bladder: Uroplakin II, GATA3, S100p
- Prostate: PSA, PSAP, prostein, NKX3.1

Neuroendocrine Differentiation

- CD56: Useful for establishing minimal degrees of neuroendocrine differentiation
- Chromogranin, synaptophysin, INSM1: Degree of positivity varies with extent of neuroendocrine differentiation

Melanoma Markers

- S100, SOX10, HMB-45, MART-1, tyrosinase, PNL2, and MITF
- High sensitivity: S100, SOX10, MART-1, tyrosinase, PNL2, and MITF; lower sensitivity: HMB-45
- High specificity: SOX10, MART-1, HMB-45, PNL2, and tyrosinase; lower specificity: S100 and MITF
- Desmoplastic melanoma: Useful markers include S100 and SOX10; most other melanoma markers can be negative
- Distinction of desmoplastic melanoma from spindle cell carcinoma and sarcoma
  o Desmoplastic melanoma: S100 and SOX10 (+); cytokeratin, p40, and p63 (-)
  o Spindle cell carcinoma: Positive for cytokeratins, especially high molecular weight cytokeratins, including CK5/6, 34βE12, CK5, CK14, p40, and p63; S100 and SOX10 (-)
  o Malignant peripheral nerve sheath tumor: Can be focally positive for S100 and SOX10
  o Synovial sarcoma: EMA and TLE3 (+); S100 and SOX10 (-)
  o All other spindle cell sarcomas are generally S100 and SOX10 (-)

Markers of Mesenchymal Cells

- Smooth muscle: SMA, desmin, H-caldesmon, calponin, MSA
- Skeletal muscle: Desmin, myogenin, MyoD1
- Endothelial cells: CD31, CD34, ERG, FLI1
- Schwann cells: S100, SOX10
- Interstitial cells of Cajal: CD117, DOG1

Panels for Work-Up of Tumors

- **Classification of non-small cell carcinoma**
  o Squamous cell carcinoma
    – Positive: p40, p63, CK5/6, and 34βE12
    – Negative: TTF-1 and napsin A; (+/-) for CK7
  o Adenocarcinoma
    – Positive: TTF-1, napsin A, and CK7
    – (+/-) for p40, p63, CK5/6, and 34βE12
  o Recommended to use starting panel with 1 marker for each differential diagnosis
- **Distinction of pulmonary small cell carcinoma from poorly differentiated squamous and basaloid carcinoma**
  o Small cell carcinoma
    – Positive: TTF-1, chromogranin, synaptophysin, CK8
    – Negative: 34βE12, p63, p40, and CK5
  o Squamous carcinoma and basaloid carcinoma
    – Positive: 34βE12, p63, p40, and CK5
    – Negative: TTF-1 and CK8
- **Distinction of lung from breast and müllerian tumors**
  o Lung
    – Positive: TTF-1 and napsin A
    – Negative: GATA3, mammaglobin, TRPS1, GCDFP-15, PAX8, WT1, and CA 125; (+/-) for ER
  o Breast
    – Positive: TRPS1, GATA3, mammaglobin, GCDFP-15, ER
    – Negative: TTF-1, napsin A, PAX8, WT1, and CA 125
  o Müllerian tract
    – Positive: PAX8, WT1, and ER
    – Negative: TTF-1, napsin A, TRPS1, GATA3, and GCDFP-15
    – (+/-) for mammaglobin
- **Distinction of hepatocellular carcinoma from cholangiocarcinoma/metastatic adenocarcinoma**
  o Hepatocellular carcinoma
    – Positive: HepPar1, glypican-3, arginase-1, pCEA (canalicular staining), AFP, and CD10 (canalicular staining)
    – Negative: MOC31 and mCEA; (+/-) for CK7
  o Adenocarcinoma
    – Positive: CK7, MOC31, mCEA (cytoplasmic staining), and pCEA (cytoplasmic staining)
    – Negative: Glypican-3, arginase-1, and AFP
    – (+/-) for HepPar1 and CD10 (cytoplasmic staining)
  o Distinction of benign mesothelial cells from mesotheliomas
    – Benign mesothelial cells
      □ Positive: Desmin, BAP1
      □ (+/-) for AE1/AE3, EMA, p63
    – Mesothelioma
      □ Positive: AE1/AE3, EMA, p53
      □ Negative: BAP1, MTAP, 5hmC
    – (+/-) for desmin

DETERMINATION OF PROGNOSTIC AND PREDICTIVE MARKERS

Metastatic/Recurrent Breast Carcinoma

- HER2, ER, PR, PD-L1, PTEN, MLH1, MSH2, PMS2, MLH6, AR

Lung Adenocarcinoma

- ALK, PD-L1, HER2, MLH1, MSH2, PMS2, MLH6, BRAF V600E, C-MET

Solid Tumors

- PD-L1, HER2, PTEN, MLH1, MSH2, PMS2, MLH6, C-MET

Immunocytochemistry

Diagnostic Immunocytochemistry Profiles in Common Renal Tumors

IHC Stain	Clear Cell	Papillary	Chromophobe	Oncocytoma	Collecting Duct	TCC
CK7	(-)	(+)	(-)	(+/-)	(+)	(+)
HMWCK	(-)	(-/+)	(-)	(-)	(+)	(+)
AE1/AE3	(+)	(+)	(+)	(-)	(+)	(+)
Vimentin	(+)	(+)	(-)	(-)	(-)	(-)
AMACR	(-)	(+)	(-)	(-)	(-)	(-)
Parvalbumin	(-)	(-)	(+)	(+)	(-)	(-)
Ksp-cadherin	(-)	(-)	(+)	(+)	(-)	(-)
RCC marker	(+)	(+)	(-)	(-)	(-)	(-)
CD10	(+)	(+)	(-/+)	(-)	(-)	(-)
C-Kit	(-)	(-)	(+)	(+)	(-)	(-)
PAX2/PAX8	(+)	(+)	(-)	(-)	(-)	(-)
GATA3	(-)	(-)	(-)	(-)	(-)	(+)
PNA	(-)	(-)	(-)	(-)	(+)	(-)
UEA-1	(-)	(-)	(-)	(-)	(+)	(-)

TCC = transitional cell carcinoma.

Distinction of Mesothelial Cells/Mesothelioma From Adenocarcinoma/Metastatic Carcinoma

Entities	Calretinin	Podoplanin /D2-40	CK5/6 and Thrombomodulin	WT1	Mesothelin	MOC31	B72.3	Ber-EP4	mCEA	CD15	Claudin-4
Mesothelial cells/ mesothelioma	(+)	(+)	(+)	(+)	(+)	(+/-)	(+/-)	(+/-)	(+/-)	(+/-)	(+/-)
Adenocarcinoma/ metastatic carcinoma	(+/-)	(+/-)	(-)	(+/-)	(-)	(+)	(+)	(+)	(+)	(+)	(+)

Small Round Blue Cell Tumor

Tumor Type	LCA (CD45)	CD99 (MIC2)	Synaptophysin	Keratin	Desmin	Myogenin	S100p
Rhabdomyosarcoma	(-)	(-)	(-)	(-)	(+)	(+)	(-)
Ewing sarcoma/PNET/Ewing-like sarcomas	(-)	(+/-)	(+)	(-/+)	(+/-)	(+/-)	(+/-)
Desmoplastic small round cell tumor	(-)	(+)	(+)	(+)	(+)	(+/-)	(-)
Lymphoma/leukemia	(+)	(+)	(-)	(-)	(-)	(-)	(-)
Small cell osteosarcoma	(-)	(+/-)	(-)	(-)	(-)	(-)	(+/-)
Small cell poorly differentiated synovial sarcoma	(-)	(-)	(-)	(+)	(-)	(-)	(+/-)
Mesenchymal chondrosarcoma	(-)	(-)	(-)	(-)	(-)	(-)	(+)

PNET = primary neuroectodermal tumor.

SELECTED REFERENCES

1. Ai D et al: TRPS1: a highly sensitive and specific marker for breast carcinoma, especially for triple-negative breast cancer. Mod Pathol. 34(4):710-9, 2021
2. Koomen BM et al: Formalin fixation for optimal concordance of programmed death-ligand 1 immunostaining between cytologic and histologic specimens from patients with non-small cell lung cancer. Cancer Cytopathol. 129(4):304-17, 2021
3. Paver EC et al: Programmed death ligand-1 (PD-L1) as a predictive marker for immunotherapy in solid tumours: a guide to immunohistochemistry implementation and interpretation. Pathology. 53(2):141-56, 2021
4. Chapel DB et al: Application of immunohistochemistry in diagnosis and management of malignant mesothelioma. Transl Lung Cancer Res. 9(Suppl 1):S3-27, 2020

Immunocytochemistry

MOC31

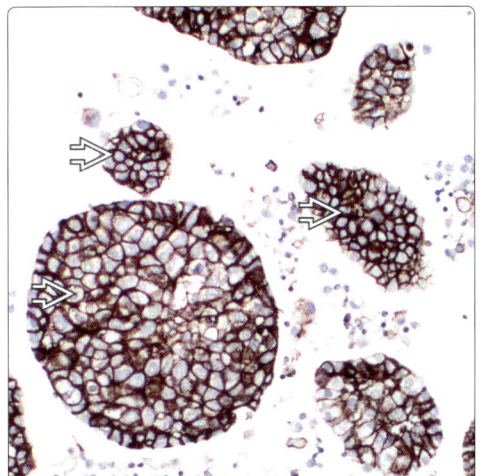

INSM1

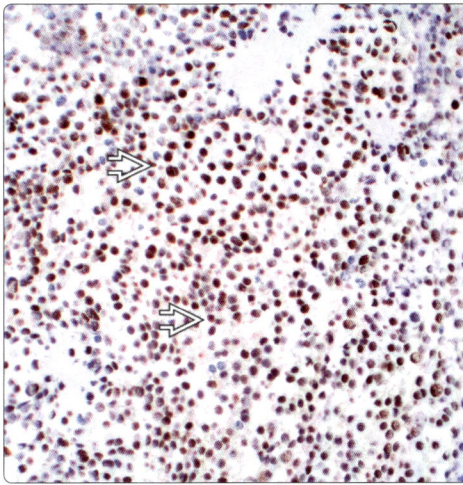

(Left) Cell block section of metastatic breast carcinoma in pleural fluid immunostained for MOC31 shows membranous staining ➔ in the tumor cells. *(Right)* Cell block section of pancreatic neuroendocrine tumor, well differentiated, immunostained for INSM1 shows nuclear staining ➔ in the tumor cells.

TTF-1

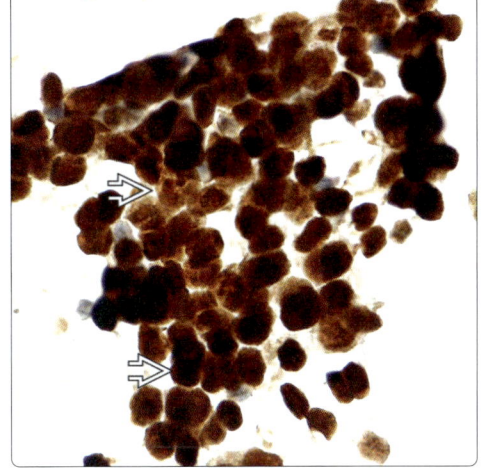

PAX8

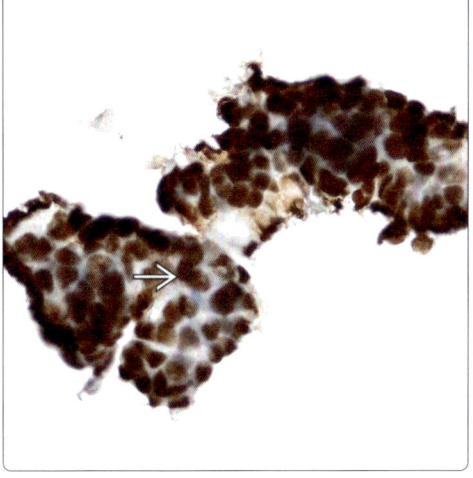

(Left) FNA smear of lung adenocarcinoma immunostained for TTF-1 shows nuclear staining ➔ in the tumor cells. *(Right)* PAX8 immunostain of an FNA of the breast shows 2 papillary clusters of tumor cells with strong nuclear positivity ➔, which supports the diagnosis of a metastatic carcinoma from the müllerian tract.

PD-L1

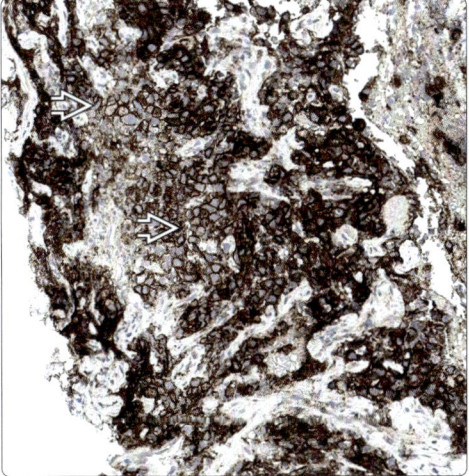

HER2

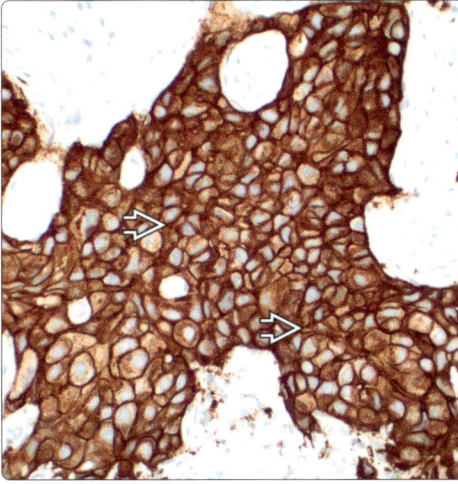

(Left) Core biopsy of metastatic breast carcinoma immunostained for PD-L1 shows complete membranous staining ➔ in the majority of the tumor cells. *(Right)* Core biopsy of an invasive ductal carcinoma of the breast immunostained for HER2 shows complete membranous staining ➔ in all of the tumor cells.

Molecular Techniques

MOLECULAR TECHNIQUES AND SMALL BIOPSY SPECIMENS

All Techniques Are Applicable

- All types of molecular techniques are applicable
  - In situ hybridization (ISH)
    - Fluorescence in situ hybridization (FISH)
    - Chromogen in situ hybridization (CISH)
  - Polymerase chain reaction (PCR)
  - Comparative genomic hybridization
  - Next-generation DNA/RNA sequencing
  - Transcriptional profiling
- Success for utilization of small biopsy specimens for molecular techniques depends on
  - Tumor cellularity: Proportion of tumor cells in comparison to other nonmalignant cells
    - Quantity of nucleic acids required varies based on selected platforms, as they dictate amount of tumor cellularity required for successful testing
  - Specimen preparation
- Core biopsies, cell blocks, stained or unstained FNA smears, cytospins, and monolayer preparation each have their own advantages and disadvantages

Advantages and Disadvantages of Different Types of Specimens for Molecular Testing

- Liquid-based preparation
  - Specimen collected directly into fixative
    - Alcohol-based fixative solution
    - Nucleic acid preservative fixative solution
  - Ease of collection
  - Specimen can be split for multiple tests
  - Specimen cellularity cannot be determined
- Direct smears/cytospin and monolayer preparations
  - Tumor cellularity can be determined accurately
  - Immediate assessment can aid in collecting adequate specimen for testing
  - Well-suited for molecular analysis because cells can be scraped from slides and used for analysis immediately
  - Alcohol-fixed and air-dried smears good for testing

Annotation of Tumor in Core Biopsy

Annotation of Tumor in Diff-Quik-Stained FNA Smear

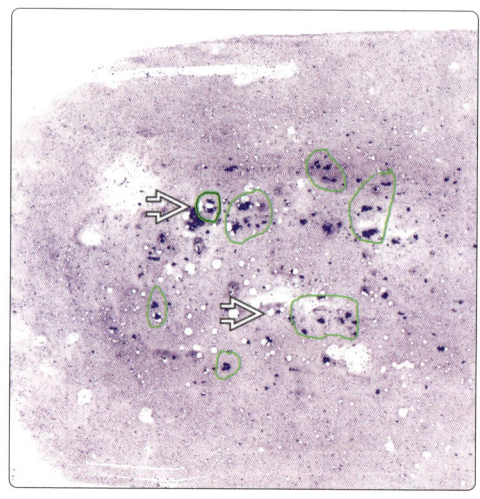

(Left) Annotation of tumor on an H&E-stained tissue section of a core biopsy ➡ permits utilization of an enriched tumor fraction from the corresponding unstained tissue sections for successful molecular testing. (Right) Annotation of tumor cells in a Diff-Quik-stained cytology smear ➡ allows scraping of the tumor cells directly from the annotated areas, thereby allowing the utilization of an enriched tumor fraction for molecular testing.

Annotation of Tumor in Cell Blocks

Annotation of Tumor in Pap-Stained Smear

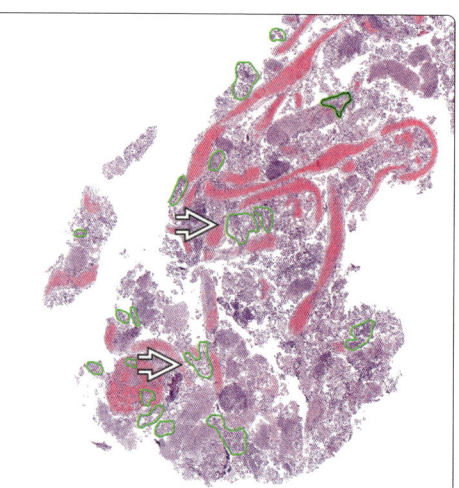
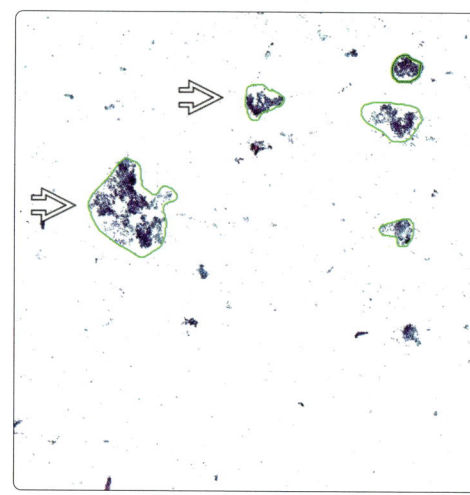

(Left) Annotation of tumor in cell blocks ➡ enriches the tumor fraction and improves the quality of nucleic acids extracted from the corresponding unstained tissue sections. (Right) Annotation of tumor cells in a Pap-stained FNA smear ➡ allows scraping of the enriched tumor fraction directly from the smear, thereby eliminating nontumor components in the smear for molecular testing.

Molecular Techniques

- o Better quality of DNA than formalin-fixed and paraffin-embedded cell blocks
- o Sample can be available for testing immediately after procurement
- Cell blocks
  - o Ease of sample collection in preservative solution
  - o Ease of sample transportation
  - o Tumor cellularity not ensured
  - o Formalin fixation can compromise quality of nucleic acids
- Core biopsy
  - o Commonly used technique
  - o Ease of sample transportation
  - o Tumor cellularity not ensured
  - o Formalin fixation can compromise quality of nucleic acids

Applications of In Situ Hybridization

- Core biopsy and cytology specimens of FNA, touch preparations of core needle biopsy, and effusions suitable for ISH testing
  - o Core biopsy, cell blocks, Diff-Quik-stained FNA smears; Diff-Quik-stained cytospins or monolayer preparation preferred
    - Availability of single cells and small sheets of tumor cells useful for counting signals
    - Absence of nuclear transection, unlike tissue sections, may lead to minor differences in signal counts
  - o Fluorescence or CISH can be used
- Validation of FISH/CISH testing before using cell blocks or direct smears for ISH recommended
- Applications of FISH/CISH using small biopsy specimens
  - o Determination of HER2 gene amplification; eligibility for therapy with trastuzumab, lapatinib, pertuzumab
    - Primary invasive mammary carcinoma; recurrent and metastatic breast carcinomas
      □ Core biopsy of primary tumor alone should be used for evaluation of HER2 gene amplification by FISH for primary breast cancer
      □ Core or FNA can be used for evaluation of HER2 gene amplification by FISH in recurrent or metastatic breast carcinoma
    - Diagnostic material obtained by FNA is particularly useful for investigation of HER2 status of bone metastasis
    - Other cancers for HER2 gene amplification by FISH: Stomach, ovary, pancreas
    - HER2 gene amplification can be evaluated by ISH preferably using dual-probe assay, including HER2 and chromosome enumeration probe (CEP17)
      □ ISH positive: HER2:CEP17 ratio > 2.0; HER2 copy numbers > 4.0 signals per cell
      □ ISH negative: HER2:CEP17 ratio < 2.0; HER2 copy numbers < 4 signals/cell
  - o Urine specimens for diagnosis of recurrent urothelial carcinoma or evaluation of macroscopic or microscopic hematuria
    - UroVysion probe kit (Abbott Laboratories)
      □ Multiprobe fluorescence ISH assay for detecting polysomy of chromosomes 3, 7, 17, and 9p21 deletion in urothelial cells from voided urine and bladder washing
      □ Cocktail of chromosome enumeration probes 3, 7, 17, and locus-specific identifier probe 9p21
      □ Evaluation of fluorescent signals in at least 25 urothelial cells that show abnormal cytomorphology
      □ Positive result: 4 or more urothelial cells showing 3 or more signals in > 2 chromosomes or > 12 urothelial cells with homozygous loss of 9p21 signals
      □ False-positive result: Tetraploidy in umbrella cells and heteroploidy in urothelial cells following human polyoma viral infection can be mistaken for malignant urothelial cells
    - Increases sensitivity of cytology alone for making diagnosis of urothelial carcinoma
  - o Determination of ALK, ROS1, MET, RET gene rearrangement; eligibility for tyrosine kinase inhibitor therapy
    - Primary or metastatic adenocarcinoma of lung
    - Other tumors: Adenocarcinomas: Colorectal, gastric; mesothelioma
  - o Determination of HPV high-risk status provides prognostic and predictive information for management of patients with head and neck squamous carcinoma
    - FNA of squamous carcinoma in neck lymph nodes from head and neck primary or unknown primary
    - CISH is generally used for this purpose
  - o Diagnosis of hematopoietic neoplasms
    - Useful when immunophenotyping by flow cytometry or immunocytochemistry leads to confusing results or cannot be performed
    - Follicular lymphoma: t(14;18)(q32;q210)
    - Mantle cell lymphoma: t(11;14)(q13;q32)
    - Anaplastic lymphoma: t(2;5)(q23;q35)
    - MYC: Burkitt lymphomas and other B-cell lymphomas, such as diffuse large B-cell lymphoma, plasmablastic lymphoma, mantle cell lymphoma, and double-hit lymphomas
  - o Diagnosis of soft tissue tumors
    - Core biopsy, touch preparation of core biopsies, cytospin, monolayer preparation, and direct smears can be used
    - Detection of specific chromosomal translocations by cytogenetic examination and fusions by RNA sequencing (Table 1)
  - o Investigation of indeterminate bile duct brushing cytology specimens
    - UroVysion probe kit: Cocktail of chromosomes 3, 7, 17, 9p21
    - Increases sensitivity of cytology alone for making diagnosis of adenocarcinoma
- Determination of Epstein-Barr virus (EBV)-encoded RNA (EBER) in EBV-related neoplasms
  - o CISH generally used for this purpose
  - o EBV-associated epithelial malignancies
    - Nasopharyngeal carcinoma
    - Gastric carcinoma
  - o EBV-associated hematopoietic neoplasms
    - Non-Hodgkin lymphoma

Molecular Techniques

- Burkitt lymphoma, diffuse large B-cell lymphoma, plasmablastic lymphoma, primary effusion lymphoma, T/NK lymphoma
  - Hodgkin lymphoma
  o EBV-associated smooth muscle tumor
- Distinction of benign mesothelial cells from mesothelioma
  o FISH using centromere 9 and CDKN2A probes for detecting homozygous deletion of 9p21 (p16)
    - 9p21 region includes genes for 2 cyclin-dependent inhibitor kinases *CDKNA2A* (p16), *CDKN2B*, methylthioadenosine phosphorylase (MTAP)
  o Can be utilized on cytology smears, cell blocks, and core biopsy
  o Sensitivity and specificity of p16 FISH
    - Effusion cytology: 56-79% and 100%
    - Histology specimens: 45-85% and 100%

Molecular Testing of Indeterminate Thyroid FNAs

- Indeterminate thyroid FNAs (constitute 10-40% of thyroid FNAs)
  o Atypical cells of undetermined significance/follicular lesions of undetermined significance
  o Follicular neoplasm/suspicious for follicular neoplasm
  o Molecular testing platforms available for further characterization
- Molecular testing platforms for investigation of indeterminate thyroid nodules
  o Afirma Genomic Sequencing Classifier (GSC) and Xpression Atlas (Veracyte, Inc.)
    - Next-generation RNA sequencing that combines gene expression and presence of DNA variants, fusions, copy number variants
    - 2 dedicated FNA passes collected in proprietary nucleic acid preservative solution required for test
    - Performance of Afirma GSC test: Prospective single center validation study showed sensitivity 94.4% and specificity 61.4% obviated surgery in 68% of patients with indeterminate thyroid cytology
  o ThyGenX thyroid oncogene panel (Interspace Diagnostics) uses next-generation sequencing (NGS) to identify DNA point mutations in *BRAF* V600E, *NRAS* codon 61, *HRAS* codon 61, *KRAS* codons 12/13, *PIK3CA* and RNA fusions *RET::PTC1*, *RET::PTC3*, and *PAX8::PPARG*
    - Requires 1 dedicated FNA pass collected in RNA preservative
    - ThyraMIR test based on analysis of 10 microRNAs available for use in conjunction with ThyGenX as reflux test for cases with negative ThyGenX result
    - ThyGenX and ThyraMIR in combination: Sensitivity and specificity for AUS/FLUS: 94% and 80%; SFN/FN: 82% and 91%
    - ThyGenX and ThyraMIR test: When both tests are negative, risk of malignancy is 6%
  o ThyroSeq v.3 test: NGS-based mutation and fusion panel, including 12,000 mutation and > 120 gene fusions [University of Pittsburgh Medical Center/Cytopathology biopsy lab (CBLPath)]
    - Bethesda II and IV categories: Sensitivity of 94%, specificity of 82%; avoid surgery in 61% of patients with indeterminate thyroid cytology
- Molecular testing of thyroid FNA
  o Promising role for diagnosis and treatment of indeterminate thyroid lesions
  o Results of molecular testing are to be used appropriately, understanding advantages and limitations of testing of each platform and in conjunction with clinical information and cytologic findings

Carcinoma of Unknown Primary

- Comprises 2-4% of all tumors
- Cytology specimens may be useful in selected cases
  o Cytology specimens are only specimens available with diagnostic material
  o Primary immunophenotyping utilizing routinely used immunomarkers does not provide indication of organ of origin of metastatic tumor
- Testing platforms
  o 92 genes RT-PCR assay using formalin-fixed and paraffin-embedded tissue (Biotheranostics CancerTYPE ID)
    - Accuracy: 79-87%

Molecular Testing for Mutations and Fusions Using NGS

- Indications
  o Lung cancer: Adenocarcinoma, adenosquamous carcinoma, large cell carcinoma, non-small cell lung cancer, not otherwise specified types; squamous cell carcinoma in light/never smokers; metastatic breast cancer, metastatic solid tumors
- Somatic mutations of *EGFR* occur in 10% of patients with non-small cell lung carcinoma
  o Asian patients, female patients, nonsmokers more likely
  o Adenocarcinoma histology
- Common alterations of *EGFR* in adenocarcinoma of lung
  o In-frame deletion in exon 19
  o Point mutation in exon 21 (L858R)
  o *EGFR* p.T790M mutations most common mechanism of resistance following 1st- and 2nd-generation tyrosine kinase inhibitors targeting *EGFR*
  o *EGFR* p.C797S, p.L292X, p.G796X, p.L718Q, p.G724S mutations major mechanism in patients receiving 3rd-generation *EGFR* inhibitors
- Targeted therapy: Presence of mutations allows selection of patients for tyrosine kinase inhibitor therapy
- Status of *KRAS* in solid tumors
- Mutation of *KRAS* noted in several types of tumor: Lung, colorectal, pancreatic, ovarian tumors
- *KRAS* is key signal transducer that plays important part in *MAPK1*, *JAK-STAT*, and *PI3K* pathways
- Clinical utility of detecting *KRAS* mutation
  o Negative predictor of benefit to anti-*EGFR* therapy in lung and colorectal tumors
    - *KRAS* p.G12C mutation in patients with non-small cell lung carcinoma can be eligible for treatment with sotorasib
- Status of *BRAF* in melanoma and other solid tumors, such as thyroid and colorectal tumors
  o Mutations of *BRAF* occur in 40-60% of metastatic melanomas
  o *BRAF* V600E mutation is most common *BRAF* mutation
- Clinical utility
  o Prognostic indicator in melanoma

Molecular Techniques

- Selects patients with metastatic melanoma and other solid tumors with *BRAF and MEK* inhibitor therapy
- Status of *KIT* mutation
  - *KIT* receptor tyrosine kinase family is important for development and progression of some tumors
    - Gastrointestinal stromal tumors, melanoma, small cell lung carcinoma, systemic mastocytosis, acute myeloid leukemia
- Clinical utility
  - Selection of patients for tyrosine kinase inhibitor therapy
- *ALK* fusions
  - Fusion of *ALK* with echinoderm microtubule-associated protein-like 4 (EML4) most common
    - Presence of *ALK* fusions is associated with responsiveness to oral ALK inhibitors
- *ROS1* fusions
  - Fusion of *ROS1* with *CD74*, *SLC34A2*, *CCDC6*, and *FIG*
    - *ROS1* fusions are associated with responsiveness to ROS1 inhibitors
- *MET* abnormalities
  - *MET* is receptor tyrosine kinase; mutations resulting in loss of exon 14 lead to dysregulation and inappropriate signaling
    - *MET* exon skipping is associated with responsiveness to *MET* inhibitors
  - High-level *MET* amplification (10 or higher copies)
    - Mutation associated with overactivation of *MET* pathway
      - Patients with this mutation respond to crizotinib or capmatinib
    - Amplification of *MET* has also been seen as secondary resistance mechanism that can emerge after treatment using other targeted agents
- *RET* fusions
  - Fusion of *RET*, receptor tyrosine kinase, with other partners *KIF5B*, *NCOA4*, CCDC6
    - *RET* fusions are associated with responsiveness to *RET* inhibitors
- NTRK (neurotrophic tyrosine kinase) 1/2/3 fusions
  - TRKA/B/C are tyrosine kinases encoded by NTRK1/2/2
    - Fusion of NTRK1/2/2 with other partners results in inappropriate signaling
- *ERBB2* (*HER2*) exon 20 insertions and point mutations
  - These mutations lead to constitutive activation of *ERBB2*; patients with these mutations respond to ado-trastuzumab
- *PIK3CA* mutations, gene-encoding phosphatidyl inositol 3-kinases (*PI3K*)
  - Activating mutations in exons 9 and 20 (mutation subtypes E542K, E545X, H1047X) are common genomic alterations in 40% of estrogen receptor positive (ER+), *HER2* breast cancer that activate PI3K enzyme activity, leading to constitutive unopposed phosphorylation of *AKT* and downstream effectors
    - PI3K inhibitor therapy in combination with endocrine therapy offered to postmenopausal patients with ER(+), *PIK3CA* mutated advanced breast cancer and metastatic breast cancer following prior endocrine therapy ± cyclin-dependent kinase (CDK) 4/6 inhibitor
- Several targets for which targeted therapy is available are under consideration in clinical trials
- Mutations in *NF2*, *GNAQ::GNA11*, *SMO::PTCH1*, *FGFR1*, *FGFR2*, *FGFR3*, *AKT1*, *NRAS*, *HER2*, *DDR2*, *PIK3CA*, *PTEN*, and *BRAF* non-V600E and amplifications in *CCND1*, *CCND2*, *CCND3*, *MET*, dMMR, *NF2* loss, and *PTEN* loss

Issues Related to Molecular Testing Using Small Biopsy Specimens

- Utilization of different types of small biopsy specimen preparations from different sources that can be selected for testing
  - Core biopsy, unstained formalin-fixed and paraffin-embedded tissue sections
  - Cell block, unstained formalin-fixed and paraffin-embedded sections
  - FNA smears
    - Pap, Diff-Quik, or unstained smears
  - Source of cytology specimens for molecular testing
    - FNA, effusions, washings, lavage
- Awareness of strengths and limitations of each type of small biopsy specimen preparation is important
- Procuring adequate material not only for diagnosis but also for ancillary molecular testing
- Immediate assessment useful for procuring adequate material for molecular testing
  - Upfront estimation of tumor cellularity in specimen for evaluation of quality of specimen for molecular testing is useful
  - Success of molecular testing depends on proper coordination between anatomic pathology and molecular pathology laboratories
  - Validation of cytology specimens for different types of molecular testing is important for routine usage
  - Minimum requirement of tumor cellularity in any type of small biopsy specimens for molecular testing is 20%
- Suitability of small biopsy specimens for different types of molecular testing should be determined on case-by-case basis
- Challenges of molecular testing not unique to small biopsy specimens to be considered
  - Biologic factors
    - Tumor heterogeneity, molecular evolution
  - Detection of mutations and alterations for which there are no effective drugs
  - Careful considerations to avoid false-positive and false-negative results
  - Adherence to evolving regulatory requirements and monitoring reimbursement issues

SELECTED REFERENCES

1. Glass RE et al: Using molecular testing to improve the management of thyroid nodules with indeterminate cytology: an institutional experience with review of molecular alterations. J Am Soc Cytopathol. 11(2):79-86, 2022
2. Ohori NP: A decade into thyroid molecular testing: where do we stand? J Am Soc Cytopathol. 11(2):59-61, 2022
3. Imyanitov EN et al: Molecular testing and targeted therapy for non-small cell lung cancer: current status and perspectives. Crit Rev Oncol Hematol. 157:103194, 2021
4. Nagai T et al: UroVysion fluorescence in situ hybridization in urothelial carcinoma: a narrative review and future perspectives. Transl Androl Urol. 10(4):1908-17, 2021
5. Savic I et al: Update on diagnosing and reporting malignant pleural mesothelioma. Acta Med Acad. 50(1):197-208, 2021
6. Huang M et al: Overview of molecular testing of cytology specimens. Acta Cytol. 64(1-2):136-46, 2020

Molecular Techniques

Cytogenetic and Molecular Alterations of Sarcomas

Sarcoma Type	Cytogenetic Alteration	Molecular Alteration
Alveolar rhabdomyosarcoma	t(2;13)(q35;q14) t(1;13)(p36;q14) t(2;2)(q35;p23) t(X;2)(q35;q13)	PAX::FOXO1 PAX7::FOXO1 PAX3::NCOA1 PAX3::AFX
Alveolar soft part sarcoma	t(X;17)(p11;q25)	TFE3::ASPSCR1
BCOR-rearranged sarcoma	Inv(X)(p11p11)	BCOR::CCNB3 BCOR::MAML3 ZC3H7B::BCOR
CIC-rearranged sarcoma	t(4;19)(q35;q13) t(X;19)(q13;q13.30)	CIC::DUX4 CIC::FOXO4
Clear cell sarcoma	t(12;22)(q13;q12) t(2;22)(q32.3;q12)	EWSR1::ATF1 CREB1::EWSR1
Dedifferentiated liposarcoma	Ring and giant marker chromosomes	Amplification of 12q13-15: MDM2, CDK4, HMGA2
Desmoplastic small round cell tumor	t(11;22)(p13;q12)	EWSR1::WT1
Epithelioid sarcoma	Deletion 22q t(8;22)(q22;q11) t(10;220	SMARCB1 inactivation
Ewing sarcoma	t(11;22)(q24;q12) t(11;22)(q12;q12)	EWSR1::FLI1 EWSR1::ERG
Extraskeletal myxoid chondrosarcoma	t(9;220(q22;q12) t(9;17)(q22;q11) t(9;15)(q22;q21) t(3;9)(q11;q22) t(9;17)(q22;q11)	EWSR1::NR4A3 TAF2N::NR4A3 TCF12::NR4A3 TFG::NR4A3 RBP56::NR4A3
Inflammatory myofibroblastic tumor	t(1;2)(q22;p23) t92;19)(p23;p13 t(2;17)(p23;q23) t(2;2)(p23;q13) t(2;2)(p23;q35) t(2;11)(p23.q35) t(2;4)(p23;q21) t(2;12)(p23;p120	TPM3::ALK TPM4::ALK CLTC::ALK RANBP2::ALK ATIC::ALK CARS::ALK SEC31L1::ALK PPFIBP1::ALK RRBP1::ALK TFG::ROS1 YWHAE::ROS1
Low-grade fibromyxoid sarcoma	t(7;16)(q33;p11) t(11;16)(p11;p11)	FUS::CREB3L2 FUS::CREB3L1
Mesenchymal chondrosarcoma	t(8;8)(q13q21)	HEY1::NCOA2
Malignant peripheral nerve sheath tumor	Complex changes	SUZ12 or EED mutation, NF1 inactivation
Myxoid liposarcoma	t(12;16)(q13;p11) t(12;22)(q13;q12)	FUS::DDIT3 EWSR1::DDIT3
Synovial sarcoma	t(X;18)(p11;q11)	SS18::SSX1/SSX2 fusion
Solitary fibrous tumor	Inv(12)(q13q13)	NAB2::STAT6 fusion
Gastrointestinal stromal tumor	Deletion 14q,22q,1p,15q	KIT or PDGFR mutation, NF1, SDHX, BRAF mutation, SDHC hypermethylation

7. Kumar N et al: Molecular testing in diagnosis of indeterminate thyroid cytology: trends and drivers. Diagn Cytopathol. 48(11):1144-51, 2020
8. Rossi ED et al: The role of molecular testing for the indeterminate thyroid FNA. Genes (Basel). 10(10), 2019
9. Lindeman NI et al: Updated molecular testing guideline for the selection of lung cancer patients for treatment with targeted tyrosine kinase inhibitors: guideline from the College of American Pathologists, the International Association for the Study of Lung Cancer, and the Association for Molecular Pathology. Arch Pathol Lab Med. 142(3):321-46, 2018
10. Rezk SA et al: Epstein-Barr virus (EBV)-associated lymphoid proliferations, a 2018 update. Hum Pathol. 79:18-41, 2018
11. Schaefer IM et al: Contemporary sarcoma diagnosis, genetics, and genomics. J Clin Oncol. 36(2):101-10, 2018
12. Zhai J: UroVysion multi-target fluorescence in situ hybridization assay for the detection of malignant bile duct brushing specimens: a comparison with routine cytology. Acta Cytol. 62(4):295-301, 2018

Molecular Techniques

Metastatic Nasopharyngeal Carcinoma, EBER(+) by Chromogen in Situ Hybridization

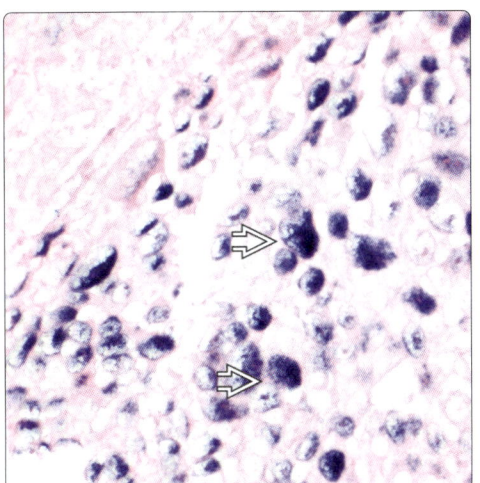

Metastatic Squamous Carcinoma, HPV(+) by Chromogen in Situ Hybridization

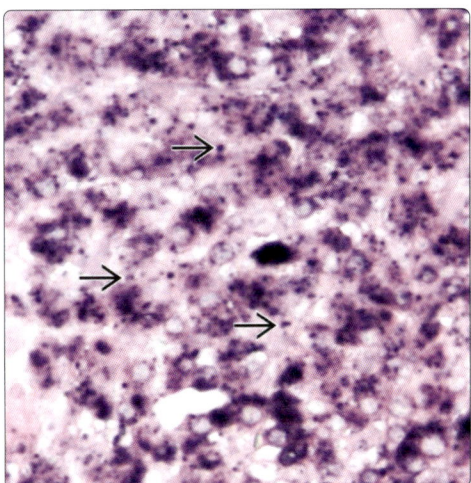

(Left) Chromogen in situ hybridization (CISH) of a cell block of a neck lymph node with metastatic nasopharyngeal carcinoma shows positive signals ➡ for EBER. *(Right)* CISH of a cell block section of a neck lymph node with metastatic squamous carcinoma shows positive signals ➡ for high-risk HPV.

Ewing Sarcoma, t(11;22)(q24;q12)

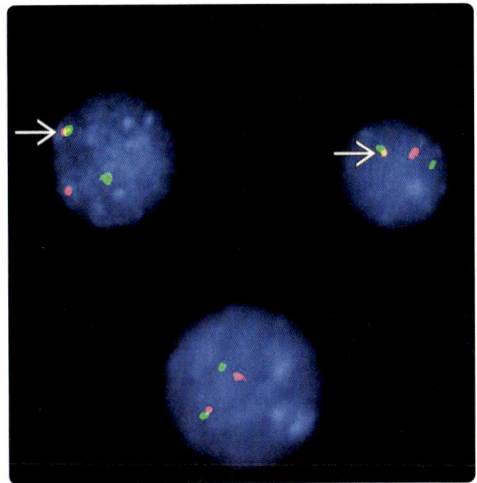

Invasive Ductal Carcinoma in Breast, *HER2* Gene Amplification by FISH

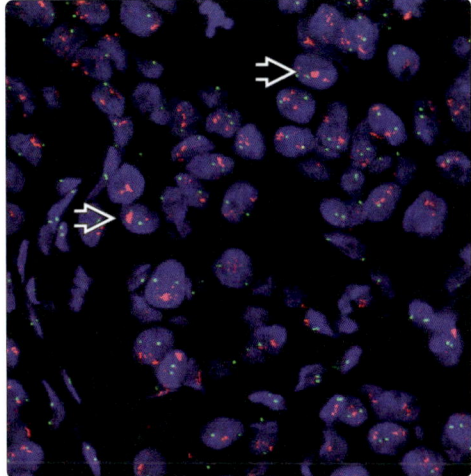

(Left) Fluorescence in situ hybridization (FISH) of an FNA smear of a case of Ewing sarcoma using the LSI-EWSR1 (22q12) dual-color probe shows yellow fusion signals ➡, indicating t(11;22)(q24;q12) chromosomal translocation. *(Right)* FISH using core biopsy of invasive breast carcinoma with the PathVysion HER2/neu probe shows a markedly increased copy numbers of HER2/neu (orange signals ➡) in comparison to signals of centromere 17 (green signals), indicating HER2/neu gene amplification.

UroVysion FISH Positive Result

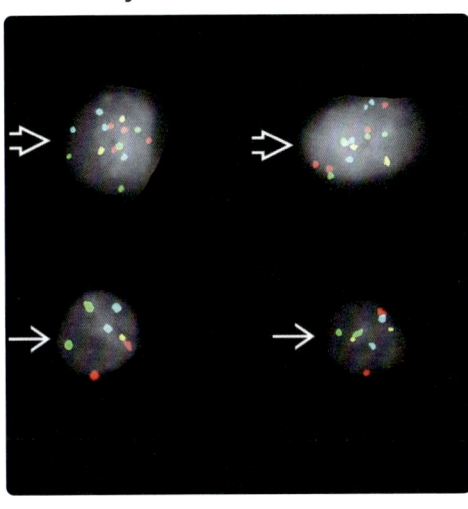

Metastatic Adenocarcinoma, *MET* Amplification

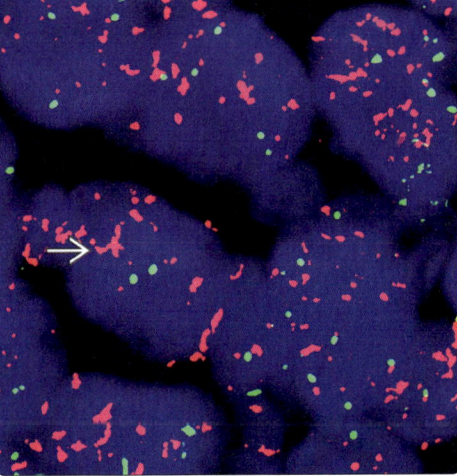

(Left) FISH of urine specimen using UroVysion probe kit (Abbott Laboratories) shows aneusomy ➡ for CEP3 (4 red signals), CEP7 (4 green signals), CEP17 (4 aqua signals), and 2 normal signals for 9p21 (gold signals) in comparison to benign urothelial cells ➡. *(Right)* FISH of a cell block of a metastatic, poorly differentiated carcinoma of the esophagus using Poseidon probes for MET shows markedly increased copy numbers of MET (red signals) ➡, thereby indicating MET amplification.

INDEX

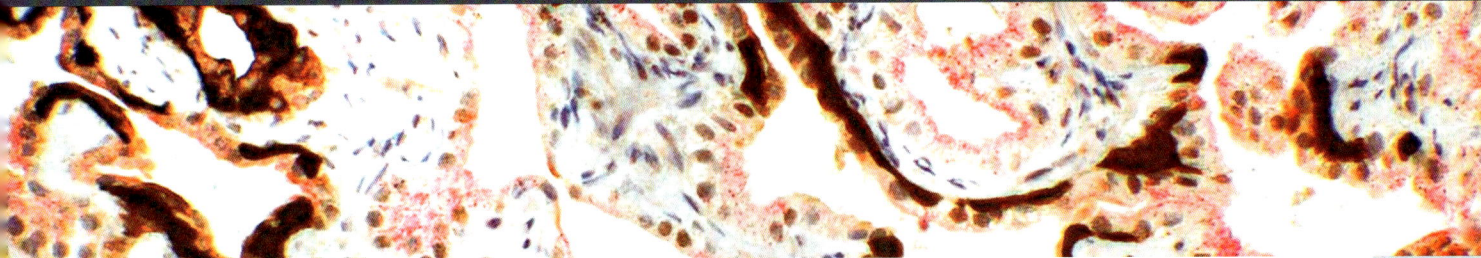

A

Abdominal fat pad aspiration
- amyloid, **665**
- superficial aspiration technique, **257**

Abdominal mass, focal nodular hyperplasia, **505**
Abdominal pain, hepatocellular adenoma, **503**
Abnormal vaginal bleeding, endocervical adenocarcinoma, variants and mimics, **53**

Abscess
- hepatic, **500, 501**
- neuropathology squash preparations, infectious, **696**
- subareolar, **420–421**

Absorptive cells, gastrointestinal cytology, **147**
Acanthamoeba keratitis, **687**
Accessory spleen, lymphoma and secondary tumors of pancreas vs., **597**

Acinar cell carcinoma, **594–595**
- differential diagnosis, **595**
- pancreatic ductal adenocarcinoma vs., **589**
- pancreatic neuroendocrine tumor vs., **587**
- prognosis, **595**
- solid pseudopapillary neoplasm of pancreas vs., **585**

Acinar cells, **571**
Acinar neoplasm, acinar cell carcinoma vs., **594**
Acinic cell carcinoma, **394–395**
- ancillary testing, **380**
- differential diagnosis, **395**
- immunohistochemistry, **395**
- secretory carcinoma vs., **409**

ACR Thyroid Imaging, Reporting and Data System (TIRADS), **261, 262**
Actinomyces species, in Pap tests, **17**
Acute lymphocytic leukemia (ALL), **191**
Acute mastitis, **420**
Acute myelogenous leukemia (AML), **191**
Adamantinoma, **610–611**
- characteristic features of classic and well-differentiated, **611**
- differential diagnosis, **611**
- immunohistochemistry, **611**
- prognosis, **611**

Adamantinoma-like Ewing sarcoma, **625, 626**
- adamantinoma vs., **611**

Adenocarcinoma, **209**
- ampulla/bile duct/pancreatic duct, **166–167**
    differential diagnosis, **167**
- basal cell, adenoid cystic carcinoma vs., **393**
- benign and reactive changes vs., **103**
- benign reactive, malignant effusion, mesothelioma vs., **205**
- breast, other malignancies in urinary cytology vs., **249**
- cribriform, **411**
    differential diagnosis, **411**
- differential stains, **223**
- ductal, pancreatic neuroendocrine tumor vs., **587**
- endometrial
    endocervical adenocarcinoma, variants and mimics vs., **53**
    endometrial cells in Pap test and glandular cells status post hysterectomy vs., **71**
- endometrioid
    endometriosis and endosalpingiosis vs.., **219**
    high-grade, **91**
    low-grade, **91**
- epithelioid hemangioendothelioma vs., **661**
- esophageal, **154–155**
    differential diagnosis, **155**
    genetic testing, **155**
    immunohistochemistry, **155**
- extrathoracic origin, respiratory adenocarcinoma vs., **124**
- extrauterine carcinomas and presentations in cervicovaginal cytopathology vs., **74–75**
- focal nodular hyperplasia vs., **505**
- gastric, **160–161**
    differential diagnosis, **161**
    immunohistochemistry, **161**
- gastritis and intestinal metaplasia vs., **159**
- high-grade, metastatic tumors to adrenal gland vs., **565**
- ICC staining patterns for benign or malignant mesothelial cells vs., **223**
- immunocytochemistry, **725**
- liver metastasis vs., **513**
- metastatic
    adenocarcinoma of urinary bladder vs., **247**
    chordoma vs., **615**
    hepatocellular carcinoma vs., **509**
- metastatic lung carcinomas, **192**
- with neuroendocrine feature, large cell neuroendocrine carcinoma vs., **77**
- noninfectious benign conditions vs., **235**
- normal pancreas cytology vs., **571**
- not otherwise specified, **402–403**
    carcinoma ex pleomorphic adenoma, **401**
    differential diagnosis, **403**
    grading, **403**
- ovarian, other malignancies in urinary cytology vs., **249**
- polymorphous, **404–405**
    adenoid cystic carcinoma vs., **393**
    cribriform adenocarcinoma vs., **411**

INDEX

differential diagnosis, **405**
immunohistochemistry, **405**
low-grade, carcinoma ex pleomorphic adenoma, **401**
prognosis, **405**
- poorly differentiated
esophageal squamous cell carcinoma vs., **157**
neuroendocrine tumor/carcinoma vs., **171**
- renal pelvic cytology, **251**
- of respiratory tract, **122–125**
diagnostic checklist, **124**
differential diagnosis, **124**
primary vs. metastasis, pulmonary metastasis, **143**
prognosis, **123**
- squamous cell carcinoma vs., **127**
of cervix, **40**
- urinary bladder, **246–247**
diagnostic checklist, **246**
differential diagnosis, **247**
- urinary cytology, **231**
Adenocarcinoma in situ. *See also* Endocervical adenocarcinoma in situ, variants and mimics.
- endometrial cells in Pap test and glandular cells status post hysterectomy vs., **71**
- high-grade squamous intraepithelial lesion and mimics vs., **31**
Adenoid basal carcinoma, uncommon malignancies in cervicovaginal cytology, **79**
Adenoid cystic carcinoma, **392–393, 451**
- basaloid neoplasms, benign and malignant vs., **399**
- carcinoma ex pleomorphic adenoma, **401**
- diagnostic checklist, **393**
- differential diagnosis, **393**
- HPV-positive head and neck squamous cell carcinoma vs., **340**
- myoepithelial carcinoma vs., **410**
- myoepithelioma vs., **390**
- pleomorphic adenoma vs., **387**
- polymorphous adenocarcinoma vs., **405**
- salivary gland analog tumors, **137**
- uncommon malignancies in cervicovaginal cytology, **79**
Adenolymphoma. *See* Warthin tumor.
Adenoma
- adenoid cystic, pleomorphic adenoma vs., **387**
- adrenal cortical, **560–561**
differential diagnosis, **561**
- basal cell. *See also* Basal cell adenoma.
adenoid cystic carcinoma vs., **393**
pleomorphic adenoma vs., **387**
- carcinoma ex pleomorphic, **400–401**
genetic testing, **401**
pleomorphic adenoma vs., **387**
- colorectal, **168–169**
differential diagnosis, **169**
- fibroadenoma vs., **436**
- hepatocellular. *See* Hepatocellular adenoma.
- metanephric, **524–525**
differential diagnosis, **525**
immunohistochemistry, **525**
nephroblastoma vs., **547**
- myoepithelial-rich pleomorphic, myoepithelial carcinoma vs., **410**

- pleomorphic. *See* Pleomorphic adenoma.
- rare benign and low malignant potential tumors, **135**
- serous microcystic, **578–579**
differential diagnosis, **579**
Adenomatous hyperplasia
- atypical, adenocarcinoma vs., **124**
- thyroid. *See* Adenomatous nodule, of thyroid gland.
Adenomatous nodule, of thyroid gland, **268–269**
- diagnostic checklist, **269**
- differential diagnosis, **268**
- follicular neoplasm/suspicious for follicular neoplasm vs., **282**
- with Hürthle cell hyperplasia, follicular neoplasm, oncocytic (Hürthle cell) type vs., **285**
- papillary thyroid carcinoma, classic subtype vs., **288**
- prognosis, **269**
Adenomyoepithelioma, fibroadenoma vs., **436**
Adenosarcoma, uncommon malignancies in cervicovaginal cytology, **79**
Adenosis, sclerosing, nonproliferative and proliferative changes in breast, **425**
Adenosquamous carcinoma, **591**
- uncommon malignancies in cervicovaginal cytology, **78–79**
Adenovirus, viral infections, **151**
Adipose tissue tumors, benign, **636–637**
- differential diagnosis, **637**
- immunohistochemistry, **637**
Adnexal cytology. *See* Cutaneous and adnexal cytology.
Adrenal cortical adenoma, **560–561**
- adrenal cortical carcinoma vs., **563**
- differential diagnosis, **561**
Adrenal cortical carcinoma, **562–563**
- conditions associated with, **563**
- differential diagnosis, **563**
- genetic testing, **563**
- metastatic tumors to kidney vs., **553**
- pheochromocytoma vs., **567**
- treatment and prognosis, **563**
- well-differentiated
adrenal cortical adenoma vs., **561**
cytology of normal adrenal gland vs., **559**
Adrenal cortical tumors, clear cell renal cell carcinoma vs., **529**
Adrenal gland, fine-needle aspiration
- adrenal cortical adenoma, **560–561**
adrenal cortical carcinoma vs., **563**
differential diagnosis, **561**
- adrenal cortical carcinoma, **562–563**
conditions associated with, **563**
differential diagnosis, **563**
genetic testing, **563**
pheochromocytoma vs., **567**
treatment and prognosis, **563**
- cytology of normal adrenal gland, **558–559**
accuracy of diagnosis, **558**
clinical indications, **558**
differential diagnosis, **559**
FNA biopsy, **558–559**
specimen collection and preparation, **558–559**

INDEX

- metastatic tumors, **564–565**
  - diagnostic checklist, **564**
  - differential diagnosis, **565**
- pheochromocytoma, **566–567**
  - adrenal cortical carcinoma vs., **563**
  - differential diagnosis, **567**
  - genetic testing, **567**
  - malignancy, **567**
  - prognosis, **567**

Adrenal nodular hyperplasia, adrenal cortical adenoma vs., **561**

Adult orbital neoplasia, **691**

Air-drying, in conventional Pap smears, atypical squamous cells, cannot rule out high-grade squamous intraepithelial lesion vs., **37**

ALK, adenocarcinoma, **124**

ALK(+) anaplastic large cell lymphoma, **368–369**
- differential diagnosis, **369**
- genetic testing, **369**
- immunohistochemistry, **369**

ALK(-) anaplastic large cell lymphoma, ALK(+) anaplastic large cell lymphoma vs., **369**

ALL. *See* Acute lymphocytic leukemia.

Alveolar macrophages
- benign and reactive changes, **103**
- respiratory cytology, **101**

Alveolar proteinosis, *Pneumocystis* pneumonia and mimics vs., **107**

Alveolar rhabdomyosarcoma, **213**
- desmoplastic small round cell tumor vs., **679**

Alveolar soft part sarcoma, **674–677**
- adult-type rhabdomyoma vs., **655**
- differential diagnosis, **675**
- genetic testing, **675**
- granular cell tumor of breast vs., **439**
- prognosis, **675**

American Society for Colposcopy and Cervical Pathology Guidelines, **11**

American Thyroid Association Guidelines Task force, **262**

Amiodarone toxicity, pulmonary alveolar proteinosis and mimics vs., **119**

AML. *See* Acute myelogenous leukemia.

Ampulla/bile duct/pancreatic duct adenocarcinoma, **166–167**
- differential diagnosis, **167**

Ampulla/bile duct/pancreatic duct reactive changes, **164–165**
- differential diagnosis, **165**

Amyloid
- abdominal fat pad aspiration, **665**
- pulmonary alveolar proteinosis and mimics vs., **119**

Amyloidosis, **683**
- rare primary thyroid lesions/neoplasms, **311**

Anal cytology, **96–97**
- diagnostic checklist, **97**
- differential diagnosis, **97**

Anal dysplasia, anal cytology, **97**

Anaplastic carcinoma
- metastatic, unusual variants of ductal carcinoma vs., **592**
- metastatic carcinoma to thyroid vs., **308**
- of thyroid, metastatic tumors of mediastinum vs., **495**

Anaplastic giant cell carcinoma, **591**

Anaplastic large cell lymphoma
- ALK(+), **368–369**
  - differential diagnosis, **369**
  - genetic testing, **369**
  - immunohistochemistry, **369**
- classic Hodgkin lymphoma vs., **375**
- mycosis fungoides vs., **365**

Anaplastic lymphoma, undifferentiated pleomorphic sarcoma vs., **651**

Anaplastic thyroid carcinoma, **304–305**
- differential diagnoses, **304**
- genetic testing, **305**
- immunohistochemistry, **305**
- poorly differentiated thyroid carcinoma vs., **303**
- prognosis, **305**

Anatomic compartments, mediastinum, **482–483**

Ancillary testing
- immunocytochemistry, **724–727**
- molecular techniques, **728–733**
- UroVysion, and others, **252–253**
  - BTA test, **253**
  - genetic tests, **253**
  - ImmunoCyt/uCyt+, **252–253**
  - nongenetic targets, **253**
  - nuclear matrix protein 22, **253**
  - sensitivity improvement considerations, **253**

Ancylostoma, parasitic infections vs., **149**

Anechoic, definition, **260**

Aneurysmal bone cyst
- giant cell tumor vs., **607**
- osteoblastoma vs., **609**
- osteosarcoma vs., **617**

Angioimmunoblastic lymphoma, **366–367**
- differential diagnosis, **367**
- genetic testing, **367**
- immunohistochemistry, **367**

Angiolipoma, angiosarcoma and other sarcomas of breast vs., **462**

Angiomyolipoma, **520–521**
- differential diagnosis, **521**
- genetic and clinical features, **521**
- immunohistochemistry, **521**
- of kidney, primary renal sarcomas vs., **544**
- prognosis, **521**

Angiomyxoma, intramuscular myxoma vs., **669**

Angiosarcoma, **213, 662–663**
- of breast, **460–463**
  - differential diagnosis, **462**
  - genetic testing, **461**
  - prognosis, **461**
- cutaneous
  - fine-needle aspiration, **472**
  - infiltrating salivary gland, adenocarcinoma, not otherwise specified vs., **403**
- differential diagnosis, **663**
- epithelioid, epithelioid hemangioendothelioma vs., **661**
- genetic testing, **663**
- hemangioma of liver vs., **507**

INDEX

- primary and metastatic nonepithelial tumors, **415**
- prognosis, **663**
- soft tissue hemangioma vs., **659**
- urinary cytology, **231**

Aniridia, nephroblastoma, **547**
Anterior chamber sample, **682**
Antipsychotic medications, rare primary thyroid lesions/neoplasms, **311**
Antithyroid medications, rare primary thyroid lesions/neoplasms, **311**
Anucleated squames/squamous cells from skin, normal cerebrospinal fluid and contamination by normal elements, differential diagnosis, **177**
Anulus fibrosus, normal cerebrospinal fluid and contamination by normal elements, differential diagnosis, **177**
Apocrine carcinoma, invasive, **451**
Apocrine metaplasia, ductal carcinoma and variants of invasive mammary carcinoma vs., **452**
Aqueous humor, **687**
Aqueous humor, triaging of, **683**
Architectural atypia, atypia of undetermined significance/follicular lesion of undetermined significance, **277**
Arias-Stella reaction
- atypical glandular cells vs., **66**
- benign mimics, gynecologic, **21**
- endocervical adenocarcinoma, variants and mimics vs., **53**
- endocervical adenocarcinoma in situ vs., **47–48**
- endometrial cancers vs., **60**

Asbestos bodies, pseudoasbestos bodies vs., miscellaneous findings including contaminants, **121**
ASC-US/LSIL Triage Study (ALTS), HPV molecular testing, **6**
Ascaris, pancreatitis, **575**
ASCCP management guidelines based on immediate and 5-year risk of CIN3+, HPV and other molecular testing in gynecologic cytology, **87**
Aseptic and Mollaret meningitis, **182–183**
- differential diagnosis, **182**

Aseptic recurrent meningitis, caused by spinal dermoid/epidermoid cyst with rupture, aseptic and Mollaret meningitis vs., **182**
Askin tumor. *See* Ewing sarcoma.
Aspergillus
- neuropathology squash preparations, infectious, **697**
- species and mimics, respiratory cytology, **109**

Aspiration biopsies
- approach to interpretation of salivary gland, **378–381**
- deep, techniques and modalities of, **476–479**
    biopsy techniques, **477**
    coaxial-needle technique, **477**
    core biopsy technique, **477**
    fine-needle technique, **477**
    postprocedure, **477**
    preprocedure, **476–477**
    procedure, **477**
    single-needle technique, **477**

Aspiration cytology, **690**

Aspiration pneumonia, miscellaneous findings including contaminants, **121**
Asteroid bodies, salivary gland aspirates, **379**
Asteroid hyalosis, **683**
Astrocytic neoplasms, oligodendroglial vs., **701**
Astrocytoma, grade 4, **701**
Atlas of Exfoliative Cytology, **5**
Atrophic endometrium, **91**
Atrophic vaginitis, benign finding, **19**
Atrophy
- with atypia, squamous cell carcinoma of cervix vs., **40**
- atypical squamous cells of undetermined significance vs., **35**
- benign finding, gynecologic, **19**
- high-grade squamous intraepithelial lesion and mimics vs., **31**

Atrophy/atrophic vaginitis, IUD cells and atypia in, atypical squamous cells, cannot rule out high-grade squamous intraepithelial lesion vs., **37**
Atrophy/bare nuclei
- endometrial cancers vs., **60**
- high-grade squamous intraepithelial lesion and mimics vs., **31**

Atypia
- cytologic
    adenocarcinoma, not otherwise specified, **403**
    reactive, viral infections vs., **151**
- not otherwise specified, atypia of undetermined significance/follicular lesion of undetermined significance, **277**
- reactive
    ampulla/bile duct/pancreatic duct adenocarcinoma vs., **167**
    gastric adenocarcinoma vs., **161**

Atypia of undetermined significance/follicular lesion of undetermined significance (AUS/FLUS), **276–279**
- different scenarios and criteria for diagnosis, **277**
- indeterminate thyroid nodules, **278**
- salivary gland aspiration biopsies and reporting terminology, **379, 380**

Atypical adenomatous hyperplasia (AAH), **123**
- adenocarcinoma vs., **124**

Atypical carcinoid, small cell carcinoma vs., **129**
Atypical cells, with extensive necrosis, mediastinal cysts and inflammatory lesions vs., **485**
Atypical cyst lining cells, atypia of undetermined significance/follicular lesion of undetermined significance, **277**
Atypical ductal hyperplasia, proliferative breast changes, **424**
Atypical endocervical cells, **65**
- favor neoplastic, **65**

Atypical endometrial cells, **65**
Atypical glandular cells (AGCs)
- endocervical adenocarcinoma, variants and mimics, **53**
- endocervicals, endometrials, and glandulars, NOS, **64–69**
    differential diagnosis, **66**
    relative distribution of malignancies in Paps reported as AGCs, **66**

INDEX

   reporting rates for AGCs, College of American Pathologists Benchmarking Data, **66**
- high-grade squamous intraepithelial lesion and mimics vs., **31**

Atypical lipomatous tumor
- benign adipose tissue tumors vs., **637**
- liposarcoma vs., **639**

Atypical lymphoid infiltrate, atypia of undetermined significance/follicular lesion of undetermined significance, **277**

Atypical (immature) metaplastic cells, atypical squamous cells, cannot rule out high-grade squamous intraepithelial lesion vs., **37**

Atypical mycobacterial lymphadenitis, granulomatous lymphadenitis, infectious and sarcoid vs., **332**

Atypical papillary neoplasms, **442**

Atypical repair
- atypical glandular cells vs., **66**
- endometrial cancers vs., **60**
- squamous cell carcinoma of cervix vs., **40**

Atypical squamous cells
- cannot rule out high-grade squamous intraepithelial lesion, **36–37**
    differential diagnosis, **37**
    prognosis, **37**
- endometrial cells in Pap test and glandular cells status post hysterectomy vs., **71**
- of undetermined significance, **34–35**
    differential diagnosis, **35**

Atypical teratoid/rhabdoid tumor (AT/RT), **189**

Atypical thymoma (WHO type B3), thymic carcinoma vs., **489**

Atypical urothelial cells, **241**
- high-grade urothelial dysplasia/carcinoma/carcinoma in situ vs., **243**

Autoimmune diseases
- granulomatous lymphadenitis, infectious and sarcoid, **331**

Autoimmune diseases, pleural, peritoneal, pericardial, and pelvic fluid, and washings
- diagnostic checklist, **203**
- differential diagnosis, **203**
- prognosis, **203**

Autoimmune pancreatitis, **575**
- lymphoma and secondary tumors of pancreas vs., **597**

Automated cell block, nongynecologic cytology, **713**
Automated coverslippers, nongynecologic cytology, **713**
Automated screening in gynecologic cytology, **8–9**
Automated stainers, nongynecologic cytology, **713**

B

B-cell lymphoma
- diffuse large, pulmonary lymphoma, **141**
- extranodal marginal zone, primary and metastatic nonepithelial tumors, **415**
- histocyte-rich large, nodular lymphocyte-predominant Hodgkin lymphoma vs., **371**
- large. *See* Large B-cell lymphoma.
- peripheral T-cell lymphoma vs., **363**
- primary mediastinal large, classic Hodgkin lymphoma vs., **375**

B-lymphoblastic leukemia/lymphoma, T-cell lymphoblastic lymphoma vs., **371**

Bacille Calmette-Guérin (BCG) therapy, **234**
Bacteria, in Pap tests, **17**
Bacterial infections
- mycobacteria, **114–115**
- neuropathology squash preparations, infectious, **696**
- ophthalmic cytopathology, **687**

Bacterial meningitis, **181**
- aseptic and Mollaret meningitis vs., **182**

Bacterial vaginosis, molecular testing in gynecologic cytology, **86**

BALT lymphoma. *See* Bronchus-associated lymphoma.

Bare nuclei of atrophy
- deep, atypical glandular cells vs., **66**
- high-grade squamous intraepithelial lesion and mimics vs., **31**

Barrett esophagus, **152–153**
- differential diagnosis, **153**
- with dysplasia, esophagitis and Barrett esophagus vs., **153**
- with high-grade dysplasia, esophageal adenocarcinoma vs., **155**

Bartonella henselae infection, granulomatous lymphadenitis, infectious and sarcoid vs., **332**

Basal cell adenocarcinoma. *See also* Basaloid neoplasms, benign and malignant, salivary gland.
- adenoid cystic carcinoma vs., **393**

Basal cell adenoma. *See also* Basaloid neoplasms, benign and malignant, salivary gland.
- adenoid cystic carcinoma vs., **393**
- ancillary testing, **380**
- pleomorphic adenoma vs., **387**

Basal cell carcinoma, fine-needle aspiration, **471**
Basal urothelial cells, urinary cytology, **229**
Basaloid carcinoma, immunocytochemistry, **725**
Basaloid cell pattern, salivary gland aspirates, **378**
Basaloid lesions, salivary gland, basaloid neoplasms, benign and malignant vs., **399**

Basaloid neoplasms, benign and malignant, salivary gland, **398–399**
- differential diagnosis, **399**
- prognosis, **399**

Basaloid squamous cell carcinoma
- adenoid cystic carcinoma vs., **393**
- HPV-positive head and neck squamous cell carcinoma vs., **340**
- variant of squamous cell carcinoma of cervix, **40**

Basic fine-needle aspiration technique, **257**
Bcl-2, follicular lymphoma, **350**

Beckwith-Wiedemann syndrome
- adrenal cortical carcinoma, **563**
- hepatoblastoma, **511**
- nephroblastoma, **547**

Behçet disease
- neurodegenerative disease vs., **187**

INDEX

- squamous cell carcinoma of cervix vs., **40**

Benign adipose tissue tumors, **636–637**
- differential diagnosis, **637**
- immunohistochemistry, **637**

Benign and infectious conditions, gynecologic cytopathology
- infectious and other organisms in Pap tests, **16–17**
    - bacteria, **17**
    - *Chlamydia trachomatis*, **17**
    - cytopathology, **16–17**
    - fungi, **16–17**
    - protozoa, **16**
    - viruses, **17**
- nonneoplastic findings, mimics, and artifacts, **18–25**
- normal Pap test, **14–15**
    - cell types, **14**
    - cytopathology, **14–15**
    - endocervical cells, **15**
    - endometrial cells, **15**
    - physiology/histology of cervix, **14**
    - squamous cells, **14–15**
    - squamous metaplastic cells, **15**

Benign artifacts, gynecologic, **21**
- cockleburs, **21**
- cornflaking, **21**
- fibers and threads, **21**
- lubricant jelly, **21**
- pollen, **21**
- starch granules, **21**

Benign cells, normal, benign and reactive changes, **103**

Benign changes, **102–105**
- diagnostic checklist, **103**
- differential diagnosis, **103**

Benign effusions, normal cellular components, **196**

Benign entities, smooth muscle tumors vs., **653**

Benign fibrous histiocytoma, giant cell tumor vs., **607**

Benign follicular nodule (Bethesda terminology). *See* Adenomatous nodule, of thyroid gland.

Benign hepatic lesions, hepatocellular carcinoma vs., **509**

Benign intracranial/intraspinal cells
- differential diagnosis, **177**
- immunochemistry, **177**

Benign lesions, granular cell tumor of breast vs., **439**

Benign lymphocytic effusion, lymphoid effusion and lymphomas vs., **215**

Benign lymphoid-rich effusions, **215**

Benign mimics, gynecologic, **18–21**
- Arias-Stella reaction, **21**
- contaminant fungal organisms, **21**
- deciduosis, **20**
- endocervical glandular hyperplasia, diffuse and lobular, **20**
- follicular cervicitis, **20**
- glycogenation, **21**
- histiocytes, **21**
- IUD-related changes, **20**
- microglandular hyperplasia, **19–20**
- multinucleated giant cells/histiocytes, **21**
- neuroendocrine carcinoma of cervix vs., **77**
- pemphigus, **21**
- rectovaginal fistula, **21**
- transitional cell metaplasia, **19**
- tubal metaplasia/tuboendometrioid metaplasia, **19**

Benign neoplasms
- inflammatory and infectious conditions of liver vs., **501**
- medullary thyroid carcinoma vs., **300**
- salivary gland aspiration biopsies and reporting terminology, **379, 380**

Benign nerve sheath tumors, smooth muscle tumors vs., **653**

Benign nonneoplastic findings, gynecologic, **18–21**
- atrophy and atrophic vaginitis, **19**
- endocervical cell inflammatory changes, **18–19**
- hyperkeratosis, **19**
- parakeratosis, **19**
- radiation changes, **19**
- repair, **19**
- squamous cell inflammatory changes, **18**

Benign papillary neoplasms, **441**

Benign peripheral nerve sheath tumors, mediastinal cysts and inflammatory lesions vs., **485**

Benign reactive effusion, carcinoma vs., **210**

Benign reactive mesothelial hyperplasia, malignant effusion, mesothelioma vs., **205**

Benign renal tubular cells, clear cell renal cell carcinoma vs., **529**

Benign respiratory epithelium, columnar cell subtype vs., papillary thyroid carcinoma subtypes, **291**

Benign spindle cell neoplasms, solitary fibrous tumor vs., **667**

Bethesda Reporting System, **6**
- Bethesda Reporting System for Cervicovaginal Cytology (2001 and 2015 Version), **6**
- National Cancer Institute Conference (1988), **6**

The Bethesda System for Reporting Thyroid Cytology (TBSRTC), **266–267**
- benign, **267**
- follicular neoplasm, **267**
- malignant/positive for malignancy, **267**
- nondiagnostic, **266–267**
- suspicious for malignancy (SM), **267**

Bile ducts
- ampulla/pancreatic duct reactive changes, **164–165**
- carcinoma, ampulla/bile duct/pancreatic duct reactive changes vs., **165**
- dysplasia, ampulla/bile duct/pancreatic duct reactive changes vs., **165**
- gastrointestinal cytology, **147**
- intraepithelial neoplasia, ampulla/bile duct/pancreatic duct adenocarcinoma vs., **167**

Biological safety cabinet, nongynecologic cytology, **713**

Biphasic synovial sarcoma, **671**

Bland hypermucinous epithelium, atypical glandular cells vs., **66**

Blastemal-predominant Wilms tumor, clear cell sarcoma of kidney vs., **549**

Blastoma
- pleuropulmonary, rare malignant tumors, **137**
- pulmonary, rare malignant tumors, **137**

Blastomyces dermatitidis, neuropathology squash preparations, infectious, **697**

INDEX

Bleeding, vaginal, endocervical adenocarcinoma in situ, **47**
Blood clots, cell block techniques, **712**
Bloody specimens, nongynecologic cytology, **713**
Bone, fine-needle aspiration
- adamantinoma, **610–611**
- approach to cytologic/small biopsy diagnosis of primary bone tumors, **600–601**
    - adequacy/rapid onsite evaluation and triage during biopsy, **600–601**
    - age range, **600**
    - initial evaluation, **601**
- bone lymphoma, **628–629**
- chondroblastoma, **604–605**
- chondromas of bone and soft tissue, **602–603**
- chondrosarcoma, **620–623**
- chordoma, **614–615**
- Ewing sarcoma, **624–627**
- giant cell tumor, **606–607**
- Langerhans cell histiocytosis, **612–613**
- metastatic tumors of bone, **630–631**
- osteoblastoma, **608–609**
- osteosarcoma, **616–619**

Bone cyst, aneurysmal
- giant cell tumor vs., **607**
- osteoblastoma vs., **609**
- osteosarcoma vs., **617**

Bone lymphoma, **628–629**
- diagnostic checklist, **629**
- differential diagnosis, **629**
- immunohistochemistry, **629**

Bone marrow cells, normal cerebrospinal fluid and contamination by normal elements, differential diagnosis, **177**

Borderline serous neoplasms, endometriosis and endosalpingiosis vs., **219**

Brain tumors, primary, **188–189**
- diagnostic checklist, **189**
- differential diagnosis, **189**

Branchial cleft cyst, **385**
- HPV-positive head and neck squamous cell carcinoma vs., **340**

Breast, fine-needle aspiration
- angiosarcoma, **460–463**
    - differential diagnosis, **462**
    - genetic testing, **462**
    - prognosis, **461**
- cytology specimens for risk assessment of breast cancer, **466–467**
    - ductal lavage, **467**
    - nipple aspiration fluid, **466–467**
    - random periareolar fine-needle aspiration, **467**
    - terminology, **466**
- ductal carcinoma and variants of invasive mammary carcinoma, **448–455**
    - differential diagnosis, **451–452**
    - invasive ductal carcinoma histologic types, **448**
    - prognosis, **449**
- fat necrosis, **422–423**
    - differential diagnosis, **423**
    - prognosis, **423**
- fibroadenoma, **434–437**
    - differential diagnosis, **436**
- granular cell tumor of breast, **438–439**
    - differential diagnosis, **439**
- gynecomastia, **430–431**
    - differential diagnosis, **431**
    - prognosis, **431**
- inflammatory and granulomatous conditions, **420–421**
    - acute mastitis, **420**
    - differential diagnosis, **421**
    - duct ectasia, **421**
    - granulomatous mastitis, **421**
    - lymphocytic mastitis, **421**
    - subareolar abscess, **420–421**
- lobular carcinoma, **456–457**
    - differential diagnosis, **457**
- lymphomas and metastatic tumors of breast, **464–465**
    - differential diagnosis, **465**
- mucocele-like lesion, **432–433**
    - differential diagnosis, **432–433**
- myofibroblastoma, **446–447**
    - differential diagnosis, **447**
    - prognosis, **447**
- nonproliferative and proliferative changes, **424–427**
    - differential diagnosis, **425**
    - prognosis, **424–425**
- papillary neoplasm, **440–445**
    - atypical, **442**
    - differential diagnosis, **442**
    - malignant, **441**
    - prognosis, **441**
- phyllodes tumor, **458–459**
    - differential diagnosis, **459**
    - prognosis, **459**
- radial scar/complex sclerosing lesion, **428–429**
    - differential diagnosis, **429**
    - prognosis, **429**
- role of, techniques and triple test, **418–419**
    - advantages, **418**
    - complications, **418**
    - current applications, **419**
    - disadvantages, **418**
    - International Academy of Cytology Yokohama System, **418**
    - interpretation, **419**
    - reporting criteria, **418–419**

Breast adenocarcinoma, other malignancies in urinary cytology vs., **249**

Breast cancer, cytology specimens for risk assessment of, **466–467**
- ductal lavage, **467**
- nipple aspiration fluid, **466–467**
- random periareolar fine-needle aspiration, **467**
- terminology, **466**

Breast carcinoma
- ductal type, **209**
- metaplastic, **450–451**
    - angiosarcoma and other sarcomas of breast vs., **462**
    - phyllodes tumor vs., **459**
- metastatic, **193**
    - prognostic and predictive markers, **725**

INDEX

with signet-ring cells, unusual variants of ductal carcinoma vs., **592**
- recurrent, prognostic and predictive markers, **725**

Breast tumors
- immunocytochemistry, **725**
- metastatic
    ductal carcinoma and variants of invasive mammary carcinoma vs., **451–452**
    granular cell tumor of breast vs., **439**
- metastatic tumors to kidney vs., **553**
- primary, metastatic tumors vs., **465**

British Thyroid Association/Royal College of Pathologists (BTA/RCP) Reporting Terminology, **267**
Bronchial brushing, respiratory cytology, **100**
Bronchial cells, benign and reactive changes, **103**
Bronchial mucosa, respiratory cytology, **101**
Bronchial washing, respiratory cytology, **100**
Bronchoalveolar lavage, respiratory cytology, **100**
Bronchus-associated lymphoma, **141**
Brooke-Spiegler syndrome, **399**
Brown tumor, giant cell tumor vs., **607**
Brucella abortus infection, granulomatous lymphadenitis, infectious and sarcoid vs., **332**
Brucella melitensis infection, granulomatous lymphadenitis, infectious and sarcoid vs., **332**
Brucella suis infection, granulomatous lymphadenitis, infectious and sarcoid vs., **332**
BTA test, urinary cytology, **253**
Burkitt-like lymphoma, with 11q aberrations, Burkitt lymphoma vs., **353**
Burkitt lymphoma, **190, 215, 352–353**
- differential diagnosis, **353**
- genetic testing, **353**
- immunohistochemistry, **353**
- large B-cell lymphoma vs., **355**
- primary effusion lymphoma vs., **217**
- T-cell lymphoblastic lymphoma vs., **371**

Butterfly technique, superficial aspiration technique, **257**

C

Calcifications, pigmented thyroid lesions and crystals, **275**
Calcium crystals, salivary gland aspirates, **379**
Calcium oxalate, salivary gland aspirates, **379**
Callus, fracture, chondrosarcoma vs., **622**
Cancer screening, respiratory cytology and adequacy criteria, **100**
Candida effect, atypical squamous cells of undetermined significance vs., **35**
Candida species
- infectious benign conditions, **237**
- molecular testing in gynecologic cytology, **86**
- respiratory cytology, **109**

Candidal esophagitis, **153**
Carcinoid, small cell carcinoma vs., **129**
Carcinoid and atypical carcinoid tumors of respiratory tract, **132–133**
- diagnostic checklist, **133**
- differential diagnosis, **133**
- large cell neuroendocrine carcinoma vs., **131**

Carcinoid tumor, **543**
- differential diagnoses, **543**
- metastatic
    carcinoid tumor vs., **543**
    lobular carcinoma vs., **457**
- metastatic tumors of mediastinum vs., **495**
- neurogenic tumors vs., **493**
- spindle cell, neurogenic tumors vs., **493**
- thymic, mediastinal thymoma vs., **487**

Carcinoma
- benign reactive effusion vs., **210**
- bile ducts, ampulla/bile duct/pancreatic duct reactive changes vs., **165**
- embryonal, metastatic tumors of mediastinum vs., **495**
- epithelioid sarcoma vs., **673**
- germ cell tumors vs., **210**
- inflammatory and granulomatous conditions vs., **421**
- malignant mesothelioma vs., **210**
- melanoma vs., **210**
- with mixed differentiation, **592**
- non-Hodgkin lymphoma vs., **210**
- nonproliferative and proliferative changes in breast vs., **425**
- pancreatic ducts, ampulla/bile duct/pancreatic duct reactive changes vs., **165**
- showing thymus-like differentiation, of thyroid gland, **310**
- small round cell sarcomas vs., **210**
- of unknown primary, molecular techniques, **730**

Carcinoma ex pleomorphic adenoma, **400–401**
- genetic testing, **401**
- pleomorphic adenoma vs., **387**

Carcinoma in situ, adenocarcinoma vs., **124**
Carcinosarcoma, **591**
- ductal carcinoma and variants of invasive mammary carcinoma, **451**

Carney complex, adrenal cortical carcinoma, **563**
Castleman disease
- multicentric, HHV(+), plasmablastic lymphoma vs., **361**
- plasma cell variant, plasmacytoma vs., **357**

Cavernous hemangioma. *See* Hemangioma, liver.
CDH11 loss of expression, lobular carcinoma of breast associated with, **457**
CDKN2A gene, mutations in, pancreatic ductal adenocarcinoma, **589**
Cell block techniques, **712**
- blood clots, **712**
- Cellient, **712**
- collodion bag, **712**
- formalin, **712**
- HistoGel (propriety gel), **712**
- nano cell block, **712**
- thrombin, **712**

Cell button assessment slide, nongynecologic cytology, **713**
Cellient, cell block techniques, **712**
Cells, anal cytology, **97**

INDEX

Cellular mesoblastic nephroma, rhabdoid tumor of kidney vs., **552**
Cellular pleomorphic adenoma, basaloid neoplasms, benign and malignant vs., **399**
Cellular stroma, fibroadenoma with, phyllodes tumor vs., **459**
Centrifuges, nongynecologic cytology, **713**
Centroblast, lymph node aspiration, **324–325**
Centrocyte, lymph node aspiration, **324**
Cerebritis, neuropathology squash preparations, infectious, **696**
Cerebrospinal fluid, exfoliative cytopathology
  - infectious meningitis, **180–181**
  - leukemia and lymphoma, **190–191**
  - metastasis in CSF, **192–193**
  - neurodegenerative disease, **186–187**
  - normal cerebrospinal fluid and contamination by normal elements, **176–179**
      differential diagnosis, **177**
      reporting criteria, **176–177**
  - primary brain tumors, **188–189**
  - septic and Mollaret meningitis, **182–183**
  - subarachnoid hemorrhage, **184–185**
Cerebrospinal fluid pleocytosis, infectious meningitis, **180**
Cervical abnormality, endocervical adenocarcinoma, variants and mimics, **53**
Cervical adenocarcinoma. *See* Endocervical adenocarcinoma, variants and mimics.
Cervical cancer screening, **4–7**
Cervical intraepithelial neoplasia grades 2 (CIN2). *See* High-grade squamous intraepithelial lesion.
Cervical intraepithelial neoplasia grades 3 (CIN3). *See* High-grade squamous intraepithelial lesion.
Cervical Intraepithelial Neoplasia Reporting System, **5**
Cervical mass, endocervical adenocarcinoma, variants and mimics, **53**
Cervical neuroendocrine tumors and their mimics, neuroendocrine carcinoma of cervix, **77**
Cervical squamous cell carcinoma, other malignancies in urinary cytology vs., **249**
Cervicitis, follicular, high-grade squamous intraepithelial lesion and mimics vs., **31**
Cervicovaginal cytology
  - extrauterine carcinomas and presentations in, **74–75**
      differential diagnosis, **74**
      extrauterine malignancies in cervicovaginal cytology, **75**
  - uncommon malignancies, **78–81**
      adenoid basal carcinoma, **79**
      adenoid cystic carcinoma, **79**
      adenosarcoma, **79**
      adenosquamous carcinoma, **78–79**
      epithelioid trophoblastic tumor, **79**
      Ewing sarcoma, **79**
      lymphoma, **78**
      melanoma, **78**
      primitive neuroectodermal tumor, **79**
      sarcomas, **79**
      small round blue cell tumors, **79**

Cervix, neuroendocrine carcinoma, **76–77**
  - differential diagnosis, **77**
  - prognosis, **77**
Charcot-Leyden crystals, **121**
Chemotherapy effect
  - high-grade urothelial dysplasia/carcinoma/carcinoma in situ vs., **243**
  - reactive urothelial changes, **239**
Chemotherapy-related esophagitis, **153**
Chief cells, gastrointestinal cytology, **147**
Chlamydia infection, granulomatous lymphadenitis, infectious and sarcoid vs., **332**
Chlamydia trachomatis
  - molecular testing in gynecologic cytology, **86**
  - in Pap tests, **17**
Chloroma, lymphomas vs., **465**
Cholangiocarcinoma
  - ampulla/bile duct/pancreatic duct adenocarcinoma, **167**
  - hepatocellular carcinoma vs., **509**
  - immunocytochemistry, **725**
Cholesterol crystals, salivary gland aspirates, **379**
Chondroblastic osteosarcoma, **616**
  - chondrosarcoma vs., **622**
Chondroblastoma, **604–605**
  - differential diagnosis, **605**
  - giant cell tumor vs., **607**
  - immunohistochemistry, **605**
  - Langerhans cell histiocytosis vs., **613**
Chondroblastoma-like osteosarcoma, chondroblastoma vs., **605**
Chondroid chordoma, **615**
Chondrolipoma, **637**
Chondromas of bone and soft tissue, **602–603**
  - differential diagnosis, **603**
  - prognosis, **603**
Chondromyxoid fibroma, chondrosarcoma vs., **622**
Chondrosarcoma, **620–623**
  - clear cell, **621**
  - dedifferentiated, **621**
      osteosarcoma vs., **617**
  - genetic testing, **622**
  - juxtacortical, **621**
  - low-grade, chondromas of bone and soft tissue vs., **603**
  - mesenchymal, **621**
      Ewing sarcoma vs., **626**
  - myxoid
      chordoma vs., **615**
      intramuscular myxoma vs., **669**
  - nonglial neoplasms vs., **705**
  - osteosarcoma vs., **617**
  - periosteal, **621**
  - primary, **621**
  - prognosis, **621**
  - secondary, **621**
Chordoma, **614–615, 704, 705**
  - chondroid, **615**
  - chondromas of bone and soft tissue vs., **603**
  - chondrosarcoma vs., **622**
  - differential diagnosis, **615**
  - immunohistochemistry, **615**
  - nonglial neoplasms vs., **705**

INDEX

- prognosis, **615**

Choriocarcinoma
- germ cell tumors, **491**
- unusual variants of ductal carcinoma vs., **592**

Choroid plexus cells
- ependymal cells vs., **177**
- normal cerebrospinal fluid and contamination by normal elements, differential diagnosis, **177**

Choroidal lymphomas, **691**

Chromophobe renal cell carcinoma, **536–537**
- carcinoid tumor vs., **543**
- clear cell renal cell carcinoma vs., **529**
- differential diagnosis, **537**
- immunohistochemistry, **537**
- kidney oncocytoma vs., **523**
- normal kidney cytology vs., **517**
- prognosis, **537**

Chromosome 9 deletions, urothelial carcinoma, **555**

Chromosome 9p13 loss, papillary renal cell carcinoma, **533**

Chromosome Y loss
- oncocytoma, **523**
- papillary renal cell carcinoma, **533**

Chronic acquired polyneuropathies, neurodegenerative disease vs., **187**

Chronic granulomatous inflammation, Rosai-Dorfman disease vs., **335**

Chronic inflammatory demyelinating polyneuropathy (CIDP), neurodegenerative disease vs., **187**

Chronic lymphocytic/Hashimoto thyroiditis, **270–271**
- differential diagnosis, **271**

Chronic lymphocytic leukemia/small lymphocytic lymphoma (CLL/SLL), **191, 215**
- mantle cell lymphoma vs., **347**
- nodal marginal zone lymphoma vs., **349**
- with plasmacytic differentiation, lymphoplasmacytic lymphoma vs., **345**

Chronic sialadenitis/sialometaplasia, mucoepidermoid carcinoma vs., **397**

CIDP. *See* Chronic inflammatory demyelinating polyneuropathy.

Cigarette smoking, HPV-positive head and neck squamous cell carcinoma, **339**

Cirrhosis
- focal nodular hyperplasia vs., **505**
- hepatocellular carcinoma, **509**

Classic Hodgkin lymphoma, **374–375**
- ALK(+) anaplastic large cell lymphoma vs., **369**
- differential diagnosis, **375**
- immunohistochemistry, **375**
- nodular lymphocyte-predominant Hodgkin lymphoma vs., **371**

Clear cell carcinoma, of primary vs. metastatic origin, pulmonary metastasis, **143**

Clear cell chondrosarcoma, **621**

Clear cell hidradenoma, fine-needle aspiration, **471**

Clear cell neoplasm, salivary gland aspirates, **378**

Clear cell papillary renal cell carcinoma, **534–535**
- differential diagnosis, **535**
- genetic testing, **535**
- immunohistochemistry, **535**
- prognosis, **535**

Clear cell renal cell carcinoma, **528–531**
- angiomyolipoma vs., **521**
- clear cell papillary renal cell carcinoma vs., **535**
- conventional, *TFE3*- and *TFEB*-rearranged renal cell carcinomas vs., **539**
- cytology-histology correlation, **529**
- diagnostic checklist, **528**
- differential diagnosis, **529**
- eosinophilic variant
    chromophobe renal cell carcinoma vs., **537**
    kidney oncocytoma vs., **523**
- with focal papillary growth, papillary renal cell carcinoma vs., **533**
- genetic testing, **529**
- immunohistochemistry, **529**
- low-grade, normal kidney cytology vs., **517**
- metastatic tumors to adrenal gland vs., **565**
- prognosis, **529**
- xanthogranulomatous pyelonephritis/malakoplakia vs., **527**

Clear cell sarcoma of kidney, **548–549**
- congenital mesoblastic nephroma vs., **551**
- differential diagnosis, **549**
- immunohistochemistry, **549**
- molecular genetics, **549**
- nephroblastoma vs., **547**
- prognosis, **549**
- rhabdoid tumor of kidney vs., **552**

Clear cell sarcoma of soft tissue, **676–677**
- differential diagnosis, **677**
- genetic testing, **677**
- prognosis, **677**

Clear cell subtype, papillary thyroid carcinoma subtypes, **292**

Clear cell tumors
- follicular neoplasm/suspicious for follicular neoplasm vs., **282**
- metastatic tumors of mediastinum vs., **495**
- metastatic tumors to adrenal gland vs., **565**
- rare benign and low malignant potential tumors vs., **135**

Clear cells
- salivary gland aspirates, **378**
- in tumors, metastatic tumors to kidney vs., **553**

CMV. *See* Cytomegalovirus.

Coaxial-needle technique, **477**

Coccidian protozoans, parasitic infections vs., **149**

Coccidioides immitis, neuropathology squash preparations, infectious, **697**

Coccobacilli, in Pap tests, **17**

Cockleburs, gynecologic artifact, **21**

Collecting duct carcinoma, **540**
- differential diagnoses, **540**
- metastatic tumors to kidney vs., **553**
- urothelial carcinoma vs., **555**

Collodion bag, cell block techniques, **712**

Colloid carcinoma, **591**

Colloid nodule. *See* Adenomatous nodule, of thyroid gland.

INDEX

Colorectal adenocarcinoma
- metastatic, direct invasion, adenocarcinoma of urinary bladder vs., 247
- other malignancies in urinary cytology vs., 249

Colorectal adenoma/carcinoma, 168–169
- differential diagnosis, 169

Colorectal neuroendocrine tumor/carcinoma, 171
Colorectum, gastrointestinal cytology, 147
Columnar cell subtype, papillary thyroid carcinoma subtypes, 291
- differential diagnosis, 291

Comet-tail artifact, definition, 260
Complex sclerosing lesion, 428–429
- differential diagnosis, 429
- prognosis, 429

Congenital adrenal hyperplasia, adrenal cortical carcinoma, 563
Congenital mesoblastic nephroma, 550–552
- clear cell sarcoma of kidney vs., 549
- differential diagnosis, 551
- genetic features, 551
- metanephric stromal tumor vs., 526

Constituent tumors, mediastinum, 482–483
Core biopsy, respiratory cytology, 100
Core biopsy technique, 477
Corneal scrapes, 687
Cornflaking, gynecologic artifact, 21
Corpora amylacea, 121
- pulmonary alveolar proteinosis and mimics vs., 119
- urinary cytology, 229

COVID-19, infectious conditions, in pleural, peritoneal, pericardial, and pelvic fluid, 200
Coxsackievirus, pancreatitis, 575
Creola bodies, benign and reactive changes, 103
Cribriform adenocarcinoma, 411
- differential diagnosis, 411

Cribriform carcinoma, 450
Cribriform-morular carcinoma, 310
Cryptococcal meningitis, 180, 181
Cryptococcus neoformans infection
- neuropathology squash preparations, infectious, 697
- *Pneumocystis* pneumonia and mimics vs., 107

Cryptosporidium
- pancreatitis, 575
- parasitic infections vs., 149

Crystals, pigmented thyroid lesions and crystals, 275
Curschmann spiral, 121
Cutaneous and adnexal cytology, 470–473
- fine-needle aspiration, 470–472
    cutaneous and adnexal neoplasms, 471–472
    nonneoplastic conditions, 470–471
- Tzanck smears, 470
    herpes, 470
    Molluscum contagiosum, 470

Cutaneous angiosarcoma, infiltrating salivary gland, adenocarcinoma, not otherwise specified vs., 403
Cyclin-D1/*CCND1*, parathyroid cyst, adenoma, and carcinoma, 319
Cyclospora, parasitic infections vs., 149

Cyst contents, atypia of undetermined significance/follicular lesion of undetermined significance, 277
Cystadenoma lymphomatosum, papillary, cysts vs., 385
Cystic carcinoma, adenoid, 392–393, 451
- basaloid neoplasms, benign and malignant vs., 399
- carcinoma ex pleomorphic adenoma, 401
- diagnostic checklist, 393
- differential diagnosis, 393
- HPV-positive head and neck squamous cell carcinoma vs., 340
- myoepithelial carcinoma vs., 410
- myoepithelioma vs., 390
- pleomorphic adenoma vs., 387
- polymorphous adenocarcinoma vs., 405
- prognosis, 393
- salivary gland analog tumors, 136, 137
- uncommon malignancies in cervicovaginal cytology, 79

Cystic lesions, salivary gland aspirates, 378
Cystic nephroma, renal cyst vs., 519
Cystic partially differentiated nephroblastoma, renal cyst vs., 519
Cystic renal cell carcinoma, renal cyst vs., 519
Cystic subtype, papillary thyroid carcinoma, 290–291
Cystic thymoma, mediastinal cysts and inflammatory lesions vs., 485
Cysticercosis, neuropathology squash preparations, infectious, 696, 697
Cystitis glandularis, 234
Cysts, 384–385
- aneurysmal bone
    giant cell tumor vs., 607
    osteoblastoma vs., 609
    osteosarcoma vs., 617
- branchial cleft, 385
- diagnostic checklist, 385
- differential diagnosis, 385
- epidermal inclusion, 385
- hydatid, 500, 501
- lymphoepithelial, 385
- mediastinal, 484–485
- nonproliferative and proliferative changes in breast, 425
- of pancreas, lymphoepithelial, 576
- parathyroid, 318–321
    differential diagnosis, 319
    genetic testing, 319
    immunohistochemistry, 319
- renal, 518–519
    diagnostic checklist, 518
- retention, 385

Cytocentrifuges, nongynecologic cytology, 713
Cytologic atypia
- adenocarcinoma, not otherwise specified, 403
- atypia of undetermined significance/follicular lesion of undetermined significance, 277
- reactive, viral infections vs., 151

INDEX

Cytologic/small biopsy diagnosis
- of primary bone tumors, approach to, **600–601**
    - adequacy/rapid onsite evaluation and triage during biopsy, **600–601**
    - age range, **600**
    - initial evaluation, **601**
- of primary soft tissue lesions, approach to, **634–635**
    - cytologic categorization of primary soft tissue tumors by cell types, **635**
    - general criteria for cytologic grading, **634–635**
    - important clinical findings, **634**
    - mesenchymal lesions: helpful cytologic features, **634**
    - proposed IAC-IARC-WHO reporting system for soft tissue cytopathology/small biopsies, **635**
    - soft tissue sarcomas (non-SRBCT): prognostic factors, **635**

Cytology
- of normal adrenal gland, **558–559**
    - differential diagnosis, **559**
    - FNA biopsy, **558–559**
        - accuracy of diagnosis, **558**
        - clinical indications, **558**
        - specimen collection and preparation, **558–559**
- of normal kidney, **516–517**
    - anatomic features, **516**
    - architectural organization, **516**
    - differential diagnosis, **517**
    - immunohistochemistry, **517**
    - misinterpretations of benign elements, **517**
    - renal FNA, **516–517**
        - accuracy of diagnosis, **516–517**
        - clinical indications, **516**
        - complications & contraindications, **517**
        - specimen collection & preparation, **517**
- of normal liver, **498–499**
    - differential diagnosis, **499**
    - inadvertently sample another organ, **499**
- of normal pancreas, **570–571**
    - anatomic features, **570**
    - architectural organization, **570**
    - clinical utility of pancreas FNA, **570–571**
    - differential diagnosis, **571**
    - pancreatic cytology reporting terminology, **572–573**
        - ancillary and molecular testing in pancreatic cysts/cystic neoplasms, **573**
        - approach to cytologic analysis of pancreatic cysts, **573**
        - role of molecular testing, **573**
        - WHO International System for Reporting Pancreatic Cytopathology, **572–573**
- specimen types, and reporting terminology, normal urinary, **228–231**
    - cytologic features, **229**
    - diagnostic checklist, **229**
    - specimen types, **228**
        - catheterization, **228**
        - ileal conduit specimens, **229**
        - urinary bladder wash (barbotage), **228**
        - voided (clean catch), **228**

Cytology processing, **710–713**
- cell block techniques, **712**
    - blood clots, **712**
    - Cellient, **712**
    - collodion bag, **712**
    - formalin, **712**
    - HistoGel (propriety gel), **712**
    - nano cell block, **712**
    - thrombin, **712**
- coverslipping, **711**
- fine-needle aspiration, **711**
- real-time telecytology, **711–712**
- specimen preparation techniques, **710**
    - cytocentrifugation, **710**
    - SurePath nongynecologic processing, **710**
    - ThinPrep and SurePath gynecologic processing, **710**
    - ThinPrep nongynecologic processing, **710**
- specimen receipt, **710**
- staining methods, **710–711**
    - destaining, **711**
    - Diff-Quik stain, **711**
    - progressive staining, **710–711**
    - rapid Pap, **711**
    - regressive staining, **710**

Cytomegalovirus (CMV), **112–113**
- diagnostic checklist, **113**
- differential diagnosis, **113**
- pancreatitis, **575**
- in Pap tests, **17**
- prognosis, **113**
- viral infections, **151**

Cytoplasmic details, anal cytology, **97**

Cytopreparation, instrumentation, and automated screening in gynecologic cytology, **8–9**
- advantages of liquid-based preparations, **9**
- automated screening, **9**
- comparison of conventional Pap smears and liquid-based Pap test, **9**
- Papanicolaou test screening sample collection, **8**
- test types, **8**

Cytopreparatory techniques, **710–715**

D

de Quervain thyroiditis. *See* Granulomatous thyroiditis.

Debris
- extraneous, fungal organisms in respiratory cytology vs., **109**
- parasitic organisms in respiratory cytology vs., **111**

Deciduosis, benign mimic, gynecologic, **20**

Dedifferentiated chondrosarcoma, **621**
- osteosarcoma vs., **617**

Dedifferentiated liposarcoma, liposarcoma vs., **639**

Dedifferentiated pleomorphic sarcoma, undifferentiated pleomorphic sarcoma vs., **651**

Deep aspiration biopsies, techniques and modalities of, **476–479**
- biopsy techniques, **477**

INDEX

- coaxial-needle technique, 477
- core biopsy technique, 477
- fine-needle technique, 477
- postprocedure, 477
- preprocedure, 476–477
- procedure, 477
- single-needle technique, 477

Deep atrophy, bare nuclei of, atypical glandular cells vs., 66

Degenerative changes, atypical urothelial cells vs., 241

Dematiaceous fungi, neuropathology squash preparations, infectious, 697

Denys-Drash syndrome, nephroblastoma, 547

Desmoid fibromatosis
- low-grade myofibroblastic sarcoma vs., 647
- smooth muscle tumors vs., 653

Desmoid tumor
- rare extrathyroidal lesions presenting as thyroid nodules, 311
- spindle cell neoplasms of gastrointestinal tract vs., 173

Desmoplastic small round cell tumor, 213, 678–679
- differential diagnosis, 679
- genetic testing, 679

Developmental anomaly
- mediastinal cysts and inflammatory lesions, 485
- nephroblastoma (Wilms tumor), 547
- squamous cell carcinoma of urinary bladder, 245

Dientamoeba fragilis, parasitic infections vs., 149

Differentiated carcinoma, poorly, angiosarcoma vs., 663

Diffuse large B-cell lymphoma, 141, 163, 191, 215. *See also* Thyroid lymphoma.
- ALK(+)
    plasmablastic lymphoma vs., 361
    plasmacytoma vs., 357
- ALK(+) anaplastic large cell lymphoma vs., 369
- Burkitt lymphoma vs., 353
- mantle cell lymphoma vs., 347
- mediastinal large B-cell lymphoma vs., 359
- pulmonary lymphoma, 141

Diffuse malignant mesothelioma (DMM), 204–207
- clinical presentation of, 205
- differential diagnosis, 205
- international system category, 205
- prognosis, 205

Diffuse sclerosing subtype, papillary thyroid carcinoma subtypes vs., papillary thyroid carcinoma subtypes, 291

Diffuse toxic goiter, 274
- differential diagnosis, 274

Diffuse-type tenosynovial giant cell tumor/pigmented villonodular synovitis, giant cell tumor of tendon sheath vs., 649

Diluted vitreous, 682

Dimorphic fungi, respiratory cytology, 109

Directly sampled endometrial cytology, 90–93
- diagnostic criteria, 90
- relative risk and management of TYS categories based on Japanese studies, 91
- Yokohama System (TYS) for Reporting Endometrial Cytology, 90

Directly sampled endometriosis
- adenocarcinoma in situ and mimics, 48
- atypical glandular cells vs., 66
- endocervical adenocarcinoma in situ vs., 47
- endometrial cancers vs., 60

Directly sampled endometrium
- atypical glandular cells vs., 66
- endometrial cancers vs., 60

Dirofilaria immitis (dog heartworm), respiratory cytology, 111

Distorted benign glomeruli, papillary renal cell carcinoma vs., 533

Dizziness, superficial aspiration technique, 257

DNA methylation, molecular testing in gynecologic cytology, 85

Duct ectasia, 421

Ductal adenocarcinoma, pancreatic neuroendocrine tumor vs., 587

Ductal carcinoma and variants of invasive mammary carcinoma, 448–455
- differential diagnosis, 451–452
- invasive ductal carcinoma histologic types, 448
- prognosis, 449

Ductal carcinoma in situ (DCIS), 441

Ductal carcinoma of breast, 449–450
- fibroadenoma vs., 436
- metastatic, lobular carcinoma vs., 457
- metastatic breast carcinomas, 192
- papillary neoplasms vs., 442
- unusual variants of, 590–593
    differential diagnosis, 592
    genetic testing, 592
    prognosis, 591

Ductal cells, 571

Ductal hyperplasia, proliferative breast changes
- atypical, 424
- usual, 424

Ductal lavage, risk assessment of breast cancer, 467

Dyshormonogenetic goiter, rare primary thyroid lesions/neoplasms, 311

Dysplasia
- Barrett esophagus with, esophagitis and Barrett esophagus vs., 153
- bile ducts, ampulla/bile duct/pancreatic duct reactive changes vs., 165
- gastric, gastric adenocarcinoma vs., 161
- high-grade
    Barrett esophagus with, esophageal adenocarcinoma vs., 155
    gastritis and intestinal metaplasia vs., 159
- high-grade squamous, esophageal squamous cell carcinoma vs., 157
- osteofibrous, adamantinoma vs., 611
- pancreatic ducts, ampulla/bile duct/pancreatic duct reactive changes vs., 165

Dysplasia Reporting System, 5

INDEX

E

EBV. *See* Epstein-Barr virus.
Eccentric nuclei, SMARCA4-deficient undifferentiated tumor vs., **139**
Eccrine carcinoma, fine-needle aspiration, **471**
Echinococcus species (hydatid disease), respiratory cytology, **111**
Echogenicity, **260**
Ectasia, duct, **421**
Ectopic thymoma, thyroid lymphoma vs., **306**
Edema
 - angiosarcoma and other sarcomas of breast, **461**
 - localized myxoid, intramuscular myxoma vs., **669**
Effusions with mixed inflammation, infectious conditions, pleural, peritoneal, pericardial, and pelvic fluid vs., **201**
EGFR, adenocarcinoma, **124**
Embryonal carcinoma
 - germ cell tumors vs., **491**
 - metastatic tumors of mediastinum vs., **495**
Embryonal rhabdomyosarcoma, **213**
 - intramuscular myxoma vs., **669**
Encapsulated papillary carcinoma, **441**
Encephalitis, neuropathology squash preparations, infectious, **696**
Enchondroma
 - chondromas of bone and soft tissue, **603**
 - chondrosarcoma vs., **622**
Endobronchial FNA and core biopsy, respiratory cytology, **100**
Endocervical adenocarcinoma
 - invasive, endocervical adenocarcinoma in situ vs., **47**
 - usual type, gastric-type adenocarcinoma vs., **57**
 - variants and mimics, **52–55**
   differential diagnosis, **53**
   immunohistochemistry, **53**
   infectious agents, **53**
Endocervical adenocarcinoma in situ
 - variants and mimics, **46–51**
   adenocarcinoma in situ and mimics, **48**
   comparison between conventional Pap smear and liquid-based technologies, **48**
   differential diagnosis, **47–48**
   immunohistochemistry, **47**
   infectious agents, **47**
Endocervical carcinoma, primary
 - cytologic distinction between endocervical and endometrial primaries, **60**
 - endometrial cancers vs., **60**
Endocervical cells
 - cytopathology, normal Pap test, **15**
 - inflammatory changes, benign finding, **18–19**
Endocervical glands, reactive, endocervical adenocarcinoma in situ vs., **47**
Endocervical glandular hyperplasia, lobular
 - atypical glandular cells vs., **66**
 - diffuse and, benign mimic, gynecologic, **20**
Endocervical/transformation zone component, Papanicolaou test, **11**
 - cellularity, **11**
 - special pointers in adequacy evaluation, **11**
Endocrine neoplasm, pancreatic
 - acinar cell carcinoma vs., **595**
 - solid pseudopapillary neoplasm of pancreas vs., **585**
Endometrial adenocarcinoma, endocervical adenocarcinoma, variants and mimics vs., **53**
Endometrial cancers, usual types, variants, and mimics, **58–63**
 - cytologic distinction between endocervical and endometrial primaries, **60**
 - differential diagnosis, **60**
 - immunohistochemistry, **60**
 - prognosis, **59**
 - type I (low-grade cancers), **59**
 - type II (high-grade cancers), **59**
Endometrial carcinoma, metastatic, columnar cell subtype vs., papillary thyroid carcinoma subtypes, **291**
Endometrial cells
 - atypical squamous cells, cannot rule out high-grade squamous intraepithelial lesion vs., **37**
 - cytopathology, normal Pap test, **15**
 - Pap test and glandular cells status post hysterectomy, **70–71**
   differential diagnosis, **71**
Endometrial hyperplasia, **91**
 - with atypia, **91**
 - endometrial cancers vs., **60**
Endometrial polyps
 - atypical glandular cells vs., **66**
 - endocervical adenocarcinoma in situ vs., **48**
Endometrial stromal sarcoma, **91**
Endometrioid adenocarcinoma
 - endometriosis and endosalpingiosis vs., **219**
 - high-grade, **91**
 - low-grade, **91**
Endometriosis, **218–219, 234**
 - diagnostic checklist, **219**
 - differential diagnosis, **219**
 - endocervical adenocarcinoma in situ vs., **47**
 - fine-needle aspiration, **470–471**
Endometrium
 - atrophic, **91**
 - menstrual
   atypical glandular cells vs., **66**
   endometrial cancers vs., **60**
   squamous cell carcinoma of cervix vs., **40**
 - proliferative, **91**
 - secretory, **91**
Endosalpingiosis, **218–219**
 - diagnostic checklist, **219**
 - differential diagnosis, **219**
Enhanced through-transmission, definition, **260**
Entamoeba histolytica
 - parasitic infections vs., **149**
 - respiratory cytology, **111**
Enteric adenocarcinomas, adenocarcinoma vs., **124**
Enterobius vermicularis, parasitic infections vs., **149**

INDEX

Environmental exposure
- hepatocellular carcinoma, **509**
- inflammatory and reactive lymphoid hyperplasia, **329**
- squamous cell carcinoma of cervix, **39**
- squamous cell carcinoma of urinary bladder, **245**
- Warthin tumor, **389**

Eosinophilic effusions, infectious conditions, pleural, peritoneal, pericardial, and pelvic fluid vs., **201**

Ependymal cells
- choroid plexus cells vs., **177**
- normal cerebrospinal fluid and contamination by normal elements, differential diagnosis, **177**
- pia-arachnoid cells vs., **177**

Ependymoma, **701**

Epidermal inclusion cyst, **385**
- extrathyroidal lesions presenting as thyroid nodules, **311**
- fine-needle aspiration, **470**

Epidermoid cyst, lymphoepithelial cyst of pancreas vs., **576**

Epithelial/epithelioid tumors, metastatic malignant, primary brain tumors vs., **189**

Epithelial-myoepithelial carcinoma
- adenoid cystic carcinoma vs., **393**
- carcinoma ex pleomorphic adenoma, **401**
- salivary gland analog tumors, **137**

Epithelial predominant Wilms tumor, metanephric adenoma vs., **525**

Epithelial tumors, categorization and typing of, **724–725**

Epithelioid angiomyolipoma/PEComa, *TFE3*- and *TFEB*-rearranged renal cell carcinomas vs., **539**

Epithelioid angiosarcoma, epithelioid hemangioendothelioma vs., **661**

Epithelioid cell neoplasm, perivascular, clear cell sarcoma of soft tissue vs., **677**

Epithelioid hemangioendothelioma, **213, 660–661**
- angiosarcoma vs., **663**
- differential diagnosis, **661**
- genetic testing, **661**
- hemangioma of liver vs., **507**
- prognosis, **661**
- soft tissue hemangioma vs., **659**

Epithelioid hemangioma
- epithelioid hemangioendothelioma vs., **661**
- metastatic tumors of bone, **631**

Epithelioid sarcoma, **672–673**
- angiosarcoma vs., **663**
- clear cell sarcoma of soft tissue vs., **677**
- differential diagnosis, **673**
- epithelioid hemangioendothelioma vs., **661**
- genetic testing, **673**
- prognosis, **673**

Epithelioid trophoblastic tumor, **79**
- squamous cell carcinoma of cervix vs., **40**

Epithelioid tumors, metastatic tumors of mediastinum vs., **495**

Epithelioid vascular tumors, metastatic tumors of bone vs., **631**

Epithelium, normal foveolar, esophagitis and Barrett esophagus vs., **153**

Epstein-Barr virus (EBV), classic Hodgkin lymphoma, **375**

Epstein-Barr virus (EBV)-associated posttransplant lymphoproliferative disorders (PTLD), renal lymphomas, **545**

Erdheim-Chester disease, fat necrosis vs., **423**

Escherichia coli, parasitic infections vs., **149**

Esophageal adenocarcinoma, **154–155**
- differential diagnosis, **155**
- genetic testing, **155**
- immunohistochemistry, **155**

Esophageal neuroendocrine tumor/carcinoma, **171**

Esophageal squamous cell carcinoma, **156–157**
- differential diagnosis, **157**

Esophagitis, **152–153**
- candidal, **153**
- differential diagnosis, **153**
- radiation, esophageal squamous cell carcinoma vs., **157**
- radiation/chemotherapy-related, **153**
- reflux, **153**
    esophageal squamous cell carcinoma vs., **157**
- viral, **153**

Esophagus
- Barrett, **152–153**
    differential diagnosis, **153**
    with dysplasia, esophagitis and Barrett esophagus vs., **153**
- cytology, **147**

ETV6-NTRK3 gene fusion, congenital mesoblastic nephroma associated with, **551**

Ewing sarcoma, **624–627**
- adamantinoma-like, adamantinoma vs., **611**
- desmoplastic small round cell tumor vs., **679**
- differential diagnosis, **626**
- immunohistochemistry, **626**
- prognosis, **625**

Ewing sarcoma/primitive neuroectodermal tumor
- bone lymphoma vs., **629**
- clear cell sarcoma of kidney vs., **549**
- mesenchymal chondrosarcoma vs., **666**
- neurogenic tumors vs., **493**
- osteosarcoma vs., **617**
- uncommon malignancies in cervicovaginal cytology, **79**

Exfoliation cytology, **682, 690**

Extensive cystitis glandularis, adenocarcinoma of urinary bladder vs., **247**

Extracranial/extraspinal contaminants, in normal cerebrospinal fluid, **177**

Extraneous debris. *See also* Debris.
- fungal organisms in respiratory cytology vs., **109**

Extranodal marginal zone B-cell lymphoma. *See also* Thyroid lymphoma.
- primary and metastatic nonepithelial tumors, **415**

Extrathyroidal lesions, presenting as thyroid nodules, **311**

Extrauterine carcinomas and other malignancies of female genital tract
- extrauterine carcinomas and presentations in cervicovaginal cytopathology, **74–75**
    differential diagnosis, **74**
    extrauterine malignancies in cervicovaginal cytology, **75**

INDEX

- neuroendocrine carcinoma of cervix, **76–77**
    - differential diagnosis, **77**
    - prognosis, **77**
- primary, endometrial cancers vs., **60**
- uncommon malignancies in cervicovaginal cytology, **78–81**
    - adenoid basal carcinoma, **79**
    - adenoid cystic carcinoma, **79**
    - adenosarcoma, **79**
    - adenosquamous carcinoma, **78–79**
    - epithelioid trophoblastic tumor, **79**
    - Ewing sarcoma, **79**
    - lymphoma, **78**
    - melanoma, **78**
    - primitive neuroectodermal tumor, **79**
    - sarcomas, **79**
    - small round blue cell tumors, **79**

F

Fainting, superficial aspiration technique, **257**
False-negative aspirates, cause of, salivary gland aspiration biopsies and reporting terminology, **379**
False-negative diagnosis/missed cases, cause for, high-grade squamous intraepithelial lesion and mimics and, **31**
Familial adenomatous polyposis, hepatoblastoma, **511**
Familial medullary thyroid carcinoma-only syndrome, **299**
Familial nephroblastoma, nephroblastoma, **547**
Familial syndromes, papillary thyroid carcinoma, classic subtype, **287**
Fasciitis, nodular
  - myofibroblastoma vs., **645**
  - primary and metastatic nonepithelial tumors, **415**
Fat necrosis, **422–423**
  - differential diagnosis, **423**
  - prognosis, **423**
Ferruginous body exposures, miscellaneous findings including contaminants, **121**
FGFR3 mutations, urothelial carcinoma, **555**
Fibers and threads, gynecologic artifact, **21**
Fibroadenolipoma, fibroadenoma vs., **436**
Fibroadenoma, **434–437**
  - with cellular stroma, phyllodes tumor vs., **459**
  - differential diagnosis, **436**
  - myxoid
      ductal carcinoma and variants of invasive mammary carcinoma vs., **451**
      mucocele-like lesion vs., **433**
  - nonproliferative and proliferative changes in breast vs., **425**
  - papillary neoplasms vs., **442**
Fibroadipose tissue, normal, benign adipose tissue tumors vs., **637**
Fibroblastic osteosarcoma, **616**
Fibroblasts, normal cerebrospinal fluid and contamination by normal elements, differential diagnosis, **177**

Fibrocystic changes. *See also* Nonproliferative and proliferative changes, in breast.
  - in breast
      fibroadenoma vs., **436**
      papillary neoplasms vs., **442**
  - with dilated ducts containing mucin, mucocele-like lesion vs., **433**
Fibroid polyp, inflammatory, spindle cell neoplasms of gastrointestinal tract vs., **173**
Fibrolipoma, **637**
Fibroma, chondromyxoid, chondrosarcoma vs., **622**
Fibroma/benign fibrous histiocytoma, nonossifying, giant cell tumor vs., **607**
Fibromatosis
  - desmoid, low-grade myofibroblastic sarcoma vs., **647**
  - fibrosarcoma vs., **643**
  - myofibroblastoma, mammary vs., **447**
  - myofibroblastoma vs., **645**
Fibromyxoid sarcoma, low-grade
  - fibrosarcoma vs., **643**
  - intramuscular myxoma vs., **669**
  - low-grade myofibroblastic sarcoma vs., **647**
Fibrosarcoma, **642–643**
  - differential diagnosis, **643**
  - genetic testing, **643**
  - immunohistochemistry, **643**
  - infantile, low-grade myofibroblastic sarcoma vs., **647**
  - smooth muscle tumors vs., **653**
Fibrous histiocytoma, benign, giant cell tumor vs., **607**
Fibrous meningioma, nonglial neoplasms vs., **705**
Fine-needle aspiration
  - deep organs and tissues
      adrenal gland. *See* Adrenal gland, fine-needle aspiration.
      bone. *See* Bone, fine-needle aspiration.
      kidney. *See* Kidney, fine-needle aspiration.
      liver. *See* Liver, fine-needle aspiration.
      mediastinum. *See* Mediastinum, fine-needle aspiration.
      pancreas. *See* Pancreas, fine-needle aspiration.
      soft tissue. *See* Soft tissue, fine-needle aspiration.
      techniques and modalities of deep aspiration biopsies, **476–479**
          biopsy techniques, **477**
          coaxial-needle technique, **477**
          core biopsy technique, **477**
          fine-needle technique, **477**
          postprocedure, **477**
          preprocedure, **476–477**
          procedure, **477**
          single-needle technique, **477**
  - sample prep and triage in evaluating suspected lymphoma, **326–327**
      adenopathy with history of lymphoma, **326**
      diagnosing lymphoma in cytopathology laboratory, **327**
      FNA processing and triage, **327**
      unexplained adenopathy, **326**
      utility and limitations of FNA, **326–327**

INDEX

- superficial
    breast. *See* Breast, fine-needle aspiration.
    lymph nodes. *See* Lymph nodes, fine-needle aspiration.
    salivary gland. *See* Salivary gland, fine-needle aspiration.
    thyroid gland. *See* Thyroid gland, fine-needle aspiration.
FNA. *See* Fine-needle aspiration.
Focal cytologic atypia, atypia of undetermined significance/follicular lesion of undetermined significance, **277**
Focal mucinosis, intramuscular myxoma vs., **669**
Focal nodular hyperplasia, **504–505**
 - differential diagnosis, **505**
 - hepatocellular adenoma vs., **503**
 - prognosis, **505**
Follicular adenoma, **281**
Follicular carcinoma, **281**
Follicular cells, Graves disease/diffuse toxic goiter, **274**
Follicular cervicitis
 - atypical glandular cells vs., **66**
 - benign mimic, gynecologic, **20**
 - high-grade squamous intraepithelial lesion and mimics vs., **31**
Follicular lesion, papillary thyroid carcinoma, classic subtype vs., **288**
Follicular lesion of undetermined significance (FLUS). *See* Atypia of undetermined significance/follicular lesion of undetermined significance.
Follicular lymphoma, **350–351**
 - differential diagnosis, **351**
 - genetic testing, **351**
 - genetics, **351**
 - grade 3, large B-cell lymphoma vs., **355**
 - grading, **351**
 - immunohistochemistry, **351**
 - mantle cell lymphoma vs., **347**
 - nodal marginal zone lymphoma vs., **349**
 - nodular lymphocyte-predominant Hodgkin lymphoma vs., **371**
 - small lymphocytic lymphoma vs., **343**
Follicular neoplasm
 - adenomatous (benign follicular) nodule vs., **268**
 - with clear cell features, metastatic carcinoma to thyroid vs., **308**
 - oncocytic (Hürthle cell) type, **284–285**
    differential diagnosis, **285**
    prognosis, **285**
 - papillary thyroid carcinoma, classic subtype vs., **288**
Follicular neoplasm/suspicious for follicular neoplasm, **280–283**
 - cytologic differences, **282**
 - differential diagnosis, **281–282**
 - follicular adenoma, **281**
 - follicular carcinoma, **281**
 - genetics, **281**
 - positive predictive value of cytologic diagnosis of, **282**
 - prognosis, **281**

Follicular or well-differentiated carcinoma, poorly differentiated thyroid carcinoma vs., **303**
Follicular subtype of papillary thyroid carcinoma (FSPTC), **282**
 - follicular neoplasm/suspicious for follicular neoplasm vs., **281**
Food particles, **121**
Foregut cysts, **485**
Foreign body granulomas, granulomatous lymphadenitis, infectious and sarcoid vs., **332**
Foreign body reaction, granulomatous lymphadenitis, infectious and sarcoid, **331**
Foreign material, pigmented thyroid lesions and crystals, **275**
Formalin, cell block techniques, **712**
Foveolar cells, gastrointestinal cytology, **147**
Foveolar epithelium, normal, esophagitis and Barrett esophagus vs., **153**
Fracture callus, chondrosarcoma vs., **622**
Francisella tularensis infection, granulomatous lymphadenitis, infectious and sarcoid vs., **332**
French technique (capillary action, no aspiration), superficial aspiration technique, **257**
Fungal infections
 - granulomatous thyroiditis, **273**
 - mycobacteria and other bacterial infections vs., **115**
 - neuropathology squash preparations, infectious, **696, 697**
 - ophthalmic cytopathology, **687**
 - other, *Pneumocystis* pneumonia and mimics vs., **107**
Fungal lymphadenitis, granulomatous lymphadenitis, infectious and sarcoid vs., **332**
Fungal organisms
 - benign mimic, gynecologic, **21**
 - in respiratory cytology, **108–109**
    diagnostic checklist, **109**
    differential diagnosis, **109**
Fungal thyroiditis, **273**
Fungi
 - in Pap tests, **16–17**
 - parasitic organisms in respiratory cytology vs., **111**

Ganglion, intramuscular myxoma vs., **669**
Ganglioneuroblastoma, **493**
Ganglioneuroma, **493, 665**
Gastric adenocarcinoma, **160–161**
 - differential diagnosis, **161**
 - immunohistochemistry, **161**
Gastric carcinoma, metastatic
 - lobular carcinoma vs., **457**
 - unusual variants of ductal carcinoma vs., **592**
Gastric dysplasia, gastric adenocarcinoma vs., **161**
Gastric epithelium, normal pancreas cytology vs., **571**
Gastric lymphoma, **162–163**
 - differential diagnosis, **163**
 - gastric adenocarcinoma vs., **161**

INDEX

Gastric neuroendocrine tumor/carcinoma, **171**
Gastric-type adenocarcinoma (GAS), **56–57**
- differential diagnosis, **57**
- genetic abnormalities, **57**
- immunohistochemistry, **57**
- prognosis, **57**

Gastritis, **158–159**
- differential diagnosis, **159**

Gastrointestinal adenocarcinomas, **209**
Gastrointestinal stromal tumor (GIST)
- angiosarcoma vs., **662**
- smooth muscle tumors vs., **653**
- solitary fibrous tumor vs., **667**
- spindle cell neoplasms of gastrointestinal tract, **172–173**
    differential diagnosis, **173**

Gastrointestinal tract, exfoliative cytopathology
- ampulla/bile duct/pancreatic duct adenocarcinoma, **166–167**
- ampulla/bile duct/pancreatic duct reactive changes, **164–165**
- colorectal adenoma/carcinoma, **168–169**
- esophageal adenocarcinoma, **154–155**
- esophageal squamous cell carcinoma, **156–157**
- esophagitis and Barrett esophagus, **152–153**
- gastric adenocarcinoma, **160–161**
- gastric lymphoma, **162–163**
- gastritis and intestinal metaplasia, **158–159**
- neuroendocrine tumor/carcinoma, **170–171**
- parasitic infections, **148–149**
- specimen types in gastrointestinal cytology and normal cellular components, **146–147**
- spindle cell neoplasms of gastrointestinal tract, including gastrointestinal stromal tumors, **172–173**
- viral infections, **150–151**

Gastrointestinal tract contamination, lymphoepithelial cyst of pancreas vs., **576**
Gastrointestinal tract mucosa, normal, mucinous cystic neoplasm of pancreas vs., **581**
Gene sequencing classifier (GSC), **278**
Genitourinary anomalies, nephroblastoma, **547**
Germ cell tumors, **490–491**
- carcinoma vs., **210**
- differential diagnosis, **491**
- immunohistochemistry, **491**
- mediastinal large B-cell lymphoma vs., **359**
- mediastinum, metastatic tumors of mediastinum vs., **495**
- NUT carcinoma vs., **138**
- SMARCA4-deficient undifferentiated tumor vs., **139**

Germinoma, germ cell tumors, **491**
Giant cell carcinoma, anaplastic, **591**
Giant cell reparative granuloma/brown tumor, giant cell tumor vs., **607**
Giant cell-rich osteosarcoma, giant cell tumor vs., **607**
Giant cell tumor, **606–607**
- chondroblastoma vs., **605**
- differential diagnosis, **607**
- immunohistochemistry, **607**
- osteosarcoma vs., **617**
- prognosis, **607**
- rare benign and low malignant potential tumors, **135**
- tenosynovial, clear cell sarcoma of soft tissue vs., **677**

Giant cell tumor of soft tissue, giant cell tumor of tendon sheath vs., **649**
Giant cell tumor of tendon sheath, **648–649**
- differential diagnosis, **649**
- immunohistochemistry, **649**
- prognosis, **649**

Giant cells/histiocytes, multinucleated, benign mimic, gynecologic, **21**
Giardia lamblia, parasitic infections vs., **149**
GIST. *See* Gastrointestinal stromal tumor.
Glandular cell abnormalities and mimics
- adenocarcinoma, gastric type, **56–57**
    differential diagnosis, **57**
    genetic abnormalities, **57**
    immunohistochemistry, **57**
    prognosis, **57**
- atypical glandular cells: endocervicals, endometrials, and glandulars, NOS, **64–69**
    differential diagnosis, **66**
- endocervical adenocarcinoma, variants and mimics, **52–55**
    differential diagnosis, **53**
    immunohistochemistry, **53**
    infectious agents, **53**
- endocervical adenocarcinoma in situ, variants and mimics, **46–51**
    adenocarcinoma in situ and mimics, **48**
    comparison between conventional Pap smear and liquid-based technologies, **48**
    differential diagnosis, **47–48**
    immunohistochemistry, **47**
    infectious agents, **47**
- endometrial cancers: usual types, variants, and mimics, **58–63**
    cytologic distinction between endocervical and endometrial primaries, **60**
    differential diagnosis, **60**
    immunohistochemistry, **60**
    prognosis, **59**
    type I (low-grade cancers), **59**
    type II (high-grade cancers), **59**
- endometrial cells in Pap test and glandular cells status post hysterectomy, **70–71**
    differential diagnosis, **71**

Glandular cells, atypical
- endocervical adenocarcinoma, variants and mimics, **53**
- high-grade squamous intraepithelial lesion and mimics vs., **31**

Glandular cells status post hysterectomy, endometrial cells in Pap test, **70–71**
- differential diagnosis, **71**

Glandular epithelial cells, gastrointestinal cytology, **147**
Glial process, reactive vs. neoplastic, **701**
Glioblastoma, **189**
- metastatic malignancies vs., **701**

Glomeruli, distorted benign, papillary renal cell carcinoma vs., **533**

INDEX

Glomus tumor, rare benign and low malignant potential tumors, **135**
Glycogen-rich carcinoma, **451**
Glycogen storage disease, hepatoblastoma, **511**
Glycogenation, benign mimic, gynecologic, **21**
Goblet cell hyperplasia, benign and reactive changes, **103**
Goblet cells, gastrointestinal cytology, **147**
Goiter
- diffuse toxic, **274**
    differential diagnosis, **274**
- dyshormonogenetic, rare primary thyroid lesions/neoplasms, **311**

Granular cell tumor
- adult-type rhabdomyoma vs., **655**
- alveolar soft part sarcoma vs., **675**
- breast, **438–439**
    differential diagnosis, **438–439**
- ductal carcinoma and variants of invasive mammary carcinoma vs., **452**
- fat necrosis vs., **423**
- rare benign and low malignant potential tumors, **135**

Granulation tissue/mesenchymal repair, angiosarcoma and other sarcomas of breast vs., **462**
Granulocytic sarcoma, lymphomas vs., **465**
Granuloma-inducing processes, Langerhans cell histiocytosis vs., **613**
Granulomas
- foreign body granulomas, granulomatous lymphadenitis, infectious and sarcoid vs., **332**
- liver, **500, 501**
- noninfectious, mycobacteria and other bacterial infections vs., **115**
- plasma cell, plasmacytoma vs., **357**
- salivary gland aspirates, **378**

Granulomatous conditions, **420–421**
- acute mastitis, **420**
- differential diagnosis, **421**
- duct ectasia, **421**
- granulomatous mastitis, **421**
- lymphocytic mastitis, **421**
- subareolar abscess, **420–421**

Granulomatous inflammation
- chronic, Rosai-Dorfman disease vs., **335**
- due to infectious etiologies, sarcoidosis and other immune-related conditions vs., **117**
- mediastinal cysts and inflammatory lesions vs., **485**

Granulomatous lymphadenitis
- infectious and sarcoid, **330–333**
    diagnostic checklist, **332**
    differential diagnosis, **332**
    immunohistochemistry, **331**
    prognosis, **331**
- peripheral T-cell lymphoma vs., **363**

Granulomatous mastitis, **421**
Granulomatous responses, sarcoidosis and other immune-related conditions vs., **117**
Granulomatous sialadenitis, **383**
Granulomatous thyroiditis, **272–273**
- diagnostic checklist, **272**
- differential diagnosis, **273**

- genetics, **273**

Graves disease, **274**
- chronic lymphocytic/Hashimoto thyroiditis vs., **271**
- differential diagnosis, **274**

Guillain-Barré syndrome (GBS), neurodegenerative disease vs., **186**

Gynecologic cytopathology
- anal cytology, **96–97**
    diagnostic checklist, **97**
    differential diagnosis, **97**
- cytopreparation, instrumentation, and automated screening, **8–9**
    advantages of liquid-based preparations, **9**
    automated screening, **9**
    comparison of conventional Pap smears and liquid-based Pap test, **9**
    Papanicolaou test screening sample collection, **8**
    test types, **8**
- directly sampled endometrial cytology, **92–95**
    diagnostic criteria, **90**
    relative risk and management of TYS categories based on Japanese studies, **91**
    Yokohama System (TYS) for Reporting Endometrial Cytology, **90**
- HPV and other molecular testing in gynecologic cytology, **84–87**
- overview, Pap test and cervical cancer screening, **4–7**
    Atlas of Exfoliative Cytology, **5**
    Bethesda Reporting System, **6**
    Cervical Intraepithelial Neoplasia Reporting System, **5**
    class reporting system, **5**
    conventional smear to liquid-based cytology, **7**
    Dysplasia Reporting System, **5**
    evolution of Pap test, **7**
    First National Cytology Conference (1948), **5**
    HPV molecular testing (ASC-US/LSIL Triage Study) (ALTS), **6–7**
- specimen adequacy in cervicovaginal cytology, **10–11**
    adequacy reporting categories, **10**
    American Society for Colposcopy and Cervical Pathology Guidelines, **11**
    endocervical/transformation zone component, **11**
        cellularity, **11**
        special pointers in adequacy evaluation, **11**
    management, **11**
    squamous cellularity criteria, **10–11**
        conventional Pap smear, **10**
        liquid-based preparations, **10–11**

Gynecomastia, **430–431**
- differential diagnosis, **431**
- prognosis, **431**

H

Hamartoma
- rare benign and low malignant potential tumors, **135**

Hamartoma, fibroadenoma vs., **436**

INDEX

Hashimoto thyroiditis
- follicular neoplasm/suspicious for follicular neoplasm vs., **282**
- Graves disease/diffuse toxic goiter vs., **274**
- papillary thyroid carcinoma, classic subtype vs., **288**

Helicobacter pylori
- gastric adenocarcinoma, **161**
- gastric lymphoma, **163**
- gastritis and intestinal metaplasia, **159**

Hemangioblastoma, nonglial neoplasms vs., **705**

Hemangioendothelioma
- epithelioid, **660–661**
    - differential diagnosis, **661**
    - genetic testing, **661**
    - hemangioma of liver vs., **507**
    - prognosis, **661**
    - soft tissue hemangioma vs., **659**
- pseudomyogenic, epithelioid hemangioendothelioma vs., **661**

Hemangioma
- angiosarcoma and other sarcomas of breast vs., **462**
- angiosarcoma vs., **663**
- epithelioid, epithelioid hemangioendothelioma vs., **661**
- juvenile variant, primary and metastatic nonepithelial tumors, **415**
- liver, **506–507**
    - differential diagnosis, **507**
- soft tissue, **658–659**
    - differential diagnosis, **659**

Hematologic malignancies, urinary cytology, **231**

Hematoma
- organizing, soft tissue hemangioma vs., **659**
- superficial aspiration technique, **257**

Hematuria, clear cell renal cell carcinoma, **529**

Hemihypertrophy, hepatoblastoma, **511**

Hemorrhage, subarachnoid, **184–185**
- differential diagnosis, **185**
- prognosis, **185**
- traumatic tap vs. pathologic bleed, **185**

Hemosiderin, pigmented thyroid lesions and crystals, **275**

Hemosiderin-laden macrophages, **121**

Hemosiderotic synovitis, giant cell tumor of tendon sheath vs., **649**

Hepatic abscess, **500**, **501**

Hepatic lesions, benign, hepatocellular carcinoma vs., **509**

Hepatoblastoma, **510–511**
- conditions associated with, **511**
- differential diagnosis, **511**
- immunohistochemistry, **511**

Hepatocellular adenoma, **502–503**
- diagnostic checklist, **503**
- differential diagnosis, **503**
- focal nodular hyperplasia vs., **505**
- inflammatory and infectious conditions of liver vs., **501**
- normal liver cytology vs., **499**

Hepatocellular carcinoma, **508–509**
- differential diagnosis, **509**
- focal nodular hyperplasia vs., **505**
- hepatoblastoma vs., **511**
- hepatocellular adenoma vs., **503**
- immunocytochemistry, **725**
- immunohistochemistry, **509**
- liver metastasis vs., **513**
- metastatic, unusual variants of ductal carcinoma vs., **592**
- metastatic tumors to kidney vs., **553**
- normal liver cytology vs., **499**

Hepatocytes, normal pancreas cytology vs., **571**

Hepatoid carcinoma, **591**

Herpes simplex virus (HSV), **696**
- molecular testing in gynecologic cytology, **86**
- pancreatitis, **575**
- in Pap tests, **17**
- Tzanck smears, **470**

Herpes simplex virus 1 (HSV1), viral infections vs., **151**

Herpes simplex virus 2 (HSV2)
- Mollaret meningitis, **182**
- viral infections vs., **151**

Herpes simplex virus (HSV) meningoencephalitis, **180**

Herpes viral infection, low-grade squamous intraepithelial lesion and mimics vs., **29**

Herpes zoster, Tzanck smears, **470**

Herpesvirus, **112–113**
- diagnostic checklist, **113**
- differential diagnosis, **113**
- infectious benign conditions, **236**
- prognosis, **113**

Herpetic keratitis, **687**

Hibernoma, **637**
- adult-type rhabdomyoma vs., **655**

Hidradenoma, clear cell, fine-needle aspiration, **472**

High-grade adenocarcinomas, metastatic tumors to adrenal gland vs., **565**

High-grade B-cell lymphoma
- large B-cell lymphoma vs., **355**
- with *MYC* and *BCL2* &/or *BCL6* rearrangements, Burkitt lymphoma vs., **353**

High-grade dysplasia, gastritis and intestinal metaplasia vs., **159**

High-grade endometrioid adenocarcinoma, **91**

High-grade malignancies, metastatic, pheochromocytoma vs., **567**

High-grade malignant neoplasms, salivary gland aspirates, **378–379**

High-grade neuroendocrine carcinomas, carcinoid and atypical carcinoid vs., **133**

High-grade pancreatic intraepithelial neoplasm, pancreatic ductal adenocarcinoma vs., **589**

High-grade renal cell carcinoma, urothelial carcinoma vs., **555**

High-grade serous carcinoma, **91**
- low-grade serous carcinoma vs., **221**

High-grade squamous dysplasia, esophageal squamous cell carcinoma vs., **157**

High-grade squamous intraepithelial lesion
- adenocarcinoma in situ and mimics, **48**
- atypical glandular cells vs., **66**
- atypical squamous cells, cannot rule out high, **36–37**
    - differential diagnosis, **37**
    - prognosis, **37**
- endocervical adenocarcinoma in situ vs., **48**

INDEX

- endometrial cells in Pap test and glandular cells status post hysterectomy vs., **71**
- and mimics, **30–33**
    - differential diagnosis, **31**
    - with inflammation, squamous cell carcinoma of cervix vs., **40**

High-grade surface osteosarcoma, **617**

High-grade urothelial carcinoma
- ancillary testing, UroVysion, and others, **253**
- atypical urothelial cells vs., **241**
- low-grade urothelial lesions vs., **240**
- reactive urothelial changes vs., **239**
- renal pelvic cytology, **251**
- suspicious, atypical urothelial cells vs., **241**
- urinary cytology, **229–231**

High-grade urothelial dysplasia/carcinoma/carcinoma in situ, **242–243**
- differential diagnosis, **243**

High-risk HPV-positive rates, by cytology interpretation, molecular testing in gynecologic cytology, **87**

Histiocytes
- atypical squamous cells, cannot rule out high-grade squamous intraepithelial lesion vs., **37**
- benign gynecologic mimic, **21**
- cytomorphology of, in pleural, peritoneal, pericardial, and pelvic fluid and washings, **197**
- lobular carcinoma vs., **457**
- lymph node aspiration, **325**
- parasitic organisms in respiratory cytology vs., **111**

Histiocytoid cells, atypia of undetermined significance/follicular lesion of undetermined significance, **277**

Histiocytoma, benign fibrous, giant cell tumor vs., **607**

Histiocytosis, Langerhans cell, **612–613**
- bone lymphoma vs., **629**
- differential diagnosis, **613**
- immunohistochemistry, **613**
- prognosis, **613**

Histocyte-rich large B-cell lymphoma, nodular lymphocyte-predominant Hodgkin lymphoma vs., **371**

HistoGel (propriety gel), cell block techniques, **712**

Histoplasma capsulatum
- neuropathology squash preparations, infectious, **697**
- *Pneumocystis* pneumonia and mimics vs., **107**

HIV neuropathy, neurodegenerative disease vs., **187**

HLA-B8, Graves disease/diffuse toxic goiter, **274**

HLA-DR3, Graves disease/diffuse toxic goiter, **274**

Hobnail subtype, papillary thyroid carcinoma subtypes, **291**

Hodgkin disease (HD) effusions, **215**

Hodgkin lymphoma, **141**
- classic, **374–375**
    - ALK(+) anaplastic large cell lymphoma vs., **369**
    - angioimmunoblastic lymphoma vs., **367**
    - differential diagnosis, **375**
    - immunohistochemistry, **375**
    - mediastinal large B-cell lymphoma vs., **359**
    - peripheral T-cell lymphoma vs., **363**
- inflammatory and infectious conditions of liver vs., **501**
- inflammatory and reactive lymphoid hyperplasia vs., **329**
- nodular lymphocyte-predominant, **372–373**
    - differential diagnosis, **373**
    - follicular lymphoma vs., **351**
    - immunohistochemistry, **373**

Hookworms, parasitic infections vs., **149**

HPV. *See* Human papillomavirus.

HPV-positive head and neck squamous cell carcinoma, **338–341**
- diagnostic checklist, **340–341**
- differential diagnosis, **340**
- immunohistochemistry, **339–340**
- mimics, **341**

HPV-related multiphenotypic sinonasal carcinoma, **340–341**

HRAS gene mutation, medullary thyroid carcinoma, **299**

HRPT2 mutation, parathyroid cyst, adenoma, and carcinoma, **319**

HSIL. *See* High-grade squamous intraepithelial lesion.

HSV. *See* Herpes simplex virus.

Human herpesvirus 8 (HHV-8), **217**

Human papillomavirus (HPV). *See also* Infectious benign conditions.
- infectious benign conditions, **237**
- molecular testing, **6–7, 84–86**
    - ASCCP management guidelines based on immediate and 5-year risk of CIN3+, **87**
    - high-risk HPV-positive rates by cytology interpretation, **87**
    - widely used HPV testing platforms, **87**
- squamous cell carcinoma of cervix, **39**
- viral infections, **151**

Hürthle cell neoplasm
- adult-type rhabdomyoma vs., **655**
- metastatic carcinoma to thyroid vs., **308**
- parathyroid cyst, adenoma, and carcinoma vs., **319**

Hürthle cell proliferation, chronic lymphocytic/Hashimoto thyroiditis vs., **271**

Hürthle cell tumors, oncocytic, oncocytic subtype vs., papillary thyroid carcinoma subtypes, **292**

Hyalinizing clear cell carcinoma, ancillary testing, **380**

Hyalinizing trabecular tumor
- medullary thyroid carcinoma vs., **300**
- papillary thyroid carcinoma, classic subtype vs., **288**
- rare primary thyroid lesions/neoplasms, **311**

Hybrid capture technique (Hybrid Capture II), molecular testing in gynecologic cytology, **85**

Hybrid oncocytic/chromophobe tumor, kidney oncocytoma vs., **523**

Hydatid cyst, inflammatory and infectious conditions of liver, **500, 501**

Hyperchromatic crowded groups (HCGs), etiologies for, high-grade squamous intraepithelial lesion and mimics vs., **31**

Hyperechoic, definition, **260**

Hyperkeratosis
- benign finding, gynecologic, **19**
- low-grade squamous intraepithelial lesion and mimics vs., **29**

INDEX

Hyperplasia
- nodular oncocytic, oncocytoma of salivary gland vs., **391**
- reactive lymphoid, nodular lymphocyte-predominant Hodgkin lymphoma vs., **371**

Hyperplastic nodule, macrofollicular subtype vs., papillary thyroid carcinoma subtype, **292**

Hypoechoic, definition, **260**

I

Ileal conduit specimens, **232–233**
- diagnostic checklist, **233**
- differential diagnosis, **233**
- prognosis, **233**

Ileal pouch. *See* Ileal conduit specimens.

Immune-related conditions
- lymphocyte-rich effusion vs., **197**
- sarcoidosis, **116–117**
    - diagnostic checklist, **117**
    - differential diagnosis, **117**

Immunoblast, lymph node aspiration, **325**

ImmunoCyt/uCyt+, urinary cytology, **252–253**
- equipment, **253**
- newer tests, **253**
- sensitivity and specificity, **253**
- type of analysis, **253**

Immunocytochemistry, **724–727**
- applications, **724–725**
    - categorization and typing of epithelial tumors, **724–725**
    - determine organ of origin of malignant tumors, **725**
    - markers of mesenchymal cells, **725**
    - melanoma markers, **725**
    - neuroendocrine differentiation, **725**
    - panels for work-up of tumors, **725**
- determination of prognostic and predictive markers, **725**
- diagnostic immunocytochemistry profiles in common renal tumors, **726**
- distinction of mesothelial cells/mesothelioma from adenocarcinoma/metastatic carcinoma, **726**
- histochemistry, and other ancillary techniques, **222–225**
    - differential stains for mesotheliomas and adenocarcinomas, **223**
    - ICC staining patterns for benign or malignant mesothelial cells vs. adenocarcinoma, **223**
    - indications for histochemical stains in body fluids, **222**
        - detection of infectious organisms, **222**
        - reactive mesothelial cells/mesotheliomas from adenocarcinoma, **222**
    - indications for IHC stains in body fluids, **222**
        - determination of primary site of malignancy, **223**
        - reactive mesothelial cells/mesotheliomas from adenocarcinoma, **222**
    - indications for use of flow cytometry in body fluids, **223**
        - lymphoma vs. reactive lymphocytic effusion, **223**
        - reactive effusions vs. metastatic carcinomas, **223**
    - use of ancillary studies in body fluid specimens, **222**
- immunostaining, **724**
- small round blue cell tumor, **726**

Immunosuppression
- HPV-positive head and neck squamous cell carcinoma, **339**
- squamous cell carcinoma of cervix, **39**

In situ hybridization
- high-grade urothelial dysplasia/carcinoma/carcinoma in situ, **243**
- molecular techniques, **729–730**

Inadvertent sampling of liver
- adrenal cortical adenoma vs., **561**
- cytology of normal adrenal gland vs., **559**
- kidney oncocytoma vs., **523**

Indiana pouch. *See* Ileal conduit specimens.

Infantile fibrosarcoma, low-grade myofibroblastic sarcoma vs., **647**

Infarcted pleomorphic adenoma, with squamous differentiation, metastatic carcinoma vs., **413**

Infection
- bacterial. *See* Bacterial infections.
- fungal. *See* Fungal infections.
- mediastinal cysts and inflammatory lesions vs., **485**
- parasitic, **148–149**
    - differential diagnosis, **149**
- renal lymphomas vs., **545**
- tight halos due to, low-grade squamous intraepithelial lesion and mimics vs., **29**
- viral, **150–151**
    - differential diagnosis, **151**

Infectious agents
- anal cytology, **97**
- Burkitt lymphoma, **353**
- endocervical adenocarcinoma, variants and mimics, **53**
- endocervical adenocarcinoma in situ, **47**
- granulomatous lymphadenitis, infectious and sarcoid, **331**
- granulomatous thyroiditis, **273**
- hepatocellular carcinoma, **509**
- HPV-positive head and neck squamous cell carcinoma, **339**
- infectious meningitis associate with, **181**
- inflammatory and reactive lymphoid hyperplasia, **329**
- neuroendocrine carcinoma of cervix, **77**
- squamous cell carcinoma of urinary bladder, **245**

Infectious benign conditions, urine cytology, **236–237**
- diagnostic checklist, **237**
- differential diagnosis, **237**

Infectious conditions, pleural, peritoneal, pericardial, and pelvic fluid, **200–201**
- diagnostic checklist, **201**
- differential diagnosis, **201**
- prognosis, **201**

Infectious meningitis, **180–181**

Infectious meningoencephalitis, **181**

Infectious vaginitis/cervicitis, molecular testing in gynecologic cytology, **86–87**

INDEX

Inflammation
- renal lymphomas vs., **545**
- tight halos due to, low-grade squamous intraepithelial lesion and mimics vs., **29**

Inflammatory and granulomatous conditions, breast, **420–421**
- acute mastitis, **420**
- differential diagnosis, **421**
- duct ectasia, **421**
- granulomatous mastitis, **421**
- lymphocytic mastitis, **421**
- subareolar abscess, **420–421**

Inflammatory and infectious conditions of liver, **500–501**
- diagnostic checklist, **501**
- differential diagnosis, **501**
- granuloma, **500**
- hepatic abscess, **500**
- hydatid cyst, **500**

Inflammatory and reactive lymphoid hyperplasia, **328–329**
- diagnostic checklist, **329**
- differential diagnosis, **329**
- immunohistochemistry, **329**

Inflammatory breast carcinoma, inflammatory and granulomatous conditions vs., **421**

Inflammatory cells, salivary gland aspirates, **378**

Inflammatory changes, atypical squamous cells of undetermined significance vs., **35**

Inflammatory fibroid polyp, spindle cell neoplasms of gastrointestinal tract vs., **173**

Inflammatory myofibroblastic tumor
- low-grade myofibroblastic sarcoma vs., **647**
- lymphomas vs., **465**
- rare benign and low malignant potential tumors, **135**

Inflammatory polyp, colorectal adenoma/carcinoma vs., **169**

Inherited neuropathies, neurodegenerative disease vs., **187**

Instrumentation, in gynecologic cytology, **8–9**

Insular thyroid carcinoma. *See also* Poorly differentiated thyroid carcinoma.
- medullary thyroid carcinoma vs., **300**

Intermediate-grade neuroendocrine tumors of lung. *See* Carcinoid and atypical carcinoid tumors of respiratory tract.

Intermediate urothelial cells, urinary cytology, **229**

Intestinal epithelium, normal pancreas cytology vs., **571**

Intestinal metaplasia, **158–159**
- differential diagnosis, **159**

Intra- and peripancreatic splenules, **577**
- differential diagnosis, **577**

Intracranial/intraspinal cells, benign
- differential diagnosis, **177**
- immunochemistry, **177**

Intraductal carcinoma, low-grade, secretory carcinoma vs., **409**

Intraductal papillary mucinous neoplasm
- branch duct type, mucinous cystic neoplasm of pancreas vs., **581**
- of pancreas, **582–583**
  - differential diagnosis, **583**
  - genetic testing, **583**
- pancreatic ductal adenocarcinoma, **589**

Intraepithelial neoplasia, pancreatic
- ampulla/bile duct/pancreatic duct adenocarcinoma vs., **167**
- intraductal papillary mucinous neoplasm of pancreas vs., **583**

Intraglandular lymph nodes, normal salivary gland and sialadenitis, **383**

Intralobular stromal cells, abnormal growth of, fibroadenoma, **435**

Intramammary lymph node, lymphomas vs., **465**

Intramuscular ganglion, intramuscular myxoma vs., **669**

Intramuscular lipoma, **637**

Intramuscular myxoma, **668–669**
- differential diagnosis, **669**
- genetic testing, **669**
- prognosis, **669**

Intraocular solid tumors, **683**

Intraosseous synovial sarcoma, adamantinoma vs., **611**

Intrathyroid parathyroid tumor, medullary thyroid carcinoma vs., **300**

Invasive apocrine carcinoma, **451**

Invasive carcinoma of breast, granular cell tumor of breast vs., **439**

Invasive ductal carcinoma (IDC), **448**

Invasive endocervical adenocarcinoma, endocervical adenocarcinoma in situ vs., **47**

Invasive micropapillary carcinoma, of breast, **450**
- papillary neoplasms vs., **442**

Invasive papillary carcinoma, **441, 450**

Invasive urothelial carcinoma, with glandular differentiation, adenocarcinoma of urinary bladder vs., **247**

Iodine deficiency, anaplastic thyroid carcinoma, **305**

Islet cells, normal pancreas cytology vs., **571**

Isoechoic, definition, **260**

Isospora, parasitic infections vs., **149**

IUD cells
- atypical glandular cells vs., **66**
- endometrial cancers vs., **60**
- high-grade squamous intraepithelial lesion and mimics vs., **31**

IUD-related changes, benign mimic, gynecologic, **20**

J

Juxtacortical chondrosarcoma, **621**

K

Kaposi sarcoma
- fine-needle aspiration, **472**
- soft tissue hemangioma vs., **659**

INDEX

Keratinizing squamous cell carcinoma, **157**
- cytopathology, squamous cell carcinoma of cervix, **39**

Keratinizing squamous metaplasia, squamous cell carcinoma of urinary bladder vs., **245**

Keratinous cyst, **385**

Kidney, fine-needle aspiration
- angiomyolipoma, **520–521**
    - differential diagnosis, **521**
    - genetic and clinical features, **521**
    - immunohistochemistry, **521**
    - prognosis, **521**
- carcinoid tumor, **543**
    - differential diagnoses, **543**
- chromophobe renal cell carcinoma, **536–537**
    - differential diagnosis, **537**
    - immunohistochemistry, **537**
    - prognosis, **537**
- clear cell papillary renal cell carcinoma, **534–535**
    - differential diagnosis, **535**
    - genetic testing, **535**
    - immunohistochemistry, **535**
    - prognosis, **535**
- clear cell renal cell carcinoma, **528–531**
    - cytology-histology correlation, **529**
    - diagnostic checklist, **528**
    - differential diagnosis, **529**
    - genetic testing, **529**
    - immunohistochemistry, **529**
    - prognosis, **529**
- clear cell sarcoma, **548–549**
    - differential diagnosis, **549**
    - immunohistochemistry, **549**
    - molecular genetics, **549**
    - prognosis, **549**
- collecting duct carcinoma, **540**
    - differential diagnoses, **540**
- congenital mesoblastic nephroma, **550–552**
    - differential diagnosis, **551**
    - genetic features, **551**
- cytology of normal kidney, **516–517**
- metanephric adenoma, **524–525**
    - differential diagnosis, **525**
    - immunohistochemistry, **525**
    - nephroblastoma vs., **547**
- metanephric stromal tumor, **526**
    - classification, **526**
    - differential diagnosis, **526**
- metastatic tumors to kidney, **553**
    - diagnostic checklist, **553**
    - differential diagnosis, **553**
- mucinous tubular and spindle cell carcinoma of kidney, **542**
    - differential diagnoses, **542**
- nephroblastoma (Wilms tumor), **546–547**
    - conditions associated, **547**
    - developmental anomaly, **547**
    - differential diagnosis, **547**
    - genetic abnormalities, **547**
    - immunohistochemistry, **547**
    - prognosis, **547**
- oncocytoma, **522–523**
    - differential diagnosis, **523**
    - immunohistochemistry, **523**
    - molecular abnormalities, **523**
- papillary renal cell carcinoma, **532–533**
    - differential diagnosis, **533**
    - immunohistochemistry, **533**
- primary renal sarcomas, **544**
- renal cysts, **518–519**
    - Bosniak classification system, **519**
    - diagnostic checklist, **518**
    - differential diagnosis, **519**
- renal lymphomas, **545**
    - diagnostic checklist, **545**
    - differential diagnoses, **545**
- renal medullary carcinoma, **541**
    - differential diagnoses, **541**
- rhabdoid tumor of kidney, **552**
    - differential diagnosis, **552**
- urothelial carcinoma, **554–555**
- xanthogranulomatous pyelonephritis/malakoplakia, **527**
    - differential diagnoses, **527**

Kikuchi lymphadenitis, Rosai-Dorfman disease vs., **335**

Koilocytes, viral infections vs., **151**

KRAS gene mutation
- adenocarcinoma, **124**
- adenosquamous carcinoma, **592**
- medullary thyroid carcinoma, **299**
- pancreatic ductal adenocarcinoma, **589**

Küttner tumor, **383**

L

Lactobacillus, in Pap tests, **17**

Langerhans cell histiocytosis, **612–613**
- bone lymphoma vs., **629**
- differential diagnosis, **613**
- immunohistochemistry, **613**
- prognosis, **613**
- Rosai-Dorfman disease vs., **335**

Large B-cell lymphoma, **354–355**
- anaplastic variant, **355**
- centroblastic variant, **355**
- differential diagnosis, **355**
- immunoblastic variant, **355**
    - plasmablastic lymphoma vs., **361**
- immunohistochemistry, **355**
- mediastinal, **358–359**
    - differential diagnosis, **359**
    - immunohistochemistry, **359**
- metastatic tumors of mediastinum vs., **495**
- primary effusion lymphoma vs., **217**
- primary mediastinal, classic Hodgkin lymphoma vs., **375**
- T-cell/histiocyte rich, **355**
- T-cell lymphoblastic lymphoma vs., **371**

Large cell carcinoma of lung, metastatic tumors of mediastinum vs., **495**

Large cell neuroendocrine carcinoma, **130–131**
- cervix, **77**

INDEX

- diagnostic checklist, **131**
- differential diagnosis, **131**
- small cell carcinoma vs., **129**

Large cell variant, Ewing sarcoma, **625, 626**
Large duct papilloma (LDP), **441**
Large-volume fluids, nongynecologic cytology, **713**
Legionella, pancreatitis, **575**
Leiomyoma
- myxoid, intramuscular myxoma vs., **669**
- rare benign and low malignant potential tumors, **135**
- smooth muscle tumors vs., **653**
- spindle cell neoplasms of gastrointestinal tract, **173**

Leiomyosarcoma, **213**
- low-grade myofibroblastic sarcoma vs., **647**
- pleomorphic, undifferentiated pleomorphic sarcoma vs., **651**
- smooth muscle tumors, **653**
- solitary fibrous tumor vs., **667**
- spindle cell neoplasms of gastrointestinal tract vs., **173**
- synovial sarcoma vs., **671**
- urinary cytology, **231**

Lepidic-pattern adenocarcinomas, adenocarcinoma vs., **124**
Leptospira, pancreatitis, **575**
Leptothrix species, in Pap tests, **17**
Lesions, round cell, bone lymphoma vs., **629**
Leukemia
- in cerebrospinal fluid, **190–191**
    - differential diagnosis, **191**
- large cell neuroendocrine carcinoma vs., **77**
- small cell neuroendocrine carcinoma vs., **77**
- T-lymphoblastic, **371**

Leukemic breast involvement, lymphomas vs., **465**
Leukemic effusions, **215**
Li-Fraumeni syndrome
- adrenal cortical carcinoma, **563**
- hepatoblastoma, **511**

Lipid-laden macrophages, **121**
Lipid-rich carcinoma, **451**
Lipofuscin, pigmented thyroid lesions and crystals, **275**
Lipoma
- cytologic/small biopsy categorization of primary soft tissue tumors, **635**
- intramuscular, **637**
- primary and metastatic nonepithelial tumors, **415**
- rare benign and low malignant potential tumors, **135**
- spindle cell, **637**

Lipomatous tumor, atypical
- benign adipose tissue tumors vs., **637**
- liposarcoma vs., **639**

Liposarcoma, **638–641**
- dedifferentiated, liposarcoma vs., **639**
- differential diagnosis, **639**
- genetic testing, **639**
- immunohistochemistry, **639**
- myxoid
    - benign adipose tissue tumors vs., **637**
    - cytologic/small biopsy categorization of primary soft tissue tumors, **635**
    - intramuscular myxoma vs., **669**
    - liposarcoma vs., **639**
- myxoid pleomorphic, liposarcoma vs., **639**
- pleomorphic
    - liposarcoma vs., **639**
    - undifferentiated pleomorphic sarcoma vs., **651**
- retroperitoneal low-grade, angiomyolipoma vs., **521**
- round cell, liposarcoma vs., **639**
- well-differentiated
    - cytologic/small biopsy categorization of primary soft tissue tumors, **635**
    - liposarcoma vs., **639**

Liquid-based pap tests, **8**
Liver, fine-needle aspiration
- cytology of normal liver, **498–499**
    - differential diagnosis, **499**
- focal nodular hyperplasia, **504–505**
    - differential diagnosis, **505**
    - hepatocellular adenoma vs., **503**
    - prognosis, **505**
- hemangioma, **506–507**
    - differential diagnosis, **507**
- hepatoblastoma, **510–511**
    - conditions associated with, **511**
    - differential diagnosis, **511**
    - immunohistochemistry, **511**
- hepatocellular adenoma, **502–503**
    - diagnostic checklist, **503**
    - differential diagnosis, **503**
    - focal nodular hyperplasia vs., **505**
    - normal liver cytology vs., **499**
- inflammatory and infectious conditions of liver, **500–501**
    - diagnostic checklist, **501**
    - differential diagnosis, **501**
- liver metastasis, **512–513**
    - diagnostic checklist, **512**
    - differential diagnosis, **513**

Liver disease, gynecomastia and, **431**
Liver metastasis, **512–513**
- diagnostic checklist, **512**
- differential diagnosis, **513**

Liver parenchyma, normal, hepatoblastoma vs., **511**
Lobular carcinoma, **209, 456–457**
- differential diagnosis, **457**
- in metastatic breast carcinomas, **192**

Lobular endocervical glandular hyperplasia
- atypical glandular cells vs., **66**
- gastric-type adenocarcinoma vs., **57**

Low-grade adenocarcinoma, polymorphous, carcinoma ex pleomorphic adenoma, **401**
Low-grade central osteosarcoma, **616**
Low-grade chondrosarcoma, chondromas of bone and soft tissue vs., **603**
Low-grade clear cell renal cell carcinoma, normal kidney cytology vs., **517**
Low-grade endometrioid adenocarcinoma, **91**
Low-grade fibromyxoid sarcoma
- fibrosarcoma vs., **643**
- intramuscular myxoma vs., **669**
- low-grade myofibroblastic sarcoma vs., **647**

Low-grade intraductal carcinoma, secretory carcinoma vs., **409**

INDEX

Low-grade liposarcoma, retroperitoneal, angiomyolipoma vs., **521**
Low-grade lymphoma, with marked plasmacytic differentiation, plasmacytoma vs., **357**
Low-grade mucoepidermoid carcinoma
  - normal salivary gland and sialadenitis vs., **383**
Low-grade myofibroblastic sarcoma, **646–647**
  - differential diagnosis, **647**
  - immunohistochemistry, **647**
  - myofibroblastoma vs., **645**
  - prognosis, **647**
Low-grade myofibrosarcoma, fibrosarcoma vs., **643**
Low-grade myxofibrosarcoma, intramuscular myxoma vs., **669**
Low-grade neuroendocrine tumors, of lung. *See* Carcinoid and atypical carcinoid tumors of respiratory tract.
Low-grade papillary neoplasms, ancillary testing, UroVysion, and others, **253**
Low-grade papillary urothelial neoplasm, reactive urothelial changes vs., **239**
Low-grade renal cell carcinomas, carcinoid tumor vs., **543**
Low-grade serous carcinoma
  - endometriosis and endosalpingiosis vs., **219**
  - high-grade serous carcinoma vs., **221**
Low-grade spindle cell neoplasms, solitary fibrous tumor vs., **667**
Low-grade squamous intraepithelial lesion and mimics, **28–29**
  - differential diagnosis, **29**
  - prognosis, **29**
Low-grade urothelial lesions, **240**
  - diagnostic checklist, **240**
  - differential diagnosis, **240**
  - high-grade urothelial dysplasia/carcinoma/carcinoma in situ vs., **243**
Low-grade urothelial neoplasm
  - renal pelvic cytology, **251**
  - urinary cytology, **231**
Lubricant jelly, gynecologic artifact, **21**
Lumbar puncture, clinical indication of, **176**
Lung, anaplastic carcinoma of, metastatic tumors to kidney vs., **553**
Lung adenocarcinoma
  - adenocarcinoma vs., **124**
  - prognostic and predictive markers, **725**
Lung carcinoma
  - large cell, metastatic tumors of mediastinum vs., **495**
  - metastatic, **193**
     thymic carcinoma vs., **489**
  - non-small cell, metastatic tumors of mediastinum vs., **495**
  - primary, pulmonary metastasis vs., **143**
  - small cell, metastatic tumors of mediastinum vs., **495**
Lung tumors
  - immunocytochemistry, **725**
  - metastatic tumors to kidney vs., **553**
Lupus mastitis, fat necrosis vs., **423**
Lupus pleuritis, systemic lupus erythematosus effusion vs., **203**
Lyme disease, neurodegenerative disease vs., **187**

Lymph nodes
  - enlarged, intra- and peripancreatic splenules vs., **577**
  - intraglandular, normal salivary gland and sialadenitis, **383**
  - metastasis, intramammary, ductal carcinoma and variants of invasive mammary carcinoma vs., **452**
  - nonmycobacterial infections of, granulomatous lymphadenitis, infectious and sarcoid vs., **332**
Lymph nodes, fine-needle aspiration
  - ALK(+) anaplastic large cell lymphoma, **368–369**
     differential diagnosis, **369**
     genetic testing, **369**
     immunohistochemistry, **369**
  - angioimmunoblastic lymphoma, **366–367**
     differential diagnosis, **367**
     genetic testing, **367**
     immunohistochemistry, **367**
  - Burkitt lymphoma, **352–353**
     differential diagnosis, **353**
     genetic testing, **353**
     immunohistochemistry, **353**
  - classic Hodgkin lymphoma, **374–375**
  - FNA sample prep and triage in evaluating suspected lymphoma, **326–327**
  - follicular lymphoma, **350–351**
     differential diagnosis, **351**
     genetic testing, **351**
     genetics, **351**
     grading, **351**
     immunohistochemistry, **351**
  - granulomatous lymphadenitis, infectious and sarcoid, **330–333**
     diagnostic checklist, **332**
     differential diagnosis, **332**
     immunohistochemistry, **331**
     prognosis, **331**
  - HPV-positive head and neck squamous cell carcinoma, **338–341**
     diagnostic checklist, **340–341**
     differential diagnosis, **340**
     immunohistochemistry, **339–340**
     mimics, **341**
  - indications for aspiration, techniques, and reporting, **324–325**
     cytologic features, **324–325**
     diagnostic checklist, **325**
     proposed 2-tiered system, **325**
     technique, **324**
     types of procedures, **324**
  - inflammatory and reactive lymphoid hyperplasia, **328–329**
     diagnostic checklist, **329**
     differential diagnosis, **329**
     immunohistochemistry, **329**
  - large B-cell lymphoma, **354–355**
     anaplastic variant, **355**
     centroblastic variant, **355**
     differential diagnosis, **355**
     immunoblastic variant, **355**
     immunohistochemistry, **355**

INDEX

T-cell/histiocyte rich, **355**
- lymphoplasmacytic lymphoma, **344–345**
    differential diagnosis, **345**
    genetic testing, **345**
    immunohistochemistry, **345**
- mantle cell lymphoma, **346–347**
    blastoid variant, Burkitt lymphoma vs., **353**
    differential diagnosis, **347**
    follicular lymphoma vs., **351**
    genetic testing, **347**
    immunohistochemistry, **347**
    nodal marginal zone lymphoma vs., **349**
    pleomorphic variant, large B-cell lymphoma vs., **355**
    small lymphocytic lymphoma vs., **343**
- mediastinal large B-cell lymphoma, **358–359**
    differential diagnosis, **359**
    immunohistochemistry, **359**
- metastatic malignancies (carcinoma, melanoma), **336–337**
    immunohistochemistry, **337**
- mycosis fungoides, **364–365**
    differential diagnosis, **365**
    genetic testing, **365**
    immunohistochemistry, **365**
- nodal marginal zone lymphoma, **348–349**
    differential diagnosis, **349**
    genetic testing, **349**
    prognosis, **349**
- nodular lymphocyte-predominant Hodgkin lymphoma, **372–373**
    differential diagnosis, **373**
    follicular lymphoma vs., **351**
    immunohistochemistry, **373**
- peripheral T-cell lymphoma, **362–363**
    differential diagnosis, **363**
    genetic testing, **363**
    immunohistochemistry, **363**
- plasmablastic lymphoma, **360–361**
    differential diagnosis, **361**
    immunohistochemistry, **361**
- plasmacytoma, **356–357**
    differential diagnosis, **357**
    immunohistochemistry, **357**
- Rosai-Dorfman disease, **334–335**
    differential diagnosis, **335**
    immunohistochemistry, **335**
    prognosis, **335**
- small lymphocytic lymphoma, **342–343**
    differential diagnosis, **343**
    immunohistochemistry, **343**
    prognosis, **343**
- T-cell lymphoblastic lymphoma, **370–371**
    differential diagnosis, **371**
    genetic testing, **371**
    immunohistochemistry, **371**
Lymphadenitis
- atypical mycobacterial lymphadenitis, granulomatous lymphadenitis, infectious and sarcoid vs., **332**
- fungal lymphadenitis, granulomatous lymphadenitis, infectious and sarcoid vs., **332**
- granulomatous, peripheral T-cell lymphoma vs., **363**
- Kikuchi lymphadenitis, Rosai-Dorfman disease vs., **335**
Lymphadenoid goiter. *See* Chronic lymphocytic/Hashimoto thyroiditis.
Lymphadenopathies, viral, nodular lymphocyte-predominant Hodgkin lymphoma vs., **371**
Lymphangioma
- lymphoepithelial cyst of pancreas vs., **576**
- serous microcystic adenoma vs., **579**
Lymphoblastic leukemia/lymphoma, Burkitt lymphoma vs., **353**
Lymphoblastic lymphoma, **190, 215**
- mantle cell lymphoma vs., **347**
- mediastinal thymoma vs., **487**
- metastatic tumors of mediastinum vs., **495**
Lymphocyte-rich effusions
- differential diagnosis, **197**
- infectious conditions, pleural, peritoneal, pericardial, and pelvic fluid vs., **201**
Lymphocytes
- cytomorphology of, in pleural, peritoneal, pericardial, and pelvic fluid and washings, **197**
- Graves disease/diffuse toxic goiter, **274**
- lymph node aspiration, **324–325**
Lymphocytic cell pattern, salivary gland aspirates, **378**
Lymphocytic/Hashimoto thyroiditis
- follicular neoplasm, oncocytic (Hürthle cell) type vs., **285**
- granulomatous thyroiditis vs., **273**
- thyroid lymphoma vs., **306**
- Warthin-like subtype vs., papillary thyroid carcinoma subtype, **292**
Lymphocytic mastitis, **421**
Lymphocytic meningitis, leukemia and lymphoma vs., **191**
Lymphoepithelial cyst
- pancreas, **576**
    differential diagnosis, **576**
- salivary gland, **385**
Lymphoid effusion and lymphomas, **214–215**
- differential diagnosis, **215**
- prognosis, **215**
Lymphoid hyperplasia, inflammatory and reactive, **328–329**
- diagnostic checklist, **329**
- differential diagnosis, **329**
- immunohistochemistry, **329**
Lymphoid proliferation, reactive, pulmonary lymphoma vs., **141**
Lymphoma, **704, 705**
- anaplastic large cell. *See* Anaplastic large cell lymphoma.
- angioimmunoblastic, **366–367**
    differential diagnosis, **367**
    genetic testing, **367**
    immunohistochemistry, **367**
- bone, **628–629**
    diagnostic checklist, **629**
    differential diagnosis, **629**
    immunohistochemistry, **629**
- breast, **464–465**
    differential diagnosis, **465**
- bronchus-associated, **141**

- in cerebrospinal fluid, **190–191**
    - differential diagnosis, **191**
- choroidal, **691**
- classic Hodgkin, **374–375**
    - differential diagnosis, **375**
    - immunohistochemistry, **375**
- cysts vs., **385**
- desmoplastic small round cell tumor vs., **679**
- diffuse large B-cell. See Diffuse large B-cell lymphoma.
- gastric, **162–163**
    - differential diagnosis, **163**
    - gastric adenocarcinoma vs., **161**
- high-grade B-cell lymphoma, with *MYC* and *BCL2* &/or *BCL6* rearrangements, Burkitt lymphoma vs., **353**
- Hodgkin. See Hodgkin lymphoma.
- inflammatory and granulomatous conditions vs., **421**
- intra- and peripancreatic splenules vs., **577**
- large cell neuroendocrine carcinoma vs., **77**
- liver metastasis vs., **513**
- low-grade, with marked plasmacytic differentiation, plasmacytoma vs., **357**
- lymphoblastic
    - Burkitt lymphoma vs., **353**
    - mantle cell lymphoma vs., **347**
    - mediastinal thymoma vs., **487**
    - metastatic tumors of mediastinum vs., **495**
- lymphocyte-rich effusion vs., **197**
- malignant, Ewing sarcoma vs., **626**
- medullary thyroid carcinoma vs., **300**
- meningeal, aseptic and Mollaret meningitis vs., **182**
- mucosa-associated lymphoid tissue, **141**
- neuroendocrine tumor/carcinoma vs., **171**
- nodular lymphocyte-predominant Hodgkin, **372–373**
    - differential diagnosis, **373**
    - follicular lymphoma vs., **351**
    - immunohistochemistry, **373**
- non-Hodgkin
    - inflammatory and reactive lymphoid hyperplasia vs., **329**
    - metastatic tumors of mediastinum vs., **495**
- nonglial neoplasms vs., **705**
- normal salivary gland and sialadenitis on aspiration vs., **383**
- other malignancies in urinary cytology vs., **249**
- pancreas, **596–597**
    - differential diagnosis, **597**
- pancreatic neuroendocrine tumor vs., **587**
- peripheral T-cell, ALK(+) anaplastic large cell vs., **369**
- plasmablastic. See Plasmablastic lymphoma.
- primary and metastatic nonepithelial tumors, **415**
- primary effusion, **216–217**
    - diagnostic checklist, **216**
    - differential diagnosis, **217**
    - prognosis, **217**
- primary/metastatic, ductal carcinoma and variants of invasive mammary carcinoma vs., **452**
- pulmonary, **140–141**
    - diagnostic checklist, **141**
    - differential diagnosis, **141**
- rare extrathyroidal lesions presenting as thyroid nodules, **311**
- renal, **545**
    - diagnostic checklist, **545**
    - differential diagnoses, **545**
- sarcoma vs., **213**
- secondary involvement of stomach by lymphoma, gastric lymphoma vs., **163**
- small cell carcinoma vs., **129, 210**
- small cell neuroendocrine carcinoma vs., **77**
- small lymphocytic, **342–343**
    - differential diagnosis, **343**
    - immunohistochemistry, **343**
    - prognosis, **343**
- suspected lymphoma, FNA sample prep and triage in evaluating, **326–327**
- T-cell lymphoblastic, **370–371**
    - differential diagnosis, **371**
    - genetic testing, **371**
    - immunohistochemistry, **371**
- T-lymphoblastic
    - mediastinal large B-cell lymphoma vs., **359**
- thyroid, **306–307**
    - differential diagnoses, **306**
    - genetic testing, **307**
    - immunohistochemistry, **307**
- urinary cytology, **231**
Lymphomatosum, papillary cystadenoma, cysts vs., **385**
Lymphoplasmacytic lymphoma, **344–345**
- differential diagnosis, **345**
- genetic testing, **345**
- with immunoglobulin inclusions, adult-type rhabdomyoma vs., **655**
- immunohistochemistry, **345**
- nodal marginal zone lymphoma vs., **349**
- small lymphocytic lymphoma vs., **343**
Lynch syndrome, medullary carcinoma associated with, **592**

M

Macrofollicular subtype, papillary thyroid carcinoma subtypes, **292**
- differential diagnosis, **292**
Male breast cancer, gynecomastia vs., **431**
Malignancies
- in cervicovaginal cytology, uncommon, **78–81**
    - adenoid basal carcinoma, **79**
    - adenoid cystic carcinoma, **79**
    - adenosarcoma, **79**
    - adenosquamous carcinoma, **78–79**
    - epithelioid trophoblastic tumor, **79**
    - Ewing sarcoma, **79**
    - lymphoma, **78**
    - melanoma, **78**
    - primitive neuroectodermal tumor, **79**
    - sarcomas, **79**
    - small round blue cell tumors, **79**
- granulomatous lymphadenitis, infectious and sarcoid, **331**

INDEX

- high-grade, renal medullary carcinoma vs., **541**
- mycobacteria and other bacterial infections vs., **115**
- nonhematologic, large B-cell lymphoma vs., **355**
- parasitic organisms in respiratory cytology vs., **111**
- recurrent, esophagitis and Barrett esophagus vs., **153**
- sarcoidosis and other immune-related conditions vs., **117**
- in urinary cytology, **248–249**
  - diagnostic checklist, **248**
  - differential diagnosis, **249**
- vegetable matter vs., miscellaneous findings including contaminants, **121**

Malignant effusion
- carcinomas, **208–211**
  - diagnostic checklist, **210**
  - differential diagnosis, **210**
  - prognosis, **209**
- mesothelioma, **204–207**
  - differential diagnosis, **205**
  - international system category, **205**
  - prognosis, **205**
- sarcomas, **212–213**
  - characteristics in body cavity fluid, **213**
  - differential diagnosis, **213**
  - prognosis, **213**

Malignant entities, smooth muscle tumors vs., **653**
Malignant fibrous histiocytoma. See Undifferentiated pleomorphic sarcoma.
Malignant lymphoma
- Ewing sarcoma vs., **626**
- HPV-positive head and neck squamous cell carcinoma vs., **340**

Malignant melanoma, sarcoma vs., **213**
Malignant mesothelioma
- carcinoma vs., **210**
- sarcoma vs., **213**

Malignant neoplasms
- inflammatory and infectious conditions of liver vs., **501**
- medullary thyroid carcinoma vs., **300**
- rare primary malignant thyroid neoplasms, **310–311**

Malignant peripheral nerve sheath tumor, **493**
- clear cell sarcoma of soft tissue vs., **677**
- fibrosarcoma vs., **643**
- pleomorphic, undifferentiated pleomorphic sarcoma vs., **651**
- smooth muscle tumors vs., **653**
- of soft tissue, intramuscular myxoma vs., **669**
- synovial sarcoma vs., **671**

Malignant phyllodes tumor, angiosarcoma and other sarcomas of breast vs., **462**
Malignant tumors, rare, **136–137**
- diagnostic checklist, **137**
- differential diagnosis, **137**
- immunohistochemistry, **137**

MALT lymphoma. See Mucosa-associated lymphoid tissue lymphoma.
Mammary analogue secretory carcinoma. See also Secretory carcinoma.
- ancillary testing, **380**

Mammary carcinoma
- angiosarcoma and other sarcomas of breast vs., **462**
- primary, lymphomas vs., **465**

Mantle cell lymphoma, **346–347**
- blastoid variant, Burkitt lymphoma vs., **353**
- differential diagnosis, **347**
- follicular lymphoma vs., **351**
- genetic testing, **347**
- immunohistochemistry, **347**
- nodal marginal zone lymphoma vs., **349**
- pleomorphic variant, large B-cell lymphoma vs., **355**
- small lymphocytic lymphoma vs., **343**

Mass, palpable, hepatocellular adenoma, **503**
Mass-forming lesions, neuropathology squash preparations, infectious, **696**
Mass lesion, clear cell renal cell carcinoma, **529**

Mastitis
- acute, **420**
- granulomatous, **421**
- lupus, fat necrosis vs., **423**
- lymphocytic, **421**

Mature cystic teratomas
- germ cell tumors, **491**
- mediastinal cysts and inflammatory lesions vs., **485**

Mediastinal cysts and inflammatory lesions, **484–485**
- developmental anomaly, **485**
- differential diagnosis, **485**

Mediastinal large B-cell lymphoma, **358–359**
- differential diagnosis, **359**
- immunohistochemistry, **359**

Mediastinum, fine-needle aspiration
- anatomic compartments and constituent tumors, **482–483**
- germ cell tumors, **490–491**
  - differential diagnosis, **491**
  - immunohistochemistry, **491**
  - mediastinal large B-cell lymphoma vs., **359**
  - mediastinum, metastatic tumors of mediastinum vs., **495**
- mediastinal cysts and inflammatory lesions, **484–485**
  - developmental anomaly, **485**
  - differential diagnosis, **485**
- metastatic tumors, **494–495**
  - differential diagnosis, **495**
  - immunohistochemistry, **495**
- neurogenic tumors, **492–493**
  - differential diagnosis, **493**
  - genetic testing, **493**
  - immunohistochemistry, **493**
- thymic carcinoma, **488–489**
  - differential diagnosis, **489**
  - immunohistochemistry, **489**
  - metastatic tumors of mediastinum vs., **495**
  - prognosis, **489**
- thymoma, **486–487**
  - differential diagnosis, **487**
  - immunohistochemistry, **487**

Medullary carcinoma, **450, 591**
- anaplastic thyroid carcinoma vs., **304**
- follicular neoplasm/suspicious for follicular neoplasm vs., **282**

- HPV-positive head and neck squamous cell carcinoma vs., 340

Medullary thyroid carcinoma, 298–301
- diagnostic checklist, 300
- differential diagnosis, 300
- follicular neoplasm, oncocytic (Hürthle cell) type vs., 285
- genetic predisposition, 299
- genetic testing, 300
- metastatic carcinoma to thyroid vs., 308
- oncocytic subtype vs., papillary thyroid carcinoma subtypes, 292
- papillary thyroid carcinoma, classic subtype vs., 288
- parathyroid cyst, adenoma, and carcinoma vs., 319
- poorly differentiated thyroid carcinoma vs., 303
- prognosis, 299

Medulloblastoma (MB), 189

Melanin, pigmented thyroid lesions and crystals, 275

Melanoma, 705
- angiosarcoma vs., 663
- carcinoma vs., 210
- clear cell sarcoma of soft tissue vs., 677
- epithelioid hemangioendothelioma vs., 661
- epithelioid sarcoma vs., 673
- fine-needle aspiration, 471–472
- liver metastasis vs., 513
- lymphoid effusion and lymphomas vs., 215
- malignant, anaplastic thyroid carcinoma vs., 304
- markers, immunocytochemistry, 725
- metastatic
    angiosarcoma and other sarcomas of breast vs., 462
    lobular carcinoma vs., 457
    lymph nodes, 336–337
    malignant, primary renal sarcomas vs., 544
    medullary thyroid carcinoma vs., 300
    metastatic tumors to kidney vs., 553
    myofibroblastoma, mammary vs., 447
    plasmacytoma vs., 357
    primary and metastatic nonepithelial tumors, 415
    unusual variants of ductal carcinoma vs., 592
    uveal melanoma vs., 683
    vs. primary origin, pulmonary metastasis, 143
- metastatic tumors of mediastinum vs., 495
- nonglial neoplasms vs., 705
- other malignancies in urinary cytology vs., 249
- plasmablastic lymphoma vs., 361
- primary effusion lymphoma vs., 217
- SMARCA4-deficient undifferentiated tumor vs., 139
- smooth muscle tumors vs., 653
- spindle cell, neurogenic tumors vs., 493
- thyroid lymphoma vs., 306
- uncommon malignancies in cervicovaginal cytology, 78–79
- undifferentiated pleomorphic sarcoma vs., 651
- urinary cytology, 231
- uveal tract, 691

MEN1 mutation, parathyroid cyst, adenoma, and carcinoma, 319

Meningeal lymphoma, aseptic and Mollaret meningitis vs., 182

Meningioma, 704, 705
- fibrous subtype, nonglial neoplasms vs., 705
- microcystic/angiomatous subtype, nonglial neoplasms vs., 705
- rare benign and low malignant potential tumors, 135

Meningitis
- aseptic and Mollaret, 182–183
    differential diagnosis, 182
- infectious, 180–181
- neuropathology squash preparations, infectious, 696

Meningothelial cells, reactive, metastasis in cerebrospinal fluid vs., 193

Menstrual endometrium
- atypical glandular cells vs., 66
- endometrial cancers vs., 60
- squamous cell carcinoma of cervix vs., 40

Merkel cell carcinoma
- fine-needle aspiration, 472
- HPV-positive head and neck squamous cell carcinoma vs., 340

Mesenchymal cells, markers of, immunocytochemistry, 725

Mesenchymal chondrosarcoma, 621, 666
- differential diagnosis, 666
- Ewing sarcoma vs., 626

Mesenchymal lesions, helpful cytologic features, 634

Mesenchymal tumors
- primary and metastatic nonepithelial tumors, 415
- rare extrathyroidal lesions presenting as thyroid nodules, 311

Mesoblastic nephroma, cellular, rhabdoid tumor of kidney vs., 552

Mesoblastic nephroma, congenital, 550–552
- clear cell sarcoma of kidney vs., 549
- differential diagnosis, 551
- genetic features, 551
- metanephric stromal tumor vs., 526

Mesothelial cells
- cytomorphology of, in pleural, peritoneal, pericardial, and pelvic fluid and washings, 197
- normal, normal liver cytology vs., 499
- reactive
    characteristics, 197
    differential diagnosis, 197

Mesothelial hyperplasia
- benign reactive, malignant effusion, mesothelioma vs., 205
- endometriosis and endosalpingiosis vs., 219
- reactive, ovarian neoplasms vs., 221

Mesothelioma
- adenocarcinoma vs., 124
- angiosarcoma vs., 662
- differential stains, 223
- endometriosis and endosalpingiosis vs., 219
- metastatic tumors of mediastinum vs., 495
- peritoneal, ovarian neoplasms vs., 221
- rare malignant tumors, 137
- reactive mesothelial cells vs., 197
- SMARCA4-deficient undifferentiated tumor vs., 139
- smooth muscle tumors vs., 653

INDEX

MET mutations, papillary renal cell carcinoma, **533**
Metabolic disorders, hepatocellular carcinoma, **509**
Metanephric adenofibroma, metanephric stromal tumor vs., **526**
Metanephric adenoma, **524–525**
- differential diagnosis, **525**
- immunohistochemistry, **525**
- nephroblastoma vs., **547**

Metanephric stromal tumor, **526**
- classification, **526**
- congenital mesoblastic nephroma vs., **551**
- differential diagnosis, **526**

Metaplasia
- intestinal, **158–159**
    differential diagnosis, **159**
- oncocytic, oncocytoma of salivary gland vs., **391**

Metaplastic carcinoma of breast, **450–451**
- angiosarcoma and other sarcomas of breast vs., **462**
- phyllodes tumor vs., **459**

Metastasis
- in cerebrospinal fluid, **192–193**
    ancillary test, **193**
    differential diagnosis, **193**
    prognosis, **193**
- fine-needle aspiration, **472**
- liver, **512–513**
    diagnostic checklist, **512**
    differential diagnosis, **513**
- parathyroid cyst, adenoma, and carcinoma vs., **319**
- parotid gland, metastatic carcinoma, **413**
- pulmonary, **142–143**
    differential diagnosis, **143**
    immunohistochemistry, **143**
    molecular testing, **143**
- rare malignant tumors vs., **137**
- small cell carcinoma vs., **129**
- submandibular gland, metastatic carcinoma, **413**

Metastatic adenocarcinoma
- adenocarcinoma of urinary bladder vs., **247**
- chordoma vs., **615**
- hepatocellular carcinoma vs., **509**
- immunocytochemistry, **725**

Metastatic anaplastic carcinoma, unusual variants of ductal carcinoma vs., **592**
Metastatic breast carcinoma, **193**
- prognostic and predictive markers, **725**
- with signet-ring cells, unusual variants of ductal carcinoma vs., **592**

Metastatic carcinoid tumor, carcinoid tumor vs., **543**
Metastatic carcinoma, **412–413, 704, 705**
- ampulla/bile duct/pancreatic duct adenocarcinoma vs., **167**
- classic Hodgkin lymphoma vs., **375**
- collecting duct carcinoma vs., **540**
- colon, columnar cell subtype vs., papillary thyroid carcinoma subtypes, **291**
- diagnostic checklist, **413**
- differential diagnosis, **413**
- endometrial, columnar cell subtype vs., papillary thyroid carcinoma subtypes, **291**
- gastric
    lobular carcinoma vs., **457**
    unusual variants of ductal carcinoma vs., **592**
- hepatocellular, unusual variants of ductal carcinoma vs., **592**
- immunohistochemistry, **413**
- lung and other organs, thymic carcinoma vs., **489**
- lymph nodes, **336–337**
    immunohistochemistry, **337**
    mediastinal large B-cell lymphoma vs., **359**
- nonglial neoplasms vs., **705**
- nongynecologic, ovarian neoplasms vs., **221**
- osteosarcoma vs., **617**
- pancreatic ductal adenocarcinoma vs., **589**
- renal cell, serous microcystic adenoma vs., **579**
- small cell
    adrenal cortical adenoma vs., **561**
    cytology of normal adrenal gland vs., **559**
- to thyroid, **308–309**
    differential diagnoses, **308**
    genetic testing, **309**
    immunohistochemistry, **309**
    prognosis, **309**
- urothelial carcinoma vs., **555**

Metastatic diseases, adenocarcinoma, not otherwise specified vs., **403**
Metastatic epithelial tumors, renal lymphomas vs., **545**
Metastatic lung carcinomas, **193**
Metastatic lymphoma, ductal carcinoma and variants of invasive mammary carcinoma vs., **452**
Metastatic malignancies
- epithelial/epithelioid tumors, primary brain tumors vs., **189**
- glioblastoma vs., **701**
- high-grade, pheochromocytoma vs., **567**
- lymph nodes, **336–337**
    immunohistochemistry, **337**
- melanoma, primary renal sarcomas vs., **544**
- normal liver cytology vs., **499**
- reactive mesothelial cells vs., **197**

Metastatic melanoma, primary and metastatic nonepithelial tumors, **415**
Metastatic neuroblastoma to orbit, **690**
Metastatic neuroendocrine carcinoma, desmoplastic small round cell tumor vs., **679**
Metastatic oncocytic malignancies, follicular neoplasm, oncocytic (Hürthle cell) type vs., **285**
Metastatic renal cell carcinoma
- acinic cell carcinoma vs., **395**
- metastatic carcinoma vs., **413**

Metastatic small cell carcinoma
- bone lymphoma vs., **629**
- small cell neuroendocrine carcinoma vs., **77**

Metastatic squamous cell carcinoma
- metastatic carcinoma vs., **413**
- squamous cell carcinoma vs., **127**

Metastatic tumors
- adrenal cortical carcinoma vs., **563**
- to adrenal gland, **564–565**
    diagnostic checklist, **564**

INDEX

  differential diagnosis, **565**
- of bone, **630–631**
  differential diagnosis, **631**
  immunohistochemistry, **631**
- of breast, **464–465**
  differential diagnosis, **465**
  granular cell tumor of breast vs., **439**
- clear cell renal cell carcinoma vs., **529**
- ductal carcinoma and variants of invasive mammary carcinoma vs., **451–452**
- to kidney, **553**
  diagnostic checklist, **553**
  differential diagnosis, **553**
- mediastinum, **494–495**
  differential diagnosis, **495**
  immunohistochemistry, **495**
- neuroendocrine
  carcinoid and atypical carcinoid vs., **133**
  large cell neuroendocrine carcinoma vs., **131**
  medullary thyroid carcinoma vs., **300**
  pancreatic neuroendocrine tumor vs., **587**

Michaelis-Gutmann bodies, **527**
Microglandular adenosis, ductal carcinoma and variants of invasive mammary carcinoma vs., **451**
Microglandular hyperplasia
- atypical glandular cells vs., **66**
- benign mimic, gynecologic, **19–20**
- endocervical adenocarcinoma, variants and mimics vs., **53**

Microliths, **121**
Micropapillary carcinoma
- of breast, invasive, papillary neoplasms vs., **442**
- invasive, **450**

Microsatellite instability, urothelial carcinoma, **555**
Microsporidial keratitis, **687**
Milan system, salivary gland aspiration biopsies, **379–380**
Mild cytologic atypia, atypia of undetermined significance/follicular lesion of undetermined significance, **277**
Minocycline, pigmented thyroid lesions and crystals, **275**
Miscellaneous findings, including contaminants, **120–121**
- differential diagnosis, **121**

Mixed medullary and follicular (follicular/parafollicular) carcinomas, medullary thyroid carcinoma vs., **300**
Molecular techniques, **728–733**
- advantages and disadvantages of different types of specimens for molecular testing, **728–729**
- applicable techniques, **728**
- applications of in situ hybridization, **729–730**
- carcinoma of unknown primary, **730**
- cytogenetics and molecular alterations of sarcomas, **732**
- issues related to, **731**
- molecular testing for mutations and fusions using NGS, **730–731**
- molecular testing of indeterminate thyroid FNAs, **730**

Molecular testing in gynecologic cytology, HPV, **84–87**
- ASCCP management guidelines based on immediate and 5-year risk of CIN3+, **87**
- high-risk HPV-positive rates by cytology interpretation, **87**
- widely used HPV testing platforms, **87**

Mollaret meningitis, **182–183**
- differential diagnosis, **182**

Molluscum contagiosum
- in Pap tests, **17**
- Tzanck smears, **470**

Monocytoid B-cells, mucosa-associated lymphoid tissue lymphoma, **163**
Monophasic synovial sarcoma, solitary fibrous tumor vs., **667**
Monotonous lymphoid infiltrate, atypia of undetermined significance/follicular lesion of undetermined significance, **277**
Mucinous carcinoma, **450**
- fibroadenoma vs., **436**
- mucocele-like lesion vs., **433**

Mucinous cystic neoplasm, of pancreas, **580–581**
- differential diagnosis, **581**
- intraductal papillary mucinous neoplasm of pancreas vs., **583**
- pancreatic ductal adenocarcinoma, **589**
- prognosis, **581**
- serous microcystic adenoma vs., **579**

Mucinous neoplasm of pancreas, normal pancreas cytology vs., **571**
Mucinous pattern, salivary gland aspirates, **379**
Mucinous tubular and spindle cell carcinoma of kidney, **542**
- differential diagnoses, **542**
- primary renal sarcomas vs., **544**

Mucocele-like lesion (MLL), **432–433**
- differential diagnosis, **433**

Mucocele-like tumor, ductal carcinoma and variants of invasive mammary carcinoma vs., **451**
Mucoepidermoid carcinoma, **396–397**
- acinic cell carcinoma vs., **395**
- ancillary testing, **380**
- carcinoma ex pleomorphic adenoma, **401**
- cysts vs., **385**
- diagnostic checklist, **397**
- differential diagnosis, **397**
- genetic testing, **397**
- low-grade, normal salivary gland and sialadenitis vs., **383**
- oncocytoma of salivary gland vs., **391**
- primary high-grade, metastatic carcinoma vs., **413**
- prognosis, **397**
- sclerosing with eosinophilia, **310–311**
  thyroid lymphoma vs., **306**

Mucor species, respiratory cytology, **109**
Mucosa-associated lymphoid tissue (MALT) lymphoma, **141, 163**
- chronic lymphocytic/Hashimoto thyroiditis vs., **271**

Mucus extravasation reaction, mucoepidermoid carcinoma vs., **397**
Müllerian tumors, immunocytochemistry, **725**
Multinucleated giant cells
- benign gynecologic mimic, **21**

INDEX

- unusual variants of ductal carcinoma vs., **592**
Multiple endocrine neoplasia type 1, adrenal cortical carcinoma, **563**
Multiple endocrine neoplasia type 2, medullary thyroid carcinoma, **299**
Multiple endocrine neoplasia type 2B, medullary thyroid carcinoma, **299**
Multiple sclerosis, neurodegenerative disease vs., **187**
Mumps virus, pancreatitis, **575**
MYC protooncogene, Burkitt lymphoma, **353**
Mycobacteria and other bacterial infections, **114–115**
- diagnostic checklist, **115**
- differential diagnosis, **115**
Mycobacterial lymphadenitis, atypical, granulomatous lymphadenitis, infectious and sarcoid vs., **332**
Mycobacterial thyroiditis, **273**
Mycobacterium avium-intracellulare (MAI), parasitic infections vs., **149**
Mycobacterium tuberculosis, mycobacteria and other bacterial infections, **115**
Mycobacterium tuberculosis lymphadenitis, granulomatous lymphadenitis, infectious and sarcoid vs., **332**
Mycosis fungoides, **364–365**
- differential diagnosis, **365**
- genetic testing, **365**
- immunohistochemistry, **365**
Myeloid sarcoma, plasmablastic lymphoma vs., **361**
Myoepithelial carcinoma, **410**
- carcinoma ex pleomorphic adenoma, **401**
- differential diagnosis, **410**
Myoepithelial-rich pleomorphic adenoma, myoepithelial carcinoma vs., **410**
Myoepithelioma, **390**
- differential diagnoses, **390**
- myoepithelial carcinoma vs., **410**
- pleomorphic adenoma vs., **387**
Myofibroblastic sarcoma, low-grade, **646–647**
- differential diagnosis, **647**
- immunohistochemistry, **647**
- myofibroblastoma vs., **645**
- prognosis, **647**
Myofibroblastic tumors, inflammatory
- low-grade myofibroblastic sarcoma vs., **647**
- lymphomas vs., **465**
- rare benign and low malignant potential tumors, **135**
Myofibroblastoma, **644–645**
- differential diagnosis, **645**
- genetic testing, **645**
- immunohistochemistry, **645**
- mammary, **446–447**
    differential diagnosis, **447**
    prognosis, **447**
- prognosis, **645**
Myofibroma/myofibromatosis, low-grade myofibroblastic sarcoma vs., **647**
Myofibromatosis, low-grade myofibroblastic sarcoma vs., **647**
Myofibrosarcoma
- low-grade, fibrosarcoma vs., **643**
- smooth muscle tumors vs., **653**

Myolipoma, **637**
Myomelanocytic tumor, alveolar soft part sarcoma vs., **675**
Myositis/fasciitis, proliferative, **664–665**
Myositis ossificans, **665**
Myxofibrosarcoma, low-grade, intramuscular myxoma vs., **669**
Myxoid chondrosarcoma
- extraskeletal, mesenchymal chondrosarcoma vs., **666**
- intramuscular myxoma vs., **669**
Myxoid edema, localized, intramuscular myxoma vs., **669**
Myxoid fibroadenoma
- ductal carcinoma and variants of invasive mammary carcinoma vs., **451**
- mucocele-like lesion vs., **433**
Myxoid leiomyoma, intramuscular myxoma vs., **669**
Myxoid liposarcoma
- benign adipose tissue tumors vs., **637**
- cytologic/small biopsy categorization of primary soft tissue tumors, **635**
- intramuscular myxoma vs., **669**
- liposarcoma vs., **639**
Myxoid nerve sheath tumors, intramuscular myxoma vs., **669**
Myxoid pleomorphic liposarcoma, liposarcoma vs., **639**
Myxolipoma, **637**
Myxoma, intramuscular, **668–669**
Myxopapillary ependymoma, **701**

N

Nano cell block, cell block techniques, **712**
Nasopharyngeal carcinoma, HPV-positive head and neck squamous cell carcinoma vs., **340**
Navicular cells, low-grade squamous intraepithelial lesion and mimics vs., **29**
Navigation bronchoscopy, respiratory cytology, **100**
Necator, parasitic infections vs., **149**
Necrosis
- extensive, atypical cells with, mediastinal cysts and inflammatory lesions vs., **485**
- fat, **422–423**
    differential diagnosis, **423**
    prognosis, **423**
- pulmonary alveolar proteinosis and mimics vs., **119**
Needle tract seeding, superficial aspiration technique, **257**
Neisseria gonorrhoeae, molecular testing in gynecologic cytology, **86**
Neoplasia
- in adults, **691**
- in children, **690–691**
Neoplasms, granulomatous thyroiditis vs., **273**
Neoplastic C-cell hyperplasia, medullary thyroid carcinoma, **299**
Neoplastic glial process, reactive vs., **701**
Nephroblastoma (Wilms tumor), **546–547**
- blastemal-predominant, clear cell sarcoma of kidney vs., **549**
- conditions associated, **547**

- congenital mesoblastic nephroma vs., **551**
- developmental anomaly, **547**
- differential diagnosis, **547**
- genetic abnormalities, **547**
- immunohistochemistry, **547**
- prognosis, **547**

Nephrogenic adenoma (metaplasia), **234**

Nephrogenic nephroma. *See* Metanephric adenoma.

Nephroma, congenital mesoblastic, clear cell sarcoma of kidney vs., **549**

Nerve sheath tumors
- malignant peripheral, fibrosarcoma vs., **643**
- myxoid, intramuscular myxoma vs., **669**
- pleomorphic malignant peripheral, undifferentiated pleomorphic sarcoma vs., **651**

Neuroblastoma, **493**
- bone lymphoma vs., **629**
- Ewing sarcoma vs., **626**
- metastatic tumors of mediastinum vs., **495**
- nephroblastoma vs., **547**
- neurogenic tumors vs., **493**

Neurodegenerative diseases, **186–187**
- differential diagnosis, **187**
- prognosis, **187**

Neuroendocrine carcinoma, **170–171**
- cervix, **76–77**
    - differential diagnosis, **77**
    - prognosis, **77**
- colorectal, **171**
- differential diagnosis, **171**
- esophageal, **171**
- etiology/pathogenesis, **171**
- gastric, **171**
- metastatic
    - desmoplastic small round cell tumor vs., **679**
    - large cell neuroendocrine carcinoma vs., **131**
- NUT carcinoma vs., **138**
- primary vs. metastasis, pulmonary metastasis, **143**
- small bowel, **171**
- SMARCA4-deficient undifferentiated tumor vs., **139**

Neuroendocrine/small cell carcinoma, of thyroid gland, **311**

Neuroendocrine tumor, **170–171**
- colorectal, **171**
- differential diagnosis, **171**
- ductal carcinoma and variants of invasive mammary carcinoma, **450**
- esophageal, **171**
- gastric, **171**
- metastatic
    - carcinoid and atypical carcinoid vs., **133**
    - medullary thyroid carcinoma vs., **300**
- metastatic tumors of mediastinum vs., **495**
- pancreatic, **586–587**
    - differential diagnosis, **587**
    - intra- and peripancreatic splenules vs., **577**
    - prognosis, **587**
- small bowel, **171**

Neurofibroma, **493**
- primary and metastatic nonepithelial tumors, **415**

Neurogenic cysts, **485**

Neurogenic tumors
- mediastinum, **492–493**
    - differential diagnosis, **493**
    - genetic testing, **493**
    - immunohistochemistry, **493**
- primary and metastatic nonepithelial tumors, **415**

Neuropathology squash preparations
- glial neoplasms, **700–703**
    - differential diagnosis, **701**
    - molecular alterations, **700**
    - WHO CNS 2021, revised integrated diagnoses, **700**
- infectious, **696–699**
    - bacterial infection, **696**
    - cysticercosis, **696, 697**
    - differential diagnosis, **697**
    - diffuse processes, **696**
    - fungal infection, **696, 697**
    - mass-forming lesions, **696**
    - toxoplasmosis, **696, 697**
    - tuberculosis, **696, 697**
    - viral infection, **696, 697**
- nonglial neoplasms, **704–707**
    - differential diagnosis, **705**

Neurosarcoidosis, neurodegenerative disease vs., **187**

Nipple aspiration fluid, risk assessment of breast cancer, **466–467**

Nocardia, mycobacteria and other bacterial infections, **115**

Nodal marginal zone B-cell lymphoma, **349**
- mantle cell lymphoma vs., **347**

Nodal marginal zone lymphoma, **348–349**
- differential diagnosis, **349**
- follicular lymphoma vs., **351**
- genetic testing, **349**
- lymphoplasmacytic lymphoma vs., **345**
- prognosis, **349**
- small lymphocytic lymphoma vs., **343**

Nodular adenosis/adenosis tumor, fibroadenoma vs., **436**

Nodular fasciitis, **664**
- intramuscular myxoma vs., **669**
- myofibroblastoma, mammary vs., **447**
- myofibroblastoma vs., **645**
- primary and metastatic nonepithelial tumors, **415**

Nodular goiter. *See* Adenomatous nodule, of thyroid gland.

Nodular hyperplasia, anaplastic thyroid carcinoma, **305**

Nodular lymphocyte-predominant Hodgkin lymphoma, **372–373**
- differential diagnosis, **373**
- follicular lymphoma vs., **351**
- immunohistochemistry, **373**

Nodular oncocytic hyperplasia, oncocytoma of salivary gland vs., **391**

Nodular sclerosis, mediastinal large B-cell lymphoma vs., **359**

Nodules, ultrasound, **261**

Non-Hodgkin lymphoma
- carcinoma vs., **210**
- effusions, **215**
- inflammatory and infectious conditions of liver vs., **501**
- inflammatory and reactive lymphoid hyperplasia vs., **329**

INDEX

- metastatic tumors of mediastinum vs., **495**

Non-small cell carcinoma
- immunocytochemistry, **725**
- large cell neuroendocrine carcinoma vs., **131**
- not otherwise specified, adenocarcinoma vs., **124**
- rare malignant tumors vs., **137**

Non-small cell lung carcinoma
- metastatic tumors of mediastinum vs., **495**
- SMARCA4-deficient undifferentiated tumor vs., **139**

Nonepithelial tumors, primary and metastatic, **414–415**

Nongynecologic cytology, cytopreparatory techniques and instrumentation, **710–715**
- cytology processing, **710–713**. *See also* Cytology processing.
- instrumentation, **713**
- troubleshooting common problems, **713**

Nongynecologic metastatic carcinoma, ovarian neoplasms vs., **221**

Nonhematologic malignancies, nonhematological, large B-cell lymphoma vs., **355**

Noninfectious benign condition, urine cytology, **234–235**
- diagnostic checklist, **235**
- differential diagnosis, **235**
- prognosis, **235**

Noninfectious granulomas, mycobacteria and other bacterial infections vs., **115**

Noninvasive follicular thyroid neoplasm with papillary-like nuclear features (NIFTP), **282, 290**
- follicular neoplasm/suspicious for follicular neoplasm vs., **281–282**
- papillary thyroid carcinoma, classic subtype vs., **288**

Nonkeratinizing squamous cell carcinoma, **157**
- cytopathology, squamous cell carcinoma of cervix, **39–40**

Nonmesenchymal neoplasms, pleomorphic, undifferentiated pleomorphic sarcoma vs., **651**

Nonmycobacterial infections, of lymph nodes, granulomatous lymphadenitis, infectious and sarcoid vs., **332**

Nonneoplastic conditions, fine-needle aspiration, **470–471**

Nonneoplastic ductal epithelium, reactive, pancreatic ductal adenocarcinoma vs., **589**

Nonneoplastic findings, mimics, and artifacts, benign and infectious conditions, gynecologic cytopathology, **18–25**

Nonossifying fibroma/benign fibrous histiocytoma, giant cell tumor vs., **607**

Nonpolio enterovirus encephalomyelitis, neurodegenerative disease vs., **187**

Nonproliferative and proliferative changes, in breast, **424–427**
- differential diagnosis, **425**
- prognosis, **424–425**

Nontuberculous mycobacteria (NTM), mycobacteria and other bacterial infections, **115**

Normal cellular components, in pleural, peritoneal, pericardial, and pelvic fluid and washings, **196–199**
- differential diagnosis, **197**
- international system for serous fluid cytopathology, **197**
- reactive mesothelial cells, differential diagnosis, **197**

Normal cerebrospinal fluid, and contamination by normal elements, **176–179**
- clinical complications, **176**
- differential diagnosis, **177**
- immunochemistry for differential diagnosis of benign intracranial/intraspinal cells, **177**
- reporting criteria, **176–177**

Normal fibroadipose tissue, benign adipose tissue tumors vs., **637**

Normal foveolar epithelium, esophagitis and Barrett esophagus vs., **153**

Normal gastrointestinal tract mucosa, mucinous cystic neoplasm of pancreas vs., **581**

Normal liver
- cytology, **498–499**
    - differential diagnosis, **499**
- hemangioma of liver vs., **507**

Normal mesothelial cells, normal liver cytology vs., **499**

Normal pancreas, cytology, **570–571**
- anatomic features, **570**
- architectural organization, **570**
- clinical utility of pancreas FNA, **570–571**
- differential diagnosis, **571**

Normal pancreatic acinar tissue, acinar cell carcinoma vs., **595**

Normal Pap test, **14–15**
- cell types, **14**
- cytopathology, **14–15**
    - endocervical cells, **15**
    - endometrial cells, **15**
    - squamous cells, **14–15**
    - squamous metaplastic cells, **15**
- physiology/histology of cervix, **14**

Normal salivary gland and sialadenitis
- acinic cell carcinoma vs., **395**
- on aspiration, **382–383**
    - diagnostic checklist, **383**
    - differential diagnosis, **383**

Normal striated muscle, adult-type rhabdomyoma vs., **655**

Normal urinary cytology, specimen types, and reporting terminology, **228–231**
- cytologic features, **229**
- diagnostic checklist, **229**
- specimen types, **228**
    - catheterization, **228**
    - ileal conduit specimens, **229**
    - urinary bladder wash (barbotage), **228**
    - voided (clean catch), **228**

NRAS gene mutation, medullary thyroid carcinoma, **299**

Nuclear details, anal cytology, **97**

Nuclear matrix protein 22, urinary cytology, **253**

Nuclear pleomorphism, **701**

Nucleus pulposus, normal cerebrospinal fluid and contamination by normal elements, differential diagnosis, **177**

NUT carcinoma, **138**
- differential diagnosis, **138**
- SMARCA4-deficient undifferentiated tumor vs., **139**

INDEX

O

Obesity, gynecomastia and, **431**
Ocular infectious diseases, **686**
- with impact on vision, **686–687**

Oligodendroglial neoplasms, astrocytic vs., **701**
Oligodendrogliomas, **701**
Oncocytic (Hürthle Cell) aspirates, atypia of undetermined significance/follicular lesion of undetermined significance, **277**
Oncocytic cell pattern, salivary gland aspirates, **378**
Oncocytic cells
- salivary gland carcinomas with, Warthin tumor vs., **389**
- in tumors
    - metastatic tumors to adrenal gland vs., **565**
    - metastatic tumors to kidney vs., **553**

Oncocytic hyperplasia, nodular, oncocytoma of salivary gland vs., **391**
Oncocytic metaplasia, oncocytoma of salivary gland vs., **391**
Oncocytic neoplasm, medullary thyroid carcinoma vs., **300**
Oncocytic papillary thyroid carcinoma, follicular neoplasm, oncocytic (Hürthle cell) type vs., **285**
Oncocytic subtype, papillary thyroid carcinoma subtypes, **291–292**
- differential diagnosis, **292**

Oncocytoma
- kidney, **522–523**
    - carcinoid tumor vs., **543**
    - chromophobe renal cell carcinoma vs., **537**
    - differential diagnosis, **523**
    - immunohistochemistry, **523**
    - molecular abnormalities, **523**
    - normal kidney cytology vs., **517**
- salivary gland, **391**
    - differential diagnosis, **391**
    - immunohistochemistry, **391**
- Warthin tumor vs., **389**

Ophthalmic cytology, **682–685**
- acellular samples, **683**
- cytologic preparation and interpretation, **682–683**
- intraocular solid tumors, **683**
- triaging of vitreous and aqueous humor, **683**
- types of samples, **682**

Ophthalmic cytopathology
- infectious, **686–689**
    - bacterial infections, **687**
    - fungal infections, **687**
    - ocular infectious diseases, **686**
    - parasitic infections, **687**
    - risk of vision loss through several mechanisms, **687**
    - specimen handling, **687**
    - viral infections, **687**
    - worldwide infectious ocular diseases, **686**
- neoplastic, **690–695**
    - aspiration cytology, **690**
    - exfoliative cytology, **690**
    - intraocular neoplasia, **691**
    - intraocular retinoblastoma, **691**
    - orbital neoplasia, **690, 691**
    - touch imprint cytology, **690**

Oral contaminant
- mycobacteria and other bacterial infections vs., **115**
- respiratory cytology, **101**

Oral contraceptive use, hepatocellular adenoma, **503**
Orbital neoplasia
- adults, **691**
- children, **690**

Oropharyngeal lesions, viral infections vs., **151**
Osteoblastic osteosarcoma, **616**
Osteoblastoma, **608–609**
- differential diagnosis, **609**
- osteosarcoma vs., **617**

Osteoblastoma-like osteosarcoma, osteoblastoma vs., **609**
Osteofibrous dysplasia, adamantinoma vs., **611**
Osteoid osteoma, osteoblastoma vs., **609**
Osteolipoma, **637**
Osteoma, osteoid, osteoblastoma vs., **609**
Osteomyelitis
- bone lymphoma vs., **629**
- Langerhans cell histiocytosis vs., **613**

Osteosarcoma, **616–619**
- chondroblastic, **616**
    - chondrosarcoma vs., **622**
- chondroblastoma-like, chondroblastoma vs., **605**
- chondromas of bone and soft tissue vs., **603**
- differential diagnosis, **617**
- fibroblastic, **616**
- giant cell-rich, giant cell tumor vs., **607**
- high-grade surface, **617**
- immunohistochemistry, **617**
- low-grade central, **616**
- mesenchymal chondrosarcoma vs., **666**
- metastatic tumors of bone vs., **631**
- osteoblastic, **616**
- osteoblastoma-like, osteoblastoma vs., **609**
- parosteal, **616**
- periosteal, **616**
- prognosis, **616**
- small cell, **616**
- telangiectatic, **616**

Ovarian adenocarcinoma, other malignancies in urinary cytology vs., **249**
Ovarian neoplasms, **220–221**
- differential diagnosis, **221**
- prognosis, **221**

P

Pain
- abdominal, hepatocellular adenoma, **503**
- clear cell renal cell carcinoma, **529**

Palpable mass, hepatocellular adenoma, **503**
Pancreas
- anaplastic carcinoma of, metastatic tumors to kidney vs., **553**

INDEX

- lymphoma of, **596–597**
  - differential diagnosis, **597**
- secondary tumors of, **596–597**
  - differential diagnosis, **597**

Pancreas, fine-needle aspiration
- acinar cell carcinoma, **594–595**
  - differential diagnosis, **595**
  - prognosis, **595**
- cytology of normal pancreas, **570–571**
  - anatomic features, **570**
  - architectural organization, **570**
  - clinical utility of pancreas FNA, **570–571**
  - differential diagnosis, **571**
- intra- and peripancreatic splenules, **577**
  - differential diagnosis, **577**
- intraductal papillary mucinous neoplasm, **582–583**
  - differential diagnosis, **583**
  - genetic testing, **583**
  - mucinous cystic neoplasm of pancreas vs., **581**
- lymphoepithelial cyst of pancreas, **576**
  - differential diagnosis, **576**
- lymphoma and secondary tumors of pancreas, **596–597**
- mucinous cystic neoplasm, of pancreas, **580–581**
  - differential diagnosis, **581**
  - prognosis, **581**
- pancreatic cytology reporting terminology, **572–573**
  - ancillary and molecular testing in pancreatic cysts/cystic neoplasms, **573**
  - approach to cytologic analysis of pancreatic cysts, **573**
  - role of molecular testing, **573**
  - WHO International System for Reporting Pancreatic Cytopathology, **572–573**
- pancreatic ductal adenocarcinoma, **588–589**
  - differential diagnosis, **589**
  - genetic testing, **589**
  - precursor lesions, **589**
- pancreatic neuroendocrine tumor, **586–587**
  - differential diagnosis, **587**
  - prognosis, **587**
- pancreatitis, **574–575**
  - autoimmune, **575**
  - differential diagnosis, **575**
  - drug induced, **575**
  - genetic testing, **575**
  - infectious agents, **575**
  - metabolic induced, **575**
  - trauma induced, **575**
  - vascular induced, **575**
- serous microcystic adenoma, **578–579**
  - differential diagnosis, **579**
- solid pseudopapillary neoplasm of pancreas, **584–585**
  - differential diagnosis, **585**
  - prognosis, **585**
- unusual variants of ductal carcinoma, **590–593**
  - differential diagnosis, **592**
  - genetic testing, **592**
  - prognosis, **591**

Pancreatic acinar tissue, normal, acinar cell carcinoma vs., **595**

Pancreatic adenocarcinoma, pancreatitis vs., **575**

Pancreatic cytology reporting terminology, **572–573**
- ancillary and molecular testing in pancreatic cysts/cystic neoplasms, **573**
- approach to cytologic analysis of pancreatic cysts, **573**
- role of molecular testing, **573**
- WHO International System for Reporting Pancreatic Cytopathology, **572–573**

Pancreatic ductal adenocarcinoma, **588–589**
- differential diagnosis, **589**
- genetic testing, **589**
- precursor lesions, **589**

Pancreatic ducts
- ampulla/bile duct reactive changes, **164–165**
- carcinoma, ampulla/bile duct/pancreatic duct reactive changes vs., **165**
- dysplasia, ampulla/bile duct/pancreatic duct reactive changes vs., **165**
- gastrointestinal cytology, **147**
- intraepithelial neoplasia, ampulla/bile duct/pancreatic duct adenocarcinoma vs., **167**

Pancreatic endocrine neoplasm
- acinar cell carcinoma vs., **595**
- pancreatic ductal adenocarcinoma vs., **589**
- solid pseudopapillary neoplasm of pancreas vs., **585**

Pancreatic intraepithelial neoplasm
- intraductal papillary mucinous neoplasm of pancreas vs., **583**
- pancreatic ductal adenocarcinoma vs., **589**

Pancreatic neuroendocrine tumor, **586–587**
- differential diagnosis, **587**
- intra- and peripancreatic splenules vs.., **577**
- prognosis, **587**

Pancreatitis, **574–575**
- autoimmune, **575**
  - lymphoma and secondary tumors of pancreas vs., **597**
- differential diagnosis, **575**
- drug induced, **575**
- genetic testing, **575**
- infectious agents, **575**
- metabolic induced, **575**
- trauma induced, **575**
- vascular induced, **575**

Pancreatoblastoma
- acinar cell carcinoma vs., **594**
- unusual variants of ductal carcinoma vs., **592**

Pap test and glandular cells status post hysterectomy, endometrial cells, **70–71**
- differential diagnosis, **71**

Papanicolaou, George Nicholas, **4**

Papanicolaou stain, **5**

Papanicolaou (Pap) test, **4, 14–15**
- adequacy reporting categories, **10**
- American Society for Colposcopy and Cervical Pathology Guidelines, **11**
- automated screening, **9**
- cell types, **14**
- cervical cancer screening and, **4–7**
  - conventional smear to liquid-based cytology, **7**
  - evolution of Pap test, **7**
  - First National Cytology Conference (1948), **5**

INDEX

HPV molecular testing (ASC-US/LSIL Triage Study) (ALTS), **6–7**
- cytopathology, **14–15**
    - endocervical cells, **15**
    - endometrial cells, **15**
    - squamous cells, **14–15**
    - squamous metaplastic cells, **15**
- endocervical/transformation zone component, **11**
    - cellularity, **11**
    - special pointers in adequacy evaluation, **11**
- infectious and other organisms in, **16–17**
    - bacteria, **17**
    - *Chlamydia trachomatis*, **17**
    - cytopathology, **16–17**
    - fungi, **16–17**
    - protozoa, **16**
    - viruses, **17**
- liquid-based Pap tests, **8**
    - advantages, **9**
- physiology/histology of cervix, **14**
- reporting system
    - Atlas of Exfoliative Cytology, **5**
    - Bethesda Reporting System, **6**
    - Cervical Intraepithelial Neoplasia Reporting System, **5**
    - class reporting system, **5**
    - Dysplasia Reporting System, **5**
- sample collection, **8**
    - broom, **8**
    - cotton swab, **8**
    - patient instructions, **8**
    - recommendations, **8**
    - slide preparation, **8**
    - spatula and brush, **8**
- squamous cellularity criteria, **10–11**
    - conventional Pap smear, **10**
    - liquid-based preparations, **10–11**
- test types
    - comparison of conventional Pap smears and liquid-based Pap test, **9**
    - conventional Pap smears, **8**
    - liquid-based Pap tests, **8**

Papillary adenoma, papillary renal cell carcinoma vs., **533**

Papillary carcinoma
- of breast, **441**
- invasive, **450**
- of primary vs. metastatic origin, pulmonary metastasis, **143**

Papillary clear cell renal cell carcinoma, papillary renal cell carcinoma vs., **533**

Papillary cystadenoma lymphomatosum. *See also* Warthin tumor.
- cysts vs., **385**

Papillary hyperplasia
- papillary thyroid carcinoma, classic subtype vs., **288**
- within renal cysts, papillary renal cell carcinoma vs., **533**

Papillary mucinous neoplasm, intraductal, of pancreas, **582–583**
- differential diagnosis, **583**
- genetic testing, **583**

Papillary neoplasms, of breast, **440–445**
- atypical, **442**
- benign, **441**
- differential diagnosis, **442**
- malignant, **441**
- prognosis, **441**

Papillary renal cell carcinoma, **532–533**
- clear cell, **534–535**
    - differential diagnosis, **535**
    - genetic testing, **535**
    - immunohistochemistry, **535**
    - prognosis, **535**
- clear cell papillary renal cell carcinoma vs., **535**
- clear cell renal cell carcinoma vs., **529**
- collecting duct carcinoma vs., **540**
- differential diagnosis, **533**
- immunohistochemistry, **533**
- metanephric adenoma vs., **525**
- mucinous tubular and spindle carcinoma vs., **542**
- normal kidney cytology vs., **517**
- *TFE3*- and *TFEB*-rearranged renal cell carcinomas vs., **539**

Papillary squamotransitional carcinoma, variant of squamous cell carcinoma of cervix, **40**

Papillary squamous carcinoma, variant of squamous cell carcinoma of cervix, **40**

Papillary thyroid carcinoma
- adenomatous (benign follicular) nodule vs., **268**
- classic subtype, **286–289**
    - diagnostic checklist, **288**
    - differential diagnosis, **288**
    - genetic testing, **288**
    - prognosis, **287**
- granulomatous thyroiditis vs., **273**
- Graves disease/diffuse toxic goiter vs., **274**
- medullary thyroid carcinoma vs., **300**
- metastatic to lymph nodes, cribriform adenocarcinoma vs., **411**
- poorly differentiated thyroid carcinoma vs., **303**
- subtypes, **290–297**
    - clear cell subtype, **292**
    - columnar cell subtype, **291**
        - differential diagnosis, **291**
    - cystic subtype, **290–291**
    - diagnostic checklist, **292**
    - diffuse sclerosing subtype, **291**
    - hobnail subtype, **291**
    - macrofollicular subtype, **292**
        - differential diagnosis, **292**
    - oncocytic subtype, **291–292**
        - differential diagnosis, **292**
    - solid subtype, **292**
        - differential diagnosis, **292**
    - tall cell subtype, **291**
    - Warthin-like subtype, **292**
        - differential diagnosis, **292**

Papillary urothelial carcinoma, papillary renal cell carcinoma vs., **533**

Papillary urothelial neoplasm, low-grade, reactive urothelial changes vs., **239**

Papilloma
- breast, **441–442**

INDEX

- ductal carcinoma and variants of invasive mammary carcinoma vs., **452**
- fibroadenoma vs., **436**
- nonproliferative and proliferative changes in breast vs., **425**
- rare benign and low malignant potential tumors, **135**

Paraganglioma, **493**
- adult-type rhabdomyoma vs., **655**
- alveolar soft part sarcoma vs., **675**
- medullary thyroid carcinoma vs., **300**
- metastatic tumors of mediastinum vs., **495**
- neurogenic tumors vs., **493**
- rare extrathyroidal lesions presenting as thyroid nodules, **311**

Paragonimus species, respiratory cytology, **111**
Parakeratosis, benign finding, gynecologic, **19**
Parasitic infections, **148–149**
- differential diagnosis, **149**
- mycobacteria and other bacterial infections vs., **115**
- ophthalmic cytopathology, **687**

Parasitic organisms, in respiratory cytology, **110–111**
- differential diagnosis, **111**

Parathyroid adenoma/carcinoma
- follicular neoplasm/suspicious for follicular neoplasm vs., **282**
- rare extrathyroidal lesions presenting as thyroid nodules, **311**

Parathyroid cyst, adenoma, and carcinoma, **318–321**
- differential diagnosis, **319**
- genetic testing, **319**
- immunohistochemistry, **319**

Parathyroid gland, fine-needle aspiration, parathyroid cyst, adenoma, and carcinoma, **318–321**
- differential diagnosis, **319**
- genetic testing, **319**
- immunohistochemistry, **319**

Parietal cells, gastrointestinal cytology, **147**
Paris system, **229–231**
- morphologic criteria, **231**
- relative risk, **231**

Parosteal osteosarcoma, **616**
Parotid gland metastasis, metastatic carcinoma, **413**
Pathogens, vegetable matter vs., miscellaneous findings including contaminants, **121**
PCR. *See* Polymerase chain reaction.
Pediatric small round blue cell sarcoma, **213**
Pelvic endometriosis, **219**
Pemphigus, benign mimic, gynecologic, **21**
Pemphigus vulgaris, squamous cell carcinoma of cervix vs., **40**
Percutaneous FNA and core biopsy, respiratory cytology, **100**
Periareolar fine-needle aspiration, risk assessment of breast cancer, **467**
Pericardial cysts, **485**
Periosteal chondromas, chondromas of bone and soft tissue, **603**
Periosteal chondrosarcoma, **621**
Periosteal osteosarcoma, **616**

Peripheral nerve sheath tumor
- benign, mediastinal cysts and inflammatory lesions vs., **485**
- malignant
  clear cell sarcoma of soft tissue vs., **677**
  fibrosarcoma vs., **643**
  pleomorphic, undifferentiated pleomorphic sarcoma vs., **651**
  smooth muscle tumors vs., **653**
  synovial sarcoma vs., **671**

Peripheral nervous system tumors
- metastatic tumors of mediastinum vs., **495**
- neurogenic tumors vs., **493**

Peripheral neuroepithelioma. *See* Ewing sarcoma.
Peripheral T-cell lymphoma, **362–363**
- ALK(+) anaplastic large cell lymphoma vs., **369**
- classic Hodgkin lymphoma vs., **375**
- differential diagnosis, **363**
- genetic testing, **363**
- immunohistochemistry, **363**
- mycosis fungoides vs., **365**
- nodal marginal zone lymphoma vs., **349**
- not otherwise specified, angioimmunoblastic lymphoma vs., **367**

Peritoneal mesothelioma, ovarian neoplasms vs., **221**
Peritoneal washings, **196**
Perivascular epithelioid cell neoplasm, clear cell sarcoma of soft tissue vs., **677**
Pheochromocytoma, **566–567**
- adrenal cortical carcinoma vs., **563**
- cytology of normal adrenal gland, **559**
- differential diagnosis, **567**
- genetic testing, **567**
- malignancy, **567**
- prognosis, **567**

Phyllodes tumor, **458–459**
- differential diagnosis, **459**
- fibroadenoma vs., **436**
- malignant
  angiosarcoma and other sarcomas of breast vs., **462**
  ductal carcinoma and variants of invasive mammary carcinoma vs., **452**
- prognosis, **459**

Pia-arachnoid cells
- ependymal cells vs., **177**
- normal cerebrospinal fluid and contamination by normal elements, differential diagnosis, **177**

Pigmented thyroid lesions and crystals, **275**
Pigmented villonodular synovitis, giant cell tumor of tendon sheath vs., **649**
Pilocytic astrocytoma, **701**
Pilomatrixoma
- cysts vs., **385**
- fine-needle aspiration, **471**

Pinworm, parasitic infections vs., **149**
Pituitary adenoma, **704, 705**
- nonglial neoplasms vs., **705**

Plasma cell granuloma, plasmacytoma vs., **357**
Plasma cell myeloma
- plasmablastic, plasmablastic lymphoma vs., **361**

INDEX

- small cell variant, lymphoplasmacytic lymphoma vs., **345**
- urinary cytology, **231**

Plasma cells, lymph node aspiration, **325**

Plasmablastic lymphoma, **360–361**
- differential diagnosis, **361**
- immunohistochemistry, **361**
- plasmacytoma vs., **357**
- primary effusion lymphoma vs., **217**

Plasmablastic plasma cell myeloma
- plasmablastic lymphoma vs., **361**
- primary effusion lymphoma vs., **217**

Plasmacytoma, **356–357**
- differential diagnosis, **357**
- immunohistochemistry, **357**
- myoepithelial carcinoma vs., **410**
- myoepithelioma vs., **390**
- pancreatic neuroendocrine tumor vs., **587**

Pleomorphic adenoma
- adenoid cystic carcinoma vs., **393**
- ancillary testing, **380**
- basaloid neoplasms, benign and malignant vs., **399**
- carcinoma ex, **400–401**
    - genetic testing, **401**
    - pleomorphic adenoma vs., **387**
- myoepithelial-rich, myoepithelial carcinoma vs., **410**
- myoepithelioma vs., **390**
- oncocytoma of salivary gland vs., **391**
- polymorphous adenocarcinoma vs., **405**
- salivary gland, **386–387**
    - diagnostic checklist, **387**
    - differential diagnosis, **387**
    - genetic testing, **387**
    - immunohistochemistry, **387**

Pleomorphic leiomyosarcoma, undifferentiated pleomorphic sarcoma vs., **651**

Pleomorphic liposarcoma
- liposarcoma vs., **639**
- undifferentiated pleomorphic sarcoma vs., **651**

Pleomorphic malignancies, pleomorphic-type rhabdomyosarcoma vs., **655**

Pleomorphic malignant peripheral nerve sheath tumor, undifferentiated pleomorphic sarcoma vs., **651**

Pleomorphic nonmesenchymal neoplasms, undifferentiated pleomorphic sarcoma vs., **651**

Pleomorphic rhabdomyosarcoma, undifferentiated pleomorphic sarcoma vs., **651**

Pleomorphic sarcoma
- dedifferentiated, undifferentiated pleomorphic sarcoma vs., **651**
- smooth muscle tumors vs., **653**
- undifferentiated, **650–651**
    - differential diagnosis, **651**
    - genetic testing, **651**
    - immunohistochemistry, **651**
    - prognosis, **651**
- undifferentiated, osteosarcoma vs., **617**

Pleomorphic tumors, metastatic tumors of mediastinum vs., **495**

Pleural, peritoneal, pericardial, and pelvic fluid and washings
- autoimmune diseases, **202–203**
    - diagnostic checklist, **203**
    - differential diagnosis, **203**
    - prognosis, **203**
- endometriosis and endosalpingiosis, **218–219**
- immunocytochemistry, histochemistry, and other ancillary techniques, **222–225**
- infectious conditions, **200–201**
    - diagnostic checklist, **201**
    - differential diagnosis, **201**
    - prognosis, **201**
- lymphoid effusion and lymphomas, **214–215**
- malignant effusion, carcinomas, **208–211**
- malignant effusion, mesothelioma, **204–207**
    - differential diagnosis, **205**
    - international system category, **205**
    - prognosis, **205**
- malignant effusion, sarcomas, **212–213**
- normal cellular components and reactive mesothelial proliferations, **196–199**
- ovarian neoplasms, **220–221**
    - differential diagnosis, **221**
    - prognosis, **221**
- primary effusion lymphoma, **216–217**

Pleural cavity endometriosis, **219**

Pleuropulmonary blastoma, rare malignant tumors, **137**

Pneumocystis, fungal organisms in respiratory cytology vs., **109**

Pneumocystis pneumonia
- and mimics, **106–107**
    - diagnostic checklist, **107**
    - differential diagnosis, **107**
- pulmonary alveolar proteinosis and mimics vs., **119**

Pneumocytes, benign and reactive changes, **103**

Pneumocytoma (sclerosing hemangioma), rare benign and low malignant potential tumors vs., **135**

Pneumothorax, superficial aspiration technique, **257**

Pollen
- gynecologic artifact, **21**

Pollen,
- parasitic infections vs., **149**

Polymerase chain reaction (PCR), **222**

Polymorphous adenocarcinoma, **404–405**
- adenoid cystic carcinoma vs., **393**
- cribriform adenocarcinoma vs., **411**
- differential diagnosis, **405**
- immunohistochemistry, **405**
- low-grade. *See also* Polymorphous adenocarcinoma. carcinoma ex pleomorphic adenoma, **401**
- prognosis, **405**

Polyomavirus. *See also* Infectious benign conditions.
- high-grade urothelial dysplasia/carcinoma/carcinoma in situ vs., **243**
- infectious benign conditions, **236**

Polyp, inflammatory, colorectal adenoma/carcinoma vs., **169**

Polyp, inflammatory fibroid, spindle cell neoplasms of gastrointestinal tract vs., **173**

INDEX

Polyps, endometrial
- atypical glandular cells vs., **66**
- endometrial cancers vs., **60**

Poorly differentiated adenocarcinoma
- esophageal squamous cell carcinoma vs., **157**
- neuroendocrine tumor/carcinoma vs., **171**

Poorly differentiated carcinoma
- angiosarcoma vs., **663**
- gastric lymphoma vs., **163**
- lymphoid effusion and lymphomas vs., **215**
- plasmacytoma vs., **357**
- primary effusion lymphoma vs., **217**
- primary renal sarcomas vs., **544**
- sarcomas, **213**

Poorly differentiated primary vs. metastasis, pulmonary metastasis, **143**

Poorly differentiated squamous cell carcinoma, **157**
- esophageal adenocarcinoma vs., **155**
- immunocytochemistry, **725**

Poorly differentiated synovial sarcoma, **671**

Poorly differentiated (high-grade) thymic epithelial neoplasm. *See* Thymic carcinoma.

Poorly differentiated thyroid carcinoma, **302–303**
- differential diagnosis, **303**
- follicular neoplasm/suspicious for follicular neoplasm vs., **282**
- genetic testing, **303**

Posterior shadowing, definition, **260**

Postinfectious encephalomyelitis, neurodegenerative disease vs., **187**

Posttrachelectomy sampling, endocervical adenocarcinoma in situ, **47**

Posttransplant lymphoproliferative disorders (PTLD), Epstein-Barr virus (EBV)-associated, renal lymphomas, **545**

Preexisting benign thyroid disease, papillary thyroid carcinoma, classic subtype, **287**

Primary brain tumors, **188–189**
- diagnostic checklist, **189**
- differential diagnosis, **189**

Primary breast tumor, metastatic tumors vs., **465**

Primary carcinoma
- endocervical
    cytologic distinction between endocervical and endometrial primaries, **60**
    endometrial cancers vs., **60**
- extrauterine, endometrial cancers vs., **60**

Primary chondrosarcoma, **621**

Primary CNS vasculitis, neurodegenerative disease vs., **187**

Primary effusion lymphoma, **216–217**
- diagnostic checklist, **216**
- differential diagnosis, **217**
- prognosis, **217**

Primary effusion lymphoma-like lymphoma, primary effusion lymphoma vs., **217**

Primary epithelial tumors, renal lymphomas vs., **545**

Primary high-grade mucoepidermoid carcinoma, metastatic carcinoma vs., **413**

Primary lymphoma, ductal carcinoma and variants of invasive mammary carcinoma vs., **452**

Primary malignant thyroid neoplasms, rare, **310–311**

Primary mammary carcinoma, lymphomas vs., **465**

Primary mediastinal large B-cell lymphoma, classic Hodgkin lymphoma vs., **375**

Primary renal sarcomas, **544**
- diagnostic checklist, **544**
- differential diagnoses, **544**
- mucinous tubular and spindle carcinoma vs., **542**

Primary sarcoma
- anaplastic thyroid carcinoma vs., **304**
- ductal carcinoma and variants of invasive mammary carcinoma vs., **452**
- phyllodes tumor vs., **459**

Primary soft tissue lesions, approach to cytologic/small biopsy diagnosis, **634–635**

Primary squamous cell carcinoma, metastatic carcinoma vs., **413**

Primary tumors
- bone, approach to cytologic/small biopsy diagnosis, **600–601**
- pancreatic, lymphoma and secondary tumors of pancreas vs., **597**

Primitive neuroectodermal tumor
- bone lymphoma vs., **629**
- osteosarcoma vs., **617**

Progressive multifocal leukoencephalopathy, **696**
- neurodegenerative disease vs., **187**

Proliferation, reactive lymphoid, pulmonary lymphoma vs., **141**

Proliferative breast changes, **424–427**
- with atypia, **425**
- differential diagnosis, **425**
- prognosis, **424–425**
- without atypia, **425**

Proliferative endometrium, **91**

Proliferative myositis/fasciitis, **664–665**

Prostate adenocarcinoma
- direct invasion by, adenocarcinoma of urinary bladder vs., **247**
- other malignancies in urinary cytology vs., **249**

Protozoa, in Pap tests, **16**

Psammoma bodies, **121, 209**
- salivary gland aspirates, **379**

Pseudoangiomatous stromal hyperplasia
- angiosarcoma and other sarcomas of breast vs., **462**
- fibroadenoma vs., **436**

Pseudoasbestos bodies, asbestos bodies vs., miscellaneous findings including contaminants, **121**

Pseudocyst
- lymphoepithelial cyst of pancreas vs., **576**
- mucinous cystic neoplasm of pancreas vs., **581**
- serous microcystic adenoma vs., **579**

Pseudogoblet cells, gastritis and intestinal metaplasia vs., **159**

Pseudogynecomastia, gynecomastia vs., **431**

Pseudomyogenic hemangioendothelioma, epithelioid hemangioendothelioma vs., **661**

Pseudopapillary neoplasm, solid, acinar cell carcinoma vs., **595**

Pseudosarcomatous myofibroblastic proliferations, **234**

INDEX

Pulmonary adenocarcinoma, other malignancies in urinary cytology vs., **249**
Pulmonary alveolar proteinosis (PAP), and mimics, **118–119**
- diagnostic checklist, **119**
- differential diagnosis, **119**

Pulmonary blastoma
- adenocarcinoma vs., **124**
- rare malignant tumors, **137**

Pulmonary lymphoma, **140–141**
- diagnostic checklist, **141**
- differential diagnosis, **141**

Pulmonary metastasis, **142–143**
- differential diagnosis, **143**
- immunohistochemistry, **143**
- molecular testing, **143**

Q

Quality assurance, **717–718**
- cytology-histology correlations, **717**
- diagnostic statistics, **718**
- examination of unknown slides, **718**
- measures of screening performance, **717–718**
- proficiency testing, **718**
- retrospective reviews, **717**
- turnaround time, **718**

Quality improvement and laboratory management for cytopathology, **716–721**
- Cytology-Specific Mandates Under CLIA 1988 (USA specific), **720**
- quality assurance, **717–718**
    - cytology-histology correlations, **717**
    - diagnostic statistics, **718**
    - examination of unknown slides, **718**
    - measures of screening performance, **717–718**
    - proficiency testing, **718**
    - retrospective reviews, **717**
    - turnaround time, **718**
- quality control, **716–717**
    - preanalytical, **717**
- quality improvement, **716**
- risk reduction, **718–719**
    - amended reports from retrospective reviews, **718**
    - dashboards for performance improvement, **719**
    - documentation of knowledge of changes, **718**
    - laboratory safety, **719**
    - quality assurance/quality control specific to FNA service, **719**
    - record keeping per CLIA '88, **718**
    - significant and unexpected findings, **719**
    - slide handling and retention, **718**
    - solid policies and procedures, **718**
    - telecytopathology for rapid on-site evaluation, **719**
    - workload limits, **718–719**
- total quality management, **716**

R

Radial scar/complex sclerosing lesion, **428–429**
- differential diagnosis, **429**
- prognosis, **429**

Radial sclerosing lesion/sclerosing adenosis, ductal carcinoma and variants of invasive mammary carcinoma vs., **451**

Radiation changes
- angiosarcoma and other sarcomas of breast vs., **462**
- benign finding, gynecologic, **19**

Radiation effect
- high-grade urothelial dysplasia/carcinoma/carcinoma in situ vs., **243**
- low-grade squamous intraepithelial lesion and mimics vs., **29**
- rare primary thyroid lesion and, **311**
- reactive urothelial changes, **239**

Radiation esophagitis, **153**
- esophageal squamous cell carcinoma vs., **157**

Radiation exposure
- anaplastic thyroid carcinoma, **305**
- angiosarcoma and other sarcomas of breast, **461**

Rare benign and low malignant potential tumors, **134–135**
- diagnostic checklist, **135**
- differential diagnosis, **135**

Rare malignant tumors, **136–137**
- diagnostic checklist, **137**
- differential diagnosis, **137**

Rare thyroid neoplasms
- primary malignant thyroid neoplasms, **310–311**
- rare extrathyroidal lesions presenting as thyroid nodules, **311**
- rare primary thyroid lesions/neoplasms, **311**

Reactive and neoplastic soft tissue entities, **664–665**
- abdominal fat pad aspiration for amyloid, **665**
- ganglioneuroma, **665**
- myositis ossificans, **665**
- nodular fasciitis, **664**
- proliferative myositis/fasciitis, **664–665**

Reactive atypia
- ampulla/bile duct/pancreatic duct adenocarcinoma vs., **167**
- gastric adenocarcinoma vs., **161**
- ulcer, esophageal adenocarcinoma vs., **155**

Reactive cells, benign and reactive changes, **103**

Reactive changes, **102–105**
- adenocarcinoma vs., **124**
- ampulla/bile duct/pancreatic duct, **164–165**
    differential diagnosis, **165**
- anal cytology vs., **97**
- atypical urothelial cells vs., **241**
- carcinoid and atypical carcinoid vs., **133**
- colorectal adenoma/carcinoma vs., **169**
- diagnostic checklist, **103**
- differential diagnosis, **103**
- esophageal squamous cell carcinoma vs., **157**
- squamous cell carcinoma vs., **127**

INDEX

- viral infections vs., **113**
Reactive cytologic atypia, viral infections vs., **151**
Reactive effect, high-grade urothelial dysplasia/carcinoma/carcinoma in situ vs., **243**
Reactive endocervical glands, endocervical adenocarcinoma in situ vs., **47**
Reactive glandular cells, benign and reactive changes, **103**
Reactive glial process, neoplastic vs., **701**
Reactive hyperplasia
- angioimmunoblastic lymphoma vs., **367**
- C-cell, medullary thyroid carcinoma, **299**
- follicular
    mantle cell lymphoma vs., **347**
- interfollicular, nodal marginal zone lymphoma vs., **349**
- mesothelial
    benign, malignant effusion, mesothelioma vs., **205**
    ovarian neoplasms vs., **221**
- mycosis fungoides vs., **365**
Reactive lymphoid hyperplasia, nodular lymphocyte-predominant Hodgkin lymphoma vs., **371**
Reactive lymphoid proliferation, pulmonary lymphoma vs., **141**
Reactive meningothelial cells, metastasis in cerebrospinal fluid vs., **193**
Reactive mesothelial cells
- characteristics, **197**
- differential diagnosis, **197**
- endometriosis and endosalpingiosis vs., **219**
- malignant effusion, mesothelioma vs., **204**
- mesothelioma vs., **197**
Reactive mesothelial hyperplasia, **196**
- benign, malignant effusion, mesothelioma, **204**
- ovarian neoplasms vs., **221**
Reactive mesothelial proliferations, in pleural, peritoneal, pericardial, and pelvic fluid and washings, **196–199**
- differential diagnosis, **197**
- international system for serous fluid cytopathology, **197**
- normal cellular components, **196**
Reactive nonneoplastic ductal epithelium, pancreatic ductal adenocarcinoma vs., **589**
Reactive process
- follicular lymphoma vs., **351**
- small lymphocytic lymphoma vs., **343**
Reactive squamous cells, benign and reactive changes, **103**
Reactive urothelial changes, **238–239**
- diagnostic checklist, **239**
- differential diagnosis, **239**
Rectovaginal fistula, benign mimic, gynecologic, **21**
Recurrent breast carcinoma, prognostic and predictive markers, **725**
Recurrent malignancy, esophagitis and Barrett esophagus vs., **153**
Recurrent urothelial carcinoma, ileal conduit specimens vs., **233**
Reflux esophagitis, esophageal squamous cell carcinoma vs., **157**
Regenerative changes, colorectal adenoma/carcinoma vs., **169**
Renal cell carcinoma
- adrenal cortical carcinoma vs., **563**
- in children, alveolar soft part sarcoma vs., **675**
- chromophobe, **536–537**
    differential diagnosis, **537**
    immunohistochemistry, **537**
    prognosis, **537**
- clear cell
    angiomyolipoma vs., **521**
    low-grade, normal kidney cytology vs., **517**
- high-grade, urothelial carcinoma vs., **555**
- low-grade, carcinoid tumor vs., **543**
- metastatic
    acinic cell carcinoma vs., **395**
    metastatic carcinoma vs., **413**
    serous microcystic adenoma vs., **579**
- metastatic tumors of mediastinum vs., **495**
- other malignancies in urinary cytology vs., **249**
- papillary
    metanephric adenoma vs., **525**
    mucinous tubular and spindle carcinoma vs., **542**
    normal kidney cytology vs., **517**
- renal pelvic cytology, **251**
- sarcomatoid
    angiomyolipoma vs., **521**
    mucinous tubular and spindle carcinoma vs., **542**
    primary renal sarcomas vs., **544**
- translocation-associated
    clear cell papillary renal cell carcinoma vs., **535**
    clear cell renal cell carcinoma vs., **529**
Renal cysts, **518–519**
- Bosniak classification system, **519**
- diagnostic checklist, **518**
- differential diagnosis, **519**
Renal lymphomas, **545**
- diagnostic checklist, **545**
- differential diagnoses, **545**
Renal medullary carcinoma, **541**
- collecting duct carcinoma vs., **540**
- differential diagnoses, **541**
- rhabdoid tumor of kidney vs., **552**
Renal pelvic cytology, **250–251**
Renal pelvis
- entities encountered, **251**
- methods for sampling, **251**
Renal sarcomas, primary, mucinous tubular and spindle carcinoma vs., **542**
Renal tubular cells, benign, clear cell renal cell carcinoma vs., **529**
Repair
- adenocarcinoma in situ and mimics, **48**
- atypical
    atypical glandular cells vs., **66**
    endometrial cancers vs., **60**
    squamous cell carcinoma of cervix vs., **40**
- squamous tissue, robust, atypical squamous cells of undetermined significance vs., **35**
Reserve cell hyperplasia
- benign and reactive changes, **103**
- small cell carcinoma vs., **129**

INDEX

Respiratory tract, exfoliative cytopathology, including lung FNAs
- adenocarcinoma, **122–125**
    - diagnostic checklist, **124**
    - differential diagnosis, **124**
    - prognosis, **123**
- benign and reactive changes, **102–105**
    - diagnostic checklist, **103**
    - differential diagnosis, **103**
- carcinoid and atypical carcinoid, **132–133**
    - diagnostic checklist, **133**
    - differential diagnosis, **133**
- fungal organisms in respiratory cytology, **108–109**
    - diagnostic checklist, **109**
    - differential diagnosis, **109**
- large cell neuroendocrine carcinoma, **130–131**
    - diagnostic checklist, **131**
    - differential diagnosis, **131**
- miscellaneous findings including contaminants, **120–121**
    - differential diagnosis, **121**
- mycobacteria and other bacterial infections, **114–115**
- NUT carcinoma, **138**
    - differential diagnosis, **138**
    - SMARCA4-deficient undifferentiated tumor vs., **139**
- parasitic organisms in respiratory cytology, **110–111**
    - differential diagnosis, **111**
- *Pneumocystis* pneumonia and mimics, **106–107**
    - diagnostic checklist, **107**
    - differential diagnosis, **107**
- pulmonary alveolar proteinosis and mimics, **118–119**
    - diagnostic checklist, **119**
    - differential diagnosis, **119**
- pulmonary lymphoma, **140–141**
    - diagnostic checklist, **141**
    - differential diagnosis, **141**
- pulmonary metastasis, **142–143**
    - differential diagnosis, **143**
    - immunohistochemistry, **143**
    - molecular testing, **143**
- rare benign and low malignant potential tumors, **134–135**
    - diagnostic checklist, **135**
    - differential diagnosis, **135**
- rare malignant tumors, **136–137**
    - diagnostic checklist, **137**
    - differential diagnosis, **137**
- sarcoidosis, and other immune-related conditions, **116–117**
    - diagnostic checklist, **117**
    - differential diagnosis, **117**
- small cell carcinoma, **128–129**
    - diagnostic checklist, **129**
    - differential diagnosis, **129**
- SMARCA4-deficient undifferentiated tumor, **139**
    - diagnostic checklist, **139**
    - differential diagnosis, **139**
- specimen types in respiratory cytology and adequacy criteria, **100–101**
    - cancer screening, **100**
    - specimen handling, **100**
    - tuberculosis screening, **100**
- squamous cell carcinoma, **126–127**
    - diagnostic checklist, **127**
    - differential diagnosis, **127**
- viral infections, **112–113**
    - diagnostic checklist, **113**
    - differential diagnosis, **113**
    - prognosis, **113**

RET mutation
- medullary thyroid carcinoma, **300**
- parathyroid cyst, adenoma, and carcinoma, **319**

Retained lens fragments, **683**

Retention cysts, **385**
- intraductal papillary mucinous neoplasm of pancreas vs., **583**

Retinoblastoma, intraocular, **690**

Retroperitoneal low-grade liposarcoma, angiomyolipoma vs., **521**

Rhabdoid sarcoma, epithelioid sarcoma vs., **673**

Rhabdoid tumor of kidney, **552**
- clear cell sarcoma of kidney vs., **549**
- congenital mesoblastic nephroma vs., **551**
- differential diagnosis, **552**

Rhabdomyoma, **655**. *See also* Skeletal muscle tumors.
- adult-type
    - differential diagnosis, **655**
    - skeletal muscle tumors vs., **655**
- alveolar soft part sarcoma vs., **675**
- differential diagnosis, **655**
- embryonal-type, skeletal muscle tumors vs., **655**
- fetal type, **655**
- genetics, **655**
- genital type, **655**

Rhabdomyosarcoma, **655**. *See also* Skeletal muscle tumors.
- alveolar-type
    - desmoplastic small round cell tumor vs., **679**
    - skeletal muscle tumors vs., **655**
- bone lymphoma vs., **629**
- differential diagnosis, **655**
- embryonal, **213**
    - differential diagnosis, **655**
    - intramuscular myxoma vs., **669**
- mesenchymal chondrosarcoma vs., **666**
- orbital, in children, **690**
- pleomorphic
    - skeletal muscle tumors vs., **655**
    - undifferentiated pleomorphic sarcoma vs., **651**
- smooth muscle tumors vs., **653**
- spindle cell/sclerosing
    - skeletal muscle tumors vs., **655**

Rheumatoid arthritis (RA) effusion, **202–203**
- differential diagnosis, **203**

Rhodococcus, mycobacteria and other bacterial infections, **115**

Riedel thyroiditis
- anaplastic thyroid carcinoma vs., **304**
- chronic lymphocytic/Hashimoto thyroiditis vs., **271**
- rare primary thyroid lesions/neoplasms, **311**

Risk reduction, cytopathology, **718–719**
- amended reports from retrospective reviews, **718**
- dashboards for performance improvement, **719**

INDEX

- documentation of knowledge of changes, **718**
- laboratory safety, **719**
- quality assurance/quality control specific to FNA service, **719**
- record keeping per CLIA '88, **718**
- significant and unexpected findings, **719**
- slide handling and retention, **718**
- solid policies and procedures, **718**
- telecytopathology for rapid on-site evaluation, **719**
- workload limits, **718–719**

Robust squamous repair, atypical squamous cells of undetermined significance vs., **35**
Romanowsky stain, rare malignant tumors, **137**
ROS1, adenocarcinoma, **124**
Rosai-Dorfman disease (RDD), **334–335**
- differential diagnosis, **335**
- immunohistochemistry, **335**
- prognosis, **335**

Rosette formation, **701**
Round cell lesions, bone lymphoma vs., **629**
Round cell liposarcoma, liposarcoma vs., **639**

S

Salivary duct carcinoma, **406–407**
- ancillary testing, **380**
- carcinoma ex pleomorphic adenoma, **401**
- differential diagnosis, **407**
- other types with high-grade transformation, salivary duct carcinoma vs., **407**
- prognosis, **407**

Salivary gland, fine-needle aspiration
- acinic cell carcinoma, **394–395**
- adenocarcinoma, not otherwise specified, **402–403**
- adenoid cystic carcinoma, **392–393**
- approach to interpretation of salivary gland aspiration biopsies and reporting terminology, **378–381**
- basaloid neoplasms, benign and malignant, **398–399**
- carcinoma ex pleomorphic adenoma, **400–401**
- cribriform adenocarcinoma, **411**
- cysts, **384–385**
- metastatic carcinoma, **412–413**
- mucoepidermoid carcinoma, **396–397**
- myoepithelial carcinoma, **410**
- myoepithelioma, **390**
- normal salivary gland and sialadenitis on aspiration, **382–383**
- oncocytoma, **391**
- pleomorphic adenoma, **386–387**
- polymorphous adenocarcinoma, **404–405**
- primary and metastatic nonepithelial tumors, **414–415**
- salivary duct carcinoma, **406–407**
- secretory carcinoma, **408–409**
  Warthin tumor, **388 389**

Salivary gland analog tumors
- rare benign and low malignant potential tumors, **135**
- rare malignant tumors, **137**

Salivary gland aspiration biopsies, approach to interpretation of, and reporting terminology, **378–381**
- Milan reporting system, **379–380**
- patterns of salivary gland aspirates, **378–379**
- statistics, **379**

Salivary gland basaloid lesions, basaloid neoplasms, benign and malignant vs., **399**
Salivary gland carcinoma, with oncocytic cells, Warthin tumor vs., **389**
Salivary gland neoplasm of uncertain malignant potential, salivary gland aspiration biopsies and reporting terminology, **379, 380**
Salivary gland oncocytoma, adult-type rhabdomyoma vs., **655**

Salivary gland tumors
- adenocarcinoma, not otherwise specified vs., **403**
- adenocarcinoma vs., **124**
- ancillary testing, **380**
- metastatic tumors to kidney vs., **553**

Salmonella, pancreatitis, **575**
Sampling of liver tissue, inadvertent
- adrenal cortical adenoma vs., **561**
- cytology of normal adrenal gland vs., **559**
- kidney oncocytoma vs., **523**

Sarcoidosis
- granulomatous lymphadenitis, infectious and sarcoid vs., **332**
- granulomatous thyroiditis, **273**
- mediastinal cysts and inflammatory lesions vs., **485**
- other immune-related conditions, **116–117**
    diagnostic checklist, **117**
    differential diagnosis, **117**

Sarcoma
- adamantinoma-like Ewing, adamantinoma vs., **611**
- adenosarcoma, uncommon malignancies in cervicovaginal cytology, **79**
- alveolar soft part, **674–677**
    differential diagnosis, **675**
    genetic testing, **675**
    prognosis, **675**
- angiosarcoma vs., **663**
- of breast, **460–463**
    differential diagnosis, **462**
    genetic testing, **461**
    prognosis, **461**
- clear cell, of kidney, congenital mesoblastic nephroma vs., **551**
- dedifferentiated pleomorphic, undifferentiated pleomorphic sarcoma vs., **651**
- epithelioid, **672–673**
    clear cell sarcoma of soft tissue vs., **677**
    differential diagnosis, **673**
    epithelioid hemangioendothelioma vs., **661**
    genetic testing, **673**
    prognosis, **673**
- Ewing, **624–627**
    desmoplastic small round cell tumor vs., **679**
    differential diagnosis, **626**
    immunohistochemistry, **626**
    osteosarcoma vs., **617**

INDEX

prognosis, **625**
uncommon malignancies in cervicovaginal cytology, **79**
- fibrosarcoma vs.
  low-grade fibromyxoid, **643**
  synovial, **643**
- granulocytic, lymphomas vs., **465**
- intraosseous synovial, adamantinoma vs., **611**
- liver metastasis vs., **513**
- low-grade fibromyxoid
  intramuscular myxoma vs., **669**
  low-grade myofibroblastic sarcoma vs., **647**
- low-grade myofibroblastic, **646–647**
  differential diagnosis, **647**
  immunohistochemistry, **647**
  myofibroblastoma vs., **645**
  prognosis, **647**
- metastatic
  angiosarcoma and other sarcomas of breast vs., **462**
  ductal carcinoma and variants of invasive mammary carcinoma vs., **452**
  vs. primary origin, pulmonary metastasis, **143**
- metastatic tumors of mediastinum vs., **495**
- myeloid, plasmablastic lymphoma vs., **361**
- myxofibrosarcoma, low-grade, intramuscular myxoma vs., **669**
- with myxoid stroma, embryonal-type rhabdomyosarcoma vs., **655**
- rare malignant tumors, **137**
- rhabdoid, epithelioid sarcoma vs., **673**
- SMARCA4-deficient undifferentiated tumor vs., **139**
- soft tissue, (non-SRBCT): prognostic factors, **635**
- synovial, **670–671**
  cytogenetics/molecular genetics, **671**
  differential diagnosis, **671**
- uncommon malignancies in cervicovaginal cytology, **79**
- undifferentiated pleomorphic, **650–651**
  differential diagnosis, **651**
  genetic testing, **651**
  immunohistochemistry, **651**
  osteosarcoma vs., **617**
  prognosis, **651**
- urinary cytology, **231**
Sarcomatoid carcinoma, **591**
- smooth muscle tumors vs., **653**
- undifferentiated pleomorphic sarcoma vs., **651**
Sarcomatoid renal cell carcinoma
- angiomyolipoma vs., **521**
- mucinous tubular and spindle carcinoma vs., **542**
- primary renal sarcomas vs., **544**
Schistosoma species, respiratory cytology, **111**
Schwannoma, **493, 704, 705**
- clear cell sarcoma of soft tissue vs., **677**
- myoepithelioma vs., **390**
- myofibroblastoma, mammary vs., **447**
- nonglial neoplasms vs., **705**
- primary and metastatic nonepithelial tumors, **415**
- solitary fibrous tumor vs., **667**
- spindle cell neoplasms of gastrointestinal tract, **172, 173**

Sclerosing adenosis, nonproliferative and proliferative changes in breast, **425**
Sclerosing hemangioma, rare benign and low malignant potential tumors vs., **135**
Sclerosing lesion, radial scar/complex, **428–429**
- differential diagnosis, **429**
- prognosis, **429**
Sclerosing mucoepidermoid carcinoma with eosinophilia
- of thyroid gland, **310–311**
- thyroid lymphoma vs., **306**
Sclerosing sialadenitis (Küttner Tumor), chronic, **383**
Sclerosing variant, Ewing sarcoma, **625, 626**
SDHx mutations, pheochromocytoma associated with, **567**
Secondary chondrosarcoma, **621**
Secondary tumors, of pancreas, **596–597**
- differential diagnosis, **597**
Secretory carcinoma, **408–409, 450**
- acinic cell carcinoma vs., **395**
- differential diagnosis, **409**
- immunohistochemistry, **409**
Secretory endometrium, **91**
Sellar region cysts, nonglial neoplasms vs., **705**
Seminoma
- germ cell tumors vs., **491**
- mediastinal cysts and inflammatory lesions vs., **485**
- mediastinal thymoma vs., **487**
Serous carcinoma, high-grade, **91**
Serous cystic neoplasm
- intraductal papillary mucinous neoplasm of pancreas vs., **583**
- mucinous cystic neoplasm of pancreas vs., **581**
Serous microcystic adenoma, **578–579**
- differential diagnosis, **579**
Serous neoplasms, borderline and low-grade, endometriosis and endosalpingiosis vs., **219**
Serous neoplasms of müllerian origin, **209**
Sialadenitis
- acinic cell carcinoma vs., **395**
- on aspiration, **382–383**
  acute, **382**
  chronic, **383**
  chronic sclerosing, **383**
  diagnostic checklist, **383**
  differential diagnosis, **383**
  granulomatous, **383**
- chronic, mucoepidermoid carcinoma vs., **397**
Sialometaplasia, mucoepidermoid carcinoma vs., **397**
Signal amplification methods, molecular testing in gynecologic cytology, **85**
Signet-ring adenocarcinomas, **210**
Signet-ring cell carcinoma, **591**
Signet-ring cells, breast carcinoma with, unusual variants of ductal carcinoma vs., **592**
Simple cyst, renal cyst vs., **519**
Simpson-Golabi-Behmel syndrome, hepatoblastoma, **511**
Single cells, etiologies for, high-grade squamous intraepithelial lesion and mimics vs., **31**
Single-needle technique, **477**
Sinus histiocytosis with massive lymphadenopathy. *See* Rosai-Dorfman disease.

INDEX

Skeletal muscle tumors, **654–657**
- differential diagnosis, **655**
- genetics, **655**

SLE. *See* Systemic lupus erythematosus.

SMAD4 gene, mutations in, pancreatic ductal adenocarcinoma, **589**

Small &/or basaloid cells, squamous cell carcinoma with, small cell neuroendocrine carcinoma vs., **77**

Small cell carcinoma, **128–129, 209**
- benign and reactive changes vs., **103**
- diagnostic checklist, **129**
- differential diagnosis, **129**
- endometrial cancers vs., **60**
- HPV-positive head and neck squamous cell carcinoma vs., **340**
- large cell neuroendocrine carcinoma vs., **131**
- lymphoid effusion and lymphomas vs., **215**
- lymphoma vs., **210**
- metastatic
    adrenal cortical adenoma vs., **561**
    bone lymphoma vs., **629**
    cytology of normal adrenal gland vs., **559**
    metastatic tumors to adrenal gland vs., **565**
    small cell neuroendocrine carcinoma vs., **77**
- other malignancies in urinary cytology vs., **249**
- pulmonary
    immunocytochemistry, **725**
    metastatic tumors of mediastinum vs., **495**
- pulmonary lymphoma vs., **141**
- squamous cell carcinoma vs., **127**
- urinary cytology, **231**

Small cell neuroendocrine carcinoma, cervix, **77**
- squamous cell carcinoma of cervix vs., **40**

Small cell osteosarcoma, **616**
- Ewing sarcoma vs., **626**

Small cell tumors, metastatic tumors of mediastinum vs., **495**

Small duct papilloma (SDP), **441**

Small intestine, gastrointestinal cytology, **147**

Small lymphocytes, lymph node aspiration, **324**

Small lymphocytic lymphoma, **342–343**
- differential diagnosis, **343**
- immunohistochemistry, **343**
- mantle cell lymphoma vs., **347**
- nodal marginal zone lymphoma vs., **349**
- prognosis, **343**

Small round blue cell tumors
- hepatoblastoma vs., **511**
- lymphoid effusion and lymphomas vs., **215**
- metastatic tumors of mediastinum vs., **495**
- NUT carcinoma vs., **138**
- others, rhabdomyosarcoma vs., **655**
- uncommon malignancies in cervicovaginal cytology, **79**

Small round cell sarcomas, carcinoma vs., **210**

Small round cell tumor, desmoplastic, **678–679**
- differential diagnosis, **679**
- genetic testing, **679**

SMARCA4-deficient undifferentiated tumor, **139**
- diagnostic checklist, **139**
- differential diagnosis, **139**

Smoking
- HPV-positive head and neck squamous cell carcinoma, **339**
- squamous cell carcinoma of cervix, **39**

Smooth muscle tumors, **652–653**
- differential diagnosis, **653**
- immunohistochemistry, **653**

Soft tissue, fine-needle aspiration
- alveolar soft part sarcoma, **674–677**
- angiosarcoma, **662–663**
- approach to cytologic/small biopsy diagnosis of primary soft tissue lesions, **634–635**
- benign adipose tissue tumors, **636–637**
- clear cell sarcoma of soft tissue, **676–677**
- desmoplastic small round cell tumor, **678–679**
- epithelioid hemangioendothelioma, **660–661**
- epithelioid sarcoma, **672–673**
- fibrosarcoma, **642–643**
- giant cell tumor of tendon sheath, **648–649**
- hemangioma, **658–659**
- intramuscular myxoma, **668–669**
- liposarcoma, **638–639**
- low-grade myofibroblastic sarcoma, **646–647**
- mesenchymal chondrosarcoma, **666**
- myofibroblastoma, **644–645**
- other reactive and neoplastic soft tissue entities, **664–665**
- skeletal muscle tumors, **654–657**
- smooth muscle tumors, **652–653**
- solitary fibrous tumor, **667**
- synovial sarcoma, **670–671**
- undifferentiated pleomorphic sarcoma, **650–651**

Solid organ biopsy, **477**

Solid pseudopapillary neoplasm of pancreas, **584–585**
- acinar cell carcinoma vs., **595**
- differential diagnosis, **585**
- intraductal papillary mucinous neoplasm of pancreas vs., **583**
- pancreatic neuroendocrine tumor vs., **587**
- prognosis, **585**

Solid subtype papillary thyroid carcinoma, **292**
- differential diagnosis, **292**

Solid tumors, prognostic and predictive markers, **725**

Solitary fibrous tumor, **667, 704, 705**
- differential diagnosis, **667**
- low-grade myofibroblastic sarcoma vs., **647**
- malignant, **213**
    mesenchymal chondrosarcoma vs., **666**
- nonglial neoplasms vs., **705**
- rare benign and low malignant potential tumors, **135**
- smooth muscle tumors vs., **653**
- spindle cell neoplasms of gastrointestinal tract vs., **173**
- synovial sarcoma vs., **671**

Somatic mutations, papillary thyroid carcinoma, classic subtype, **287**

Specimen adequacy in cervicovaginal cytology, **10–11**
- adequacy reporting categories, **10**
- American Society for Colposcopy and Cervical Pathology Guidelines, **11**
- endocervical/transformation zone component, **11**
    cellularity, **11**

xlvii

INDEX

  special pointers in adequacy evaluation, **11**
 - management, **11**
 - squamous cellularity criteria, **10–11**
    conventional Pap smear, **10**
    liquid-based preparations, **10–11**
Specimen preparation techniques, cytology processing, **710**
 - cytocentrifugation, **710**
 - SurePath nongynecologic processing, **710**
 - ThinPrep and SurePath gynecologic processing, **710**
 - ThinPrep nongynecologic processing, **710**
Specimen types in gastrointestinal cytology and normal cellular components, **146–147**
 - normal cellular components
    esophagus, **147**
    pancreatic and bile ducts, **147**
    small intestine and colorectum, **147**
    stomach, **147**
 - specimen types
    brushing, **146**
    endoscopic ultrasound-guided fine-needle aspiration, **147**
    washing, **146–147**
Specimen types in respiratory cytology and adequacy criteria, **100–101**
 - cancer screening, **100**
 - specimen handling, **100**
 - tuberculosis screening, **100**
Spermatozoa, urinary cytology, **229**
Spherulosis, **683**
Spindle cell carcinoid tumor, neurogenic tumors vs., **493**
Spindle cell carcinoma
 - ductal carcinoma and variants of invasive mammary carcinoma, **450–451**
 - metaplastic, myofibroblastoma, mammary vs., **447**
 - squamous cell carcinoma, variant of squamous cell carcinoma of cervix, **40**
 - synovial sarcoma vs., **671**
Spindle cell lipoma, **637**
Spindle cell malignancies, spindle cell/sclerosing rhabdomyosarcoma vs., **655**
Spindle cell melanoma, neurogenic tumors vs., **493**
Spindle cell neoplasms
 - of gastrointestinal tract, including gastrointestinal stromal tumors, **172–173**
    differential diagnosis, **173**
 - neurogenic tumors vs., **493**
 - solitary fibrous tumor vs., **667**
 - xanthogranulomatous pyelonephritis/malakoplakia vs., **527**
Spindle cell sarcoma-like variant, Ewing sarcoma, **625, 626**
Spindle cell squamous cell carcinoma, esophageal squamous cell carcinoma vs., **157**
Spindle cell thymoma, neurogenic tumors vs., **493**
Spindle cell tumor
 - of breast, fat necrosis vs., **423**
 - mediastinal thymoma vs., **487**
 - metastatic, phyllodes tumor vs., **459**
 - metastatic tumors of mediastinum vs., **495**
Spindle cells, salivary gland aspirates, **379**

Spindle epithelial tumor with thymus-like differentiation, **310**
Spleen, accessory, lymphoma and secondary tumors of pancreas vs., **597**
Sputum, respiratory cytology, **100**
Squamous carcinoma in situ. *See* High-grade squamous intraepithelial lesion.
Squamous cell abnormalities and mimics, gynecologic
 - atypical squamous cells, cannot rule out high-grade squamous intraepithelial lesion, **36–37**
    differential diagnosis, **37**
    prognosis, **37**
 - atypical squamous cells of undetermined significance, **34–35**
    differential diagnosis, **35**
 - high-grade squamous intraepithelial lesion and mimics, **30–33**
    differential diagnosis, **31**
 - low-grade squamous intraepithelial lesion and mimics, **28–29**
    differential diagnosis, **29**
    prognosis, **29**
 - squamous cell carcinoma of cervix, variants and mimics, **38–43**
    basaloid squamous cell carcinoma, **40**
    differential diagnosis, **40**
    human papillomavirus, **39**
    immunohistochemistry, **40**
    papillary squamotransitional carcinoma, **40**
    papillary squamous carcinoma, **40**
    spindle cell squamous cell carcinoma, **40**
    verrucous carcinoma, **40**
Squamous cell carcinoma, **126–127, 209**
 - adenocarcinoma vs., **124**
 - basaloid
    adenoid cystic carcinoma vs., **393**
    HPV-positive head and neck squamous cell carcinoma vs., **340**
    variant of squamous cell carcinoma of cervix, **40**
 - benign and reactive changes vs., **103**
 - of cervix, variants and mimics, **38–43**
    basaloid squamous carcinoma, **40**
    differential diagnosis, **40**
    immunohistochemistry, **40**
    morphologic variants, **40**
    papillary squamotransitional carcinoma, **40**
    papillary squamous carcinoma, **40**
    spindle cell squamous cell carcinoma, **40**
    verrucous carcinoma, **40**
 - conventional, HPV-positive head and neck squamous cell carcinoma vs., **340**
 - cysts vs., **385**
 - diagnostic checklist, **127**
 - differential diagnosis, **127**
 - direct extension of
    from adjacent organs, squamous cell carcinoma of urinary bladder vs., **245**
    metastatic carcinoma to thyroid vs., **308**
 - ductal carcinoma and variants of invasive mammary carcinoma, **450**

INDEX

- endometrial cells in Pap test and glandular cells status post hysterectomy vs., **71**
- esophageal, **156–157**
    - differential diagnosis, **157**
- fine-needle aspiration, **471**
- immunocytochemistry, **725**
- inflammatory and infectious conditions of liver vs., **501**
- keratinizing, **157**
    - cytopathology, **39**
- metastatic
    - metastatic carcinoma vs., **413**
    - metastatic tumors to kidney vs., **553**
    - to parotid area, salivary duct carcinoma vs., **407**
    - squamous cell carcinoma vs., **127**
    - unusual variants of ductal carcinoma vs., **592**
- metastatic tumors of mediastinum vs., **495**
- mucoepidermoid carcinoma vs., **397**
- nonkeratinizing, **157**
    - cytopathology, **39–40**
- normal salivary gland and sialadenitis vs., **383**
- NUT carcinoma vs., **138**
- papillary, variant of squamous cell carcinoma of cervix, **40**
- papillary squamotransitional carcinoma, variant of squamous cell carcinoma of cervix, **40**
- poorly differentiated, **157**
    - esophageal adenocarcinoma vs., **155**
- primary
    - metastatic carcinoma vs., **413**
    - pulmonary metastasis vs., **143**
- renal pelvic cytology, **251**
- with small &/or basaloid cells, small cell neuroendocrine carcinoma vs., **77**
- spindle cell
    - esophageal squamous cell carcinoma vs., **157**
    - variant of squamous cell carcinoma of cervix, **40**
- of urinary bladder, **244–245**
    - diagnostic checklist, **245**
    - differential diagnosis, **245**
    - prognosis, **245**
- urinary cytology, **231**
- verrucous carcinoma, variant of squamous cell carcinoma of cervix, **40**
- Warthin tumor vs., **389**

Squamous cell inflammatory changes, benign finding, gynecologic, **18**

Squamous cells
- atypical, cannot rule out high-grade squamous intraepithelial lesion, **36–37**
    - differential diagnosis, **37**
    - prognosis, **37**
- cytopathology, normal Pap test, **14–15**
- of undetermined significance, atypical, **34–35**
    - differential diagnosis, **35**

Squamous cellularity criteria, Papanicolaou test, **10–11**
- conventional Pap smear, **10**
- liquid-based preparations, **10–11**

Squamous dysplasia, high-grade, esophageal squamous cell carcinoma vs., **157**

Squamous epithelial cells, gastrointestinal cytology, **147**

Squamous intraepithelial lesion and mimics
- high-grade, **30–33**
    - differential diagnosis, **31**
- low-grade, **28–29**
    - differential diagnosis, **29**
    - prognosis, **29**

Squamous metaplasia
- benign and reactive changes, **103**
- keratinizing, squamous cell carcinoma of urinary bladder vs., **245**

Squamous metaplastic cells
- with benign inflammatory changes, atypical squamous cells, cannot rule out high-grade squamous intraepithelial lesion vs., **37**
- cytopathology, normal Pap test, **15**

Squamous repair, robust, atypical squamous cells of undetermined significance vs., **35**

Staining methods, cytology processing, **710–711**
- destaining, **711**
- Diff-Quik stain, **711**
- progressive staining, **710–711**
- rapid Pap, **711**
- regressive staining, **710**

Starch granules
- gynecologic artifact, **21**
- normal cerebrospinal fluid and contamination by normal elements, differential diagnosis, **177**

STK11 gene mutations, gastric-type adenocarcinoma, **57**

Stomach
- gastrointestinal cytology, **147**
- secondary involvement, by lymphoma, gastric lymphoma vs., **163**

Striated muscle, normal, adult-type rhabdomyoma vs., **655**

Stroma patterns, in neoplasm, salivary gland aspirates, **378**

Stromal hyperplasia, pseudoangiomatous
- angiosarcoma and other sarcomas of breast vs., **462**
- fibroadenoma vs., **436**

Stromal tumor, metanephric, **526**
- classification, **526**
- congenital mesoblastic nephroma vs., **551**
- differential diagnosis, **526**

Strongyloides, parasitic infections vs., **149**

Strongyloides stercoralis (threadworm), respiratory cytology, **111**

Subacute thyroiditis. *See* Granulomatous thyroiditis.

Subarachnoid hemorrhage (SAH), **184–185**
- differential diagnosis, **185**
- prognosis, **185**
- traumatic tap vs. pathologic bleed, **185**

Subareolar abscess, **420–421**

Submandibular gland metastasis, metastatic carcinoma, **413**

Sugar tumor, rare benign and low malignant potential tumors vs., **135**

SUMP. *See* Salivary gland neoplasm of uncertain malignant potential.

Superficial aspiration technique, **256–257**
- abdominal fat pad aspiration, **257**
- butterfly technique, **257**
- complications, **257**

INDEX

- examination and patient consent, **256**
- French technique (capillary action, no aspiration), **257**
- supplies, **256**

Superficial umbrella cells, urinary cytology, **229**

SurePath, nongynecologic cytology, **713**

Suspected lymphoma, FNA sample prep and triage in evaluating, **326–327**
- adenopathy with history of lymphoma, **326**
- diagnosing lymphoma in cytopathology laboratory, **327**
- FNA processing and triage, **327**
- unexplained adenopathy, **326**
- utility and limitations of FNA, **326–327**

Suspicious for follicular neoplasm, **282**. *See also* Follicular neoplasm/suspicious for follicular neoplasm.

Suspicious for malignancy, salivary gland aspiration biopsies and reporting terminology, **379, 380**

Synchesis scintillans, **683**

Synovial sarcoma, **213, 670–671**
- cytogenetics/molecular genetics, **671**
- differential diagnosis, **671**
- fibrosarcoma vs., **643**
- inflammatory and infectious conditions of liver vs., **501**
- intraosseous, adamantinoma vs., **611**
- mesenchymal chondrosarcoma vs., **666**
- smooth muscle tumors vs., **653**

Systemic lupus erythematosus (SLE) effusion, **202–203**
- differential diagnosis, **203**

T

t(10;17)(q22;p13), clear cell sarcoma of kidney, **549**

t(11;14)(q13;q32), mantle cell lymphoma, **347**

t(12;15)(p13;q25), congenital mesoblastic nephroma associated with, **551**

t(14;18), follicular lymphoma, **351**

T-cell lymphoblastic lymphoma, **370–371**
- differential diagnosis, **371**
- genetic testing, **371**
- immunohistochemistry, **371**

T-cell lymphoma, **363**
- , nodular lymphocyte-predominant Hodgkin lymphoma vs., **371**
- peripheral, **362–363**
  - differential diagnosis, **363**
  - genetic testing, **363**
  - immunohistochemistry, **363**
  - mycosis fungoides vs., **365**
  - not otherwise specified, angioimmunoblastic lymphoma vs., **367**
- peripheral, ALK(+) anaplastic large cell lymphoma vs., **369**
- peripheral, classic Hodgkin lymphoma vs., **375**
- peripheral T-cell lymphoma vs., **363**

T-lymphoblastic leukemia, **371**
- mediastinal large B-cell lymphoma vs., **359**

Tall cell subtype, papillary thyroid carcinoma, **291**
- Warthin-like subtype vs., papillary thyroid carcinoma subtype, **292**

Target amplification methods, molecular testing in gynecologic cytology, **84–85**

Telangiectatic osteosarcoma, **616**

Tendon sheath, giant cell tumor of, **648–649**
- differential diagnosis, **649**
- immunohistochemistry, **649**
- prognosis, **649**

Tenosynovial giant cell tumor
- clear cell sarcoma of soft tissue vs., **677**
- localized. *See* Giant cell tumor of tendon sheath.

Teratomas
- germ cell tumors vs., **491**
- mature cystic
  - germ cell tumors, **491**
  - mediastinal cysts and inflammatory lesions vs., **485**

Terminal duct carcinoma. *See* Polymorphous adenocarcinoma.

TFE3-rearranged renal cell carcinomas, **538–539**
- diagnostic checklist, **539**
- differential diagnosis, **539**
- immunohistochemistry, **539**
- prognosis, **539**

TFEB-rearranged renal cell carcinomas, **538–539**
- diagnostic checklist, **539**
- differential diagnosis, **539**
- immunohistochemistry, **539**
- prognosis, **539**

Thin layer preparations, nongynecologic cytology, **713**

ThinPrep, nongynecologic cytology, **713**

Thrombin, cell block techniques, **712**

Thrombus, organizing, soft tissue hemangioma vs., **659**

Thymic carcinoid tumor, mediastinal thymoma vs., **487**

Thymic carcinoma, **488–489**
- differential diagnosis, **489**
- immunohistochemistry, **489**
- metastatic tumors of mediastinum vs., **495**
- prognosis, **489**

Thymic cysts, **485**

Thymoma, **486–487**
- atypical (WHO type B3), thymic carcinoma vs., **489**
- cystic, mediastinal cysts and inflammatory lesions vs., **485**
- differential diagnosis, **487**
- ectopic, thyroid lymphoma vs., **306**
- immunohistochemistry, **487**
- metastatic tumors of mediastinum vs., **495**
- spindle cell, neurogenic tumors vs., **493**
- T-cell lymphoblastic lymphoma vs., **371**
- WHO type C. *See* Thymic carcinoma.

Thyroglossal duct cyst, rare extrathyroidal lesions presenting as thyroid nodules, **311**

Thyroid carcinoma
- papillary, metastatic to lymph nodes, cribriform adenocarcinoma vs., **411**
- poorly differentiated, **302–303**
  - anaplastic thyroid carcinoma vs., **304**
  - differential diagnosis, **303**
  - genetic testing, **303**
  - solid subtype vs., papillary thyroid carcinoma subtype, **292**
- showing thymus-like differentiation, **310**

INDEX

Thyroid follicular neoplasm
- metastatic carcinoma to thyroid vs., **308**
- parathyroid cyst, adenoma, and carcinoma vs., **319**

Thyroid gland
- anatomy, **260**
- normal, **260**

Thyroid gland, fine-needle aspiration
- adenomatous (benign follicular) nodule, **268–269**
   - diagnostic checklist, **269**
   - differential diagnosis, **268**
   - prognosis, **269**
- anaplastic thyroid carcinoma, **304–305**
- atypia of undetermined significance/follicular lesion of undetermined significance, **276–279**
- chronic lymphocytic/Hashimoto thyroiditis, **270–271**
- follicular neoplasm, oncocytic (Hürthle cell) type, **284–285**
- follicular neoplasm/suspicious for follicular neoplasm, **280–283**
- granulomatous thyroiditis, **272–273**
- Graves disease/diffuse toxic goiter, **274**
- lymphoma, **306–307**
- medullary thyroid carcinoma. See Medullary thyroid carcinoma.
- metastatic carcinoma, to thyroid, **308–309**
- molecular testing of indeterminate, **730**
- other nonneoplastic and neoplastic thyroid lesions, **310–315**
- papillary thyroid carcinoma, classic subtype, **286–289**
- papillary thyroid carcinoma subtypes, **290–297**
- pigmented thyroid lesions and crystals, **275**
- reporting terminology and specimen adequacy, **266–267**
   - The Bethesda System for Reporting Thyroid Cytology (TBSRTC), **266–267**
   - British Thyroid Association/Royal College of Pathologists (BTA/RCP) Reporting Terminology, **267**
   - molecular testing, guidelines, **267**
- ultrasound-guided thyroid fine-needle aspiration, **260–265**

Thyroid lesions, other nonneoplastic and neoplastic, **310–315**
- rare extrathyroidal lesions presenting as thyroid nodules, **311**
- rare primary malignant thyroid neoplasms, **310–311**
- rare primary thyroid lesions/neoplasms, **311**

Thyroid lymphoma, **306–307**
- differential diagnoses, **306**
- genetic testing, **307**
- immunohistochemistry, **307**

Thyroid neoplasms, rare
- extrathyroidal lesions presenting as thyroid nodules, **311**
- primary malignant thyroid neoplasms, **310–311**
- primary thyroid lesions/neoplasms, **311**

Thyroid nodules, extrathyroidal lesions presenting as thyroid nodules, **311**

Thyroiditides
- chronic lymphocytic/Hashimoto thyroiditis vs., **271**
- granulomatous thyroiditis vs., **273**

Tight halos due to inflammation/infections, low-grade squamous intraepithelial lesion and mimics vs., **29**

Tissue alterations, superficial aspiration technique, **257**

Touch imprint cytology, **690**

Toxic multinodular goiter, Graves disease/diffuse toxic goiter vs., **274**

Toxin exposure, urothelial carcinoma, **555**

Toxoplasma
- fungal organisms in respiratory cytology vs., **109**
- pancreatitis, **575**

Toxoplasma gondii, **687**
- respiratory cytology, **111**

Toxoplasmosis, neuropathology squash preparations, infectious, **696, 697**

TP53 gene, mutations in, pancreatic ductal adenocarcinoma, **589**

Transcription-mediated amplification (TMA) (Aptima), molecular testing in gynecologic cytology, **85**

Transducer types, ultrasound, definition, **260**

Transitional cell metaplasia, benign mimic, gynecologic, **19**

Translocation-associated renal cell carcinoma
- clear cell papillary renal cell carcinoma vs., **535**
- clear cell renal cell carcinoma vs., **529**

Traumatic tap
- pathologic bleed vs., **185**
- subarachnoid hemorrhage vs., **184**

Treponema pallidum infection, granulomatous lymphadenitis, infectious and sarcoid vs., **332**

Trichomonas
- infectious benign conditions, **237**
- parasitic infections vs., **149**

Trichomonas vaginalis, molecular testing in gynecologic cytology, **86**

Trichuris trichiura, parasitic infections vs., **149**

Triple test, **419**

Trisomy 7, papillary renal cell carcinoma, **533**
Trisomy 12, papillary renal cell carcinoma, **533**
Trisomy 16, papillary renal cell carcinoma, **533**
Trisomy 17, papillary renal cell carcinoma, **533**
Trisomy 18, hepatoblastoma, **511**
Trisomy 20, papillary renal cell carcinoma, **533**

Tropheryma whipplei, parasitic infections vs., **149**

Trophoblastic tumor, epithelioid, squamous cell carcinoma of cervix vs., **40**

TSC1 and *TSC2* gene mutations, angiomyolipoma, **521**

Tubal metaplasia
- adenocarcinoma in situ and mimics, **48**
- atypical glandular cells vs., **66**
- endocervical adenocarcinoma in situ vs., **47**

Tuberculosis
- granulomatous thyroiditis, **273**
- infectious conditions, in pleural, peritoneal, pericardial, and pelvic fluid, **200**
- lymphocyte-rich effusion vs., **197**
- neuropathology squash preparations, infectious, **696, 697**

Tuberculosis screening, respiratory cytology and adequacy criteria, **100**

Tuberous sclerosis complex, angiomyolipoma, **521**

INDEX

Tubular adenoma, fibroadenoma vs., **436**
Tubular carcinoma, **450**
- radial scar/complex sclerosing lesion vs., **429**

Tyrosine crystals, salivary gland aspirates, **379**
Tzanck smears, **470**
- herpes, **470**
- *Molluscum contagiosum*, **470**

U

Ulcer
- colorectal adenoma/carcinoma vs., **169**
- with reactive atypia
    esophageal adenocarcinoma vs., **155**
    gastric adenocarcinoma vs., **161**

Ultrasound-guided thyroid fine-needle aspiration, **260–265**
- ACR Thyroid Imaging, Reporting and Data System (TIRADS), **261, 262**
- American Thyroid Association Guidelines Task force, **262**
- biopsy, **261–262**
- ultrasound, **260–261**

Undifferentiated anaplastic carcinoma, **591–592**
Undifferentiated carcinoma
- medullary thyroid carcinoma vs., **300**
- with osteoclast-like giant cells, **592**

Undifferentiated pleomorphic sarcoma, **213, 650–651**
- differential diagnosis, **651**
- genetic testing, **651**
- immunohistochemistry, **651**
- osteosarcoma vs., **617**
- prognosis, **651**

Undifferentiated thyroid carcinoma, thyroid lymphoma vs., **306**
Undifferentiated tumor, SMARCA4-deficient, **139**
Undiluted vitreous, **682**
Unusual variants of ductal carcinoma, **590–593**
- differential diagnosis, **592**
- genetic testing, **592**
- prognosis, **591**

Ureteropyeloscopic brushings and washings, renal pelvic cytology, **251**
Urinary cytology
- adenocarcinoma of urinary bladder, **246–247**
    diagnostic checklist, **246**
    differential diagnosis, **247**
- atypical urothelial cells, **241**
- high-grade urothelial dysplasia/carcinoma/carcinoma in situ, **242–243**
    differential diagnosis, **243**
- ileal conduit specimens, **232–233**
    diagnostic checklist, **233**
    differential diagnosis, **233**
    prognosis, **233**
- infectious benign conditions, **236–237**
    diagnostic checklist, **237**
    differential diagnosis, **237**
- low-grade urothelial lesions, **240**
- noninfectious benign condition, **234–235**
    diagnostic checklist, **235**
    differential diagnosis, **235**
    prognosis, **235**
- other malignancies in urinary cytology, **248–249**
    diagnostic checklist, **248**
    differential diagnosis, **249**
- reactive urothelial changes, **238–239**
- renal pelvic cytology, **250–251**
- specimen types, and reporting terminology, normal, **228–231**
    cytologic features, **229**
    diagnostic checklist, **229**
    specimen types, **228**
        catheterization, **228**
        ileal conduit specimens, **229**
        urinary bladder wash (barbotage), **228**
        voided (clean catch), **228**
- squamous cell carcinoma of urinary bladder, **244–245**
    diagnostic checklist, **245**
    differential diagnosis, **245**
    prognosis, **245**

Urinary diversion. *See* Ileal conduit specimens.
Urinary tract cancer, urothelial carcinoma, **555**
Urolithiasis, low-grade urothelial lesions vs., **240**
Urothelial carcinoma, **554–555**
- collecting duct carcinoma vs., **540**
- differential diagnosis, **555**
- high-grade
    low-grade urothelial lesions vs., **240**
    reactive urothelial changes vs., **239**
- infectious benign conditions vs., **237**
- molecular features, **555**
- noninfectious benign conditions vs., **235**
- other malignancies in urinary cytology vs., **249**
- prognosis, **555**
- recurrent, ileal conduit specimens vs., **233**
- risk factors, **555**
- with squamous differentiation, invasive, squamous cell carcinoma of urinary bladder vs., **245**

Urothelial cells, atypical, **241**
Urothelial changes, reactive, **238–239**
- diagnostic checklist, **239**
- differential diagnosis, **239**

Urothelial lesions, low-grade, **240**
- diagnostic checklist, **240**
- differential diagnosis, **240**
- high-grade urothelial dysplasia/carcinoma/carcinoma in situ vs., **243**

Urothelial neoplasm, low-grade papillary, reactive urothelial changes vs., **239**
UroVysion, urinary cytology, **252**
- equipment, **252**
- fluorescence in situ hybridization (FISH) results, **252**
- sensitivity and specificity, **252**
- type of analysis, **252**

Usual ductal hyperplasia, proliferative breast changes, **424**
Uterus, directly sampled lower uterine segment, endocervical adenocarcinoma in situ vs., **47**
Uveal melanoma, metastatic vs., **683**

INDEX

V

Vaccination, HPV molecular testing, **7**
Vaginal bleeding
- abnormal, endocervical adenocarcinoma, variants and mimics, **53**
- endocervical adenocarcinoma in situ, **47**

Vaginosis, bacterial, molecular testing in gynecologic cytology, **86**
Varicella-Zoster virus, viral infections vs., **151**
Vascular lesions
- atypical, angiosarcoma vs., **663**
- soft tissue hemangioma vs., **659**

Vascular tumors, epithelioid, metastatic tumors of bone vs., **631**
Vegetable matter
- low-grade squamous intraepithelial lesion and mimics vs., **29**
- miscellaneous findings including contaminants
    malignancy vs., **121**
    pathogens vs., **121**

Verrucous carcinoma, variant of squamous cell carcinoma of cervix, **40**
VHL gene, mutations, clear cell renal cell carcinoma, **528**
Villonodular synovitis, pigmented, giant cell tumor of tendon sheath vs., **649**
Viral esophagitis, **153**
Viral infections, **112–113, 150–151**
- diagnostic checklist, **113**
- differential diagnosis, **113, 151**
- herpes, low-grade squamous intraepithelial lesion and mimics vs., **29**
- mycobacteria and other bacterial infections vs., **115**
- neuropathology squash preparations, infectious, **696, 697**
- ophthalmic cytopathology, **687**
- prognosis, **113**

Viral lymphadenopathies, nodular lymphocyte-predominant Hodgkin lymphoma vs., **371**
Viral meningitis, **181**
Viruses, in Pap tests, **17**
Vitreous biopsy, **682**
Vitreous humor, **687**
- triaging, **683**

von Hippel-Lindau-associated pancreatic cysts, serous microcystic adenoma vs., **579**

W

WAGR syndrome, nephroblastoma (Wilms tumor), **547**
Warthin-like subtype, papillary thyroid carcinoma subtypes, **292**
- differential diagnosis, **292**

Warthin tumor, **388–389**
- acinic cell carcinoma vs., **395**
- cysts vs., **385**
- differential diagnosis, **389**
- with extensive squamous differentiation, metastatic carcinoma vs., **413**
- mucoepidermoid carcinoma vs., **397**
- normal salivary gland and sialadenitis vs., **383**
- oncocytoma of salivary gland vs., **391**

Well-differentiated adrenal cortical carcinoma
- adrenal cortical adenoma vs., **561**
- cytology of normal adrenal gland vs., **559**

Well-differentiated liposarcoma, **213**
- cytologic/small biopsy categorization of primary soft tissue tumors, **635**
- liposarcoma vs., **639**

Well-differentiated neuroendocrine neoplasm/serous microcystic adenoma, combined, serous microcystic adenoma vs., **579**
Wilms tumor
- congenital mesoblastic nephroma vs., **551**
- cystic partially differentiated, renal cyst vs., **519**
- epithelial predominant, metanephric adenoma vs., **525**
- renal medullary carcinoma vs., **541**

WT1 gene deletions, nephroblastoma, **547**
WT2 gene alterations, nephroblastoma, **547**

X

Xanthogranulomatous pyelonephritis/malakoplakia, **527**
- differential diagnoses, **527**

Y

Yokohama System (TYS), reporting endometrial cytology, directly sampled endometrial cytology, **90**
Yolk sac tumor
- germ cell tumors vs., **491**
- renal medullary carcinoma vs., **541**

Z

Zenker (esophageal) diverticulum, rare extrathyroidal lesion presenting as thyroid nodules, **311**
Zygomycetes
- neuropathology squash preparations, infectious, **697**
- respiratory cytology, **109**

Zymogen-poor acinic cell carcinoma. *See* Secretory carcinoma.